CLINICAL PHARMACY

Volume 10, Number 1
January 1991

Treatment of systemic scleroderma
Angiotensin-converting-enzyme inhibitors in the management of renal disease
Nondepolarizing neuromuscular blocking agents in mechanically ventilated patients

AMERICAN SOCIETY OF HOSPITAL PHARMACISTS

January 1991 Volume 10, Number 1

Coden: CPHADV ISSN: 0278-2677

CLINICAL PHARMACY

4 **News**

New method of analyzing health data stirs debate, Lawrence K. Altman . . . Changes in federal programs for reporting suspected adverse reactions to vaccines announced . . . Transdermal fentanyl approved for chronic pain management . . . Doxazosin approved as antihypertensive agent

12 **Therapy Consultation**

Use of ketoconazole in the treatment of Cushing's syndrome

Therapy Reviews

14 **Current options for the treatment of systemic scleroderma**
Barbara A. McGee, Michael D. Barnett, and Ralph E. Small

25 **Use of angiotensin-converting-enzyme inhibitors in the management of renal disease**
John P. Asher and Kim M. Murray

32 **Use of nondepolarizing neuromuscular blocking agents in mechanically ventilated patients**
Marcia L. Buck and Michael D. Reed

Research

49 **Intravenous ciprofloxacin versus ceftazidime for treatment of nosocomial pneumonia and urinary tract infection**
Robert P. Rapp, Marianne Billeter, Jimmi Hatton, A. Bryon Young, Phillip A. Tibbs, and Robert J. Dempsey

Drug Experience

56 **Pancreatitis during pentamidine therapy in patients with AIDS**
Michael G. O'Neil, Steven E. Selub, and Lawrence J. Hak

ASHP Reports

60 **Procedure for submission of manuscripts to journals published by the American Society of Hospital Pharmacists**

62 **Instructions for submitting computer disks with revised manuscripts**

DUE Criteria

63 **Criteria for use of enalapril maleate in adults**
Allison L. Coley

68 **CP Continuing Education**

71 **FDA Adverse Reaction Report Form and Instructions**

74 **Current Literature**

Drug Reaction Alerts . . . Book Review: *Field Drug Reference for Emergency Care Providers* (Gonzalez, Ornato), Judith Jacobi

80 **Advertising Index**

Editorial Office
4630 Montgomery Avenue
Bethesda, MD 20814
301-657-3000
FAX 301-657-1615

Advertising Representative
William McCausland Associates, Inc.
P.O. Box 189
Pitman, NJ 08071
609-589-5454
FAX 609-582-7611

Printed on acid-free paper effective with Volume 8, January 1989

Instructions to Authors

CLINICAL PHARMACY, a forum for the drug therapeutics information that pharmacists need to perform their clinical roles, gives priority to (1) studies that objectively evaluate drug effects in human trials, (2) evaluative review articles on the clinical uses of new drugs, and (3) evaluations of the current status of drug therapy in selected diseases. Contributions to the following sections are invited:

Drug Reviews: Detailed, analytical reviews on the clinical use of specific drugs, with preference given to new drugs and to evaluative rather than descriptive literature reviews.

Therapy Reviews: Articles that focus primarily on a disease state and its treatment.

Clinical Frontiers: Articles that review important, ongoing research on disease processes, drug mechanisms, or new technologies and project the likely implications for therapy.

Research: Reports of well-conducted original research on drug effects in humans.

Research Notes: Short research reports, such as updates on previously published work, confirmations of previous findings, or original research of modest scope.

Grand Rounds: Patient case reports and literature reviews combined in a way that gives them high educational value.

Drug Experience: Straightforward reports, with selected literature references, of unusual drug experiences.

Therapy Consultation: Brief advice, in a question-and-answer format, on how to handle specific drug-therapy problems. Readers are invited to submit questions, which the editor will forward to consultants for answering.

Letters: Short comments on previously published work or about potential problems, apparent trends, or controversies in drug therapy or clinical research.

Commentaries: Well-reasoned expressions of opinion on drug-therapy or clinical-research issues.

The editors have the sole authority to decide in which section to publish an accepted manuscript.

Manuscripts are subject to review by qualified outside reviewers, as well as by the editors, and will be accepted for publication only if they are believed to represent an important contribution to the literature. All papers submitted for publication must be accompanied by a completed copy of a manuscript checklist. The checklist, which generally conforms to the Uniform Requirements for Manuscripts Submitted to Biomedical Journals, appears on pages 60–61 of the January 1991 issue. Authors of especially important original work may request "fast-track" review of their papers. Authors may suggest appropriate reviewers for their papers.

Accepted materials become the permanent and sole property of ASHP and may not be published or reprinted elsewhere without written permission from both the author and the editor.

The editors reserve the right to revise all materials submitted, if necessary. The publisher assumes no responsibility for the statements and opinions advanced by contributors to CLINICAL PHARMACY.

Under the terms of the Copyright Revision Act of 1976 (Public Law 94-553) it is necessary to have the rights of the authors transferred to the publisher in order to provide for the widest possible dissemination of professional and scientific literature. Accordingly, all transmittal letters accompanying manuscripts submitted for publication, including contributions for the Letters column, must contain the following language: "In consideration of the American Society of Hospital Pharmacists (ASHP) taking action in reviewing and editing my (our) submission, the author(s) undersigned hereby transfer(s), assign(s), or otherwise convey(s) all ownership rights in the submission and all copyright ownership to ASHP. In the event that such work is not published by ASHP, all said rights shall be released." We regret that we cannot consider manuscripts for publication that are not accompanied with transmittal letters containing the above language signed by all authors.

Authors must certify in their letter of transmittal that none of the material in their manuscript has been published previously nor is under consideration or been accepted for publication elsewhere. If this certification cannot be made, suitable explanation must be offered.

Eight copies of all manuscripts should be submitted. Manuscripts should be typewritten with double spacing (including tables) on one side of good quality, 21.6 × 27.9-cm white paper, and with margins of at least 2.5 cm. For guidance on style, authors should consult the manuscript checklist, recent issues of CLINICAL PHARMACY, and the *Council of Biology Editors Style Manual*, fifth edition. *The American Heritage Dictionary of the English Language* and the AMA's *Manual for Authors and Editors* contain helpful advice on correct usage.

Galley proofs or final edited manuscripts are sent to authors for inspection against the original manuscript and for correction. Unnecessary alterations at this stage must be avoided. An order form for reprints is sent to the corresponding author at the time of publication.

CLINICAL PHARMACY (ISSN 0278-2677) is published monthly by the American Society of Hospital Pharmacists, 4630 Montgomery Avenue, Bethesda, MD 20814. Joseph A. Oddis, Executive Vice President. Second class postage is paid at Bethesda, MD, and at additional mailing offices. **Postmaster: Send address changes to: *Clinical Pharmacy,* 4630 Montgomery Avenue, Bethesda, MD 20814.**

Annual Subscription Rate:	*USA*	*Non-USA*
ASHP Members	$45	$60
ASHP Student Members and Residents	$35	$50
Institutions and Nonmembers	$75	$90

The cost of single copies of current issues is $6. The cost of single copies of issues from 1985 and earlier is $10. Airmail delivery outside of the continental United States is available for an additional charge of $90 per year. Requests to replace missing issues free of charge are honored only up to six months after date of issue.

Payments to ASHP are not deductible as charitable contributions for federal income tax purposes. However, they may be deductible under other provisions of the Internal Revenue Code.

Advertising for CLINICAL PHARMACY is accepted in accordance with the Statement of Advertising Policy of the American Society of Hospital Pharmacists (see *Am J Hosp Pharm.* 1987; 44:1146). For additional information, contact the Advertising Representative (William McCausland Associates, Inc., P.O. Box 189, Pitman, NJ 08071. Phone 609-589-5454, FAX 609-582-7611.)

All articles published, including editorials, letters, and book reviews, represent the opinions of the authors and do not reflect the official policy of the American Society of Hospital Pharmacists or the institution with which the author is affiliated, unless this is specified.

Microfilm and microfiche editions are available for purchase. Contact University Microfilms, 300 N. Zeeb Road, Ann Arbor, MI 48106.

Articles in CLINICAL PHARMACY are abstracted and indexed in *Current Contents, Clinical Sciences, Excerpta Medica, Index Medicus, Inpharma, International Pharmaceutical Abstracts*, and *Reactions*.

February 1991 Volume 10, Number 2 Coden: CPHADV ISSN: 0278-2677

CLINICAL PHARMACY

88 **News**

Consensus panel considers uses of botulinum toxin . . . FDA bans 223 ingredients in nonprescription drug products . . . Report on pain management in childhood cancer published . . . Consensus report focuses on hypertension during pregnancy

Drug Reviews

95 **Levamisole in the adjuvant treatment of colon cancer**
Rebecca S. Mutch and Paul R. Hutson

110 **Recombinant interleukin-2: A biological response modifier**
P. E. Kintzel and Karim Anton Calis

Research Notes

129 **Prospective evaluation of a vancomycin dosage guideline for neonates**
Mariane Hardenbrook Gabriel, Carl W. Kildoo III, Jane L. Gennrich, Houchang D. Modanlou, and Shelly Rainforth Collins

132 **Effect of ultrafiltration product and ultrafiltration–freezing sequence on free phenytoin determination**
Leanne B. Smith, Bruce D. Anderson, and Carol B. Pugh

136 **Hypoprothrombinemic effect of warfarin not influenced by ciprofloxacin**
Joseph P. Rindone, Catherine L. Keuey, William N. Jones, and Harinder S. Garewal

138 **Acceptability of cholestyramine and colestipol formulations in three common vehicles**
Matthew K. Ito and Anthony P. Morreale

Editorial

141 **Recombinant interleukin-2 and the quest for FDA approval**
Joseph A. Tami

DUE Criteria

143 **Criteria for use of epoetin**
Teresa A. Bennett, Mark W. Todd, and Stephen Sandroni

147 **CP Continuing Education**

151 **FDA Adverse Reaction Report Form and Instructions**

154 **Current Literature**

Drug Reaction Alerts . . . Book Review: *Clinical Pharmacology of Psychotherapeutic Drugs, Third Edition (Hollister, Csernansky)*, Timothy E. Welty

160 **Advertising Index**

Editorial Office
4630 Montgomery Avenue
Bethesda, MD 20814
301-657-3000
FAX 301-657-1615

Advertising Representative
William McCausland Associates, Inc.
P.O. Box 189
Pitman, NJ 08071
609-589-5454
FAX 609-582-7611

Printed on acid-free paper effective with Volume 8, January 1989

Instructions to Authors

CLINICAL PHARMACY, a forum for the drug therapeutics information that pharmacists need to perform their clinical roles, gives priority to (1) studies that objectively evaluate drug effects in human trials, (2) evaluative review articles on the clinical uses of new drugs, and (3) evaluations of the current status of drug therapy in selected diseases. Contributions to the following sections are invited:

Drug Reviews: Detailed, analytical reviews on the clinical use of specific drugs, with preference given to new drugs and to evaluative rather than descriptive literature reviews.

Therapy Reviews: Articles that focus primarily on a disease state and its treatment.

Clinical Frontiers: Articles that review important, ongoing research on disease processes, drug mechanisms, or new technologies and project the likely implications for therapy.

Research: Reports of well-conducted original research on drug effects in humans.

Research Notes: Short research reports, such as updates on previously published work, confirmations of previous findings, or original research of modest scope.

Grand Rounds: Patient case reports and literature reviews combined in a way that gives them high educational value.

Drug Experience: Straightforward reports, with selected literature references, of unusual drug experiences.

Therapy Consultation: Brief advice, in a question-and-answer format, on how to handle specific drug-therapy problems. Readers are invited to submit questions, which the editor will forward to consultants for answering.

Letters: Short comments on previously published work or about potential problems, apparent trends, or controversies in drug therapy or clinical research.

Commentaries: Well-reasoned expressions of opinion on drug-therapy or clinical-research issues.

The editors have the sole authority to decide in which section to publish an accepted manuscript.

Manuscripts are subject to review by qualified outside reviewers, as well as by the editors, and will be accepted for publication only if they are believed to represent an important contribution to the literature. All papers submitted for publication must be accompanied by a completed copy of a manuscript checklist. The checklist, which generally conforms to the Uniform Requirements for Manuscripts Submitted to Biomedical Journals, appears on pages 60–61 of the January 1991 issue. Authors of especially important original work may request "fast-track" review of their papers. Authors may suggest appropriate reviewers for their papers.

Accepted materials become the permanent and sole property of ASHP and may not be published or reprinted elsewhere without written permission from both the author and the editor.

The editors reserve the right to revise all materials submitted, if necessary. The publisher assumes no responsibility for the statements and opinions advanced by contributors to CLINICAL PHARMACY.

Under the terms of the Copyright Revision Act of 1976 (Public Law 94-553) it is necessary to have the rights of the authors transferred to the publisher in order to provide for the widest possible dissemination of professional and scientific literature. Accordingly, all transmittal letters accompanying manuscripts submitted for publication, including contributions for the Letters column, must contain the following language: "In consideration of the American Society of Hospital Pharmacists (ASHP) taking action in reviewing and editing my (our) submission, the author(s) undersigned hereby transfer(s), assign(s), or otherwise convey(s) all ownership rights in the submission and all copyright ownership to ASHP. In the event that such work is not published by ASHP, all said rights shall be released." We regret that we cannot consider manuscripts for publication that are not accompanied with transmittal letters containing the above language signed by all authors.

Authors must certify in their letter of transmittal that none of the material in their manuscript has been published previously nor is under consideration or been accepted for publication elsewhere. If this certification cannot be made, suitable explanation must be offered.

Eight copies of all manuscripts should be submitted. Manuscripts should be typewritten with double spacing (including tables) on one side of good quality, 21.6 × 27.9-cm white paper, and with margins of at least 2.5 cm. For guidance on style, authors should consult the manuscript checklist, recent issues of CLINICAL PHARMACY, and the *Council of Biology Editors Style Manual*, fifth edition. *The American Heritage Dictionary of the English Language* and the AMA's *Manual for Authors and Editors* contain helpful advice on correct usage.

Galley proofs or final edited manuscripts are sent to authors for inspection against the original manuscript and for correction. Unnecessary alterations at this stage must be avoided. An order form for reprints is sent to the corresponding author at the time of publication.

CLINICAL PHARMACY (ISSN 0278-2677) is published monthly by the American Society of Hospital Pharmacists, 4630 Montgomery Avenue, Bethesda, MD 20814. Joseph A. Oddis, Executive Vice President. Second class postage is paid at Bethesda, MD, and at additional mailing offices. **Postmaster: Send address changes to: *Clinical Pharmacy,* 4630 Montgomery Avenue, Bethesda, MD 20814.**

Annual Subscription Rate:	*USA*	*Non-USA*
ASHP Members	$45	$60
ASHP Student Members and Residents	$35	$50
Institutions and Nonmembers	$80	$95

The cost of single copies of current issues is $6. The cost of single copies of issues from 1985 and earlier is $10. Airmail delivery outside of the continental United States is available for an additional charge of $90 per year. Requests to replace missing issues free of charge are honored only up to six months after date of issue.

Payments to ASHP are not deductible as charitable contributions for federal income tax purposes. However, they may be deductible under other provisions of the Internal Revenue Code.

Advertising for CLINICAL PHARMACY is accepted in accordance with the Statement of Advertising Policy of the American Society of Hospital Pharmacists (see *Am J Hosp Pharm.* 1987; 44:1146). For additional information, contact the Advertising Representative (William McCausland Associates, Inc., P.O. Box 189, Pitman, NJ 08071. Phone 609-589-5454, FAX 609-582-7611.)

All articles published, including editorials, letters, and book reviews, represent the opinions of the authors and do not reflect the official policy of the American Society of Hospital Pharmacists or the institution with which the author is affiliated, unless this is specified.

Microfilm and microfiche editions are available for purchase. Contact University Microfilms, 300 N. Zeeb Road, Ann Arbor, MI 48106.

Articles in CLINICAL PHARMACY are abstracted and indexed in *Current Contents, Clinical Sciences, Excerpta Medica, Index Medicus, Inpharma, International Pharmaceutical Abstracts,* and *Reactions.*

March 1991 Volume 10, Number 3

Coden: CPHADV ISSN: 0278-2677

CLINICAL PHARMACY

167 **News**

Year-end review shows 23 new drugs approved, 14 important biologic licensing actions taken by FDA . . . New recommendations for prevention of bacterial endocarditis include amoxicillin use . . . Report assesses use of blood pressure monitoring devices for ambulatory patients

177 **Letters**

Interferon for genital warts, Celine M. Stahl-Bayliss

Drug Review

179 **Fluconazole: A new antifungal agent**
Steven F. Kowalsky and Dennis M. Dixon

Therapy Review

195 **Evaluation and treatment of ventricular arrhythmias: An update**
Patrick L. McCollam and Robert B. Parker

Research

206 **Comparison of MS-DOS and Macintosh pharmacokinetic analysis programs using a two-compartment, two-infusion dosing scheme**
Edward M. Hampton, Kyle Hrdlicka, and David W. A. Bourne

Editorials

210 **Trials and tribulations of evaluating ventricular arrhythmias**
Jean Nappi

211 **Antiarrhythmic monitoring: Misplaced emphasis**

Grand Rounds

213 **Elemental mercury poisoning**
Mauro J. Florentine and Dominic J. Sanfilippo II

DUE Criteria

222 **Criteria for use of fluconazole in adult and pediatric inpatients and outpatients**
Kimberly M. Bourne and S. Diane Goodwin

228 **CP Continuing Education**

233 **FDA Adverse Reaction Report Form and Instructions**

235 **Current Literature**

Drug Reaction Alerts . . . Book Reviews: *Cancer Chemotherapy by Infusion, Second Edition* (*Lokich*), James H. Keller . . . *Poisoning and Drug Overdose* (*Olson, Becker, Benowitz et al.*), James J. Kresel . . . Books Received

246 **Advertising Index**

Editorial Office
4630 Montgomery Avenue
Bethesda, MD 20814
301-657-3000
Fax 301-657-1615

Advertising Representative
William McCausland Associates, Inc.
P.O. Box 189
Pitman, NJ 08071
609-589-5454
Fax 609-582-7611

Printed on acid-free paper effective with Volume 8, January 1989.

Instructions to Authors

CLINICAL PHARMACY, a forum for the drug therapeutics information that pharmacists need to perform their clinical roles, gives priority to (1) studies that objectively evaluate drug effects in human trials, (2) evaluative review articles on the clinical uses of new drugs, and (3) evaluations of the current status of drug therapy in selected diseases. Contributions to the following sections are invited.

Drug Reviews: Detailed, analytical reviews on the clinical use of specific drugs, with preference given to new drugs and to evaluative rather than descriptive literature reviews.

Therapy Reviews: Articles that focus primarily on a disease state and its treatment.

Clinical Frontiers: Articles that review important, ongoing research on disease processes, drug mechanisms, or new technologies and project the likely implications for therapy.

Research: Reports of well-conducted original research on drug effects in humans.

Research Notes: Short research reports, such as updates on previously published work, confirmations of previous findings, or original research of modest scope.

Grand Rounds: Patient case reports and literature reviews combined in a way that gives them high educational value.

Drug Experience: Straightforward reports, with selected literature references, of unusual drug experiences.

Therapy Consultation: Brief advice, in a question-and-answer format, on how to handle specific drug-therapy problems. Readers are invited to submit questions, which the editor will forward to consultants for answering.

Letters: Short comments on previously published work or about potential problems, apparent trends, or controversies in drug therapy or clinical research.

Commentaries: Well-reasoned expressions of opinion on drug-therapy or clinical-research issues.

The editors have the sole authority to decide in which section to publish an accepted manuscript.

Manuscripts are subject to review by qualified outside reviewers, as well as by the editors, and will be accepted for publication only if they are believed to represent an important contribution to the literature. All papers submitted for publication must be accompanied by a completed copy of a manuscript checklist. The checklist, which generally conforms to the Uniform Requirements for Manuscripts Submitted to Biomedical Journals, appears on pages 60-61 of the January 1991 issue. Authors of especially important original work may request "fast-track" review of their papers. Authors may suggest appropriate reviewers for their papers.

Accepted materials become the permanent and sole property of ASHP and may not be published or reprinted elsewhere without written permission from both the author and the editor.

The editors reserve the right to revise all materials submitted, if necessary. The publisher assumes no responsibility for the statements and opinions advanced by contributors to CLINICAL PHARMACY.

Under the terms of the Copyright Revision Act of 1976 (Public Law 94-553) it is necessary to have the rights of the authors transferred to the publisher in order to provide for the widest possible dissemination of professional and scientific literature. Accordingly, all transmittal letters accompanying manuscripts submitted for publication, including contributions for the Letters column, must contain the following language: "In consideration of the American Society of Hospital Pharmacists (ASHP) taking action in reviewing and editing my (our) submission, the author(s) undersigned hereby transfer(s), assign(s), or otherwise convey(s) all ownership rights in the submission and all copyright ownership to ASHP. In the event that such work is not published by ASHP, all said rights shall be released." We regret that we cannot consider manuscripts for publication that are not accompanied by transmittal letters containing the above language signed by all authors.

Authors must certify in their letter of transmittal that none of the material in their manuscript has been published previously nor is under consideration or been accepted for publication elsewhere. If this certification cannot be made, suitable explanation must be offered.

Eight copies of all manuscripts should be submitted. Manuscripts should be typewritten with double spacing (including tables) on one side of good-quality, 21.6 x 27.9-cm white paper, and with margins of at least 2.5 cm. For guidance on style, authors should consult the manuscript checklist, recent issues of CLINICAL PHARMACY, and the *Council of Biology Editors Style Manual, fifth edition. The American Heritage Dictionary of the English Language and the AMA's Manual of Style* contain helpful advice on correct usage.

Galley proofs or final edited manuscripts are sent to authors for inspection against the original manuscript and for correction. Unnecessary alterations at this stage must be avoided. An order form for reprints is sent to the corresponding author at the time of publication.

CLINICAL PHARMACY (ISSN 0278-2677) is published monthly by the American Society of Hospital Pharmacists, 4630 Montgomery Avenue, Bethesda, MD 20814. Joseph A. Oddis, Executive Vice President. Second-class postage is paid at Bethesda, MD, and at additional mailing offices. **Postmaster: Send address changes to: *Clinical Pharmacy*, 4630 Montgomery Avenue, Bethesda, MD 20814.**

Annual Subscription Rate:	*USA*	*Non-USA*
ASHP Members	$45	$60
ASHP Student Members and Residents	$35	$50
Institutions and Nonmembers	$80	$95

The cost of single copies of current issues is $6. The cost of single copies of issues from 1985 and earlier is $10. Airmail delivery outside the continental United States is available for an additional charge of $90 per year. Requests to replace missing issues free of charge are honored only up to six months after date of issue.

Payments to ASHP are not deductible as charitable contributions for federal income tax purposes. However, they may be deductible under other provisions of the Internal Revenue Code.

Advertising for CLINICAL PHARMACY is accepted in accordance with the Statement of Advertising Policy of the American Society of Hospital Pharmacists (see *Am J Hosp Pharm.* 1987; 44:1146). For additional information, contact the Advertising Representative (William McCausland Associates, Inc., P.O. Box 189, Pitman, NJ 08071. Phone 609-589-5454, Fax 609-582-7611).

All articles published, including editorials, letters, and book reviews, represent the opinions of the authors and do not reflect the official policy of the American Society of Hospital Pharmacists or the institution with which the author is affiliated, unless this is specified.

Microfilm and microfiche editions are available for purchase. Contact University Microfilms, 300 N. Zeeb Road, Ann Arbor, MI 48106.

Articles in CLINICAL PHARMACY are abstracted and indexed in *Current Contents, Clinical Sciences, Excerpta Medica, Index Medicus, Inpharma, International Pharmaceutical Abstracts,* and *Reactions.*

April 1991 Volume 10, Number 4 Coden: CPHADV ISSN: 0278-2677

CLINICAL PHARMACY

249 **News**

Ondansetron granted marketing approval . . . Rubella prevention guidelines updated by CDC . . . Two reports on hypertension available from National Heart, Lung, and Blood Institute

257 **Letters**

Pentamidine-induced facial numbness, Anne Y. F. Lin, Candace Smith

261 **Corrections**

Therapy Reviews

268 **Neutropenia in patients infected with human immunodeficiency virus**
Deb S. Israel and Karen I. Plaisance

280 **Current and investigational therapies for AIDS-associated *Mycobacterium avium* complex disease**
R. Chris Rathbun, Emory S. Martin III, Virginia E. Eaton, and Earl B. Matthew

Drug Experience

292 **Continuous subcutaneous infusion of terbutaline for suppression of preterm labor**
Janet R. Fischer and Brian L. Kaatz

297 **Vancomycin half-life in a patient with hepatic and renal dysfunction**
Robert E. Pachorek and Frederick Wood

301 **Preventing recurrent varicella and herpes zoster with oral acyclovir in HIV-seropositive patients**
Pierre Dellamonica, Michel Carles, François Lokiec, Véronique Mondain, Evelyne Bernard, and Franck Johanson

DUE Criteria

303 **Criteria for use of epoetin**
Teresa A. Bennett, Mark W. Todd, and Stephen Sandroni

307 **Criteria for use of misoprostol**
Mark W. Todd

309 **CP Continuing Education**

311 **FDA Adverse Reaction Report Form and Instructions**

313 **Current Literature**

Drug Reaction Alerts . . . Book Reviews: *Drugs in Pregnancy and Lactation, Third Edition (Briggs, Freeman, Yaffe)*, Don R. Porter . . . *Goodman and Gilman's The Pharmacological Basis of Therapeutics, 8th edition (Gilman, Rall, Nies et al.)*, Burgunda W. Volger . . . Books Received

318 **Advertising Index**

Editorial Office
4630 Montgomery Avenue
Bethesda, MD 20814
301-657-3000
Fax 301-657-1615

Advertising Representative
William McCausland Associates, Inc.
P.O. Box 189
Pitman, NJ 08071
609-589-5454
Fax 609-582-7611

Printed on acid-free paper effective with Volume 8, January 1989.

Instructions to Authors

Clinical Pharmacy, a forum for the drug therapeutics information that pharmacists need to perform their clinical roles, gives priority to (1) studies that objectively evaluate drug effects in human trials, (2) evaluative review articles on the clinical uses of new drugs, and (3) evaluations of the current status of drug therapy in selected diseases. Contributions to the following sections are invited.

Drug Reviews: Detailed, analytical reviews on the clinical use of specific drugs, with preference given to new drugs and to evaluative rather than descriptive literature reviews.

Therapy Reviews: Articles that focus primarily on a disease state and its treatment.

Clinical Frontiers: Articles that review important, ongoing research on disease processes, drug mechanisms, or new technologies and project the likely implications for therapy.

Research: Reports of well-conducted original research on drug effects in humans.

Research Notes: Short research reports, such as updates on previously published work, confirmations of previous findings, or original research of modest scope.

Grand Rounds: Patient case reports and literature reviews combined in a way that gives them high educational value.

Drug Experience: Straightforward reports, with selected literature references, of unusual drug experiences.

Therapy Consultation: Brief advice, in a question-and-answer format, on how to handle specific drug-therapy problems. Readers are invited to submit questions, which the editor will forward to consultants for answering.

Letters: Short comments on previously published work or about potential problems, apparent trends, or controversies in drug therapy or clinical research.

Commentaries: Well-reasoned expressions of opinion on drug-therapy or clinical-research issues.

The editors have the sole authority to decide in which section to publish an accepted manuscript.

Manuscripts are subject to review by qualified outside reviewers, as well as by the editors, and will be accepted for publication only if they are believed to represent an important contribution to the literature. All papers submitted for publication must be accompanied by a completed copy of a manuscript checklist. The checklist, which generally conforms to the Uniform Requirements for Manuscripts Submitted to Biomedical Journals, appears on pages 60-61 of the January 1991 issue. Authors of especially important original work may request "fast-track" review of their papers. Authors may suggest appropriate reviewers for their papers.

Accepted materials become the permanent and sole property of ASHP and may not be published or reprinted elsewhere without written permission from both the author and the editor.

The editors reserve the right to revise all materials submitted, if necessary. The publisher assumes no responsibility for the statements and opinions advanced by contributors to Clinical Pharmacy.

Under the terms of the Copyright Revision Act of 1976 (Public Law 94-553) it is necessary to have the rights of the authors transferred to the publisher in order to provide for the widest possible dissemination of professional and scientific literature. Accordingly, all transmittal letters accompanying manuscripts submitted for publication, including contributions for the Letters column, must contain the following language: "In consideration of the American Society of Hospital Pharmacists (ASHP) taking action in reviewing and editing my (our) submission, the author(s) undersigned hereby transfer(s), assign(s), or otherwise convey(s) all ownership rights in the submission and all copyright ownership to ASHP. In the event that such work is not published by ASHP, all said rights shall be released." We regret that we cannot consider manuscripts for publication that are not accompanied by transmittal letters containing the above language signed by all authors.

Authors must certify in their letter of transmittal that none of the material in their manuscript has been published previously nor is under consideration or been accepted for publication elsewhere. If this certification cannot be made, suitable explanation must be offered.

Eight copies of all manuscripts should be submitted. Manuscripts should be typewritten with double spacing (including tables) on one side of good-quality, 21.6 x 27.9-cm white paper, and with margins of at least 2.5 cm. For guidance on style, authors should consult the manuscript checklist, recent issues of Clinical Pharmacy, and the *Council of Biology Editors Style Manual, fifth edition. The American Heritage Dictionary of the English Language and the AMA's Manual of Style* contain helpful advice on correct usage.

Galley proofs or final edited manuscripts are sent to authors for inspection against the original manuscript and for correction. Unnecessary alterations at this stage must be avoided. An order form for reprints is sent to the corresponding author at the time of publication.

Clinical Pharmacy (ISSN 0278-2677) is published monthly by the American Society of Hospital Pharmacists, 4630 Montgomery Avenue, Bethesda, MD 20814. Joseph A. Oddis, Executive Vice President. Second-class postage is paid at Bethesda, MD, and at additional mailing offices. **Postmaster: Send address changes to: *Clinical Pharmacy*, 4630 Montgomery Avenue, Bethesda, MD 20814.**

Annual Subscription Rate:	*USA*	*Non-USA*
ASHP Members	$45	$60
ASHP Student Members and Residents	$35	$50
Institutions and Nonmembers	$80	$95

The cost of single copies of current issues is $6. The cost of single copies of issues from 1985 and earlier is $10. Airmail delivery outside the continental United States is available for an additional charge of $90 per year. Requests to replace missing issues free of charge are honored only up to six months after date of issue.

Payments to ASHP are not deductible as charitable contributions for federal income tax purposes. However, they may be deductible under other provisions of the Internal Revenue Code.

Advertising for Clinical Pharmacy is accepted in accordance with the Statement of Advertising Policy of the American Society of Hospital Pharmacists (see *Am J Hosp Pharm.* 1987; 44:1146). For additional information, contact the Advertising Representative (William McCausland Associates, Inc., P.O. Box 189, Pitman, NJ 08071. Phone 609-589-5454, Fax 609-582-7611).

All articles published, including editorials, letters, and book reviews, represent the opinions of the authors and do not reflect the official policy of the American Society of Hospital Pharmacists or the institution with which the author is affiliated, unless this is specified.

Microfilm and microfiche editions are available for purchase. Contact University Microfilms, 300 N. Zeeb Road, Ann Arbor, MI 48106.

Articles in Clinical Pharmacy are abstracted and indexed in *Current Contents, Clinical Sciences, Excerpta Medica, Index Medicus, Inpharma, International Pharmaceutical Abstracts,* and *Reactions*.

June 1991 Volume 10, Number 6 Coden: CPHADV ISSN: 0278-2677

CLINICAL PHARMACY

411 **News**

Marketing of recombinant granulocyte–macrophage colony-stimulating factor approved by FDA . . . Etodolac approved for marketing in United States . . . Anabolic steroids reclassified as Schedule III controlled substances . . . Latex in medical devices may cause severe reactions; extra care advised . . . CDC revises mefloquine dosage recommendations

427 **Therapy Consultation**

Treatment of nocturnal leg cramps and restless leg syndrome

429 **Letters**

Cryoprecipitate for uremic bleeding, Robertson Davenport; Patricia Couch

429 **Correction**

Drug Review

430 **Ondansetron—the first of a new class of antiemetic agents**
Betty J. Chaffee and Roberta M. Tankanow

Therapy Reviews

447 **Alternatives in the treatment of memory loss in patients with Alzheimer's disease**
Burgunda W. Volger

456 **Treatment of delirium in the critically ill patient**
Douglas N. Fish

Therapy Update

467 **Ethnicity and psychotropic drugs**
William S. Bond

DUE Criteria

471 **Criteria for use of ondansetron hydrochloride in adult and pediatric inpatients and adult outpatients**
Steven C. Hartwig

474 **CP Continuing Education**

478 **Current Literature**

Drug Reaction Alerts . . . Books Received

479 **FDA Adverse Reaction Report Form and Instructions**

482 **Advertising Index**

Editorial Office
4630 Montgomery Avenue
Bethesda, MD 20814
301-657-3000
Fax 301-657-1615

Advertising Representative
William McCausland Associates, Inc.
P.O. Box 189
Pitman, NJ 08071
609-589-5454
Fax 609-582-7611

Printed on acid-free paper effective with Volume 8, January 1989.

Instructions to Authors

Clinical Pharmacy, a forum for the drug therapeutics information that pharmacists need to perform their clinical roles, gives priority to (1) studies that objectively evaluate drug effects in human trials, (2) evaluative review articles on the clinical uses of new drugs, and (3) evaluations of the current status of drug therapy in selected diseases. Contributions to the following sections are invited.

Drug Reviews: Detailed, analytical reviews on the clinical use of specific drugs, with preference given to new drugs and to evaluative rather than descriptive literature reviews.

Therapy Reviews: Articles that focus primarily on a disease state and its treatment.

Clinical Frontiers: Articles that review important, ongoing research on disease processes, drug mechanisms, or new technologies and project the likely implications for therapy.

Research: Reports of well-conducted original research on drug effects in humans.

Research Notes: Short research reports, such as updates on previously published work, confirmations of previous findings, or original research of modest scope.

Grand Rounds: Patient case reports and literature reviews combined in a way that gives them high educational value.

Drug Experience: Straightforward reports, with selected literature references, of unusual drug experiences.

Therapy Consultation: Brief advice, in a question-and-answer format, on how to handle specific drug-therapy problems. Readers are invited to submit questions, which the editor will forward to consultants for answering.

Letters: Short comments on previously published work or about potential problems, apparent trends, or controversies in drug therapy or clinical research.

Commentaries: Well-reasoned expressions of opinion on drug-therapy or clinical-research issues.

The editors have the sole authority to decide in which section to publish an accepted manuscript.

Manuscripts are subject to review by qualified outside reviewers, as well as by the editors, and will be accepted for publication only if they are believed to represent an important contribution to the literature. All papers submitted for publication must be accompanied by a completed copy of a manuscript checklist. The checklist, which generally conforms to the Uniform Requirements for Manuscripts Submitted to Biomedical Journals, appears on pages 60-61 of the January 1991 issue. Authors of especially important original work may request "fast-track" review of their papers. Authors may suggest appropriate reviewers for their papers.

Accepted materials become the permanent and sole property of ASHP and may not be published or reprinted elsewhere without written permission from both the author and the editor.

The editors reserve the right to revise all materials submitted, if necessary. The publisher assumes no responsibility for the statements and opinions advanced by contributors to Clinical Pharmacy.

Under the terms of the Copyright Revision Act of 1976 (Public Law 94-553) it is necessary to have the rights of the authors transferred to the publisher in order to provide for the widest possible dissemination of professional and scientific literature. Accordingly, all transmittal letters accompanying manuscripts submitted for publication, including contributions for the Letters column, must contain the following language: "In consideration of the American Society of Hospital Pharmacists (ASHP) taking action in reviewing and editing my (our) submission, the author(s) undersigned hereby transfer(s), assign(s), or otherwise convey(s) all ownership rights in the submission and all copyright ownership to ASHP. In the event that such work is not published by ASHP, all said rights shall be released." We regret that we cannot consider manuscripts for publication that are not accompanied by transmittal letters containing the above language signed by all authors.

Authors must certify in their letter of transmittal that none of the material in their manuscript has been published previously nor is under consideration or been accepted for publication elsewhere. If this certification cannot be made, suitable explanation must be offered.

Eight copies of all manuscripts should be submitted. Manuscripts should be typewritten with double spacing (including tables) on one side of good-quality, 21.6 x 27.9-cm white paper, and with margins of at least 2.5 cm. For guidance on style, authors should consult the manuscript checklist, recent issues of Clinical Pharmacy, and the *Council of Biology Editors Style Manual, fifth edition. The American Heritage Dictionary of the English Language and the AMA's Manual of Style* contain helpful advice on correct usage.

Galley proofs or final edited manuscripts are sent to authors for inspection against the original manuscript and for correction. Unnecessary alterations at this stage must be avoided. An order form for reprints is sent to the corresponding author at the time of publication.

Clinical Pharmacy (ISSN 0278-2677) is published monthly by the American Society of Hospital Pharmacists, 4630 Montgomery Avenue, Bethesda, MD 20814. Joseph A. Oddis, Executive Vice President. Second-class postage is paid at Bethesda, MD, and at additional mailing offices. **Postmaster: Send address changes to: *Clinical Pharmacy*, 4630 Montgomery Avenue, Bethesda, MD 20814.**

Annual Subscription Rate:	*USA*	*Non-USA*
ASHP Members	$45	$60
ASHP Student Members and Residents	$35	$50
Institutions and Nonmembers	$80	$95

The cost of single copies is $10. Airmail delivery outside the continental United States is available for an additional charge of $90 per year. Requests to replace missing issues free of charge are honored only up to six months after date of issue.

Payments to ASHP are not deductible as charitable contributions for federal income tax purposes. However, they may be deductible under other provisions of the Internal Revenue Code.

Advertising for Clinical Pharmacy is accepted in accordance with the Statement of Advertising Policy of the American Society of Hospital Pharmacists (see *Am J Hosp Pharm.* 1987; 44:1146). For additional information, contact the Advertising Representative (William McCausland Associates, Inc., P.O. Box 189, Pitman, NJ 08071. Phone 609-589-5454, Fax 609-582-7611).

All articles published, including editorials, letters, and book reviews, represent the opinions of the authors and do not reflect the official policy of the American Society of Hospital Pharmacists or the institution with which the author is affiliated, unless this is specified.

Microfilm and microfiche editions are available for purchase. Contact University Microfilms, 300 N. Zeeb Road, Ann Arbor, MI 48106.

Articles in Clinical Pharmacy are abstracted and indexed in *Current Contents, Clinical Sciences, Excerpta Medica, Index Medicus, Inpharma, International Pharmaceutical Abstracts*, and *Reactions*.

July 1991 Volume 10, Number 7 Coden: CPHADV ISSN: 0278-2677

CLINICAL PHARMACY

486 **News**

Conference attendees told ISIS-3 shows equal efficacy, safety differences among thrombolytics, William A. Check . . . Fludarabine approved for marketing . . . Enzyme replacement therapy approved for Gaucher's disease

500 **Letters**

Labetalol for treatment of hypertension in a child, Denis Y. Ishisaka, Charles D. Yonan, Ben F. Housel . . . Antimicrobial dosages in guidelines for prevention of bacterial endocarditis, Julie McMorrow, Paul R. Jones, Milap C. Nahata

501 **Correction**

Therapy Reviews

503 **Therapy of acute thromboembolism with heparin and warfarin**
Barry L. Carter

518 **Pharmacologic management of endometriosis**
Emmanuel Saltiel and Susan M. Garabedian-Ruffalo

Research

532 **Pharmacokinetics and pharmacodynamics of glyburide in young and elderly nondiabetic adults**
Terry L. Schwinghammer, Edward J. Antal, Reneé T. Kubacka, Mary E. Hackimer, and Jann M. Johnston

539 **Effect of ranitidine on the disposition of orally and intravenously administered triazolam**
R. Pete Vanderveen, Jana L. Jirak, Gary R. Peters, Steven R. Cox, and Paul A. Bombardt

544 **Susceptibility of *Xanthomonas maltophilia* and amikacin-resistant gram-negative bacteria to newer antimicrobials**
Joy R. Matsuyama, Barbara Beail, Carolyn Wallis, Dee Zeleznik, and Teresa Tartaglione

DUE Criteria

549 **Criteria for use of hetastarch**
Sharon A. Basile

552 **CP Continuing Education**

555 **FDA Adverse Reaction Report Form and Instructions**

558 **Current Literature**

Drug Reaction Alerts

558 **Advertising Index**

Editorial Office
4630 Montgomery Avenue
Bethesda, MD 20814
301-657-3000
Fax 301-657-1615

Advertising Representative
William McCausland Associates, Inc.
P.O. Box 189
Pitman, NJ 08071
609-589-5454
Fax 609-582-7611

Printed on acid-free paper effective with Volume 8, January 1989.

Instructions to Authors

Clinical Pharmacy, a forum for the drug therapeutics information that pharmacists need to perform their clinical roles, gives priority to (1) studies that objectively evaluate drug effects in human trials, (2) evaluative review articles on the clinical uses of new drugs, and (3) evaluations of the current status of drug therapy in selected diseases. Contributions to the following sections are invited.

Drug Reviews: Detailed, analytical reviews on the clinical use of specific drugs, with preference given to new drugs and to evaluative rather than descriptive literature reviews.

Therapy Reviews: Articles that focus primarily on a disease state and its treatment.

Clinical Frontiers: Articles that review important, ongoing research on disease processes, drug mechanisms, or new technologies and project the likely implications for therapy.

Research: Reports of well-conducted original research on drug effects in humans.

Research Notes: Short research reports, such as updates on previously published work, confirmations of previous findings, or original research of modest scope.

Grand Rounds: Patient case reports and literature reviews combined in a way that gives them high educational value.

Drug Experience: Straightforward reports, with selected literature references, of unusual drug experiences.

Therapy Consultation: Brief advice, in a question-and-answer format, on how to handle specific drug-therapy problems. Readers are invited to submit questions, which the editor will forward to consultants for answering.

Letters: Short comments on previously published work or about potential problems, apparent trends, or controversies in drug therapy or clinical research.

Commentaries: Well-reasoned expressions of opinion on drug-therapy or clinical-research issues.

The editors have the sole authority to decide in which section to publish an accepted manuscript.

Manuscripts are subject to review by qualified outside reviewers, as well as by the editors, and will be accepted for publication only if they are believed to represent an important contribution to the literature. All papers submitted for publication must be accompanied by a completed copy of a manuscript checklist. The checklist, which generally conforms to the Uniform Requirements for Manuscripts Submitted to Biomedical Journals, appears on pages 60-61 of the January 1991 issue. Authors of especially important original work may request "fast-track" review of their papers. Authors may suggest appropriate reviewers for their papers.

Accepted materials become the permanent and sole property of ASHP and may not be published or reprinted elsewhere without written permission from both the author and the editor.

The editors reserve the right to revise all materials submitted, if necessary. The publisher assumes no responsibility for the statements and opinions advanced by contributors to Clinical Pharmacy.

Under the terms of the Copyright Revision Act of 1976 (Public Law 94-553) it is necessary to have the rights of the authors transferred to the publisher in order to provide for the widest possible dissemination of professional and scientific literature. Accordingly, all transmittal letters accompanying manuscripts submitted for publication, including contributions for the Letters column, must contain the following language: "In consideration of the American Society of Hospital Pharmacists (ASHP) taking action in reviewing and editing my (our) submission, the author(s) undersigned hereby transfer(s), assign(s), or otherwise convey(s) all ownership rights in the submission and all copyright ownership to ASHP. In the event that such work is not published by ASHP, all said rights shall be released." We regret that we cannot consider manuscripts for publication that are not accompanied by transmittal letters containing the above language signed by all authors.

Authors must certify in their letter of transmittal that none of the material in their manuscript has been published previously nor is under consideration or been accepted for publication elsewhere. If this certification cannot be made, suitable explanation must be offered.

Eight copies of all manuscripts should be submitted. Manuscripts should be typewritten with double spacing (including tables) on one side of good-quality, 21.6 x 27.9-cm white paper, and with margins of at least 2.5 cm. For guidance on style, authors should consult the manuscript checklist, recent issues of Clinical Pharmacy, and the *Council of Biology Editors Style Manual, fifth edition. The American Heritage Dictionary of the English Language and the AMA's Manual of Style* contain helpful advice on correct usage.

Galley proofs or final edited manuscripts are sent to authors for inspection against the original manuscript and for correction. Unnecessary alterations at this stage must be avoided. An order form for reprints is sent to the corresponding author at the time of publication.

Clinical Pharmacy (ISSN 0278-2677) is published monthly by the American Society of Hospital Pharmacists, 4630 Montgomery Avenue, Bethesda, MD 20814. Joseph A. Oddis, Executive Vice President. Second-class postage is paid at Bethesda, MD, and at additional mailing offices. **Postmaster: Send address changes to: *Clinical Pharmacy*, 4630 Montgomery Avenue, Bethesda, MD 20814.**

Annual Subscription Rate:	*USA*	*Non-USA*
ASHP Members	$45	$60
ASHP Student Members and Residents	$35	$50
Institutions and Nonmembers	$80	$95

The cost of single copies is $10. Airmail delivery outside the continental United States is available for an additional charge of $90 per year. Requests to replace missing issues free of charge are honored only up to six months after date of issue.

Payments to ASHP are not deductible as charitable contributions for federal income tax purposes. However, they may be deductible under other provisions of the Internal Revenue Code.

Advertising for Clinical Pharmacy is accepted in accordance with the Statement of Advertising Policy of the American Society of Hospital Pharmacists (see *Am J Hosp Pharm.* 1987;44:1146). For additional information, contact the Advertising Representative (William McCausland Associates, Inc., P.O. Box 189, Pitman, NJ 08071. Phone 609-589-5454, Fax 609-582-7611).

All articles published, including editorials, letters, and book reviews, represent the opinions of the authors and do not reflect the official policy of the American Society of Hospital Pharmacists or the institution with which the author is affiliated, unless this is specified.

Microfilm and microfiche editions are available for purchase. Contact University Microfilms, 300 N. Zeeb Road, Ann Arbor, MI 48106.

Articles in Clinical Pharmacy are abstracted and indexed in *Current Contents, Clinical Sciences, Excerpta Medica, Index Medicus, Inpharma, International Pharmaceutical Abstracts,* and *Reactions.*

August 1991 Volume 10, Number 8 Coden: CPHADV ISSN: 0278-2677

CLINICAL PHARMACY

569 **News**

Guidelines for *Pneumocystis carinii* pneumonia prophylaxis in children issued . . . Gallium marketed for treatment of cancer-related hypercalcemia . . . Two cardiovascular agents, ramipril and isradipine, approved for U.S. market

Drug Review

581 **Clinical uses of fentanyl, sufentanil, and alfentanil**
Michael A. Clotz and Milap C. Nahata

Therapy Review

594 **Drug use during breast-feeding**
Philip O. Anderson

Research

625 **Determination of sedative and amnestic doses of lorazepam in children**
David W. Henry, Joseph W. Burwinkle, and Neil E. Klutman

Research Note

630 **Infusion failure caused by phlebitis and extravasation**
Alex Wright and John Hecker

DUE Criteria

635 **Criteria for use of fentanyl citrate, sufentanil citrate, and alfentanil hydrochloride**
Grant B. Satterlee and Irene A. Skora

638 **CP Continuing Education**

641 **FDA Adverse Reaction Report Form and Instructions**

644 **Current Literature**

Drug Reaction Alerts . . . Book Reviews: *Biopharmaceutics and Clinical Pharmacokinetics, Fourth Edition (Gibaldi)*, Donald G. Floriddia . . . *Drug Safety in Pregnancy (Folb, Dukes)*, Don Uden . . . Books Received

650 **Advertising Index**

Editorial Office
4630 Montgomery Avenue
Bethesda, MD 20814
301-657-3000
Fax 301-657-1615

Advertising Representative
William McCausland Associates, Inc.
P.O. Box 189
Pitman, NJ 08071
609-589-5454
Fax 609-582-7611

Printed on acid-free paper effective with Volume 8, January 1989.

Instructions to Authors

CLINICAL PHARMACY, a forum for the drug therapeutics information that pharmacists need to perform their clinical roles, gives priority to (1) studies that objectively evaluate drug effects in human trials, (2) evaluative review articles on the clinical uses of new drugs, and (3) evaluations of the current status of drug therapy in selected diseases. Contributions to the following sections are invited.

Drug Reviews: Detailed, analytical reviews on the clinical use of specific drugs, with preference given to new drugs and to evaluative rather than descriptive literature reviews.

Therapy Reviews: Articles that focus primarily on a disease state and its treatment.

Clinical Frontiers: Articles that review important, ongoing research on disease processes, drug mechanisms, or new technologies and project the likely implications for therapy.

Research: Reports of well-conducted original research on drug effects in humans.

Research Notes: Short research reports, such as updates on previously published work, confirmations of previous findings, or original research of modest scope.

Grand Rounds: Patient case reports and literature reviews combined in a way that gives them high educational value.

Drug Experience: Straightforward reports, with selected literature references, of unusual drug experiences.

Therapy Consultation: Brief advice, in a question-and-answer format, on how to handle specific drug-therapy problems. Readers are invited to submit questions, which the editor will forward to consultants for answering.

Letters: Short comments on previously published work or about potential problems, apparent trends, or controversies in drug therapy or clinical research.

Commentaries: Well-reasoned expressions of opinion on drug-therapy or clinical-research issues.

The editors have the sole authority to decide in which section to publish an accepted manuscript.

Manuscripts are subject to review by qualified outside reviewers, as well as by the editors, and will be accepted for publication only if they are believed to represent an important contribution to the literature. All papers submitted for publication must be accompanied by a completed copy of a manuscript checklist. The checklist, which generally conforms to the Uniform Requirements for Manuscripts Submitted to Biomedical Journals, appears on pages 60-61 of the January 1991 issue. Authors of especially important original work may request "fast-track" review of their papers. Authors may suggest appropriate reviewers for their papers.

Accepted materials become the permanent and sole property of ASHP and may not be published or reprinted elsewhere without written permission from both the author and the editor.

The editors reserve the right to revise all materials submitted, if necessary. The publisher assumes no responsibility for the statements and opinions advanced by contributors to CLINICAL PHARMACY.

Under the terms of the Copyright Revision Act of 1976 (Public Law 94-553) it is necessary to have the rights of the authors transferred to the publisher in order to provide for the widest possible dissemination of professional and scientific literature. Accordingly, all transmittal letters accompanying manuscripts submitted for publication, including contributions for the Letters column, must contain the following language: "In consideration of the American Society of Hospital Pharmacists (ASHP) taking action in reviewing and editing my (our) submission, the author(s) undersigned hereby transfer(s), assign(s), or otherwise convey(s) all ownership rights in the submission and all copyright ownership to ASHP. In the event that such work is not published by ASHP, all said rights shall be released." We regret that we cannot consider manuscripts for publication that are not accompanied by transmittal letters containing the above language signed by all authors.

Authors must certify in their letter of transmittal that none of the material in their manuscript has been published previously nor is under consideration or been accepted for publication elsewhere. If this certification cannot be made, suitable explanation must be offered.

Eight copies of all manuscripts should be submitted. Manuscripts should be typewritten with double spacing (including tables) on one side of good-quality, 21.6 x 27.9-cm white paper, and with margins of at least 2.5 cm. For guidance on style, authors should consult the manuscript checklist, recent issues of CLINICAL PHARMACY, and the *Council of Biology Editors Style Manual, fifth edition. The American Heritage Dictionary of the English Language and the AMA's Manual of Style* contain helpful advice on correct usage.

Galley proofs or final edited manuscripts are sent to authors for inspection against the original manuscript and for correction. Unnecessary alterations at this stage must be avoided. An order form for reprints is sent to the corresponding author at the time of publication.

CLINICAL PHARMACY (ISSN 0278-2677) is published monthly by the American Society of Hospital Pharmacists, 4630 Montgomery Avenue, Bethesda, MD 20814. Joseph A. Oddis, Executive Vice President. Second-class postage is paid at Bethesda, MD, and at additional mailing offices. **Postmaster: Send address changes to: *Clinical Pharmacy*, 4630 Montgomery Avenue, Bethesda, MD 20814.**

Annual Subscription Rate:	*USA*	*Non-USA*
ASHP Members	$45	$60
ASHP Student Members and Residents	$35	$50
Institutions and Nonmembers	$80	$95

The cost of single copies is $10. Airmail delivery outside the continental United States is available for an additional charge of $90 per year. Requests to replace missing issues free of charge are honored only up to six months after date of issue.

Payments to ASHP are not deductible as charitable contributions for federal income tax purposes. However, they may be deductible under other provisions of the Internal Revenue Code.

Advertising for CLINICAL PHARMACY is accepted in accordance with the Statement of Advertising Policy of the American Society of Hospital Pharmacists (see *Am J Hosp Pharm.* 1987;44:1146). For additional information, contact the Advertising Representative (William McCausland Associates, Inc., P.O. Box 189, Pitman, NJ 08071. Phone 609-589-5454, Fax 609-582-7611).

All articles published, including editorials, letters, and book reviews, represent the opinions of the authors and do not reflect the official policy of the American Society of Hospital Pharmacists or the institution with which the author is affiliated, unless this is specified.

Microfilm and microfiche editions are available for purchase. Contact University Microfilms, 300 N. Zeeb Road, Ann Arbor, MI 48106.

Articles in CLINICAL PHARMACY are abstracted and indexed in *Current Contents, Clinical Sciences, Excerpta Medica, Index Medicus, Inpharma, International Pharmaceutical Abstracts,* and *Reactions.*

September 1991 Volume 10, Number 9 Coden: CPHADV ISSN: 0278-2677

CLINICAL PHARMACY

653 **News**

CDC publishes guidelines for anergy testing in HIV-infected persons . . . Intravenous quinidine recommended for severe *Plasmodium falciparum* malaria; injectable quinine discontinued by CDC Drug Service . . . Single large dose of intravenous immune globulin more effective than four-day regimen in patients with Kawasaki disease, investigators report

658 **Therapy Consultation**

Analgesic selection when the patient is allergic to codeine

664 **Letters**

Dosage of antimycobacterial agents, Charles A. Peloquin . . . Valproic acid hepatotoxicity in adults and older children, Jamie T. Gilman

Therapy Reviews

667 **Management of acute pain in children**
Varsha Bhatt-Mehta and David A. Rosen

685 **Treatment of asthma in children**
Christine M. Murphy, Shannon L. Coonce, and Pamela A. Simon

Research Notes

704 **Prediction of serum albumin concentration after albumin supplementation in pediatric patients receiving parenteral nutrition**
Emily B. Cochran and Susan L. Hogue

706 **A nonexponential, nonlogarithmic pharmacokinetic dosing method for gentamicin**
Thomas E. Lackner, Weeranuj Yamreudeewong, and Peter D. Weiss

Drug Experience

711 **Multiple-dose activated charcoal as adjunct therapy after chronic phenytoin intoxication**
Paul J. Weidle, Daniel J. Skiest, and Alan Forrest

DUE Criteria

715 **Criteria for use of ketorolac tromethamine in adult inpatients and outpatients**
Michele F. Shepherd

718 **CP Continuing Education**

726 **Current Literature**

Drug Reaction Alerts . . . Book Reviews: *Diseases of the Nose, Throat, Ear, Head, and Neck, Fourteenth Edition (Ballenger)*, Elaine R. Green . . . *Handbook of Psychiatric Emergencies (Dubin, Weiss)*, Susan S. Fish

727 **FDA Adverse Reaction Report Form and Instructions**

730 **Advertising Index**

Editorial Office
4630 Montgomery Avenue
Bethesda, MD 20814
301-657-3000
Fax 301-657-1615

Advertising Representative
William McCausland Associates, Inc.
P.O. Box 189
Pitman, NJ 08071
609-589-5454
Fax 609-582-7611

Printed on acid-free paper effective with Volume 8, January 1989.

Instructions to Authors

CLINICAL PHARMACY, a forum for the drug therapeutics information that pharmacists need to perform their clinical roles, gives priority to (1) studies that objectively evaluate drug effects in human trials, (2) evaluative review articles on the clinical uses of new drugs, and (3) evaluations of the current status of drug therapy in selected diseases. Contributions to the following sections are invited.

Drug Reviews: Detailed, analytical reviews on the clinical use of specific drugs, with preference given to new drugs and to evaluative rather than descriptive literature reviews.

Therapy Reviews: Articles that focus primarily on a disease state and its treatment.

Clinical Frontiers: Articles that review important, ongoing research on disease processes, drug mechanisms, or new technologies and project the likely implications for therapy.

Research: Reports of well-conducted original research on drug effects in humans.

Research Notes: Short research reports, such as updates on previously published work, confirmations of previous findings, or original research of modest scope.

Grand Rounds: Patient case reports and literature reviews combined in a way that gives them high educational value.

Drug Experience: Straightforward reports, with selected literature references, of unusual drug experiences.

Therapy Consultation: Brief advice, in a question-and-answer format, on how to handle specific drug-therapy problems. Readers are invited to submit questions, which the editor will forward to consultants for answering.

Letters: Short comments on previously published work or about potential problems, apparent trends, or controversies in drug therapy or clinical research.

Commentaries: Well-reasoned expressions of opinion on drug-therapy or clinical-research issues.

The editors have the sole authority to decide in which section to publish an accepted manuscript.

Manuscripts are subject to review by qualified outside reviewers, as well as by the editors, and will be accepted for publication only if they are believed to represent an important contribution to the literature. All papers submitted for publication must be accompanied by a completed copy of a manuscript checklist. The checklist, which generally conforms to the Uniform Requirements for Manuscripts Submitted to Biomedical Journals, appears on pages 60-61 of the January 1991 issue. Authors of especially important original work may request "fast-track" review of their papers. Authors may suggest appropriate reviewers for their papers.

Accepted materials become the permanent and sole property of ASHP and may not be published or reprinted elsewhere without written permission from both the author and the editor.

The editors reserve the right to revise all materials submitted, if necessary. The publisher assumes no responsibility for the statements and opinions advanced by contributors to CLINICAL PHARMACY.

Under the terms of the Copyright Revision Act of 1976 (Public Law 94-553) it is necessary to have the rights of the authors transferred to the publisher in order to provide for the widest possible dissemination of professional and scientific literature. Accordingly, all transmittal letters accompanying manuscripts submitted for publication, including contributions for the Letters column, must contain the following language: "In consideration of the American Society of Hospital Pharmacists (ASHP) taking action in reviewing and editing my (our) submission, the author(s) undersigned hereby transfer(s), assign(s), or otherwise convey(s) all ownership rights in the submission and all copyright ownership to ASHP. In the event that such work is not published by ASHP, all said rights shall be released." We regret that we cannot consider manuscripts for publication that are not accompanied by transmittal letters containing the above language signed by all authors.

Authors must certify in their letter of transmittal that none of the material in their manuscript has been published previously nor is under consideration or been accepted for publication elsewhere. If this certification cannot be made, suitable explanation must be offered.

Eight copies of all manuscripts should be submitted. Manuscripts should be typewritten with double spacing (including tables) on one side of good-quality, 21.6 x 27.9-cm white paper, and with margins of at least 2.5 cm. For guidance on style, authors should consult the manuscript checklist, recent issues of CLINICAL PHARMACY, and the *Council of Biology Editors Style Manual, fifth edition. The American Heritage Dictionary of the English Language and the AMA's Manual of Style* contain helpful advice on correct usage.

Galley proofs or final edited manuscripts are sent to authors for inspection against the original manuscript and for correction. Unnecessary alterations at this stage must be avoided. An order form for reprints is sent to the corresponding author at the time of publication.

CLINICAL PHARMACY (ISSN 0278-2677) is published monthly by the American Society of Hospital Pharmacists, 4630 Montgomery Avenue, Bethesda, MD 20814. Joseph A. Oddis, Executive Vice President. Second-class postage is paid at Bethesda, MD, and at additional mailing offices. **Postmaster: Send address changes to: *Clinical Pharmacy*, 4630 Montgomery Avenue, Bethesda, MD 20814.**

Annual Subscription Rate:	*USA*	*Non-USA*
ASHP Members	$45	$60
ASHP Student Members and Residents	$35	$50
Institutions and Nonmembers	$80	$95

The cost of single copies is $10. Airmail delivery outside the continental United States is available for an additional charge of $90 per year. Requests to replace missing issues free of charge are honored only up to six months after date of issue.

Payments to ASHP are not deductible as charitable contributions for federal income tax purposes. However, they may be deductible under other provisions of the Internal Revenue Code.

Advertising for CLINICAL PHARMACY is accepted in accordance with the Statement of Advertising Policy of the American Society of Hospital Pharmacists (see *Am J Hosp Pharm.* 1987; 44:1146). For additional information, contact the Advertising Representative (William McCausland Associates, Inc., P.O. Box 189, Pitman, NJ 08071. Phone 609-589-5454, Fax 609-582-7611).

All articles published, including editorials, letters, and book reviews, represent the opinions of the authors and do not reflect the official policy of the American Society of Hospital Pharmacists or the institution with which the author is affiliated, unless this is specified.

Microfilm and microfiche editions are available for purchase. Contact University Microfilms, 300 N. Zeeb Road, Ann Arbor, MI 48106.

Articles in CLINICAL PHARMACY are abstracted and indexed in *Current Contents, Clinical Sciences, Excerpta Medica, Index Medicus, Inpharma, International Pharmaceutical Abstracts,* and *Reactions.*

October 1991 Volume 10, Number 10 Coden: CPHADV ISSN: 0278-2677

CLINICAL PHARMACY

733 **News**

Haemophilus b immunization recommendations updated by American Academy of Pediatrics . . . American Academy of Pediatrics issues recommendations on treatment of Lyme disease . . . Benazepril approved for treatment of hypertension

740 **Therapy Consultation**

Treatment options for a patient with osteoarthritis and a history of ulcer disease

742 **Letters**

Hyperthyroidism associated with mercury poisoning, Michael McCann, Stuart Scheckner . . . Ethnicity and clozapine-induced agranulocytosis, Karen Overstreet Price

Therapy Reviews

745 **Management of postoperative pain by continuous epidural infusion of analgesics**
Amy L. Shafer and Andrew J. Donnelly

765 **Assessment and treatment of acetaminophen overdose**
Richard K. Lewis and Frank P. Paloucek

775 **Treatment of chronic iron overload**
Marilyn H. Kirking

Research Note

784 **Altered aminoglycoside volume of distribution in patients with acquired immunodeficiency syndrome**
Joyce M. Longley, Donald G. Pittman, and F. David Newby

DUE Criteria

787 **Criteria for stress ulcer prophylaxis in intensive-care patients**
Mark D. Peters II, Katherine A. Michael, Julie A. Sjolander, Keith A. Swanson, and Richard A. Medina

792 **CP Continuing Education**

801 **FDA Adverse Reaction Report Form and Instructions**

803 **Current Literature**

Drug Reaction Alerts . . . Book Reviews: *Drug Interactions & Updates, 1991 (Hansten, Horn),* Mary Lea Gora . . . *Infections in Intravenous Drug Abusers (Levine, Sobel),* Stephen Mendel . . . Books Received

806 **Advertising Index**

Editorial Office
4630 Montgomery Avenue
Bethesda, MD 20814
301-657-3000
Fax 301-657-1615

Advertising Representative
William McCausland Associates, Inc.
P.O. Box 189
Pitman, NJ 08071
609-589-5454
Fax 609-582-7611

Printed on acid-free paper effective with Volume 8, January 1989.

Instructions to Authors

CLINICAL PHARMACY, a forum for the drug therapeutics information that pharmacists need to perform their clinical roles, gives priority to (1) studies that objectively evaluate drug effects in human trials, (2) evaluative review articles on the clinical uses of new drugs, and (3) evaluations of the current status of drug therapy in selected diseases. Contributions to the following sections are invited.

Drug Reviews: Detailed, analytical reviews on the clinical use of specific drugs, with preference given to new drugs and to evaluative rather than descriptive literature reviews.

Therapy Reviews: Articles that focus primarily on a disease state and its treatment.

Therapy Update: Concise analytical reviews of narrowly defined, important topics in pharmacotherapy.

Clinical Frontiers: Articles that review important, ongoing research on disease processes, drug mechanisms, or new technologies and project the likely implications for therapy.

Research: Reports of well-conducted original research on drug effects in humans.

Research Notes: Short research reports, such as updates on previously published work, confirmations of previous findings, or original research of modest scope.

Grand Rounds: Patient case reports and literature reviews combined in a way that gives them high educational value.

Drug Experience: Straightforward reports, with selected literature references, of unusual drug experiences.

Therapy Consultation: Brief advice, in a question-and-answer format, on how to handle specific drug-therapy problems. Readers are invited to submit questions, which the editor will forward to consultants for answering.

Letters: Short comments on previously published work or about potential problems, apparent trends, or controversies in drug therapy or clinical research.

Commentaries: Well-reasoned expressions of opinion on drug-therapy or clinical-research issues.

The editors have the sole authority to decide in which section to publish an accepted manuscript.

Manuscripts are subject to review by qualified outside reviewers, as well as by the editors, and will be accepted for publication only if they are believed to represent an important contribution to the literature. All papers submitted for publication must be accompanied by a completed copy of a manuscript checklist. The checklist, which generally conforms to the Uniform Requirements for Manuscripts Submitted to Biomedical Journals, appears on pages 60-61 of the January 1991 issue. Authors of especially important original work may request "fast-track" review of their papers. Authors may suggest appropriate reviewers for their papers.

Accepted materials become the permanent and sole property of ASHP and may not be published or reprinted elsewhere without written permission from both the author and the editor.

The editors reserve the right to revise all materials submitted, if necessary. The publisher assumes no responsibility for the statements and opinions advanced by contributors to CLINICAL PHARMACY.

Under the terms of the Copyright Revision Act of 1976 (Public Law 94-553) it is necessary to have the rights of the authors transferred to the publisher in order to provide for the widest possible dissemination of professional and scientific literature. Accordingly, all transmittal letters accompanying manuscripts submitted for publication, including contributions for the Letters column, must contain the following language: "In consideration of the American Society of Hospital Pharmacists (ASHP) taking action in reviewing and editing my (our) submission, the author(s) undersigned hereby transfer(s), assign(s), or otherwise convey(s) all ownership rights in the submission and all copyright ownership to ASHP. In the event that such work is not published by ASHP, all said rights shall be released." We regret that we cannot consider manuscripts for publication that are not accompanied by transmittal letters containing the above language signed by all authors.

Authors must certify in their letter of transmittal that none of the material in their manuscript has been published previously nor is under consideration or been accepted for publication elsewhere. If this certification cannot be made, suitable explanation must be offered.

Eight copies of all manuscripts should be submitted. Manuscripts should be typewritten with double spacing (including tables) on one side of good-quality, 21.6 x 27.9-cm white paper, and with margins of at least 2.5 cm. For guidance on style, authors should consult the manuscript checklist, recent issues of CLINICAL PHARMACY, and the *Council of Biology Editors Style Manual, fifth edition. The American Heritage Dictionary of the English Language and the AMA's Manual of Style* contain helpful advice on correct usage.

Galley proofs or final edited manuscripts are sent to authors for inspection against the original manuscript and for correction. Unnecessary alterations at this stage must be avoided. An order form for reprints is sent to the corresponding author at the time of publication.

CLINICAL PHARMACY (ISSN 0278-2677) is published monthly by the American Society of Hospital Pharmacists, 4630 Montgomery Avenue, Bethesda, MD 20814. Joseph A. Oddis, Executive Vice President. Second-class postage is paid at Bethesda, MD, and at additional mailing offices. **Postmaster: Send address changes to: *Clinical Pharmacy*, 4630 Montgomery Avenue, Bethesda, MD 20814.**

Annual Subscription Rate:	*USA*	*Non-USA*
ASHP Members	$45	$60
ASHP Student Members and Residents	$35	$50
Institutions and Nonmembers	$80	$95

The cost of single copies is $10. Airmail delivery outside the continental United States is available for an additional charge of $90 per year. Requests to replace missing issues free of charge are honored only up to six months after date of issue.

Payments to ASHP are not deductible as charitable contributions for federal income tax purposes. However, they may be deductible under other provisions of the Internal Revenue Code.

Advertising for CLINICAL PHARMACY is accepted in accordance with the Statement of Advertising Policy of the American Society of Hospital Pharmacists (see *Am J Hosp Pharm.* 1987; 44:1146). For additional information, contact the Advertising Representative (William McCausland Associates, Inc., P.O. Box 189, Pitman, NJ 08071. Phone 609-589-5454, Fax 609-582-7611).

All articles published, including editorials, letters, and book reviews, represent the opinions of the authors and do not reflect the official policy of the American Society of Hospital Pharmacists or the institution with which the author is affiliated, unless this is specified.

Microfilm and microfiche editions are available for purchase. Contact University Microfilms, 300 N. Zeeb Road, Ann Arbor, MI 48106.

Articles in CLINICAL PHARMACY are abstracted and indexed in *Current Contents, Clinical Sciences, Current Awareness in Biologic Sciences, Excerpta Medica, Index Medicus, Inpharma, International Pharmaceutical Abstracts*, and *Reactions*.

November 1991 Volume 10, Number 11 Coden: CPHADV ISSN: 0278-2677

CLINICAL PHARMACY

809 **News**

Highlights of the Seventh International Conference on AIDS, Roberta J. Wong . . . Study raises safety questions about β-agonist inhaler overuse

823 **Letters**

Retreatment with digoxin immune Fab, Nancy M. Allen . . . Laboratory monitoring of heparin therapy, Ann K. Wittkowsky

824 **Correction**

Therapy Reviews

825 **Advances in the treatment of unstable angina pectoris**
Sarah A. Spinler and Lisa E. Davis

839 **Pathophysiology and treatment of Wilson's disease**
Roberta M. Tankanow

Clinical Frontiers

850 **Diastolic dysfunction in congestive heart failure**
Julie A. Johnson

Therapy Update

862 **Calcium-channel blockers for treatment of diabetic nephropathy**
Kim M. Murray

Research

866 **Modification of gastric pH with oral glutamic acid hydrochloride**
Margaret J. Knapp, Rosemary R. Berardi, Jennifer B. Dressman, Joan M. Rider, and Peggy L. Carver

Research Note

870 **Effects of misoprostol or ranitidine on ibuprofen pharmacokinetics**
Ralph E. Small, Melody G. Wilmot-Pater, Barbara A. McGee, and Hayes E. Willis

DUE Criteria

873 **Criteria for use of moricizine in adult inpatients and outpatients**
Teresa A. Bennett, J. Mark Trotter, and Alan B. Miller

876 **CP Continuing Education**

880 **Current Literature**

Drug Reaction Alerts . . . Book Reviews: *Handbook of Drug Therapy in Liver and Kidney Disease* (Schrier, Gambertoglio), J. Russell May . . . *Manual of Clinical Microbiology, Fifth Edition* (Balows, Hausler, Herrmann *et al.*), Patricia L. Orlando . . . *Pharmacological Treatment of Endocrinopathies: Bone Disease, Kidney Stones and Related Disorders* (Pak), Thomas J. Comstock . . . Books Received

881 **FDA Adverse Reaction Report Form and Instructions**

890 **Advertising Index**

Editorial Office
4630 Montgomery Avenue
Bethesda, MD 20814
301-657-3000
Fax 301-657-1615

Advertising Representative
William McCausland Associates, Inc.
P.O. Box 189
Pitman, NJ 08071
609-589-5454
Fax 609-582-7611

Printed on acid-free paper effective with Volume 8, January 1989.

Instructions to Authors

Clinical Pharmacy, a forum for the drug therapeutics information that pharmacists need to perform their clinical roles, gives priority to (1) studies that objectively evaluate drug effects in human trials, (2) evaluative review articles on the clinical uses of new drugs, and (3) evaluations of the current status of drug therapy in selected diseases. Contributions to the following sections are invited.

Drug Reviews: Detailed, analytical reviews on the clinical use of specific drugs, with preference given to new drugs and to evaluative rather than descriptive literature reviews.

Therapy Reviews: Articles that focus primarily on a disease state and its treatment.

Therapy Update: Concise analytical reviews of narrowly defined, important topics in pharmacotherapy.

Clinical Frontiers: Articles that review important, ongoing research on disease processes, drug mechanisms, or new technologies and project the likely implications for therapy.

Research: Reports of well-conducted original research on drug effects in humans.

Research Notes: Short research reports, such as updates on previously published work, confirmations of previous findings, or original research of modest scope.

Grand Rounds: Patient case reports and literature reviews combined in a way that gives them high educational value.

Drug Experience: Straightforward reports, with selected literature references, of unusual drug experiences.

Therapy Consultation: Brief advice, in a question-and-answer format, on how to handle specific drug-therapy problems. Readers are invited to submit questions, which the editor will forward to consultants for answering.

Letters: Short comments on previously published work or about potential problems, apparent trends, or controversies in drug therapy or clinical research.

Commentaries: Well-reasoned expressions of opinion on drug-therapy or clinical-research issues.

The editors have the sole authority to decide in which section to publish an accepted manuscript.

Manuscripts are subject to review by qualified outside reviewers, as well as by the editors, and will be accepted for publication only if they are believed to represent an important contribution to the literature. All papers submitted for publication must be accompanied by a completed copy of a manuscript checklist. The checklist, which generally conforms to the Uniform Requirements for Manuscripts Submitted to Biomedical Journals, appears on pages 60-61 of the January 1991 issue. Authors of especially important original work may request "fast-track" review of their papers. Authors may suggest appropriate reviewers for their papers.

Accepted materials become the permanent and sole property of ASHP and may not be published or reprinted elsewhere without written permission from both the author and the editor.

The editors reserve the right to revise all materials submitted, if necessary. The publisher assumes no responsibility for the statements and opinions advanced by contributors to Clinical Pharmacy.

Under the terms of the Copyright Revision Act of 1976 (Public Law 94-553) it is necessary to have the rights of the authors transferred to the publisher in order to provide for the widest possible dissemination of professional and scientific literature. Accordingly, all transmittal letters accompanying manuscripts submitted for publication, including contributions for the Letters column, must contain the following language: "In consideration of the American Society of Hospital Pharmacists (ASHP) taking action in reviewing and editing my (our) submission, the author(s) undersigned hereby transfer(s), assign(s), or otherwise convey(s) all ownership rights in the submission and all copyright ownership to ASHP. In the event that such work is not published by ASHP, all said rights shall be released." We regret that we cannot consider manuscripts for publication that are not accompanied by transmittal letters containing the above language signed by all authors.

Authors must certify in their letter of transmittal that none of the material in their manuscript has been published previously nor is under consideration or been accepted for publication elsewhere. If this certification cannot be made, suitable explanation must be offered.

Eight copies of all manuscripts should be submitted. Manuscripts should be typewritten with double spacing (including tables) on one side of good-quality, 21.6 x 27.9-cm white paper, and with margins of at least 2.5 cm. For guidance on style, authors should consult the manuscript checklist, recent issues of Clinical Pharmacy, and the *Council of Biology Editors Style Manual, fifth edition. The American Heritage Dictionary of the English Language and the AMA's Manual of Style* contain helpful advice on correct usage.

Galley proofs or final edited manuscripts are sent to authors for inspection against the original manuscript and for correction. Unnecessary alterations at this stage must be avoided. An order form for reprints is sent to the corresponding author at the time of publication.

Clinical Pharmacy (ISSN 0278-2677) is published monthly by the American Society of Hospital Pharmacists, 4630 Montgomery Avenue, Bethesda, MD 20814. Joseph A. Oddis, Executive Vice President. Second-class postage is paid at Bethesda, MD, and at additional mailing offices. **Postmaster: Send address changes to: *Clinical Pharmacy*, 4630 Montgomery Avenue, Bethesda, MD 20814.**

Annual Subscription Rate:	*USA*	*Non-USA*
ASHP Members	$45	$60
ASHP Student Members and Residents	$35	$50
Institutions and Nonmembers	$80	$95

The cost of single copies is $10. Airmail delivery outside the continental United States is available for an additional charge of $90 per year. Requests to replace missing issues free of charge are honored only up to six months after date of issue.

Payments to ASHP are not deductible as charitable contributions for federal income tax purposes. However, they may be deductible under other provisions of the Internal Revenue Code.

Advertising for Clinical Pharmacy is accepted in accordance with the Statement of Advertising Policy of the American Society of Hospital Pharmacists (see *Am J Hosp Pharm.* 1987; 44:1146). For additional information, contact the Advertising Representative (William McCausland Associates, Inc., P.O. Box 189, Pitman, NJ 08071. Phone 609-589-5454, Fax 609-582-7611).

All articles published, including editorials, letters, and book reviews, represent the opinions of the authors and do not reflect the official policy of the American Society of Hospital Pharmacists or the institution with which the author is affiliated, unless this is specified.

Microfilm and microfiche editions are available for purchase. Contact University Microfilms, 300 N. Zeeb Road, Ann Arbor, MI 48106.

Articles in Clinical Pharmacy are abstracted and indexed in *Current Contents, Clinical Sciences, Current Awareness in Biologic Sciences, Excerpta Medica, Index Medicus, Inpharma, International Pharmaceutical Abstracts*, and *Reactions*.

December 1991 Volume 10, Number 12 Coden: CPHADV ISSN: 0278-2677

CLINICAL PHARMACY

893 **News**

Consensus panel stresses need for greater awareness of panic disorder and its treatment . . . E5 antiendotoxin antibody reduces mortality among subset of patients with gram-negative sepsis, study finds . . . CAST II halted because of mortality trends . . . Bristol discontinues sales of encainide . . . Study shows effect of postmenopausal estrogen therapy on cardiovascular risk . . . CDC offers recommendations for folic acid prevention of neural tube defects

909 **Therapy Consultation**

Comparing surfactant products

912 **Letters**

Inverse relationship between desmopressin dosage and antidiuresis, Robert E. Ariano, Beverly Seymour . . . Correction to *AHFS Drug Information 91*, Stephanie L. Scholten

913 **Corrections**

Drug Review

914 **Succimer, an oral lead chelator**
Katherine V. Mann and John D. Travers

Research

923 **Nomogram for dosing warfarin at steady state**
Dean A. Fredriks and Robert W. Coleman

Research Notes

928 **Estimating phenytoin dosages in black African and Indian children**
Julia H. Botha, Raymond Miller, and Manikum Moodley

931 **Use of gentamicin clearance in estimating renal function**
Randall K. Nakahiro, Mark P. Okamoto, Alfred Chin, Mark A. Gill, Joanne S. Chae, and David A. Sclar

935 **Effect of flurbiprofen and aspirin on platelet aggregation**
Kelly T. Pincus, William J. Spruill, and Roy C. Parish

938 **Effect of use of generic thioridazine products on clinical outcome and quality of life**
Elena Bablenis, Stanley S. Weber, and Robert L. Dufresne

Editorial

942 **Succimer: Controversial issues involving the release of a new product**
William Banner, Jr.

Commentary

943 **Which lipid-lowering agent should be used first?**
David R. Rutledge

ASHP Report

946 **Acknowledgment to reviewers—October 1, 1990, to September 30, 1991**

DUE Criteria

947 **Criteria for use of sargramostim (granulocyte–macrophage colony-stimulating factor)**
J. Michael Burr and Bruce B. McCall

950 **Criteria for use of filgrastim (granulocyte colony-stimulating factor)**
J. Michael Burr and Bruce B. McCall

953 **CP Continuing Education**

955 **ASHP journal continuing-education instructions and enrollment form**

959 **FDA Adverse Reaction Report Form and Instructions**

966 **Current Literature**

Drug Reaction Alerts . . . Book Reviews: *Patient Compliance in Medical Practice and Clinical Trials* (*Cramer, Spilker*), David A. Graves . . . *Regional Antineoplastic Drug Delivery in the Management of Malignant Disease* (*Markman*), J. Kelly Martin, Jr. . . . Books Received

976 **Advertising Index**

980 **Annual Index**

Instructions to Authors

CLINICAL PHARMACY, a forum for the drug therapeutics information that pharmacists need to perform their clinical roles, gives priority to (1) studies that objectively evaluate drug effects in human trials, (2) evaluative review articles on the clinical uses of new drugs, and (3) evaluations of the current status of drug therapy in selected diseases. Contributions to the following sections are invited.

Drug Reviews: Detailed, analytical reviews on the clinical use of specific drugs, with preference given to new drugs and to evaluative rather than descriptive literature reviews.

Therapy Reviews: Articles that focus primarily on a disease state and its treatment.

Therapy Update: Concise analytical reviews of narrowly defined, important topics in pharmacotherapy.

Clinical Frontiers: Articles that review important, ongoing research on disease processes, drug mechanisms, or new technologies and project the likely implications for therapy.

Research: Reports of well-conducted original research on drug effects in humans.

Research Notes: Short research reports, such as updates on previously published work, confirmations of previous findings, or original research of modest scope.

Grand Rounds: Patient case reports and literature reviews combined in a way that gives them high educational value.

Drug Experience: Straightforward reports, with selected literature references, of unusual drug experiences.

Therapy Consultation: Brief advice, in a question-and-answer format, on how to handle specific drug-therapy problems. Readers are invited to submit questions, which the editor will forward to consultants for answering.

Letters: Short comments on previously published work or about potential problems, apparent trends, or controversies in drug therapy or clinical research.

Commentaries: Well-reasoned expressions of opinion on drug-therapy or clinical-research issues.

The editors have the sole authority to decide in which section to publish an accepted manuscript.

Manuscripts are subject to review by qualified outside reviewers, as well as by the editors, and will be accepted for publication only if they are believed to represent an important contribution to the literature. All papers submitted for publication must be accompanied by a completed copy of a manuscript checklist. The checklist, which generally conforms to the Uniform Requirements for Manuscripts Submitted to Biomedical Journals, appears on pages 60-61 of the January 1991 issue. Authors of especially important original work may request "fast-track" review of their papers. Authors may suggest appropriate reviewers for their papers.

Accepted materials become the permanent and sole property of ASHP and may not be published or reprinted elsewhere without written permission from both the author and the editor.

The editors reserve the right to revise all materials submitted, if necessary. The publisher assumes no responsibility for the statements and opinions advanced by contributors to CLINICAL PHARMACY.

Under the terms of the Copyright Revision Act of 1976 (Public Law 94-553) it is necessary to have the rights of the authors transferred to the publisher in order to provide for the widest possible dissemination of professional and scientific literature. Accordingly, all transmittal letters accompanying manuscripts submitted for publication, including contributions for the Letters column, must contain the following language: "In consideration of the American Society of Hospital Pharmacists (ASHP) taking action in reviewing and editing my (our) submission, the author(s) undersigned hereby transfer(s), assign(s), or otherwise convey(s) all ownership rights in the submission and all copyright ownership to ASHP. In the event that such work is not published by ASHP, all said rights shall be released." We regret that we cannot consider manuscripts for publication that are not accompanied by transmittal letters containing the above language signed by all authors.

Authors must certify in their letter of transmittal that none of the material in their manuscript has been published previously nor is under consideration or been accepted for publication elsewhere. If this certification cannot be made, suitable explanation must be offered.

Eight copies of all manuscripts should be submitted. Manuscripts should be typewritten with double spacing (including tables) on one side of good-quality, 21.6 x 27.9-cm white paper, and with margins of at least 2.5 cm. For guidance on style, authors should consult the manuscript checklist, recent issues of CLINICAL PHARMACY, and the *Council of Biology Editors Style Manual, fifth edition. The American Heritage Dictionary of the English Language and the AMA's Manual of Style* contain helpful advice on correct usage.

Galley proofs or final edited manuscripts are sent to authors for inspection against the original manuscript and for correction. Unnecessary alterations at this stage must be avoided. An order form for reprints is sent to the corresponding author at the time of publication.

CLINICAL PHARMACY (ISSN 0278-2677) is published monthly by the American Society of Hospital Pharmacists, 4630 Montgomery Avenue, Bethesda, MD 20814. Joseph A. Oddis, Executive Vice President. Second-class postage is paid at Bethesda, MD, and at additional mailing offices. **Postmaster: Send address changes to: *Clinical Pharmacy*, 4630 Montgomery Avenue, Bethesda, MD 20814.**

Annual Subscription Rate:	*USA*	*Non-USA*
ASHP Members	$45	$60
ASHP Student Members and Residents	$35	$50
Institutions and Nonmembers	$80	$95

The cost of single copies is $10. Airmail delivery outside the continental United States is available for an additional charge of $90 per year. Requests to replace missing issues free of charge are honored only up to six months after date of issue.

Payments to ASHP are not deductible as charitable contributions for federal income tax purposes. However, they may be deductible under other provisions of the Internal Revenue Code.

Advertising for CLINICAL PHARMACY is accepted in accordance with the Statement of Advertising Policy of the American Society of Hospital Pharmacists (see *Am J Hosp Pharm*. 1987; 44:1146). For additional information, contact the Advertising Representative (William McCausland Associates, Inc., P.O. Box 189, Pitman, NJ 08071. Phone 609-589-5454, Fax 609-582-7611).

All articles published, including editorials, letters, and book reviews, represent the opinions of the authors and do not reflect the official policy of the American Society of Hospital Pharmacists or the institution with which the author is affiliated, unless this is specified.

Microfilm and microfiche editions are available for purchase. Contact University Microfilms, 300 N. Zeeb Road, Ann Arbor, MI 48106.

Articles in CLINICAL PHARMACY are abstracted and indexed in *Current Contents, Clinical Sciences, Current Awareness in Biologic Sciences, Excerpta Medica, Index Medicus, Inpharma, International Pharmaceutical Abstracts*, and *Reactions*.

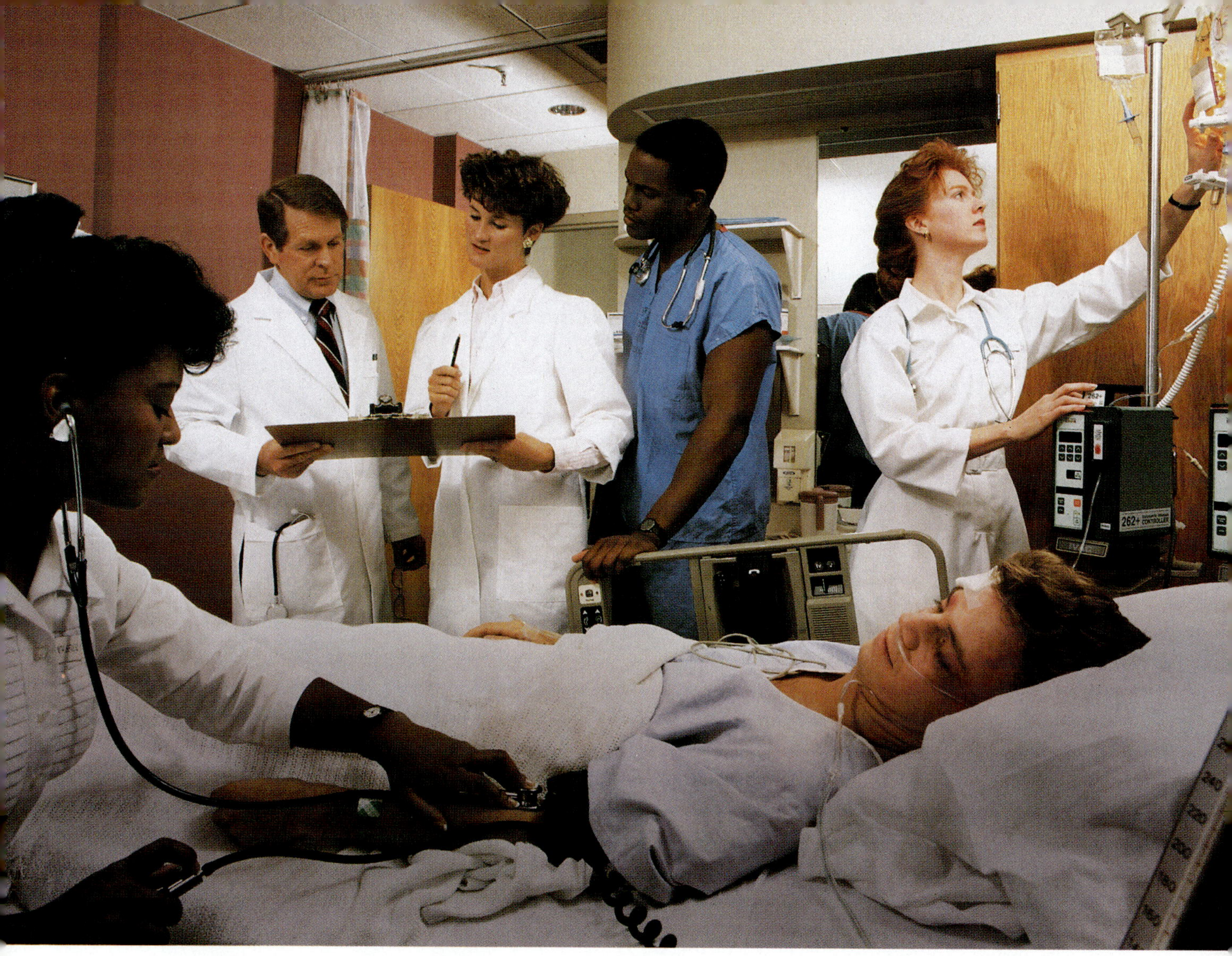

News

New method of analyzing health data stirs debate 4
Lawrence K. Altman

Changes in federal programs for reporting suspected adverse reactions to vaccines announced 9

Transdermal fentanyl approved for chronic pain management 9

Doxazosin approved as antihypertensive agent 9

News Briefs 10

Upcoming Specialty Meetings 11

New method of analyzing health data stirs debate

Editor's note: The following article was originally published in The New York Times, *August 21, 1990.*

Increasing use of a controversial statistical method to evaluate medical therapies and surgical procedures is beginning to affect profoundly the care of pregnant women and patients with cancer, heart disease, and many other common conditions.

The method, known as meta-analysis, promises to play an increasingly important role in determining health risks, environmental hazards, and national policy on payment for medical care.

Meta-analysis is a term derived from the Greek meaning an analysis that is more comprehensive. The larger numbers obtained by combining studies provide a greater statistical power than any of the individual studies. Researchers are often able to draw more reliable inferences or new conclusions from the combined results than from smaller studies that may be inconclusive individually.

In earlier applications of meta-analysis, researchers evaluated intelligence quotients, government social welfare programs, and many other topics. Meta-analysis has come to medicine late, but "it is now undergoing a boom in popularity," said Dr. Thomas C. Chalmers, a distinguished physician with the Department of Veterans Affairs in Boston and a pioneer in the methodology.

The method involves an analysis of previous analyses. It combines the results of a wide range of existing smaller studies and then applies one of several statistical techniques to discover more precisely what is known from previous research. It may also produce a unified result from diverse, apparently contradictory studies.

The technique has already shed new light on the effectiveness of medical therapies. Although it has not, in itself, revolutionized any medical treatment, it has helped to clear away the confusion caused by studies with scattered and apparently conflicting findings and has strengthened and confirmed findings from traditional clinical trials.

Continued on page 7

News *Continued from page 4*

Critics charge that poorly done meta-analyses can yield the wrong answers, although none interviewed could cite an example. Critics also say even well-done meta-analyses have been oversold in that they underemphasize the degree of uncertainty in the findings.

Experts themselves debate various methodological problems such as whether to include flawed studies in the meta-analysis along with well-done ones.

Meta-analyses provide a quantitative, systematic statistical alternative to the traditional scientific review article in which an expert assesses the meaning of a range of studies. Meta-analyses are intended to avoid the simplistic methods of review authors who often reach a conclusion by intuition, or by tallying the number of studies showing benefits and those failing to do so or on the basis of subjective biases.

"The issue is the increasing recognition that scientists don't apply the rules of science when they do traditional reviews," said Dr. Iain Chalmers, a British expert on the new approach who is not related to Dr. Thomas C. Chalmers. His team from the National Perinatal Epidemiology Unit at Oxford University has written a two-volume summary of more than 300 meta-analyses that are credited for beginning to change the practice of obstetrics.

Their work has shown that scientists "apply the rules of science in their laboratory and their studies, but when

Backers say technique can draw big, reliable conclusions from small, inconsistent findings.

they come to do a review they throw those rules out the window, and they don't use proper statistical techniques," Dr. Iain Chalmers said.

The Findings: Old Wisdom Overturned. The work of Dr. Iain Chalmers's team has rejected the value of many traditional obstetrical practices such as restricting movement of a woman during labor, trying to turn a baby around in the womb before the pregnancy reaches its full term, and making a routine incision called an episiotomy during childbirth. One meta-analysis by the team has led some American and Canadian obstetricians to substitute polyglycolic acid sutures for others, including chromic catgut, nylon, and silk, which are more painful, Dr. Iain Chalmers said.

Meta-analyses have re-established the value of some therapies that had fallen from favor, like electroshock therapy for mental depression, which had been criticized as ineffective and dangerous but is now undergoing a revival.

After performing a meta-analysis on three new studies of breast cancer in 1988, the National Cancer Institute issued an alert that the drug tamoxifen vastly improved the prognosis for women whose cancer was confined to the breast. Earlier studies had been inconclusive about the benefit of tamoxifen for such patients.

Continued on page 8

Continued from page 7

About 60% of the doctors who responded to a questionnaire from the National Cancer Institute said the alert led them to prescribe the drug.

The impact of meta-analysis on medical practice cannot be distinguished precisely from the cumulative effect of individual studies. But meta-analysis has become a frequent topic at meetings throughout the world and medical journals regularly report meta-analyses of a widening array of perplexing health problems.

Among the new targets for meta-analyses are epidemiological studies of the relationship between electromagnetic fields and cancer, adverse reactions to drugs, and the effectiveness of diagnostic tests.

"Whether you will get a certain scan or surgery from your doctor in 10 years will be based on cost-effectiveness and that decision will be based largely on meta-analyses," said Dr. Steven R. Cummings, an epidemiologist and specialist in internal medicine at the University of California at San Francisco Medical Center.

Results of meta-analyses compete with or could even replace the huge, definitive clinical trials that are often used to evaluate drugs and other therapies. Volunteers for such studies agree to receive a drug being tested or a dummy pill according to a choice made by lot.

The perceived publication bias in favor of things that work has fueled debate over whether to analyze only published studies or to include all that can be found.

In helping to reconcile conflicting results from such studies, some meta-analyses have avoided the need for conducting yet another one.

But other meta-analyses have only reinforced the inconclusive nature of the evidence concerning a therapy or procedure, largely because even when combined, most of the studies that the method evaluates are still too small to provide definitive answers.

Debate now centers around whether it is better to do a huge randomized trial or to do many smaller ones and then to perform a meta-analysis.

Rare are the penicillins and other major advances that are so startlingly beneficial that the results are obvious without a meta-analysis.

Medicine mostly progresses in small steps. It is in measuring them that meta-analysis plays its greatest role, said Richard Peto, a statistician who is a pioneer of the method and who heads the cancer studies unit at Oxford University in England.

The randomized clinical trials achieved striking results when they were introduced about 50 years ago. But in the 1960s and 1970s, such "trials bogged down because what was being studied didn't have such striking effects and the studies were incapable of answering the questions they were trying to address" because of their size and design, Mr. Peto said.

Meanwhile, researchers began advancing the techniques used since the 1930s by researchers in physics and agriculture to pool data. Credit is given to Gene V. Glass, a psychologist now at Arizona State University in Tempe, for coining the term meta-analysis in 1976.

For several years meta-analysis was used almost exclusively by researchers in psychology and education, and the method was often scorned. Writing in a medical journal, one British psychologist called it "an exercise in mega-silliness."

Not until the 1980s did meta-analysis begin to gain acceptance in medicine. Experts now say that earlier use of meta-analyses would have shown

- The lack of any scientific basis for prescribing the hormone stilbestrol during pregnancy, thus preventing its use and an epidemic of vaginal cancers that resulted;
- The benefit of prescribing antibiotics for patients before colon surgery;
- That the widespread prophylactic use of a drug, lidocaine, in coronary-care units to prevent heart attack victims from developing potentially fatal heart rhythms did not actually reduce deaths and may have been harmful in other ways.

In 1982, a meta-analysis confirmed earlier studies showing that a clot-dissolving drug, streptokinase, reduced the death rate from heart attacks. Yet the practice of prescribing streptokinase remained unchanged in the United States until large studies involving tens of thousands of patients were done in Europe to prove its value conclusively.

"During that time, thousands of deaths might have been prevented if more doctors had accepted the data from the early meta-analysis," Dr. Thomas Chalmers said.

The Method: A Combination of Evidence. Researchers do not study new groups of people in a meta-analysis, but they carry it out like a scientific experiment. First they pose a research question, such as whether a treatment or procedure works.

Then, before starting the process, the researchers specify the criteria they intend to follow in identifying the relevant studies in the medical literature and in determining which they will include or exclude.

Amongteps that researchers generally consider are the time that will be covered, the language in which the study is written, and the criteria for combining the data from the selected studies.

The dispute that swirls around meta-analyses reflects the difficulties in deciding how to do one.

"You cannot simply dump numbers in and turn a crank," said Dr. John C. Bailar III, a professor of epidemiology and biostatistics at McGill University in Montreal who was granted a MacArthur Foundation fellowship last month.

Dr. Bailar described himself as a healthy skeptic about the value of meta-analysis. He said the method has not provided the results that could be achieved from other types of careful scientific studies.

"While a meta-analysis looks objective and fairly straightforward, both terms are wrong," Dr. Bailar said. Meta-analyses are partly subjective due to decisions about how to carry them out, he said.

"It is not straightforward because a really thoughtful combination of evidence from multiple studies, whether it is a meta-analysis or something else, requires a great deal of deep professional judgment about how and what to combine," Dr. Bailar said.

The precision claimed for meta-analysis, he said, "can often be a false precision."

The Problems: An Urgent Need for Improvement. Although the nature of meta-analyses does not permit a single rigid set of rules and there is no single correct method to perform one, there is general recognition of the need to strengthen the techniques used in carrying them out.

Even experts who favor the method say there is an urgent need to improve ways to search for studies and to evaluate the quality of those that are found to reduce the problems of comparing data collected in different studies.

Proponents say much of the criticism is misdirected or shooting the messenger. It is meta-analysis, they say, that has pointed out many seriously flawed studies published in medical journals.

Dr. Gordon H. Guyatt, an epidemiologist at McMaster University School of Medicine in Hamilton, Ontario, said the controversy resembles that involved in analyzing any individual trial. "The enormous difference in meta-analysis is that the sources of disagreement become explicit."

It is by highlighting the conflicts that meta-analysis can yield its biggest payoffs; researchers are then spurred to resolve them by doing additional studies.

Meta-analysis has highlighted the tendency of editors of medical journals to favor publishing studies that show benefits from a therapy or procedure and to reject studies that show none.

The perceived publication bias in favor of things that work has fueled a debate over whether to analyze only published studies or to include all that can be found.

But the unanswered question is how far to go to find the unpublished studies in authors' files.

To help correct the problem many leaders have urged government and other agencies not to pay for studies unless the researchers agree to register them and to provide the crucial raw data that allow other researchers to do meta-analyses.

Another problem is the reluctance of medical journals to publish updates of meta-analyses, although they are needed to determine whether new studies have altered previous conclusions. Some meta-analyses that initially showed no clear advantage of a therapy have shown benefits when later studies were included. One example is a drug, fluorouracil, used in the treatment of bowel cancer.

Experts also agree that it is unrealistic to expect that meta-analyses and the randomized controlled studies upon which they are based can answer all questions in medical practice.

"One must be concerned that although even the best meta-analysis may represent all available trials and relevant studies, it may not represent clinical practice because of the nature of how and where research is conducted," Dr. Stephen B. Thacker, the chief epidemiologist at the federal Centers for Disease Control, wrote in 1988 in the *Journal of the American Medical Association*.

Everyone recognizes that the method has hidden problems common to all types of research. One is that statistical precision cannot substitute for conceptual clarity. Another is that results based on sound biological reasoning may be more convincing than those with strong statistical associations that lack plausible biological explanations.

LAWRENCE K. ALTMAN

Changes in federal programs for reporting suspected adverse reactions to vaccines announced

The types of vaccine-related adverse reactions that can be reported through the U.S. Department of Health and Human Services Vaccine Adverse Event Reporting System (VAERS) were expanded on November 1, 1990, to include any suspected adverse event after the administration of any vaccine. Before November 1, health-care providers and vaccine manufacturers were required by law to report suspected cases of the reactions listed in the table on page 10; other reactions were not considered reportable.

VAERS will serve as the sole system for monitoring reports of vaccine-related adverse events. It will replace the monitoring systems run by FDA and the Centers for Disease Control. Reporting forms and information about reporting requirements can be obtained by calling VAERS at 800-822-7967.

Transdermal fentanyl approved for chronic pain management

A transdermal fentanyl system (Duragesic, Alza Corporation, distributed by Janssen Pharmaceutica) has been approved for the management of chronic pain in patients who require opioid analgesia. Use in the management of postoperative pain is not recommended because of marked interpatient variability in absorption and disposition. Hypoventilation, the most serious reaction reported in clinical trials of transdermal fentanyl, was reported in 2% of cancer patients and 4% of postoperative patients.

The patches provide continuous delivery of fentanyl for 72 hours. Patients who experience adverse reactions should be monitored for at least 12 hours after he patch is removed. About 17 hours after patch removal, serum fentanyl concentrations will have decreased by 50%.

Dosage must be individualized. The product labeling provides tables that can be used in determining initial dosage for patients currently receiving oral or injectable opioid analgesics. If other central nervous system depressants are given concomitantly, the dosage of one or both agents should be reduced by at least 50%.

Doxazosin approved as antihypertensive agent

Doxazosin mesylate (Cardura, Pfizer Inc.), an α_1-adrenergic-receptor inhibitor, was approved in November for use alone or in combination with diuretics or β-adrenergic-receptor blockers as a first-line treatment for hypertension.

Doxazosin undergoes first-pass metabolism and is about 65% bioavailable. The drug is about 98% bound to plasma proteins. It is extensively metabolized in the liver. Although several metabolites are active, the antihypertensive effect rests primarily with the parent drug. Elimination is biphasic. The terminal elimination half-life is about 22 hours.

The maximum reduction in blood pressure occurs two

Table 1.
Reportable Events after Immunization[a,b]

Vaccine or Toxoid[c]	Event	Interval from Immunization
DTP, P, DTP poliovirus combined	Anaphylaxis or anaphylactic shock	24 hr
	Encephalopathy (or encephalitis)[d]	7 days
	Shock collapse or hypotonic–hyporesponsive collapse[e]	7 days
	Residual seizure disorder[f]	. . .[f]
	Any acute complication or sequela (including death) of above events	No limit
	(See package insert)[g]	. . .[g]
Measles, mumps, and rubella; DT, Td, T	Anaphylaxis or anaphylactic shock	24 hr
	Encephalopathy (or encephalitis)[d]	15 days for measles, mumps, and rubella vaccines; 7 days for DT, Td, and T toxoids
	Residual seizure disorder[f]	. . .[f]
	Any acute complication or sequela (including death) of above events	No limit
	(See package insert)[g]	. . .[g]
Oral poliovirus vaccine	Paralytic poliomyelitis in a nonimmunodeficient recipient or an immunodeficient recipient or a vaccine-associated community case	30 days 6 months No limit
	Any acute complication or sequela (including death) of above events	No limit
	(See package insert)[g]	. . .[g]
Inactivated poliovirus vaccine	Anaphylaxis or anaphylactic shock	24 hr
	Any acute complication or sequela (including death) of above event	No limit
	(See package insert)[g]	. . .[g]

[a] Adapted from National Vaccine Program, Food and Drug Administration, Centers for Disease Control. Vaccine Adverse Event Reporting System—United States. *MMWR.* 1990; 39:730–3.

[b] Events listed are required by law to be reported to the U.S. Department of Health and Human Services; VAERS will accept all reports of suspected adverse events after the administration of any vaccine.

[c] DTP = diphtheria and tetanus toxoids and pertussis vaccine adsorbed, P = pertussis vaccine adsorbed, DT = diphtheria and tetanus toxoids adsorbed, Td = tetanus and diphtheria toxoids adsorbed for adult use, T = tetanus toxoid.

[d] Encephalopathy means any substantial acquired abnormality of, injury to, or impairment of brain function. Among the frequent manifestations of encephalopathy are focal and diffuse neurologic signs, increased intracranial pressure, or changes lasting ≥6 hours in level of consciousness, with or without convulsions. The neurologic signs and symptoms of encephalopathy may be temporary with complete recovery, or they may result in various degrees of permanent impairment. Signs and symptoms such as high-pitched and unusual screaming, persistent unconsolable crying, and bulging fontanel are compatible with an encephalopathy, but in and of themselves are not conclusive evidence of encephalopathy. Encephalopathy usually can be documented by slow wave activity on an electroencephalogram.

[e] Shock collapse or hypotonic–hyporesponsive collapse may be evidenced by signs or symptoms such as decrease in or loss of muscle tone, paralysis (partial or complete), hemiplegia, hemiparesis, loss of color or change of color to pale white or blue, unresponsiveness to environmental stimuli, depression of or loss of consciousness, prolonged sleeping with difficulty arousing, or cardiovascular or respiratory arrest.

[f] Residual seizure disorder may be considered to have occurred if (1) no other seizure or convulsion unaccompanied by fever or accompanied by a fever of <102 °F occurred before the first seizure or convulsion after the administration of the vaccine involved, and (2) if in the case of measles-, mumps-, or rubella-containing vaccines, the first seizure or convulsion occurred within 15 days after vaccination or in the case of any other vaccine, the first seizure or convulsion occurred within 3 days after vaccination, and (3) if two or more seizures or convulsions unaccompanied by fever or accompanied by a fever of <102 °F occurred within one year after vaccination. The terms seizure and convulsion include grand mal, petit mal, absence, myoclonic, tonic–clonic, and focal motor seizures and signs.

[g] Refer to the contraindication section of the manufacturer's package insert for each vaccine.

to six hours after a dose. As is true of other α_1-adrenergic-receptor blockers, effects on heart rate and blood pressure are more pronounced in the standing position.

The initial recommended dosage of doxazosin mesylate is 1 mg once daily. If required for blood pressure control, the daily dose may be increased to 2, 4, 8, and then 16 mg. Cardura is supplied as 1-, 2-, 4-, and 8-mg scored tablets in bottles of 100.

News Briefs

• A ready-to-use **rice-based electrolyte solution** for oral rehydration therapy (Ricelyte) has been marketed by Mead Johnson.

• Free single copies of the report of the **NIH Consensus Development Conference on Treatment of Early Stage Breast Cancer** can be obtained by writing to William H. Hall, Director of Communications, Office of Medical Applications of Research, National Institutes of Health, Building 1, Room 259, Bethesda, MD 20892.

• Recommendations for **preventing and controlling tuberculosis** in nursing homes and other facilities that provide long-term care to the elderly have been issued by the Centers for Disease Control. The statement is published in *Morbidity and Mortality Weekly Report* (*MMWR.* 1990; 39(RR-10):7-13.).

Upcoming Specialty Meetings

Focus on Fungal Infections. Phoenix, AZ, February 21–22; contact Imedex U.S.A., Inc., 1060 Cambridge Square, Suite D, Alpharetta, GA 30201-9885; 404-751-7332.

Congress of the International Anesthesia Research Society (65th). San Antonio, TX, March 8–12; contact IARS, 3645 Warrensville Center Road, Cleveland, OH 44122; 216-295-1124 or 1130.

Society for Adolescent Medicine. Denver, CO, March 14–17; contact SAM, 19401 East Highway 40, Suite 120, Independence, MO 64055; 816-795-8336.

American College of Preventive Medicine. Baltimore, MD, March 15–19; contact ACPM, 1015 K Street N.W., Suite 403, Washington, DC 20005; 202-789-0003.

First International Congress on Biological Response Modifiers, organized by the Inter-American Society for Chemotherapy. Québec City, Canada, March 22–24; contact Michel G. Bergeron, M.D., BRM Congress Coordinator, C. H. Université Laval, 2705 Boul. Laurier, Québec City, Québec, Canada G1V 4G2; 418-654-2705.

Update: Controversies in Emergency and Primary Care. Kauai, HI, March 23–30; contact AIPE, P.O. Box 2586, La Jolla, CA 92038.

American Association of Immunologists. Atlanta, GA, April 21–26; contact AAI, 9650 Rockville Pike, Bethesda, MD 20814; 301-301-7178.

American Pediatric Society. New Orleans, LA, April 29–May 3; contact APS, 1650 Yale Boulevard S.E., Suite 104, Albuquerque, NM 87106; 505-764-0068.

Cytokines in Hemopoiesis, Oncology, and AIDS. Hannover, Germany, June 19–22; contact PD Dr. M. Freund, Department of Hematology and Oncology, Hannover Medical School, P.O. Box 610180, D-3000 Hannover 61, Federal Republic of Germany; 49511-5323610.

Therapy Consultation

The Therapy Consultation *section provides brief advice, in question-and-answer format, on how to handle specific drug-therapy problems. Readers are invited to submit questions, which will be referred to a consultant for an answer. The problems should not be highly specialized or unusual, nor should they be mundane. Questions are answered briefly, based largely on the judgment and personal experience of the consultant, although selected references may be cited to substantiate the consultant's advice.*

Assistance in identifying Therapy Consultation *topics is provided by the drug information centers at Medical College of Virginia Hospitals, Richmond; University of California Medical Center, San Diego; and University of Michigan Medical Center, Ann Arbor.*

Use of ketoconazole in the treatment of Cushing's syndrome

Question: Ketoconazole has been prescribed for a patient with Cushing's syndrome who is scheduled to undergo surgery for removal of an ACTH-producing pituitary tumor. What is the rationale for using ketoconazole in this patient?

Answer: Cushing's syndrome is caused by prolonged exposure to inappropriately high concentrations of cortisol. Cortisol secretion by the adrenal gland is stimulated by pituitary adrenocorticotropic hormone (ACTH), which in turn is under the control of hypothalamic corticotropin-releasing hormone (CRH). Normally, adrenal cortisol feeds back to the pituitary gland and the hypothalamus to inhibit the secretion of ACTH and CRH so that cortisol overproduction is prevented. In patients with endogenous Cushing's syndrome, there is increased production of cortisol that may be due to secretion by an adrenal tumor, excessive pituitary ACTH production (Cushing's disease), or ectopic ACTH secretion from a neoplasm.[1,2]

The primary treatment of Cushing's syndrome involves surgical resection of the tumor. Pharmacologic therapy to inhibit cortisol production has had limited use in the adjunctive management of Cushing's syndrome. Drugs that lower plasma cortisol concentrations are used before surgery in an effort to improve the patient's clinical and metabolic status. Drug therapy is also useful when surgery is unsuccessful or contraindicated.[1,2]

Metyrapone, aminoglutethimide, and mitotane have been the drugs most widely used to inhibit the synthesis and secretion of adrenal steroids. Mitotane also destroys adrenocortical cells by a cytolytic action. The clinical use of these drugs is limited, however, by unpredictable and unsatisfactory therapeutic responses, undesirable adverse effects, and poor tolerability.[3]

Ketoconazole has recently found use in the medical management of Cushing's syndrome. In vitro studies have demonstrated that ketoconazole inhibits ACTH-stimulated cortisol production; substantial inhibition is achieved at drug concentrations of 1 to 5 μg/dL.[4] Radiolabeling studies have shown that ketoconazole blocks the synthesis of adrenal steroids at two enzyme steps, (1) 11-β-hydroxylase and (2) cholesterol side-chain cleavage of the adrenal steroid synthesis pathway.[5] The inhibitory effect on cortisol production has led to trials evaluating the clinical efficacy of ketoconazole against hypercortisolism in patients with Cushing's syndrome.

Sonino et al.[6] studied the effects of ketoconazole in five patients with pituitary-dependent Cushing's disease. All had recurrent hypercortisolism after having undergone unsuccessful pituitary surgery. Ketoconazole was administered at a dosage of 400 mg every 12 hours for four weeks. Thereafter, the dosage was reduced according to individual patient response and was 600 mg/day for all subjects at six weeks. Within 24 hours of the start of ketoconazole therapy, urinary cortisol concentrations markedly declined in all patients and remained within the normal range throughout the four- to six-month study. Concomitantly, there was a decline in plasma cortisol, and all patients showed substantial symptomatic improvement. At the dosages used, ketoconazole produced no adverse effects. Similar beneficial results have been reported by other investigators who used ketoconazole to treat patients with Cushing's disease.[7,8] The dosage in these trials ranged from 600 to 800 mg/day.

Ketoconazole has been associated with potentially serious adverse effects. In a trial of six patients with Cushing's disease who received ketoconazole 400 mg twice daily, adverse effects were reported in four patients. Acute hypoadrenalism occurred in one subject, and three patients had lethargy, fever, and nausea. Of the six patients, three developed hepatotoxicity within 7 to 12 days of starting ketoconazole therapy. The drug was withdrawn in these three patients, and the abnormalities of liver function resolved within 15 days.[9]

Ketoconazole has also been used to treat hypercortisolism secondary to ectopic ACTH-producing tumors. Farwell et al.[10] treated a 50-year-old patient with a metastatic, ACTH-producing carcinoid tumor of the thymus. Ketoconazole 400 mg/day given in divided doses totally suppressed urinary cortisol excretion and produced marked clinical improvement. Optimal control in this patient was achieved with 200 to 400 mg/day.

These findings show that ketoconazole inhibits cortisol synthesis and is effective in treating hypercortisolism in patients with Cushing's syndrome. Ketoconazole appears to be a good alternative to other adrenal steroid inhibitors, whose use is limited by inadequate therapeutic responses and severe toxicity.

Patients receiving ketoconazole should be monitored closely for signs of hepatotoxicity, and the drug should be given at the lowest effective dosage that will control hypercortisolism. Further controlled trials are needed to define the place of ketoconazole in the treatment of Cushing's syndrome.

1. Williams GH, Dluhy RG. Diseases of the adrenal cortex. In: Braunwald E, Isselbacher, KJ, Petersdorf RG, eds. Harrison's principles of internal medicine. 11th ed. New York: McGraw-Hill; 1987:1753–64.
2. Schteingart DE. Cushing's syndrome. *Endocrinol Metab Clin North Am.* 1989; 18:311–38.
3. Carpenter PC. Cushing's syndrome; update of diagnosis and management. *Mayo Clin Proc.* 1986; 61:49–58.
4. Pont A, Williams PL, Loose DS et al. Ketoconazole blocks adrenal steroid synthesis. *Ann Intern Med.* 1982; 97:370–2.
5. Loose DS, Kan PB, Hirst MA et al. Ketoconazole blocks adrenal steroidogenesis by inhibiting cytochrome P450-dependent enzymes. *J Clin Invest.* 1983; 71:1495–9.
6. Sonino N, Boscaro M, Merola G et al. Prolonged treatment of Cushing's disease by ketoconazole. *J Clin Endocrinol Metab.* 1985; 61:718–22.
7. Terzolo M, Panarelli M, Piovesan A. Ketoconazole treatment in Cushing's disease. Effect on the circadian profile of plasma ACTH and cortisol. *J Endocrinol Invest.* 1988; 11:717–21.
8. Loli P, Berselli MA, Tagliaferri M. Use of ketoconazole in the treatment of Cushing's syndrome. *J Clin Endocrinol Metab.* 1986; 63:1365–71.
9. McCance DR, Hadden DR, Kennedy L et al. Clinical experience with ketoconazole as a therapy for patients with Cushing's syndrome. *Clin Endocrinol.* 1987; 27:593–9.
10. Farwell AP, Devlin JT, Steward JA. Total suppression of cortisol excretion by ketoconazole in the therapy of the ectopic adrenocorticotropic hormone syndrome. *Am J Med.* 1988; 84:1063–6.

UJJAINI KHANDERIA, M.S., PHARM.D., Clinical Assistant Professor
College of Pharmacy
The University of Michigan
Clinical Pharmacist, The University of Michigan Hospitals
Ann Arbor, MI 48109-0008

Current options for the treatment of systemic scleroderma

BARBARA A. MCGEE, MICHAEL D. BARNETT, AND RALPH E. SMALL

Abstract: The epidemiology, pathology, diagnosis, and clinical manifestations of systemic scleroderma (SSc) are described, and therapeutic options are discussed.

SSc is a rare condition of unknown etiology that occurs in a subset of scleroderma patients. It is distinguished by involvement of the small arteries, microvessels, and diffuse connective tissue. The degree of internal organ involvement is the main determinant of morbidity and mortality.

Management of SSc may entail supportive, palliative, remittive, and immunosuppressive therapies. Supportive therapy involves maintaining the affected extremities at warm temperatures and the use of emollient creams. Results of palliative treatment are mixed. Toxic reactions may be associated with many of these medications. Dermatologic manifestations have been treated with nonsteroidal anti-inflammatory agents, low-dose corticosteroids, dimethyl sulfoxide, and edetate disodium; peripheral and internal-organ vascular obstruction, with α-adrenergic blockers, angiotensin-converting-enzyme inhibitors, and calcium-channel blockers. Antacids with alginic acid, histamine H_2-receptor antagonists, sucralfate, and cholinergic-acting agents may be used to relieve GI symptoms. Lung infections should be treated promptly with antibiotics. No drug therapy has been successful in reducing the incidence of fatal cardiac arrhythmias or in preventing cardiac fibrosis. Captopril and enalapril are essential in the control of SSc renal crisis. Penicillamine may hold promise as a remittive therapy. The immunosuppressive agents fluorouracil, cyclosporine, and methotrexate, which have shown limited effectiveness in preliminary studies, merit further investigation.

No therapeutic agent has yet been shown to alter the course of SSc on a consistent or long-term basis. Toxicity and drug interactions remain a major concern in patient management, and aggressive monitoring is essential.

Index terms: Anti-inflammatory agents; Gastrointestinal drugs; Immunosuppressive agents; Scleroderma; Sympatholytic agents
Clin Pharm. 1991; 10:14–25

Scleroderma is a general diagnosis that encompasses several complex diseases such as localized scleroderma, systemic scleroderma (ranging from limited to diffuse), and mixed connective-tissue syndromes, all of which display similar histopathologic characteristics.[1,2] Systemic scleroderma, or systemic sclerosis (SSc), occurs in a subset of scleroderma patients and is distinguished by disease involvement of small arteries, microvessels, and diffuse connective tissue. Characteristics of SSc include fibrosis and vascular destruction within the skin as well as any connective-tissue-containing organ, including the gastrointestinal (GI) tract, lungs, kidneys, and heart.[2] The clinical hallmark of SSc is symmetrical stiffness and thickening of the skin, accompanied by vascular insufficiency.[3]

Localized scleroderma (also called morphea or

BARBARA A. MCGEE, PHARM.D., is Clinical Pharmacy Fellow in Rheumatology, Allergy, and Immunology, School of Pharmacy, Medical College of Virginia (MCV)/Virginia Commonwealth University (VCU), Richmond, Virginia. MICHAEL D. BARNETT, PHARM.D., is Chief, Inpatient Pharmacy Services, Keesler Medical Center, Keesler Air Force Base, Biloxi, MS; at the time this article was written, he was a doctor of pharmacy degree candidate, School of Pharmacy, MCV/VCU. RALPH E. SMALL, PHARM.D., is Associate Professor of Pharmacy and Pharmaceutics and Associate Professor of Medicine (Rheumatology, Allergy, and Immunology), MCV/VCU.

Address reprint requests to Dr. Small at Box 533, MCV Station, Medical College of Virginia/Virginia Commonwealth University, Richmond, VA 23298-0533.

This is **article 680-204-9101 in the ASHP Continuing Education System;** it qualifies for 1.0 hour of continuing-education credit. See page 68 for learning objectives and test questions.

linear scleroderma), by contrast, has no effects on the internal organs or vasculature; its manifestations are limited to the skin. Scleroderma can occur as part of an overlap syndrome, in which sclerodactyly and vascular changes occur in conjunction with myositis, polyarthritis, or leukopenia, all of which are features of other connective-tissue diseases. This article will focus on SSc and its treatment.

Epidemiology

SSc is relatively rare, with an incidence of 4 to 12 new cases per million population per year.[4] The five-year survival rate from onset of SSc is reported to be between 34% and 73%.[5,6] The presence of internal organ involvement is the principal determinant of morbidity and mortality, and internal manifestations of the disease seem to closely parallel the rate of progression and extent of skin involvement.[7] The peak time of onset of SSc in the general population is between the ages of 30 and 50 years; in women, onset is most common between the ages of 30 and 39 years.[6] Women are three times more likely to have SSc than men. The female-to-male ratio is thought to be greater in nonwhite populations than among Caucasians.[3,5]

The etiology of SSc is unknown. Several environmental, genetic, immunological, and neoplastic conditions have been associated with scleroderma and scleroderma-like syndromes (Table 1).[8–10]

Table 1.
Causes or Possible Associations of Scleroderma Syndromes[a]

Environmental or Pharmacological
Vibration (e.g., jackhammer)
Pneumococcosis
Polyvinyl chloride
Chlorinated hydrocarbons
Benzene
Meta-phenylenediamine
Silica dust
Epoxy resins
Rapeseed oil
Carbidopa
Bleomycin
Tryptophan
Silicon augmentation mammoplasty
Genetic
Progeria
Werner's syndrome
Phenylketonuria
Porphyria
Neoplastic Disease-Related
Bronchoalveolar carcinoma
Carcinoid syndrome
Immunological
Graft-versus-host disease
Lupus erythematosus
Dermatomyositis
Sjögren's syndrome
Hashimoto's thyroiditis
Vasculitis

[a] Compiled from references 7–10.

Pathogenesis

The reason for the development of fibrosis in patients with SSc is not understood; however, histologic findings have led to hypotheses about the etiology and pathogenesis of the disease. Three mechanisms have been implicated in the development of fibrosis: alterations in the vascular wall, alterations in the immune system, and disturbed control of collagen metabolism. Each of these pathways leads to fibrotic changes within structures containing connective tissue.[1]

Diagnosis and Classification

The diagnosis of SSc is based on the presence of clinical signs and symptoms. Several sets of criteria have been developed to increase specificity and sensitivity of diagnosis. Patients with digital sclerodactyly and internal organ involvement other than the lungs, who appear to have clinical manifestations of SSc, do not meet the American Rheumatism Association (ARA)[11] criteria for a definite diagnosis. These patients are generally diagnosed as having scleroderma. Over time, the disease may progress until it fulfills ARA criteria for a definite diagnosis of SSc. Criteria by the ARA are compared with those proposed by Barnett et al.[3] in Table 2.

Because of the large variation in mortality in SSc patients, subclassification may be helpful in determining prognosis. Lack of knowledge about the pathogenesis of the disease makes such classifications difficult. Several SSc classification systems are based on the degree of cutaneous and internal

Table 2.
Two Sets of Criteria for Diagnosis of Scleroderma

American Rheumatism Association[a]
Major criterion
Skin sclerosis proximal to the metacarpophalangeal joints
Minor criteria
Sclerodactyly
Digital pitting scars (pitting of finger tips)
Bilateral basal pulmonary fibrosis
Barnett et al.[b]
Typical scleroderma
Symmetrical skin thickening
Raynaud's phenomenon; acrocyanosis
Characteristic nail-fold capillary changes
Typical antinuclear antibodies
Characteristic systemic organ involvement
Atypical scleroderma
Various combinations of last four criteria listed above
No skin changes or finger swelling only

[a] Adapted from reference 11. The ARA criteria for diagnosis of scleroderma require the presence of the major criterion or at least two of the minor criteria.

[b] Adapted from reference 3.

organ involvement.[2] The most commonly used system divides SSc into either limited or diffuse disease. Limited SSc is characterized by cutaneous involvement of the hands and feet and peripheral vascular manifestations; some investigators include patients with cutaneous involvement of the face and forearms in this group. Patients may have limited disease for many years before developing internal organ involvement. Patients with diffuse SSc have more abrupt and extensive cutaneous symptoms including the trunk as well as the extremities. Internal organ involvement occurs earlier in the course of the disease. The distinction between these two categories is not always clear. Some investigators label the limited-disease category as CREST (calcinosis cutis, Raynaud's phenomenon, esophageal dysfunction, sclerodactyly, telangiectasia). This causes problems when categorizing patients who do not have generalized involvement of the skin, yet do not have all five characteristics of CREST. Because of difficulty in developing a common disease-classification system, it is difficult to interpret the results of epidemiologic and drug therapy studies.

Some investigators have recently proposed a method of classifying SSc into three categories based on early extent of skin sclerosis (Table 3). Patients with limited disease are subdivided into those with hand involvement only and those with involvement of the proximal extremities.[12] Patients with diffuse cutaneous involvement constitute the third category. Not included in this system is a fourth category of SSc patients who have internal organ manifestations without skin sclerosis. Their disease is known as sine, or atypical, scleroderma.[3,7]

Clinical Manifestations and Treatment

At the time of diagnosis, SSc patients may display a diversity of symptoms involving one organ system or many systems. The degree of functional limitation caused by SSc is likewise diverse. Virtually any organ may be involved; sites that must be monitored for alterations in function include the skin, peripheral vascular and cardiovascular systems, GI tract, lungs, and kidneys.

There are no clear-cut guidelines concerning the introduction of drug therapy aimed at altering the progression of the disease. Chronological staging of the disease by assessing the extent of organ involvement may help in indicating when therapy is appropriate.[8] The most common stages of organ involvement are listed in Table 4; as a patient advances from one stage to the next, prognosis becomes poorer. Other indicators of a poor prognosis are listed in Table 5. Some clinicians prescribe treatment to relieve symptoms of patients in stages I or II, even when their condition is apparently stable. Therapy is targeted to the clinically involved organs. Treatment for the alteration of disease progression is frequently reserved for clinically unstable patients in stages II and III. Many of the agents used for patients in stages II and III have poorly documented activity and are highly toxic; as a result, physicians may be reluctant to prescribe them.

Environmental control and physical medicine may be all that is needed for patients in stage I of SSc. Maintaining a warm temperature in the extremities through heated gloves, socks, and headgear will alleviate symptoms. Application of heat and massage, along with careful attention to skin care, is essential. Smoking should be strongly discouraged in all scleroderma patients because nicotine will exacerbate vasoconstriction. Provider support and positive attitude, reassurance, and patient education are vital in helping all SSc patients cope with their disease.[8,15]

Table 3.
Classification of SSc

Classification	Area Affected
Limited (Type I, Digital)	Fingers or toes, but not the proximal extremities or trunk; some classifications include lower eyelids, neck, and axillae
Moderate (Type II, Proximal Extremity)	Proximal extremities or face, but not the trunk
Diffuse (Type III, Truncal)	Thorax or abdomen

[a] Adapted from reference 12, with permission.

Table 4.
Chronological Stages of SSc by Organ Involvement[a]

Stage	Organs Involved
I	Skin, peripheral vascular system (Raynaud's phenomenon), esophagus
II	Lungs, gastrointestinal tract beyond the esophagus
III	Cardiovascular and renal systems

[a] Adapted from reference 8, with permission.

Table 5.
Unfavorable Prognostic Signs for SSc[a]

Extensive and diffuse (Type III) skin involvement
Rapid progression of disease over last six months
Multiple organ involvement
Increased age
Male gender
Elevated Westergren erythrocyte sedimentation rate
Hypergammaglobulinemia
Stage III disease
Hypertension

[a] Compiled from references 1, 7, 8, 13, and 14.

Dermatologic. Development of the dermatologic manifestations of SSc can be divided into three phases: edematous, sclerotic, and atrophic. During the edematous phase, the skin appears thick, edematous, and erythematous, indicating an inflammatory response. The symptoms usually start in the fingers and hands; later, they may appear on the face. The fingers are usually swollen with a nonpitting edema and cannot be fully extended. During the sclerotic phase, the skin hardens and painful ulcers develop around the finger tips or knuckles. The ulcers heal slowly and may lead to infections and gangrene. Mottled or diffuse hyperpigmentation or focal hypopigmentation may develop, probably as postinflammatory responses. During the atrophic phase, osseous resorption may cause articular deformities of the hands and, at times, complete dissolution of terminal phalanges.

Loss of hand function is common, particularly during the sclerotic phase. Progressive thickening of the skin and connective tissue involvement may result in immobility of the underlying joints, or "clawhand," with arthralgias caused by contractures. Muscle and tendon involvement leads to myalgias and tendon friction rubs. Several authors suggest using nonsteroidal anti-inflammatory drugs (NSAIDs) or low-dose corticosteroids (daily physiological doses) for symptomatic relief of the myalgias and arthralgias.[1,7,8]

Generalized skin care, massage, exercise, regular movement, emollient creams, and ointments should be used to keep the skin pliable and prevent immobility.[7] No therapy is available to soften the hidebound skin of scleroderma or alter progression of the disease. Numerous agents have been tried, but objective evidence of beneficial changes in skin or visceral areas has not been demonstrated in prospective, controlled trials. Agents tested exclusively for dermatologic activity include edetate disodium and dimethyl sulfoxide. Colchicine and aminobenzoic acid have been studied for dermatologic as well as other systemic effects in SSc.[13,16–22]

Olszewer and Carter,[16] reporting a large, retrospective analysis of the use of edetate disodium in various chronic degenerative diseases, noted subjective improvement of skin manifestations in four patients with SSc. The patients received edetate disodium 50 mg/kg of body weight by i.v. infusion over 3 to 3.5 hours, two to three times a week, for an unreported period of time. Ascorbic acid, vitamin B complex, and magnesium were added to the infusions. No controls were examined, and detailed information on evaluation of the SSc patients was not available from the data presented. The authors concluded that further study of edetate disodium may be warranted.

Several authors have assessed the usefulness of dimethyl sulfoxide in the treatment of the cutaneous manifestations of SSc. Tuffanelli[17] evaluated 24 patients with extensive cutaneous disease involvement and Raynaud's phenomenon. Dimethyl sulfoxide 90% was applied to one hand and arm of each patient twice daily for two to five months; the other hand and arm served as controls. An investigator who was blinded to which arm was treated found no difference in cutaneous sclerosis or joint mobility between the two limbs. He also found no difference in the rate of progression or healing of digital ulcers between the treated and untreated arms and hands of these patients.

Scherbel et al.[18] studied 42 patients treated with dimethyl sulfoxide for 3 to 23 months. Eighteen patients had only cutaneous and esophageal involvement, 19 patients had more severe dermatologic and GI involvement, and 5 patients had involvement of the skin, GI tract, and other internal organs. Each patient was considered to be his or her own control because previous therapy had failed. Dimethyl sulfoxide was applied topically to all affected areas in concentrations ranging from 30% to 100% and in doses of 60 to 100 g/day. After two to three weeks, application was limited to hands, forearms, feet, and face, for a total dose of 50 to 75 g/day. Therapy was initially applied three times a day, and frequency of application was decreased over time or as improvement was seen. Immersion technique was used for the hands, wrists, and feet of 10 patients in whom topical therapy produced no results. Nine patients with tendon contractures, interstitial calcinosis, or capsular adhesions were treated with subcutaneous dimethyl sulfoxide in 1% to 5% concentrations, 0.1 to 5 g/day, four days each week, for two to four weeks. A good-to-excellent response (an improvement in greater than 50% of symptoms) occurred in 26 patients; a fair-to-poor response in 16 patients. The patients with milder disease responded best to therapy. While the reports of decreases in ischemic ulcers, calcinosis, and skin thickness in some patients were promising, the lack of controls in this study makes it difficult to reach definitive conclusions on efficacy. The natural course of the disease may in fact result in alleviation of dermatologic manifestations.

In a more recent study, Williams et al.[19] examined the efficacy of dimethyl sulfoxide versus sodium chloride solution for the treatment of digital ulcers in a double-blind, multicenter, controlled trial involving 84 patients. Patients were randomly divided into three treatment groups and received dimethyl sulfoxide 70%, dimethyl sulfoxide 2%, or 0.9% sodium chloride solution by immersion technique three times a day for 12 weeks. Only the more severely affected hand of each patient was treated. Patients were evaluated at 2, 4, 8, and 12 weeks by the same observer. There was no significant difference in the total number of ulcers or in the number of infected or inflamed ulcers. The total surface area of open ulcers decreased in all study groups. Differences in outcome between the treated and untreated hand were evident only in the group treated with 70% dimethyl sulfoxide. These patients reported increased pain in the untreated hand and decreased pain in the treated hand. More than 25% of the patients using 70% dimethyl sulfoxide developed severe cracking, blistering, sloughing, or burning of the skin and were withdrawn from the study. The authors concluded that dimethyl sulfoxide is not effective in enhancing the healing of digital ulcers.

Vascular. Many factors contribute to the small artery obstruction that occurs in the peripheral vasculature and sometimes in the internal-organ vasculature of SSc patients.[7] Marked intimal hyperplasia and adventitial fibrosis cause severe narrowing of the arterial lumen. Ongoing endothelial cell injury increases the potential for platelet aggregation and the release of substances with potent local effects on vascular smooth muscle tone. SSc patients are also thought to have hematologic changes such as thrombocytosis, decreased red blood cell filterability, and increased plasma viscosity, all of which may exacerbate the already-compromised vascular perfusion. When vasoconstriction occurs, these changes render SSc patients susceptible to Raynaud's phenomenon, both peripherally and within the cardiac, pulmonary, and renal vasculature.

More than 95% of scleroderma patients have peripheral Raynaud's phenomenon. Its presence, however, is not diagnostic of SSc. Patients with SSc usually develop nonpitting edema, which is not a manifestation of primary Raynaud's disease. The two diseases can be distinguished by testing with wide-field nail-fold capillaroscopy.[2] Drug treatment of SSc-associated Raynaud's phenomenon and peripheral vascular disease has included α-adrenergic-receptor blockers,[23] angiotensin-converting-enzyme (ACE) inhibitors,[24] calcium-channel blockers,[25-27] ketanserin,[28,29] prostaglandin E_1 (PGE_1),[30] prostacyclin (PGI_2),[31] and plasmapheresis.[32] Response to therapy is dependent on the degree of fixed obstructive change in the digital vasculature. Drugs that block sympathetic vasoconstriction (reserpine, methyldopa, phenoxybenzamine, prazosin, and guanethidine) may protect the extremities from some of the effects of cold and stress[7]; however, high doses may produce adverse vascular effects. These drugs may be more tolerable if low doses of several drugs are used.[8] ACE inhibitors have been shown to reverse renal crisis in SSc patients. They also have been implicated as having some beneficial effects on sclerodermatous involvement of the skin and peripheral vasculature.[33] These additional benefits have yet to be determined in a controlled trial. Nifedipine and diltiazem are thought to be useful in SSc patients for their vasodilatory and antiplatelet-aggregation effects.[7] They have been shown to be effective in primary Raynaud's disease; however, their effectiveness in scleroderma-associated Raynaud's phenomenon is limited to patients with less severe disease. Nifedipine has been shown to promote healing of digital ulcers,[25,26] but this benefit may be offset by marked worsening of lower esophageal sphincter tone, which results in reflux esophagitis.[24] Diltiazem may produce fewer adverse effects on lower esophageal function.[27]

The possible role of serotonin in the induction or amplification of platelet aggregation and vasoconstriction in patients with peripheral vascular disease has prompted studies of ketanserin, a selective serotonin type 2 receptor antagonist, in the treatment of Raynaud's phenomenon.[20,28,29,34,35] Evidence of the effectiveness of ketanserin when used for SSc is mixed.[28,29] In one open-label study of 30 patients, ketanserin 40 mg three times a day for one month provided subjective improvement of Raynaud's symptoms in patients with SSc but no improvement in patients with primary Raynaud's disease.[34] There was no objective improvement in either group. In another open-label study, Altomare et al.[28] found ketanserin 20 mg three times daily in 10 patients with SSc to provide subjective improvement. No quantitative objective data were reported to support these findings. More recently, authors of an international, double-blind, placebo-controlled study involving 222 patients with SSc[35] reported that patients receiving ketanserin 40 mg three times a day had marked improvement in Raynaud's symptoms, as subjectively assessed by both patients and physicians. The study failed to demonstrate any improvement over placebo in functional or objective assessments. There was no significant difference in the number of adverse events between the groups; however, there was a trend toward increased headache, weakness, and dizziness in patients receiving ketanserin.

PGE_1 and PGI_2 have been shown to produce objective and subjective improvement in SSc-associated Raynaud's symptomatology in a small number of patients. Their efficacy is thought to be due both to vasodilation and platelet inhibition that can last up to several weeks after one dose. Use of these agents is severely limited by adverse effects, which include hypotension, headache, nausea, and vomiting, and by the need to administer them by i.v. infusion.[30,31]

Pentoxifylline has been investigated for use in the treatment of Raynaud's phenomenon associated with SSc. The results were similar to those seen with nifedipine.[36] Therapy with 400 mg three times a day for one year did not decrease the number or severity of Raynaud's attacks, although patients reported a decrease in the number of finger tip ulcerations.

Impotence and erectile dysfunction are among the complications thought to result from vascular changes in SSc.[37] There is no current recommendation for treatment of this complication. Several patients receiving treatment for peripheral Raynaud's phenomenon noted that the medication had no effect on their impotence.

Gastrointestinal. The GI tract is the most common, and usually the first, internal organ system to be affected by SSc. Histologic changes in the GI tract include atrophy or fibrous replacement of the muscularis and increased collagen deposition in the lamina propria and submucosa. These changes cause decreased motility and reduced peristaltic activity in the lower two thirds of the esophagus. Esophageal hypomotility and reflux are noted in approximately 80% of SSc patients. Complications stemming from esophageal hypomotility and reflux are dysphagia, peptic esophagitis, and esophageal stricture. Decreased motility and increased gastric emptying time are complications of stomach involvement, which affects 5% of SSc patients.[7,36] Symptomatic treatment is recommended in these patients. Careful chewing, eating multiple small meals, and elevating the head of the patient's bed or couch may be helpful.[7,8,38] Drug therapy for esophageal symptoms of SSc includes antacids with alginic acid for symptomatic dysphagia,[39] histamine H_2-receptor antagonists to decrease gastric acidity,[8,37] sucralfate for cytoprotection,[40] and cholinergic-acting agents (cisapride[41] and metoclopramide[42]) to decrease gastric emptying time (Table 6). Of these agents, only cisapride and metoclopramide have been studied in SSc patients.

Horowitz et al.[41] studied the effects of cisapride on esophageal and gastric emptying in eight SSc patients with upper GI symptoms. Compared with placebo, a single 10-mg i.v. dose of cisapride produced a statistically significant improvement in gastric emptying time for both solids and liquids. The effect on esophageal emptying time was not statistically significant; there was still some retardation of the food bolus (both liquid and solid) in the esophagus. After the i.v. cisapride dose, the patients received cisapride 10 mg orally four times a day for one month. No radiologic studies were performed after oral therapy, but there was a marked subjective improvement in GI symptomatology in patients evaluated for the presence of heartburn, constipation, dysphagia, and nocturnal acid secretion.

Johnson et al.[42] studied the effect of metoclopramide on esophageal and gastric motility in 12 SSc patients with esophageal involvement. Patients treated with metoclopramide had improved lower-esophageal-sphincter pressure, less gastroesophageal reflux, and a shorter gastric emptying time. The inconsistent effects on esophageal motility were similar to those seen in the cisapride study. The effects of metoclopramide on gastroesophageal reflux make it a viable option for symptomatic treatment in SSc patients.

Small-bowel dysfunction occurs in 40% to 50% of SSc patients. Malabsorption and duodenal hypomotility result in bacterial overgrowth, which may lead to diarrhea.[7] Unexplained weight loss may be caused by malabsorption. Diet can be altered to provide low-residue, low-lactose intake and an increased concentration of vitamins and minerals. Diarrhea has been reported to be successfully treated with two- to four-week courses of low-dose tetracycline hydrochloride or ampicillin (250 to 500 mg per day), confirming the theory that such diarrhea is caused by the overgrowth of normal flora. Antimicrobial therapy should be alternated be-

Table 6.
Pharmacologic Therapy of SSc Esophageal Symptoms[a]

Drug	Usual Dosage	Mode of Action
Antacids with alginic acid (Gaviscon)[b]	30 mL p.r.n. up to seven times daily	May protectively coat esophagus or mechanically impair reflux
Histamine H_2-receptor antagonists[c]		
Cimetidine	300 mg q.i.d.	Blocks H_2 receptors, decreasing gastric acid secretion through a reduction in cyclic adenosine monophosphate
Ranitidine (as the hydrochloride salt)	150 mg b.i.d.	
Nizatidine	150 mg b.i.d.	
Famotidine	20 mg q.d.	
Sucralfate[d]	1 g q.i.d.	Forms cytoprotective barrier that increases mucus and PGE_2 production
Cisapride	10 mg q.i.d.	Indirect cholinergic action of increased acetylcholine release in mesenteric plexus, resulting in increased gastric emptying
Metoclopramide (as the hydrochloride salt)	10 mg q.i.d. before meals and at bedtime	Sensitizes acetylcholine receptors in GI tract, exerts direct effect on smooth muscle, or both; is a dopamine antagonist; end result is increased gastric motility

[a] Compiled from references 37–41.
[b] Gaviscon (Marion Merrell Dow) contains magnesium trisilicate and should be used with caution if renal disease is suspected.
[c] The dosages given are for treatment of active symptoms of reflux esophagitis; dosage for maintenance therapy would be same as bedtime dosages for duodenal ulcer treatment.
[d] Sucralfate may be used as a "slurry," mixed with water before intake. (Other formulas have sorbitol, cherry flavoring, or both added.) Sucralfate has not been studied in SSc patients.

tween these two agents to prevent the development of resistant gut flora.[7,8]

The colon is affected in approximately 33% of SSc patients, but it rarely causes symptoms. Abnormal colonic motility may cause constipation, obstipation, or pseudo-obstruction.[7]

Pulmonary. The pulmonary effects of SSc include pleurisy, pulmonary hypertension, diffuse interstitial lung disease, and, in rare cases, pleural effusion.[7] Histologic lung changes in SSc patients include dense, acellular fibrotic replacement of the connective tissue within the alveolar wall.[43] This may include infiltration of lymphocytes and plasma cells. Pulmonary vascular changes also occur, resulting in pulmonary hypertension and cor pulmonale.

Clinical signs and symptoms of pulmonary involvement include progressive shortness of breath and cough. Breathing may be rapid and shallow, and patients may have bibasilar crackles. Symptoms result from decreases in diffusing capacity and lung compliance. Pulmonary function tests (PFTs) often reveal a restrictive defect. Roentgenographic studies demonstrate diffuse reticulonodular changes, predominantly in the lower lungs. Minor degrees of pleural thickening may be evident over the bases, and the heart may be enlarged. Lung changes develop quite gradually, and mortality is generally caused by infectious complications rather than decreased pulmonary function. Prompt use of low-dose antimicrobials (tetracycline hydrochloride or ampicillin 250 mg twice daily) for bronchitis-like symptoms will clear the infection.[7]

Colchicine and corticosteroids have failed to demonstrate any beneficial effect on the evolution of lung fibrosis in SSc patients.[21,44] The effects of penicillamine on pulmonary function as well as on other organ systems have been evaluated. Results are discussed below under "Remittive Therapy."

Cardiovascular. Four types of cardiac involvement occur in SSc patients: abnormalities of rhythm and conduction, pericardial disease, myocardial disease, and congestive heart failure (CHF). CHF is usually right sided and is thought to be a result of lung disease.[45] The cardiovascular abnormalities are due to fibrosis of the myocardium or conduction system and to vascular and microvascular damage.[45] Acute vasospastic reactions may occur upon exposure to cold temperatures. The cardiovascular complications of SSc are associated with a high mortality rate.

SSc patients have been observed to have a higher incidence of abnormal electrocardiograms (ECGs) than age-matched controls.[46] Kostis et al.[47] studied ECGs as a potential prognostic indicator of disease in SSc patients and found an association between arrhythmias and mortality during a 33-month follow-up. Cause of death is not mentioned, and it is unclear whether death was due to cardiac complications or other problems associated with advanced disease. Twenty-four-hour ECG monitoring has been shown to be more sensitive than either a resting or an exercise ECG.[48] Successful use of drug therapy in reducing the incidence of fatal arrhythmias has not been reported.

No drug therapy has been shown to prevent cardiac fibrosis. Thallium scan has revealed that nifedipine,[49] i.v. dipyridamole,[50] and captopril[51] acutely increase perfusion of the myocardium in SSc patients after defects have been detected. These studies did not reveal if the ischemic areas were reperfused or if collateral circulation increased.

Nifedipine also has been reported to protect SSc patients from cold-induced decreases in myocardial perfusion. In one small study, nifedipine did prevent cold-induced changes in left ventricular wall motion, but few patients were studied, and the results did not achieve statistical significance.[52] The need for this therapy is questionable, because although wall motion was altered upon exposure to cold, the patients had no decrease in left ventricular ejection fraction. The long-term effects of these drugs on cardiac function in SSc patients require further study.

Corticosteroids and NSAIDs have been suggested as beneficial in SSc patients with pericarditis.[7,53] CHF may be treated with diuretics; however, this must be done cautiously to prevent renal failure. Digoxin and salt-restricted diets also have been suggested for symptomatic relief.[8]

Renal. Renal involvement in SSc is caused by ischemia from the vascular changes within the kidney. In addition to this chronic effect, a Raynaud-type vasospasm in the renal vasculature that is caused by cold temperatures, sudden loss of fluid, or glucocorticoid therapy is believed to occur.[54] The clinical effects of SSc on the renal system occur suddenly, with the development of hypertension, elevated plasma renin levels, hypertensive retinopathy, and rapid deterioration of renal function. Patient complaints may include severe headache, blurred vision, or symptoms of CHF. Seizures may occur. Before 1980, renal crisis in an SSc patient was almost always fatal.

Steen et al.[54] looked for common characteristics in patients who developed renal crisis and found that diffuse skin involvement, rapid progression of skin thickening early in the course of the disease, pericardial effusion, and CHF were present significantly more often in these patients than in those who did not experience a renal crisis. Six months before the onset of the renal crisis, there were no significant differences in creatinine clearance, serum creatinine, hematocrit, blood pressure, hematuria, urine protein, or plasma renin levels between patients who did and did not develop renal crisis.

The most common manifestations of renal crisis

are malignant or accelerated hypertension and hyperreninemia.[55] The ACE inhibitors captopril and enalapril have been essential in controlling the hyperreninemia and renal crisis.[20,33,56,57] In addition to decreasing renin (angiotensin II) formation and lowering blood pressure, ACE inhibitors are thought to indirectly increase bradykinin and prostaglandins, thereby improving renal perfusion. No controlled trials have been done to determine the best treatment for renal crisis. Controlling blood pressure is important, and sympatholytic agents (reserpine, methyldopa, phenoxybenzamine, prazosin, guanethidine) or minoxidil may be needed when ACE inhibitors alone cannot maintain normotension.[8]

Retrospective studies and case reports indicate that a small percentage of patients who experience acute renal failure caused by SSc suffer from nonhypertensive renal crisis.[58,59] Characteristics common to these patients during crisis include rapid decrease in hematocrit, microangiopathy, and thrombocytopenia. These patients are thought to have a higher mortality rate at one year after renal crisis than SSc patients with hypertensive renal crisis. Little information is available on the treatment of these patients; however, there is one report of two patients successfully treated with captopril.[58]

Remittive Therapy

Several therapies that aim at altering the course of SSc, rather than treating specific organ systems, have been studied. Their efficacy is difficult to assess because of the variable course of the disease. Because the etiology of SSc is unknown, it is also difficult to determine what physiologic activity should be targeted to interrupt progression of the disease.

Colchicine has been considered as a treatment for SSc because it may disrupt microtubule formation and prevent extrusion of collagen fibers from fibroblasts. It also may enhance the action of collagenase and increase collagen degradation. In an uncontrolled, prospective trial, Alarcon-Segovia et al.[19] examined the long-term effects of colchicine in 19 patients with SSc. Patients received colchicine orally for at least 18 months at the highest dosage they could tolerate. Dosages ranged from 6 to 21 mg per week, with an average of 10.1 mg/week. Changes in skin manifestations of the disease served as the basis for evaluating therapy. All but two patients showed improvement in at least one objective measurement. The patients whose disease was of shorter duration and who received larger dosages of colchicine had greater improvement than those whose disease had a longer course and whose dosages were smaller. Interpretation of these results is difficult, because with time and disease progression the superficial dermis of many SSc patients becomes more lax.[1,7]

Steigerwald,[22] in a double-blind, crossover study, observed worsening or no improvement in visceral symptoms in patients who had received colchicine compared with placebo.[22] Improvement in skin symptoms was noted in 6 of 22 colchicine-treated patients and in 3 of 22 placebo-treated patients. Other investigators, who found that patients could not tolerate the high dosages (approximately 10 mg/week), have questioned the usefulness of colchicine in SSc.[18]

Some authors have associated the use of penicillamine with stabilization, or even improvement, of pulmonary fibrosis, GI involvement, and skin changes in SSc patients.[60,61] Penicillamine increases the soluble collagen (type IV) in the skin and increases the turnover of insoluble collagen (type I and III).[62] It may also have some immunomodulatory effects.

Steen et al.[60] evaluated results of PFTs in a retrospective study of patients who met the ARA criteria for SSc. Patients were divided into two groups. The treatment group had received penicillamine for at least six months and had their first PFT within three months of starting the drug and the second PFT at least 18 months later. The control group had two PFTs done at least 18 months apart and had not received penicillamine. The investigators reported an improvement in carbon monoxide diffusion capacity (DLCO) in the treatment group. After the regression coefficient was adjusted for possible confounding variables, this difference was statistically significant. No difference was found between the treatment and control groups in vital capacity (VC) or in the forced expiratory volume in one second (FEV_1). Although the study indicates that there may be some benefit from penicillamine therapy, the comparability of the two groups is questionable because of the retrospective design of the study.

DeClerck et al.[61] reported a retrospective study of 23 SSc patients whose therapy was followed for an average of 4.7 years. Sixteen patients received penicillamine for 0.75 to 11 years (average, 3.9 years). The control group received no therapy or low-dose prednisone. A statistically significant difference in the change in DLCO from the first evaluation to the last was noted between the study group and the control group. The average DLCO decreased in the control group but did not change in the treatment group. There was considerable variation within the groups. The changes in VC and FEV_1 in the treatment group were not significantly different from those of the control group.

In an 18-month prospective, open trial, Wollheim and Akesson[20] compared penicillamine 750 mg/day with cyclofenil, a weak estrogenic and antiestrogenic compound. Sixteen patients were included in each group. Cutaneous, pulmonary, and esophageal manifestations of SSc were assessed objectively. Neither therapy appeared to affect progression of the disease. A higher rate of withdrawal (mainly due to hepatotoxicity) was observed in the cyclofenil group than in the control group.

Toxic effects of penicillamine are a major concern in the treatment of SSc. A retrospective evaluation of 259 patients treated with penicillamine for an average of 1.8 years found that 47% had adverse reactions (rash, proteinuria, GI symptoms, dysgeusia, stomatitis, thrombocytopenia, and neutropenia).[63] Twenty-nine percent of the patients stopped treatment because of these adverse reactions. Many of the toxicities were dose related, a finding that has led a number of authors to conclude that if penicillamine is used for treatment of SSc, therapy should include aggressive monitoring and conservative dosing (250 to 500 mg/day).[8,63] Prospective controlled trials are needed to adequately assess the usefulness of penicillamine therapy in SSc.

Zarafonetis et al.[13] examined the effect of aminobenzoate potassium (Potaba, Glenwood) on survival in 390 SSc patients diagnosed between 1948 and 1980. The rate of survival in patients who received aminobenzoate potassium 4 g three times daily was significantly higher than that in patients who never received this drug. When the authors adjusted for demographic and clinical differences between the treatment and control groups, the difference was no longer statistically significant. The average age of the control patients was significantly higher than that of study group patients, and the symptoms of the former indicated a poorer prognosis at the time of entry in the study.

Immunosuppressant Therapy

A number of immunosuppressive agents have been studied in the treatment of SSc. They include chlorambucil,[64,65] azathioprine,[66] fluorouracil,[67,68] cyclosporine,[69,70] and methotrexate.[71] Plasmapheresis, combined with immunosuppression induced by prednisone and cyclophosphamide, also has been studied.[72]

In an open-label trial involving 27 patients, Steigerwald[64] found no benefit in the use of chlorambucil for SSc patients. Furst et al.[65] examined the efficacy of chlorambucil for SSc in a three-year prospective, placebo-controlled trial involving 58 patients, all of whom met ARA criteria for the diagnosis of SSc. The groups were well matched, and evaluation included assessment of the skin and internal organs. Chlorambucil demonstrated no effect on disease progression over a three-year period.

Jansen et al.[66] studied the effect of azathioprine in an open-label trial involving 21 patients with various stages of SSc. Patients received 150 mg/day for 5 to 23 months. Some subjective dermatological improvements were noted, but most patients had no improvement, worsening of disease, or serious adverse effects. Azathioprine is not recommended for the treatment of SSc.

Casas et al.[67] reported the use of fluorouracil in 12 SSc patients with diffuse disease. Each patient received an induction phase of fluorouracil 12.5 mg/kg/day i.v. for four to five doses, then four additional doses of 8 to 10 mg/kg i.v. given every two days. This was followed by a weekly maintenance dose of 10 to 20 mg/kg i.v. for 1.5 to 20 weeks. Objective improvements in hand and arm function were noted in all patients, as was improvement in Raynaud's symptoms. One patient died during the study from aspiration pneumonia, and four patients were lost to follow-up. Adverse effects included mild GI upset (seven patients), transient leukopenia (two), and severe headache (one).

Malaviya et al.[68] reported the toxic effects of fluorouracil in 11 SSc patients receiving doses similar to those used by Casas et al.[67] The investigators noted serious toxicity in three of the patients. Two patients developed bloody diarrhea, stomatitis, alopecia, and rash after the fifth daily dose of fluorouracil. One other patient developed the same symptoms as well as pancytopenia after a total of seven doses. Six other patients demonstrated minor toxicity. These studies indicate that fluorouracil may alleviate some of the symptoms of SSc; additional studies are needed to find an effective dose with limited toxicity.

A number of cases have been reported of the use of cyclosporine in SSc. Yocum and Wilder[69] used cyclosporine in an 18-year-old woman with progressive SSc and extensive skin involvement. The initial dosage was 10 mg/kg/day. After six months of treatment, a skin biopsy demonstrated marked decreases in thickness and healed digital ulcerations. After 10 months of treatment at a dosage of 4 mg/kg/day, the serum creatine phosphokinase (CPK) level tripled, and the cyclosporine was discontinued for 18 days. The skin disease worsened. Cyclosporine was carefully reinstated, and the CPK gradually declined. Amor and Dougados[70] reported two cases of cyclosporine use in SSc patients. Both patients received 2.5 mg/kg/day. Each developed a life-threatening hypertensive renal crisis within four to eight weeks of initiation of therapy. If cyclosporine is to be investigated further for use in SSc, a population that will be least affected by its renal effects must be targeted.

Van den Hoogen et al.[71] reported two cases of methotrexate use in patients with scleroderma (one with overlap syndrome and the other with SSc). The authors noted a marked decrease in the total skin score, signifying an improvement in both patients. The patient with overlap syndrome received methotrexate (as the sodium salt) 15 mg/week i.m.; because of compromised renal function, the other patient was given methotrexate 5 mg/week orally. The patient receiving the i.m. methotrexate developed an aspergillosis lung infection at six months, and therapy was discontinued. Duration of treatment in the patient receiving oral methotrexate was not reported. Methotrexate warrants further investigation in larger numbers of patients.

Plasmapheresis may have some short-term benefit in Raynaud's phenomenon; however, no long-term effects have been demonstrated.[32] Placebo plasma exchange has been shown to be as effective as plasmapheresis in Raynaud's phenomenon, possibly because of reflex release of PGE_1. Dau et al.[72] examined the use of plasmapheresis with prednisone and cyclophosphamide in patients with various types of scleroderma. One patient received azathioprine instead of cyclophosphamide, and three others had to be switched to chlorambucil after developing leukopenia and cystitis from a few months of cyclophosphamide therapy. Clinical improvement was observed in 14 of 15 patients studied. The one patient who had no improvement withdrew. Ten of the patients had skin biopsies before and after plasmapheresis; all patients demonstrated objective improvement in swelling of collagen and narrowing of the fibrillar distance. Further studies are needed to determine the long-term effects of plasmapheresis and an immunosuppressant drug.

Recommendations for Therapy

The treatment of SSc requires an individualized approach in which general supportive therapy and patient education are essential. Therapy is directed toward the alleviation of the signs and symptoms of the disease. No treatment has demonstrated consistent, long-term benefit in reversing or preventing disease progression.

Current therapeutic choices in the treatment of SSc patients, as listed in Tables 6 and 7, are based primarily on published reports of clinical experience. Clinical experience supports penicillamine as the initial choice for remittive therapy. Immunosuppressant medications may hold promise for treatment of SSc. Further study must be done with methotrexate, cyclosporine, and fluorouracil before their use can be recommended. Additional prospective, double-blind studies are needed in order to evaluate drug use in SSc patients.

Conclusion

No currently available therapy has consistently demonstrated the ability to arrest or alter the progression of SSc. Therapies aimed at symptomatic improvement must be individualized and carefully monitored to prevent adverse effects and interactions.

References

1. Krieg T, Meurer M. Systemic scleroderma: clinical and pathophysiological aspects. *Am Acad Dermatol*. 1988; 18:457–81.
2. Leroy EC, Krieg T, Black C et al. Scleroderma (systemic

Table 7.
Current Recommendations for the Treatment of Systemic Scleroderma

Indication and Treatment	Usual Dosage	Proposed Effect
Cutaneous Thickening		
Emollient creams	Once to several times daily	Maintain pliability and blood flow; prevent immobility
Massage		
Exercise		
Digital Ulcers		
Nifedipine	10–30 mg t.i.d.	Improve blood flow
Raynaud's Phenomenon		
Nifedipine	10–30 mg t.i.d.	Dilate vessels; prevent platelet aggregation
Diltiazem hydrochloride	30–60 mg t.i.d.	
Diarrhea		
Tetracycline hydrochloride	250–500 mg q.d.	Decrease overgrowth of normal flora
Ampicillin	250–500 mg q.d.	
Bronchitis		
Antimicrobials		Treat infection
Cardiovascular Complications		
Sodium-restricted diet		Decrease fluid load
Pericarditis		
NSAIDs[a]	Anti-inflammatory dosage levels	Decrease inflammation
Corticosteroids		
Renal Complications		
Captopril[b]		Dilate renal vessels; decrease renin level
Antihypertensives		Lower blood pressure
Remittive Therapy		
Penicillamine	250–750 mg q.d.	Produce immunomodulation; increase turnover of insoluble collagen

[a] NSAIDs = nonsteroidal anti-inflammatory drugs.
[b] Insufficient data available to recommend dosage. Start at low dosage and increase to control blood pressure if patient is hypertensive.

sclerosis): classification, subsets and pathogenesis. *J Rheumatol.* 1988; 15:202–5.
3. Barnett AJ, Miller M, Littlejohn GO. The diagnosis and classification of scleroderma (systemic sclerosis). *Postgrad Med J.* 1988; 64:121–5.
4. Medsger TA. Epidemiology of progressive systemic sclerosis. *Clin Rheum Dis.* 1979; 5:15–25.
5. Medsger TA. Epidemiology of progressive systemic sclerosis. In: Black C, Myers AR, eds. Systemic sclerosis (scleroderma). New York: Gower; 1985:53–5.
6. Medsger TA, Masi AT. The epidemiology of systemic sclerosis (scleroderma). *Ann Intern Med.* 1971; 74:714–21.
7. Seibold JR. Scleroderma. In: Kelly WN, Harris ED, Ruddy S et al. eds. Textbook of rheumatology. 3rd ed. Philadelphia: Saunders; 1989:1215–44.
8. Oliver GF, Winkelmann RK. The current treatment of scleroderma. *Drugs.* 1989; 39:87–96.
9. Owens GR, Medsger TA. Systemic sclerosis secondary to occupational exposure. *Am J Med.* 1988; 85:114–6.
10. Spiera H. Scleroderma after silicon augmentation mammoplasty. *JAMA.* 1988; 260:236–8.
11. American Rheumatism Association Subcommittee for Scleroderma Criteria of the Diagnostic and Therapeutic Criteria Committee. Preliminary criteria for the classification of systemic sclerosis (scleroderma). *Arthritis Rheum.* 1980; 23:581–90.
12. Masi AT. Classification of systemic sclerosis (scleroderma): relationship of cutaneous subgroups in early disease to outcome and serologic reactivity. *J Rheumatol.* 1988; 15:894–7.
13. Zarafonetis CJD, Dabich L, Negri D et al. Retrospective studies in scleroderma: effect of potassium para-aminobenzoate on survival. *J Clin Epidemiol.* 1988; 41:193–205.
14. Akesson A, Wollheim FA. Organ manifestations in 100 patients with progressive systemic sclerosis: a comparison between the CREST syndrome and diffuse scleroderma. *Br J Rheumatol.* 1989; 28:281–6.
15. Barnett AJ. The "neck sign" in scleroderma. *Arthritis Rheum.* 1989; 32:209–11.
16. Olszewer E, Carter JP. EDTA chelation therapy in chronic degenerative disease. *Med Hypotheses.* 1988; 27:41–9.
17. Tuffanelli DL. A clinical trial with dimethyl sulfoxide in scleroderma. *Arch Dermatol.* 1966; 93:724–5.
18. Scherbel AL, McCormack LJ, Layle JK. Further observations on the effect of dimethyl sulfoxide in patients with generalized scleroderma. *Ann NY Acad Sci.* 1967; 141:613–29.
19. Williams HJ, Furst DE, Dahl SL et al. Double-blind, multicenter controlled trial comparing topical dimethyl sulfoxide and normal saline for treatment of hand ulcers in patients with systemic sclerosis. *Arthritis Rheum.* 1985; 28:308–14.
20. Wollheim FA and Akesson A. Treatment of systemic sclerosis in 1988. *Semin Arthritis Rheum.* 1989; 18:181–8.
21. Alarcon-Segovia D, Ramos-Niembro F, Ibnanez deKasep G et al. Long-term evaluation of colchicine in the treatment of scleroderma. *J Rheumatol.* 1979; 6:705–12.
22. Steigerwald JC. Colchicine vs placebo in the treatment of progressive systemic sclerosis. In: Black C, Myers AR, eds. Systemic sclerosis (scleroderma). New York: Gower; 1985: 415–7.
23. Surwit RS, Gilgor RS, Allen LM et al. A double blind study of prazosin in the treatment of Raynaud's phenomenon in scleroderma. *Arch Dermatol.* 1984; 120:329–31.
24. Rustin MHA, Almond NE, Beacham JA et al. The effect of captopril on cutaneous blood flow in patients with primary Raynaud's phenomenon. *Br J Dermatol.* 1987; 117:751–8.
25. Woo TY, Wong RC, Campbell JP et al. Nifedipine in scleroderma ulcerations. *Int J Dermatol.* 1984; 23:678–80.
26. Czirjak L, Szegedi GY. Nifedipine treatment for progressive systemic sclerosis. *Arthritis Rheum.* 1986; 29:1053–4.
27. Jean F, Aubert A, Bloch F et al. Effects of diltiazem versus nifedipine on lower esophageal sphincter pressure in patients with progressive systemic sclerosis. *Arthritis Rheum.* 1986; 29:1054–5.
28. Altomare GF, Pigatto PD, Polenghi MM. Ketanserin in the treatment of progressive systemic sclerosis. *Angiology.* 1988; 39:583–6.
29. Ortonne JP, Torzuoli C, Dujardin P et al. Ketanserin in the treatment of systemic sclerosis: a double blind controlled trial. *Br J Dermatol.* 1989; 120:261–6.
30. Martin MFR, Dowd PM, Ring EFJ et al. Prostaglandin E_1 infusions for vascular insufficiency in progressive systemic sclerosis. *Ann Rheum Dis.* 1981; 40:350–4.
31. Dowd PM, Martin MFR, Cooke ED et al. Treatment of Raynaud's phenomenon by intravenous infusion of prostacyclin (PGI_2). *Br J Dermatol.* 1982; 106:81–9.
32. McCune MA, Winkelmann RK, Osmundson PJ et al. A controlled study of plasmapheresis in scleroderma. *J Clin Apheresis.* 1983; 1:206–14.
33. Wasner C, Cooke RC, Fries JF. Successful medical treatment of scleroderma renal crisis. *N Engl J Med.* 1978; 299:873–5.
34. Seibold JR, Jageneau AHM. Treatment of Raynaud's phenomenon with ketanserin, a selective antagonist of the serotonin$_2$ (5-HT_2) receptor. *Arthritis Rheum.* 1984; 27:139–46.
35. Coffman JD, Clement DL, Creager MA et al. International study of ketanserin in Raynaud's phenomenon. *Am J Med.* 1989; 87:264–8.
36. Seibold JR, O'Byrne M, Harris JN. Open trial of pentoxifylline in the prophylaxis of digital ulceration in systemic sclerosis. *Arthritis Rheum.* 1987; 30(Suppl 4):S120.
37. Nowlin NS, Brick JE, Weaver DJ et al. Impotence in scleroderma. *Ann Intern Med.* 1986; 104:794–8.
38. Richter JE, Castell DO. Gastroesophageal reflux. Pathogenesis, diagnosis and therapy. *Ann Intern Med.* 1982; 97:93–103.
39. Stanciu C, Bennett JR. Alginate/antacid in the reduction of gastro-oesophageal reflux. *Lancet.* 1974; 1:109–11.
40. Elsborg L, Beck B, Stubgaard M. Effect of sucralfate on gastroesophageal reflux in esophagitis. *Hepatogastroenterology.* 1985; 32:181–4.
41. Horowitz M, Maddern GH, Maddox A et al. Effects of cisapride on gastric and esophageal emptying in progressive systemic sclerosis. *Gastroenterology.* 1987; 93:311–5.
42. Johnson DA, Drane WE, Curran J et al. Metoclopramide response in patients with progressive systemic sclerosis. Effect on esophageal and gastric motility abnormalities. *Arch Intern Med.* 1987; 147:1597–601.
43. Rodnan GP, Black RL, Bollet AJ et al. Observations on the use of prednisone in patients with progressive systemic sclerosis (diffuse scleroderma). *Ann Intern Med.* 1956; 44:16–29.
44. McCarthy DS, Baragar FD, Dhingra S et al. The lungs in systemic sclerosis (scleroderma): a review and new information. *Semin Arthritis Rheum.* 1988; 17:271–83.
45. Owens GR, Follansbee WP. Cardiopulmonary manifestations of systemic sclerosis. *Chest.* 1987; 91:118–27.
46. Follansbee WP, Curtiss EI, Rahko PS et al. The electrocardiogram in systemic sclerosis (scleroderma). *Am J Med.* 1985; 79:183–92.
47. Kostis JB, Seibold JR, Turkevick D et al. Prognostic importance of cardiac arrhythmias in systemic sclerosis. *Am J Med.* 1988; 84:1007–15.
48. Geirsson AJ, Bolm-Bulow B, Pahlm O et al. Cardiac involvement in systemic sclerosis. *Semin Arthritis Rheum.* 1989; 19: 110–6.
49. Kahan A, Devaux JY, Amor B et al. Nifedipine and thallium-201 myocardial perfusion in progressive systemic sclerosis. *N Engl J Med.* 1986; 314:1397–402.
50. Kahan A, Devaux JY, Amor B et al. Pharmacodynamic effect of dipyridamole on thallium-201 myocardial perfusion in progressive systemic sclerosis with diffuse scleroderma. *Ann Rheum Dis.* 1986; 45:718–25.
51. Kahan A, Amor B, Menkes CJ et al. Captopril in the long-term treatment of myocardial perfusion abnormalities in systemic sclerosis. *Arthritis Rheum.* 1986; 29(Suppl 4):S27.
52. Ellis WW, Baer AN, Robertson RM et al. Left ventricular dysfunction induced by cold exposure in patients with systemic sclerosis. *Am J Med.* 1986; 80:385–92.

53. Medsger TA. Progressive systemic sclerosis. *Clin Rheum Dis.* 1983; 9:655–70.
54. Steen VD, Medsger TA, Osial TA. Factors predicting development of renal involvement in progressive systemic sclerosis. *Am J Med.* 1984; 76:779–86.
55. Cannon PJ, Hassar M, Case DB et al. The relationship of hypertension and renal failure in scleroderma (progressive systemic sclerosis) to structural and functional abnormalities of renal cortical circulation. *Medicine.* 1974; 53:1–46.
56. Zawada ET, Clements PJ, Furst DA et al. Clinical course of patients with scleroderma renal crisis treated with captopril. *Nephron.* 1981; 27:74–8.
57. Chapman PJ, Pascoe MD, Van Syl-Smith R. Successful use of captopril in the treatment of "scleroderma renal crisis." *Clin Nephrol.* 1986; 26:106–8.
58. Helfrich DJ, Banner B, Steen VD et al. Normotensive renal failure in systemic sclerosis. *Arthritis Rheum.* 1989; 32:1128–34.
59. Kagan A, Nissim F, Green L et al. Scleroderma renal crisis without hypertension. *J Rheumatol.* 1989; 16:707–8.
60. Steen VD, Owens GR, Redmond C et al. The effect of D-penicillamine on pulmonary findings in systemic sclerosis. *Arthritis Rheum.* 1985; 28:882–8.
61. DeClerck LS, Dequeker J, Francx L et al. D-penicillamine therapy and interstitial lung disease in scleroderma: a long-term follow-up study. *Arthritis Rheum.* 1987; 30:643–50.
62. Nimni ME. Penicillamine and collagen metabolism. *Scand J Rheumatol* 1979; 28(Suppl):71–8.
63. Steen VD, Blair S, Medsger TA. The toxicity of D-penicillamine in systemic sclerosis. *Ann Intern Med.* 1986; 104:699–705.
64. Steigerwald JC. Chlorambucil in the treatment of progressive systemic sclerosis. In: Black C, Myers AR, eds. Systemic sclerosis (scleroderma). New York: Gower; 1985:415–7.
65. Furst DE, Hillis S, Lachenbruch PA et al. Preliminary results of the double-blind parallel, randomized trial of chlorambucil vs placebo in progressive systemic sclerosis (PSS). *Arthritis Rheum.* 1986; 29(Suppl 4):S29.
66. Jansen GT, Barraza DF, Ballard JL et al. Generalized scleroderma: treatment with an immunosuppressive agent. *Arch Dermatol.* 1968; 97:690–8.
67. Casas JA, Subauste CP, Alarcon GS. A new promising treatment in systemic sclerosis: 5-fluorouracil. *Ann Rheum Dis.* 1987; 46:763–7.
68. Malaviya AN, Singh RR, Dhar A et al. 5-fluorouracil in progressive systemic sclerosis: is it safe? *Ann Rheum Dis.* 1988; 47:964–5.
69. Yocum DE, Wilder RL. Cyclosporin A in a progressive systemic sclerosis. *Am J Med.* 1987; 83:369–70.
70. Amor B, Dougados M. Cyclosporin: therapeutic effects in rheumatic diseases. *Transplant Proc.* 1988; 20(Suppl 4):218–23.
71. Van den Hoogen FHJ, Boerbooms AMT, van de Putte LBA. Methotrexate treatment in scleroderma. *Am J Med.* 1989; 87:116–7.
72. Dau PC, Kahaleh MB, Sagebiel RW. Plasmapheresis and immunosuppressive drug therapy in scleroderma. *Arthritis Rheum.* 1981; 24:1128–36.

Use of angiotensin-converting-enzyme inhibitors in the management of renal disease

John P. Asher and Kim M. Murray

Abstract: The role of angiotensin-converting-enzyme inhibitors (ACEIs) in the treatment of progressive renal disease is described.

Researchers have evaluated the use of ACEIs in patients with two types of progressive kidney disease: diabetic nephropathy and renal insufficiency associated with connective-tissue disease. When introduced early in the course of diabetic nephropathy, ACEIs appear to produce greater reductions in urinary protein concentrations than do other antihypertensive agents, even when systemic blood pressure does not decrease. They also slow the rate of decline of renal plasma flow and glomerular filtration rate. Results are less impressive when ACEIs are initiated at a later stage of disease. Captopril has been shown to be associated with a decline in serum creatinine level in patients with systemic scleroderma, and with reductions in blood pressure and increases in the glomerular filtration rate in patients with systemic lupus erythematosus. Because these patients were receiving other agents that might have influenced study outcome, specific conclusions about the efficacy of ACEIs in connective-tissue disease cannot yet be drawn. They may, however, be recommended as adjunctive agents in treatment of this condition.

The relative safety of the ACEIs, combined with their ability to arrest or slow the progression of renal failure, makes them primary options in the management of selected renal diseases.

Index terms: Angiotensin-converting-enzyme inhibitors; Captopril; Enalapril maleate; Kidney diseases; Lisinopril

Clin Pharm. 1991; 10:25–31

John P. Asher is a doctor of pharmacy degree candidate, College of Pharmacy, University of South Carolina, and Staff Pharmacist, Department of Pharmaceutical Services, Richland Memorial Hospital, Columbia, SC. Kim M. Murray, Pharm.D., is Clinical Assistant Professor, College of Pharmacy, and Adjunct Assistant Professor, Department of Medicine, School of Medicine, University of South Carolina, Columbia.

Address reprint requests to Dr. Murray at the Department of Pharmaceutical Services, Richland Memorial Hospital, 5 Richland Medical Park, Columbia, SC 29203.

Angiotensin-converting-enzyme inhibitors (ACEIs) have been available for the treatment of hypertension in the United States since the introduction of captopril in 1980. Enalapril followed in 1985, and lisinopril was introduced in 1988. The primary therapeutic effects of the ACEIs are related to their action on the renin–angiotensin–aldosterone system.[1] Angiotensin II is thought to be both a systemic and a local intrarenal hormone.[2] Its formation is catalyzed by the action of circulating angiotensin-converting enzyme on angiotensin I. The synthesis of angiotensin I is stimulated by the release of the hormone renin, primarily from juxtaglomerular cells located in the afferent renal arterioles.[1]

Angiotensin II increases renal vascular tone and alters renal blood flow, glomerular dynamics, and the filtration coefficient, which is a function of capillary surface area and permeability per unit of surface area.[2] It promotes the release of aldosterone from the adrenal gland, increasing tubular reabsorption of sodium. Researchers have evaluated the use of ACEIs in pathologies associated with compromised renal function, including diabetic nephropathy and renal insufficiency resulting from connective-tissue diseases. The purpose of this review is to discuss the role of ACEIs in preventing or slowing the progression of renal disease.

Diabetic Nephropathy

Diabetic nephropathy is a major cause of mortality in insulin-dependent diabetic patients.[3] Death generally occurs within seven years of the onset of persistent proteinuria.[4] Glomerular filtration of macromolecules can be influenced by capillary permeability, capillary plasma flow rate, and transcapillary hydraulic pressure.[5] Hyperfiltration is caused by metabolic changes that occur in the diabetic patient,[5] such as hyperglycemia-induced expansion of the extracellular fluid volume, structural hypertrophy of the kidney, altered glucoregulatory or vasoregulatory hormone action, or a combination thereof. The typical alterations are enhanced transcapillary hydraulic pressure and glomerular plasma flow rate.[3] Dialysis and renal transplantation have been shown to be effective invasive treatments for the uremic diabetic patient. ACEIs have been reported to reduce urinary protein excretion in patients with diabetic nephropathy and other diseases.[6]

Parving et al.[4] studied the effects of early, aggressive antihypertensive therapy on albuminuria and glomerular filtration rates in young, insulin-dependent diabetic patients with diabetic nephropathy and hypertension. The antihypertensive regimens included metoprolol, hydralazine, and furosemide or a thiazide diuretic. The authors reported significant decreases in blood pressure and albumin excretion; changes in glomerular filtration rates, however, were not significant.[4] These results confirm those of an earlier study by Mogensen,[7] which reported that antihypertensive treatment in this patient population can impede the progressive deterioration of kidney function.

One of the earlier studies of the effects of ACE inhibition on heavy proteinuria in azotemic diabetic patients was conducted by Taguma et al.[5] Included in the study were 10 patients with a clinical diagnosis of diabetic nephropathy, all of whom were on antihypertensive regimens. Urinary protein excretion, blood pressure, serum creatinine, serum electrolytes, and total serum protein concentrations were evaluated in each patient before and after captopril therapy. During the two-week control period, urinary protein excretion and renal function were stable. During the eight-week study period, captopril 37.5 mg was administered to each patient orally three times daily. By the end of two weeks, the urinary protein concentration decreased significantly, from 10.6 ± 2.2 g/24 hr to 6.1 ± 1.4 g/24 hr, and it remained stable during the following weeks. At eight weeks, the concentrations were 4.9 ± 1.0 g/24 hr. Systolic or diastolic blood pressure decreased by more than 10 mm Hg in 7 of 10 patients, but blood pressure readings before and after captopril therapy did not differ significantly. However, a Type II statistical error is possible because the sample was small. The decrease in proteinuria may have been due to changes induced by ACE inhibition rather than to alterations of systemic blood pressure. The authors attributed the changes to captopril-induced reductions in intrarenal hypertension and resulting alterations in intrarenal hemodynamics; no renal hemodynamic studies were performed to confirm this hypothesis.

Bjorck et al.[8] evaluated the short-term (nine days) and long-term (two years) effects of captopril in patients with diabetic nephropathy and hypertension. Short-term results showed significant increases in renal plasma flow, from 265 to 302 mL/min/1.73 sq mm, and decreases in the filtration fraction (fraction of plasma perfusing the kidney that is filtered), from 14.3% to 12.8%, without changes in the glomerular filtration rate. During long-term treatment, significant decreases occurred in arterial blood pressures; mean arterial blood pressure decreased by 5 mm Hg, and the rate of deterioration in glomerular filtration was slower (10.3 mL/min/yr at baseline versus 2.4 mL/min/yr after six months of therapy). The degree of reduction in blood pressure did not correlate with the rate of deterioration of glomerular filtration rate.

Heeg et al.[9] evaluated the effects of lisinopril on blood pressure, renal hemodynamics, and proteinuria in 13 patients with impaired renal function, hypertension, and proteinuria. Various etiologies were responsible for the renal disease in this population. Three patients had diabetic nephropathy. All patients had been receiving antihypertensive therapy (diuretics, β blockers, or vasodilators) for at least one year. Comparisons and measurements were made during conventional antihypertensive therapy, a 2-week control period without antihypertensive agents, and a 12-week lisinopril regimen. Furosemide was added to the lisinopril regimen if the maximum dose of 40 mg per day did not reduce the diastolic blood pressure to 95 mm Hg or less. During the period in which patients were receiving lisinopril, systolic and diastolic blood pressures were significantly decreased at week 12, but not at weeks 4 and 8, compared with blood pressures during conventional antihypertensive therapy. Urinary protein excretion rates were not significantly different from those recorded during conventional therapy and the control period. Proteinuria decreased significantly during lisinopril therapy compared with both the control and conventional-therapy phases. Changes in blood pressures did not correlate with decreases in protein excretion, whereas ACE inhibition did correlate with decreased proteinuria. ACE activity decreased from 30.5 ± 9.5 to 4.6 ± 3.5 units/L at four weeks and remained at this low level. Peripheral renin activity increased significantly, from 1.35 ± 1.23 to 20.1 ± 19.7 nmol AI/L/hr, with a significant fall in plasma aldosterone concentration (1.30 ± 0.67 to 0.71 ± 0.53 nmol/L). Other significant changes seen during ACE inhibition included increased serum urea concentration (15.1 ± 6.5 to 21.9 ± 14.4 mmol/L), decreased creatinine clearance (28.7 ± 16.1 to 24.5 ± 12.8 mL/min), decreased filtration fraction (16.5 ± 10.3%), decreased glomerular filtration rate (mean 21 ± 10%) and increased serum potassium (4.9 ± 0.8 to 5.1 ± 0.5 mmol/L). No significant differences were seen in serum creatinine, serum albumin, and effective renal plasma flow.

Blood pressure was most difficult to control in the three patients with diabetic nephropathy; all required furosemide. These patients had the lowest initial filtration fraction and the smallest decrease during lisinopril therapy. They also had less improvement in protein excretion and renal vascular resistance. The benefits of ACE inhibition in diabetic nephropathy were not confirmed in these three patients with advanced renal disease.

Parving et al.[10] evaluated the effects of a combination of captopril and a diuretic in patients with diabetic nephropathy over a two-and-one-half-year period. Compared with untreated controls, the treatment group had significant decreases in mean arterial pressure (mean decrease, 8.7 ± 1.3 mm Hg), decreases in albumin excretion (decrease to 390 ± 1.1 μg/min versus increase to 1367 ± 1.3 μg/min in the captopril and control groups, respectively), and a decreased rate of decline in the glomerular filtration rate (5.8 ± 0.7 mL/yr versus 10.0 ± 1.3 mL/yr).

In the normal kidney, angiotensin II produces efferent arteriolar vasoconstriction and a reduction in glomerular ultrafiltration. These changes lead to an increase in capillary and transcapillary hydraulic pressure. Glomerular filtration is maintained despite alterations in plasma flow and the reduction of filtration surface area caused by structural damage to nephrons.[11-12] In the diseased kidney, locally generated angiotensin II may preserve filtration despite renal structural damage. Filtration rates are decreased in damaged nephrons but are above normal in the best-preserved nephrons.[7,9,12]

Antihypertensive therapy can impede the progression of kidney failure.[12] The extent of the decrease in blood pressure correlates neither with the degree of reduction in proteinuria nor with the rate of decline in the glomerular filtration rate.[13,14] ACEIs appear to effect a greater reduction in proteinuria and in the rate of fall of the glomerular filtration rate than do other antihypertensive therapies, even when systemic blood pressure does not decrease. This suggests the decrease in urinary protein excretion is due to reductions in intrarenal hypertension and changes in intrarenal hemodynamics, creatinine clearance, and filtration fraction produced by ACEI therapy.[15]

Early studies with ACEIs demonstrated an association of proteinuria with captopril[16] and enalapril[17] (1.2% and 0.6%, respectively). One factor that may have contributed to these findings are the high doses of the ACEIs administered to patients in early research. No association has yet been reported between proteinuria and lisinopril.[18]

Captopril, enalapril, and lisinopril are effective (Table 1) and should be considered as a component of the antihypertensive regimen to decrease proteinuria in diabetic nephropathy. Results may be less impressive when ACEI therapy is initiated in patients with advanced renal dysfunction and low filtration fractions than in those with early disease. Although all antihypertensive therapies are beneficial in reducing the rate of progression of proteinuria in diabetic nephropathy, the ACEIs appear to be more beneficial than other treatments. ACEIs decrease proteinuria, establishing them as the preferred agents with which to institute therapy.

Renal Impairment Related to Connective-Tissue Disease

Systemic Scleroderma. Systemic scleroderma, or systemic sclerosis, is a complex, generalized connective-tissue disease marked by inflammatory immunological reactivity, vascular lesions, and widespread fibrosis of multiple organ systems.[19] Women tend to be affected more than men. Symptoms typically appear in the third to fifth decade of life.[20] Renal failure is a major determinant of a poor prognosis; it usually develops gradually and is

Table 1.
Effects of Angiotensin-Converting-Enzyme Inhibitors (ACEIs) on Renal Function in Patients with Diabetic Nephropathy

Reference	Diagnosis[a]	Antihypertensive Therapy	Follow-up	Effect of Therapy[b,c] UAE	BP	SCr	CL_{cr}	GFR	RDGFR	RPF	FF
5	DN (n = 10)	Captopril added to antihypertensive regimen	2 wk	Dec							
			4 wk	Dec	Unc						
			8 wk	Dec	Unc	Unc					
8	DN and HTN (n = 13)	Captopril plus diuretic	9 days					Unc		Inc	Dec
			2 yr		Dec				Dec		
9	HTN and DN or OP (n = 13)	Lisinopril	4 wk	Dec							
			8 wk	Dec							
			12 wk	Dec	Dec	Unc	Dec		Dec	Unc	Dec
10	DN and HTN (n = 18)	Captopril plus diuretic	27–36 mo	Dec	Dec				Dec		
14	DN (n = 22)	Captopril (n = 8)	6 wk	Dec[c]	Dec						
		Nifedipine (n = 7)		Inc	Inc						
		Placebo (n = 7)									
15	DN (n = 11)	Enalapril maleate	2 wk	Dec[d]				Dec[d]		Variable[d]	Dec[d]
				Unc[e]				Unc[e]			Unc[e]

[a] DN = diabetic nephropathy, HTN = hypertension, OP = causes of proteinuria other than diabetic nephropathy.
[b] Reported as increased (Inc) or decreased (Dec) if mean values before and after ACEI therapy were significantly different (references 4, 5, 7, 8, 14, and 15) or if mean values for ACEI treatment group and control group were significantly different (references 9 and 10); Unc = unchanged. UAE = urinary albumin excretion, BP = blood pressure, SCr = serum creatinine concentration, CL_{cr} = creatinine clearance, GFR = glomerular filtration rate, RDGFR = rate of decline of GFR, RPF = renal plasma flow, FF = filtration fraction.
[c] Also decreased at six months.
[d] Patients with an elevated baseline GFR (n = 6).
[e] Patients with normal baseline GFR (n = 5).

characterized by mild to moderately severe vascular lesions.[21,22] The onset of renal involvement may also be abrupt, heralded by scleroderma renal crisis (SRC), a severe process associated with a sudden development of malignant arterial hypertension and a subsequent accelerated decline of renal function.[20] SRC is life threatening and can result in death within one month.[19] Elevated peripheral renin levels have been noted in patients with systemic sclerosis.[22-25] This finding, along with the severe hypertension observed in SRC, is the basis for the use of ACEIs in patients with systemic scleroderma.

Several investigators have explored the use of captopril to treat hypertension in patients with systemic scleroderma.[22,25-28] Lopez-Ovejero et al.[25] demonstrated the positive effect of captopril therapy on the control of elevated blood pressure associated with SRC in two patients, a 33-year-old woman and a 25-year-old man. Both patients had increased plasma renin activity. Dosages titrated to 150 mg orally every six hours produced favorable blood pressure control in both patients. Improvement of renal function was documented by the decline of serum creatinine (from 1.6 to 1.2 mg/dL over two weeks in the woman and from 3.0 to 2.3 mg/dL over seven days in the man) and an increase in creatinine clearance rates (from 39 to 65 mL/min over two weeks in the woman and from 15 to 33 mL/min over seven days in the man). The female patient continued to receive 600 mg per day at a 29-week follow-up visit; the male patient's dose was reduced to 200 mg per day after 20 weeks of captopril therapy.

Zawada et al.[26] evaluated the use of captopril in four patients who displayed the sudden deterioration of renal function characteristic of SRC. In some cases, treatment with captopril controlled blood pressure and slowed the progression of renal insufficiency, as determined through serum creatinine levels. In one patient, captopril therapy was begun with 50 mg orally three times daily when the serum creatinine concentration reached 7.5 mg/dL. The patient required hemodialysis. Despite its beneficial effect on blood pressure and urine output, the drug was discontinued because the patient developed a persistent rash. Although hemodialysis continued, the patient died 46 days after the onset of SRC. The other three patients began to receive captopril therapy earlier in the course of their renal disease, when serum creatinine levels were much lower than those of the first patient. One of these three patients received captopril 25 mg orally two times daily until death from cardiomyopathy 73 days after the diagnosis of SRC. The remaining two patients received captopril 150 mg orally three times a day, along with other antihypertensives. These patients were followed for more than 300 days, and renal hypertension was successfully controlled. The authors suggest that stabilization of renal function at lower serum creatinine levels is associated with an improved outcome.

Beckett et al.[27] concluded that the early initiation

of captopril therapy for scleroderma-related hypertension and renal insufficiency may prevent the development of advanced and potentially irreversible renal changes. This information needs to be interpreted cautiously. The prospective study involved seven patients who had received percutaneous renal biopsies and were followed up to 34 months. All antihypertensive medications were discontinued before the start of captopril treatment. The final dosage range of captopril in these patients was 32 to 100 mg per day; furosemide was administered concurrently to six of the patients. Blood pressure control was achieved in all seven patients. Although serum creatinine concentrations improved in six of the seven patients, only three patients had follow-up renal biopsies. The histologic lesions were similar to those present at the beginning of the study but showed evidence of increased glomerular fibrosis and vascular sclerosis.

Thurm et al.[28] reviewed the records of 23 scleroderma patients treated with captopril under a compassionate-use protocol. Patients had proteinuria (1+ or greater), blood pressure >140/90 mm Hg, and azotemia (blood urea nitrogen >25 mg/dL). The therapeutic goal was to reduce supine diastolic blood pressure by at least 10 mm Hg or to a value of less than 105 mm Hg. Serum creatinine levels were also monitored. All previous antihypertensive therapy except diuretics was discontinued. Captopril was started at a dosage of 25 mg orally three times daily, and the dosage was gradually increased until the therapeutic goal was achieved. Goal blood pressures were reached within the first day of captopril therapy by 15 patients and within the first five days by five additional patients. Despite the early favorable responses, some captopril dosages were increased substantially, resulting in a range of 75 to 750 mg per day (mean, 350 mg per day). Eleven patients required additional antihypertensive agents, and seven patients required hemodialysis for adequate blood pressure control. Eleven of 23 patients remained on captopril for 21 to 36 months; 4 of the 11 were managed with captopril alone and continued to demonstrate favorable blood pressure control. Serum creatinine concentrations measured at a follow-up visit for seven patients were lower than baseline values, suggesting stabilized or improved renal function. This review demonstrates that captopril used as monotherapy or combined with other antihypertensive agents may be effective in some scleroderma patients who develop hypertension.

Chapman et al.[22] described the successful use of captopril to control elevated blood pressure (230/150 mm Hg) and a rising serum creatinine concentration in a 53-year-old man with SRC. Laboratory tests revealed evidence of hyperreninemia. Treatment with prazosin, furosemide, and atenolol failed to control blood pressure or halt progression of renal failure. Hemodialysis was instituted, and captopril 50 mg orally twice daily was added, resulting in blood pressure control. Prazosin was stopped at this point, and hemodialysis was discontinued after the patient had received captopril for 13 days. The serum creatinine concentration decreased from 589 μmol/L to 150 μmol/L after seven months of captopril therapy. At seven months, a total daily captopril dosage of 400 mg was required for blood pressure control. This case report supports the potential value of captopril in an antihypertensive regimen for control of the accelerated hypertension and renal failure of SRC.

A body of evidence demonstrates that ACEIs are reasonable therapeutic choices to improve survival in patients with scleroderma-associated hypertension and renal failure. Early treatment may improve patient outcome, although renal failure may progress, necessitating hemodialysis.

Systemic Lupus Erythematosus. Systemic lupus erythematosus (SLE) is a chronic inflammatory disease that can involve all organ systems. Rapid deterioration of kidney function is the clinical manifestation that is most closely associated with a poor prognosis.[29,30] Approximately one half of SLE patients have renal involvement early in the course of their disease, and progression is generally slow.[20] Wallace et al.[31] reported 10-year survival rates of 65% and 87% for SLE patients with and without renal involvement, respectively. Ninety percent of these patients were female, which is consistent with the overall prevalence of the disease.[32] In the United States, black women with SLE outnumber white women with the condition by a three-to-one margin.[20] Renal involvement can be described under the broad heading of lupus nephritis.

Drug therapy of lupus nephritis is not curative, but it often appears to reduce proteinuria and renal inflammation. Corticosteroids are commonly used to lessen inflammation and modify the immune response. They also have been combined with cytotoxic agents such as azathioprine and cyclophosphamide. ACEIs can be used concurrently with these drugs to manage the hypertension frequently associated with lupus nephritis. Long-term hemodialysis and renal transplantation are options for the management of end-stage disease.[30,32]

Herlitz et al.[33] investigated the effectiveness of captopril in the treatment of hypertension associated with lupus nephritis in 14 patients. Renal involvement was defined as elevated serum creatinine levels and reduced glomerular filtration rates, which were measured using edetate sodium labeled with chromium 51 as a filtration marker. Diagnosis was confirmed by renal biopsy in nine patients. Immunosuppressive therapy with prednisolone and azathioprine was continued in 13 patients, while 1 patient received prednisolone alone. Twelve of the patients had received three or more antihypertensives before receiving captopril. After an initial oral dose of 12.5–25 mg, the captopril dosage was adjusted until the diastolic blood pressure was less than 95 mm Hg. At dosages of 153 ± 31 mg/day, captopril improved blood pressure control in 11 of the 14 patients studied. These patients were followed for six months, by which time their blood pressures had dropped to a mean of 145/92 ± 5/3 mm Hg from a baseline mean of 178/110 ± 7/4 mm Hg. Mean captopril dosage was 110 ± 17 mg/day at six months. At 12 months, blood pressure levels in 10 of the 11 patients were maintained with a mean captopril dosage of 70 ± 15 mg/day; mean blood pressure at this point was 146/91 ± 8/3 mm Hg. Eight of the ten patients received furosemide, and four of these eight patients also received a β-adrenergic-receptor antagonist. Although only one of the eight patients followed for at least six months showed a significant improvement in glomerular filtration rate, progressive renal deterioration was not evident in the other seven patients.

This information implies that ACEIs may help in preventing a continued decline of renal function in patients with SLE. An increase in glomerular filtration rate is one consequence of ACEI therapy that may influence recovery from renal failure.[34] Arresting deterioration of renal function also may be related to blood pressure control. Specific conclusions about the therapeutic efficacy of ACEIs in patients with lupus nephritis cannot be derived from this study, because the patients were receiving other agents that might have influenced outcome. ACEIs might be a reasonable adjunctive therapy for the control of hypertension in patients with lupus nephritis.

Undifferentiated Connective-Tissue Disease. Undifferentiated connective-tissue disease (UCTD) is an early pattern of rheumatic disease that can progress to scleroderma, SLE, polymyositis, or a combination of clinical manifestations of these distinct entities, referred to as mixed connective-tissue disease. Like scleroderma and SLE, UCTD may be associated with acute renal failure and accelerated hypertension.

Strongwater et al.[35] report a single case involving a 27-year-old woman diagnosed as having UCTD and treated with ACEIs. The patient had hypertension and progressive renal failure and eventually required dialysis. Corticosteroids were introduced and tapered over an 18-month period. Blood pressure control was achieved with i.v. nitroprusside, which was gradually tapered as oral antihypertensive therapy was initiated and maintained with captopril 25 mg orally three times daily and clonidine. The patient developed a pruritic, maculopapular rash that was attributed to captopril; enalapril maleate 10 mg orally daily was introduced as a substitute. Renal function improved, and dialysis was discontinued six months after the start of captopril therapy (four months after the change to enalapril). The patient's renal function, as measured by decreased serum creatinine levels, improved over the subsequent two-and-one-half years. The enalapril maleate dosage was eventually increased to 15 mg daily.

Summary. Captopril has been studied more extensively than any ACEI in the treatment of connective-tissue disease. Previous reports have indicated that patients with renal insufficiency related to collagen vascular diseases such as scleroderma and SLE may be at increased risk for neutropenia and agranulocytosis as a result of captopril therapy.[19,36] Although none of the patients followed in the scleroderma and SLE reviews had evidence of these adverse effects, white blood cell counts should be monitored carefully at the start of captopril therapy and periodically thereafter. ACEIs other than captopril may show equally beneficial therapeutic effects. These agents should be considered as options, used alone or in combination with other antihypertensive agents, to impede the potentially fatal renal and hypertensive complications of scleroderma, SLE, and UCTD.

Conclusion

The literature supports the use of all ACEIs currently marketed in the United States for the treatment of proteinuria due to diabetic nephropathy. Indications for the use of ACEIs in patients with connective-tissue diseases are not as well defined. Captopril has been shown to have beneficial effects on renal function in patients with scleroderma or SLE. Studies of the use of other ACEIs in patients with these conditions are limited. Early initiation of ACEI treatment can result in improved clinical efficacy.

The relative safety of ACEIs, along with the beneficial alterations in renal hemodynamics they have been shown to produce, positions these agents as primary therapeutic options in the management of selected renal diseases.

References

1. Ujhelyi MR, Ferguson RK, Vlasses PH. Angiotensin-converting-enzyme inhibitors: mechanistic controversies. *Pharmacotherapy*. 1989; 9:351–62.
2. Johnston CI, Jackson B. Overview: angiotensin-converting-enzyme inhibition in renovascular hypertension. *Kidney Int*. 1987; 31(Suppl 20):S154–6.
3. Reddi AS, Camerini-Davalos RA. Diabetic nephropathy; an update. *Arch Intern Med*. 1990; 150:31–43.
4. Parving HH, Smidt UM, Anderson AR et al. Early aggressive antihypertensive treatment reduces rate of decline in kidney function in diabetic nephropathy. *Lancet*. 1983; 1:1175–8.
5. Taguma Y, Kitamoto Y, Futaki G et al. Effect of captopril on heavy proteinuria in azotemic diabetics. *N Engl J Med*. 1985; 313:1617–20.
6. Traindl O, Pohanka E, Kovanrik J. Progression of chronic renal failure. *Lancet*. 1988; 2:962–3.
7. Mogensen CE. Long-term antihypertensive treatment in-

hibiting progression of diabetic nephropathy. *Br Med J.* 1982; 285:685–8.
8. Bjorck S, Nyberg G, Mulec H et al. Beneficial effects of angiotensin-converting-enzyme inhibition on renal function in patients with diabetic nephropathy. *Br Med J.* 1986; 293:471–4.
9. Heeg JE, de Jong PE, van der Hem GK et al. Reduction of proteinuria by angiotensin-converting-enzyme inhibition. *Kidney Int.* 1987; 32:78–83.
10. Parving HH, Hommel E, Smidt UM. Protection of kidney function and decrease in albuminuria by captopril in insulin-dependent diabetics with nephropathy. *Br Med J.* 1988; 297:1086–91.
11. Keane WF, Anderson S, Aurell M et al. Angiotensin-converting-enzyme inhibitors and progressive renal insufficiency. *Ann Intern Med.* 1989; 111:503–16.
12. Ledingham JGG. Effects of angiotensin II and of angiotensin-converting-enzyme inhibition in chronic renal failure. *Kidney Int.* 1987; 31(Suppl 20):S112–6.
13. Takeda R, Morimoto S, Uchida K et al. Effects of captopril on both hypertension and proteinuria. *Arch Intern Med.* 1980; 140:1531–3.
14. Mimran A, Insua A, Ribstein J et al. Comparative effect of captopril and nifedipine in normotensive patients with incipient diabetic nephropathy. *Diabetes Care.* 1988; 11:850–3.
15. Abu-Romeh SH, Nawaz MK, Ali JH et al. Short-term effect of angiotensin-converting-enzyme inhibitor enalapril in incipient diabetic nephropathy. *Clin Nephrol.* 1989; 31:18–21.
16. E. R. Squibb & Sons, Inc. Captopril package insert. Princeton, NJ; 1985 Sep.
17. Davis RO, Irvin JD, Kramsch DK et al. Enalapril worldwide experience. *Am J Med.* 1984; 77(suppl 2A):25–35.
18. Noble TA, Murray KM. Lisinopril: a nonsulfhydryl angiotensin-converting-enzyme inhibitor. *Clin Pharm.* 1988; 7:659–69.
19. Oliver GF, Winkelmann RK. The current treatment of scleroderma. *Drugs.* 1989; 37:87–96.
20. Rodnan GP, Schumacher HR, eds. Primer on the rheumatic diseases. 8th ed. Atlanta: Arthritis Foundation; 1983.
21. Cannon PJ. Medical management of renal scleroderma. *N Engl J Med.* 1978; 299:886–7. Editorial.
22. Chapman PJ, Pascoe MD, vanZyl-Smit R. Successful use of captopril in the treatment of "scleroderma renal crisis." *Clin Nephrol.* 1986; 26:106–8.
23. Gevras H, Gevras I, Cannon PJ et al. Is elevated plasma renin activity of prognostic importance in progressive systemic sclerosis? *Arch Intern Med.* 1977; 137:1554–8.
24. Kovalchik MT, Guggenheim SJ, Silverman MH et al. The kidney in progressive systemic sclerosis: a prospective study. *Ann Intern Med.* 1978; 89:881–7.
25. Lopez-Ovejero JA, Saal SD, D'Angelo WA et al. Reversal of vascular and renal crisis of scleroderma by oral angiotensin-converting-enzyme blockade. *N Engl J Med.* 1979; 300:1417–9.
26. Zawada ET, Clements PJ, Furst DA et al. Clinical course of patients with scleroderma renal crisis treated with captopril. *Nephron.* 1981; 27:74–8.
27. Beckett VL, Donadio JV, Brennan LA et al. Use of captopril as early therapy for renal scleroderma: a prospective study. *Mayo Clin Proc.* 1985; 60:763–71.
28. Thurm RH, Alexander JC. Captopril in the treatment of scleroderma renal crisis. *Arch Int Med.* 1984; 144:733–5.
29. Keller F, Oehlenberg B, Kunzendorf U et al. Long-term treatment and prognosis of rapidly progressive glomerulonephritis. *Clin Nephrol.* 1989; 31:190–7.
30. Burlingame MB, Delafuente JC. Treatment of systemic lupus erythematosus. *Drug Intell Clin Pharm.* 1988; 22:283–9.
31. Wallace DJ, Podell T, Weiner J et al. Systemic lupus erythematosus—survival patterns: experience with 609 patients. *JAMA.* 1981; 245:934–8.
32. Robinson DR. Systemic lupus erythematosus. In: Rubenstein E, Federman DD, eds. Scientific American Medicine. New York: Scientific American; 1988:1–15.
33. Herlitz H, Edeno C, Mulec H et al. Captopril treatment of hypertension and renal failure in systemic lupus erythematosus. *Nephron.* 1984; 38:253–6.
34. Schlueter WA, Battle DC. Renal effects of antihypertensive drugs. *Drugs.* 1989; 37:900–25.
35. Strongwater SL, Galvanek EG, Stoff JS. Control of hypertension and reversal of renal failure in undifferentiated connective tissue disease by enalapril. *Arch Intern Med.* 1989; 149:582–5.
36. Cooper RA. Captopril-associated neutropenia: who is at risk? *Arch Intern Med.* 1983; 143:659–60. Editorial.

"

Antihypertensive Drug Response

It has been an almost universal experience with antihypertensive drugs that the doses used in established practice are significantly lower than the doses used in early studies and the regimens recommended when the drugs were first introduced. Doses of β-blockers and thiazides used nowadays very rarely reach the levels recommended in earlier years. ACE inhibitors and calcium antagonists are also used in much lower doses than those recommended initially. This in part reflects a failure to recognize the limitations of trial design including forced dose titration, time versus drug effects, and above all, the wider variability in response in the general population. Until very recently information on the dose-effect relations of antihypertensive drugs was limited or absent, and many drugs were claimed to have "flat" dose-response curves. This is probably incorrect and originated because early studies used high doses that produced drug concentrations on the upper plateau of a maximal effective dose (E_{max}) relation so that the lower part of the dose-response curve was not adequately explored. Similar misunderstandings led to conclusions that there was no relation between the plasma level of antihypertensive drugs and their pharmacological effect. As discussed below, individual variability in drug plasma levels (i.e., pharmacokinetics) is probably the largest source of variability in response to many antihypertensive drugs.

—Reid JL, Meredith PA. Concentration–effect analysis of antihypertensive drug responses. *Hypertension.* 1990; 16:12–8.

"

Use of nondepolarizing neuromuscular blocking agents in mechanically ventilated patients

MARCIA L. BUCK AND MICHAEL D. REED

Abstract: The pharmacology and history of development of nondepolarizing neuromuscular blocking agents are presented, and the pharmacokinetics and pharmacodynamics of these agents, administration guidelines for mechanically ventilated patients, adverse effects, factors affecting paralysis, and methods for blockade reversal are reviewed.

Nondepolarizing neuromuscular blocking agents (tubocurarine, metocurine, pancuronium, vecuronium, and atracurium) are frequently used to induce prolonged pharmacologic paralysis in patients in the intensive-care unit (ICU). These agents are poorly absorbed after oral administration and must be administered by injection, preferably by the i.v. route. Individualized adjustment of the dose is necessary to maintain the desired degree of paralysis. Dosing modifications may be necessary in patients with underlying renal or hepatic diseases and in pediatric and geriatric patients. Patients with thermal burns require larger doses of these drugs than other patients.

These agents can cause several important adverse effects, including histamine release, cardiovascular changes, and muscle atrophy. Pathophysiologic variables and drug interactions can affect the degree of paralysis. Generally, patients no longer requiring paralysis in the ICU will be allowed to spontaneously regain muscle function after drug therapy has been discontinued. If the effects of the nondepolarizing neuromuscular blocking agents must be reversed more rapidly, acetylcholinesterase-inhibiting agents such as physostigmine, neostigmine, pyridostigmine, and edrophonium can be used.

Nondepolarizing neuromuscular blocking agents can be used to paralyze mechanically ventilated patients, facilitating optimal oxygenation and ventilation.

Index terms: Dosage; History; Paralysis; Pharmacokinetics; Skeletal muscle relaxants; Toxicity; Ventilators

Clin Pharm. 1991; 10:32–48

Compromised pulmonary function requiring the use of mechanical ventilatory support is common in critically ill patients. There are various methods of temporarily augmenting pulmonary function or giving complete artificial ventilation to patients, and these methods serve as a foundation of modern critical-care practice.[1] The current practice of using positive-pressure ventilatory therapies to overcome compromised pulmonary function contrasts with the earlier use of negative-pressure ventilation (the iron lung). Positive-pressure ventilation and positive end-expiratory pressure alter airway pressures and are used to improve pulmonary mechanics and gas exchange.[2] These techniques permit patient-specific tailoring of ventilatory support based on the need for either full or intermittent support, the latter of which allows for spontaneous respiration.[1,2]

Despite the immense therapeutic importance of these ventilatory treatment modalities, controversy persists as to their optimal use (i.e., initiation, duration, and weaning). There is also controversy over the optimal use of drugs that can be administered concurrently to facilitate patient compliance with artificial ventilatory support. Active or spontaneous respiratory muscle contractions that oppose mechanical ventilation will increase intrathoracic pressure and reduce alveolar ventilation. "Fighting the ventilator" is one of the most common reasons for the initiation of drug therapy. In addition to improving patient compliance and acceptance of ventilator therapy, sedation and pharmacologic paralysis can relax the patient and possibly permit improved oxygenation.[3,4]

The use of analgesia and sedation as supplemental therapy in the mechanically ventilated patient has been reviewed recently.[5] Sedation may be provided with a number of different agents, including opioids, benzodiazepines, barbiturates, and anesthetics.[6–11] The newer synthetic opioids, including fentanyl and alfentanil, are frequently administered to patients receiving intensive care. Al-

MARCIA L. BUCK, PHARM.D., is Pediatric Clinical Pharmacy Specialist, Department of Pharmacy, University of Virginia Health Sciences Center, Charlottesville, VA. MICHAEL D. REED, PHARM.D., is Associate Professor of Pediatrics, Department of Pediatrics, Division of Pediatric Pharmacology/Critical Care, University of Virginia Health Sciences Center.

Address reprint requests to Dr. Buck at the Department of Pharmacy, Box 274-11, University of Virginia Health Sciences Center, Charlottesville, VA 22908.

The assistance of the following individuals in reviewing this manuscript before submission for publication is acknowledged: James B. Besunder, D.O., Jeffrey L. Blumer, M.D., Ph.D., Jill M. Luer, Pharm.D., and Madolin K. Witte, M.D.

This is **article 680-204-9102** in the **ASHP Continuing-Education System;** it qualifies for 1.0 hour of continuing-education credit. See page 69 for learning objectives and test questions.

though these agents are effective in sedating and relaxing these patients, the development of tolerance and opioid-related adverse effects continue to limit their overall usefulness.[6,7] Midazolam, a short-acting benzodiazepine, is useful in the mechanically ventilated patient; however, withdrawal symptoms after discontinuation of midazolam therapy have been reported in the intensive-care unit (ICU).[8,9] Which opioid, benzodiazepine, or combination of these agents is preferable for use in mechanically ventilated patients remains to be determined. Propofol[10] and ketamine,[11] used most frequently as general anesthetics, have been successfully used to provide sedation for ICU patients. Further study is necessary to better define the optimal role of these drugs as therapeutic adjuncts in critically ill patients.

In patients who fail to respond to sedation alone, or when patients develop tolerance to sedatives, paralysis with nondepolarizing neuromuscular blocking agents is frequently used to provide added relaxation and to permit optimal ventilatory support.[12] In addition to its use to relax mechanically ventilated patients, pharmacologic paralysis may improve compliance with ventilation in adults with various pulmonary diseases including the adult respiratory distress syndrome and status asthmaticus and in infants with respiratory diseases.[13-17] The patients most likely to benefit from pharmacologic paralysis are those whose respiratory muscles maintain spontaneous and vigorous activity that is counterproductive to ventilation. Patients who exhibit little inherent muscle activity while receiving mechanical ventilation are less likely to experience further improvement in ventilation or oxygenation as the result of pharmacologic paralysis.[16,17]

The frequent need for pharmacologic paralysis in the intensive-care setting makes it important for the physician, pharmacist, and nurse working in the ICU to be familiar with the clinical pharmacology of paralyzing agents. We will focus on the use of nondepolarizing neuromuscular blocking agents to facilitate mechanical ventilation of critically ill patients. The basic pharmacology and a brief history of the development of these compounds will be presented, followed by a review of their pharmacokinetic and pharmacodynamic principles, administration guidelines, adverse effects, factors affecting neuromuscular blockade, and methods for blockade reversal.

Pharmacology

The neuromuscular blocking agents (or skeletal muscle relaxants) can be divided, based on their primary mechanism of action, into two categories: the depolarizing agents and the nondepolarizing, or reversible, agents. The only depolarizing agent in widespread clinical use today is succinylcholine, which is used to assist intubation procedures and during surgery. The development of tachyphylaxis as a result of desensitization of the neuromuscular receptors, the drug's adverse-effect profile, and the inability to reverse succinylcholine-induced paralysis prevent it from being useful for long-term paralysis in the ICU.[18] The nondepolarizing agents, including tubocurarine, metocurine, pancuronium, vecuronium, and atracurium, are used in the management of mechanically ventilated patients to produce controlled, prolonged paralysis.

Site of Action. The neuromuscular junction consists of a presynaptic motor-neuron terminal and the postsynaptic muscle fiber, or endplate. Acetylcholine acts as a neurotransmitter at the neuromuscular junction as well as at the autonomic ganglia and postganglionic parasympathetic nerve endings and within the central nervous system.[19] Upon stimulation of the presynaptic motor neuron, acetylcholine is released from vesicles in the membrane of the motor-neuron terminal. The neurotransmitter then crosses the synaptic cleft, binds to receptor proteins on the postsynaptic muscle fiber, and causes ion channels to open.[18,20] The entry of positively charged ions (i.e., sodium, calcium, and potassium) into the muscle membrane causes depolarization. This depolarization may then trigger an action potential, which can propagate along the muscle fiber in both directions and cause the release of calcium ions from intracellular stores. Calcium is necessary for the interaction of the actin and myosin filaments of the fiber, which results in muscle contraction.

Once acetylcholine, a quaternary ammonium compound, crosses the synaptic cleft and binds to its receptor, it is hydrolyzed into choline and acetate by acetylcholinesterase, and the muscle fiber returns to a resting state. To prevent repeated stimulation of the motor-neuron terminal from depleting acetylcholine, a positive feedback system allows low acetylcholine concentrations to trigger increased production.[14,18,20]

Nondepolarizing neuromuscular blocking agents affect both presynaptic and postsynaptic sites. These agents compete with acetylcholine for receptor-binding sites. If enough sites are occupied, they completely inhibit acetylcholine binding and thus prevent depolarization. In addition, these drugs may block presynaptic receptors, preventing positive feedback and decreasing the amount of acetylcholine produced.[14,20]

Drug Development

The effects of curare have been recognized for centuries. Curare encompasses a variety of natural alkaloids that can paralyze skeletal muscle. South American Indians have used curare as arrow poison for hunting. It is believed that early British explorers of South America brought samples of these native alkaloids to Europe, where investigation of their neuromuscular blocking effects began. In the twentieth century, the initial development of methods to isolate and purify curare stimulated clinical research.[21]

In 1932, West[22] reported the successful use of curare to treat patients with tetanus and spastic disorders. After Griffith and Johnson[23] first used curare in 1942 to relax skeletal muscles during surgery, the use of neuromuscular blockers as part of anesthesia rapidly became widespread. It was recognized that these agents not only aided in relaxing muscles for surgical procedures, but also facilitated artificial ventilation of the patient.[21]

The chemical structure of tubocurarine was established in 1935[21] (Figure 1). Identification of an active component of curare created a great deal of interest in this class of compounds. The limited availability of the natural compound led to the development of a synthetic derivative, metocurine, which is approximately three times more potent than tubocurarine. During the 1940s many synthetic compounds with neuromuscular blocking properties were developed. Gallamine is the only synthetic compound of this group other than metocurine still in clinical use in the United States.[21] Although gallamine is still used in surgical procedures, its adverse cardiovascular effects, most notably tachycardia, prevent it from being useful in mechanically ventilated patients.[3] Other synthetic methonium compounds developed during the 1940s are no longer used in clinical practice.

In the 1960s, research began to focus on agents that possessed neuromuscular blocking properties but were associated with fewer adverse effects.[21] In 1964 pancuronium was formulated. Although it had a long duration of action, the drug also possessed vagolytic and sympathomimetic effects, which can adversely affect the heart. Exploration of the chemical properties of pancuronium as they related to specific actions led to the development of compounds with various neuromuscular blocking and vagolytic effects.[24] An agent that possesses few cardiovascular effects, vecuronium, was introduced into clinical use by researchers at the University of California, San Francisco, in 1979. Atracurium was developed in the early 1980s through collaboration between the University of Strathclyde and Wellcome Research Laboratories. This compound possesses few pharmacologic effects other than its neuromuscular blocking action. Its metabolism is unique, as it undergoes elimination by means of Hofmann degradation.[25]

In addition to these agents, several other new compounds are currently undergoing clinical trials. Mivacurium possesses a short duration of action and appears to be particularly useful for surgical procedures. Adverse cardiovascular effects, including a decrease in arterial blood pressure, have been associated with its use in preliminary studies.

Figure 1. Structures of nondepolarizing neuromuscular blocking agents used during mechanical ventilation.

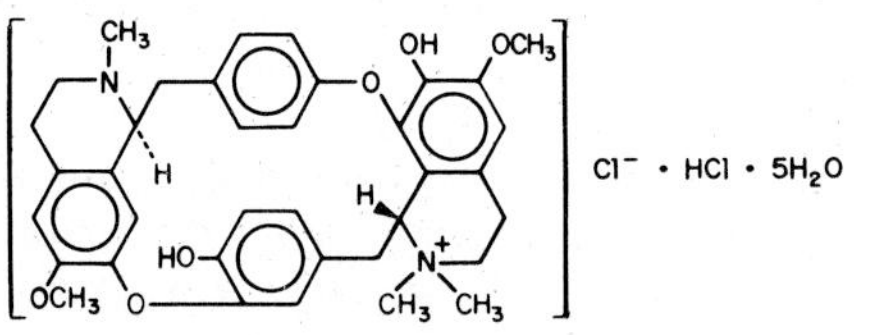

Tubocurarine chloride

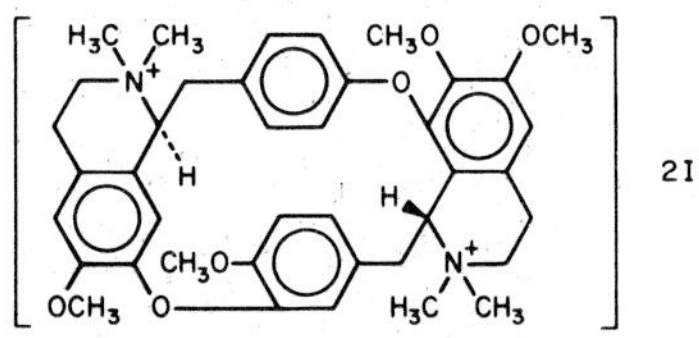

Metocurine iodide

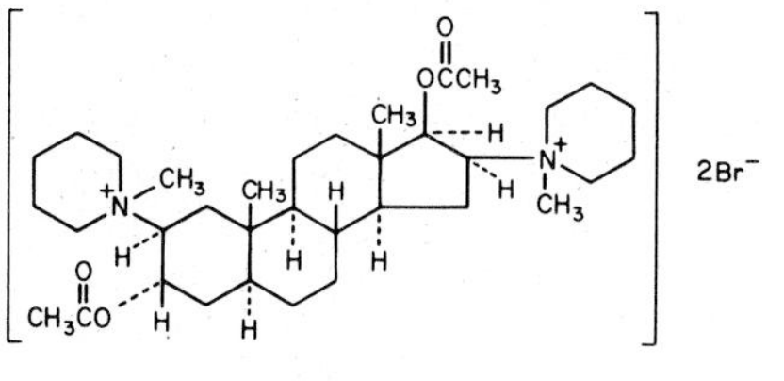

Pancuronium bromide

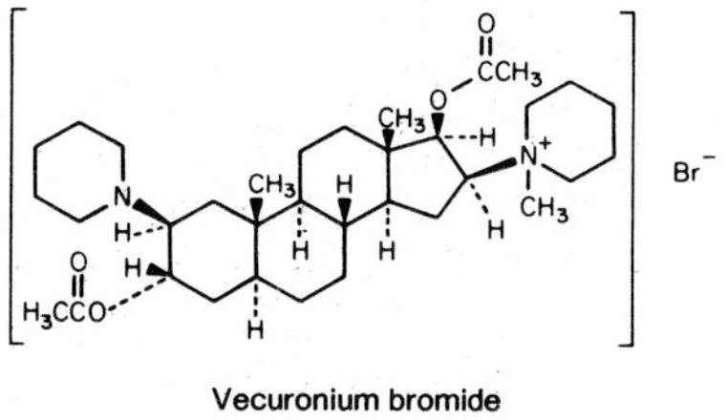

Vecuronium bromide

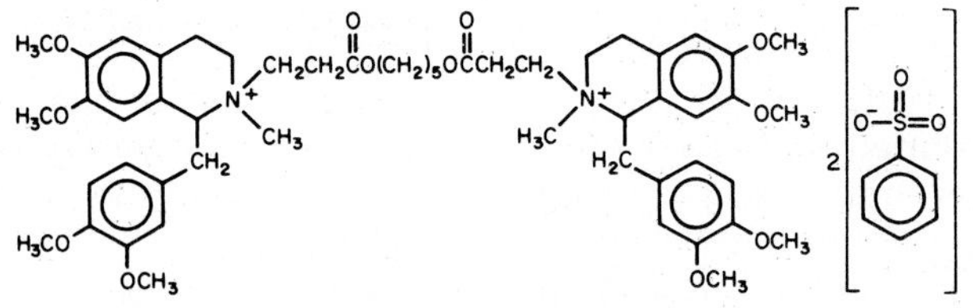

Atracurium besylate

Pipecuronium and doxacurium are long-acting neuromuscular blocking agents that have little effect on the heart.[26] To date, none of these agents have been evaluated for use in the mechanically ventilated patient, although it is anticipated that they may be useful in this setting.

Pharmacokinetics

The pharmacokinetic profiles of these drugs in surgery have been well documented, but few data are available describing their pharmacokinetic characteristics after long-term administration in mechanically ventilated patients. Moreover, mechanical ventilation may reduce cardiac output, as well as blood flow to the kidneys and liver, which could affect the pharmacokinetics of drugs given to these patients.[27-29] Further studies performed specifically in intubated patients will be necessary to determine the effects of ventilator therapy on the pharmacokinetics of nondepolarizing neuromuscular blocking agents. Table 1 lists mean pharmacokinetic values for agents that are often used in mechanically ventilated patients. These data were obtained from adult patients with normal renal and hepatic function who were undergoing surgery or receiving pharmacologic paralysis during mechanical ventilation.[30-43] All of these agents undergo a relatively rapid distribution followed by a slower elimination phase; as a result, two-compartment and three-compartment models have been used to determine the estimates of pharmacokinetic values presented in Table 1.

Absorption. All agents in this class possess one to three quaternary ammonium groups and as a result are ionized and positively charged, regardless of pH (Figure 1). Thus, neuromuscular blocking agents are poorly absorbed from the gastrointestinal tract and must be administered by injection.[44]

Distribution. The volume of distribution of the nondepolarizing neuromuscular blocking agents in adults ranges from approximately 0.2 L/kg to 0.3 L/kg, a volume approximate to the extracellular fluid space (Table 1).[19] As ionized molecules, nondepolarizing neuromuscular blocking agents have negligible intracellular penetration. These drugs are variably bound to serum proteins, primarily albumin and gamma globulin. Tubocurarine is 30–50% bound, with no changes described in patients with renal or hepatic dysfunction.[45-47] Metocurine exhibits 30–40% protein binding.[48] Pancuronium appears to be 10–30% protein bound.[47,49] Controversy persists over the extent of vecuronium binding. Duvaldestin and Henzel[47] reported 30% binding, whereas Foldes and Deery[50] reported 90% binding of vecuronium to plasma proteins. Differences in ultracentrifugation methods, concentrations of drugs studied, and methods for determining the loss due to binding of drug to analytical equipment may account for this variation in study results. In addition, Foldes and Deery[50] also reported the protein binding of atracurium as 82%. Because of the limited data describing the extent to which these drugs are bound to plasma proteins, and the discrepancies in these studies, further investigation based on more standardized methodology is necessary to determine and compare the extent of protein binding of these two agents.

Elimination. Tubocurarine, metocurine, pancuronium, and vecuronium are eliminated by both hepatic and renal routes. Tubocurarine is primarily eliminated by renal filtration, with animal models demonstrating approximately 10% biliary excretion and 1–2% hepatic metabolism.[51] More than 90% of a given metocurine dose is excreted in the urine unchanged; however, a small amount (less than 10%) is excreted in the bile.[47]

Renal excretion of pancuronium accounts for 30–40% of a given dose, with approximately 11% eliminated via the bile. The remaining drug is metabolized in the liver. The 3-hydroxypancuronium metabolite identified in humans is pharmacologically active, but the amount present in patients with normal renal and hepatic function appears to have no important clinical effect.[52] Other metabolites have not been identified in human subjects. The 3-hydroxy metabolite is excreted in the urine and in bile.

Vecuronium is hydrolyzed to active 3-hydroxyvecuronium and 3-desacetylvecuronium in the liver, but the clinical importance of these metabolites in human subjects with normal renal and hepatic function is unknown. As is the case with pancuro-

Table 1.
Pharmacokinetic Values for Nondepolarizing Neuromuscular Blocking Agents in Adult Patients with Normal Renal and Hepatic Function[a]

Drug	V_1 (L/kg)	V (L/kg)	$t_{1/2}$ (min)	CL (mL/kg/min)	References
Tubocurarine	0.11–0.15	0.3–0.4	89–172	1.6–3.0	30–32
Metocurine	0.04–0.09	0.35–0.45	121–269	1.1–2.1	33–35
Pancuronium	0.05–0.12	0.26–0.28	114–140	1.8–1.9	36–38
Vecuronium	0.05–0.11	0.19–0.25	58–80	3.0–5.2	37, 39, 40
Atracurium	0.04–0.06	0.16–0.18	20–21	5.3–6.1	41–43

[a] V_1 = volume of the central compartment; V = volume of distribution; $t_{1/2}$ = elimination half-life; CL = body clearance. Data are presented as the range of the mean values for the studies cited.

nium, other metabolites may exist. Renal excretion accounts for 15–25% of a given dose of vecuronium. Of the remaining 75–85%, most is excreted in the bile, and the rest is metabolized.[53,54]

The pathway of metabolic disposition for atracurium is different from the primary routes described for the agents above. Atracurium is cleared primarily by Hofmann degradation and also undergoes hydrolysis by nonspecific blood esterases.[55] Hofmann degradation is a spontaneous "self-destroying" mechanism that involves nonenzymatic degradation of atracurium to less complex compounds at physiologic pH and temperature. The products of Hofmann degradation are laudanosine, which is a weakly active compound, and a quaternary monoacrylate. Because of the presence of an ester grouping on atracurium, atracurium also is degraded by blood esterases to a quaternary alcohol and a quaternary acid. Conversion to all of these metabolites is rapid; the elimination half-life of atracurium is approximately 20 minutes. The products of this degradation are eliminated in the bile and urine.

Concern persists over the ability of laudanosine to cross the blood-brain barrier and accumulate in the central nervous system (CNS). Chapple et al.[56] reported seizures in dogs that had a plasma laudanosine concentration of >17 mg/L. However, a bolus dose of atracurium besylate 0.3–0.5 mg/kg given to healthy adults produced plasma laudanosine concentrations of less than 0.4 mg/L.[43] Patients receiving atracurium infusions for 38 to 219 hours during mechanical ventilation in an ICU had laudanosine serum concentrations of 1.9–5 mg/L with no evidence of cerebral excitation.[57] Until further data are available, the possibility of laudanosine accumulation resulting in CNS excitation and seizures should be considered in patients with compromised renal or hepatic function who are receiving atracurium for prolonged periods. The difficulty of assessing seizure activity in pharmacologically paralyzed patients should be considered, particularly in those patients receiving prolonged administration of atracurium. Continuous electroencephalogram recordings may be useful in monitoring these patients.[58]

Pharmacodynamics

Assessment of the efficacy of a nondepolarizing neuromuscular blocking agent in the intubated patient is difficult. Information is available regarding time of onset and recovery time, but because this information is derived from the use of these agents during surgery, it may not be applicable to their use during mechanical ventilation. Onset of effect is rapid, as determined before surgery, averaging only 2–10 minutes until maximal effect is reached.[22,34,59–67] Onset of effect depends on cardiac output and blood flow to muscle tissue, which may be altered in the ICU patient.[64]

The duration of pharmacologic effect varies among the nondepolarizing neuromuscular blocking agents. Duration also depends on the amount and the number of doses administered, renal and hepatic function, and the presence of active metabolites.[19,65] Recovery time from 25% to 75% of muscle twitch control can be used during surgical procedures to compare durations of effect. This test involves stimulation of the ulnar nerve at the wrist in a pattern often referred to as "train of four" (two cycles of two stimulations) and monitoring the resultant force of thumb adduction.[60] The range of recovery times associated with these drugs is shown in Table 2.

Less is known about recovery from the effects of these agents when they are used for prolonged periods in the ICU setting. The equipment used to test muscle twitch control in pharmacodynamic studies is not available in most ICUs. Clinical assessment of gross motor movement is the most frequently used method of determining the effect of these drugs in the ICU. After an infusion, the average time to spontaneous recovery for mechanically ventilated patients with normal renal and hepatic function has been reported as 28 minutes for vecuronium,[66] as evaluated by clinical assessment, and 40 minutes for atracurium,[67] as determined by nerve stimulation. The data on these patient groups appear to show a great deal of interpatient variability. In addition, these studies have not fully accounted for the effects of concurrent sedation.

Table 2.
Durations of Effect of Selected Nondepolarizing Neuromuscular Blocking Agents

Drug and I.V. Dose (mg/kg)	No. Patients	Duration of Effect (min)[a]	Reference
Tubocurarine chloride			
0.3	8	48 (45–51)	32
0.3	7	48 (36–60)	33
0.6	12	80.5 (73.6–87.4)	59
Metocurine iodide			
0.15	7	47 (37–57)	33
0.2	7	70 (10–130)	34
0.3	15	82.4 (70.4–94.4)	59
Pancuronium bromide			
0.1	13	99.3 (84.3–114.3)	59
0.03	10	26 (18–34)	60
0.1	6[b]	28 (22–34)	61
Vecuronium bromide			
0.02	7	14.1 (11.2–17)	60
0.1	6[b]	7 (5–9)	61
0.1	8	11.6 (10.5–12.7)	62
Atracurium besylate			
0.5	10	10.5 (9.4–11.6)	43
0.2	5	11.8 (10.7–12.9)	63
0.4	5	10.7 (10.1–11.3)	63

[a] Time required for recovery of twitch control from 25% to 75%. Data are presented as the mean (range).

[b] Determined in children three to six years of age.

Determination of pharmacodynamics based on subjective clinical assessment of movement alone is frequently inaccurate. However, this is often the only mechanism available in the ICU to clinically assess the need for adjustments in dosage or to determine the time to recovery of spontaneous ventilation. Further objective evaluation of muscle twitch control, similar to the "train of four" testing used during surgery, is needed to compare the durations of effect of these agents in mechanically ventilated patients. Once these pharmacodynamic values are determined, routine use of this equipment may become standard ICU practice. Clearly, more data describing the pharmacokinetic–pharmacodynamic correlates of these drugs are needed to refine their use during mechanical ventilation in the ICU setting.

Drug Administration

As previously discussed, these drugs are poorly absorbed after oral administration and thus must be administered by injection. The i.v. route is preferred because surgery or mechanical ventilation could affect drug absorption from i.m. sites. The i.v. route also permits a more rapid and complete onset of action, allowing close adjustment of the drug dose to the effect. Those agents that have a longer duration of action (recovery time from 25% to 75% of muscle function of >1 hr), including tubocurarine and metocurine, are generally administered every two to three hours.[68] Vecuronium and pancuronium, which have intermediate durations of action (recovery time of 10–30 minutes), are administered either every one to three hours or as a continuous infusion.[13,66,69–73] Atracurium is most often administered as a continuous infusion because of its short duration of action (recovery time of approximately 10 minutes).[57,67,72,74–76]

Because of the primary pathways by which these drugs are cleared from the body, dosing modifications may be necessary in patients with underlying renal or hepatic diseases. In addition, disposition profiles for these agents that differ from profiles obtained for adults have been described in the pediatric and geriatric patient populations, as well as in patients who have suffered substantial thermal injuries. These patient populations will be discussed in the following sections.

Table 3 provides guidelines for the dosing of these agents in mechanically ventilated patients who have normal renal and hepatic function. Individualized adjustment of the dose is necessary to maintain the desired degree of paralysis. In several case reports, dosing requirements have increased after prolonged use.[73,77,78] This increased requirement has not been adequately explained or consistently reported. It may relate to the patient's disease, altered pharmacokinetics due to prolonged mechanical ventilation, or other unrecognized factors that could affect the efficacy of nondepolarizing neuromuscular blocking agents.

Infusion through a central venous catheter is preferred for long-term administration. Atracurium has been associated with phlebitis in a small number of patients receiving infusions through peripheral catheters.[67] Pain during injection of vecuronium has been reported and may be the result of the drug's acidity (pH approximately 4.5).[79]

Use in Patients with Renal Dysfunction

With the exception of vecuronium and atracurium, the majority of the clinically useful nondepolarizing neuromuscular blocking agents are eliminated unchanged from the body via the kidney. As a result, a change in renal function may necessitate alterations in the patient's dosing requirements of these agents.

Miller et al.[80] and Hunter et al.[81] reported an expected increase in elimination half-life and duration of action for patients with renal disease who received tubocurarine. Metocurine exhibited a similar increase in elimination half-life and dura-

Table 3.
Recommendations for Initial I.V. Dosing of Nondepolarizing Neuromuscular Blocking Agents[a]

Drug	Intermittent Dosing	Continuous Infusion	References
Tubocurarine chloride[b]	0.25–0.50 mg/kg q 2–3 hr	. . .	68
Metocurine iodide[b]	0.25–0.50 mg/kg q 3 hr	. . .	68
Pancuronium bromide	0.1–0.2 mg/kg q 1–3 hr	Loading dose[c] = 0.03–0.1 mg/kg Infusion = 0.06–0.1 mg/kg/hr	13, 69
Vecuronium bromide	0.1–0.2 mg/kg q 1 hr	Loading dose[c] = 0.1 mg/kg Infusion = 0.05–0.1 mg/kg/hr	66, 70–73
Atracurium besylate	. . .	Loading dose[c] = 0.4–0.5 mg/kg Infusion = 0.4–1.0 mg/kg/hr	57, 67, 72, 74–76

[a] These are reasonable initial starting doses for use in the facilitation of mechanical ventilation. Patients receiving these agents require close clinical monitoring. Subsequent dosage adjustments are based on clinical effect. Drug dosages may need to be adjusted in patients with underlying organ disease (see the text).

[b] Limited information is available on the dosage of these agents for mechanically ventilated patients.

[c] Loading dose usually administered over 5–10 minutes.

tion of action.[82] McLeod et al.[83] reported a marked increase in the volume of distribution of pancuronium in patients who had renal dysfunction (0.236 ± 0.025 L/kg [mean ± S.D.]) compared with patients who had normal renal function (0.148 ± 0.014 L/kg). They also reported a decrease in plasma clearance (20 ± 2 mL/min for patients with renal dysfunction versus 74 ± 8 mL/min for patients with normal renal function) and a concurrent decrease in the elimination rate constant (0.085 ± 0.013 hr^{-1} versus 0.414 ± 0.014 hr^{-1}). Pancuronium, as well as its active metabolite, will accumulate in patients with renal dysfunction, and the duration of effect will be prolonged.[84]

These data underscore the importance of careful clinical monitoring of drug effects and the integrity of the patient's renal function when these agents are used for prolonged periods in the ICU. Because tubocurarine, metocurine, and pancuronium depend on the renal route for elimination from the body, it would appear prudent to either measure or estimate a patient's glomerular filtration rate before and during therapy. We adjust the dosage of nondepolarizing neuromuscular blocking agents to directly reflect the degree of renal insufficiency (e.g., a patient with a creatinine clearance half that expected for his or her age would initially receive half the normal dosage). Most important, however, drug dosing in these patients should be modified to achieve the desired clinical effect.

In contrast to the agents described above, the disposition of vecuronium and atracurium appears to be less affected by changes in renal function during short-term use. Fahey and colleagues[39] found no significant differences in the pharmacokinetic profiles of vecuronium in patients with and without compromised renal function. In addition, no differences in pharmacodynamic effects were noted. Also, no differences between anephric and normal subjects were noted with respect to onset and recovery time.[81] Similarly, Lynam and coworkers[85] reported no difference in pharmacokinetic values, but they did observe a prolonged duration of action in patients with renal disease. This longer duration has also been observed in mechanically ventilated patients receiving long-term infusions of vecuronium.[66] As is the case with pancuronium, the accumulation of vecuronium and its active metabolites may result in this prolonged pharmacodynamic effect.[54]

Atracurium pharmacokinetics and pharmacodynamics do not appear to be affected by changes in a patient's renal function.[42,43,74,81,86] However, elevated laudanosine concentrations have been reported in patients with renal dysfunction who received atracurium during surgery and during mechanical ventilation.[74,75,87] As discussed above, the accumulation of this metabolite to a plasma concentration of >17 mg/L has resulted in seizures in an animal model.[56] The potential for accumulation of metabolites that have paralyzing activity or other adverse effects must be considered when the therapeutic need for these agents is assessed. Further study is necessary to ascertain the effects of these metabolites after long-term repeated doses or continuous infusion of the nondepolarizing neuromuscular blocking agents during mechanical ventilation.

Use in Patients with Hepatic Dysfunction

The disposition and pharmacodynamic characteristics of hepatically metabolized neuromuscular blocking agents would be expected to be influenced by changes in a patient's liver function. Patients with hepatic dysfunction have exhibited a resistance to usual therapeutic doses of tubocurarine and pancuronium.[36,88] This resistance is manifested as an increased initial dose requirement and appears to be caused by an increase in the volume of distribution.[36] Subsequent paralytic drug doses must be administered to these patients with caution because of the expected prolongation of the observed elimination half-life. Because these drugs are excreted in bile, cholestasis in patients with liver dysfunction may also result in reduced clearance and prolonged duration of action.[88]

The pharmacokinetic profile of vecuronium has also been shown to be altered in patients with hepatic dysfunction. Significant decreases in clearance and a longer elimination half-life have been described in patients with cirrhosis and cholestasis.[40,89] No differences were observed in the volume of distribution. Comparison of pharmacodynamic variables has shown that, at higher doses, vecuronium has a significantly longer duration of action in patients with cirrhosis than in patients who have normal hepatic function.[40,90]

As described above, atracurium is not eliminated by hepatic metabolism but is cleared by Hofmann degradation and hydrolysis by blood esterases. Numerous studies of atracurium have shown that the pharmacokinetic profiles and clinical responses of patients with moderate hepatic disease are similar to those of patients with normal hepatic function.[41,91,92] Prolonged neuromuscular blockade by atracurium has been described in a monkey model of hepatic vascular occlusion. These data suggest that total occlusion of the hepatic circulation will substantially affect recovery time; thus, patients with severe hepatic disease may require dosage adjustment.[93] Ward and Weatherley[42] reported a significant decrease in laudanosine clearance in patients with hepatic dysfunction who received atracurium (6 ± 4 mL/kg/min [mean ± S.E.M.] versus 10 ± 1 mL/kg/min in control subjects). Parker and Hunter[94] found no change in laudanosine clearance, but an increased volume of distribution and prolonged elimination half-life in patients with hepatic cirrhosis. The potential for increased tissue and CNS accumulation of laudanosine should be considered when this agent is used in ICU patients who have liver disease.

Use in Patients with Thermal Injuries

The pharmacodynamic response to neuromuscular blocking agents has been reported to be markedly blunted in patients with thermal injuries. Numerous reports document an increased dosage requirement in these patients for each of the agents used for paralysis during mechanical ventilation.[95-106] This blunted response or relative resistance to these agents is typically described in patients with burns involving more than 10% of the body surface area. In patients with more than 40% body surface area involvement, doses of these drugs may need to be 2.5–5 times the usual dose.[96] This alteration in drug effect may continue for up to a year after the initial thermal trauma.[100]

Burn trauma can alter the disposition of drugs through changes in blood flow patterns, alteration of hepatic and renal function, and changes in protein-binding capacity.[95,96] Recovery from thermal injuries can be divided into two metabolic phases. In the initial (acute) phase, blood flow to organs and tissues is decreased. Drugs administered during this phase may not be well distributed within the body. During the second (hypermetabolic) phase, blood flow to organs and tissues increases, possibly resulting in an increased clearance of drug.[96]

Martyn and co-workers[99] evaluated the pharmacokinetic profile of tubocurarine in burn patients to determine whether differences in clearance could at least partially explain the increased dosage requirement. Eight patients with 15–80% burns and six control subjects were given a single intravenous dose of tubocurarine. Intrinsic clearance in the burn patients (1.62 ± 0.59 mL/kg/min [mean ± S.D.]) was not significantly different from that observed in control subjects (1.56 ± 0.41 mL/kg/min). Similarly, the pharmacokinetic characteristics of atracurium (i.e., volume of distribution, distribution and elimination half-lives, body clearance) have been shown to be unchanged in patients with thermal injuries compared with matched control subjects.[104] In this latter study,[104] burn patients required 3.4 times the serum concentration of atracurium required in control subjects to achieve a similar degree of paralysis.

Alterations in plasma proteins may occur after burn trauma, affecting the binding capability of neuromuscular blocking agents. Leibel and colleagues[98] evaluated the protein-binding capacity of burn patients and control subjects receiving tubocurarine. These authors found 5.7 ± 0.9 nmol (mean ± S.D.) of tubocurarine per gram of plasma protein in the serum of burn patients compared with 3.4 ± 0.7 nmol of tubocurarine per gram of plasma protein in the control subjects. Although this difference was significant ($p < 0.0005$), it does not appear to be responsible for the degree of resistance observed in burn patients when it is evaluated in relation to these agents' low affinity for protein binding. These investigators also found that, although serum albumin concentrations were reduced in patients with thermal injuries, concentrations of α_1-acid glycoprotein were increased. Nondepolarizing neuromuscular blocking agents may exhibit increased binding to α_1-acid glycoprotein, which could result in a reduced amount of free drug available to bind to the receptor at the neuromuscular junction.

Other factors in the plasma of burn patients that may compete for neuromuscular receptors, result in changes in receptor sensitivity, or produce an increase in receptor number have all been suggested as possible mechanisms for the blunted response to nondepolarizing neuromuscular blocking agents. Storella et al.[107] performed an in vitro study of the effects of tubocurarine and pancuronium when added to plasma samples obtained from both burn patients and control subjects. Isolated rat neuromuscular tissue was exposed to the prepared plasma samples, and the response to nerve stimulation was measured. The plasma samples from the burn patients did not elicit as great a response as the samples from the control subjects did. The authors concluded that circulating plasma factors may be responsible for the decreased potency of the neuromuscular blocking agents in patients with thermal injury. Further research is needed to identify the reason for this blunted response to nondepolarizing neuromuscular blocking agents. ICU patients with thermal injuries who require mechanical ventilation may exhibit this resistance to pharmacologic paralysis, and drug doses should be adjusted to clinical response.

Use in Elderly Patients

As the percentage of elderly people in our society increases, the use of mechanical ventilation in this patient population will also likely increase. Information about the changes in pharmacokinetics and pharmacodynamic responses caused by increasing age will be necessary for optimal management of these patients. In addition to the effects of age on renal and hepatic function, decreases in body muscle, fat stores, and plasma proteins can affect the disposition of nondepolarizing neuromuscular blocking agents. It has also been suggested that the functional capacity of the neuromuscular junction declines with increasing age.[19,33]

Specific differences in the pharmacokinetics of these drugs relative to increasing age were first reported by McLeod et al.[108] These authors examined pancuronium pharmacokinetics in the elderly and found that, although the drug's apparent volume of distribution was similar to that reported in younger patients, plasma clearance decreased with advancing age. Matteo and colleagues[33] assessed the pharmacokinetics of tubocurarine in a group of 21 patients aged 70 to 87 years and in 21 younger, healthy subjects. After a single 0.3 mg/kg bolus dose of tubocurarine chloride, plasma tubocurarine concentrations were consistently higher throughout the study period in the elderly patients compared with the control subjects. These investigators also described a smaller apparent volume of distribution (0.281 ± 0.04 L/kg [mean ± S.D.] in elderly patients versus 0.425 ± 0.06 L/kg in control subjects) and a lower body clearance rate (0.79 ± 0.18 mL/kg/min versus 1.71 ± 0.32 mL/kg/min), as well as a prolonged elimination half-life (268 ± 51 minutes versus 173 ± 38 minutes) and a prolonged recovery time from 25% to 75% of muscle control (94 ± 32 minutes versus 48 ± 12 minutes).

Although Duvaldestin et al.[109] found no difference in the apparent volume of distribution in elderly patients and control subjects receiving pancuronium, these investigators did describe a decrease in body clearance, as well as increases in elimination half-life and time to recovery similar to those reported by Matteo et al.[33] for tubocurarine. Aging has been shown to have similar effects on metocurine disposition: a decrease in the apparent volume of distribution, decreased plasma clearance, and a prolonged elimination half-life, without a difference in recovery time.[33]

A study of vecuronium administered by continuous infusion during surgery to patients over 60 years of age showed that these patients required substantially lower doses to maintain adequate paralysis compared with a group of patients younger than 40 years. Recovery times in the elderly patients were more than twice those of the control group (44.94 ± 6.91 minutes [mean ± S.E.M.] versus 16.24 ± 4 minutes).[110] Rupp et al.[111] found a smaller volume of distribution and a reduction in plasma clearance in elderly patients compared with younger patients when both groups received a vecuronium bromide infusion of 0.15 mg/kg/hr.

Atracurium clearance does not appear to be affected by age. Thus, atracurium may be an alternative to other nondepolarizing neuromuscular blocking agents in elderly patients.[112] It has been observed that elderly patients may require lower doses by infusion than younger patients for paralysis during mechanical ventilation.[67] Studies involving a larger number of patients will be necessary before more definitive recommendations can be made regarding atracurium doses and the likelihood of accumulation of the laudanosine metabolite. As has been observed with other pharmacologic agents used in elderly patients, initial doses of the nondepolarizing neuromuscular blocking agents should be lower than those used in younger patients because of potential differences in both volume of distribution and body clearance.

Use in Children

Nondepolarizing neuromuscular blocking agents have been widely used in children to induce paralysis during surgical procedures and during mechanical ventilation. Several reviews of their use in infants and children have been published.[14,20,113]

In 1963, Heese and colleagues[114] reported the successful recovery of neonates with respiratory distress syndrome in response to therapy that included paralysis during mechanical ventilation. Use of therapeutic paralysis during mechanical ventilation in the neonatal ICU soon became widespread.[115-119] Additional research has demonstrated the potential benefit of pharmacologic paralysis in the prevention of mechanical ventilator-associated pneumothorax and pulmonary interstitial emphysema.[120,121] Use of these agents has also been shown to minimize fluctuations in cerebral blood flow, an important variable associated with the development of intraventricular hemorrhage in neonates.[122,123] Prolonged use of nondepolarizing neuromuscular blocking agents, however, has been associated with fluid retention and negative effects on neonatal pulmonary mechanics.[124,125] Bhutani and colleagues[125] reported that significant decreases in pulmonary dynamic compliance and increased pulmonary resistance resulting in increased ventilatory support were observed in infants during treatment with pharmacologic paralysis. Caution should be used in asphyxiated infants, as paralysis can mask symptoms of seizure activity.[58]

Tubocurarine, metocurine, pancuronium, vecuronium, and atracurium have all been used for paralysis in infants and children. Tubocurarine was used in children during surgery as early as 1943. The pharmacokinetic and pharmacodynamic properties of tubocurarine have been described for infants and children.[31,32] Matteo and colleagues[32] evaluated tubocurarine pharmacokinetics and pharmacodynamics in infants, children, and adults. These authors reported a decrease in clearance and a prolonged elimination half-life in infants compared with children and adults, reflecting normal physiologic differences in extracellular fluid volume and renal function of this population. Pharmacokinetic values in children older than one year did not differ significantly from those observed in adults. Pharmacodynamic responses to tubocurarine did not differ among the age groups. Similar results were observed in an evaluation of metocurine pharmacokinetics and pharmacodynamics in infants, children, and adults.[34,126]

A study of tubocurarine and metocurine dose requirements in neonates who were pharmacologically paralyzed during mechanical ventilation showed an increasing requirement for metocurine iodide over a week of treatment, up to 115–780% of the initial dose of 0.25–0.50 mg/kg. In contrast, tubocurarine requirements did not dramatically increase.[68] The authors were unable to explain these differences. Patient response, as well as factors that could influence the effect of nondepolarizing neuromuscular blocking agents, should be considered when dosing requirements rise dramatically.

Pancuronium use in infants and children has also been well studied.[114–119,121–125] The pharmacokinetic and pharmacodynamic profile of pancuronium in children appears similar to that described in adults.[61] Vecuronium has been used in infants and children undergoing surgical procedures and for paralysis during mechanical ventilation.[61,71,127–131] Eldadah and Newth[71] compared vecuronium bromide given by intermittent infusion (100 μg/kg) and continuous infusion (loading dose of 150 μg/kg and maintenance dosage of 1 μg/kg/min) in 12 infants and children. Patients receiving continuous infusion required less vecuronium to maintain the same degree of paralysis. These investigators described no change from baseline in heart rate and mean arterial blood pressure for either group. Children with liver dysfunction required a lower total vecuronium dose than children with normal hepatic function. Careful titration of dosage appears to be essential. The use of a higher dosage (1.67 μg/kg/min) in one infant resulted in a prolonged, profound neuromuscular blockade.[127] Although it has not been studied, the potential exists for accumulation of vecuronium in children paralyzed during mechanical ventilation. Pharmacokinetic and pharmacodynamic analysis of vecuronium used during surgery has shown a larger volume of distribution in infants compared with older children, but no difference in body clearance or elimination half-life.[61,129] Recovery time for infants appears to be longer than that reported for older children and adults.[129–131]

Atracurium besylate has been used for paralysis during surgical procedures in infants and children.[132–135] Goudsouzian[132] reported effective paralysis during surgery with dosages of 0.46 ± 0.02 mg/kg/hr (mean ± S.E.M.) in infants and 0.50 ± 0.02 mg/kg/hr in older children.[133] Time to spontaneous recovery has been reported to be markedly longer in infants than in older children and adults.[134] Atracurium was also reported to reduce fluctuation in intracranial pressure in a seven-year-old child with a severe head injury.[15] Successful paralysis was achieved with a loading dose of 0.3 mg/kg followed by an infusion of 0.6 mg/kg/hr for 72 hours. No adverse effects were reported. Pharmacokinetic values for atracurium in children are similar to those established for adults; however, infants appear to have a larger volume of distribution (210 ± 118 mL/kg [mean ± S.D.] versus 100 ± 22 mL/kg in adults) and a more rapid total body clearance (7.9 ± 2.0 mL/kg/hr versus 5.3 ± 0.9 mL/kg/hr).[136]

Reports of the long-term use of nondepolarizing neuromuscular blocking agents in children are limited. Current recommendations are based on a relatively small number of patients. Therapy may be initiated with the doses shown in Table 3, with adjustment according to clinical response. The possibility of a prolonged recovery time should be taken into account when discontinuation of therapy is being considered.

Adverse Effects

The nondepolarizing neuromuscular blocking agents can cause a number of important adverse effects. During drug administration, histamine release[137–145] and cardiovascular changes[68,69,71,71,139,140,144,146–152] may affect therapy. Muscle atrophy[153–157] may also occur during long-term drug use and may persist after drug therapy has been discontinued. Along with these adverse effects, it is important to monitor the integrity of eyelid movement (the blink reflex) so that doses of paralytic or sedative agents can be adjusted to either maintain the reflex or allow closure of the eyes. Other measures to protect against corneal abrasions (e.g., taping shut the eyelids, using artificial tears) can be instituted as needed. As previously mentioned, i.v. infusion of atracurium has caused phlebitis,[67] and vecuronium may cause pain during injection.[79]

In addition to the adverse effects related to the use of nondepolarizing neuromuscular blocking agents, a number of other complications can arise in the mechanically ventilated, critically ill patient. These complications may include decubitus ulcers requiring frequent, scheduled repositioning, accumulation of pulmonary secretions requiring pulmonary suction, and the risk of development of deep vein thromboses with subsequent embolism.

Histamine Release. All nondepolarizing neuromuscular blocking agents can provoke the release of histamine from mast cells. Histamine release may be manifested clinically as bronchospasm and vasodilatation, resulting in transient hypotension and cutaneous flushing.[137] Equipotent doses of nondepolarizing neuromuscular blocking agents have been tested in vitro using isolated human tissue samples and in vivo with intradermal injection to establish the agents' relative histamine-releasing activity.[137,138] Galletly[137] measured wheal response to intradermal injection of equipotent doses of nondepolarizing neuromuscular blocking agents. With pancuronium assigned a baseline value of 1, the relative histamine-releasing potential for the other agents was 172 for tubocurarine, 52 for atracurium, and 1.1 for vecuronium. Measurement of plasma histamine after administration of nondepolarizing neuromuscular blocking agents has shown results similar to those observed with skin testing.[139–144] From these studies, the histamine-releasing properties of metocurine appear to be similar to those of pancuronium and vecuronium.[144]

A dose-dependent increase in plasma histamine has been reported in patients receiving tubocurarine during surgery.[140] The release of histamine in that study correlated with a decrease in blood pressure. Although atracurium administration can also cause an increase in plasma histamine, the amount secreted typically results in cutaneous flushing without further important clinical symptoms.[141–143] Slowing the rate of drug administration may lessen the clinical manifestations of histamine release. When choosing a nondepolarizing neuromuscular blocking agent, clinicians should consider its histamine-releasing potential relative to the dose and the rate of administration in mechanically ventilated patients. If symptoms are present, a distinction should be made between anaphylaxis and histamine release. Although true anaphylactic reactions involving an immunologically mediated response are rare, cases have been reported.[145]

Cardiovascular Effects. The cardiovascular effects of the nondepolarizing neuromuscular blocking agents may result from their direct activity at cholinergic receptors of the autonomic ganglia and the adrenal medulla. The resulting physiologic effects include a vagolytic effect on the heart (producing tachycardia) and an increase in arterial blood pressure. The extent of the effect is related to the selectivity of the drug for the neuromuscular junction.[21]

In a study by Cabel et al.,[146] pancuronium administered to infants for ventilatory control caused a transient increase in heart rate and a sustained increase in mean arterial blood pressure. The authors also measured an increase in blood epinephrine and norepinephrine concentrations and postulated that the increase in blood pressure resulted from excess sympathetic activity. Similar hemodynamic changes have been observed in adults and older children receiving pancuronium[139,147] and in patients receiving tubocurarine.[148]

In contrast, metocurine has been shown to have little effect on cardiac function.[144,149] Vecuronium and atracurium, which have greater specificity for binding at the neuromuscular junction, also appear to have minimal effects on heart rate or blood pressure. Vecuronium has been shown by in vitro analysis to have a negligible effect on isolated vagal nerve.[150] This finding is consistent with the lack of cardiovascular effects observed in clinical studies performed during surgical procedures[151] and in studies of vecuronium's use for paralysis during mechanical ventilation.[68,71,72] Atracurium has also been shown in clinical trials to have little effect on cardiovascular function.[69,148,152]

Unlike the other nondepolarizing neuromuscular blocking agents used in mechanically ventilated patients, tubocurarine has more histamine-related effects than direct cardiac effects. Use of tubocurarine is frequently associated with a decrease in arterial blood pressure.[139,140]

Muscular Effects. In patients receiving these agents over a prolonged period of time, there is the potential for development of disuse atrophy and weakness of skeletal muscles. This condition has been documented in both adults and infants receiving these agents during mechanical ventilation.[153–156] Op de Coul et al.[155] reported on 12 adult patients who experienced diffuse muscle atrophy after prolonged use (one to three weeks) of pancuronium during mechanical ventilation. Within six months after discontinuation of pancuronium therapy, seven patients had full recovery of muscle function, two had partial recovery, and three patients had died of their primary disease. Joint contractures have also been reported in newborns receiving repeated doses of pancuronium.[157] The possibility for muscle atrophy must be periodically assessed in patients requiring long-term pharmacologic paralysis during mechanical ventilation. Physical therapy and range-of-motion exercises have been recommended to lessen the potential for disuse atrophy in paralyzed patients.[157]

Factors Affecting Paralysis

Many factors can influence the degree of paralysis induced by these agents.[19,146–152,158–195] Effects may be antagonistic or may potentiate muscular blockade. The resulting clinical manifestations depend on the degree of blockade induced, the agent used, and individual patient characteristics. Table 4 lists pathophysiologic variables and drug interactions capable of altering the effects of nondepolarizing neuromuscular blocking agents.

Discontinuing Therapy and Reversal of Blockade

In most instances, patients no longer requiring paralysis in the ICU will be allowed to spontaneously regain muscle function after drug therapy has been discontinued. Adequate ventilation of the patient must be continued until all effects of the nondepolarizing neuromuscular blocking agent have dissipated. There may be rare instances, however, when the effects of a neuromuscular blocking agent must be reversed more rapidly. This need may arise when rapid clinical deterioration of the patient makes it necessary to assess and monitor those muscle functions eliminated by pharmacologic paralysis to determine the appropriate therapeutic intervention. Reversal can be accomplished with the use of acetylcholinesterase-inhibiting agents. These drugs prevent the breakdown of ace-

Table 4.
Clinical Variables Affecting Pharmacodynamics of Nondepolarizing Neuromuscular Blocking Agents[a]

Clinical Variable	Possible Effect	References
Pathophysiologic Variable		
Hypothermia	Potentiate blockade	158
Acid-base balance[b]		
Acidosis	Potentiate blockade: tubocurarine and vecuronium; no effect or antagonism: metocurine and pancuronium	159–162
Alkalosis	Antagonize blockade: tubocurarine and vecuronium; no effect or potentiation: metocurine and pancuronium	
Electrolyte status		
Increased potassium	Decreased sensitivity to blockade	163–165
Increased calcium	Decreased sensitivity to blockade	
Increased magnesium	Potentiate blockade	
Decreased blood flow to muscles	Delay in onset	166
Neuromuscular disease (e.g., myasthenia gravis)	Increased sensitivity	167–169
Collagen diseases (e.g., polymyositis)	Increased sensitivity	170
Cardiovascular disease	Effect on heart rate and blood pressure	146–152
Pregnancy	Increased drug clearance; potential for decreased blockade	171
Burns	Increased drug clearance	95–106
Drug Interactions		
Other nondepolarizing neuromuscular blocking agents	Additive or possible synergistic effect	172–174
Antimicrobial agents		
Aminoglycosides	Potentiate blockade	175–178
Polymyxin	Potentiate blockade	
Tetracyclines	Potentiate blockade	
Clindamycin, lincomycin	Potentiate blockade	
Vancomycin	Potentiate blockade	
Sedative-anesthetics		
Midazolam	May potentiate blockade	179
Ketamine	May potentiate blockade	180
Cardiovascular drugs		
Furosemide[c]	Antagonize blockade of pancuronium; potentiate blockade of tubocurarine	181–185
Beta-blocking agents	Potentiate blockade	
Procainamide	Potentiate blockade	
Quinidine	Potentiate blockade	
Calcium-channel blockers	Potentiate blockade	
Methylxanthines	Antagonize blockade	186, 187
Antiepileptic drugs		
Phenytoin	Increased resistance to blockade; no effect with atracurium	181–191
Carbamazepine	Increased resistance to blockade	
Psychotropic drugs		
Lithium carbonate	Potentiate blockade of pancuronium	192
Immunosuppressive agents		
Azathioprine	Mild antagonism	193
Cyclosporine	Potentiate blockade	194
Corticosteroids	Antagonize blockade	188, 195

[a] The use of nondepolarizing neuromuscular blocking agents in the presence of these clinical variables is not contraindicated, but it may require closer patient monitoring and adjustment of the dose necessary to achieve paralysis.

[b] The effect may depend on the chemical structure: tubocurarine and vecuronium are monoquaternary compounds, whereas the others are bisquaternary compounds. The effect on atracurium has not been reported.

[c] Antagonism of pancuronium has been reported in patients with normal renal function. Potentiation of tubocurarine has been reported in anephric patients.

tylcholine by tissue-bound acetylcholinesterase, allowing the neurotransmitter to accumulate at the neuromuscular junction. Because of the law of mass action, the effect of the neuromuscular blocking agent will be counteracted by shifting the balance between acetylcholine and the blocking agent to favor acetylcholine binding at the postsynaptic muscle fiber, allowing muscle function to resume.[196,197] Acetylcholinesterase inhibitors may also act at the postsynaptic muscle fiber by altering acetylcholine ion-channel function.[198]

Physostigmine, neostigmine, pyridostigmine,

and edrophonium are acetylcholinesterase inhibitors in clinical use. The more lipophilic compound, physostigmine, is the only clinically available acetylcholinesterase inhibitor that crosses the blood–brain barrier. As a result, physostigmine can reverse central anticholinergic symptoms, but it is less efficient in reversing neuromuscular blockade.[196] Neostigmine, pyridostigmine, and edrophonium are used more often to reverse the effects of pharmacologic paralysis during surgery. Of the three, edrophonium has the most rapid onset and the shortest duration of action, and pyridostigmine has the slowest onset and the longest duration of action.[196,199]

Recommended intravenous doses of these agents to reverse pharmacologic paralysis after surgery are edrophonium chloride 0.3–1.0 mg/kg, pyridostigmine bromide 0.1–0.25 mg/kg, and neostigmine methylsulfate 0.01–0.035 mg/kg. These agents can reversibly bind to any cholinergic receptor, nicotinic (such as the motor neuron terminal) or muscarinic (located in the heart, salivary glands, and gut). For this reason, these agents are frequently administered concomitantly with atropine sulfate (0.008–0.018 mg/kg) or glycopyrrolate (0.002–0.016 mg/kg) to prevent possible bradycardia, increased salivation, and hyperperistalsis caused by acetylcholine interaction at muscarinic receptors.[196,200]

Little is known about the use of these agents for reversing the effects of long-term paralysis during mechanical ventilation. Use of neostigmine to reverse the effects of up to 3.5 hours of continuous atracurium infusion resulted in a rate of return of muscle function no different than that seen in patients receiving no reversal agent.[200] It has been suggested that patients with total paralysis be allowed to recover some degree of muscle response spontaneously before attempting full reversal with an acetylcholinesterase-inhibiting agent.[196]

Sedation during Paralysis

It is important to recognize the need for adequate sedation during pharmacologic muscle paralysis. There is a common misconception that administration of a nondepolarizing neuromuscular blocking agent also provides sedation and analgesia. In a report published in 1947,[201] Smith, an anesthesiologist, allowed his colleagues to paralyze him with tubocurarine without administering sedation. Smith was able to provide details of his experience to his colleagues as soon as the effects of the blocking agent had been reversed. He reported sensations of choking during the period that he was unable to swallow and shortness of breath, even though he was aware that he was receiving mechanical ventilation. Throughout the experience, Smith was completely aware of his surroundings. The authors concluded that nondepolarizing neuromuscular blocking agents have no effect on sensorium. Unfortunately, this lesson has often been overlooked or forgotten.

As recently as 1984, the experiences of a nurse who was a patient in an ICU showed the lack of understanding of the need for frequent assessment of the adequacy of sedation.[202] In 1989, a survey of nurses and physicians showed that 10–25% mistakenly believed that pancuronium provided analgesia, and another 5–10% did not know what effect pancuronium had on analgesia.[203] Sedation, and if necessary analgesia, should be provided throughout the period of paralysis. Timing and administration of doses should receive special attention because it is frequently impossible to ascertain the level of sedation experienced by the patient.

Conclusion

Nondepolarizing neuromuscular blocking agents can be used to paralyze mechanically ventilated patients, facilitating optimal oxygenation and ventilation. Choice and administration of an agent should reflect consideration of patient characteristics and the potential for pharmacokinetic changes, drug interactions, and adverse effects.

References

1. Shapiro B. General principles of airway pressure therapy. In: Shoemaker WC, Ayres S, Grenvik A et al., eds. Textbook of critical care. 2nd ed. Philadelphia: Saunders; 1989:505–15.
2. Gioia FR, Stephenson RL, Alterwitz SA. Principles of respiratory support and mechanical ventilation. In: Rogers MC, ed. Textbook of pediatric intensive care. Baltimore: Williams & Wilkins; 1987:113–69.
3. Levesque PR. Use of muscle relaxants in the intensive care unit. In: MacDonnell KF, Fahey PJ, Segal MS, eds. Respiratory intensive care. Boston: Little, Brown; 1987:125–30.
4. Flynn P. Muscle relaxation. *Acta Anaesthesiol Scand*. 1988; 32 (Suppl 87):21–4.
5. Aitkenhead AR. Analgesia and sedation in intensive care. *Br J Anaesth*. 1989; 63:196–206.
6. Shafer A, White PF, Schuttler J et al. Use of a fentanyl infusion in the intensive care unit: tolerance to its anesthetic effects? *Anesthesiology*. 1983; 59:245–8.
7. Sinclair ME, Sear JW, Summerfield RJ et al. Alfentanil infusions on the intensive therapy unit. *Intensive Care Med*. 1988; 14:55–9.
8. Byatt CM, Lewis LD, Dawling S et al. Accumulation of midazolam after repeated dosage in patients receiving mechanical ventilation in an intensive care unit. *Br Med J*. 1984; 289:799–800.
9. Finley PR, Nolan PE. Precipitation of benzodiazepine withdrawal following sudden discontinuation of midazolam. *DICP*. 1989; 23:151–2.
10. Harris CE, Grounds RM, Murray AM et al. Propofol for long-term sedation in the intensive care unit: a comparison with papaveretum and midazolam. *Anaesthesia*. 1990; 45:366–72.
11. Rock MJ, de la Rocha SR, L'Hommedieu et al. Use of ketamine in asthmatic children to treat respiratory failure refractory to conventional therapy. *Crit Care Med*. 1986; 14:514–6.
12. Miller-Jones CMH, Williams JH. Sedation for ventilation: a retrospective study of fifty patients. *Anaesthesia*. 1980;

35:1104–7.
13. Light RW, Bengfort JL, George RB. The adult respiratory distress syndrome and pancuronium bromide. *Anesth Analg*. 1975; 54:219–23.
14. Costarino AT, Polin RA. Neuromuscular relaxants in the neonate. *Clin Perinatol*. 1987; 14:965–89.
15. Hutchinson JD, Pinock CA. A use of atracurium infusion. *Anaesthesia*. 1984; 39:72. Letter.
16. Bishop MJ. Hemodynamic and gas exchange effects of pancuronium bromide in sedated patients with respiratory failure. *Anesthesiology*. 1984; 60:369–71.
17. Coggeshall JW, Marini JJ, Newman JH. Improved oxygenation after muscle relaxation in adult respiratory distress syndrome. *Arch Intern Med*. 1985; 145:1718–20.
18. Lingle CJ, Steinbach JH. Neuromuscular blocking agents. *Int Anesthesiol Clin*. 1988; 26:288–301.
19. Bevan DR, Bevan JC, Donati F. Muscle relaxants in clinical anesthesia. Chicago: Year Book Medical Publishers; 1988.
20. Nugent SK, Laravuso R, Rogers MC. Pharmacology and use of muscle relaxants in infants and children. *J Pediatr*. 1979; 94:481–7.
21. Taylor P. Neuromuscular blocking agents. In: Goodman and Gilman's the pharmacological basis of therapeutics. 7th ed. Gilman AG, Goodman LS, Rall TW et al., eds. New York: Macmillan; 1985:222–34.
22. West R. Curare in man. *Proc R Soc Med*. 1932; 25:1107–16.
23. Griffith HR, Johnson GE. The use of curare in general anesthesia. *Anesthesiology*. 1942; 3:418–20.
24. Reilly CS, Nimmo WS. New intravenous anaesthetics and neuromuscular blocking drugs: a review of their properties and clinical use. *Drugs*. 1987; 34:98–135.
25. Torda TA. The "new" relaxants. A review of the clinical pharmacology of atracurium and vecuronium. *Anaesth Intensive Care*. 1987; 15:72–82.
26. Shanks CA. What's new in skeletal muscle relaxants and their antagonists? *Anesth Clin North Am*. 1988; 6:335–55.
27. Richard C, Berdeaux A, Delion F et al. Effect of mechanical ventilation on hepatic drug pharmacokinetics. *Chest*. 1986; 90:837–41.
28. Pinsky MR. The influence of positive-pressure ventilation on cardiovascular function in the critically ill. *Crit Care Clin*. 1985; 1:699–717.
29. Perkins MW, Dasta JF, DeHaven B. Physiologic implications of mechanical ventilation on pharmacokinetics. *DICP*. 1989; 23:316–23.
30. Ramzan MI, Shanks CA, Triggs EJ. Pharmacokinetics of tubocurarine administered by combined IV bolus and infusion. *Br J Anaesth*. 1980; 52:893–9.
31. Fisher DM, O'Keeffe C, Stanski DR et al. Pharmacokinetics and pharmacodynamics of d-tubocurarine in infants, children, and adults. *Anesthesiology*. 1982; 57:203–8.
32. Matteo RS, Lieberman IG, Salanitre E et al. Distribution, elimination, and action of d-tubocurarine in neonates, infants, children, and adults. *Anesth Analg*. 1984; 63:799–804.
33. Matteo RS, Backus WW, McDaniel DD et al. Pharmacokinetics and pharmacodynamics of d-tubocurarine and metocurine in the elderly. *Anesth Analg*. 1985; 64:23–9.
34. Weinstein JA, Matteo RS, Ornstein E et al. Pharmacokinetics and pharmacodynamics of metocurine in infants, children and adults. *Anesthesiology*. 1987; 67:A615. Abstract.
35. Avram MJ, Shanks CA, Henthorn TK et al. Metocurine kinetics in patients undergoing operations requiring cardiopulmonary bypass. *Clin Pharmacol Ther*. 1987; 42:576–81.
36. Duvaldestin P, Agoston S, Henzel D et al. Pancuronium pharmacokinetics in patients with liver cirrhosis. *Br J Anaesth*. 1978; 50:1131–6.
37. Cronnelly R, Fisher DM, Miller RD et al. Pharmacokinetics and pharmacodynamics of vecuronium (ORG NC45) and pancuronium in anesthetized humans. *Anesthesiology*. 1983; 58:405–8.
38. Somogyi AA, Shanks CA, Triggs EJ. Clinical pharmacokinetics of pancuronium bromide. *Eur J Clin Pharmacol*. 1976; 10:367–72.
39. Fahey MR, Morris RB, Miller RD et al. Pharmacokinetics of ORG NC45 (Norcuron) in patients with and without renal failure. *Br J Anaesth*. 1981; 53:1049–53.
40. Lebrault C, Berger JL, D'Hollander AA et al. Pharmacokinetics and pharmacodynamics of vecuronium (ORG NC45) in patients with cirrhosis. *Anesthesiology*. 1985; 62:601–5.
41. Ward S, Neill EAM. Pharmacokinetics of atracurium in acute hepatic failure (with acute renal failure). *Br J Anaesth*. 1983; 55:1169–72.
42. Ward S, Weatherley BC. Pharmacokinetics of atracurium and its metabolites. *Br J Anaesth*. 1986; 58:6S–10S.
43. Fahey MR, Rupp SM, Fisher DM et al. The pharmacokinetics and pharmacodynamics of atracurium in patients with and without renal failure. *Anesthesiology*. 1984; 61:699–702.
44. Ramzan MJ, Somogyi AA, Walker JS et al. Clinical pharmacokinetics of the non-depolarizing muscle relaxants. *Clin Pharmacokinet*. 1981; 6:25–60.
45. Ghoneim MM, Kramer E, Bannow R et al. Binding of d-tubocurarine to plasma proteins in normal man and in patients with hepatic or renal disease. *Anesthesiology*. 1973; 39:410–5.
46. Ghoneim MM, Pandya H. Binding of tubocurarine to specific serum protein fractions. *Br J Anaesth*. 1975; 47:853–6.
47. Duvaldestin P, Henzel D. Binding of tubocurarine, fazadinium, pancuronium and ORG NC45 to serum proteins in normal man and in patients with cirrhosis. *Br J Anaesth*. 1982; 54:513–6.
48. Meijer DKF, Weitering JG, Vermeer GA et al. Comparative pharmacokinetics of d-tubocurarine and metocurine in man. *Anesthesiology*. 1979; 51:402–7.
49. Wood M, Stone WJ, Wood AJJ. Plasma binding of pancuronium: effects of age, sex, and disease. *Anesth Analg*. 1983; 62:29–32.
50. Foldes FF, Deery A. Protein binding of atracurium and other short-acting neuromuscular blocking agents and their interaction with human cholinesterases. *Br J Anaesth*. 1983; 55:31S–34S.
51. Cohen EN, Brewer HW, Smith D. The metabolism and elimination of d-tubocurarine-H^3. *Anesthesiology*. 1967; 28:309–17.
52. Agoston S, Vermeer GA, Kersten UW et al. The fate of pancuronium bromide in man. *Acta Anaesthesiol Scand*. 1973; 17:267–75.
53. Bencini AF, Scaf AHJ, Agoston S et al. Disposition of vecuronium bromide in the cat. *Br J Anaesth*. 1985; 57:782–8.
54. Segredo V, Matthay MA, Sharma ML et al. Prolonged neuromuscular blockade after long-term administration of vecuronium in two critically ill patients. *Anesthesiology*. 1990; 72:566–70.
55. Hughes R. Atracurium: an overview. *Br J Anaesth*. 1986; 58:2S–5S.
56. Chapple DJ, Miller AA, Wheatley PL. Neurological and cardiovascular effects of laudanosine in conscious and anaesthetized dogs. *Anesthesiology*. 1985; 63:A311. Abstract.
57. Yate PM, Flynn PJ, Arnold RW et al. Clinical experience and plasma laudanosine concentrations during the infusion of atracurium in the intensive care unit. *Br J Anaesth*. 1987; 59:211–7.
58. Coen RW, McCutchen CB, Wermer D et al. Continuous monitoring of the electroencephalogram following perinatal asphyxia. *J Pediatr*. 1982; 100:628–30.
59. Savarese JJ, Ali HH, Antonio RP. The clinical pharmacology of metocurine: dimethyltubocurarine revisited. *Anesthesiology*. 1977; 47:277–84.
60. Fahey MR, Morris RB, Miller RD et al. Clinical pharmacology of ORG NC45 (Norcuron): a new depolarizing muscle relaxant. *Anesthesiology*. 1981; 55:6–11.
61. Meistelman C, Agoston S, Kersten UW et al. Pharmacokinetics and pharmacodynamics of vecuronium and pancuronium in anesthetized children. *Anesth Analg*. 1986; 65:1319–23.
62. Agoston S, Salt P, Newton D et al. The neuromuscular blocking action of ORG NC45, a new pancuronium deriva-

tive, in anaesthetized patients: a pilot study. *Br J Anaesth.* 1980; 52:53S–59S.
63. Sokoll MD, Gergis SD, Mehta M et al. Safety and efficacy of atracurium (BW33A) in surgical patients receiving balanced or isoflurane anesthesia. *Anesthesiology.* 1983; 58:450–5.
64. Donati F. Onset of action of relaxants. *Can J Anaesth.* 1988; 35:S52–S58.
65. Fisher DM, Rosen JI. A pharmacokinetic explanation for increasing recovery time following larger or repeated doses of nondepolarizing muscle relaxants. *Anesthesiology.* 1986; 65:286–91.
66. Darrah WC, Johnston JR, Mirakhur RK. Vecuronium infusions for prolonged muscle relaxation in the intensive care unit. *Crit Care Med.* 1989; 17:1297–300.
67. Wadson AJ, Dogra S, Anand S. Atracurium infusion in the intensive care unit. *Br J Anaesth.* 1986; 58:64S–67S.
68. Nussmeier N, Henry GW, Stevens DC et al. Dose requirements for d-tubocurarine and metocurine used for chronic respiratory paralysis in neonates. *J Pediatr Surg.* 1981; 16:700–3.
69. Clyburn PA, Marshall RD. Control of ventilation by continuous infusion of pancuronium bromide. *Anaesthesia.* 1981; 36:860–2.
70. Smith CL, Hunter JM, Jones RS. Vecuronium infusions in patients with renal failure in an ITU. *Anaesthesia.* 1987; 42:387–93.
71. Eldadah MK, Newth CJL. Vecuronium by continuous infusion for neuromuscular blockade in infants and children. *Crit Care Med.* 1989; 17:989–92.
72. Hunter JM. Infusions of atracurium and vecuronium in patients with multisystem organ failure in the intensive therapy unit. *Insights Anaesthesiol.* 1987; 1:23–7.
73. Coursin DB, Klasek G, Goelzer SL. Increased requirements for continuously infused vecuronium in critically ill patients. *Anesth Analg.* 1989; 69:518–21.
74. Griffiths RB, Hunter JM, Jones RS. Atracurium infusions in patients with renal failure on an ITU. *Anaesthesia.* 1986; 41:375–81.
75. Parker CJR, Jones JE, Hunter JM. Disposition of infusions of atracurium and its metabolite, laudanosine, in patients in renal and respiratory failure in an ITU. *Br J Anaesth.* 1988; 61:531–40.
76. Pollard BJ, Harper NJN, Doran BRH. Use of continuous prolonged administration of atracurium in the ITU to a patient with myasthenia gravis. *Br J Anaesth.* 1989; 62:95–7.
77. Callanan DL. Development of resistance to pancuronium in adult respiratory distress syndrome. *Anesth Analg.* 1985; 64:1126–8.
78. Haas JL, Shaefer MS, Miwa LJ et al. Prolonged paralysis associated with long-term pancuronium use. *Pharmacotherapy.* 1989; 9:154–7.
79. Kent AP, Bricker SRW, Coleman P. Pain during injection of vecuronium. *Anaesthesia.* 1988; 43:334. Letter.
80. Miller RD, Matteo RS, Benet LZ et al. The pharmacokinetics of d-tubocurarine in man with and without renal failure. *J Pharmacol Exp Ther.* 1977; 202:1–7.
81. Hunter JM, Jones RS, Utting JE. Comparison of vecuronium, atracurium and tubocurarine in normal patients and in patients with no renal function. *Br J Anaesth.* 1984; 56:941–51.
82. Brotherton WP, Matteo RS. Pharmacokinetics and pharmacodynamics of metocurine in humans with and without renal failure. *Anesthesiology.* 1981; 55:273–6.
83. McLeod K, Watson MJ, Rawlins MD. Pharmacokinetics of pancuronium in patients with normal and impaired renal function. *Br J Anaesth.* 1976; 48:341–5.
84. Vandenbrom RHG, Wierda JMKH. Pancuronium bromide in the intensive care unit: a case of overdose. *Anesthesiology.* 1988; 69:996–7.
85. Lynam DP, Cronnelly R, Arden J et al. The pharmacodynamics and pharmacokinetics of vecuronium in patients with and without renal failure. *Anesthesiology.* 1986; 65:A296. Abstract.
86. Hunter JM, Jones RS, Utting JE. Use of atracurium in patients with no renal function. *Br J Anaesth.* 1982; 54:1251–8.
87. Fahey MR, Rupp SM, Canfell C et al. Effect of renal failure on laudanosine excretion in man. *Br J Anaesth.* 1985; 57:1049–51.
88. Somogyi AA, Shanks CA, Triggs EJ. Disposition kinetics of pancuronium bromide in patients with total biliary obstruction. *Br J Anaesth.* 1977; 49:1103–8.
89. Lebrault C, Strumza P, Henzel D et al. Pharmacokinetics and pharmacodynamics of vecuronium in patients with cholestasis. *Anesthesiology.* 1985; 63:A314. Abstract.
90. Hunter JM, Parker CJR, Bell CF et al. The use of different doses of vecuronium in patients with liver dysfunction. *Br J Anaesth.* 1985; 57:758–64.
91. Cook DR, Brandom BW, Stiller RL et al. Pharmacokinetics of atracurium in normal and liver failure patients. *Anesthesiology.* 1984; 61:A433. Abstract.
92. Miller RD. Pharmacokinetics of atracurium and other nondepolarizing neuromuscular blocking agents in normal patients and those with renal or hepatic dysfunction. *Br J Anaesth.* 1986; 58:11S–13S.
93. Tsai SK, Lee C, Mok MS. Atracurium induced neuromuscular block is prolonged in hepatic vascular occlusion. *Anesthesiology.* 1987; 67:A605. Abstract.
94. Parker CJR, Hunter JM. Pharmacokinetics of atracurium and laudanosine in patients with hepatic cirrhosis. *Br J Anaesth.* 1989; 62:177–83.
95. Martyn J. Clinical pharmacology and drug therapy in the burned patient. *Anesthesiology.* 1986; 65:67–75.
96. Martyn J, Goldhill DR, Goudsouzian NG. Clinical pharmacology of muscle relaxants in patients with burns. *J Clin Pharmacol.* 1986; 26:680–5.
97. Martyn JAJ, Szyfelbein SK, Ali HH et al. Increased d-tubocurarine requirement following major thermal injury. *Anesthesiology.* 1980; 52:352–5.
98. Leibel WS, Martyn JAJ, Szyfelbein SK et al. Elevated plasma binding cannot account for the burn-related d-tubocurarine hyposensitivity. *Anesthesiology.* 1981; 54:378–82.
99. Martyn JAJ, Matteo RS, Greenblatt DJ et al. Pharmacokinetics of d-tubocurarine in patients with thermal injury. *Anesth Analg.* 1982; 61:241–6.
100. Martyn JAJ, Matteo RS, Szyfelbein SK et al. Unprecedented resistance to neuromuscular blocking effects of metocurine with persistence after complete recovery in a burned patient. *Anesth Analg.* 1982; 61:614–7.
101. Hagen J, Martyn J, Szyfelbein SK et al. Cardiovascular and neuromuscular responses to high-dose pancuronium-metocurine in pediatric burned and reconstructive patients. *Anesth Analg.* 1986; 65:1340–4.
102. Yamashita M, Shiga T, Matsuki A et al. Unusual resistance to pancuronium in severely burned patients: case reports. *Can Anaesth Soc J.* 1982; 29:630–1.
103. Martyn JAJ, Liu LMP, Szyfelbein SK et al. The neuromuscular effects of pancuronium in burned children. *Anesthesiology.* 1983; 59:561–4.
104. Marathe PH, Dwersteg JF, Pavlin EG et al. Effect of thermal injury on the pharmacokinetics and pharmacodynamics of atracurium in humans. *Anesthesiology.* 1989; 70:752–5.
105. Mills AK, Martyn JAJ. Evaluation of atracurium neuromuscular blockade in paediatric patients with burn injury. *Br J Anaesth.* 1988; 60:450–5.
106. Mills A, Martyn JAJ. Evaluation of vecuronium neuromuscular blockade in pediatric patients with thermal injury. *Anesth Analg.* 1987; 66:S119. Abstract.
107. Storella RJ, Martyn JAJ, Bierkamper GG. Anti-curare effect of plasma from patients with thermal injury. *Life Sci.* 1988; 43:35–40.
108. McLeod K, Hull CJ, Watson MJ. Effects of ageing on the pharmacokinetics of pancuronium. *Br J Anaesth.* 1979; 51:435–8.
109. Duvaldestin P, Saada J, Berger JL et al. Pharmacokinetics, pharmacodynamics, and dose-response relationships of

pancuronium and elderly subjects. *Anesthesiology.* 1982; 56:36–40.
110. D'Hollander A, Massaux F, Nevelsteen M et al. Age-dependent dose-response relationship of ORG NC45 in anaesthetized patients. *Br J Anaesth.* 1982; 54:653–7.
111. Rupp SM, Fisher DM, Miller RD et al. Pharmacokinetics and pharmacodynamics of vecuronium in the elderly. *Anesthesiology.* 1983; 59:A270. Abstract.
112. Rowlands DE. Atracurium in the elderly. *Br J Anaesth.* 1986; 58:39S.
113. Cook DR. Muscle relaxants in infants and children. *Anesth Analg.* 1981; 60:335–43.
114. Heese H, Wittmann W, Malan AF. The management of the respiratory distress syndrome of the newborn with positive-pressure respiration. *S Afr Med J.* 1963; 37:123–6.
115. Stark AR, Bascom R, Frantz ID. Muscle relaxation in mechanically ventilated infants. *J Pediatr.* 1979; 94:439–43.
116. Henry GW, Stevens DC, Schreiner RL et al. Respiratory paralysis to improve oxygenation and mortality in large newborn infants with respiratory distress. *J Pediatr Surg.* 1979; 14:761–6.
117. Crone RK, Favorito J. The effects of pancuronium bromide on infants with hyaline membrane disease. *J Pediatr.* 1980; 97:991–3.
118. Pollitzer MJ, Reynolds EOR, Shaw DG et al. Pancuronium during mechanical ventilation speeds recovery of lungs of infants with hyaline membrane disease. *Lancet.* 1981; 1:346–8.
119. Runkle B, Bancalari E. Acute cardiopulmonary effects of pancuronium bromide in mechanically ventilated newborn infants. *J Pediatr.* 1984; 104:614–7.
120. Greenough A, Morley C, Davis J. Interaction of spontaneous respiration with artificial ventilation in preterm babies. *J Pediatr.* 1983; 103:769–73.
121. Greenough A, Wood S, Morley CJ et al. Pancuronium prevents pneumothoraces in ventilated premature babies who actively expire against positive pressure ventilation. *Lancet.* 1984; 1:1–3.
122. Perlman JM, Goodman S, Kreusser JL et al. Reduction in intraventricular hemorrhage by elimination of fluctuating cerebral blood-flow velocity in preterm infants with respiratory distress syndrome. *N Engl J Med.* 1985; 312:1353–7.
123. Finer NN, Tomney PM. Controlled evaluation of muscle relaxation in the ventilated neonate. *Pediatrics.* 1981; 67:641–6.
124. Greenough A, Gamsu HR, Greenall F. Investigation of the effects of paralysis by pancuronium on heart rate variability, blood pressure and fluid balance. *Acta Paediatr Scand.* 1989; 78:829–34.
125. Bhutani VK, Abbasi S, Sivieri EM. Continuous skeletal muscle paralysis: effect on neonatal pulmonary mechanics. *Pediatrics.* 1988; 81:419–22.
126. Goudsouzian NG, Liu LMP, Savarese JJ. Metocurine in infants and children: neuromuscular and clinical effects. *Anesthesiology.* 1978; 49:266–9.
127. Sinclair JF, Malcolm GA, Stephenson JBP et al. Prolonged neuromuscular blockade in an infant. *Anaesthesia.* 1987; 42:1020. Letter.
128. Meistelman C, Loose JP, Saint-Maurice C et al. Clinical pharmacology of vecuronium in children: studies during nitrous oxide and halothane in oxygen anaesthesia. *Br J Anaesth.* 1986; 58:996–1000.
129. Fisher DM, Castagnoli K, Miller RD. Vecuronium kinetics and dynamics in anesthetized infants and children. *Clin Pharmacol Ther.* 1985; 37:402–6.
130. Kalli I, Meretoja OA. Duration of action of vecuronium in infants and children anaesthetized without potent inhalation agents. *Acta Anaesthesiol Scand.* 1989; 33:29–33.
131. Harwood TN, Moorthy SS. Prolonged vecuronium-induced neuromuscular blockade in children. *Anesth Analg.* 1989; 68:534–6.
132. Goudsouzian NG. Atracurium infusion in infants. *Anesthesiology.* 1988; 68:267–9.
133. Goudsouzian NG, Martyn J, Rudd GD et al. Continuous infusion of atracurium in children. *Anesthesiology.* 1986; 64:171–4.
134. Meretoja OA, Kalli I. Spontaneous recovery of neuromuscular function after atracurium in pediatric patients. *Anesth Analg.* 1986; 65:1042–6.
135. Goudsouzian NG, Liu LMP, Cote' CJ et al. Safety and efficacy of atracurium in adolescents and children anesthetized with halothane. *Anesthesiology.* 1983; 59:459–62.
136. Fisher DM, Canfell PC, Spellman MJ et al. Pharmacokinetics and pharmacodynamics of atracurium in infants and children. *Anesthesiology.* 1990; 73:33–7.
137. Galletly DC. Comparative cutaneous histamine release by neuromuscular blocking agents. *Anaesth Intensive Care.* 1986; 14:365–9.
138. North FC, Kettelkamp N, Hirshman CA. Comparison of cutaneous and in vitro histamine release by muscle relaxants. *Anesthesiology.* 1987; 66:543–6.
139. Montgomery CJ, Steward DJ. A comparative evaluation of intubating doses of atracurium, d-tubocurarine, pancuronium and vecuronium in children. *Can J Anaesth.* 1988; 35:36–40.
140. Moss J, Rosow CE, Savarese JJ et al. Role of histamine in the hypotensive action of d-tubocurarine in humans. *Anesthesiology.* 1981; 55:19–25.
141. Barnes PK, de Renzy-Martin N, Thomas VJE et al. Plasma histamine levels following atracurium. *Anaesthesia.* 1986; 41:821–4.
142. Watkins J. Histamine release and atracurium. *Br J Anaesth.* 1986; 58:19S–22S.
143. Goudsouzian NG, Young ET, Moss J et al. Histamine release during the administration of atracurium or vecuronium in children. *Br J Anaesth.* 1986; 58:1229–33.
144. McCullough LA, Stone WA, Delaunois AL et al. The effect of dimethyl tubocurarine iodide on cardiovascular parameters, postganglionic sympathetic activity, and histamine release. *Anesth Analg.* 1972; 51:554–9.
145. Holt AW, Vedig AE. Anaphylaxis following vecuronium. *Anaesth Intensive Care.* 1988; 16:378–9. Letter.
146. Cabel LA, Siassi B, Artal R et al. Cardiovascular and catecholamine changes after administration of pancuronium in distressed neonates. *Pediatrics.* 1985; 75:284–7.
147. Kelman GR, Kennedy BR. Cardiovascular effects of pancuronium in man. *Br J Anaesth.* 1971; 43:335–8.
148. Barnes PK, Thomas VJE, Boyd I et al. Comparison of the effects of atracurium and tubocurarine on heart rate and arterial pressure in anaesthetized man. *Br J Anaesth.* 1983; 55:91S–94S.
149. Zaidan JR, Kaplan JA. Cardiovascular effects of metocurine in patients with aortic stenosis. *Anesthesiology.* 1982; 56:395–7.
150. Lee Son S, Waud BE, Waud DR. A comparison of the neuromuscular blocking and vagolytic effects of ORG NC45 and pancuronium. *Anesthesiology.* 1981; 55:12–8.
151. Kristensen J, Helbo-Hansen HS, Toft P et al. The cardiovascular effects of vecuronium during halothane anaesthesia. *Anaesthesiol Scand.* 1989; 33:494–7.
152. Savarese JJ, Basta SJ, Ali HH et al. Neuromuscular and cardiovascular effects of BW 33A (atracurium) in patients under halothane anesthesia. *Anesthesiology.* 1982; 57:A262. Abstract.
153. Rutledge ML, Hawkins EP, Langston C. Skeletal muscle growth failure induced in premature newborn infants by prolonged pancuronium treatment. *J Pediatr.* 1986; 109:883–6.
154. Torres CF, Maniscalco WM, Agostinelli T. Muscle weakness and atrophy following prolonged paralysis with pancuronium bromide in neonates. *Ann Neurol.* 1985; 18:403. Abstract.
155. Op de Coul AAW, Lambregts PCLA, Koeman T et al. Neuromuscular complications in patients given Pavulon (pancuronium bromide) during artificial ventilation. *Clin Neurol Neurosurg.* 1985; 87:17–22.

156. Kupfer Y, Okrent DG, Twersky RA et al. Disuse atrophy in a ventilated patient with status asthmaticus receiving neuromuscular blockade. *Crit Care Med*. 1987; 15:795–6.
157. Sinha SK, Levene MI. Pancuronium bromide induced joint contractures in the newborn. *Arch Dis Child*. 1984; 59:73–5.
158. Ham J, Miller RD, Benet LZ et al. Pharmacokinetics and pharmacodynamics of d-tubocurarine during hypothermia in the cat. *Anesthesiology*. 1978; 49:324–9.
159. Baraka A. The influence of carbon dioxide on the neuromuscular block caused by tubocurarine chloride in the human subject. *Br J Anaesth*. 1964; 36:272–8.
160. Funk DI, Crul JF, Pol FM. Effects of changes in acid-base balance on neuromuscular blockade produced by ORG-NC45. *Acta Anaesthesiol Scand*. 1980; 24:119–24.
161. Ono K, Ohta Y, Morita K et al. The influence of respiratory-induced acid-base changes on the action of non-depolarizing muscle relaxants in rats. *Anesthesiology*. 1988; 68:357–62.
162. Gencarelli PJ, Swen J, Koot HWJ et al. The effects of hypercarbia and hypocarbia on pancuronium and vecuronium neuromuscular blockades in anaesthetized humans. *Anesthesiology*. 1983; 59:376–80.
163. Waud BE, Waud DR. Interaction of calcium and potassium with neuromuscular blocking agents. *Br J Anaesth*. 1980; 52:863–6.
164. Gramstad L, Hysing ES. Effect of ionized calcium on the neuromuscular blocking actions of atracurium and vecuronium in the cat. *Br J Anaesth*. 1990; 64:199–206.
165. Baraka A, Yazigi A. Neuromuscular interaction of magnesium with succinylcholine-vecuronium sequence in the eclamptic parturient. *Anesthesiology*. 1987; 67:806–9.
166. Goat VA, Yeung ML, Blakeney C et al. The effect of blood flow upon the activity of gallamine triethiodide. *Br J Anaesth*. 1976; 48:69–73.
167. Buzello W, Noeldge G, Krieg N et al. Vecuronium for muscle relaxation in patients with myasthenia gravis. *Anesthesiology*. 1986; 64:507–9.
168. Nilsson E, Meretoja OA. Vecuronium dose-response and maintenance requirements in patients with myasthenia gravis. *Anesthesiology*. 1990; 73:28–32.
169. Gyermek L. Increased potency of nondepolarizing relaxants after poliomyelitis. *J Clin Pharmacol*. 1990; 30:170–3.
170. Flusche G, Unger-Sargon J, Lambert DH. Prolonged neuromuscular paralysis with vecuronium in a patient with polymyositis. *Anesth Analg*. 1987; 66:188–90.
171. Thomas D, Windsor JRW. Prolonged sedation and paralysis in a pregnant patient: delivery of an infant with a normal Apgar score. *Anaesthesia*. 1985; 40:465–7.
172. Lebowitz PW, Ramsey FM, Savarese JJ et al. Potentiation of neuromuscular blockade in man produced by combinations of pancuronium and metocurine or pancuronium and d-tubocurarine. *Anesth Analg*. 1980; 59:604–9.
173. Rashkovsky OM, Agoston S, Ket JM. Interaction between pancuronium bromide and vecuronium bromide. *Br J Anaesth*. 1985; 57:1063–6.
174. Ornstein E, Matteo RS, Weinstein JA et al. The effect of maintenance doses of vecuronium on pre-established metocurine- or vecuronium-induced neuromuscular blockade. *Anesthesiology*. 1988; 69:954–5.
175. Sokollo MD, Gergis SD. Antibiotics and neuromuscular function. *Anesthesiology*. 1981; 55:148–59.
176. Singh YN, Marshall IG, Harvey AL. Pre- and postjunctional blocking effects of aminoglycosides, polymyxin, tetracycline and lincosamide antibiotics. *Br J Anaesth*. 1982; 54:1295–306.
177. Kronenfeld MA, Thomas SJ, Turndorf H. Recurrence of neuromuscular blockade after reversal of vecuronium in a patient receiving polymyxin/amikacin sternal irrigation. *Anesthesiology*. 1986; 65:93–4.
178. Huang KC, Heise A, Shrader AK et al. Vancomycin enhances the neuromuscular blockade of vecuronium. *Anesth Analg*. 1990; 71:194–6.
179. Driessen JJ, Crul JF, Vree TB et al. Benzodiazepines and neuromuscular blocking drugs in patients. *Acta Anaesthesiol Scand*. 1986; 30:642–6.
180. Toft A, Helbo-Hansen S. Interaction of ketamine with atracurium. *Br J Anaesth*. 1989; 62:319–20.
181. Azar I, Cottrell J, Gupta B et al. Furosemide facilitates recovery of evoked twitch response after pancuronium. *Anesth Analg*. 1980; 59:55–7.
182. Miller RD, Sohn YJ, Matteo RS. Enhancement of d-tubocurarine neuromuscular blockade by diuretics in man. *Anesthesiology*. 1976; 45:442–5.
183. Argov Z, Mastaglia FL. Disorders of neuromuscular transmission caused by drugs. *N Engl J Med*. 1979; 301:409–13.
184. Chang CC, Chiou LC, Hwang LL et al. Mechanisms of the synergistic interactions between organic calcium channel antagonists and various neuromuscular blocking agents. *Jpn J Pharmacol*. 1990; 53:285–92.
185. Jelen-Esselborn S, Blobner M. Potentiation of nondepolarizing muscle relaxants by nifedipine during isoflurane anesthesia. *Anaesthesist*. 1990; 39:173–8.
186. Azar I, Kumar D, Betcher AM. Resistance to pancuronium in an asthmatic patient treated with aminophylline and steroids. *Can Anaesth Soc J*. 1982; 29:280–2.
187. Doll DC, Rosenberg H. Antagonism of neuromuscular blockage by theophylline. *Anesth Analg*. 1979; 58:139–40.
188. Ornstein E, Matteo RS, Schwartz AE et al. The effect of phenytoin on the magnitude and duration of neuromuscular block following atracurium or vecuronium. *Anesthesiology*. 1987; 67:191–6.
189. Hickey DR, Sangwan S, Bevan JC. Phenytoin-induced resistance to pancuronium: use of atracurium infusion in management of a neurosurgical patient. *Anaesthesia*. 1988; 43:757–9.
190. Gray H, Slater RM, Pollard BJ. The effect of acutely administered phenytoin on vecuronium-induced neuromuscular blockade. *Anaesthesia*. 1989; 44:379–81.
191. Roth S, Ebrahim ZY. Resistance to pancuronium in patients receiving carbamazepine. *Anesthesiology*. 1987; 66:691–3.
192. Borden H, Clarke MT, Katz H. The use of pancuronium bromide in patients receiving lithium carbonate. *Can Anaesth Soc J*. 1974; 21:79–82.
193. Gramstad L. Atracurium, vecuronium and pancuronium in end-stage renal failure: dose-response properties and interactions with azathioprine. *Br J Anaesth*. 1987; 59:995–1003.
194. Crosby E, Robblee JA. Cyclosporine-pancuronium interaction in a patient with a renal allograft. *Can J Anaesth*. 1988; 35:300–2.
195. Meyers EF. Partial recovery from pancuronium neuromuscular blockade following hydrocortisone administration. *Anesthesiology*. 1977; 46:148–50.
196. Buzello W. Postoperative care: antagonism of drugs used in anaesthesia: muscle relaxants. *Acta Anaesthesiol Scand*. 1988; 32(Suppl 87):25–7.
197. Cronnelly R, Morris RB. Antagonism of neuromuscular blockade. *Br J Anaesth*. 1982; 54:183–94.
198. Wachtel RE. Comparison of anticholinesterases and their effects on acetylcholine-activated ion channels. *Anesthesiology*. 1990; 72:496–503.
199. Kopman AF. Recovery times following edrophonium and neostigmine reversal of pancuronium, atracurium, and vecuronium steady-state infusions. *Anesthesiology*. 1986; 65:572–8.
200. Engbaek J, Ostergaard D, Skovgaard LT et al. Reversal of intense neuromuscular blockade following infusion of atracurium. *Anesthesiology*. 1990; 72:803–6.
201. Smith SM, Brown HO, Toman JEP et al. The lack of cerebral effects of d-tubocurarine. *Anesthesiology*. 1947; 8:1–14.
202. Parker MM, Schubert W, Shelhamer JH et al. Perceptions of a critically ill patient experiencing therapeutic paralysis in an ICU. *Crit Care Med*. 1984; 12:69–71.
203. Loper KA, Butler S, Nessly M et al. Paralyzed with pain: the need for education. *Pain*. 1989; 37:315–6.

Research

Intravenous ciprofloxacin versus ceftazidime for treatment of nosocomial pneumonia and urinary tract infection

ROBERT P. RAPP, MARIANNE BILLETER, JIMMI HATTON, A. BRYON YOUNG, PHILLIP A. TIBBS, AND ROBERT J. DEMPSEY

Abstract: Intravenous ciprofloxacin and ceftazidime were compared for efficacy in the treatment of nosocomial pneumonia and urinary tract infection (UTI).

Patients with nosocomial pneumonia were randomized to receive ciprofloxacin (as the lactate salt) 300 mg i.v. every 12 hours or ceftazidime (with sodium carbonate) 2 g i.v. every eight hours. Patients with UTI were randomized to receive ciprofloxacin 200 mg i.v. every 12 hours or ceftazidime 1 g i.v. every eight hours. Sputum and urine specimens were collected before, during, and after therapy.

For patients with pneumonia, the organisms most frequently isolated before treatment began were *Escherichia coli, Haemophilus influenzae, Klebsiella pneumoniae*, and *Proteus mirabilis*. Of the 17 pneumonia patients who completed ciprofloxacin treatment, 15 (88%) had resolution of signs and symptoms or improvement. Of the 15 ceftazidime-treated pneumonia patients, 13 (87%) had resolution or improvement. *Staphylococcus aureus, Streptococcus* species, *Acinetobacter* species, and *K. pneumoniae* infections persisted for the ciprofloxacin treatment failures. Infections by *Enterobacter cloacae* and *Acinetobacter* species persisted for the ceftazidime treatment failures. For UTI patients, *E. coli* was the organism most frequently isolated before treatment. All 14 UTI patients who completed treatment showed resolution or improvement. In the ciprofloxacin group two patients were superinfected by *Enterococcus* species, and in the ceftazidime group there were two superinfections by *Enterococcus* species and one by *Enterobacter cloacae*.

Intravenous ciprofloxacin was as effective as ceftazidime in the treatment of nosocomial pneumonia and urinary tract infection. Caution should be exercised when treating serious infections by streptococci or staphylococci.

Index terms: *Acinobacter* species; Ceftazidime; Cephalosporins; Ciprofloxacin lactate; *Enterobacter cloacae*; *Klebsiella pneumoniae*; Pneumonia; Quinolones; Resistance; *Staphylococcus aureus*; *Streptococcus* species; Urinary tract infections
Clin Pharm. 1991; 10:49–55

Patients with severe head injuries have prolonged hospital stays that put them at risk for nosocomial infections. Therapies for nosocomial infections include the combination of an aminoglycoside and a broad-spectrum penicillin, a third-generation cephalosporin with or without an aminoglycoside, and a carbapenem. When infection with *Pseudomonas aeruginosa* is suspected, combination therapy is recommended.[1] The renal toxicity and ototoxicity associated with the aminoglycosides and the continuing problems with β-lactam-resistant bacteria make the treatment of

ROBERT P. RAPP, PHARM.D., is Professor and Director, Division of Pharmacy Practice and Science, College of Pharmacy, University of Kentucky (UK), Lexington. MARIANNE BILLETER, PHARM.D., is Assistant Clinical Professor, College of Pharmacy, Xavier University of Louisiana, New Orleans; at the time of this study she was Fellow in Infectious Disease, A. B. Chandler Medical Center, UK. JIMMI HATTON, PHARM.D., is Assistant Professor, Division of Pharmacy Practice and Science, College of Pharmacy, UK. A. BRYON YOUNG, M.D., is Professor and Chairman, Department of Surgery, and Chief, Division of Neurosurgery, and PHILLIP A. TIBBS, M.D., and ROBERT J. DEMPSEY, M.D., are Associate Professors, Department of Surgery, Division of Neurosurgery, A. B. Chandler Medical Center, UK.

Address reprint requests to Dr. Rapp at the A. B. Chandler Medical Center, University Hospital, Room C-117, 800 Rose Street, Lexington, KY 40536.

The assistance of the residents in neurosurgery and the residents in clinical pharmacy at the A. B. Chandler Medical Center, Lexington, KY, is acknowledged.

Supported by a grant from Miles Inc., West Haven, CT.

Presented at the 24th Annual ASHP Midyear Clinical Meeting, Atlanta, GA, December 4, 1989.

nosocomial infections a continuing challenge.

The fluorinated quinolone antimicrobials offer an alternative for the treatment of nosocomial infections. Ciprofloxacin, a potent fluorinated quinolone, has excellent activity against most gram-negative bacteria and moderate activity against *Ps. aeruginosa* and methicillin-sensitive and methicillin-resistant *Staphylococcus aureus*.[2] The small molecular size and zwitterionic structure of ciprofloxacin promote extensive tissue penetration. The concentrations of ciprofloxacin in body fluids and tissues are equal to or in some cases greater than the concentration in serum. The kidney is one site where the concentration in tissue is several times greater than the serum concentration. Ciprofloxacin reaches therapeutic concentrations in urine, making it an alternative for treating nosocomial urinary tract infection (UTI), including that caused by *Ps. aeruginosa*.[3] Ciprofloxacin also has excellent penetration into bronchial secretions, making it an attractive option for treating nosocomial pneumonia.[4]

Oral ciprofloxacin was first marketed in 1988 for the treatment of a wide variety of gram-positive and gram-negative infections. Ciprofloxacin offers the first successful oral alternative for treating a variety of infections that have previously required intravenous antimicrobial therapy. However, the need for an injectable product still exists for those patients unable to take oral medications.

The purpose of this Phase III study was to compare the efficacy of intravenous ciprofloxacin with that of the third-generation cephalosporin ceftazidime in the treatment of nosocomial pneumonia and UTI.

Methods

Patient Selection. This was a prospective, controlled, randomized, double-blind study conducted at a single center. Patients admitted to the neurosurgery service who were 18 years of age or older and had clinical evidence of nosocomial pneumonia or UTI were eligible for participation. Clinical evidence of pneumonia had to include fever, leukocytosis, increased production of sputum that in culture grew one or more organisms susceptible to the study drugs, and roentgenographic evidence of pulmonary infiltration. Clinical evidence of UTI had to include fever, leukocyturia, and a positive culture result of $>10^5$ colony-forming units (CFU) per milliliter for a catheter-obtained urine specimen. Patients were not eligible for participation if they had a history of an allergy to cephalosporins or carboxyquinolone antimicrobials, mild infection not requiring intravenous therapy, the need for concomitant antimicrobials with a spectrum of activity similar to that of the study drugs, renal insufficiency (serum creatinine concentration, ≥ 2 mg/dL), or an anticipated survival time of less than 30 days after treatment. Pregnant or lactating women were also excluded. The study was approved by the institutional review board, and informed consent was obtained from participants in advance.

Treatment. Patients with pneumonia were randomized to receive either ciprofloxacin (as the lactate salt) 300 mg i.v. every 12 hours or ceftazidime (with sodium carbonate) 2 g i.v. every eight hours. UTI was treated with ciprofloxacin (as the lactate salt) 200 mg i.v. every 12 hours or ceftazidime (with sodium carbonate) 1 g i.v. every eight hours. Doses of ciprofloxacin (Miles Inc., West Haven, CT, lot 315254) were diluted in 100 mL of 5% dextrose injection or 0.9% sodium chloride injection. Doses of ceftazidime (Glaxo Inc., Research Triangle Park, NC, lot B3405-LA) were reconstituted with sterile water and then further diluted with 100 mL of 5% dextrose injection or 0.9% sodium chloride injection. All doses were administered over 30 minutes.

The duration of treatment was based on each patient's clinical course and outcome. A minimum of four days of therapy was required for the evaluation of efficacy. Concomitant antimicrobial therapy was permitted if one or more of the infecting organisms were resistant to the study drug and if the spectrum of the antimicrobial did not overlap that of the study drug. Metronidazole could be administered with the study drug if pulmonary infection by an anaerobic organism was suspected.

Bacteriologic Assays. Specimens of sputum and urine were obtained before, during (at 72 hours of therapy), and after therapy. Sputum was obtained after deep coughing or by endotracheal aspiration. Sputum samples were considered evaluable if they contained ≥ 25 white blood cells and ≤ 10 epithelial cells per microscopic field at high magnification and grew at least one organism in culture that was susceptible to the study drugs and considered to be a pathogen by the investigator. Urine specimens were obtained by catheter. Sputum and urine samples were processed in the hospital's clinical microbiology laboratory by using standard procedures.

Susceptibility testing was performed by the modified Kirby–Bauer procedure with a 5-μg ciprofloxacin disk and a 30-μg ceftazidime disk. Isolates were considered susceptible to ciprofloxacin if the zone of inhibition was ≥ 21 mm in width, of intermediate susceptibility if the zone was 16–20 mm, and resistant if the zone was ≤ 15 mm. Isolates were considered susceptible to ceftazidime if the zone of inhibition measured ≥ 18 mm, of intermediate susceptibility if the zone measured 15–17 mm, and resistant if the zone measured ≤ 14 mm. Minimum inhibitory concentrations (MICs) were determined by the standard twofold-serial-dilution tube procedure with Mueller–Hinton medium and an inoculum size of approximately 10^5 CFU/mL. Organisms were deemed susceptible to ciprofloxacin if the MIC was <1 μg/mL, of intermediate susceptibility if the MIC was 1–2 μg/mL, and resistant if the MIC was >2 μg/mL. For ceftazidime, isolates were considered susceptible, of intermediate susceptibility, and resistant if the MIC was ≤8, 16, and ≥32 μg/mL, respectively.

Assessment of Response to Treatment. Clinical and bacteriologic responses were assessed separately. Patients were considered evaluable if they had received a minimum of four days of therapy. Clinical responses were graded as complete resolution (disappearance of all signs and symptoms related to the infection), improvement (marked or moderate reduction in the severity or number of the signs and symptoms), or treatment failure (insufficient lessening of the signs and symptoms to qualify as improvement). Bacteriologic responses were graded as eradication (absence of the infecting organism at the end of therapy), persistence (presence of the infecting organism at the end of therapy), or superinfection (presence of a new organism at the end of therapy judged to be causing infection). The bacteriologic response was classified as indeterminate when cultures were not established after therapy.

Statistical Analysis. The significance of differences in age and duration of therapy between the treatment groups in each patient subset was determined by Student's *t* test. The significance of differences in clinical outcomes was measured with the chi-square test. A p value of <0.05 was considered significant.

Results

Fifty-five patients (27 ciprofloxacin-treated patients and 28 ceftazidime-treated patients) were entered into the study between September 1986 and June 1988; 46 completed treatment (22 with ciprofloxacin and 24 with ceftazidime). Thirty-two of the patients who completed treatment were treated for nosocomial pneumonia (17 ciprofloxacin and 15 ceftazidime), and 14 received treatment for UTI (five ciprofloxacin and nine ceftazidime). Nine patients did not complete the study (five ciprofloxacin and four ceftazidime). In four of these patients (three ciprofloxacin and one ceftazidime), consulting physicians recommended treatment with standard therapy; in two patients (both ceftazidime), bacterial isolates were resistant to the study drug; in one patient (ciprofloxacin), a sample of ventricular fluid obtained before therapy began yielded a positive culture result after one day of therapy, and meningitis was diagnosed; in one patient (ciprofloxacin), pretreatment cultures did not grow an organism; and one patient (ceftazidime) was transferred to another facility before completing therapy.

Pneumonia. The mean ages and durations of therapy of the groups with nosocomial pneumonia were not significantly different (Table 1). Of the 32 patients treated for pneumonia, 21 were mechanically ventilated through an endotracheal tube or a tracheostomy.

The organisms identified in sputum samples obtained before therapy started are listed in Table 2. The most frequently isolated organisms were *Escherichia coli, Haemophilus influenzae, Klebsiella pneumoniae,* and *Proteus mirabilis.*

Fifteen (88.2%) of the 17 patients with pneumonia who were treated with ciprofloxacin had complete resolution of their signs and symptoms or had improvement; similarly, 13 (86.7%) of the 15 ceftazidime-treated patients showed complete resolution or improvement ($p > 0.10$) (Table 3). Infection by *Staph. aureus, Streptococcus* species, *Acinetobacter* species, and *K. pneumoniae* was persistent in the two patients who failed to respond to ciprofloxacin. The two patients who failed to respond to ceftazidime included one with an *Enterobacter cloacae* infection that became resistant; persistent infection by *Acinetobacter* species was observed in both patients.

Five of the 17 pneumonia patients receiving ciprofloxacin responded with eradication of the infecting organisms. Persistent infection was found in eight patients, superinfection by resistant *Ps. aeruginosa* was seen in three, and the bacteriologic response was indeterminate in three (cultures not done). Eight of the 15 patients receiving ceftazidime had an eradication response, five showed persistent infection, and two developed superinfection (Table 3). The superinfections were due to resistant *Pseudomonas maltophilia* and *Staph. aureus.*

UTI. The mean ages and durations of therapy of the groups with UTI were not significantly different (Table 1). Fourteen patients (five ciprofloxacin and nine ceftazidime) were treated for UTI. Ten patients had an indwelling urinary catheter.

E. coli was the organism most frequently isolated in each group before treatment started (Table 2). Patients receiving either drug had complete resolution or improvement of the signs and symptoms of UTI (Table 3).

All the infecting organisms were eradicated in both groups (Table 3). However, there were five superinfections, two (both due to *Enterococcus* species) in ciprofloxacin-treated patients and three (two by *Enterococcus* species and one by ceftazidime-resistant *E. cloacae*) in patients given ceftazidime.

MICs. The MICs of ciprofloxacin and ceftazidime for the organisms isolated from sputum and urine samples taken before therapy began are listed in Table 4.

Adverse Effects. Adverse reactions were minimal in all the patients. Of the 22 patients who received ciprofloxacin, one developed eosinophilia and one had elevated liver enzyme levels, which

Table 1.
Demographic Data for the Study Patients

Characteristic	Patients with Pneumonia: Ciprofloxacin Therapy (*n* = 17)	Patients with Pneumonia: Ceftazidime Therapy (*n* = 15)	Patients with Urinary Tract Infection: Ciprofloxacin Therapy (*n* = 5)	Patients with Urinary Tract Infection: Ceftazidime Therapy (*n* = 9)
Sex ratio (m/f)	14/3	10/5	1/4	2/7
Age (yr)				
Mean ± S.D.	45.5 ± 19.9	42.4 ± 20.6	42.4 ± 28.1	65.8 ± 10.9
Range	19–81	22–84	18–79	54–83
Neurosurgical diagnosis (no. patients)				
Brainstem injury	0	2	0	0
Brain tumor	1	0	0	1
Cerebrovascular accident	2	2	0	3
Closed head injury	3	4	0	1
Cervical laminectomy	1	0	0	0
Gunshot wound	1	0	0	0
Herrington rod placement	0	0	0	1
Intracranical hemorrhage	5	4	1	0
Lumbar disk disease	0	0	1	0
Paralysis	4	1	2	0
Pseudotumor cerebri	0	1	0	0
Seizures	0	0	1	0
Skull fracture	0	1	0	1
Ventriculoperitoneal shunt placement	0	0	0	1
Unknown	0	0	0	1
Tracheostomy or endotracheal tube (no. patients)	10	11	0	0
Foley catheter (no. patients)	0	0	3	7
Duration of therapy (days)				
Mean ± S.D.	10.1 ± 3.3	10.2 ± 2.6	7.8 ± 1.7	6.8 ± 0.8
Range	5–17	7–14	7–11	5–8

returned to normal after therapy ended. Two of the 24 patients who received ceftazidime had eosinophilia, and one developed a rash.

Discussion

Pneumonia is one of the most common hospital-acquired infections. Patients at greatest risk for nosocomial pneumonia are those who are mechanically ventilated with an endotracheal or tracheostomy tube. The pneumonias are usually mixed infections caused by aerobic gram-negative bacilli.[5] Nosocomial pneumonia is difficult to treat and is associated with a significant rate of mortality. The two ceftazidime treatment failures occurred in patients with tracheostomy tubes. The bacteria responsible for the persistent infections, *E. cloacae* and *Acinetobacter* species, are known to develop resistance to third-generation cephalosporins because of the induction and hyperproduction of Richmond and Sykes type I β-lactamases.[6] Presumably, this mechanism of resistance was present for both ceftazidime treatment failures. The ceftazidime-resistant organisms did remain susceptible to ciprofloxacin. The two ciprofloxacin treatment failures were not in mechanically ventilated patients. However, these patients had persistent infections by *Staph. aureus* and a *Streptococcus* species. The MIC of ciprofloxacin for *Staph. aureus* tends to be close to the break point, and the organism is difficult to eradicate with this agent. Ciprofloxacin has marginal activity against most streptococci.[7]

Several investigators have successfully treated serious infections with intravenous ciprofloxacin.[8–14] Giamarellou and Galanakis[8] treated 54 critically ill patients with ciprofloxacin 200 mg i.v. every 12 hours. Thirty of the patients were later switched to oral ciprofloxacin (750 mg b.i.d.). The most frequently isolated pathogens were *Ps. aeruginosa, Acinetobacter* species, and *E. cloacae*. Forty-nine patients had a successful clinical outcome, and five patients did not show improvement.

Lode et al.[12] compared the efficacy of intravenous ciprofloxacin with that of imipenem–cilastatin in 66 patients with serious bacterial infections, primarily of the lower respiratory tract, and found no significant difference. Bacterial isolates identified before treatment started were eradicated in 67% of the ciprofloxacin group and 79% of the imipenem–cilastatin group. Two patients (6.7%) treated with ciprofloxacin and six patients (20%) in the imipenem–cilastatin group failed to respond.

When Peloquin et al.[13] treated 55 patients with gram-negative infection of the lower respiratory tract with ciprofloxacin 200 mg i.v. every 12 hours, those individuals infected by *Enterobacteriaceae* species or *H. influenzae* responded well. Most of the bacteria isolated were eradicated within one day. Resistant *Ps. aeruginosa* was isolated for 10 treatment failures. Ciprofloxacin 200 mg i.v. seems to be effective in treating nosocomial lower respiratory tract infection caused by the more susceptible Enterobacteriaceae species and *H. influenzae;* higher doses may be necessary in treating *Ps. aeruginosa* infection of the respiratory tract.

Levine et al.[14] treated 113 seriously infected patients with ciprofloxacin 200 mg i.v. every 12 hours or ceftazidime 2 g i.v. every eight hours in a randomized, double-blind trial. Infections in the 68 patients who were evaluated included UTI, pneumonia, and sepsis. There was no difference in clinical outcome between the ciprofloxacin-treated and ceftazidime-treated groups. The bacteria that persisted in the patients who did not respond to ciprofloxacin were *K. pneumoniae, Ps. aeruginosa, Proteus vulgaris, Staph. aureus,* and *Streptococcus pneumoniae.* Patients with indwelling urinary catheters have a 5–10% daily risk of UTI caused by gram-negative bacilli.[15] Many of the patients in this study who were treated for UTI had an indwelling urinary catheter. All the patients were treated successfully with ciprofloxacin or ceftazidime. Five patients did develop superinfection. Four of the superinfections (in two ciprofloxacin-treated patients and two ceftazidime-treated patients) were due to *Enterococcus* species, and one *E. cloacae* isolate was identified in a patient receiving ceftazidime.

Oral ciprofloxacin has been used extensively to treat UTI. Ryan et al.[16] treated 32 patients with UTI caused by organisms resistant to trimethoprim-sulfamethoxazole. The patients were treated with ciprofloxacin 500 mg p.o. every 12 hours for at least five days. Twenty-eight patients (93%) were treated successfully. However, eight patients developed superinfections by *Candida* species (four patients), *Enterococcus* species (three patients), or *Providencia* species (one patient). Ciprofloxacin, like other broad-spectrum antimicrobials, predisposes the patient to superinfection.

The neurosurgical patients in the present study had nosocomial pneumonia or UTI. There was no significant difference in clinical or bacteriologic outcome when these patients were treated with intravenous ciprofloxacin or ceftazidime. However, because of the sample size, the possibility of a Type II statistical error cannot be eliminated.[17]

Table 2.
Microorganisms Isolated from Sputum and Urine Samples Obtained before Therapy Began

Organism(s)	No. Isolates: Patients Who Received Ciprofloxacin	No. Isolates: Patients Who Received Ceftazidime
Sputum		
Beta-hemolytic streptococci	1	0
Group B streptococci	1	0
Group F streptococci	0	2
Streptococcus pneumoniae	1	0
Staphylococcus aureus	3	2
Citrobacter freundii	1	0
Enterobacter aerogenes	1	2
Enterobacter cloacae	2	2
Escherichia coli	2	5
Haemophilus influenzae	6	4
Haemophilus parainfluenzae	2	0
Klebsiella oxytoca	0	1
Klebsiella pneumoniae	5	2
Morganella morganii	0	1
Proteus mirabilis	3	5
Pseudomonas aeruginosa	1	0
Pseudomonas maltophilia	1	0
Serratia marcescens	0	2
Urine		
Enterococcus species	2	0
Staphylococcus epidermidis	0	1
Enterobacter aerogenes	0	1
Enterobacter cloacae	0	1
Escherichia coli	5	5
Gardnerella vaginalis	0	1
Klebsiella pneumoniae	0	1
Pseudomonas aeruginosa	2	2

Table 3.
Clinical and Bacteriologic Outcomes in Patients Who Completed Therapy

Outcome	Patients with Pneumonia: Ciprofloxacin Therapy (*n* = 17)	Patients with Pneumonia: Ceftazidime Therapy (*n* = 15)	Patients with Urinary Tract Infection: Ciprofloxacin Therapy (*n* = 5)	Patients with Urinary Tract Infection: Ceftazidime Therapy (*n* = 9)
Clinical				
Complete resolution	9	10	4	5
Improvement	6	3	1	4
Failure	2	2	0	0
Bacteriologic				
Eradication	5	8	3	6
Persistence	8	5	0	0
Superinfection	1	2	2	3
Indeterminate	3	0	0	0

Table 4.
Minimum Inhibitory Concentrations (MICs) of Study Drugs for Bacteria Isolated from Sputum and Urine Samples Obtained before Therapy Began

Organism	No. Isolates	MIC (μg/mL)[a]	
		Ciprofloxacin	Ceftazidime
Beta-hemolytic streptococci	1	N.D.	N.D.
Group B streptococci	1	0.5	≤0.25
Enterococcus species	2	0.75–1.0	16–32
Group F streptococci	2	0.015–2.0	≤0.25–8.0
Streptococcus pneumoniae	1	0.03	0.5
Staphylococcus aureus	5	0.03–0.125	4.0–128
Staphylococcus epidermidis	1	0.5	16
Citrobacter freundii	1	0.03	64
Enterobacter aerogenes	4	≤0.015–0.125	≤0.25–>64
Enterobacter cloacae	5	0.125–0.25	1.0–64
Escherichia coli	17	≤0.015–0.75	0.5–4.0
Gardnerella vaginalis	1	N.V.	N.V.
Haemophilus influenzae	10	≤0.015–0.03	≤0.25–1.0
Haemophilus parainfluenzae	2	0.03–0.06	0.25–0.5
Klebsiella oxytoca	1	0.125	2.0
Klebsiella pneumoniae	8	≤0.015–0.75	≤0.25–1.0
Morganella morganii	1	0.125–1.0	1.0–>64
Proteus mirabilis	8	0.03–0.5	0.5–1.0
Pseudomonas aeruginosa	5	≤0.015–1.5	0.5–32
Pseudomonas maltophilia	1	0.5–1.5	4.0–32
Serratia marcescens	2	0.5	0.5–2.0

[a] N.D. = not done, N.V. = not viable.

In no other study in the literature has a 300-mg dose of intravenous ciprofloxacin been used to treat serious infections. The high dose used in this study had an efficacy comparable to that observed in other studies with lower doses of intravenous ciprofloxacin and did not produce an increased rate of adverse effects. The cause of persistent infections in patients in this study was limited to gram-positive organisms. Researchers using 200-mg doses of intravenous ciprofloxacin have reported persistent infections due to a mixture of gram-positive and gram-negative organisms. Higher doses may be needed to treat difficult gram-negative infections, such as those caused by *Ps. aeruginosa*.

Ciprofloxacin, with its broad spectrum of activity and low propensity to induce bacterial resistance during therapy, is an excellent addition to the antimicrobial armamentarium. The drug's activity is particularly good against most gram-negative organisms. Oral ciprofloxacin has been shown to be highly effective in treating numerous infections, including UTI, pneumonia, and skin and soft tissue infections. The availability of an oral dosage form allows for home treatment of patients who would normally require intravenous antimicrobials and hospitalization.[18] Nevertheless, an intravenous formulation is needed.

Conclusion

Intravenous ciprofloxacin was as effective as ceftazidime in the treatment of nosocomial pneumonia and urinary tract infection. Caution should be exercised, however, when treating serious infections by streptococci or staphylococci. Ciprofloxacin dosages of 300 mg or greater i.v. every 12 hours may be required for treating *Pseudomonas aeruginosa* infection.

References

1. Anon. The choice of antimicrobial drugs. *Med Lett Drug Ther.* 1990; 32:41–8.
2. Sanders CC. In vitro activity, mechanism of action, and resistance. *Rev Infect Dis.* 1988; 10:516–27.
3. LeBel M. Ciprofloxacin: chemistry, mechanism of action, resistance, antimicrobial spectrum, pharmacokinetics, clinical trials, and adverse reactions. *Pharmacotherapy.* 1988; 8:3–33.
4. Berre J, Thy J, Husson M et al. Penetration of ciprofloxacin in bronchial secretions after intravenous administration. *J Antimicrob Chemother.* 1988; 22:499–504.
5. Craven DE, Steger KA. Nosocomial pneumonia in the intubated patient: new concepts on pathogenesis and prevention. *Infect Dis Clin North Am.* 1989; 3:843–66.
6. Sanders WE, Sanders CC. Inducible beta-lactamases: clinical and epidemiologic implication for use of newer cephalosporins. *Rev Infect Dis.* 1988; 10:830–8.
7. Drusano GL. An overview of the pharmacology of intravenously administered ciprofloxacin. *Am J Med.* 1987; 82(Suppl 4A):339–45.
8. Giamarellou HG, Galanakis N. Use of intravenous ciprofloxacin in difficult-to-treat infections. *Am J Med.* 1987; 82(Suppl 4A):346–51.
9. Nix DE, Sands MF, Peloquin CA et al. Dual individualization of intravenous ciprofloxacin in patients with nosocomial lower respiratory tract infections. *Am J Med.* 1987; 82(Suppl 4A):352–6.
10. Chrysanthopoulos CJ, Skoutelis AT, Starakis JC et al. Use of intravenous ciprofloxacin in respiratory tract infections and

biliary sepsis. *Am J Med*. 1987; 82(Suppl 4A):357–9.
11. Scully BE, Neu HC. Treatment of serious infections with intravenous ciprofloxacin. *Am J Med*. 1987; 82(Suppl 4A):369–75.
12. Lode H, Wiley R, Hoffken G et al. Prospective randomized controlled study of ciprofloxacin versus imipenem–cilastatin in severe clinical infections. *Antimicrob Agents Chemother*. 1987; 31:1491–6.
13. Peloquin CA, Cumbo TJ, Nix DE et al. Evaluation of intravenous ciprofloxacin in patients with nosocomial lower respiratory tract infections. *Arch Intern Med*. 1989; 149:2269–73.
14. Levine DP, McNeil P, Lerner SA. Randomized, double-blind comparative study of intravenous ciprofloxacin versus ceftazidime in the treatment of serious infections. *Am J Med*. 1989; 87(Suppl 5A):160s–3s.
15. Sugarman B, Young EJ. Infections associated with prosthetic devices: magnitude of the problem. *Infect Dis Clin North Am*. 1989; 3:187–98.
16. Ryan JL, Berenson CS, Greco TP et al. Oral ciprofloxacin in resistant urinary tract infection. *Am J Med*. 1987; 82(Suppl 4A):303–6.
17. Freiman JA, Chalmers TC, Smith H et al. The importance of beta, the type II error and sample size in the design and interpretation of the randomized control trial. *N Engl J Med*. 1978; 299:690–4.
18. Fass RJ. Efficacy and safety of oral ciprofloxacin for treatment of serious urinary tract infections. *Antimicrob Agents Chemother*. 1987; 31:148–50.

“

Priorities in AIDS Clinical Trials

Since most HIV-infected homosexual men in the United States were infected from 1979 to 1985, before the routes of transmission of the virus were identified and the viral cause of the disease widely understood, the window of opportunity for conducting large-scale clinical trials in this population is closing. In most of these patients disease will occur on average approximately 11 years after infection. Hence, many symptomatic patients will be identified in the next three to six years, and we must develop effective therapies for them soon. We need information about new agents, both alone and in combination, regarding their short-term effects on viral load and their ability to hold back the progression of disease. Since drug resistance is likely to be a problem with all antiviral agents if they are used for very long periods, we must also find out which agents or combinations are best for primary therapy and which are best for rescue regimens. For example, if one of the dideoxy drugs fails to suppress HIV infection, perhaps we should use new strategies at fixed times after starting a given approach, when in vitro resistance can be demonstrated, or when certain surrogate markers show drug failure, rather than wait for disease complications to show drug failure. A basic uncertainty today is whether clinical drug failure is due to inadequate viral suppression from the first day of treatment (whether early or late in disease) or to the development of drug resistance late in treatment. New and better starting regimens would be the way to deal with inadequate suppression, whereas drug resistance demands new rescue regimens or combination therapy at the onset.

—Merigan TC. You *can* teach an old dog new tricks: how AIDS trials are pioneering new strategies. *N Engl J Med*. 1990; 323:1341–3.

”

Drug Experience

Straightforward reports of unusual drug experiences are included in this section. These may be confirmations of previously reported drug experiences or brief apparent first reports. While selected references may be cited, the purpose of a Drug Experience *report is not to present an extensive review of the literature.*

A related section, Grand Rounds, *includes papers that are well-documented patient case reports with a thorough review of the important literature to help put the case in perspective.*

Pancreatitis during pentamidine therapy in patients with AIDS

MICHAEL G. O'NEIL, STEVEN E. SELUB, AND LAWRENCE J. HAK

Clin Pharm. 1991; 10:56–9

Pneumocystis carinii pneumonia (PCP) is the most common infection identified in patients with AIDS when they are first seen by the physician. Trimethoprim–sulfamethoxazole is often effective in treating PCP, but many patients experience severe adverse effects.[1-6] Intravenous pentamidine isethionate is the alternative treatment of choice in these patients. However, pentamidine also has adverse effects, including nephrotoxicity,[7-10] hypoglycemia,[9,11-13] and hypotension.[14,15] Although pentamidine-associated pancreatitis has been reported, there are only six cases in the literature.[16-19] We report here a series of five cases of pancreatitis that occurred during pentamidine therapy at one institution from October 1, 1986, to October 31, 1987. Specific patient characteristics and treatment data are listed in Table 1.

Case Reports. *Case 1.* An 18-year-old man with hemophilia A was hospitalized because of a two-week history of increasing dyspnea, fever, and chills. PCP was diagnosed after bronchoalveolar lavage. Intravenous pentamidine was administered when the patient failed to improve with trimethoprim–sulfamethoxazole. On day 7 of pentamidine therapy, the serum amylase and lipase concentrations were 173 and 625 units/L, respectively. The patient developed shock on day 9; blood cultures grew *Streptococcus viridans* and *Staphylococcus aureus*, for which intravenous vancomycin therapy was started. On day 14 of pentamidine therapy, the patient complained of epigastric pain, and his serum amylase concentration was 280 units/L and his lipase concentration 1259 units/L. The pentamidine was discontinued, and three days later the patient's abdominal pain diminished; the amylase and lipase concentrations fell to 103 and 617 units/L, respectively. The patient died after klebsiella-related pneumonia supervened.

Case 2. A 32-year-old woman who had become infected with the human immunodeficiency virus through heterosexual intercourse was admitted for treatment of PCP and cytomegalovirus-associated pneumonitis. She received intravenous trimethoprim–sulfamethoxazole, as well as erythromycin. On hospital day 5, the patient required mechanical ventilatory support because of respiratory failure; two days later, the trimethoprim–sulfamethoxazole was discontinued and intravenous pentamidine treatment was started. The patient complained of abdominal pain after nine days of pentamidine therapy; the serum amylase concentration was 264 units/L. Her abdominal pain worsened, and her amylase and lipase concentrations reached maxima of 414 and 796 units/L, respectively. The pentamidine therapy was stopped, and treatment with trimethoprim and dapsone was begun. Abdominal ultrasonography showed a boggy pancreas. Her clinical condition improved; after 18 hospital days she was discharged with no abdomi-

MICHAEL G. O'NEIL, PHARM.D., is Critical Care Pharmacist/Nutrition Support Team Coordinator, Department of Pharmacy, Wesley Long Community Hospital, Greensboro, NC. STEVEN E. SELUB, M.D., is Gastroenterology Fellow, Department of Gastroenterology, North Carolina Memorial Hospital, Chapel Hill, NC. LAWRENCE J. HAK, PHARM.D., is Associate Professor of Pharmacology, School of Pharmacy, The University of North Carolina at Chapel Hill.

Address reprint requests to Dr. O'Neil at the Department of Pharmacy, Wesley Long Community Hospital, 501 N. Elam Avenue, Drawer X-3, Greensboro, NC 27402.

Table 1.
Characteristics of Five Patients with Pentamidine-Associated Pancreatitis

Characteristic	Patient 1	Patient 2	Patient 3	Patient 4	Patient 5
Age (yr)	18	32	46	24	63
Sex	M	F	M	M	M
AIDS risk factor	Hemophilia A	Heterosexual contact	Hemophilia A	Hemophilia A	Hemophilia A
Pentamidine isethionate dosage (mg/day)	220	228	220	240	240
Cumulative pentamidine isethionate dose (mg)	1320	2052	1540	5040	1920
No. days of therapy before detection of pancreatitis	6	9	7	21	8
Concurrent diseases and complications	Pneumothorax, hemophilia A, bacterial pneumonia, hepatomegaly, sepsis	Cytomegalovirus-associated pneumonitis, anemia, ileus, herpesvirus type 1 infection, bacterial pneumonia	Hemophilia A, bacterial pneumonia, herpesvirus type 1 infection	Bacterial pneumonia, sinusitis, hepatitis B surface antigen positivity, adult respiratory distress syndrome, hemophilia A, tuberculosis	Bacterial pneumonia, chronic active hepatitis, hemophilia A, herpes zoster
Concurrent drugs (starting day[a])	Pentamidine (6), cefuroxime (1), TMP–SMX[b] (1), Mylanta (1), aluminum carbonate (1), factor VIII (1), sucralfate (1), lorazepam (1), dopamine (9), vancomycin (9)	Pentamidine (5), vancomycin (7), dopamine (7), TMP–SMX (1), erythromycin (1), calcium carbonate (1), morphine (1), ceftriaxone (7)	Pentamidine (8), clindamycin (9), ceftriaxone (9), factor VIII (1), nystatin (1), TMP–SMX (1), acyclovir (1)	Pentamidine (1), cefuroxime (1), rifampin (4), ethambutol (4), isoniazid (4), Mylanta (1), ceftriaxone (1), factor VIII (1), zidovudine (1), erythromycin (1), dopamine (2), metaproterenol (3), lorazepam (1)	Pentamidine (1), cefuroxime (1), ranitidine (1), tobramycin (6), factor VIII (1), ketoconazole (1), zidovudine (1), acetaminophen (1), aminocaproic acid (?), vancomycin (4)
Basis for diagnosis of pancreatitis[c]	Abdominal pain; amylase conc., 280 units/L; lipase conc., 1259 units/L	Abdominal pain; amylase conc., 414 units/L; lipase conc., 796 units/L; abdominal ultrasonography	Amylase conc., 310 units/L; postmortem examination	Abdominal pain; amylase conc., 1749 units/L	Abdominal pain; amylase conc., 595 units/L
Serum creatinine conc. (mg/dL)[d]	1.7	1.5	0.6	3.5	2.1
Outcome	Died	Survived	Died	Died	Died

[a] Hospital day when therapy was started.
[b] TMP–SMX = trimethoprim–sulfamethoxazole.
[c] Serum amylase and lipase concentrations are the highest concentrations measured during pentamidine therapy.
[d] Highest concentration during pentamidine therapy.

nal pain, although her serum amylase concentration was 244 units/L.

Case 3. A 46-year-old man with hemophilia A and AIDS diagnosed two years earlier was admitted with a one-week history of dyspnea, chills, and fevers. Chest roentgenography revealed bilateral lung infiltration, and *Pneumocystis carinii* was detected in silver-stained bronchoalveolar washings. Therapy was begun with intravenous trimethoprim–sulfamethoxazole, along with nystatin for oral candidiasis. Pulmonary function worsened, and mechanical ventilation was required. After eight days of this therapy without improvement, the patient was switched to intravenous pentamidine. On hospital day 14, the patient complained of abdominal pain, and his serum amylase concentration was 310 units/L. The pentamidine therapy was continued for a total of 14 days, but because of poor therapeutic response, the patient was switched to eflornithine. His pancreatitis resolved several days later. However, his respiratory status worsened, and he died 39 days after admission. An autopsy revealed a pancreas with diffusely scattered small white foci of saponification and fibrosis consistent with resolving pancreatitis.

Case 4. A 24-year-old man with hemophilia A and AIDS that was diagnosed two years earlier was hospitalized because of dyspnea and a worsening cough. Chest roentgenography showed infiltration of the left lower lobe. A silver-stained sputum sample was positive for *Pneumocystis carinii.* Pentamidine therapy was begun because the patient had a history of developing hives after treatment with trimethoprim–sulfamethoxazole. The patient became hypotensive and was transferred to the intensive-care unit. Isoniazid, rifampin, and ethambutol were administered after a sputum sample stained positive for acid-fast bacilli; cefuroxime was added to treat branhamella that grew in the culture. Antituberculosis agents and antibiotics were continued throughout the patient's hospital course.

During the next week, the patient's leukocyte count fell, his serum creatinine concentration rose from 0.9 mg/dL to 1.7 mg/dL, and his serum potassium concentration increased to 5.6 meq/L. His respiratory status was marginal, and he continued to have occasional episodes of hypotension. On hospital day 21, the patient developed pain in the right upper quadrant; the serum amylase concentration was 1190 units/L. The pentamidine therapy was discontinued. The amylase concentration continued to rise to 1749 units/L over the next two days, and the serum creatinine concentration reached 3.0 mg/dL. The abdominal pain improved slowly, and the amylase level decreased. The patient's respiratory status deteriorated, however, and he developed adult respiratory distress syndrome on day 27 and subsequently died. The serum amylase concentration at the time of death was 140 units/L.

Case 5. A 63-year-old man with hemophilia A and a diagnosis of AIDS made one year previously was admitted to the hospital with worsening dyspnea, fever, chills, and night sweats. His medical history included chronic active hepatitis, herpes zoster, and chronic fatigue. The patient was allergic to trimethoprim–sulfamethoxazole and cephalexin; both drugs caused a rash. Dense bilateral infiltration and decreased lung volume were seen on chest roentgenography. The serum amylase and creatinine concentrations were 40 units/L and 0.8 mg/dL, respectively. Ketoconazole, cefuroxime, and pentamidine were administered. The following day, *Pneumocystis carinii* was identified in the sputum. Cultures of blood drawn on admission grew *Staphylococcus epidermidis,* for which the patient received vancomycin. His respiratory status deteriorated, requiring mechanical ventilation. The serum amylase concentration was 75 units/L on hospital day 8. On the next day, the patient showed slight abdominal guarding, and the serum amylase concentration was 98 units/L. On day 11, the total bilirubin concentration was 4.4 mg/dL, the direct-reacting bilirubin concentration was 3.6 mg/dL, and the serum amylase concentration was 167 units/L. Serum bilirubin levels began to decline, while amylase concentrations continued to rise to a maximum of 595 units/L. The patient was switched from intravenous pentamidine to the aerosolized form, and trimethoprim and dapsone were added. The patient continued to deteriorate, and on day 37 he died. The serum amylase concentration at the time of death was 74 units/L.

Discussion. During a 13-month period, 13 patients with AIDS and PCP were treated with intravenous pentamidine at North Carolina Memorial Hospital (NCMH). Five of these patients developed pancreatitis. None had a history of pancreatitis, biliary disease, or hyperlipidemia or had previously been treated with pentamidine. Two of the patients (in cases 3 and 5) reported that they did not use ethanol; the other three described their ethanol use as minimal. Although pentamidine-associated pancreatitis has been reported previously,[16–19] it is uncommon, and pancreatitis was not reported as an adverse reaction in several studies comparing pentamidine with other medications in the treatment of PCP.[1,12–13,20]

One possible explanation for the pentamidine-associated pancreatitis in our patients is that four of them had received trimethoprim–sulfamethoxazole earlier. Both sulfonamides and trimethoprim–sulfamethoxazole have been associated with pancreatitis.[21–23] However, the patients all developed pancreatitis after one or two weeks of therapy and improved when the sulfa-containing medication was discontinued. Our patients developed pancreatitis 5–21 days after trimethoprim–sulfamethoxazole was discontinued rather than while still being treated with it. Thus, trimethoprim–sulfamethoxazole probably did not cause our patients' pancreatitis. It may, on the other hand, predispose patients receiving pentamidine to pancreatitis. Four of the six patients previously reported in the literature received trimethoprim–sulfamethoxazole; if our patients are included, then 8 of 11 patients with pentamidine-associated pancreatitis had been treated earlier with trimethoprim–sulfamethoxazole, suggesting that that combination agent may play a permissive role. Still, most AIDS patients who are treated with pentamidine have received trimethoprim–sulfamethoxazole earlier, and pancreatitis remains a rare reported adverse effect of pentamidine.

Murphey et al.[16] suggested that renal insufficiency may result in elevated serum pentamidine levels and that this could play a role in the development of pancreatitis. The patients described by Murphey et al. had elevated serum creatinine and received about 2500 mg of pentamidine isethionate before they developed pancreatitis. One of our patients had a serum creatinine concentration of 3.5 mg/dL but did not develop pancreatitis until after 21 days of therapy, when his cumulative dose was 5040 mg. Our other patients received 1320–2052 mg of pentamidine isethionate before developing pancreatitis. Given the wide variation in cumulative doses and the lack of an association between development of pancreatitis and level of renal function, we do not think that these are primary factors in pentamidine-related pancreatitis.

Pentamidine has also been found to cause hypoglycemia and hyperglycemia. Hypoglycemia is thought to be caused by initial damage to beta cells in the islets of Langerhans. Insulin is released, causing hypoglycemia. Once enough beta cells are damaged, normal insulin production is limited and hyperglycemia develops. All five patients had multiple episodes of hyperglycemia and hypoglycemia. All patients were receiving either total parenteral nutrition or tube feeding. Three of the patients were treated with pressor agents, which may affect glucose utilization. Sepsis was a common problem in these patients. Because of the multiple factors affecting blood glucose status, it was not possible to associate pentamidine therapy and dysglycemic effects.

Of the 48 AIDS patients who were treated for PCP at NCMH during the 13-month period, 18 had hemophilia A as their sole risk factor for AIDS. Five of these patients received pentamidine; of these, four developed pancreatitis during pentamidine treatment. None of the eight hemophiliac patients who received trimethoprim–sulfamethoxazole showed any signs of pancreatitis. Of the 35 nonhemophiliac patients with AIDS who received pentamidine or trimethoprim–sulfamethoxazole, only one had an episode of pancreatitis. This episode was believed to be secondary to biliary disease. The pancreatitis in this patient occurred several months before the development of PCP, and this individual did not receive pentamidine. To date, an association between hemophilia A and pancreatic disease has not been reported. In view of the high incidence of pancreatitis we observed in hemophilia A patients treated with pentamidine, we suggest that there may be an interaction between pentamidine and patients with hemophilia A that predisposes them to pancreatitis.

Conclusion. Studies are needed to determine whether there is a relationship between hemophilia A and the development of pancreatitis during pentamidine therapy.

References

1. Gordin FM, Simon GL, Wofsy CB et al. Adverse reactions to trimethoprim–sulfamethoxazole in patients with acquired immunodeficiency syndrome. *Ann Intern Med.* 1984; 100:495–9.
2. Kovacs JA, Hiemenz JW, Macher AM et al. *Pneumocystis carinii* pneumonia: a comparison between patients with the acquired immunodeficiency syndrome and patients with other immunodeficiencies. *Ann Intern Med.* 1984; 100:663–71.
3. Engleberg LA, Lerner CW, Tapper ML. Clinical features of pneumocystis pneumonia in the acquired immunodeficiency syndrome. *Am Rev Respir Dis.* 1984; 130:689–94.
4. Small CB, Harris CA, Friedland GH et al. The treatment of *Pneumocystis carinii* pneumonia in the acquired immunodeficiency syndrome. *Arch Intern Med.* 1985; 145:837–40.
5. Haverkos HW. Assessment of therapy for *Pneumocystis carinii* pneumonia. *Am J Med.* 1984; 76:501–8.
6. Jaffe HS, Abrams DI, Ammann AJ et al. Complications of co-trimoxazole in treatment of AIDS associated *Pneumocystis carinii* in homosexual men. *Lancet.* 1983; 2:1109–11.
7. Fitzsimmons WE, Luskin S. Pentamidine therapy in renal failure: case report and literature review. *Drug Intell Clin Pharm.* 1988; 22:25–8.
8. Makulu DR, Waalkes PT. Interaction between aromatic diamidines and nucleic acids: possible implications for chemotherapy. *J Natl Cancer Inst.* 1975; 54:305–9.
9. Walzer PD, Perl DP, Krogstad DJ et al. *Pneumocystis carinii* pneumonia in the United States. *Ann Intern Med.* 1974; 80:83–93.
10. Stehr-Green JK, Helmick CG. Pentamidine and renal toxicity. *N Engl J Med.* 1985; 313:694–5. Letter.
11. Murdoch JK, Keystone JS. Pentamidine and hypoglycemia. *Ann Intern Med.* 1983; 99:879. Letter.
12. Hughs WT, Feldman S, Chaudhary JC et al. Comparison of pentamidine isethionate and trimethoprim–sulfamethoxazole in the treatment of *Pneumocystis carinii* pneumonia. *J Pediatr.* 1978; 92:285–91.
13. Anderson R, Boedicker M, Ma M et al. Adverse reactions associated with pentamidine isethionate in AIDS patients. Recommendations for monitoring therapy. *Drug Intell Clin Pharm.* 1986; 20:867–8.
14. Helmick CG, Green JK. Pentamidine associated hypotension and route of administration. *Ann Intern Med.* 1985; 103:480. Letter.
15. Navin TR, Fontaine RE. Intravenous versus intramuscular administration of pentamidine. *N Engl J Med.* 1984; 311:1701–2. Letter.
16. Murphey SA, Joseph AS. Acute pancreatitis associated with pentamidine therapy. *Arch Intern Med.* 1981; 14:565.
17. Salmeron S, Petitpretz P, Katlama C et al. Pentamidine and pancreatitis. *Ann Intern Med.* 1986; 105:140–1. Letter.
18. Zuger A, Wolf BZ, El-sadr W et al. Pentamidine-associated fatal acute pancreatitis. *JAMA.* 1986; 256:2383–5.
19. Echinard E, Dupon M, Malou M et al. Acute fatal pancreatitis following treatment with pentamidine. *Therapie.* 1986; 41:520. Letter.
20. Wharton JM, Lewis-Coleman D, Wofsy CB et al. Trimethoprim–sulfamethoxazole or pentamidine for *Pneumocystis carinii* pneumonia in the acquired immunodeficiency syndrome. *Ann Intern Med.* 1986; 105:37–44.
21. Barrett PVD, Their SO. Meningitis and pancreatitis associated with sulfamethizole. *N Engl J Med.* 1963; 268:36–7.
22. Block MB, Genant HK, Kirsner JB. Pancreatitis as an adverse reaction to salicylazosulfapyridine. *N Engl J Med.* 1970; 282:380–2.
23. Antonow DR. Acute pancreatitis associated with trimethoprim–sulfamethoxazole. *Ann Intern Med.* 1986; 104:363–5.

Procedure for submission of manuscripts to journals published by the American Society of Hospital Pharmacists

—Detach or copy these pages and mail with manuscript—

To expedite manuscript review, the American Society of Hospital Pharmacists requires that a copy of this form be completed and enclosed with each paper submitted for publication to the *American Journal of Hospital Pharmacy* (*AJHP*) or *Clinical Pharmacy*. Authors thereby certify that their papers comply with the major stylistic requirements of ASHP's journals, which are generally in conformance with the Uniform Requirements for Manuscripts Submitted to Biomedical Journals (*Ann Intern Med.* 1988; 108:258-65 and *Br Med J.* 1988; 296:401-5). ASHP exceptions to the Uniform Requirements are noted with an asterisk (*). Authors must comply with and check each point on the list (or mark "NA" for not applicable). If a manuscript is received without a completed form, the editor will mail a blank form to the author and will not process the paper until the form has been completed. *The procedure applies to all manuscripts except letters, book reviews, therapy consultations, management consultations, and similar column material. (For letters to the editor, see the instructions on the first page of the Letters column in most issues.)*

Authors are requested to include with each manuscript a letter of transmittal, the minimum content of which is noted in the checklist below. Authors are encouraged to suggest appropriate reviewers for a manuscript. For exceptionally important work, the editors will consider requests by the authors for expedited ("fast track") review.

Unsolicited manuscripts are acknowledged within one week of their receipt with a letter from the editors. The letter includes a code number that should be cited in all communications regarding the manuscript.

Manuscripts should be submitted to the editor of the appropriate journal at the following address: 4630 Montgomery Avenue, Bethesda, MD 20814.

Letter of Transmittal

_____Summarizes in no more than two sentences the nature of the manuscript.

_____Includes information on prior or duplicate publication or submission elsewhere of any part of the work.

_____Includes a statement of financial or other relationships (e.g., stock ownership, advisory board, speaker's bureau, honoraria) that might lead to a conflict of interests.

General

_____The corresponding author for this manuscript is

____

_____The preferred mailing address for the corresponding author is (please include a complete street address in case it is necessary for us to use overnight mail)

____

____

____

____

____

_____The corresponding author can be reached during business hours at the following telephone and fax numbers:

____

_____Eight complete copies (including photostatic copies of all figures) of the manuscript are submitted. One set of camera-ready figures is

_____submitted. The authors understand that the editors are not obligated to return any of this material.

_____Manuscript is typed double-spaced *throughout* (including tables, references, footnotes, figure captions, and author identification) on 21.6 x 27.9-cm white paper with margins of at least 2.5 cm all around.

_____Manuscript is not typed using all upper-case letters.

_____All pages are numbered consecutively (in the upper right-hand corner), beginning with the title page and including tables.

_____Each of the following elements begins on a separate page, in this sequence: title page, author identification page, abstract, text, footnotes, references, tables, figure captions, and figures.*

_____Abbreviations are in accordance with the *CBE Style Manual*, 5th ed. (pages 241-68). No drug or chemical names are abbreviated.

_____Pharmacokinetic abbreviations agree with those given in the following article: Rowland M, Tucker G. Symbols in pharmacokinetics. *J Pharmacokinet Biopharm.* 1980; 8:497-507.

_____If the manuscript reports the results of a survey, three copies of the survey instrument should be sent for use in the review process (not for publication).

_____Manuscript is accompanied by copies of any permission to reproduce published material, to use illustrations of identifiable persons, or to name persons for their contributions.

_____A copy of any *closely related* manuscript that may aid in the review of the submitted paper (e.g., another paper that reports a separate portion of a study submitted to ASHP) is included.

Title Page

_____Contains concise, informative title and no other information.

Author Identification Page

_____Lists as authors only those individuals who have participated sufficiently in the work to take public responsibility for the content. (Participation solely in the collection of data does not justify authorship. See *Clin Pharm.* 1986; 5:33 for elaboration.)

_____Lists the authors near the top of the page, giving first name, middle initial, and last name of each.

_____Identifies each author in the format used in the author identification section of papers published in *AJHP* and *Clinical Pharmacy*, giving highest academic degree, position, department, and institution.

_____Denotes address for reprint requests.

_____Identifies in one or more paragraphs, as appropriate, (a) contributions that need acknowledging but do not justify authorship, (b) acknowledgments of technical help, (c) acknowledgments of material and financial support (including grant numbers), and (d) financial relationships that may constitute a conflict of interest.

_____If the paper was presented in whole or in part at a meeting, includes name of meeting, location, and date paper was presented.

Abstract (not required for Letters, Notes, Research Notes, Drug Experience, Commentaries, or Reflections)

_____Is less than 150 words.

_____For research reports, concisely states objectives, methods (procedures), main results (including specific data and their statistical significance, if possible), and principal conclusions.

_____For *AJHP* descriptive reports, concisely states purposes of program, how the program works, and conclusions.

_____For review articles and primers, concisely identifies main topics covered in the review, summary of major points, and conclusion.

Text

_____When reporting experiments on humans, indicates whether the procedures followed were in accord with the ethical standards of the institution's committee on human experimentation or in accord with the Helsinki Declaration of 1975.

_____When reporting experiments on animals, indicates whether the institution's or the National Research Council's guide for the care and use of laboratory animals was followed.

_____Names of authors, institutions, or patients are not mentioned, except in descriptive reports where institution identification is essential to understanding the program.

_____For Drug Experience papers, patient's age, gender, race, weight, pertinent past medical history, and baseline laboratory values are included, as well as the generic names, manufacturers, trade names, formulations, and routes of administration of all drug products used.

_____Descriptive headings are used to identify major sections of the paper;

subheadings also may be used.

_____For stability studies, complies with guidelines for such studies (see *Am J Hosp Pharm.* 1983; 40:1159-60 and *Am J Hosp Pharm.* 1988; 45:1569-71), including documentation that the assay used is stability indicating.

_____Identifies in the Methods section all statistical tests used and the a priori level of significance; unusual or complex statistical methods are explained briefly or referenced.

_____If more than one statistical test is used, the data evaluated by each test are clearly identified in the Methods section.

_____Mean values for study results are accompanied by some measure of variability or precision (e.g., standard deviations); the use of confidence intervals, when appropriate, is encouraged.

_____Identifies precisely all drugs and chemicals used by generic name (with salt, if applicable). Trade names are used only to identify that a specific brand of drug was used. For reports of clinical research, identification of drugs as being racemic mixtures of single isomers is encouraged.

_____Measurements are reported in the units in which they were made. Volume, distance, and weight measurements should be expressed in metric units.*

_____For commercial products important to the paper, denotes, in parentheses, the trade name or model number; the manufacturer's name, city, state, and zip code; and the lot number. If such designations are numerous, they are listed as footnotes at the end of the text.

_____Every reference, figure, table, and appendix is cited in the text in numerical order. (Order of mention in text determines the number given to each.)

_____Footnotes are identified consecutively in the text by superscript, lower-case letters.*

References

_____Are identified in text, tables, and legends by superscript* Arabic umbers.

_____Are typed double-spaced on sheets separate from the text and numbered consecutively as they appear in the text. References that appear in tables should receive consecutive numbers based on the placement of the table in the text.

_____Do not include any "unpublished observations" and "personal communications." (References to written, not oral, communications may be inserted, in parentheses, in the text or included as footnotes.)

_____Have been verified by the author(s) against the original documents.

_____Abbreviations of journal titles conform to those used in *Index Medicus* (January issue).

_____Include inclusive page numbers.

_____Are in the style adopted by the U.S. National Library of Medicine and used in *Index Medicus* with the exception that only the first three authors (last name and two initials, if available) are ever listed. Examples of this style follow:

(a) Standard journal article—(list all authors when three or less; when four or more, list only first three and add et al.*):
1. Roberts LW, O'Donnell J, Matsuda T et al. Pharmacy-assisted burn unit skin bank program. Am J Hosp Pharm. 1977; 34:1353-4.

(b) Article from journal paginated by issue:
2. Goldschmidt L. Remodeling on a shoe-string improves pharmacy's efficiency. Hospitals. 1979; 53(May 1):115-6.

(c) Letter, editorial, or abstract:
3. Wightkin WT, Buckhammer CR. Simple method for intravenous-to-oral theophylline dose conversion. Clin Pharm. 1982; 1:300-1. Letter.
4. Zellmer, WA. Prescribing pharmacists. Am J Hosp Pharm. 1982; 39:1481. Editorial.
5. Bartle WR, Walker SE, Shapero T. Effect of cimetidine on phenytoin metabolism. Clin Pharmacol Ther. 1982; 31:202. Abstract.

(d) Book—personal author(s):
6. Osler AG. Complement: mechanisms and functions. Englewood Cliffs, NJ: Prentice-Hall; 1976.

(e) Chapter or article in a book:
7. Weinstein L, Swartz MN. Pathogenic properties of invading microorganisms. In: Sodeman WA Jr, Sodeman WA, eds. Pathologic physiology: mechanisms of disease. Philadelphia: Saunders; 1974:457-72.

(f) Editor, compiler, or chairman as author of book:
8. Wertheimer AI, Smith MC, eds. Pharmacy practice: social and behavioral aspects. 7th ed. Baltimore: University Park Press; 1981.

(g) Governmental agency publication:
9. National Center for Health Statistics. Acute conditions: incidence and associated disability, United States July 1968–June 1969. Rockville, MD: National Center for Health Statistics, 1972; DHEW publication no. (HSM) 72-1036. (Vital and health statistics; series 10: Data from the National Health Survey; no. 69.)

(h) Package insert:
10. Roche Laboratories. Accutane package insert. Nutley, NJ: 1982 May.

(i) Paper presented at a meeting:
11. Stern NB, Millburg WJ, Steckel SD. Managing proper disposal of antineoplastic agents. Paper presented at 17th Annual ASHP Midyear Clinical Meeting. Los Angeles, CA: 1982 Dec 7.

Tables

_____Are typed double-spaced, each (complete with title and footnotes) on a separate page (not submitted as photographs).

_____Are submitted in the original typed size, not photo-reduced.

_____Do not contain information duplicated in the text or figures.

_____Are in the style used in ASHP's journals.

_____Do not contain horizontal or vertical rules within the tabulated information.

_____Use superscript letters for footnote designations.*

_____If use data from another published or unpublished source, permission is obtained from the source (proof submitted with paper) and the source is acknowledged.

Figure Captions

_____Are typed double-spaced on a sheet separate from the text.

_____Are numbered consecutively as they are cited in the text.

_____All abbreviations and symbols used in the figure are defined; when appropriate, the measure of variability or precision represented is identified (e.g., do error bands represent standard deviation(s) or a confidence interval?).

Figures

_____Are professionally drawn and photographed. (Freehand or typewritten lettering is unacceptable.) Computer-generated figures are acceptable only if produced on letter-quality printers.

_____Are submitted as sharp, glossy, black-and-white photographic prints, usually 12.7 x 17.3 cm but no larger than 20.3 x 25.4 cm.

_____Are designed such that, when reduced to one-column width (8 cm), are legible and occupy no more than 10 cm of column length.

_____Axis labels appear outside the axes.

_____Titles and detailed explanations (including keys to symbols used) are in the captions, not the illustrations themselves.

_____If previously published, the original source is acknowledged, and written permission from the copyright holder to reproduce the material is submitted.

_____Each photographic print has a label pasted on its back indicating the figure number and title of the paper. (Do not note authors' names.* Do not write on the back.)

_____Copies of all figures are included with each copy of manuscript.

Copyright and Authorship

_____The following copyright transferal and authorship statements are submitted on a separate sheet identified with the title of the paper and signed and dated by each author.

In consideration of the American Society of Hospital Pharmacists (ASHP) taking action in reviewing and editing my (our) submission, the author(s) undersigned hereby transfer(s), assign(s), or otherwise convey(s) all ownership rights in the submission and all copyright ownership to ASHP. In the event that such work is not published by ASHP, all said rights shall be released.

_____I have participated sufficiently in the conception, design, data analysis (where applicable), and writing of this manuscript to take public responsibility for the content. I have read the final version of the paper and find it suitable for publication.

If this paper has been presented at a meeting other than one sponsored by ASHP, a copy of a release from the sponsors of that meeting, permitting publication elsewhere, is enclosed.

Exclusive Publication Statement

I certify that none of the material in this manuscript has been previously published and none of this material or substantially similar material is under consideration or has been accepted for publication elsewhere, except as described in the attachment. This includes journal articles, letters to the editor, symposia, editorials, proceedings, transactions, books, articles published by invitation, news reports, and preliminary publication of any kind except an abstract of 400 words or less.

____

(Signature of Corresponding Author) (Date)

_____If you have not complied with the item immediately above, please include an explanation in your letter of transmittal.

Instructions for submitting computer disks with revised manuscripts

—Detach or copy this page and mail with revised manuscript—

When your paper has been accepted for publication in *AJHP* or *Clinical Pharmacy* and revised as requested, follow these specifications for preparing a word processing disk containing the manuscript. Tables and figures do not need to be put on the disk; all other parts of the manuscript, including captions, should be. Disks will not be returned to authors.

- Disk must be in an **IBM-PC file format.**
- 3½ and 5 inch disks are acceptable.
- The following word processing software formats are acceptable on IBM-PC formatted disks:

ASCII text
DCA-RFT and FFT
Displaywrite 2, 3, 4, 4.2, and 5
Enable (version 1)
Freestyle/Select
IBM Writing Assistant (version 1)
Leading Edge WP
Lotus Manuscript
Mass-11
Microsoft Word PC/Mac (versions PC, 1.05, 3.01)
Multimate, Multimate Advantage I and II
NBI
Officewriter
Palantir (version 3)
PC-Write
PeachText
pfs: Write, Professional Write, and First Choice
PMate (up to 4.0)
Samna Word I, II, and III
Spellbinder (up to 5.6)
Volkswriter
Wang
Word Perfect 4.1 through 5.1
WordMarc Composer
Wordstar (up to version 6.0) and Wordstar-2000
Xerox 860, Xerox Writer II
Xywrite

If your word processor version is not listed, use the ASCII file format (same as printing to a file).

If you need further assistance, call Carol Cavanaugh at ASHP headquarters, 301-657-3000, ext 225.

- **Wang- or Macintosh-formatted disks cannot be used, but Wang or Macintosh files on IBM-file-formatted disks are acceptable.**

Please check each point below to indicate compliance:

___ 1. Manuscript is all one document.
___ 2. All headers and footers have been deleted.
___ 3. Footnotes and references are listed at end of the text. (Footnotes are not located at ends of pages on which they are mentioned.)
___ 4. I have listed below the name, phone number, and office hours of the person who can give specific information about how the disk was produced.

Name: ____________________

Phone: (____) ________ __________ ext ________

Office hours: ______________ Days: __________

Time zone: ____________________

___ 5. Each disk is labeled with the following information:

Manuscript reference code number
Name of corresponding author
Word processing file format with version number (e.g., Microsoft Word 4.0)
Disk density, if known
Date disk sent

___ 6. For mailing, disk is enclosed in appropriate protective container.
___ 7. Two copies of a printout from the disk are included; the content of the disk is identical to what appears on the paper copies.
___ 8. By signing below, I certify that the revised manuscript has been prepared according to these specifications.

____

(Signature of Corresponding Author) (Date)

DUE Criteria

The DUE Criteria section of Clinical Pharmacy features model drug-use evaluation criteria that may be employed as a component of a comprehensive quality assurance program. The criteria sets are presented in the format used in the ASHP book Criteria for Drug Use Evaluation. Some of the criteria sets will have been originally published in that book; others will be presented here for the first time and published in future volumes of the ASHP book. The practitioners who developed a criteria set are acknowledged.

In selecting drug products for coverage in DUE Criteria, priority is given to products that have been recently marketed, those that are frequently prescribed, those that have high potential risk associated with their use, and those that are expensive. When feasible, a criteria set will be linked with a Drug Review that appears in the same issue.

These criteria sets are a starting point for the development of DUE criteria for a specific practice setting. Readers are encouraged to modify the model criteria to fit their own circumstances.

Criteria for use of enalapril maleate in adults[a]

Element	Standard 100%	Standard 0%	Exception[b] or Critical Preventive/Responsive Measure[c]	Sources of Information
Justification for Use				
1. Mild to severe essential hypertension (systolic blood pressure of >160 mm Hg or diastolic blood pressure of >90 mm Hg)[1–6]	X		1A. None	1. History and physical (H&P), progress notes, nursing notes
or				
2. Renovascular hypertension (unilateral or bilateral renal artery stenosis and systolic blood pressure of >160 mm Hg or diastolic blood pressure of >90 mm Hg)[7–9]	X		2A. None	2. H&P, progress notes, nursing notes, renal arteriography or renography reports
or				
3. Refractory congestive heart failure (CHF)[4–6,10–14]: a. Dyspnea on exertion, paroxysmal nocturnal dyspnea, orthopnea, or pedal edema with at least one of the following: chest roentgenogram showing cardiomegaly or pulmonary vascular congestion, echocardiogram showing left ventricular systolic dysfunction, gallop rhythm, or jugular venous distention and b. Failed therapy with digoxin and a diuretic	X		3A. Patient unable to tolerate digoxin or diuretic	3. H&P, progress notes, nursing notes, radiology reports, echocardiogram reports, physician orders, medication administration record (MAR) 3A. Progress notes, nursing notes, physician orders, MAR
Critical (Process) Indicators				
4. Baseline serum creatinine (SCr) concentration, blood urea nitrogen	X		4A. None	4. Physician orders, laboratory reports, progress notes

Prepared by Allison L. Coley, Pharm.D., Clinical Pharmacist, Family Practice, Department of Pharmacy, University Medical Center, and Clinical Assistant Professor, College of Pharmacy, University of Florida Health Science Center/Jacksonville.

Element	Standard 100%	Standard 0%	Exception[b] or Critical Preventive/ Responsive Measure[c]	Sources of Information
(BUN) concentration, serum potassium concentration, hemoglobin (Hb) concentration, hematocrit (Hct), white blood cell (WBC) count with differential, and platelet count determined; results of liver function tests (aspartate aminotransferase [AST], alanine aminotransferase [ALT], and alkaline phosphatase [ALP]) obtained; and urinalysis (with 24-hr urinary protein analysis) performed[4–6,15,16]				
5. Diuretic therapy or sodium restriction discontinued 2–3 days before initial enalapril dose[4–6,15]	X		5A. If patient must continue taking diuretic, enalapril started at lower dosage[4–6,15]	5. Physician orders, progress notes, nursing notes, MAR 5A. H&P, progress notes, nursing notes, MAR
6. Blood pressure monitored three times daily while inpatient and monthly when outpatient	X		6A. None	6. Physician orders, nursing notes, progress notes, nursing flow sheets, discharge summary
7. SCr and BUN concentrations monitored every 2 weeks for 3 months and then every 6 months[15,16]	X		7A. In patient with severe CHF, unilateral or bilateral renal artery stenosis, or pre-existing renal impairment (creatinine clearance [CL_{cr}], <30 mL/min), SCr and BUN concentrations monitored weekly for 1 month and then every 3 months	7. Physician orders, laboratory reports, progress notes 7A. H&P, progress notes, radiology reports, echocardiogram reports, renal arteriography or renography reports, laboratory reports
8. WBC count with differential, platelet count, Hb concentration, and Hct monitored every 2 weeks for 3 months and then at least every 6 months[15,16]	X		8A. None	8. Physician orders, laboratory reports, progress notes
9. Urinary protein (24 hr) monitored every 2 weeks for 3 months and then every 6 months[15,16]	X		9A. None	9. Physician orders, laboratory reports, progress notes
10. Serum potassium concentration monitored every 2 weeks for 3 months and then every 3 months[15,16]	X		10A. Patient with renal insufficiency (CL_{cr}, <30 mL/min) or diabetes mellitus or taking potassium-sparing diuretic monitored daily for 1 week and then monthly[15]	10. Physician orders, laboratory reports, progress notes 10A. H&P, laboratory reports, progress notes, physician orders, MAR
11. AST, ALT, and ALP levels monitored every 6 months[4–6,15]	X		11A. None	11. Laboratory reports, progress notes
12. Appropriate initial adult oral dosage for hypertension: 5 mg once daily[4–6,15]	X		12A. If patient taking diuretic that cannot be discontinued, initial dose should be 2.5 mg administered under medical supervision for at least 2 hr and until blood pressure has stabilized for at least one additional hour[15] 12B. Renal impairment (see element 13)	12. Physician orders, MAR 12A. Physician orders, MAR, progress notes, nursing notes 12B. Laboratory reports
13. Appropriate initial adult oral dosage for hypertension in renally impaired patient[4–6,15]: a. Moderate to severe renal impairment (CL_{cr}, <30 mL/min): 2.5 mg once daily b. Dialysis patient: 2.5 mg after dialysis on dialysis days; dosage on nondialysis days adjusted de-	X		13A. None	13. Physician orders, MAR, laboratory reports

Element	Standard 100%	Standard 0%	Exception[b] or Critical Preventive/ Responsive Measure[c]	Sources of Information
pending on blood pressure response[15]				
14. Appropriate maintenance adult oral dosage for hypertension (normal or impaired renal function): 10–40 mg as single daily dose or divided b.i.d.[4–6,15]	X		14A. None	14. Physician orders, MAR
15. Recommended adult i.v. dosage for hypertension: 1.25 mg every 6 hr; can be administered undiluted over 5 min or diluted with up to 50 mL of diluent[17]	X		15A. If ineffective, consider 5 mg every 6 hr[17] 15B. Initial dose reduced to 0.625 mg for patient taking diuretic; if inadequate response after 1 hr, give another 0.625 mg; may give additional 1.25-mg doses at 6-hr intervals[17] 15C. Renal impairment (see element 16)	15. Physician orders, MAR 15A, B. Progress notes, physician orders, MAR 15C. Laboratory reports
16. Appropriate adult i.v. dosage for hypertension in renally impaired patient[17]: a. Moderate to severe renal impairment (CL_{cr}, <30 mL/min): 0.625 mg; if inadequate response after 1 hr, give another 0.625 mg; may give additional 1.25-mg doses at 6-hr intervals b. Dialysis patient: 0.625 mg every 6 hr	X		16A. None	16. Progress notes, laboratory reports, physician orders, MAR
17. Appropriate initial adult oral dosage for CHF: 2.5 mg once or twice daily (once daily for renally impaired patient)[11–15]	X		17A. None	17. Physician orders, MAR
18. Appropriate maintenance adult oral dosage for CHF (normal or impaired renal function): 5–20 mg/day in two divided doses[11–15]	X		18A. None	18. Physician orders, MAR
Complications				
19. Transient hypotension or dizziness[6–8,15,16]		X	19A. Identify other drug and nondrug causes 19B. Place patient in supine position[15] 19C. Consider volume expansion with 0.9% sodium chloride solution 19D. Consider dosage reduction[15]	19. Progress notes, nursing notes 19A. Progress notes, nursing notes, MAR 19B, C. Physician orders, progress notes, nursing notes 19D. Physician orders, MAR
20. Angioedema (face, extremities, lips, tongue, or larynx)[6–8,15,16]		X	20A. Identify other drug and nondrug causes 20B. Discontinue enalapril immediately 20C. Consider antihistamines 20D. If tongue or larynx involved, give epinephrine 1:1000 (0.3–0.5 mL) s.c. immediately[15]	20. Progress notes, nursing notes 20A. Progress notes, nursing notes, MAR 20B–D. Physician orders, progress notes, MAR
21. Declining renal function (SCr and BUN concentrations increasing above baseline)[6–8,15,16]		X	21A. Identify other drug and nondrug causes 21B. Reduce dosage of enalapril[15] 21C. Discontinue diuretic[15] 21D. If renal function does not improve, discontinue enalapril[15]	21. Laboratory reports, progress notes 21A. Progress notes, nursing notes, MAR, laboratory reports 21B–D. Physician orders, progress notes, MAR
22. Cough[6–8,15,16]		X	22A. Identify other drug and nondrug causes 22B. If cough persists and is intolerable, discontinue enalapril[15]	22. Progress notes, nursing notes 22A. Progress notes, nursing notes, MAR 22B. Physician orders, MAR

Element	Standard 100%	Standard 0%	Exception[b] or Critical Preventive/ Responsive Measure[c]	Sources of Information
23. Headache[6–8,15,16]		X	23A. Identify other drug and nondrug causes 23B. If headache is severe or intolerable, discontinue enalapril[15]	23. Progress notes, nursing notes, MAR 23A. Progress notes, nursing notes, physician orders, MAR 23B. Physician orders, MAR
24. Nausea, vomiting, or diarrhea[6–8,15,16]		X	24A. Identify other drug and nondrug causes 24B. Administer with meals 24C. If adverse effects are severe or intolerable, discontinue enalapril[15]	24. Progress notes, nursing notes, MAR 24A, B. Progress notes, nursing notes, physician orders, MAR 24C. Physician orders, MAR
25. Nephrotic syndrome (proteinuria of >3 g/day; serum albumin concentration, ≤3 g/dL; and peripheral edema)[6–8,14,15]		X	25A. Identify other drug and nondrug causes 25B. Discontinue enalapril	25. Laboratory reports, progress notes, nursing notes 25A. Laboratory reports, progress notes, nursing notes, MAR 25B. Physician orders, progress notes, MAR
26. Neutropenia (neutrophil count, <300/cu mm)[6–8,15,16]		X	26A. Identify other drug and nondrug causes 26B. Discontinue enalapril	26. Laboratory reports, progress notes 26A. Laboratory reports, progress notes, nursing notes, MAR 26B. Physician orders, MAR
27. Agranulocytosis[6–8,15,16]		X	27A. Identify other drug and nondrug causes 27B. Discontinue enalapril	27. Laboratory reports, progress notes 27A. Laboratory reports, progress notes, nursing notes, MAR 27B. Physician orders, MAR
28. Hyperkalemia (serum potassium concentration, >5.7 meq/L)[6–8,15,16,18]		X	28A. Identify other drug and nondrug causes 28B. Discontinue any potassium supplementation 28C. Discontinue concomitant use of potassium-sparing diuretics 28D. Reduce potassium level with sodium polystyrene sulfonate, if necessary 28E. If potassium level continues to increase after all other measures have been taken, discontinue enalapril	28. Laboratory reports, progress notes 28A. Laboratory reports, progress notes, nursing notes, MAR 28B–D. Physician orders, MAR 28E. Physician orders, progress notes, MAR
Outcome Measures				
29. Blood pressure, ≤160/90 mm Hg[1–5,7–9]	X		29A. None	29. Progress notes, nursing notes, nursing flow sheets
30. Improved CHF symptoms (decreased dyspnea on exertion, paroxysmal nocturnal dyspnea, or orthopnea); improved exercise tolerance; decreased rales, pedal edema, and jugular venous distention; and increased left ventricular ejection fraction[10–14]	X		30A. None	30. Progress notes, nursing notes, echocardiogram reports

[a] Criteria address justification for use (indications), critical (process) indicators, complications of therapy, and patient outcome. Each criterion consists of an element, a standard, exceptions to the standard, and sources of information. The element is the minimum level of evidence needed to show that patient care was optimal. The standard defines the deviation from an element that is acceptable. If no deviation is acceptable, the standard is 100%. Exceptions are circumstances in which deviation is allowable. Sources of information listed are the most reliable sources. Sources pertaining to an element or exception are identified by the number assigned to the element or exception (e.g., 14, 14A).

[b] For justification for use and critical (process) indicators.

[c] For complications and outcome measures.

References

1. Helgelan A, Hagelund CH, Strommen R et al. Enalapril, atenolol and hydrochlorothiazide in mild to moderate hypertension. *Lancet*. 1986; 1:872–5.
2. Ayers CR, Baker KM, Weaver BA et al. Enalapril maleate versus captopril: a comparison of the hormonal and antihypertensive effects. *Drugs*. 1985; 30(Suppl 1):70–3.
3. Joint National Committee on Detection, Evaluation and Treatment of High Blood Pressure. The 1988 report of the Joint National Committee on Detection, Evaluation and Treatment of High Blood Pressure. *Arch Intern Med*. 1988; 148:1023–38.
4. Borek M, Charlap S, Frishman W. Enalapril: a long-acting angiotensin-converting enzyme inhibitor. *Pharmacotherapy*. 1987; 7(5):133–48.
5. Todd PA, Heel C. Enalapril: a review of its pharmacodynamic and pharmacokinetic properties and therapeutic use in hypertension and congestive heart failure. *Drugs*. 1986; 31:198–248.
6. Vlasses PH, Larijani GE, Conner DP et al. Enalapril, a nonsulfhydryl angiotensin-converting enzyme inhibitor. *Clin Pharm*. 1985; 4:27–40.
7. Karlberg BE, Fyhrquist F, Gronhagen-Risha C et al. Enalapril and lisinopril in renovascular hypertension—antihypertensive and hormonal effects of two new angiotensin converting enzyme inhibitors. *Scand J Urol Nephrol*. 1984; 79 (Suppl):103–6.
8. Franklin SS, Smith RD. A comparison of enalapril plus hydrochlorothiazide with standard triple therapy in renovascular hypertension. *Nephron*. 1986; 44(Suppl 1):73–82.
9. Hodsman GP, Brown JJ, Cumming AM et al. Enalapril in the treatment of hypertension with renal artery stenosis. *Br Med J*. 1983; 287:1413–7.
10. DiCarlo L, Chatterjee K, Parmley WW et al. Enalapril: a new angiotensin enzyme inhibitor in chronic heart failure: acute and chronic hemodynamic evaluation. *J Am Coll Cardiol*. 1983; 2:865–71.
11. Levine BT, Olwari MJ, Cohn JN. Angiotensin converting enzyme inhibitors in congestive heart failure: overview in comparison of captopril and enalapril. *Am J Med*. 1986; 81 (Suppl 4C):36–9.
12. Sharpe DN, Murphy J, Coxon R et al. Enalapril in patients with chronic heart failure: a placebo-controlled, randomized, double-blind study. *Circulation*. 1984; 70:271–8.
13. Consensus (Cooperative North Scandinavian Enalapril Survival Study) Trial Study Group. Effects of enalapril on mortality in severe congestive heart failure. *N Engl J Med*. 1987; 316:1429–35.
14. Packer M, Lee WH, Yushak M et al. Comparison of captopril and enalapril in patients with severe chronic heart failure. *N Engl J Med*. 1986; 315:847–53.
15. Merck, Sharp & Dohme. Enalapril package insert. West Point, PA; 1988.
16. Stumpe KO, Kolloch R, Overlack A. Captopril and enalapril: evaluation of therapeutic efficacy and safety. *Pract Cardiol*. 1984; 10:111–24.
17. Merck, Sharp & Dohme. Enalaprilat package insert. West Point, PA; 1988.
18. Izzo JL, Larrabee PS, Scandling JD et al. Hyperkalemia with enalapril in advanced renal failure. *JAMA*. 1986; 255: 2605–6.

CP Continuing Education

The ASHP Continuing-Education system gives readers a self-assessment mechanism for selected articles in Clinical Pharmacy *and the* American Journal of Hospital Pharmacy. *It also allows readers to obtain continuing-education credit for these articles.*

For the purpose of CE-credit enrollment a blank answer sheet is published at the end of each installment of the column for the CE articles in that issue. An enrollee accumulates these answer sheets until the enrollment is submitted, using the form that is published in the June and December issues of Clinical Pharmacy *and in the June and December issues of* AJHP. *Any combination of tests within an 18-month period, from both* Clinical Pharmacy *and* AJHP, *may be included in an enrollment. More complete details about enrollment in the system will appear in the semiannual enrollment form.*

Article 680-204-9101 (see page 14)
Qualifies for 1 hour of CE credit.

Current options for the treatment of systemic scleroderma

Learning Objectives

After studying this article, the reader should be able to

1. Compare the major subclasses of systemic scleroderma (SSc).
2. Identify signs and symptoms associated with SSc renal disease.
3. Name the major organs that are affected by SSc.
4. Identify major causes of morbidity and mortality in SSc patients.
5. Describe the efficacy of remittive, immunosuppressive, and palliative drug therapies that have been tested in patients with SSc.
6. Recommend drug therapy for a patient with SSc renal crisis.
7. Identify three treatment options for patients with SSc suffering from Raynaud's phenomenon.

Self-assessment Questions

For each question there is only one best answer.

1. All of the following organs or organ systems must be monitored for the pathologic effects of SSc except the

   a. Heart.
   b. Kidneys.
   c. Spleen.
   d. Lungs.
   e. Gastrointestinal tract.

2. Systemic scleroderma is different from localized scleroderma because only SSc

   a. Affects just one side of the body.
   b. Is characterized by thickening of the skin.
   c. Affects small arteries and microvessels.
   d. Can be prevented with early medical treatment.

3. Which of the following is not a minor criterion for the American Rheumatism Association diagnosis of scleroderma?

   a. Elevated serum creatinine.
   b. Sclerodactyly.
   c. Digital pitting scars.
   d. Bilateral basal pulmonary fibrosis.

4. SSc disease involvement of the following organs is associated with a high rate of mortality

   a. Gastrointestinal tract and spleen.
   b. Lungs and gastrointestinal tract.
   c. Kidneys and skin.
   d. Kidneys and heart.

5. Which of the following is the medication of choice in treating Raynaud's phenomenon associated with SSc?

   a. Edetate disodium.
   b. Alginic acid.
   c. Dimethyl sulfoxide.
   d. Nifedipine.
   e. Penicillamine.

6. Which of the following is not a major subclass of systemic scleroderma?

Current Literature

Drug Reaction Alerts

Drug Reaction Alerts focuses primarily on serious, unlabeled reactions to new chemical entities. The citations are compiled monthly from International Pharmaceutical Abstracts, *which covers over 800 pharmacy and health-related journals worldwide. An address for reprints (when available) follows the name of the corresponding author in each citation.*

Pharmacists may use the FDA Adverse Reaction Report form that appears in most issues of Clinical Pharmacy *for submitting reports of adverse drug reactions directly to FDA.*

Androgens

Punch MR, Ansbacher R (Department of Obstetrics and Gynecology, University of Michigan Medical Center, Medical Professional Building, D-2206, Box 0718, Ann Arbor, MI 48019). Autogenic masculinization. *Am J Obstet Gynecol.* 1990; 163:114-6. Case. (27-year-old woman with lichen sclerosus; self-treated with topical **testosterone** up to 60 mg daily for a prolonged period of time; developed marked masculinization, possible secondary amenorrhea, and elevated serum testosterone levels; withdrawal of testosterone led to a normal menstrual period one month later and serum testosterone levels within normal range for a female adult two months later; regular menstrual cycling reported one year later)

Anti-anemia Drugs

Rogers S, Russell NH, Morgan AG (Department of Hematology and Renal Medicine, City Hospital, Nottingham NG5 1PB, England). Effect of **erythropoietin** in patients with myeloma. *Br Med J.* 1990; 301:667. Case. (51-year-old man with anemia; received erythropoietin 4000 units twice weekly; developed increased activity of multiple myeloma as shown by increase in lambda light chain urinary excretion from 1.56 g/L to 10.75 g/L; withdrawal of erythropoietin led to pretreatment levels of lambda light chain urinary excretion)

Antilipemic Agents

Aebi U, Reinhart WH (University of Bern, Inselspital, CH-3010 Bern, Switzerland). **Beclobrate** and liver disease. *Ann Intern Med.* 1990; 113:483. Case. (63-year-old woman with moderate hyperlipidemia; received beclobrate 100 mg daily for four months; developed hepatic failure; withdrawal of beclobrate did not stop progression of hepatic failure; patient died; evidence of hepatic necrosis found at autopsy)

Drug Abuse

Burkett C (Department of Obstetrics and Gynecology, R-136, University of Miami, School of Medicine, P.O. Box 01690, Miami, FL 33103), Bandstra ES, Cohen J et al. **Cocaine**-related maternal death. *Am J Obstet Gynecol.* 1990; 163:40-1. Case. (26-year-old woman, seven or eight months pregnant, who abused cocaine; found unconscious and without pulse, respirations, and blood pressure; electrocardiogram showed severe bradycardia; both patient and fetus died; cocaine and its metabolites detected in urine and in nasal secretions)

Drug Interactions

Yeh J, Soo SC, Summerton C (Richardson C, Addenbrooke's Hospital, Cambridge CB2 2QQ, England). Potentiation of action of **warfarin** by **itraconazole**. *Br Med J.* 1990; 301:669. Case. (61-year-old woman who was stabilized on warfarin 5 mg daily for one year; received itraconazole 200 mg twice daily; developed intractable bleeding and increased generalized bruising; concomitant ipratropium bromide, albuterol, budesonide, quinine sulfate, and omeprazole; withdrawal of warfarin and itraconazole and therapy with fresh frozen plasma led to normal international normalized ratio within two days; warfarin resumed without incident)

Excipients

Al-Mudallal R, Rosenbaum H, Schwartz HJ (Boyle J, Case Western Reserve University School of Medicine, Cleveland, OH 44106). Anaphylactic reaction to **barium** enema. *Am J Med.* 1990; 89:251. Case. (51-year-old woman; received rectal enema containing barium sulfate; developed anaphylaxis; therapy with epinephrine, corticosteroids, dopamine, diphenhydramine, and i.v. fluids led to resuscitation; skin prick testing with sodium benzoate, potassium sorbate, and diluted liquid barium suspension was negative; reaction attributed to one of the excipients in the enema)

Gastrointestinal Drugs

Kornbluth A (Division of Gastroenterology, Box 1069, Mount Sinai Medical Center, One Gustave L. Levy Pl., New York, NY 10029), Gupta R, Gerson CD. Life-threatening diarrhea after short-term **misoprostol** use in a patient with Crohn ileocolitis. *Ann Intern Med.* 1990; 113:474-5. Case. (56-year-old woman with osteoarthritis; received misoprostol 200 μg four times daily for six doses; developed severe diarrhea attributed to reactivation of Crohn's disease; concomitant naproxen; withdrawal of misoprostol and therapy with clindamycin and aztreonam led to gradual resolution of diarrhea; patient received therapy with sulfasalazine and oral ciprofloxacin for treatment of Crohn's disease)

Hypotensive Agents

Sieber C, Grimm E, Follath F (Division of Clinical Pharmacolo-

Continued on page 80

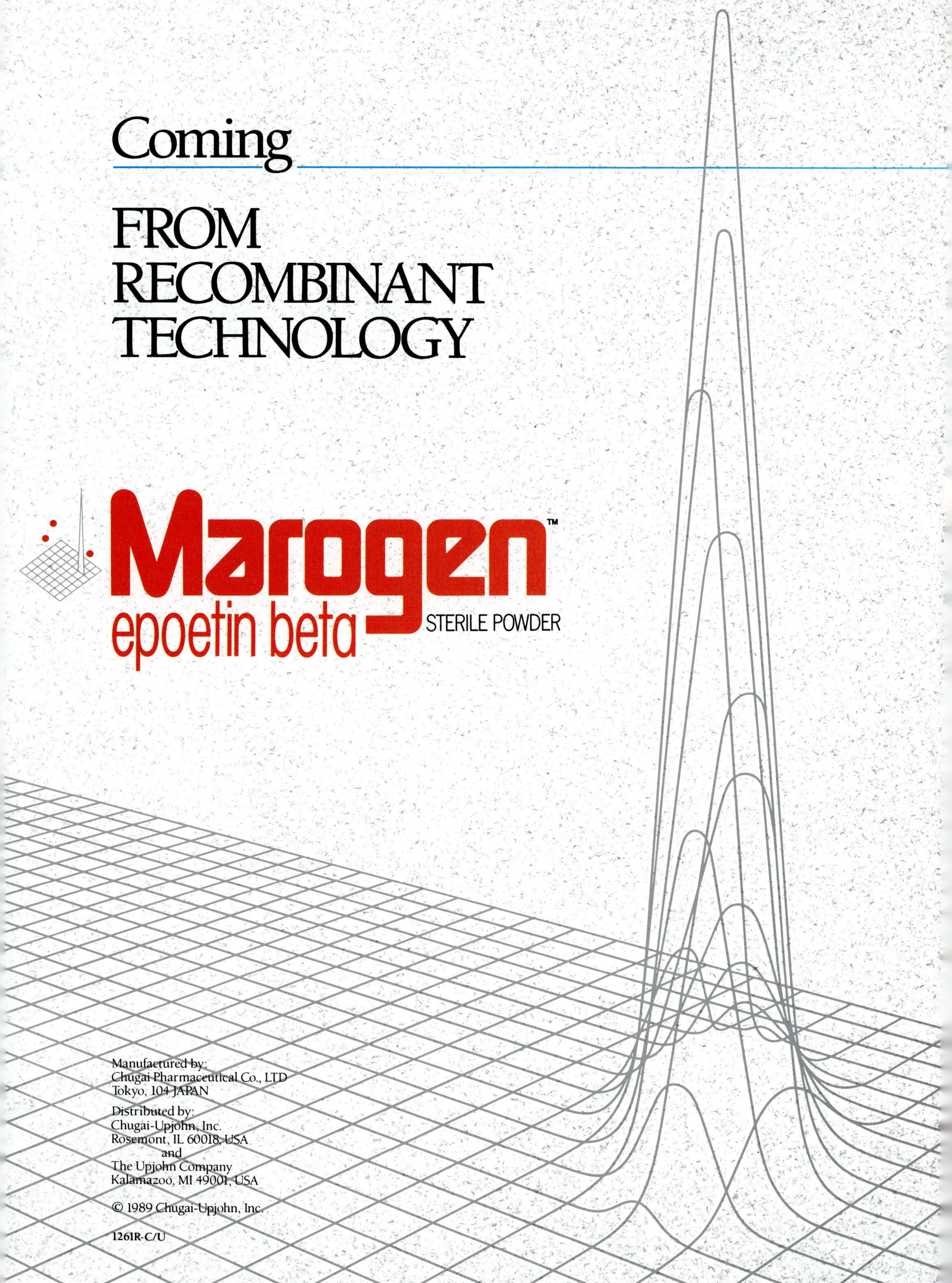

Coming
FROM RECOMBINANT TECHNOLOGY
Marogen™
epoetin beta
STERILE POWDER
Manufactured by:
Chugai Pharmaceutical Co., LTD
Tokyo, 104 JAPAN
Distributed by:
Chugai-Upjohn, Inc.
Rosemont, IL 60018, USA
and
The Upjohn Company
Kalamazoo, MI 49001, USA
© 1989 Chugai-Upjohn, Inc.
1261R-C/U

Continued from page 74

gy, University Hospital, Basel, Switzerland). **Captopril** and systemic lupus erythematosus syndrome. *Br Med J.* 1990; 301:669. Case. (53-year-old man with hypertension and congestive heart failure; received captopril initially 50 mg daily for seven months then increasing to 125 mg daily for six weeks; developed systemic lupus erythematosus; concomitant furosemide, isosorbide dinitrate, and digoxin; withdrawal of captopril led to complete resolution of symptoms and laboratory values returned to normal)

Keratolytic Agents

Meurehg CC, Amelio PX (American British Cowdray Hospital, Mexico City D.F. 01710, Mexico). Vaginal bleeding and **tretinoin** cream. *Ann Intern Med.* 1990; 113:483. Case. (64-year-old woman; applied topical cream containing tretinoin 0.05% daily to her face for five weeks; developed premenstrual symptoms and vaginal bleeding; withdrawal of tretinoin led to resolution of symptoms within three days; positive rechallenge)

Tranquilizers

Stones M, Kennie DC, Fulton JD (Stirling Royal Infirmary, Stirling, England). Dystonic dysphagia associated with **fluspirilene**. *Br Med J.* 1990; 301:668-9. Case. (80-year-old woman; received fluspirilene 3 mg weekly; developed dystonic dysphagia; premedication for endoscopy with glycopyrrolate 2 mg by intramuscular injection led to some improvement that deteriorated rapidly; therapy with benztropine 2 mg by intravenous injection led to sustained resolution of symptoms; patient was discharged and reported no recurrence of symptoms)

Book Review

Field Drug Reference for Emergency Care Providers

Edited by Edgar R. Gonzalez and Joseph P. Ornato.
Published by Drug Intelligence Publications, Inc., 1241 Broadway, Hamilton, IL 62341, 1990. vii + 231 p. Price $26.

Field Drug Reference for Emergency Care Providers is a pocket-sized book designed for providers of advanced life support (ALS) who treat patients before or during their hospitalizations.

The initial chapters review pharmacokinetic principles and pharmacology using emergency-drug examples and graphs. One chapter contains a compatibility table for i.v. solutions, examples of calculations, and several helpful reference tables (ideal body weight, Fahrenheit-to-Celsius conversion, and infusion rates for dopamine, dobutamine, nitroprusside, and nitroglycerin); the last section of this chapter presents easy-to-use tables for determining doses for neonatal and pediatric emergencies. Another chapter reviews autonomic pharmacology and emphasizes the differences in receptor activity by comparing the effects of sympathomimetic drugs.

The body of the *Field Drug Reference for Emergency Care Providers* details information needed frequently for 51 drugs used during ALS and emergency care. The authors limit the information to drugs carried by emergency medical providers and provide a comprehensive list of these drugs. However, toxicological emergency treatments other than naloxone are excluded (e.g., activated charcoal, cyanide antidote kits, physostigmine, and ipecac). Each drug monograph includes trade names, drug class, clinical action (with pharmacological and clinical results), indications, contraindications, adverse reactions, and if known, pharmacokinetic information. Also listed are drug product availability and dosage and administration guidelines including pediatric dosing. The section for special situations highlights warnings and considerations for pregnant or lactating patients and patients with organ dysfunction. The last portion of each monograph details drug interactions and overdose management.

The last sections of the book provide tables of abbreviations, a glossary of pharmacological terms, the American Heart Association's algorithms for cardiopulmonary resuscitation, and an extensive guide to identifying drugs; the drug list is very useful as a quick reference.

In general, *Field Guide Reference for Emergency Care Providers* achieves its goal as a pocket reference; however, the pharmacology review is not likely to be needed on a regular basis. Using common emergency drugs to describe pharmacologic and pharmacokinetic parameters makes the basic science of emergency care more understandable. Although fairly detailed, the drug monographs are readable and understandable. The information in the book is pertinent to paramedical practice but is useful also to emergency-care providers, such as nurses and pharmacists, in any setting.

Reviewed by Judith Jacobi, Pharm.D., Pharmacy Services, St. Vincent Hospital and Health Care Center, 2001 West 86th Street, Indianapolis, IN 46240.

Advertising Index

Adria Laboratories
Idamycin, 5–7
American Diabetes Association
Institutional, 13
American Society of Hospital Pharmacists
Aseptic Preparation of Parenteral Products, 67
Concepts in Immunology and Immunotherapeutics, 13
Criteria for Drug Use Evaluation, Volumes 1 and 2, inside front cover
Pocket Guide to Injectable Drugs, 1991 Edition, 70
Burroughs Wellcome Company
Zovirax IV, 76–78
Department of Veterans Affairs (Richmond)
Positions Available, 73
Harrisburg Hospital
Position Available, 11
Eli Lilly and Company
Hospital Division, 3
San Francisco VA Medical Center
Position Available, 13
SmithKline Beecham
Tagamet, inside back cover, outside back cover
St. Jude Children's Research Hospital
Institutional, 11
The University of Rhode Island
Position Available, 11
The Upjohn Company and Chugai-Upjohn, Inc.
Marogen, 79

News

Consensus panel considers uses of botulinum toxin 88

FDA bans 223 ingredients in nonprescription drug products 88

Report on pain management in childhood cancer published 93

Consensus report focuses on hypertension during pregnancy 93

News Briefs 94

Upcoming Specialty Meetings 94

Consensus panel considers uses of botulinum toxin

Local injections of botulinum neurotoxin type A are useful in the treatment of selected disorders characterized by muscle hyperactivity, concluded the expert panel of a National Institutes of Health Consensus Development Conference on Clinical Use of Botulinum Toxin, held in Bethesda, Maryland, November 12–14. These disorders include various neurological, ophthalmic, and voice and speech disorders.

Panelists considered botulinum toxin to be safe and effective for symptomatic management of essential blepharospasm, strabismus, hemifacial spasm, predominantly adductor spasmodic dysphonia, jaw-closing oromandibular dystonia, and cervical dystonia. The toxin was described as a promising therapy for other oromandibular dystonias, focal and segmental limb dystonias, abductor spasmodic dysphonia, stuttering, and vocal tremors. Preliminary data suggest possible uses in the management of urinary and anal sphincter dysfunction, spasticity, and dynamic deformities associated with some cases of cerebral palsy.

According to the panel's statement, botulinum toxin may be the treatment of choice for focal dystonias, which typically respond poorly to conventional therapy. When generalized disorders are treated with botulinum toxin, injections should be limited to severely affected muscle groups to avoid excessive doses of toxin. Relative contraindications to therapy include diseases of neuromuscular transmission and coagulopathy, including anticoagulant therapy.

Efficacy is related primarily to the toxin's ability to block peripheral neuromuscular transmission. Effects include muscle paralysis, atrophy, and electromyographic abnormalities. Single doses larger than 500 mouse units can produce symptoms of botulism. No drugs that counteract the neuromuscular blockade produced by the toxin are currently available. Concurrent administration of agents that potentiate neuromuscular blockade (e.g., aminoglycosides) should be avoided. Information on the chronic effects of long-term therapy are lacking; thus, long-term follow-up is needed.

Most of the recognized uses of botulinum toxin dictate management by an interdisciplinary team appropriately trained in the use of the toxin.

FDA bans 223 ingredients in nonprescription drug products

FDA has banned 223 substances included as active ingredients in 19 classes of nonprescription drug products.

Continued on page 93

Continued from page 88

Proof of efficacy for the labeled indications is lacking. The rule goes into effect May 7, 1991. Among the products cited by FDA as requiring reformulation are Donnagel (Robins), which can no longer contain atropine sulfate, hyoscyamine sulfate, and scopolamine hydrobromide; and Tegrin lotion (Block), which can no longer contain allantoin. The following ingredients are covered by the rule:

- **Topical acne drug products:** alcloxa, alkyl isoquinolinium bromide, aluminum chlorohydrex, aluminum hydroxide, benzocaine, benzoic acid, boric acid, calcium polysulfide, calcium thiosulfate, camphor, chlorhydroxyquinoline, chloroxylenol, coal tar, dibenzothiophene, estrone, magnesium aluminum silicate, magnesium sulfate, phenol, phenolate sodium, phenyl salicylate, pyrilamine maleate, resorcinol, resorcinol monoacetate, sodium borate, sodium thiosulfate, tetracaine hydrochloride, vitamin E, zinc oxide, zinc stearate, zinc sulfide, povidone–iodine, salicylic acid (>2% to 5%), and thymol
- **Anticaries drug products:** acidulated sodium phosphate, sodium carbonate, sodium monofluorophosphate (6% rinse), sodium phosphate, and hydrogen fluoride
- **Antidiarrheal drug products:** glycine, scopolamine hydrobromide, aluminum hydroxide, atropine sulfate, calcium carbonate, carboxymethylcellulose, homatropine methylbromide, hyoscyamine sulfate, *Lactobacillus acidophilus*, *Lactobacillus bulgaricus*, powdered opium, opium tincture, paregoric, phenyl salicylate, and zinc phenolsulfonate
- **Antiperspirant drug products:** aluminum bromohydrate, aluminum chloride (alcoholic solutions), alum–potassium, aluminum chloride (aqueous solution) (aerosol only), aluminum sulfate, buffered aluminum sulfate (aerosol only), and sodium aluminum chlorohydroxy lactate
- **Boil treatment drug products:** aminacrine hydrochloride, bismuth subnitrate, calomel, cholesterol, ergot fluidextract, hexachlorophene, isobutamben, lanolin, menthol, methyl salicylate, oxyquinoline sulfate, petrolatum, pine tar, rosin, rosin cerate, sassafras oil, thymol, zinc oxide, camphor, juniper tar, magnesium sulfate, and phenol
- **Cold, cough, allergy, bronchodilator, and antiasthmatic drug products:** *Antihistamine drug products:* methapyrilene hydrochloride, methapyrilene fumarate, and thenyldiamine; *Nasal decongestant drug products:* allyl isothiocyanate, turpentine oil, camphor (lozenge), creosote–beechwood (oral), eucalyptol (lozenge), eucalyptol (mouthwash), eucalyptus oil (lozenge), eucalyptus oil (mouthwash), menthol (mouthwash), peppermint oil (mouthwash), thenyldiamine, thymol, thymol (lozenge), and thymol (mouthwash)
- **Dandruff, seborrheic dermatitis, and psoriasis drug products:** boric acid, colloidal oatmeal, cresol saponated, mercury oleate, resorcinol, sodium borate, alkyl isoquinolinium, allantoin, benzalkonium chloride, benzethonium chloride, calcium undecylenate, captan, chloroxylenol, ethohexadiol, eucalyptol, juniper tar, lauryl isoquinolinium, menthol, methylbenzethonium, methyl salicylate, phenol, phenolate sodium, pine tar, povidone–iodine, sodium salicylate, thymol, and undecylenic acid
- **Digestive aid drug products:** bismuth sodium tartrate, cellulase, dehydrocholic acid, duodenal substance, dehydrated garlic, glutamic acid, homatropine, ox bile extract, pancreatin, pancrelipase, papain, pepsin, sorbitol, calcium carbonate, dihydroxyaluminum, hemicellulase, magnesium hydroxide, magnesium trisilicate, peppermint oil, sodium bicarbonate, and sodium citrate
- **Exocrine pancreatic insufficiency drug products:** hemicellulase
- **External analgesic drug products:** *Analgesic and anesthetic drug products:* chloral hydrate, methapyrilene hydrochloride, aspirin, chlorobutanol, cyclomethycaine sulfate, eugenol, hexylresorcinol, salicylamide, and thymol; *Counterirritant drug products:* chloral hydrate and eucalyptus oil; *Male genital desensitizer drug products:* benzyl alcohol, camphorated metacresol, and ephedrine hydrochloride
- **Ingrown toenail relief drug products:** chloroxylenol and urea
- **Laxative drug products:** *Bulk laxatives:* carrageenan (degraded), agar, carrageenan (native), and guar gum; *Saline laxatives:* tartaric acid; *Stool softeners:* poloxamer 188; *Stimulant laxatives:* calomel, colocynth, elaterin resin, gamboge, ipomea, jalap, podophyllum resin, aloin, bile salts or acids, calcium pantothenate, frangula, ox bile, prune concentrate, prune powder, Chinese rhubarb, and sodium oleate
- **Nail-biting and thumb-sucking deterrent drug products:** denatonium benzoate
- **Oral health-care drug products (nonantimicrobial):** antipyrine, camphor, cresol, dibucaine, dibucaine hydrochloride, lidocaine, lidocaine hydrochloride, myrrh tincture, pyrilamine maleate, tetracaine, tetracaine hydrochloride, eucalyptol, methyl salicylate, sorbitol, sugars, and thymol
- **Topical otic drug products for the prevention of swimmer's ear:** acetic acid
- **Poison treatment drug products:** ipecac fluidextract, ipecac tincture, zinc sulfate
- **Skin bleaching drug products:** ammoniated mercury
- **Skin protectant drug products:** *General:* sulfur and tannic acid; *Wound healing products:* allantoin and zinc acetate
- **Smoking deterrent drug products:** clove, coriander, eucalyptus oil, ginger Jamaica, terpeneless lemon oil, licorice root extract, menthol, methyl salicylate, quinine ascorbate, silver nitrate, and thymol

Report on pain management in childhood cancer published

The report of a consensus conference on the management of pain in childhood cancer has been published.[1] Included in the report are statements on pain assessment techniques, pharmacologic and nonpharmacologic management of disease-related pain, and management of pain associated with medical procedures; a list of research priorities in each of these areas; a summary of the conference recommendations; and a list of suggested readings. The conference, held October 19–20, 1988, was sponsored by the World Health Organization Collaborating Center for Symptom Evaluation, Madison, Wisconsin; the University of Connecticut Children's Cancer Fund, Farmington, Connecticut; and Saint Francis Hospital and Medical Center, Hartford, Connecticut.

1. Report of the Consensus Conference on the Management of Pain in Childhood Cancer. *Pediatrics.* 1990; 86:813–34.

Consensus report focuses on hypertension during pregnancy

The consensus report of the National High Blood Pressure Education Program Working Group on High Blood Pressure in Pregnancy has been released.[1] The report focuses on chronic (pre-existing) hypertension, preeclampsia, preeclampsia superimposed on chronic hypertension, and transient hypertension during pregnancy. The pathophysiology of hypertensive disorders during pregnancy is described, and guidelines for diagnosis and management are presented.

Continued on page 94

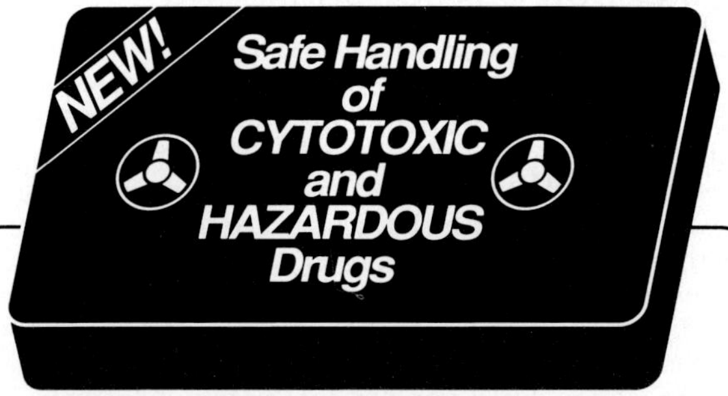

News *Continued from page 93*

1. National High Blood Pressure Education Program Working Group Report on High Blood Pressure in Pregnancy. *Am J Obstet Gynecol.* 1990; 163:1689–712.

News Briefs

• Labeled indications for **alprazolam** (Xanax, The Upjohn Company) have been expanded to include panic disorder with or without agoraphobia. The recommended starting dosage is 0.5 mg three times daily. A mean daily dosage of 5–6 mg was required in clinical trials. Upjohn has agreed to conduct postmarketing studies of the effects of drug withdrawal.

• **Toxicity warnings for sodium nitroprusside products** have been strengthened. The revised labeling draws attention to the potential for cyanide toxicity and the need for patient monitoring during therapy.

• FDA has advised consumers to discontinue use of **γ-hydroxybutyric acid** because symptoms ranging from nausea and vomiting to respiratory distress, seizures, and coma have been associated with its use. The chemical is being promoted for body building, strength training, and weight loss and as a replacement for L-tryptophan.

Upcoming Specialty Meetings

American Society for Clinical Nutrition. Seattle, WA, May 2–3; contact ASCN, 9650 Rockville Pike, Bethesda, MD 20814; 301-530-7110.

Society of General Internal Medicine. Arlington, VA, May 2–4; contact E. M. Rhodes, 655 15th Street N.W., Suite 425, Washington, DC 20005; 202-393-1662.

Society for Academic Emergency Medicine. Washington, DC, May 11–14; contact SAEM, 900 West Ottawa, Lansing. MI 48915; 517-485-5484.

American Gastroenterological Association. New Orleans, LA, May 18–24; contact S. M. Szmaciasz, 69600 Grove Road, Thorofare, NJ 08086; 609-848-9218.

International Symposium on Recent Advances in Otitis Media (5th). Bal Harbour, FL, May 20–23; contact D. J. Lim, M.D., 4331 University Hospitals Clinic, 456 West 10th Avenue, Columbus, OH 43210; (fax) 614-293-5506.

Trends in the Management of Systemic Fungal Infections. Nijmegen, the Netherlands, September 5–7; contact Imedex, Bruistensingel 144, P.O. Box 3283, 5203 DG 's-Hertogenbosch, the Netherlands; +31-73-408304 or (fax) +31-73-414766.

Fifth European Congress of Clinical Microbiology and Infectious Diseases. Oslo, Norway, September 9–11; contact Congress Secretariat, Congress–Conference, P.O. Box 7609 Skillebekk, N-0205 Oslo 2, Norway; +47-2-561930 or (fax) +47-2-560541.

Drug Reviews

Levamisole in the adjuvant treatment of colon cancer

REBECCA S. MUTCH AND PAUL R. HUTSON

Abstract: The chemistry, pharmacology, pharmacokinetics, assay methodologies, adverse effects, and dosage of levamisole are described, and the clinical studies of levamisole therapy in patients with colorectal carcinoma are reviewed.

Levamisole is a synthetic, orally active agent that has antihelmintic and immunomodulatory properties. It is capable of inducing T-cell differentiation and restoring depressed effector functions of peripheral lymphocytes and phagocytes to normal. The drug is well absorbed from the gastrointestinal tract after oral administration and is extensively metabolized by the liver. Gas chromatography and high-performance liquid chromatography are the most common methods used to measure concentrations of levamisole in biologic fluids.

Levamisole combined with fluorouracil has been associated with a one-third reduction in recurrence and risk of death in patients with surgically resected Dukes stage C colon cancer; this combination is now recommended as standard therapy in these patients. Uses in patients with rectal carcinoma, Dukes stage B colon cancer, metastatic colon cancer, other malignancies, or nonmalignant disorders remain investigational. Common adverse effects include nausea, abdominal pain, vomiting, diarrhea, metallic or altered taste, flu-like symptoms, mood elevation, insomnia, hyperalertness, dizziness, and headache. The most serious adverse effect associated with levamisole is granulocytopenia. The FDA-approved dosage of levamisole is 50 mg orally every eight hours for three days every two weeks. Levamisole therapy is to be initiated no earlier than 7 and no later than 30 days after surgery and is to be continued for one year.

Levamisole combined with fluorouracil has been associated with a one-third reduction in recurrence and risk of death in patients with resected stage C colon cancer. Further research is needed to more clearly define the mechanism of action, optimum dose and scheduling, and clinical efficacy of levamisole in treating other malignancies.

Index terms: Antineoplastic agents; Colonic neoplasms; Colorectal neoplasms; Combined therapy; Dosage; Fluorouracil; Levamisole; Pharmacokinetics; Toxicity
Clin Pharm. 1991; 10:95–109

Levamisole is the result of Janssen Pharmaceutica's 1960s efforts to design a synthetic antihelmintic agent for veterinary and human use that would be active against both parasitic worms and their larvae.[1,2] Scientific interest in the immunotherapeutic effect of this drug was sparked in 1971 when Renoux and Renoux showed that the protective effect of a *Brucella* vaccine in mice could be augmented by levamisole.[3-5] A host immune response was postulated because levamisole alone had no effect on the *Brucella abortus* organism.

Chemoimmunotherapy regimens in conjunction with complete surgical resection have long been investigated in colorectal carcinoma.[6-9] Although some trials have reported favorable results with levamisole, low patient numbers, varied methodology, and improper patient stratification have hampered conclusions regarding the overall effect of levamisole therapy on this disease. Recently a large cooperative group study involving more than

REBECCA S. MUTCH, PHARM.D., is Coordinator, Investigational Drug Services, University of Wisconsin Hospital and Clinics, Madison; when this manuscript was prepared, she was Fellow in Oncology Pharmacy, School of Pharmacy, University of Wisconsin–Madison. PAUL R. HUTSON, PHARM.D., is Assistant Professor, School of Pharmacy, University of Wisconsin–Madison.

Address reprint requests to Dr. Hutson at the School of Pharmacy, University of Wisconsin–Madison, 425 North Charter Street, Madison, WI 53706.

The assistance of Audrey Fish in manuscript preparation is acknowledged.

This is article **680-204-9104** in the **ASHP Continuing-Education System;** it qualifies for 1.0 hour of continuing-education credit. See page 147 for learning objectives and test questions.

1200 patients reported unequivocal benefit in patients with Dukes stage C colon cancer who were treated after surgery with the adjuvant therapy of fluorouracil and levamisole.[10] This report led the National Cancer Institute to issue a position statement that the combination of fluorouracil and levamisole should be considered standard adjuvant therapy for Dukes C colon carcinoma.[11]

The purpose of this paper is to review the pharmacology, pharmacokinetics, adverse effects, and clinical efficacy of levamisole in patients who have colorectal carcinoma. For the purposes of this review, only those clinical trials pertaining to levamisole's use in colorectal carcinoma will be discussed. The reader is referred to references 12–23 for reviews and information regarding the investigational use of levamisole in patients with other malignant diseases or disease states.

Chemistry

Levamisole ((−)-(*S*)-2,3,5,6-tetrahydro-6-phenylimidazo (2,1-*b*) thiazole monohydrochloride) (Figure 1) is the biologically active levoisomer of the synthetic drug tetramisole. Levamisole possesses two active moieties, an imidazole ring and thiazolidine ring, and has a molecular weight of 240.75 and a formula of $C_{11}H_{12}N_2S{\cdot}HCl$. Levamisole hydrochloride is soluble in water and stable in acid aqueous media, but it hydrolyzes in alkaline or neutral solutions.[16,24]

Pharmacology

Antihelmintic Activity. Levamisole has been used for over 20 years to treat intestinal nematodes in both human and veterinary medicine.[16,20,22,25] Antihelmintic activity is accomplished through one or both of two disparate mechanisms. Levamisole stimulates parasympathetic and sympathetic ganglia, causing spastic contractions of nematode neuromusculature and depolarizing paralysis. Additionally, levamisole interferes with nematode energy metabolism. Many species of nematodes have fumarate-dependent anaerobic metabolism and are highly susceptible to inhibition of fumarate reductase by levamisole.

Immunologic Activity. The mechanism by which levamisole affects the human immune system is complex and not yet fully understood. The majority of in vivo and in vitro data suggest that levamisole acts as an immunorestorative agent; it is capable of augmenting a depressed host immune system but is incapable of hyperstimulating an intact system.[3–5,15,26,27] Table 1 summarizes the immunologic effects of levamisole. Levamisole has been shown to stimulate precursor T lymphocytes to differentiate into mature T cells and to restore depressed effector functions of peripheral lymphocytes and phagocytes to normal. Effector lymphocyte functions stimulated by levamisole include mitogen-induced T-cell proliferation, E-rosette-forming capacity, T-cell cytotoxicity, lymphokine and interferon production, and restoration of delayed-type hypersensitivity reactions in anergic patients. Exposure of effector phagocytes to levamisole has resulted in enhanced migration, adherence, chemotaxis, phagocytosis, peroxidase activity, and intracellular killing by monocytes, macrophages, and neutrophils. Levamisole does not appear to have any direct effect on B lymphocytes or antibody production, does not possess direct antitumor effects, and does not enhance natural killer or killer cell activity.[29,30]

Although the mechanisms by which levamisole induces the above effects on the immune system are not known, several theories have been proposed. Renoux and others[3,4,16,31–33] have suggested

Figure 1. Structures of (a) levamisole, (b) 4-hydroxylevamisole, and (c) D,L-oxo-3-(2-mercapto-ethyl)-5-phenyl-imidazolidine (OMPI).

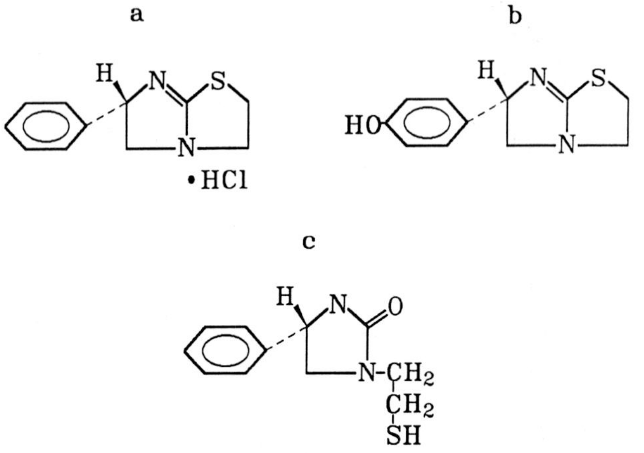

Table 1.
Immunomodulatory Properties of Levamisole[a]

- Increased E-rosette capacity (total and active)
- Increased spontaneous, mitogen-induced, or antigen-induced proliferation of T cells
- Enhanced T-cell cytotoxicity
- Enhanced phagocyte proliferation
- Enhanced antibody plaque cell formation
- Stimulation of lymphokine and interferon production
- Restoration of delayed-type hypersensitivity reactions
- Stimulation of DNA synthesis in murine splenocytes
- In vitro stimulation of blastogenesis of murine splenocytes in response to phytohemagglutinin challenge
- Enhanced antibody and complement receptor activity
- Enhanced release of colony-stimulating factor by monocytes (increased granulopoiesis)
- Increased neutrophil motility, adherence, and chemotaxis
- Increased phagocytosis
- Stimulation of neutrophil nitro blue tetrazolium reduction and phosphodiesterase and peroxidase activities
- Enhanced host resistance to infections

[a] Adapted from reference 28. Used with permission.

that at least some of the in vivo effects of levamisole are mediated through an undefined dialyzable serum factor that emulates the thymic hormone. Animal studies have demonstrated that levamisole is capable of inducing T-cell differentiation of precursor spleen cells of congenitally athymic mice in vivo but not in vitro. When injected into untreated animals, serum from levamisole-treated animals can produce the same T-cell differentiation effects as well as in vitro thymocyte maturation, an ability shared with thymic hormones. Transfer of residual levamisole, a metabolite, or serum complement was ruled out as a confounding factor in these phenomena. These effects can be explained by a thymus-independent serum factor released by an unidentified cell. This serum factor is not found in animals that fail to respond to levamisole or in untreated animals.

Levamisole may also modify intracellular concentrations of the cyclic nucleotides adenosine monophosphate (cAMP) and guanosine monophosphate (cGMP).[3,4,5,16,34,35] Changes in lymphocyte and macrophage cyclic nucleotide levels can be demonstrated during normal immune responses. Elevated cGMP within lymphocytes and phagocytes is correlated with increased cellular proliferation, enhanced cell-surface antigen expression and receptor activity, granulocyte chemotaxis, and macrophage activity. In contrast, augmentation of intracellular levels of cAMP reduces such leukocyte function. Levamisole induces a rise in cGMP levels or a decline in cAMP levels, or both, within lymphocytes and macrophages. The immunostimulatory effects of levamisole in vivo may therefore be explained by an increase of the intracellular cGMP:cAMP ratio within effector cells of the immune system.

The structure of levamisole is the basis for two additional theories. Cholinergic effects of the imidazole ring elevate cGMP levels in lymphocytes in vitro, resulting in an enhanced proliferative response to mitogens and foreign cells.[3,4] Partial hydrolysis of the sulfur ring of levamisole, thought to occur spontaneously under alkaline conditions in vitro and probably in vivo, exposes a free thiol group with antioxidant effects.[3,4,12,36] The resulting compound, D,L-2-oxo-3-(2-mercapto-ethyl)-5-phenyl-imidazolidine (OMPI), is one of the major metabolites of levamisole identified in various animal studies. Both levamisole and OMPI protect glutathione-depleted cells from auto-oxidative necrosis, although OMPI is nearly 100 times more active in this respect. Additionally, polymerization of tubulin and functional microtubule integrity in cultured cells appear to be enhanced more by OMPI than by levamisole. It has thus been proposed that levamisole or its metabolite, or both, may enhance normal cell function by reduction of intracellular peroxides, enhancement of microtubule integrity and function, and scavenging of deleterious oxidative radicals. It should be noted that OMPI has not been identified as a metabolite of levamisole in humans. Other pharmacologic effects of levamisole not clearly related to immunomodulator function include alkaline phosphatase inhibition,[37] cholinergic activity, mild mood elevation, and an anticonvulsant effect.[4]

The positive interaction between fluorouracil and levamisole observed in the most recent colorectal cancer studies remains mechanistically unclear, but it may be due to the restorative effects of levamisole on depressed cell-mediated immune responses.[38] Patients with colorectal cancer have been shown to have depressed cellular immunity immediately after surgery and in cases of advanced disease.[4,15,38] Additionally, fluorouracil itself has immunosuppressive properties.[39] The rationale for using levamisole has been based on the general observation that positive delayed-hypersensitivity (cell-mediated) reactions correlate with a more favorable prognosis after surgery in cancer patients.[40] Other investigators have suggested that levamisole hastens recovery from myelosuppression, allowing the maximum dose intensity of fluorouracil chemotherapy.[16,34,41] The positive interaction of fluorouracil and levamisole may also arise from direct inhibition of alkaline phosphatase by levamisole.[38] Resistance to fluorouracil in some cancer cells has been reported to result from accelerated catabolism of active metabolites, such as fluorodeoxyuridine monophosphate (FdUMP), by enhanced phosphatase activity.[42] Theoretically, levamisole might enhance fluorouracil activity by inhibiting the enzyme alkaline phosphatase and prolonging the intracellular half-life of the active metabolites, such as FdUMP. The therapeutic synergism of fluorouracil and levamisole cannot be explained by direct cytotoxicity of levamisole. Grem et al.[38] studied the cytotoxicity of levamisole, alone and in combination with fluorouracil, against three colorectal carcinoma cell lines at clinically relevant concentrations. The results of this study showed no evidence of direct toxicity by levamisole, and an additive interaction with fluorouracil was achieved only at suprapharmacologic doses of levamisole. Finally, measurement of immunologic variables in vivo before and after levamisole treatment has revealed no single immunologic factor that is useful in monitoring levamisole treatment in cancer patients.[16,28]

Although little is known about the mechanism of immunomodulation by levamisole, several general points have emerged from immunopharmacologic studies: (1) immunostimulant effects are dose and schedule dependent; (2) levamisole appears to be more active against metastases than against primary tumors; and (3) levamisole is more effective when combined with chemotherapy (e.g., fluorouracil) than when used alone.[15,28] Target immune effector cells remain unidentified, and the process

Table 2.
Reported Pharmacokinetic Values for Levamisole in Healthy Subjects[a]

Variable[b]	Adams[43,c]	Kouassi et al.[36,d]	Luyckx et al.[44,d]
Dose	150 mg	150 mg	2.5 mg/kg
C_{max} (mg/L)	0.76 ± 0.12	0.72 ± 0.22	0.71 ± 0.05
t_{max} (hr)	1.27 ± 0.12	1.52 ± 0.49	1.94 ± 0.16
$t_{1/2_{abs}}$ (hr)		0.55 ± 0.24	0.37 ± 0.07
$t_{1/2}$ (hr)	4.4 ± 0.7	5.56 ± 2.46	5.06 ± 0.88
AUC (mg·hr/L)	4.15 ± 1.04[e]	3.07 ± 1.32	6.83 ± 1.10
F		0.62 ± .10	0.68 ± 0.3
V (L)		266.3 ± 120.3	109.7 ± 10.2
CL_{tot} (L/hr)		33.8 ± 9.0	17.8 ± 1.9
CL_{renal} (L/hr)		1.75 ± 1.71	
Unchanged levamisole in urine (% dose administered)	~6.0	3.17 ± 2.92	

[a] Most values are reported as mean ± S.D.
[b] C_{max} = peak plasma concentration; t_{max} = time of peak plasma concentration; $t_{1/2_{abs}}$ = absorption half-life; AUC = area under the plasma concentration–time curve extrapolated to infinity; $t_{1/2}$ = elimination half-life; F = bioavailability (estimated); V = apparent volume of distribution; CL_{tot} = total body clearance; CL_{renal} = renal clearance.
[c] Radiometric assay.
[d] Gas–liquid chromatographic assay.
[e] Area under the plasma concentration–time curve from 0 to 24 hours.

by which levamisole potentiates the effect of fluorouracil in colon cancer is not known.

Pharmacokinetics

Information on the pharmacokinetic properties and metabolic fate of levamisole is limited, with much of the data derived from animal studies. Table 2 summarizes the pharmacokinetic values from three pharmacokinetic studies of levamisole in humans.

Absorption. Levamisole is reported to undergo rapid and complete absorption, with oral doses of 150 mg producing peak plasma concentrations of 0.5–0.8 μg/mL within one to three hours.[45] The absolute bioavailability of levamisole has not yet been experimentally determined in humans. Although two human studies reported similar bioavailability data (fraction absorbed, approximately 0.6–0.7),[36,44] both values were based on oral dose data and were estimated by the method of Gibaldi et al.[46] which requires an assumption about hepatic blood flow.

Pharmacokinetic values of levamisole may vary between men and women. Levamisole is absorbed approximately twice as rapidly in women as in men according to Kouassi et al.,[36] who found no other marked gender differences. Luyckx et al.[44] noted gender differences in the fraction absorbed and in the area under the plasma concentration–time curve extrapolated to infinity; however, these differences were not statistically significant in all cases. Neither group could conclude that gender differences influenced the elimination of levamisole.

Distribution. Levamisole is widely distributed in animals, with the highest tissue concentrations occurring in the liver and kidneys.[43] The distribution volume of the drug in humans is large (100–266 L), indicating extensive binding to tissue.[45] No information describing binding of levamisole to human plasma proteins is currently available.

Metabolism. Four principal routes of metabolism have been identified in studies of levamisole in rats.[43] Type I metabolism includes the 4-hydroxylation of the phenyl ring and hydrolysis of the thiazolidine ring to expose a primary thiol, yielding OMPI. The parent drug and identified metabolites also undergo glucuronidation.[43]

Levamisole is extensively metabolized by the liver in humans, with less than 6% of the administered dose appearing unchanged in the urine and feces.[45] Only one urinary metabolite, 4-hydroxylevamisole, has been identified in humans. Kouassi et al.[36] detected two unidentified urinary products in their study of healthy volunteers given oral levamisole. Twenty-four-hour urinary excretion of 4-hydroxylevamisole accounted for 1.6% of the levamisole dose administered.[36] Recovery values rose to 12.4% when conjugates in urine were hydrolyzed with β-glucuronidase. Therefore, hydroxylation and subsequent glucuronidation of levamisole constitute an important metabolic pathway for levamisole in humans. Antihelmintic and immunotherapeutic effects of hydroxylevamisole have not been reported.

Elimination. Levamisole disappears from plasma rapidly, with a terminal elimination half-life of approximately four hours. Systemic clearance is reported to be 17.8 to 33.8 L/hr, whereas the renal clearance averages 1.8 L/hr. Acidified urine increases the renal clearance of levamisole because of the weakly basic nature of the drug and its metabolites.[36]

The elimination of levamisole is reported to be best described by a monoexponential equation.[36,44] Inspection of the concentration versus time plots reported in the literature strongly suggests that a second elimination phase may exist. The weighting of data used in curve fitting was not described, nor were the criteria used to determine the optimal model. No human pharmacokinetic studies were found that evaluated plasma levamisole concentrations beyond 24 hours.

The pharmacokinetics of levamisole in patients with renal or hepatic failure has not been studied. The relatively low renal clearance of the drug suggests that dosage adjustments are not necessary in patients with impaired renal function. Luyckx et al.[44] found no significant differences in levamisole pharmacokinetics between healthy volunteers and cancer patients. There are no reports describing the effect of levamisole on the activity of the hepatic mixed-function oxidase (cytochrome P-450) enzyme system.

Assay Methodologies

Gas chromatography (GC) and high-performance liquid chromatography (HPLC) are the most common methods used to measure concentrations of levamisole in biologic fluids. Polarography has been used in the past, but its use is uncommon today.[47] There is little difference between the two most recently described GC assays.[48,49] Alkali flame ionization detection of nitrogen after separation on 3% OV-17 packing is used in both assays, with sensitivity reported to be 5–10 ng/mL from 1 mL of plasma.

Trimipramine, flurazepam, and the *p*-methyl analogue of levamisole have been used as internal standards for GC and HPLC assays.[36,48,50] The detection limit of the Alvinernie HPLC method (50 ng/mL from 0.5 mL of plasma) is approximately three times higher than that reported for GC methods.[50] Increased sensitivity may be possible by measuring ultraviolet absorption at 214 nm (the wavelength at which absorption of light is maximal for levamisole).[51]

Most published assay methods involve sample preparation with alkaline extraction into hexane and ether or hexane and isoamyl alcohol, acidic back-extraction, another alkaline extraction into an organic phase, and subsequent concentration or drying. Woestenborghs et al.[49] reported a levamisole recovery rate of 86% using solid-phase extraction.

Levamisole has been shown to bind to glass, necessitating silanization of glassware and GC column packing.[44,48,49] Although not specifically addressed, end-capping silanization of reverse-phase HPLC columns would also be prudent.

4-Hydroxylevamisole is the only metabolite of levamisole identified in humans. Kouassi et al.[36] found no 4-hydroxylevamisole in the plasma of patients, although it was found in urine. 4-Hydroxylevamisole is extracted with levamisole in a single, alkaline extraction into an organic phase, but it is not coextracted when the more typical double back-extraction is performed. In contrast, the double back-extraction of urine did yield two unidentified compounds that are apparently metabolites of levamisole.[36] The extent to which these unidentified metabolites may be glucuronidated apparently was not examined.

Levamisole is known to undergo thiazolidine ring opening under alkaline conditions to form OMPI. No mention is made of any attempts to identify OMPI or its conjugate in published assays of levamisole in human plasma or urine. The two alkaline extractions of levamisole used in several published assay methods could conceivably result in hydrolysis and ring opening, leading to in vitro formation of OMPI.

Clinical Use and Efficacy

Currently, the only indication for levamisole is as adjuvant treatment combined with fluorouracil in patients with surgically resected Dukes stage C colon cancer. Other uses discussed in this section remain investigational.

Colon and Rectal Cancer. Cancer of the colon affects approximately 110,000 persons in the United States annually and is second only to cancer of the lung as the most common cause of cancer deaths.[52] Surgical excision is the primary treatment of colon cancer, because approximately 80% of patients are diagnosed at a stage when all gross tumor can be surgically removed.[53] Despite apparent curative resection, nearly 50% of patients with operable colon cancer develop recurrent disease and die from metastatic disease.

The prognosis of patients with colon cancer is closely related to the degree of tumor penetration through the colonic wall at the time of diagnosis.[6,53–55] Most commonly this penetration is assessed by the Dukes classification system or its later modifications (Table 3). However the TNM (Primary Tumor Size, Regional Lymph Nodes, Distant Metastasis) system of the American Joint Committee on the Staging of Cancer is now being advocated for classifying stages of colon cancer (Table 4).[56] Patients with regional lymph node involvement (Dukes stage C: any T, N1–3, M0) are at high risk of recurrence after curative surgical resection of primary and nodal lesions, and they have an overall survival rate of approximately 33%.[53] Surgical failure is often due to small, often microscopic metastases present at the time of surgery, and it has prompted the search for more effective postsurgical therapies, including chemotherapy and immunotherapy. Treatment directed at occult disease after apparently complete removal of disease is

Table 3.
Dukes Classification of Adenocarcinoma of the Colon[a]

Stage	Tumor Properties	Five-Year Patient Survival (%)
A	Invasion into submucosa or into	95
	muscularis propria	90
B	B_1: invasion through muscularis propria into subserosa	60–80
	B_2: invasion through serosa	50
	B_3: involvement of adjacent structures	30
C	Involvement of regional nodes	
	1–4 nodes	56
	>4 nodes	26
D	Distant metastatic disease	5

[a] Originally published in: Grem JL. Levamisole as a therapeutic agent for colorectal carcinoma. *Cancer Cells.* 1990; 2:131–7. Reprinted with permission.

Table 4.
Tumor/Node/Metastasis (TNM) Staging and Dukes Classification[56]

Stage	Tumor/Node/Metastasis Staging: Tumor[a]	Node[b]	Metastasis[c]	Dukes Classification
0	Tis	N0	M0	
I	T1	N0	M0	A
	T2	N0	M0	A
II	T3	N0	M0	B
	T4	N0	M0	B
III	Any T	N1	M0	C
	Any T	N2, N3	M0	C
IV	Any T	Any N	M1	

[a] Staging system for primary tumor: TX = primary tumor cannot be assessed; T0 = no evidence of primary tumor; Tis = carcinoma in situ; T1 = tumor invades submucosa; T2 = tumor invades muscularis propria; T3 = tumor invades through the muscularis propria into the subserosa, or into nonperitonealized pericolic or perirectal tissues; T4 = tumor perforates the visceral peritoneum or directly invades other organs or structures.

[b] Staging system for regional lymph nodes: NX = regional lymph nodes cannot be assessed; N0 = no regional lymph node metastasis; N1 = metastasis in one to three pericolic or perirectal lymph nodes; N2 = metastasis in four or more pericolic or perirectal lymph nodes; N3 = metastasis in any lymph node along the course of a named vascular trunk.

[c] Staging system for distant metastases: MX = presence of distant metastasis cannot be assessed; M0 = no distant metastasis; M1 = distant metastasis.

termed adjuvant therapy. The most commonly used adjuvant chemotherapeutic agent, fluorouracil, has produced a small therapeutic benefit in terms of overall survival (i.e., a 3.4% higher five-year survival rate than that achieved with surgery alone).[6,55] Various forms of immunotherapy, including levamisole, have been explored in adjuvant therapy as a means of improving the clinical outcome of patients with colon cancer.

It is important to note that rectal carcinoma, which affects nearly 45,000 persons in the United States annually, differs from colon cancer in its natural course and patterns of failure.[56] Because of anatomic constraints in obtaining wide radial margins during rectal resection, local or regional failure as the only or first site of recurrence is common. Local recurrence occurs in approximately 25% of patients with Dukes B_2 rectal cancer and 50% of patients with Dukes C rectal cancer.[54] Patients with locally invasive rectal cancer may experience systemic relapse similar to that experienced by patients with advanced colon cancer. In contrast, colon cancer has fewer surgical limitations and tends to recur in the peritoneal cavity, the liver, or distant sites.[56] The location of the primary tumor may also be prognostic for ultimate survival, with rectal cancer patients generally having a lower five-year survival rate than colon cancer patients whose disease is at the same stage.[53] Inherent differences between rectal and colon cancers have resulted in separate adjuvant approaches: local control with radiotherapy and systemic chemotherapy for rectal cancer and chemotherapy versus chemoimmunotherapy for colon cancer. To appropriately evaluate the efficacy of these therapies, colon cancer and rectal cancer should be studied separately.[56] Of note, early colorectal cancer trials of levamisole frequently accrued patients with either rectal or colonic lesions, and in some trials the distribution of the primary lesion (colon versus rectal) within the treatment groups was not known.

Clinical Trials of Adjuvant Therapy in Colorectal Cancer. The results of eight clinical trials using levamisole in the adjuvant treament of surgically resectable colorectal cancer have been published and are summarized in Table 5.

Evaluating the efficacy of levamisole as adjuvant monotherapy was the primary objective of three clinical trials. Verhaegen et al.[57] enrolled 60 patients who had surgical resection of colorectal lesions and were subsequently nonrandomly assigned to either a control group (observation only) or a levamisole treatment group. The distribution of Dukes staging classification, percentage of rectal versus colonic lesions, and other patient characteristics were comparable for the two groups. The results of the survival analysis and the median disease-free interval both strongly favored the levamisole group. Seventy percent of the patients treated with levamisole were alive after five years compared with only 43% of the patients in the control group ($p = 0.028$). The median disease-free interval was 47 months for the levamisole group and 35 months for the control group. Subset analysis based on tumor location in 34 patients with primary colonic lesions revealed five-year survival rates of 62% (levamisole group) and 39% (observation only). The difference in the treatment groups reached statistical significance ($p < 0.05$) only in patients whose disease was at stages B_2 and C, with 65% of the levamisole-treated patients surviving five years compared with 35% in the observation-only group.

Table 5.
Levamisole in Adjuvant Therapy of Colorectal Cancer[a]

Reference	Dukes Stage and Primary Site	Treatment[b]	Dosage	% DFS	% Survival
57	*Dukes A, B, and C* Colon = 34 Rectum = 26	Surgery alone (*n* = 30)			43(a) (35 for B_2 and C)
		Levamisole (*n* = 30)	50 mg three times daily for 3 days every other week for 2 years		70 (65 for B_2 and C)
58	*Dukes B and C* Colon = 65 Rectum = 13	Placebo (*n* = 26)			79 B colon (b) 55 C colon
		Levamisole (*n* = 52)	2.5 mg/kg/day in 3 divided doses on days 1–2 every week for 18 months		84 B colon 46 C colon
59	*Dukes C* Colon = 287	Placebo (*n* = 145)		35(a)	39(a)
		Levamisole (*n* = 142)	Administered on days 1–2 every week for 1 year on the following body weight basis: 100 mg daily for <50 kg; 150 mg for 51–70 kg; 200 mg for 71–90 kg; and 250 mg for >90 kg	38	51
60	*Dukes B_2, B_3, and C* Colon = 373 Rectum = 28	Surgery alone (*n* = 135)		45(a) All 60 B 38 C	55(a) All 78 B 42 C
		Levamisole (*n* = 130)	50 mg every 8 hours for 3 days every 2 weeks for 1 year	58 All 77 B 50 C	59 All 78 B 52 C
		Fluorouracil plus levamisole (*n* = 136)	Same levamisole regimen as above plus fluorouracil 450 mg/sq m/day for 5 days, followed by weekly injections of 450 mg/sq m starting on day 28 for 1 year	59 All 79 B 50 C	62 All 82 B 54 C
61	*Dukes B and C* NA	Surgery alone (*n* = 19)			89(c)
		Fluorouracil (*n* = 16)	12 mg/kg orally for 5 days every 4 weeks for 12 cycles		81
		Fluorouracil plus levamisole (*n* = 17)	Same fluorouracil dosage as above plus levamisole 200 mg/day in divided doses for 2 days per week during the 3 weeks off fluorouracil		76
62	*Dukes C* Colon = 14 Rectum = 15	Semustine plus fluorouracil (*n* = 14)	325 mg/sq m of fluorouracil for 5 days every 5 weeks plus semustine 150 mg/sq m every 10 weeks for 14 cycles	50(d)	49(d)
		Semustine, fluorouracil, and levamisole (*n* = 15)	Same regimen as above plus 150 mg of levamisole for 3 days in the second and fourth weeks of the chemotherapy cycles	39	37
63	*Dukes B and C* Colon = 76 Rectum = 55	Surgery alone (*n* = 45)			48(a,e)
		Fluorouracil (*n* = 42)	1 g after surgery and on the first 2 postoperative days, then 1 g orally weekly for 6 months		56
		Fluorouracil plus levamisole (*n* = 44)	Same fluorouracil regimen as above plus 150 mg of levamisole on first 3 postoperative days		68
10	*Dukes C* Colon = 929	Surgery (*n* = 315)		47(f)	52(f)
		Levamisole (*n* = 304)	50 mg every 8 hours for 3 days every 2 weeks for 1 year	50	56
		Fluorouracil plus levamisole (*n* = 310)	Same levamisole regimen as above plus fluorouracil 450 mg/sq m/day for 5 days followed 28 days later by 450 mg/sq m every week for 48 weeks	63	71

[a] Abbreviations: % DFS = percentage of surviving patients free of disease after noted period (a–f); NA = not available; a = 5 years; b = 7 years; c = 6 months; d = 8 years; e = censored noncancer deaths; f = 3.5 years.
[b] Number of evaluable patients receiving each treatment is in parentheses.

One should interpret cautiously the dramatic results of this study, which spurred a flurry of subsequent clinical trials. Common to most of the early trials of levamisole is the criticism of small sample size. Furthermore, the use of only one surgeon to perform all of the resections and the unspecified criteria used to nonrandomly assign patients to treatment groups suggests potential bias within the study design. Others have expressed concern over the unusual survival curve, which shows no deaths in the levamisole group over a two-year period and limited data for interpretation.[55]

Two randomized double-blind studies failed to confirm the benefit of levamisole monotherapy observed by Verhaegen et al. Chlebowski et al.[58] stratified 78 patients on the basis of tumor location and Dukes classification and then randomized them to receive either levamisole or placebo. Although an initial disease-free advantage was reported for the levamisole group after 3.5 years of follow-up, no long-term survival advantage was detected at 7.5 years. Similarly Arnaud et al.[59] found no difference between levamisole-treated patients (n = 142) and placebo-treated patients (n = 145) in terms of disease-free survival or overall survival at a three-year median follow-up. In this study levamisole was administered on a weight-adjusted basis, but patients received a minimum of 2 mg/kg/day on two consecutive days each week for one year.

The remaining clinical trials addressed the efficacy of combining cytotoxic drugs with levamisole in patients with operable colorectal carcinoma. A well-designed study by Laurie et al.[60] enrolled 408 (401 evaluable) patients, stratified them according to stage of disease and tumor location, and then randomized them to the following treatment groups: (1) observation only, (2) levamisole, or (3) fluorouracil plus levamisole. Two thirds of the patients had stage C disease, and all but 21 had primary colonic lesions. At a median follow-up of 7.5 years, patients treated with fluorouracil plus levamisole and, to a lesser extent, those treated with levamisole alone were observed to have fewer recurrences than those assigned to receive observation alone. After correcting for the influence of prognostic determinants (tumor stage, primary location, and anaplasia grade), the differences in disease-free survival between the treatment groups were only suggestive for levamisole alone (p = 0.05) but were significant for the combination regimen (p = 0.003). Although survival analysis showed an overall trend for improved survival associated with both treatment regimens, these improvements reached significance only for stage C patients treated with fluorouracil plus levamisole (p = 0.03).

Bancewicz and coworkers[61] compared three treatment groups in their study of 72 patients who had surgical resection of Dukes stage B or C colorectal lesions. Treatment was initiated four to eight weeks after surgery and consisted of oral fluorouracil with or without levamisole. A third group of patients who received surgery alone served as the control group. Patients were treated for 12 months. Of the patients entered in the study, 52 were followed for 6–24 months; preliminary results were based on data from this group. The recurrence rates ranged from 16% to 29%, whereas the mean time to recurrence was 9.8 to 11.5 months. Statistically, no benefit from the use of chemotherapy and immunotherapy was detected. Concluding remarks by the authors implied continued entry of patients into the study; however, no further information is available.

Little information can be extracted from a study by Sertoli et al.,[62] which attempted to verify whether the addition of levamisole to postoperative chemotherapy (semustine [methyl-CCNU] and fluorouracil) could increase the survival or disease-free survival of patients with Dukes stage C colorectal cancer. Patients were randomly assigned to one of two treatment groups after surgical resection: (1) fluorouracil plus semustine or (2) fluorouracil, semustine, and levamisole. The authors elected to end patient accrual after entering only 29 patients. Although preliminary analysis at 18 months reported a survival benefit with levamisole, no survival difference was evident after eight years of follow-up. The small sample size is a limitation of this study.

A significant survival advantage for colorectal cancer patients treated postoperatively with levamisole and fluorouracil was reported by Windle et al.[63] After surgery, 141 patients were randomized to one of three treatment groups: control (supportive care only), fluorouracil, or fluorouracil plus levamisole. Fluorouracil was administered intravenously after surgery and on the first two postoperative days. Thereafter, fluorouracil was given orally at a dose of 1 g weekly for six months. Levamisole was given at a dose of 150 mg orally on the first three postoperative days only. All treatment groups were well matched for site of primary lesion, tumor stage, and differentiation. At a five-year minimum follow-up, the short postoperative course of levamisole combined with six months of fluorouracil therapy was found to have reduced the tumor recurrence rate. As a result, the cancer-associated death rate of patients treated with levamisole and fluorouracil was significantly lower than that reported for patients who received supportive care only (p = 0.046) or fluorouracil alone (p = 0.022). Five-year disease-specific survival rates were 68%, 56%, and 48% for fluorouracil plus levamisole, fluorouracil, and observation, respectively.

It is remarkable that three postoperative doses of levamisole in combination with fluorouracil were sufficient to confer a survival advantage, whereas fluorouracil alone produced no observable benefit over surgery alone.[63] The authors postulated that surgically induced immune suppression permits the establishment or promotion of micrometastases. In this study in vitro leukocyte migration in response to bacillus Calmette–Guérin vaccine (an indicator of cellular immunity) was suppressed below normal for 3–7 days with fluorouracil plus levamisole, 7–42 days (median, 21 days) with observation, and 7–56 days (median, 27 days) with fluorouracil alone, suggesting that levamisole substantially shortens the duration of surgical impairment of cell-mediated immunity. This study has been criticized for considering only cancer-specific survival, in that all deaths from other causes are censored.[55] The study, therefore, demonstrates a survival advantage for fluorouracil plus levamisole with respect to cancer deaths only.

These clinical trials suggest a possible benefit of levamisole either alone or in combination with fluorouracil as adjuvant therapy in patients with colorectal cancer. Clearly missing was a study that had a large sample size and a good statistical design. The promising results of the North Central Cancer Treatment Group (Laurie et al.[60]) prompted a larger national intergroup study to confirm the efficacy of adjuvant chemoimmunotherapy with levamisole or fluorouracil plus levamisole. The results of this trial were recently reported by Moertel et al.[10] A total of 1296 patients with resected adenocarcinoma of the colon, Dukes stage B_2 or C, were randomized separately to receive supportive care alone or therapy with fluorouracil and levamisole. Patients with stage C lesions could also be assigned to a third treatment group consisting of levamisole therapy alone. At the time of this report, the median follow-up was three years. The results in patients with stage B_2 disease ($n = 318$) were considered too premature to permit analysis, and an additional two years of observation appear to be required before definite conclusions can be made regarding this disease stage.

The combination therapy of fluorouracil plus levamisole significantly reduced the risk of cancer recurrence by 41% ($p < 0.0001$) and reduced the overall death rate by 33% among the 929 patients with stage C disease. Therapy with levamisole alone produced no detectable effect. Prognostic factors for recurrence included depth of invasion, number of positive regional lymph nodes, and histologic differentiation. After correction for the influence of prognostic variables, therapy with fluorouracil plus levamisole retained its significant advantage over observation in terms of recurrence ($p = 0.002$) and survival ($p = 0.005$), whereas levamisole alone had no significant advantage. These differences are clinically important, because they represent approximately a one-third reduction in recurrence and death rates in patients with stage C disease. The majority of patients were treated in the outpatient setting and generally tolerated the therapy well.

The results of this study convincingly show that adjuvant therapy with fluorouracil plus levamisole benefits patients with stage C colon carcinoma and argue for its incorporation as the standard treatment for these patients. The failure to demonstrate an outcome difference in patients with stage B_2 disease may be related to statistical limitations or to the natural course of the disease.[55] Nine hundred twenty-nine patients who had stage C disease were evaluable compared with 318 patients who had stage B_2 disease. Additionally, the five-year survival rate for patients with stage B_2 disease is generally higher than that for patients with stage C disease, implying that a longer observation time may be required to detect a difference in death rates or recurrences. One criticism of this study was the failure to incorporate a fluorouracil-only treatment group.[28,64] Such a treatment group would have allowed direct assessment of the contribution of levamisole to the beneficial effect of the combination therapy.

In summary, these studies indicate that levamisole as a single agent is of limited or no value for adjuvant treatment of colon cancer. In contrast, levamisole combined with fluorouracil has been associated with about a one-third reduction in recurrence and risk of death in patients with resected stage C colon carcinoma, and this combination is now being recommended as standard therapy for these patients. The role of levamisole therapy in patients with rectal carcinoma or Dukes stage B colon cancer has not yet been determined, and the importance of the timing of levamisole therapy in relation to surgical resection can only be partially addressed. Adjuvant therapy in all but one of the clinical trials commenced within five weeks of surgery, with Bancewicz's group allowing a delay of four to eight weeks postoperatively. The landmark study by Moertel et al.[10] initiated adjuvant therapy within three to five weeks after surgery. Theoretical considerations, animal data, and clinical trials argue for initiating adjuvant levamisole therapy shortly after surgery, because there is no evidence that starting therapy more than five to six weeks after surgery will produce any benefit.[10,15,56] Currently, fluorouracil and levamisole constitute the standard regimen to which future therapies in stage C colon cancer will be compared. Clinical trials are currently under way to evaluate a variety of regimens, including fluorouracil, levamisole, and leucovorin.[55] Leucovorin has been used in numerous clinical trials to enhance fluorouracil's activity. Because fluorouracil and leucovorin are generally considered more effective than fluorouracil alone,[54] it will be interesting to see whether the three-drug regimen of fluorouracil, leucovorin, and levamisole proves to be superior to adjuvant fluorouracil and levamisole in patients with colon cancer.

Clinical Trials in Advanced Metastatic Colorectal Cancer. Several clinical trials evaluating the efficacy of levamisole in patients with metastatic colorectal cancer have been conducted (Table 6). Favorable results were reported in a trial conducted by Borden et al.,[65,66] which showed that patients with metastatic colorectal cancer who were treated with fluorouracil and levamisole survived significantly longer than those who received fluorouracil alone ($p = 0.02$). Patients were stratified according to measurable disease, hepatic involvement, performance status, and time from diagnosis to entry, and they were randomized to one of two treatment groups: fluorouracil alone or fluorouracil plus levamisole. Of 85 patients entered, 66 were evaluable for survival and time to disease progression in the preliminary report.[65] The median survival of patients who received fluorouracil alone was 306 days compared with 566 days in patients who received fluorouracil and levamisole. The initial presence of objectively measurable disease significantly decreased the median duration of survival (188 days versus 541 days). The significance of the different treatments decreased but persisted ($p = 0.05$) when analysis was adjusted for the influence of measurable disease. Additional information on this trial appeared in abstract form with 82 patients evaluable for analysis.[66] The median survival time after fluorouracil therapy alone was 291 days, whereas that after fluorouracil plus levamisole therapy was 465 days. No information regarding antitumor response or overall survival analysis was provided. Some have criticized this study for its exclusion from analysis of early deaths, imbalance of fluorouracil ($n = 38$) and fluorouracil plus levamisole ($n = 28$) treatment groups, unknown distribution of measurable disease within treatment groups, and low patient numbers.[55]

Also limited by its small sample size is the study by Bedikian et al.,[67] which evaluated two chemotherapeutic regimens with and without levamisole in 52 previously untreated patients with metastatic colon cancer. Patients were first randomized to receive fluorouracil alternating with either methotrexate or Baker's antifol and then were independently randomized to receive or not to receive le-

Table 6.
Levamisole in Therapy of Advanced Metastatic Colorectal Cancer[a]

Reference	No. Evaluable Patients	Primary Site (Colon:Rectum)	Treatment (No. Patients)	Dosage	% Response (PR + CR)	Median Survival (months)
65, 66	82	NA	FU (NA)	FU given as 5-day loading dose of 12 mg/kg/day, then 6 mg/kg/day until toxicity, followed by 6-week cycles of the same loading dose, then 6 mg/kg/day every other day for a maximum of 3 days	NA	9.7
			FU + Lev (NA)	Same FU regimen as above plus Lev 2.5 mg/kg (to nearest 50 mg) on days 28, 29, 35, and 36 of each cycle	NA	15.5
67	52	NA	FU + MTX or BAF (25)	FU 500 mg/sq m/day on days 1–5; MTX or BAF daily for 3 days beginning 3–4 weeks after FU at 15 mg/sq m/day or 250 mg/sq m/day, respectively; cycle repeated every 6–7 weeks	10	10.5
			FU + MTX or BAF + Lev (27)	Same FU + MTX or BAF regimen as above plus Lev on days 7, 8, 14, 15, 21, and 22 of treatment with each agent at a dose of 150 mg/sq m/day	10.5	9.0
68	335	264:71	FU (69)	FU 500 mg/sq m/day on days 1–5 repeated every 5 weeks	29.7	9.0
			FU + Lev (66)	Same FU regimen as above plus Lev 50 mg every 8 hours on days 14, 15, and 16 and days 21, 22, and 23 of each FU cycle	22.5	9.5

[a] Abbreviations: PR = partial response; CR = complete response; NA = not available; FU = fluorouracil; Lev = levamisole; MTX = methotrexate; BAF = Baker's antifol.

vamisole. Results of this study found that neither the response rate nor the overall survival was influenced by levamisole administration.

A well-designed, large, cooperative group trial showed no difference in time to progression, response rate, or median survival in patients randomized to receive fluorouracil plus levamisole or fluorouracil alone.[68] After stratification, patients were randomized to receive one of five regimens: fluorouracil alone; fluorouracil plus levamisole, high-dose thymidine, or *N*-(phosphonacetyl)-L-aspartic acid (PALA); or fluorouracil plus semustine, vincristine, and streptozocin. Of the 347 patients randomized, 335 were deemed eligible for analysis. There was no evidence that any of the combination regimens produced a higher objective response rate or increased survival over that observed with fluorouracil alone.

Collectively, these trials indicate that levamisole does not add to the effect of cytotoxic chemotherapy in the adjuvant treatment of patients with metastatic colon cancer. Other trials are currently under way and may more clearly define the usefulness of levamisole in patients with disseminated disease.

Use in Other Types of Cancer. The recent encouraging results of levamisole therapy in patients with colon carcinoma cannot be directly extended to other neoplastic disease.[28] Historically, levamisole has been investigated as a treatment for a number of malignant conditions, including breast cancer, gastric cancer, non-small-cell lung carcinoma, Hodgkin's disease, non-Hodgkin's lymphoma, melanoma, and multiple myeloma.[13–15,69] Adjuvant studies of levamisole in patients with breast cancer, non-small-cell lung cancer, and melanoma have had favorable outcomes, but randomized trials involving the same disease states have often failed to confirm levamisole's efficacy or have shown the benefit not to be durable. In many studies, levamisole has been used to treat metastatic or bulky disease instead of as adjuvant therapy. It has often been used alone or with radiation therapy instead of in combination with chemotherapy, and the delay in starting levamisole therapy after surgery varies. Further well-defined clinical research based on the success in treating stage C colon cancer is needed to determine what role levamisole may have in the treatment of other malignancies.

Uses in Nonmalignant Disorders. In addition to its established use as an antihelmintic agent, levamisole has been studied as a treatment for numerous unrelated disorders, although claims of effectiveness have been poorly substantiated.[12,16–23] These disease states include immunodeficiency and allergic diseases (e.g., asthma, atopic dermatitis), chronic and recurrent viral and bacterial infections, leprosy, chronic inflammatory diseases (e.g., rheumatic diseases, systemic lupus erythematosus), neurologic diseases (e.g., multiple sclerosis), recurrent aphthous stomatitis, Crohn's disease, ulcerative colitis, and numerous dermatologic diseases.

Adverse Drug Reactions

Preclinical animal studies found levamisole to be neither teratogenic nor carcinogenic.[4,55,69] At antihelmintic doses (i.e., 150 mg given once), levamisole is virtually devoid of toxicity.[70] A variety of dosage regimens have been used for nonhelmintic conditions and have been similarly well tolerated. Common adverse effects have included the gastrointestinal symptoms of nausea, abdominal pain, vomiting, and diarrhea; metallic or altered taste; flu-like symptoms with fever and malaise; and the neurologic symptoms of mood elevation, insomnia, hyperalert state, dizziness, and headache. Other less frequently experienced adverse effects include blood dyscrasias (granulocytopenia, leukopenia, and thrombocytopenia), mucositis, proteinuria, and skin rashes. Adverse reactions to levamisole appear to be dose related and are reversible when therapy is stopped.

In 1978 Symoens et al.[70] analyzed the adverse effects of levamisole mentioned in 267 reports. These reports represent more than 6000 patients treated with levamisole for various nonhelmintic diseases. The presence or absence of adverse effects was specifically mentioned in 65% of the cases. Eighty percent of the patients whose adverse effects were reported had been receiving levamisole for more than three months. The authors descriptively categorized levamisole reactions into three groups: idiosyncratic or allergic, neurologic, and gastrointestinal. Table 7 summarizes the adverse reactions that occurred in at least 1% of the patients analyzed. Patients with rheumatic disorders reported significantly more idiosyncratic or allergic reactions, whereas gastrointestinal adverse effects predominated in the cancer patients. Common to all patients reporting symptoms were the neurologic adverse effects, fever, and gastrointestinal intolerance. The overall dropout rate because of toxicity was less than 5%.

The most serious adverse effect associated with levamisole is granulocytopenia, characterized by a dramatic drop in granulocytes with less than 20% neutrophils. Although this condition is observed most frequently in patients with rhematoid arthritis or similar connective tissue disorders,[70,71] it has been reported in the cancer literature as well.[70,72–79] Symoens et al.[70] reported leukopenia and granulocytopenia as a complication of levamisole treatment in 2.0% of cancer patients reviewed in 58 clinical trials. Since then, several published studies of levamisole therapy in patients with cancer have suggested that the incidence may actually be higher, approaching 4–10%.[74–79] Some breast cancer studies have observed no levamisole-induced granulocytopenia.[80] Among the colorectal cancer

Table 7.
Adverse Reactions Occurring in at Least 1% of Patients[70,a]

Adverse Reaction	Cancer (1179 patients)	Infectious (888 patients)	Inflammatory (601 patients)	Rheumatic (989 patients)	Various Others (243 patients)
Idiosyncratic					
Skin rash	2.6 (0.9)	1.5 (0.3)	1.7 (0.2)	14.8 (7.0)	2.1 (0.4)
Leukopenia and agranulocytosis	2.0 (1.4)	0.2 (0.3)	1.0 (0.3)	4.9 (4.5)	0.8
Febrile illness	4.8 (1.4)	1.9 (0.5)	2.8 (1.5)	3.9 (1.5)	0.4
Mouth ulcers	0.3	0.1	0.0	1.9 (0.3)	0.0
Neurologic					
Sensory stimulation	3.0 (0.1)	6.1	4.8	6.2 (0.5)	0.4
Hyperalert state	1.2	1.2	0.2	1.8	0.0
Insomnia	2.5 (0.1)	0.3	0.3	1.4	0.0
Headache	2.1	2.3	2.2	1.3 (0.2)	0.0
Dizziness	1.2	0.5	0.3	2.9	4.5
Fatigue	4.4	1.5 (0.1)	0.8	0.9	0.0
Gastrointestinal					
Nausea	13.1 (0.4)	5.0 (0.5)	4.8 (0.3)	5.0 (1.3)	5.8
Gastric intolerance	4.8 (0.4)	4.2 (0.3)	3.5 (0.2)	5.7 (0.8)	2.5
Anorexia	2.8	0.0	0.2	2.7	0.0
Vomiting	7.2	2.3	0.8	2.1 (0.2)	0.4 (0.4)
Diarrhea	2.6	0.5	0.8	0.3 (0.1)	0.0
Miscellaneous	4 (0.3)	6 (0.7)	5 (0.8)	16 (1.6)	0
Total percentage withdrawn	5.0	2.7	3.3	18.0	0.8

[a] Percentage of patients with adverse effects (% withdrawn due to specific adverse reaction).

trials, four cases (2%) of granulocytopenia were observed in 194 levamisole-treated patients in two clinical trials comparing monotherapy with placebo.[58,59] When levamisole was administered with cytotoxic therapy in the colorectal cancer trials, the predominant adverse effects were consistent with those that might be anticipated with cytotoxic therapy alone, with the occasional exception of a slight accentuation of myelosuppression.[60,62,63,65,68] The explanation for the observed variation in the incidence of granulocytopenia is not known, but it may relate to concomitant radiation, the type and intensity of chemotherapy, the levamisole dose and schedule, or unidentified individual patient characteristics.

Besides its association with specific disease states, granulocytopenia has also been reported to occur most frequently in women and in HLA B27 genotypes.[70,71] Of the granulocytopenia cases analyzed by Symoens et al.,[70] half occurred within the first three months of therapy and were often accompanied by flu-like symptoms. Because levamisole-associated granulocytopenia is frequently accompanied by flu-like symptoms, patients should be counseled to contact their physician when such symptoms appear.[24] The granulocytopenia appears to be mediated by antibodies and complement rather than by a stem-cell defect, and it is reversible after discontinuation of levamisole therapy. There is no evidence that corticosteroids or granulocyte transfusions hasten recovery.[70] Monitoring levamisole-associated granulocytopenia in patients receiving levamisole plus fluorouracil may be difficult, because fluorouracil itself is a myelosuppressive agent, especially when given as an i.v. bolus injection. When myelosuppression arises in patients receiving combination therapy with levamisole and fluorouracil, consideration should be given first to fluorouracil as the causative agent, and modifications in the fluorouracil dosage should be made accordingly. Should granulocytopenia persist or worsen despite modifications in the fluorouracil dosage, levamisole therapy should then be discontinued. Reinstitution of levamisole therapy at a lower dose cannot be recommended at this time because its therapeutic benefit has not been tested below 150 mg/day. The reader is referred to the Ergamisol package insert for specific hematologic dosage guidelines.

Leukopenia, defined as <3000 leukocytes/cu mm but with more than 20% neutrophils, is a condition also encountered during treatment with levamisole. However, it differs from granulocytopenia in numerous ways, as summarized in Table 8. Leukopenia is not considered prodromal to granulocytopenia and therefore does not appear to warrant discontinuation of therapy.[70]

Dosage and Administration

The dosage regimen of levamisole for eradicating nematode infestations is fairly well established. Adults generally receive a one-time dose of 150 mg or 1–5 mg/kg with one repeat dose sometimes required in severe cases one to seven days later.[20,22,81] Children have been given 3 mg/kg.

Examination of the cancer literature reveals two predominant oral dosage regimens: (1) 150 mg (or

Table 8.
Differences between Levamisole-Associated Granulocytopenia and Leukopenia[a]

Variable	Granulocytopenia	Leukopenia
White blood cell count	<2000 cells/cu mm	<3000 cells/cu mm
Neutrophils	<20%	<50% and >20%
HLA B27 prevalence	Increased	Normal
Bone marrow	Hypocellular during granulocytopenia (maturation arrest at promyelocyte stage); hyperreactive during recovery	Normal
Symptoms	Generally present (influenza-like illness with general feeling of malaise, fever, and chills or other nonspecific symptoms)	Absent
Continued levamisole treatment	Persisting granulocytopenia	Restoration of leukocyte count
Challenge	Positive	Negative

[a] Adapted from reference 70.

2.5 mg/kg) daily for two consecutive days every week or (2) 150 mg (or 2.5 mg/kg) daily for three consecutive days every two weeks. A review by Amery and Butterworth[82] of 46 controlled studies of adjuvant levamisole in cancer therapies focused attention on dosage regimens as they related to efficacy and the incidence of toxicity, especially granulocytopenia. Of the two standard dosage regimens, fewer adverse effects were noted with the latter schedule, something that has been suggested in other literature as well. The FDA-approved dosage regimen is 50 mg orally every eight hours for three days every two weeks. Levamisole therapy is to be initiated no earlier than 7 and no later than 30 days after surgery and is to be continued for one year.[24] The rationale for recommending initiation of levamisole between 7 and 30 days after tumor resection is not explicitly stated, but it reflects the dosage schedule of levamisole used in the national intergroup study.[10]

Classical Phase I pharmacology and immunology studies correlating levamisole dose, effect, and toxicity are lacking. The maximum tolerated dose and minimum immunopotentiating dose and schedule of levamisole have not been defined. The dose and schedule of levamisole used in clinical colon cancer trials and approved by the FDA are apparently empirically derived from antihelmintic experience with the drug.[10,55] Serendipitously, peak plasma concentrations achieved after a 2.5–5 mg/kg dose of levamisole are similar to concentrations capable of producing immunostimulatory effects in vitro.[16,43]

It has been suggested that a minimum effective dose of levamisole is required for an immunotherapeutic effect and that an excessive dose may be immunosuppressive.[4,15,16,83,84] In a placebo-controlled study of postsurgical lung cancer patients, Amery[85] administered a fixed dose of levamisole (150 mg/day) regardless of body weight. When adjusted for body weight, daily doses ranged from 1.1 to 3.8 mg/kg. Benefits from levamisole therapy occurred only in patients who received at least 2 mg/kg of levamisole daily. This observation led the author to advocate a dose of 2.5 mg/kg/day rather than the standard 150 mg/day in cancer patients. Further studies are needed to define the optimal dose and schedule of levamisole.

Cost and Availability

FDA approval of levamisole for adjuvant treatment in combination with fluorouracil of Dukes stage C colon cancer was given on June 20, 1990. Before this time, levamisole was commercially available in the United States only for veterinary use. Levamisole is manufactured by Janssen Pharmaceutical, NV Beerse, Belgium, and is distributed by Janssen Pharmaceutica, Inc., Piscataway, New Jersey, under the trade name Ergamisol.[24] Levamisole is supplied as a white, coated tablet for oral administration. Each tablet contains levamisole 50 mg (as the hydrochloride salt). Levamisole is available in blister packages of 36 tablets (9 tablets per card/four cards per box). This two-month supply has an average wholesale price of approximately $170. No injectable form of the product is currently available in the United States.

Conclusion

Compared with surgery alone, the adjuvant combination of levamisole plus fluorouracil has produced dramatic effects on disease-free survival and overall survival in patients with Dukes stage C colon cancer. Therapy with levamisole and fluorouracil has been associated with a one-third reduction in the recurrence rate and the overall death rate and is now recommended as standard therapy in these patients.

Despite years of extensive research and a long history of use in clinical colorectal cancer trials, many important properties of levamisole remain unidentified. Pharmacokinetic and pharmacodynamic studies are incomplete. Interestingly, levamisole received FDA approval without bioavailability studies or definition of the optimal dose, schedule, and time of therapy relative to surgery. Other unknowns of levamisole include its full immunologic effects, target effector cells, mechanisms of action, and mechanisms of interaction with fluorouracil. Clinical questions also remain, including the effect of levamisole and fluorouracil or other combinations in patients with Dukes stage B_2 or metastatic colon cancer and the role of levamisole therapy in rectal carcinoma and other cancers. These questions provide ample opportunities for future laboratory research and clinical trials.

References

1. Thienpont D, Vanparijs OFJ, Raeymaekers AHM et al. Tetramisole (R8299) a new potent broad spectrum anthelminthic. *Nature*. 1966; 209:1084–6.
2. Schnieden H. Levamisole. A general pharmacological perspective. *Int J Immunopharmacol*. 1981; 3:9–13.
3. Goldstein G. Mode of action of levamisole. *J Rheumatol*. 1978; 5(Suppl 4):143–8.
4. Renoux G. The general immunopharmacology of levamisole. *Drugs*. 1980; 20:89–99.
5. Janssen PA. The levamisole story. *Prog Drug Res*. 1976; 20:347–83.
6. Buyse M, Zeleniuch-Jacquotte A, Chalmers T. Adjuvant therapy of colorectal cancer: why we still don't know. *JAMA*. 1988; 259:3571–8.
7. Friedman MA, Hamilton JM. Progress in the adjuvant therapy of large bowel cancer. In: DeVita VT, Hellman S, Rosenberg SA, eds. Important advances in oncology, 1988. Philadelphia: Lippincott; 1988:273–96.
8. Mavligit GM, Guttermann JV, Malany MA. Adjuvant immunotherapy and chemoimmunotherapy in colorectal cancer (Dukes' C). *Cancer*. 1977; 40:2726–30.
9. Wolmark N, Fisher B, Rockette H et al. Postoperative adjuvant chemotherapy or BCG for colon cancer: results from NSABP protocol C-01. *J Natl Cancer Inst*. 1988; 80:30–6.
10. Moertel CG, Fleming TR, MacDonald JS et al. Levamisole and fluorouracil for adjuvant therapy of resected colon carcinoma. *N Engl J Med*. 1990; 322:352–8.
11. Anon. Trial confirms the benefit of drug therapy for Dukes' C colon cancer patients. Cancer fact sheet. Bethesda, MD: Office of Cancer Communication, National Cancer Institute; 1990 Feb.
12. Amery WK, Gough DA. Levamisole and immunotherapy: some theoretic and practical considerations and their relevance to human disease. *Oncology*. 1981; 38:168–81.
13. Amery WK, Verhaegen H. Effects of levamisole treatment in cancer patients. *J Rheumatol*. 1978; 5(Suppl 4):123–34.
14. Borden EC, Hawkins MJ. Biologic response modifiers as adjuncts to other therapeutic modalities. *Semin Oncol*. 1986; 13:144–52.
15. Spreafico F. Use of levamisole in cancer patients. *Drugs*. 1980; 20:105–16.
16. Symoens J, DeCree J, VanBever WFM et al. Levamisole. In: Goldberg ME, ed. Pharmacological and biochemical properties of drug substances. Vol. 2. Washington, DC: American Pharmaceutical Association; 1979:408–64.
17. Huskisson EC, Adams JG. An overview of the current status of levamisole in the treatment of rheumatic diseases. *Drugs*. 1980; 20:100–4.
18. Rosenthal M. A critical review of the effect of levamisole in rheumatic diseases other than rheumatoid arthritis. *J Rheumatol*. 1978; 5(Suppl 4):97–100.
19. Wilton JMA. Levamisole in chronic inflammatory diseases. *J Rheumatol*. 1978; 5(Suppl 4):101–13.
20. Brugmans J. Levamisole in infectious diseases—a review of the literature. *J Rheumatol*. 1978; 5(Suppl 4):115–21.
21. Russell AS. Use of levamisole in viral infections. *Drugs*. 1980; 20:117–21.
22. Miller MJ. Use of levamisole in parasitic infections. *Drugs*. 1980; 20:122–30.
23. Miller MF. Use of levamisole in recurrent aphthous stomatitis. *Drugs*. 1980; 20:131–6.
24. Janssen Pharmaceutica. Ergamisol package insert. Piscataway, NJ: 1990 Jun.
25. Harris BG. Levamisole: mode of action. *Biochem Soc Trans*. 1987; 15:61.
26. Bardana EJ. Recent developments in immunomodulatory therapy. *J Allergy Clin Immunol*. 1985; 75:423–40.
27. Haskell CM. Immunologic aspects of cancer chemotherapy. *Annu Rev Pharmacol Toxicol*. 1977; 17:179–95.
28. Grem JL. Levamisole as a therapeutic agent for colorectal carcinoma. *Cancer Cells*. 1990; 2:131–7.
29. Liberati M, Borden EC, McBain JA et al. Effects of levamisole on human natural killer and killer cell activity and production of interferons. *Immunopharmacology*. 1982; 5:11–8.
30. Tempero M, Haga Y, Sivinski C et al. Absence of biologic effects with levamisole treatment. *Proc Am Soc Clin Oncol*. 1990; 9:121. Abstract.
31. Amery WK, Horig C. Levamisole. In: Fenichel RL, Chirigos MA, eds. Immune modulation agents and their mechanisms. New York: Marcel Dekker; 1984: 383–408.
32. Hersh EM, Gutterman JU, Mavligit GM. Immunotherapy of human cancer. *Adv Intern Med*. 1977; 22:145–85.
33. Renoux G, Renoux M. Thymus-like activities of sulphur derivatives on T-cell differentiation. *J Exp Med*. 1977; 145:466–71.
34. Chirigos MA, Amery WK. Combined levamisole therapy: an overview of its protective effects. Immunotherapy of human cancer. New York: Raven Press; 1978:181–95.
35. Lewinski UH, Mavligit GM, Hersh EM. Cellular immune modulation after a single high dose of levamisole in patients with carcinoma. *Cancer*. 1980; 45:2185–94.
36. Kouassi E, Caille G, Lery L et al. Novel assay and pharmacokinetics of levamisole and p-hydroxylevamisole in human plasma and urine. *Biopharm Drug Dispos*. 1986; 7:71–89.
37. VanBelle H. Alkaline phosphatase: I. Kinetics and inhibition by levamisole of purified isoenzymes from humans. *Clin Chem*. 1976; 22:972–6.
38. Grem JL, Allegra CS. Toxicity of levamisole and 5-fluorouracil in human colon carcinoma cells. *J Natl Cancer Inst*. 1989; 81:1413–7.
39. Mitchell MS, DeConti RC. Immunosuppression by 5-fluorouracil. *Cancer*. 1970; 26:884–9.
40. Rao H. Wanebo HJ, Pinsky C et al. Delayed hypersensitivity reactions in patients with carcinoma of the colon and rectum. *Surg Gynecol Obstet*. 1977; 144:677–81.
41. Dujardin P, Lods JC, Cassato JP et al. Action of levamisole on recovery of bone marrow in patients receiving antineoplastic drug therapy. *Therapie*. 1976; 31:733–8.
42. Fernandes CJ, Cranford SK. Resistance of CCRF-CEM cloned sublines of 5-fluorodeoxyuridine associated with enhanced phosphatase activities. *Biochem Pharmacol*. 1985; 34:125–32.
43. Adams JG. Pharmacokinetics of levamisole. *J Rheumatol*. 1978; 5(Suppl 4):137–42.
44. Luyckx M, Rousseau F, Cazin M et al. Pharmacokinetics of levamisole in healthy subjects and cancer patients. *Eur J Drug Metab Pharmacokinet*. 1982; 7:247–54.
45. Edwards G, Breckenridge AM. Clinical pharmacokinetics of anthelmintic drugs. *Clin Pharmacokinet*. 1988; 15;67–93.
46. Gibaldi M, Boyes RN, Feldman S. Influence of first pass effect on availability of drugs on oral administration. *J Pharm Sci*. 1971; 60:1338–40.
47. Holbrook A, Scales B. Polarographic determination of tetramisole hydrochloride in extracts of animal tissue. *Anal Biochem*. 1967; 18:46–53.
48. Rousseau F, Haguenoer JM, Lesieur D, Gamot AP. Gas chromatographic determination of levamisole in human plasma—normalization and reliability of the method. *Eur J Drug Metab Pharmacokinet*. 1981; 7:281–8.
49. Woestenborghs R, Michielsen L, Heykants J. Determination of levamisole in plasma and animal tissues by gas chromatography with thermionic specific detection. *J Chromatogr*. 1981; 224:25–32.
50. Alvinerie M, Galtier P, Escoula G. Ion pair high-perfor-

mance liquid chromatographic assay of levamisole in biological fluids. *J Chromatogr*. 1981; 223:445–448.
51. Mourot D, Delepine B, Boisseau J et al. High-pressure liquid chromatographic analysis of veterinary antihelmintics: I. Quantitative determination of tetramisole. *J Pharm Sci*. 1979; 68:796–7.
52. Silverberg E, Boring CC, Squires TS. Cancer statistics, 1990. *CA*. 1990; 40:9–26.
53. Cohen AM, Shank B, Friedman MA. Colorectal cancer. In: DeVita VT, Hellman S, Rosenberg SA, eds. Cancer: principles and practice of oncology. 3rd ed. Philadelphia: Lippincott; 1989:895–964.
54. Mayer RJ, O'Connell MJ, Tepper JE et al. Status of adjuvant therapy for colorectal cancer. *J Natl Cancer Inst*. 1989; 81:1359–64.
55. Hamilton JM, Sznol M, Friedman MA. 5-Fluorouracil plus levamisole: effective adjuvant treatment for colon cancer. In: DeVita VT, Hellman S, Rosenberg SA, eds. Important advances in oncology, 1990. Philadelphia: Lippincott; 1990:115–30.
56. Adjuvant therapy for patients with colon and rectal cancer. Bethesda, MD: National Institutes of Health. Report of consensus development conference held April 16–18, 1990.
57. Verhaegen H, DeCree J, DeCock W et al. Levamisole therapy in patients with colorectal cancer. In: Terry WD, Rosenberg SA, eds. Immunotherapy of human cancer. New York: Excerpta Medica; 1982:225–9.
58. Chlebowski RT, Nystrom S, Reynolds R et al. Long-term survival following levamisole or placebo adjuvant treatment of colorectal cancer: a Western cancer study group trial. *Oncology*. 1988; 45:141–3.
59. Arnaud JP, Buyse M, Nordlinger B et al. Adjuvant therapy for poor prognosis colon cancer with levamisole: results of an EORTC double-blind randomized clinical trial. *Br J Surg*. 1989; 76:284–9.
60. Laurie JA, Moertel CG, Fleming TR et al. Surgical adjuvant therapy of large-bowel carcinoma: an evaluation of levamisole and the combination of levamisole and fluourouracil. *J Clin Oncol*. 1989; 7:1447–56.
61. Bancewicz J, Macpherson S, McVie J et al. Adjuvant chemotherapy and immunotherapy for colorectal cancer: preliminary communication. *J R Soc Med*. 1980; 73:197–9.
62. Sertoli MR, Guarneri D, Rubagotti A et al. Adjuvant immunochemotherapy in colorectal cancer Dukes C. *Oncology*. 1987; 44:78–81.
63. Windle R, Bell PRF, Shaw D. Five-year results of a randomized trial of adjuvant 5-fluorouracil and levamisole in colorectal cancer. *Br J Surg*. 1987; 74:569–72.
64. Mayer RJ. Does adjuvant therapy work in colon cancer? *N Engl J Med*. 1990; 322:399–401. Editorial.
65. Borden EC, Davis TE, Crowley JJ et al. Interim analysis of a trial of levamisole and 5-fluouracil in metastatic colorectal carcinoma. In: Terry WD, Rosenberg SA, eds. Immunotherapy of human cancer. New York: Excerpta Medica; 1982:231–5.
66. Davis T, Borden E, Wolberg W et al. Levamisole and 5-fluorouracil in metastatic colorectal carcinoma. *Proc Am Soc Clin Oncol*. 1982; 1:102. Abstract.
67. Bedikian AY, Valdivieso M, Mavligit GM et al. Sequential chemoimmunotherapy of colorectal cancer: evaluation of methotrexate, Baker's antifol and levamisole. *Cancer*. 1978; 42:2169–76.
68. Buroker TR, Moertel CG, Fleming TR et al. A controlled evaluation of recent approaches to biochemical modulation of enhancement of 5-fluorouracil therapy in colorectal carcinoma. *J Clin Oncol*. 1985; 3:1624–31.
69. Division of Cancer Treatment, National Cancer Institute. Levamisole NSC 177023 IND 13266. Clinical brochure. Bethesda, MD; 1989 Feb.
70. Symoens J, Veys E, Mielants M et al. Adverse reactions to levamisole. *Cancer Treat Rep*. 1978; 62:1721–30.
71. Hodinka L, Geher P, Meretey K et al. Levamisole-induced neutropenia and agranulocytosis: association with HLA B27 leukocyte agglutinating and lymphocytotoxic antibodies. *Int Arch Allergy Appl Immunol*. 1981; 65:460–4.
72. Parkinson DR, Cano PO, Jerry LM et al. Complications of cancer immunotherapy with levamisole. *Lancet*. 1977; 1:1129–32.
73. Willoughby MLN, Baird GM, Campbell AM. Levamisole and neutropenia. *Lancet*. 1977; 1:657.
74. Retsas S, Phillips RH, Hanham IW et al. Agranulocytosis in breast cancer patients with levamisole. *Lancet*. 1978; 2:324–5. Letter.
75. Vogel CL, Lipscomb DL, Silverman MA et al. Levamisole granulocytopenia in patients receiving an adjuvant chemoimmunotherapy program after surgery for breast carcinoma with axillary lymph node involvement. *Cancer Treat Rep*. 1978; 62:1587–9.
76. Teerenhovi L, Heinonen E, Grohn P et al. High frequency of agranulocytosis in breast-cancer patients treated with levamisole. *Lancet*. 1978; 2:151–2. Letter.
77. Danish Breast Cancer Cooperative Group. Increased breast-cancer recurrence rate after adjuvant therapy with levamisole. *Lancet*. 1980; 2:824–7.
78. Klefstrom P, Holsti P, Grohn P et al. Levamisole in the treatment of stage II breast cancer: five-year follow-up of a randomized double-blind study. *Cancer*. 1985; 55:2753–7.
79. Treurniet-Donker AD, Meischke-de Johgh ML, VanPutten WLJ. Levamisole as adjuvant immunotherapy in breast cancer. *Cancer*. 1987; 59:1590–3.
80. Carpenter JT, Smalley RV, Raney M. Ineffectiveness of levamisole in prolonging remission or survival of women treated with cyclophosphamide, doxorubicin, and 5-fluorouracil for good-risk metastatic breast carcinoma: a Southeastern cancer study group trial. *Cancer Treat Rep*. 1986; 70:1073–9.
81. Anon. Levamisole. In: Dorr RT, Fritz WL, eds. Cancer chemotherapy handbook. New York: Elsevier Science Publishing; 1980:480–5.
82. Amery WK, Butterworth BS. The dosage regimen of levamisole in cancer: is it related to efficacy and safety? *Int J Immunopharmacol*. 1983; 5:1–9.
83. Wajsman Z, Williams PD, Murphy GP et al. The value of levamisole in a Wilms tumor animal model. *Oncology*. 1978; 35:212–3.
84. Kalafut F, Kusenda J, Novotna L et al. Restoration of immune response by levamisole in B77 virus induced tumor bearing rats. *Neoplasma*. 1988; 35:369–78.
85. Amery WK. Final results of a multicenter placebo controlled levamisole study of resectable lung cancer. *Cancer Treat Rep*. 1978; 62:1677–83.

Recombinant interleukin-2: A biological response modifier

P. E. KINTZEL AND KARIM ANTON CALIS

Abstract: The chemical properties, pharmacology, immunology, pharmacokinetics, clinical trials, adverse effects, and dosage and administration of recombinant interleukin-2 are reviewed.

Recombinant interleukin-2 is an immunomodulating agent that stimulates the proliferation, activation, and differentiation of T and B cells, natural killer cells, and thymocytes. Two recombinant interleukin-2 products, aldesleukin and teceleukin, have been extensively studied. Most clinical experience with recombinant interleukin-2 has involved the treatment of renal cell carcinoma, melanoma, and colorectal cancer with a National Cancer Institute protocol. Patients with renal cell cancer and melanoma, who historically respond poorly to conventional therapy, have responded to therapy with recombinant interleukin-2. Recombinant interleukin-2 has been administered alone and in combination with lymphokine-activated killer cells, tumor-infiltrating lymphocytes, and interferons alfa and beta. In addition, the effect of dosage, administration rate, dosage schedule, route of administration, and cyclophosphamide pretreatment have been investigated. The adverse effects of recombinant interleukin-2 are generally reversible but are frequently severe and dose-related. Dose-limiting adverse effects include hypotension, edema, and renal dysfunction. Since hemodynamic monitoring and supportive care are essential, recombinant interleukin-2 should be administered in a critical-care setting by trained personnel.

Recombinant interleukin-2 represents an advance in the therapy of renal cell cancer and melanoma and offers a new approach to the treatment of other refractory or recurrent malignancies.

Index terms: Antineoplastic agents; Carcinoma; Colorectal neoplasms; Dosage; Immunotherapy; Interleukin 2; Melanoma; Pharmacokinetics; Toxicity
Clin Pharm. 1991; 10:110–28

Interleukin-2 is one of many interleukins that have been identified and cloned. Interleukins are so named because they provide a molecular mechanism for communication among leukocytes. In this capacity they are an integral component of immune regulation, which requires dynamic, complex communication among cells and tissues.[1] The characteristics of interleukins 1 through 8 are presented in Table 1.

Interleukin-2 promotes the proliferation, differentiation, and recruitment of T and B cells, natural killer (NK) cells, and thymocytes.[5] In addition, interleukin-2 causes cytolytic activity in a subset of lymphocytes and subsequent interactions between the immune system and malignant cells.[1] These biological activities make interleukin-2 attractive for use as a biological response modifier. This article reviews the chemical properties, pharmacology, immunology, pharmacokinetics, clinical trials, adverse effects, and dosage and administration of recombinant interleukin-2.

Background

Initially termed T-cell growth factor, interleukin-2 was first described in 1976 when it was discovered that the supernatant from cultures of mitogen-stimulated human peripheral blood mononuclear cells (PBMC) contained a factor that supported the in vitro proliferation of T cells.[6] In addition, interleukin-2 was found to stimulate B cells, NK cells, and lymphokine-activated killer (LAK) cells.[1,5] In 1983 Taniguchi et al.[7] reported the isolation of complete complementary DNA for interleukin-2. This made possible the efficient production of recombinant interleukin-2 in *Escherichia coli*, and enough became available for use in clinical trials. Several forms of recombinant interleukin-2 are in various stages of preclinical development and clinical investigation; aldesleukin (Proleukin, Cetus Corporation, Emeryville, CA) and teceleukin (Tecin, Hoffmann-La Roche Inc., Nutley, NJ) have been the most extensively studied.

P. E. KINTZEL, PHARM.D., is Oncology Specialty Resident, Audie L. Murphy Memorial Veterans Hospital, San Antonio, TX, and Clinical Instructor, University of Texas Health Sciences Center, San Antonio; when this article was written she was Pharmacy Resident, Department of Pharmacy, Warren G. Magnuson Clinical Center, National Institutes of Health (NIH), Bethesda, MD. KARIM ANTON CALIS, PHARM.D., is Clinical Pharmacy Specialist, Drug Information Services and Endocrinology, Department of Pharmacy, Warren G. Magnuson Clinical Center, NIH, and Clinical Assistant Professor, School of Pharmacy, University of Maryland, Baltimore.

Address reprint requests to Dr. Calis at the Drug Information Service, National Institutes of Health, Building 10, Room 1N-257, Bethesda, MD 20892.

The contributions of Joshua T. Rubin, M.D., Jim Koeller, M.S., and many other individuals are acknowledged.

This is **article 680-204-9105** in the **ASHP Continuing Education System;** it qualifies for 2 hours of CE credit. See page 148 for learning objectives and test questions.

Table 1.
Characteristics of Interleukins[a]

Interleukin (kDa)	Principal Origin(s)	Principal Site(s) of Activity	Major Effect(s)
Interleukin-1 (13–17)	Monocytes, macrophages	T cells, B cells, endothelium, fibroblasts, chondrocytes, hepatocytes, osteoclasts, synovial cells	Pyrogenesis, proinflammation, cellular proliferation, lymphokine synthesis, lymphokine receptor synthesis
Interleukin-2 (15.5)	T cells	T cells, natural killer cells, lymphokine-activated killer cells, tumor-infiltrating lymphocytes	Cellular proliferation and differentiation
Interleukin-3 (28)	T cells	Hematopoietic precursors	Hematopoiesis, cellular differentiation
Interleukin-4 (20)	T cells	B cells	Celllular proliferation and differentiation
Interleukin-5 (4)	T cells	B cells, eosinophils	Cellular proliferation and differentiation
Interleukin-6 (20–30)	Monocytes, macrophages	B cells, T cells	Pyrogenesis, cellular proliferation and differentiation
Interleukin-7 (25)	Bone marrow stromal cells	B-cell precursors	Cellular proliferation
Interleukin-8 (8–11)	Monocytes	Neutrophils	Chemotaxis, respiratory bursting

[a] Adapted from references 1–4.

Native and recombinant interleukin-2 can stimulate the generation of LAK cells[8–10] and tumor-infiltrating lymphocytes (TIL).[11–13] The first description of LAK-cell activity in humans was provided by Lotze et al.,[14] who identified lymphocytes with antitumor activity in the peripheral blood of cancer patients. Fox and Rosenberg[15] incubated peripheral blood lymphocytes (PBL) with interleukin-2 and discovered that the PBL became activated and were able to lyse fresh autologous or allogeneic tumor cells without developing lytic activity against most fresh normal host tissues. The cytotoxicity was distinct from that mediated by NK cells or cytotoxic T lymphocytes, as shown by the ability of LAK cells to lyse NK-cell-resistant fresh tumors and several NK-cell-resistant cultured tumor lines.[10,15] Morphological and kinetic studies have shown that LAK cells directly infiltrate tumor spheroids and adhere tightly to the tumor cells.[16] Tumor destruction becomes evident as the individual cells degenerate.[16,17] There is evidence that the cytolytic effect of LAK cells may be mediated or enhanced by exocytosis of cytokines.[17]

TIL have specific immunoreactivity with the tumors they occupy. They are obtained by removing cancerous tissue or a nodule from a patient and forming a cell suspension by enzymatic digestion or chopping the sample into small fragments. Interleukin-2-stimulated TIL express highly specific cytolytic activity against autologous tumors in about 40% of patients.[18,19] In mice, TIL have a 50–100 times greater antitumor effect than do LAK cells on a cell-to-cell basis.[8,20] Migration of TIL to sites of metastases has been observed in patients within 24 hours after the infusion of ^{111}In-labeled cells.[21,22] Since therapy with LAK cells or TIL involves the transfer of immune cells into the host, it is, by definition, adoptive immunotherapy.

Chemical Properties

Interleukin-2 is a 15.5-kilodalton (kDa) protein.[5,7] Native interleukin-2 is a glycosylated protein secreted by a subset of antigen-activated T lymphocytes. Deletion of amino acid residues 1–20 at the amino terminus, deletion of amino acid residues 121–133 at the carboxyl terminus, or mutation of the cysteine residue at position 58 or 105 has resulted in greater than 99% loss of mitogenic activity.[23] Complementary DNA and genomic DNA clones of interleukin-2 have been isolated and their amino acid sequences fully determined.[7,24,25]

Native interleukin-2 can be purified from a human leukemic T-cell line (Jurkat).[26] Recombinant interleukin-2 has been purified from *E. coli*,[27] *Spodoptera frugiperda* (insect) cells,[28] and monkey cells[7] that contain complementary DNA. Recombinant forms of interleukin-2 synthesized by *E. coli* differ from native interleukin-2 in that they are not glycosylated.[29] Teceleukin also differs from native interleukin-2 in the addition of a methionine residue at the amino terminus.[5] Aldesleukin (des-alanyl-1 serine-125 human interleukin-2) differs from native interleukin-2 at amino acid position 125, where a serine residue replaces a cysteine residue. In addition, aldesleukin lacks an amino-terminal alanine that is present in the native form.[30] Yet another form of recombinant interleukin-2, methionyl alanine-125 human interleukin-2 (Amgen Inc., Thousand Oaks, CA; Ortho Pharmaceutical Corp., Raritan, NJ) differs from native interleukin-2 in the addition of a methionyl residue at the amino terminus and the replacement at amino acid position 125 of a cysteine residue by an alanine residue.[31]

In vitro studies have shown that both the native and recombinant forms of interleukin-2 induce short-term proliferation and sustained long-term growth of mitogen- and alloantigen-stimulated PBMC. The native and recombinant forms of interleukin-2 have also been shown to be comparable in their ability to stimulate the growth of cytotoxic PBMC.[29,32] In no published study have the various recombinant products been compared in vitro or in vivo; nor has a comparison been made of the clinical effects.

The activity of interleukin-2 is expressed in international units, Biological Response Modifiers Program (BRMP) units,[33] Nutley units,[a] and Cetus units.[30] In the literature, aldesleukin activity has generally been expressed in Cetus units and teceleukin activity in Nutley units or BRMP units. An international standard for expressing recombinant interleukin-2 activity was authorized by the World Health Organization (WHO) in 1988.[33] Aldesleukin is currently expressed in international units, and it is predicted that in the future the activity of all generic forms of recombinant interleukin-2 will be expressed in international units. The amount of activity of recombinant interleukin-2 per milligram of protein is 1.8×10^7 IU, 1.5×10^7 Nutley units, or 3×10^6 Cetus units; 1 IU = 1 BRMP unit.

Pharmacology

The effects of interleukin-2 on responsive cells are initiated by the binding of this lymphokine to a receptor glycoprotein or glycoprotein complex on the plasma membrane of these cells.[34] The interleukin-2 receptor on immunologically stimulated cells is composed of two proteins,[35,36] the α chain (55 kDa)[37] and the β chain (75 kDa).[38] These protein chains are not linked covalently by disulfide bonds.[38] Resting T cells, large granular lymphocytes, and NK cells constitutively express the β chain on their plasma membranes. Cells that have the α chain on their surfaces are referred to as Tac positive (Tac^+).[36] Interleukin-2 binds to two distinct sites on the α and β chains. While the molecular association is initiated at the lower-affinity α chain, the signal that induces cellular proliferation is associated with the binding of interleukin-2 to the β chain.[39] There is evidence that internalization of the interleukin-2–receptor complex and tyrosine phosphorylation are components underlying activity.[39–41]

Immunologic Effects

Recombinant interleukin-2 (aldesleukin, teceleukin) stimulates T-cell proliferation and antibody-dependent cellular cytotoxicity in cancer patients.[42–45] Immunologic modulation, as measured by the number of circulating lymphocytes, the proportion of Tac^+ cells, LAK-cell activity, and NK-cell activity, correlates directly with the dosage and duration of infusion of teceleukin.[46] Patients exhibit a rapid decrease in the number of PBMC, including NK cells, within 15 minutes after intravenous injection of native or recombinant interleukin-2 (aldesleukin).[43,47] NK cells adhere to blood vessel endothelial cells and show cytolytic activity against them in the presence of recombinant interleukin-2; this may account for some of the toxicity seen during recombinant interleukin-2 therapy.[48] Recovery of PBMC counts begins 24–48 hours after the initial dose and is characterized by an increase in the proportion of Tac^+ cells.[43,47,49] Generation of NK and LAK cells has been demonstrated in cancer patients during treatment with aldesleukin or teceleukin.[44,50]

Alteration in the expression of neutrophil cell-surface receptors has been observed in association with the administration of recombinant interleukin-2.[51] This change is accompanied by a diminished neutrophil chemotactic response to the chemoattractant formylmethionylleucylphenylalanine and by a diminished ability to generate superoxide free radicals. Although neutrophils retain the ability to phagocytize *Staphylococcus aureus*, the changes in neutrophils during recombinant interleukin-2 administration may contribute to the increased susceptibility of patients to bacterial infections.

Administration of aldesleukin to patients is associated with elevated levels of other cytokines in the blood,[52,53] some of which have been shown to act synergistically with recombinant interleukin-2 in mice.[54,55] These cytokines include interferon gamma, tumor necrosis factors alpha and beta, and interleukin-6.[52–55] The endpoints for measuring synergy with these other cytokines in vivo include greater regression of tumor, increased cure rates, and prolonged survival.[54,55]

There is evidence that pretreatment with cyclophosphamide enhances the antitumor activity of recombinant interleukin-2. Papa et al.[56] reported a dose-related survival advantage in mice with pulmonary metastases that were treated with cyclophosphamide 24 hours before the start of a six-day cycle of recombinant interleukin-2; enhanced survival was not observed in mice pretreated with doxorubicin or bischloroethylnitrosourea. This effect may be due to a reduction in tumor burden by the cytotoxic agent, an increase in the susceptibility of tumor to cellular immune-modulated lysis, or a decrease in suppressor-cell activity.[57,58] Irradiation has been found to act synergistically with the combination of recombinant interleukin-2 and TIL.[59]

Antibodies to recombinant interleukin-2 have been detected in patients receiving this agent. These antibodies have not shown any interaction with native interleukin-2 nor an ability to neutralize the biological activity of recombinant interleukin-2.[60]

Pharmacokinetics

The pharmacokinetics of purified native interleukin-2 and recombinant interleukin-2 after administration to normal volunteers,[47] cancer patients,[30,43,47] or AIDS patients[61] can be described by a two-compartment model. After intravenous administration, recombinant interleukin-2 disappears from the plasma with a distribution-phase half-life of 6–13 minutes; the plasma half-life during beta-phase elimination is 30–120 minutes.[30,43,47,61] The distribution of recombinant interleukin-2 from the vascular compartment may represent binding of the lymphokine to lymphocytes or soluble interleukin-2 receptors in the plasma.[62,63]

The half-life of recombinant interleukin-2 in nude (athymic) mice was not found to differ significantly from that in immune-competent mice.[64] In addition, pretreatment of mice with cyclophosphamide or irradiation did not affect the half-life of recombinant interleukin-2. Distribution of recombinant interleukin-2 may represent its migration from the vascular space to the extracellular space.[30] The half-life of recombinant interleukin-2 is significantly increased when the lymphokine is chemically modified by the addition of polyethylene glycol (PEG).[65] Aldesleukin conjugated with PEG is undergoing Phase I trials.[66]

Konrad et al.[30] reported the pharmacokinetics of aldesleukin given to cancer patients by various routes. After intravenous administration of aldesleukin, a central volume of distribution of 4.3 L and a steady-state volume of distribution of 7.9 L were measured. A steady-state concentration in plasma of 41 U/mL was reported during intravenous infusion of 10^6 U/sq m over six hours. Area under the plasma concentration–time curve was 1.45×10^4 U·min/mL per 10^6 U/kg for 52 patients who received a bolus dose of 2.5×10^5–1.4×10^7 U/sq m given over five minutes. After intravenous administration of interleukin-2 10^5 U/kg every eight hours, activity was measured in the cerebrospinal fluid of patients.[67]

Konrad et al.[30] also reported the mean peak concentration in plasma after intramuscular administration of 10^6 U/sq m to be 14 U/mL. A peak plasma concentration of 1.3–160 U/mL was observed 90–240 minutes after intramuscular injection of 2.5×10^5–4.0×10^6 U. Bioavailability after intramuscular administration was 37% (range, 15–64%). The mean peak plasma level after subcutaneous administration of 10^6 U/sq m was 10.4 U/mL. After intraperitoneal infusion, interleukin-2 activity in the peritoneal fluid was 430 times greater than the activity in plasma. Intraperitoneal administration greatly increased the half-life of recombinant interleukin-2 in the peritoneal fluid (22 hours) and the plasma (6.3 hours).[30,68]

Detectable amounts of interleukin-2 have been measured in the urine of patients with elevated levels of endogenous serum interleukin-2 during acute renal allograft rejection or active cytomegalovirus infection.[69] Total body clearance of recombinant interleukin-2 is reportedly 120 mL/min,[30] which suggests that renal filtration is a major route of clearance (the human glomerulus can freely filter proteins smaller than 30 kDa). Preclinical evaluations in mice provided evidence that the kidneys are the major site of elimination of this lymphokine; degradation or catabolism in the renal tubules may follow filtration.[64]

Assays of Activity

The activity of recombinant interleukin-2 is usually expressed as units of activity that reflect the ability of the agent to promote proliferation in a responsive cell line. Cellular proliferation is measured by the amount of ^{3}H-thymidine incorporated into the DNA. Cells are harvested after incubation with ^{3}H-thymidine, and uptake is measured with a liquid scintillation counter. Activity is quantified as the percent uptake of ^{3}H-thymidine. The original definition of 1 U of interleukin-2 per milliliter was the concentration of interleukin-2 that caused half-maximum incorporation of ^{3}H-thymidine.[30] However, the World Health Organization has authorized a standard interleukin-2 preparation that may be used to generate a calibration curve for quantifying activity.[33]

Assays used by different laboratories may vary in terms of cell lines, culture media, and incubation times.[30,33,61] Some authors have reported the presence of "inhibitors" in serum that are related to the dilution and temperature of the sample[47]; others report that such inhibitors are absent.[64] The enzyme-linked immunosorbent assay (ELISA) and radioimmunoassay have been used to measure the concentration of recombinant interleukin-2 in serum and urine samples.[69] The ELISA, however, does not address whether the recombinant interleukin-2 being measured is physiologically functional.

Bioassays that measure the activity of interleukin-2 do not differentiate between exogenous interleukin-2 and the endogenous interleukin-2 that is produced by a stimulated immune system.[64] Elevated endogenous interleukin-2 has been observed in certain disease states, including systemic lupus erythematosus,[70] chronic progressive multiple sclerosis,[71] cytomegalovirus infection, and renal allograft rejection.[69] Therapy with recombinant interleukin-2 may lead to immunologic and physiological changes that affect its pharmacokinetic behavior. Receptor-mediated metabolism of interleukin-2 may be increased by lymphocyte proliferation and increased receptor density at the cell surface.[30,34] The pharmacokinetic behavior of interleukin-2 in the presence of decreased renal function, edema, and positive fluid balance has not been evaluated, although these conditions commonly occur during therapy with this agent[72-75] and can be predicted to influence its clearance and volume of distribution.[30,64]

Clinical Trials

Recombinant Interleukin-2 plus LAK Cells. Figure 1 diagrams one course of therapy with the initial regimen of recombinant interleukin-2 plus LAK cells as used at the Surgery Branch of the National Cancer Institute (NCI). The lymphokine is first administered as an intravenous bolus of 10^5 U/kg every eight hours on days 1-5. The goal of this priming phase is to induce rebound lymphocytosis in order to increase the yield of leukapheresis, which is the next phase of treatment.[76] Patients rest on days 6 and 7 before undergoing leukapheresis sessions of four to five hours on days 8–12.[77] Cells harvested are often separated with a Ficoll-Hypaque density gradient.[9,14] Cell recovery and lytic activity are not compromised when a more simplified procedure is used that does not include Ficoll-Hypaque separation.[78] Mononuclear cells are then incubated with 1×10^3–1.5×10^3 U of recombinant interleukin-2 per milliliter, thereby generating LAK cells from the mononuclear fraction.[9,14] LAK cells are reinfused into patients on days 12, 13, and 15, starting immediately after the end of leukapheresis. Concurrent with the infusion of LAK cells, patients also receive five days of treatment with recombinant interleukin-2 as described for the priming phase. Dose-limiting adverse reactions associated with recombinant interleukin-2 include hypotension, edema, and renal dysfunction.[76] Since patients require hemodynamic monitoring and support during this therapy, all are treated in the intensive-care unit.[73]

Figure 1. Diagrammatic representation of one course of therapy with recombinant interleukin-2 plus lymphokine-activated killer (LAK) cells as used at the National Cancer Institute. The arrows point to days on which LAK cells are reinfused after incubation with recombinant interleukin-2. IVB = intravenous bolus (10^5 U/kg every eight hours), L(*n*) = leukapheresis session.

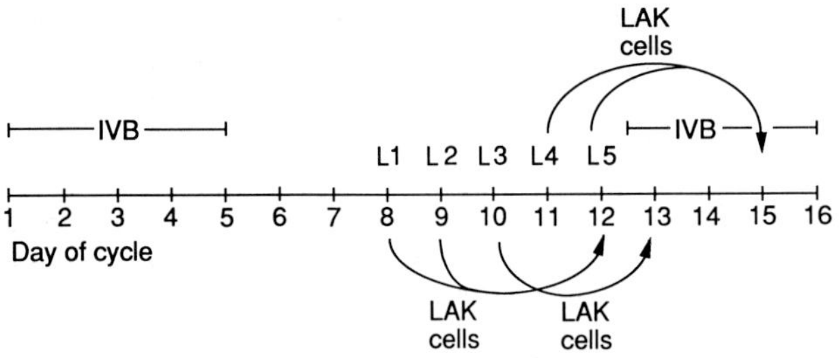

The NCI established the IL-2/LAK Working Group (ILWG) in 1985 to expand research with adoptive immunotherapy. The ILWG represents six extramural cancer centers.[79] The majority of patients being treated have had renal cell carcinoma, melanoma, and colon cancer.[77,80]

Renal Cell Cancer. The objective response rate in patients with renal cell cancer who received the initial NCI regimen[81] was 21% (Table 2). The objective response rate represents the sum of partial

Table 2.
Summary of Clinical Trials of High-Dose Recombinant Interleukin-2 with or without Lymphokine-Activated Killer Cells

References	Regimen and Cancer Type	No. Patients	No. Patients with Complete Response	No. Patients with Partial Response	Objective Response Rate (%)	Duration of Response (mo)
80, 82, 83, 86, 87	Recombinant interleukin-2 with LAK[a] cells					
	Renal cell cancer	161	10	23	21	1–36+
	Melanoma	90	5	16	23	2–52+
	Colorectal cancer	43	1	4	12	2–11
	Other	38	1	8	24	8–31+
	Total	332	17	51	20	1–52+
80, 86	Recombinant interleukin-2 without LAK cells					
	Renal cell cancer	86	6	12	21	3–34+
	Melanoma	42	0	10	24	2–41+
	Colorectal cancer	12	0	0	0	0
	Other	22	0	0	0	0
	Total	162	6	22	17	2–41+

[a] LAK = lymphokine-activated killer.

responses and complete responses. A complete response is conventionally defined as the disappearance of all clinical evidence of disease. A partial response is defined as a ≥50% decrease in the sum of the products of the longest perpendicular diameters of all lesions, without any new lesions developing.

Tumor response, including complete response, has been reported after one cycle of therapy,[76,82] and durations of response ranging from nine months to longer than 36 months have been reported.[80,82] Patients with intra-abdominal masses of >100 sq cm or with an intact primary tumor have generally not responded to therapy.[82] Sites of response have included the lungs, soft tissues, lymph nodes, and bones.[76,81,82] The total dose of recombinant interleukin-2 plus LAK cells administered has not differed significantly between responders and nonresponders; however, a positive correlation between patients' baseline performance status (ability to perform activities of daily life) and response to treatment has been reported.[82]

Melanoma. The objective response rate reported in patients with malignant melanoma after treatment with the initial NCI regimen was 23% (Table 2). Objective response was observed after one cycle of therapy; however, the time to achieve the maximum response was six months in one complete responder.[83] Dutcher et al.[83] reported a median response time of five months, and durable response times ranging from 31 months to longer than 52 months have been reported.[80,83] Sites of response have included the lungs, lymph nodes, subcutaneous tissue, and visceral sites.[76,81,83] The total dose of recombinant interleukin-2 plus LAK cells administered has not differed significantly between responders and nonresponders.[83]

Colorectal Cancer. The objective response rate in patients with colorectal cancer was 12% (Table 2). In general, the responses achieved with this regimen in colon cancer have not been as durable as those in renal cell cancer or melanoma.[80]

Recombinant Interleukin-2 Alone versus Recombinant Interleukin-2 plus LAK Cells. Responses to aldesleukin or teceleukin administered without LAK cells have been demonstrated (Table 2).[76,80,84–86] The data in Table 2 for therapy without LAK cells represent studies in which recombinant interleukin-2 was given as shown in Figure 1 or as a 120-hour continuous infusion of aldesleukin 1×10^6–5×10^6 U/sq m/24 hours followed by a break of four to six days, during which some patients underwent three sessions of leukapheresis. This was followed by a 108–120-hour continuous infusion of recombinant interleukin-2 3×10^6–5×10^6 U/sq m/24 hours, during which some patients received infusions of LAK cells.[80,86,87] One study included a cohort of 28 patients who received an additional cycle of leukapheresis and a 120-hour continuous infusion of recombinant interleukin-2 with LAK cells.[87] Recombinant interleukin-2 has been compared with recombinant interleukin-2 plus LAK cells in randomized[86] and nonrandomized[76] trials. Although a significant difference in response was not observed between the groups, there was a larger proportion of complete responses in the group that also received LAK cells.[76,86]

Recombinant Interleukin-2 plus TIL. The efficacy of cyclophosphamide pretreatment and aldesleukin with TIL has been investigated. The initial NCI protocol included cyclophosphamide 25–50 mg/kg administered 36 hours before the infusion of TIL.[88] Patients received a total of one to seven infusions (4×10^{10}–2.05×10^{11} TIL per infusion) over one to two days. After the first infusion of TIL, patients began treatment with recombinant interleukin-2 10^5 U/kg administered intravenously every eight hours until dose-limiting toxicity occurred.[19,88] The effect of pretreatment with cyclophosphamide remains controversial, and cyclophosphamide is no longer used in the current NCI protocol for interleukin-2 plus TIL.

The results of therapy with recombinant interleukin-2 plus TIL are listed in Table 3. Rosenberg et al.[88] reported that of 20 patients with melanoma, 1 responded completely to this therapy and 10 achieved a partial response. Five of the 20 patients had failed to respond in a previous trial of recombinant interleukin-2 or recombinant interleukin-2 plus LAK cells. Two of these five had a partial response after receiving recombinant interleukin-2 plus TIL. Measurable response was observed after one course of therapy; the duration of response ranged from two months to longer than 13 months. Sites of response included the lungs, liver, spleen, lymph nodes, bones, and subcutaneous tissues. Partial responses were also observed in one of four renal cell cancer patients treated with recombinant interleukin-2 plus TIL.[19]

Effect of Infusion Rate. The rate of infusion of recombinant interleukin-2 has been adjusted in an attempt to decrease treatment-related toxicity while maintaining efficacy. West et al.[87] reported the effects of administering aldesleukin 1×10^6–7×10^6 U/sq m/24 hours as a continuous infusion for a total of 120 hours (days 1–5). After the infusion, patients were allowed 36 hours of rest, which was followed by leukapheresis on days 7–10. Cycle 2 began on day 10. On days 10, 11, and 13, harvested LAK cells were reinfused, and on days 10–15 aldesleukin was concurrently administered as described for days 1–5. The patients received a total of two to four cycles of therapy; the dosage of aldesleukin was increased at the start of each cycle.

The daily dosage of aldesleukin used in this protocol was substantially lower than that described by Rosenberg.[84] However, since recombinant interleukin-2 has a short plasma half-life, continuous infusion may provide a means of optimizing delivery.[43] The minimum dosage used by West et al.[87]

Table 3.
Summary of Clinical Trials of Recombinant Interleukin-2 in Various Regimens

Reference(s)	Regimen[a]	No. Patients	No. Patients with Complete Response	No. Patients with Partial Response	Objective Response Rate (%)	Duration of Response (mo)
80	HDB rIL-2	130	4	18	17	3–41+
80, 82, 83	HDB rIL-2 + LAK cells	241	17	38	23	1–52+
88	HDB rIL-2 + TIL	20	1	10	55	2–13+
86	CI rIL-2	32	2	4	19	3–13+
86, 87	CI rIL-2 + LAK	91	5	22	30	1.5–11+
31, 89	LD rIL-2 + LAK	55	2	13	27	1–10+
90	CYC pre-Tx + rIL-2	27	1	5	22	1.5–12+
80, 92	IFN alfa + rIL-2	113	7	25	28	3–14+
97	IFN beta + rIL-2	22	1	5	27	4–24+
99	Intrasplenic rIL-2 + i.v. rIL-2	31	0	4	13	NR

[a] HDB = high-dose bolus, rIL-2 = recombinant interleukin-2, LAK = lymphokine-activated killer, TIL = tumor-infiltrating lymphocytes, CI = continuously infused, LD = low-dose, CYC = cyclophosphamide, pre-Tx = pretreatment, IFN = interferon, NR = not reported.

that yielded the desired level of lymphocytosis was 3×10^6 Cetus units/sq m/day. Thirteen of the 28 patients who received a priming dose of this size responded to treatment.

The reported objective response rate for this regimen, 22% (Table 3), is similar to the objective response rate reported for recombinant interleukin-2 plus LAK cells when high-dose recombinant interleukin-2 was administered every eight hours as a bolus injection[80]; however, no complete responses were observed by West et al. They observed partial responses in patients with melanoma (5 of 10 patients), renal cancer (3 of 6), Hodgkin's disease (1 of 1), non-Hodgkin's lymphoma (1 of 1), ovarian cancer (1 of 1), lung cancer (1 of 2), and parotid cancer (1 of 2). No complete or partial responses were achieved in the 13 patients with colon cancer who were enrolled. A duration of response exceeding seven months was reported in one patient.[87]

Effect of Dosage and Schedule. Lower dosages of recombinant interleukin-2 have been given for prolonged periods to patients with metastatic cancer.[31,89] Inpatients received 14 consecutive doses of 3×10^4 BRMP units of recombinant interleukin-2 per kilogram every eight hours on days 1–5. The patients were discharged on day 6 and underwent leukapheresis for three hours daily during outpatient visits on five consecutive days (days 8–12). The patients were then readmitted to the hospital on day 12 for infusion of LAK cells on days 12, 13, and 15 and concurrent intravenous administration of recombinant interleukin-2 3×10^4 BRMP units/kg every eight hours through day 19.[31,89]

The objective response rate for this regimen was 33% (range, 15–38%) (Table 3). The range of complete and partial response rates was 0–7% and 15–31%, respectively. The duration of response ranged from one month to longer than 10 months. Sites of response included the lungs, lymph nodes, soft tissue, liver, and bones.[31]

Effect of Pretreatment with Cyclophosphamide. The efficacy of cyclophosphamide pretreatment followed by once-daily intravenous administration of recombinant interleukin-2 in the treatment of melanoma has been investigated, since there is evidence that this approach has an increased antitumor effect.[56–58] Mitchell et al.[90] administered intravenous low-dose cyclophosphamide (350 mg/sq m) to 27 patients. Beginning three days later, aldesleukin 3.6×10^6 U/sq m was administered daily for five days. After two days without treatment, the five-day course of aldesleukin was repeated. The scheduling of aldesleukin administration was designed to facilitate the use of this regimen in a day-hospital setting in which patients could be treated and observed for eight hours.[90] The objective response rate was 23% (Table 3).

Concurrent Administration of Interferon Alfa. Phase I and Phase II trials of recombinant interleukin-2 in combination with recombinant interferon alfa have been undertaken to assess the additive or synergistic potential of this combination.[91,92] Interferon alfa is associated with increased expression of the cell surface antigens used by TIL to recognize tumor cells. This approach to therapy is supported by reports of marked synergistic antitumor activity in tumor-bearing mice treated with recombinant interleukin-2 plus recombinant interferon alfa.[54,93]

Rosenberg et al.[92] treated patients with progressively larger doses of teceleukin (1×10^6, 3×10^6, and 4.5×10^6 U/sq m) and recombinant interferon alfa (3×10^6 and 6×10^6 U/sq m). Each agent was infused intravenously over 15 minutes every eight hours. The patients received an equal number of doses of each agent. Of the 91 patients evaluated, 37% had renal cell cancer and 41% had melanoma. The objective response rate was 41% in the patients who received teceleukin 4.5×10^6 U/sq m plus recombinant interferon alfa 6×10^6 U/sq m and 23%, 20%, and 17% in the patients who received teceleukin 4.5×10^6, 3×10^6, and 1×10^6 U/sq m, respectively, along with recombinant interferon alfa 3×10^6 U/sq m—a clear dose–response relationship.

The overall objective response rate in studies of this regimen was 28% (Table 3). Sites of response included the lungs, lymph nodes, subcutaneous tissue, liver, bones, and adrenal glands. The duration of response ranged from three months to longer than 10 months. The objective response rate of patients with metastatic renal cell cancer to interferon alfa averaged 15% (range, 0–29%), with a median duration of response of eight months.[94]

Concurrent Administration of Interferon Beta. Recombinant interferon beta has been combined with recombinant interleukin-2 in an attempt to increase the response to therapy. Two studies of the use of recombinant interferon beta in the treatment of renal cell cancer showed a partial response in 3 of 31 patients.[95] The maximum tolerated dosages of aldesleukin and recombinant interferon beta as combination therapy were determined during Phase I evaluation to be aldesleukin 5×10^6 U/sq m given as an intravenous bolus injection three times weekly and interferon beta 10^7 U/sq m given as an intravenous bolus injection three times weekly.[96]

The objective response rate for this therapy in a study of 22 patients with renal cell cancer was 27% (Table 3).[97] Responses occurred within eight weeks of the initiation of treatment. Sites of response included the lungs, soft tissue, lymph nodes, and bones. Sites that did not respond included the kidneys, renal fossae, adrenal glands, and liver.

Intrasplenic Administration. Because of evidence that the spleen is rich in LAK-cell precursors,[98] intrasplenic administration of recombinant interleukin-2 was investigated as a method of enhancing LAK-cell generation.[99,100] The hope was that the use of this route of administration would circumvent the logistical difficulties of obtaining LAK cells and result in effective LAK-cell activity while requiring fewer high doses of recombinant interleukin-2. Thatcher et al.[99] administered aldesleukin 1.1×10^7 U/sq m (the previously determined maximum tolerated dose) as a one-hour infusion into the splenic artery of 31 patients with melanoma. The patients also received a total of four doses of aldesleukin 1.1×10^7 U/sq m given as one-hour intravenous infusions. The first intravenous dose was administered four hours after the start of the intrasplenic infusion, and the remaining three doses were administered on an every-other-day schedule. Four patients had partial responses, yielding an objective response rate of 13% (Table 3).

Intracranial Administration. In a Phase I study, Jacobs et al.[101] looked at the feasibility of intracranial adoptive immunotherapy for patients with malignant gliomas. These investigators injected progressively larger doses of aldesleukin 10^4–10^6 U with or without LAK cells (10^7–10^{10}) directly into the brain tissue surrounding the cavities left by surgical debulking of malignant gliomas. There was no marked systemic or neurological toxicity. Subsequent studies are summarized in Table 4.

Potential Treatment of Minimal Residual Disease. Gottlieb et al.[105] conducted a Phase I trial of the use of recombinant interleukin-2 in patients who had undergone bone marrow-ablative antineoplastic therapy or ablative therapy and autologous bone marrow transplantation. The purpose was to evaluate the possibility of using recombinant interleukin-2 to prevent relapse from minimal residual disease after ablative therapy. Minimal residual disease is believed to be responsible for the vast majority of cases of recurrent disease following bone marrow transplantation.[106] Patients with acute myelogenous leukemia (10 patients) or multiple myeloma (3 patients) received recombinant interleukin-2 0.4×10^6–1.8×10^6 IU/sq m daily for three to five days after ablative therapy or following ablative therapy and autologous bone marrow transplantation. The greatest toxicity occurred in two patients who began therapy with recombinant interleukin-2 immediately after ablative therapy and were administered this agent for 11 or 12 days. Treatment with recombinant interleukin-2 was initiated in the remaining patients when their neutrophil count reached 500 per microliter and was administered for two to five days. The incidence of hypotension, dyspnea, and edema was 20%, 13%, and 27%, respectively. None of the patients required support in the intensive-care unit.

Adverse Drug Reactions

Adverse effects during treatment with recombinant interleukin-2 are generally related to the dosage,[46,85,107] dosage interval,[107] rate of infusion,[46,87] and duration of therapy.[108] Patients appear to become less tolerant with successive courses of treatment, and this progressive decrease in tolerance cannot be circumvented by delaying retreatment.[108] The adverse effects of recombinant interleukin-2 tend to disappear after therapy is discontinued, however.[72–74,81,109–112] The incidence of adverse reactions may vary among medical centers, in part because of disparities in experience with this complex therapy. The incidence of treatment-related mortality is 1–1.5%.[74,80] Table 5 summarizes the adverse effects of recombinant interleukin-2 administered alone or in combination with cells or other agents.

Fever, rigors, chills, and malaise occur commonly within hours of the administration of aldesleukin or teceleukin.[81,85,107] Prophylaxis with acetaminophen (650 mg orally every four to six hours) and nonsteroidal anti-inflammatory agents (indo-

Table 4.
Summary of Clinical Trials of Intracranially Administered Recombinant Interleukin-2 with Lymphokine-Activated Killer Cells

Reference	Regimen	No. Patients	Outcome
102	rIL-2 10^5 Cetus units after surgery in some but not all patients plus 10^9 LAK[a] cells	55	Positive response[b] in 50 patients after 2 months, no response in 5 patients, survival advantage relative to historical controls in 19 patients, acceptable levels of toxicity
103	rIL-2 10^6 Cetus units after surgery and every other day for a total of 4 doses plus 10^9 LAK cells	13	Response durations of 70+ and 67+ mo in 2 patients, no overall survival advantage in 11 patients, acceptable levels of toxicity
104	rIL-2 10^4 Cetus units/kg/day on days 1–5 after surgery plus 10^9 LAK cells daily for 2 days	9	Partial response in 1 patient, new onset or worsening of pre-existing focal neurological deficits in all patients, new neurological deficits that were not reversible in 5 patients

[a] LAK = lymphokine-activated killer.
[b] Postive response = either no evidence of tumor enlargement or evidence of a decrease in tumor size in a patient who remains clinically stable or improves.[102]

methacin 25–50 mg orally or rectally every six to eight hours)[74,113] decreases the incidence and severity of these symptoms.[81] Rigors tend to respond to intravenous meperidine hydrochloride 25–50 mg repeated as needed for relief of symptoms and as tolerated.[73] The mechanism responsible for these constitutional symptoms and for certain changes in cardiovascular status that occur during treatment with recombinant interleukin-2 may be related to elevated serum levels of tumor necrosis factor alpha.[53,74,114]

The most common dose-limiting adverse reactions associated with high-dose bolus administration of recombinant interleukin-2 as described for the initial NCI regimen are hypotension, edema, and renal dysfunction.[76] Regimens involving administration of the agent as a continuous infusion[87] or in lower doses given over extended periods[31,89] were intended to maintain efficacy and decrease toxicity. A low incidence of hypotension requiring support with vasopressors was reported by West et al.,[87] who administered recombinant interleukin-2 as a continuous infusion. Therapy was provided in a conventional oncology nursing unit, although 6 of the 40 patients were transferred to the intensive-care unit during therapy for management of hypotensive episodes (five patients) or bacterial sepsis (one patient). Toxicity associated with the low-dose regimen described by Eberlein et al.[31] was more acceptable than that associated with high-dose recombinant interleukin-2.[80] The most frequent adverse reactions reported by Eberlein et al. were fever, chills, malaise, fatigue, anorexia, diarrhea, nausea, vomiting, rash, and stomatitis. In addition, elevation of serum creatinine ($\geq$ 2 mg/dL), elevation of serum bilirubin ($\geq$ 2 mg/dL), and anemia requiring blood transfusions were reported in 47%, 37%, and 17% of patients, respectively. None of the 29 patients required vasopressors to maintain blood pressure. On the other hand, when Stahel et al.[89] used the same low-dose regimen and the same form of recombinant interleukin-2 as Eberlein et al., patients reacted with dose-limiting toxicities like those seen with high-dose bolus administration. Hypotension with impaired renal function and central nervous system toxicity were reported. Twenty-one of the 26 patients (81%) required support with vasopressors because of decreased urinary output or hypotension. Further investigation is needed to clarify the adverse-effect profile of the low-dose approach.

Pretreatment with low-dose cyclophosphamide followed by once-daily intravenous administration of recombinant interleukin-2 was a regimen designed for the day-hospital setting, where patients can be treated and observed for eight hours. In a study by Mitchell et al.,[90] the most frequently reported adverse effects of this regimen were fatigue, fever, nausea, vomiting, rigors, and chills. Mild to moderate hypotension was observed in more than half of the 26 patients, and a decrease in blood pressure of up to 40 mm Hg was reported in

Table 5.
Summary of Adverse Effects Observed in Clinical Trials of Recombinant Interleukin-2[a]

Study Variable and Adverse Effect(s)	HDB rIL-2 + LAK Cells	HDB rIL-2 + TIL	CI rIL-2	LD rIL-2 + LAK Cells	CYC pre-Tx + rIL-2	IFN alfa + rIL-2
Reference(s)	80, 82, 83	80	87	31, 90	89	80, 92
No. patients	278	66	40	55	27	128
No. treatment courses	412	95	40	56	27	210
Fever	++++	NR	++++	++++	++++	+++
Chills and rigors	++++	++	NR	++++	++++	NR
Fatigue and somnolence	+++	++	++++	++++	++++	+
Rash and pruritus	++	+	++++	++++	++	+
Mucositis	+	+	++	+++	−	+
Gastrointestinal problems	++++	+++	+++	++++	+++	++++
Elevated serum bilirubin (>2 mg/dL)	++++	++++	+[b]	++	−	++++
Elevated serum creatinine (>2 mg/dL)	++++	++++	++[b]	+++	−	++++
Dyspnea	+	++	+	++	++	+
Intubation required	+	+	−	+	−	+
Vasopressors required	++++	+++	+	++	−	++
Oliguria	+++	++	++++	++	−	++++
Angina	+	−	NR	−	−	+
Myocardial infarction	+	−	−	−	−	+
Increase in actual body weight (≥10%)	++	++	+	++	NR	++++
Anemia						
≤5 units blood transfused	+++	++	++++[c]	+	++[d]	
>5 units blood transfused	++	+		−		++[e]
Thrombocytopenia						
<2 × 10⁴ platelets/cu mm	++	++	NR	−	++	+
≥2 × 10⁴ platelets/cu mm	++++	++++		++	++++	++++
Central venous line sepsis	+	+	+	+	+	+
Death	+	+	+	−	−	+

[a] HDB = high-dose bolus, rIL-2 = recombinant interleukin-2, LAK = lymphokine-activated killer, TIL = tumor-infiltrating lymphocytes, CI = continuously infused, LD = low-dose, CYC = cyclophosphamide, pre-Tx = pretreatment, IFN = interferon, NR = not reported, ++++ = 76–100% incidence, +++ = 51–75%, ++ = 26–50%, + = ≤25%, − = 0%.
[b] >3 mg/dL.
[c] Number of transfusions required not specified.
[d] A mild to moderate decrease in hemoglobin concentration was observed in 11 of 27 patients; no transfusions were reported.
[e] Includes transfusions of 1–5 units.

four patients (15%). Two patients required overnight hospitalization for repletion of fluids or for fatigue.

The adverse-effect profile seen when interferon alfa,[92] interferon beta,[96] or interferon gamma[115] is administered concurrently with recombinant interleukin-2 is consistent with the toxicities predicted from the dosages and scheduling of the individual biological agents administered. A more pronounced cardiotoxicity, evidenced by an increased incidence of asymptomatic elevation of creatinine kinase (MB isoenzyme fraction), may occur when interferon alfa and recombinant interleukin are used concurrently.[92] Further evaluation is needed.

The infusion of LAK cells or TIL may cause rigors or chills that tend to respond to intravenous meperidine hydrochloride 25–50 mg repeated as needed to control symptoms and as tolerated.[73] The addition of LAK cells or TIL does not otherwise increase treatment-related toxicity over that associated with recombinant interleukin-2 alone.[74,77] Hepatitis A virus seroconversion has been reported after the administration of LAK cells that were incubated in medium containing contaminated human AB serum.[76,116] LAK cells are now cultured in serum-free medium.[78]

In most studies, adverse effects occurring when recombinant interleukin-2 was administered with or without LAK-cell therapy by routes other than the intravenous have been mild to moderate. After intrasplenic administration of aldesleukin, commonly reported adverse effects included fever, nausea, emesis, and hypotension; the incidence of hypotension that required fluid support was 17%.[99] One patient in a Phase II study developed temporary respiratory arrest after the intrasplenic catheter was removed[117]; otherwise, no life-threatening toxicity has been reported for intrasplenic administration of this agent. Common adverse effects reported during and immediately after intracranial administration were fever, headache, nausea, and lethargy,[102,103] reactions that are common in neurosurgical patients after procedures.[102] Superficial wound infections were reported in four patients, but there were no reports of intracranial infections.[102] However, new onset or worsening of neurological deficits occurred in all patients who were treated with a more intensive regimen of intracranial recombinant interleukin-2 plus LAK cells (Table 4).[104]

Cardiovascular Effects

Intravenous administration of recombinant interleukin-2 causes dose-limiting hemodynamic changes that resemble those seen in septic shock.[73,111,112,118] Mean arterial pressure decreases within two hours after administration begins. As treatment proceeds, mean arterial pressure decreases by 20–30 mm Hg, necessitating the administration of intravenous fluids and pressors in 65–75% of patients.[73,74,111,112] This change is accompanied by an increase in heart rate of 35–40 beats/min.[73,111,112] Supraventricular arrhythmias responsive to conventional treatment (digoxin or verapamil) have been reported in 6.4–16% of patients.[73,74,80] Sustained supraventricular tachycardia with hypotension has been reported in 1.7% of patients.[73]

The incidence of angina with electrocardiographic evidence of ischemic changes during therapy is 2.6–6%, and the incidence of acute myocardial infarction is <1–4%.[73,74,80] The level of MB isoenzyme increased 3-6% in 2 of 10 patients whose enzyme levels were being monitored daily.[73] Both patients remained asymptomatic, and cardiac catheterization revealed no evidence of coronary artery disease.

Cardiac index increases and systemic vascular resistance decreases during therapy.[73,111,112] Mild cardiac dysfunction is evidenced by a decrease in left ventricular ejection fraction to 6–20% below pretreatment values,[73,112] accompanied by a decreased left ventricular stroke work index.[73] Pulmonary capillary wedge pressure may increase during therapy, although the change is not clinically significant.[73,111]

Hemodynamic changes persist throughout recombinant interleukin-2 treatment but tend to reverse within 24 hours after therapy ends.[73,111,112] Approaches to managing the hemodynamic changes are presented in Table 6.

Table 6.
Management of Hemodynamic Adverse Effects of Recombinant Interleukin-2[a]

A. Systolic blood pressure is <90 mm Hg or diastolic blood pressure is <50 mm Hg.
   1. Administer intravenous fluids; rate is determined by patient response and tolerance. Frequently used intravenous fluids include 0.9% sodium chloride injection, 0.45% sodium chloride injection, and 10–20 meq of potassium chloride per liter of 5% dextrose and 0.45% sodium chloride injection.
   2. If patient is anemic, transfuse blood to keep hemoglobin concentration >11 mg/dL.
   3. If necessary, administer dopamine hydrochloride 2–4 μg/kg/min to maintain renal blood flow and urine output.
B. Systolic blood pressure remains <90 mm Hg, diastolic blood pressure remains <50 mm Hg, or patient cannot tolerate fluids.
   1. Administer dopamine hydrochloride 5–10 μg/kg/min to maintain blood pressure.
C. Patient becomes tachycardic (heart rate, >150 beats/min), systolic blood pressure remains <90 mm Hg, or diastolic blood pressure remains <50 mm Hg.
   1. Give phenylephrine 5–10 μg/kg/min to maintain blood pressure.

[a] Adapted from references 73, 74, 111, and 113.

Increase in Vascular Permeability

Vascular leak syndrome (VLS), also referred to as capillary leak syndrome, is a prominent adverse effect during recombinant interleukin-2 therapy; it resolves after therapy ends.[73,119] The syndrome is manifested primarily by severe peripheral edema, (with symptomatic involvement of nerves or vessels), ascites, and pleural effusion; the incidence of these reactions is 1.8%,[73,80] 2.8%,[73] and 1.9–3.1%,[73,80] respectively. Actual body weight increases more than 10% above pretreatment values in 23–32% of patients.[73,80] Pulmonary infiltration may become evident by day 4 of treatment and is associated with a decreased ratio of oxygen partial pressure to fraction of inspired oxygen.[73] Dyspnea at rest was observed in 22% of patients receiving recombinant interleukin-2 plus LAK cells.[74] The incidence of severe respiratory distress requiring supplemental oxygen was reported to be 9.2%,[73] with intubation being required in 4.9–6.4% of patients.[73,74,80]

Approaches to the management of adverse effects related to VLS are presented in Table 7.

VLS is characterized by the leakage of proteinaceous fluid from the vascular space into the interstitium of most body tissues.[119] Consistent with this, the rate of disappearance of iodinated I 125 albumin from the plasma is elevated in patients treated with recombinant interleukin-2.[73] Analysis of the in vivo distribution of iodinated I 125 bovine serum albumin after the intraperitoneal administration of recombinant interleukin-2 in mice

Table 7.
Management of Symptoms Related to Vascular Leak Syndrome[a]

A. Actual body weight increases >10% above baseline, or rales or rhonchi are audible.
   1. Administer furosemide at dosage determined by patient response.
   2. Administer dopamine hydrochloride 2–4 μg/kg/min to maintain renal blood flow and urine output.
B. Patient has dyspnea at rest.
   1. Give supplemental oxygen by face mask.
C. Patient has severe respiratory distress.
   1. Intubate patient and provide mechanical ventilation. Administer ranitidine (as the hydrochloride salt) 50 mg i.v. every 8–12 hours as prophylaxis against stress ulcers.

[a] Adapted from reference 74.

showed that the most pronounced infiltration of fluid occurred in the thymus, spleen, lungs, liver, kidneys, and mesenteric lymph nodes; the amount of infiltration was related to the dosage and duration of treatment.[119,120] The coadministration of recombinant interferon alfa and recombinant interleukin-2 in mice exacerbates VLS.[121] There is evidence that this effect is immune mediated.[119,122,123]

Renal Effects

Reversible nephrotoxicity, consistent with a prerenal syndrome of oliguria, azotemia, elevated serum creatinine,[74,80] urinary acidification,[75] and low urinary fractional excretion of sodium,[74,75,113] has been reported during therapy with interleukin-2. This adverse effect may be exacerbated by the administration of nonsteroidal anti-inflammatory agents during recombinant interleukin-2 therapy.[107] In one study, the relative increase in serum creatinine concentration was greater in patients who continued to receive cycles of therapy with recombinant interleukin-2.[124] Patients with a baseline serum creatinine concentration of >1.5 mg/dL had a higher mean peak serum creatinine concentration and a greater percent increase in serum creatinine above baseline than did patients with pretreatment serum creatinine measurements of <1.4 mg/dL. Pretreatment serum creatinine values of ≥1.5 mg/dL have also been associated with a slower return to normal renal function.[113] The severity of nephrotoxicity in renal cell cancer patients is not greater than that in patients with other malignancies.[113]

Belldegrun et al.[124] treated 41 renal cell cancer patients with recombinant interleukin-2 at various intervals after nephrectomy and measured the effect on peak serum creatinine concentration and mean percent increase in serum creatinine concentration. The patients were grouped according to the number of months that had elapsed between nephrectomy and treatment with the lymphokine. Differences in all results among the groups were not significant.

Metabolic Effects

Hypophosphatemia, hypocalcemia, and hypomagnesemia have been reported to occur during recombinant interleukin-2 therapy and to resolve promptly after the discontinuation of treatment.[72,75] Decreased plasma phosphate concentrations may result from the incorporation of phosphate into rapidly proliferating T cells. These changes of serum chemistry are consistent with a dilutional effect secondary to the edema and positive fluid balance present during therapy. Because these abnormalities are transient and asymptomatic, aggressive supplementation of serum electrolytes is not indicated. An electrolyte should be replenished if its serum level becomes moderately to severely low or the patient becomes symptomatic. There is no evidence of acute renal tubular dysfunction, as a decreased urinary fractional excretion of calcium, magnesium, and phosphorus has not been observed during therapy.[72,75] The administration of intravenous fluids to maintain blood pressure may also contribute to the positive fluid balance and related symptoms. Conversely, an overly conservative approach to fluid administration may accelerate the increase in the serum creatinine concentration.

Neuropsychiatric Effects

Reversible dose-related neuropsychiatric adverse effects have been associated with the administration of recombinant interleukin-2.[74,80,109] Cognitive changes that meet the DSM-III-R[125] criteria for delirium have been reported in 33–50% of patients, even when administration of the agent was discontinued at the first indication of neuropsychiatric symptoms.[74,109] The cognitive changes have been accompanied by severe behavioral changes and perceptual changes in 86% and 14% of patients, respectively.[109]

Denicoff et al.[109] reported that 7 of 47 patients (15%) developed severe cognitive changes associated with delusions during recombinant interleukin-2 therapy; of these patients, five developed paranoid delusions. Neuropsychiatric symptoms usually appear only after several days of therapy.

Mental status changes do not appear to be correlated with the degree of multiple-organ compromise that occurs during therapy. Treatment-associated cerebral edema, however, may contribute to lethargy and confusion in some patients. Using magnetic resonance imaging, Saris et al.[126] found that the water content of the cerebral gray and white matter was increased in patients with extracranial cancer who were receiving intravenous recombinant interleukin-2. The patients' scores on baseline mood and cognitive tests were not predictive of neuropsychiatric symptoms. Patient counseling with respect to the potential for reversible psychiatric adverse effects has been reported to be beneficial.[109] Behavioral changes that require more than minimal supervision have responded well to a low dosage of haloperidol (≤10 mg/day).[109]

Hepatic Effects

Reversible hepatotoxicity has been observed during recombinant interleukin-2 therapy.[74,76,77,88,110] Hepatotoxicity is manifested by an increase in the serum bilirubin concentration[80] and serum aspartate aminotransferase level.[88,110] These indices have been reported to increase by a factor of 5–10 over pretreatment levels in 13–56% of patients.[74,110] Moderate elevations in serum lactate dehydrogenase, alanine aminotransferase, and alkaline phosphatase have been noted. The clinical presentation and the results of radionuclide studies of the liver are generally indicative of reversible cholestasis.[110] Decreased plasma levels of total protein,[85] total cholesterol,[85,127] albumin,[85,110,127] and γ-globulin[85] have been observed.

Hematologic Effects

Anemia, thrombocytopenia, lymphopenia, eosinophilia, mild neutropenia, and rebound lymphocytosis have been observed during and immediately after recombinant interleukin-2 therapy.[128] Anemia has been reported in up to 100% of patients,[85] and 50–96% have required blood transfusions.[74,128] During therapy, transfusion of 1–5 units, 6–10 units, and ≥11 units of blood has been necessary in 42–70%, 10–26%, and ≤15% of patients, respectively.[80,88,128] The loss of 1–1.5 units of blood during treatment is due to phlebotomy.[127] Platelet counts of less than 6×10^4 per microliter (normal range, 1.45×10^5–4.5×10^5 per microliter) have been reported in 32–53% of patients, and counts below 2×10^4 per microliter have been reported in 13–25% of patients.[80,88,128] Ettinghausen et al.[128] reported the incidence of lymphocytopenia during the administration of recombinant interleukin-2 to be 98%, and lymphocyte counts below 2×10^2 per microliter (normal range, 1×10^3–4×10^3 per microliter) were reported in 81% of patients. Lymphocytosis has been identified from the peripheral lymphocyte count after the end of therapy.[43,128] A two- to seven-fold increase above the upper limit of the normal range was reported in 17–71% of patients.[128]

Eosinophilia is a common hematologic event during recombinant interleukin-2 therapy. The onset tends to be near the end of therapy or during the first five days thereafter.[85,128] The incidence of a peak value in excess of 2×10^3 eosinophils per microliter (normal range, 1.45×10^2–4.5×10^2 per microliter) was reported to be 67%, while values exceeding 5×10^3 and 1×10^4 per microliter were reported in 38% and 12% of patients, respectively.[128] Neutrophil counts below 1×10^3 per microliter occur in 7–15% of patients, while neutropenia ($<5 \times 10^2$ neutrophils per microliter) occurs in 2–5% of patients.[128]

Clonogenic assays for hematopoietic progenitors have been used in an attempt to understand how recombinant interleukin-2 induces anemia, thrombocytopenia, and neutropenia. A depression in counts of erythroid progenitors and granulocyte–macrophage progenitors has been observed during therapy.[128] This effect was markedly more pronounced for erythroid progenitors than granulocyte–macrophage progenitors. A rebound in the counts of erythroid and granulocyte–macrophage precursors to levels significantly above baseline occurred after the discontinuation of therapy. Another factor that may contribute to the hematologic changes is the dilutional effect from the positive fluid balance that occurs during therapy.[128]

Endocrine Effects

Atkins et al.[129] reported laboratory evidence of hypothyroidism in 21% of patients receiving recombinant interleukin-2. Decreases in the serum thyroxine concentration to <35 nM (normal range, 65–148 nM) and increases in the concentration of thyroid-stimulating hormone to 7.2–166 mU/L (normal range, 0.5–5.5 mU/L) were observed. A decreased serum free thyroxine index has also been calculated in patients receiving recombinant interleukin-2.[129] Elevated or high-normal levels of serum antibodies to microsomes have been measured in patients who have symptoms consistent with hypothyroidism (e.g., fatigue, cold intolerance, thinning of hair, decreased mental capacity).[129] A subpopulation of patients who were symptomatic also had antibodies to thyroglobulin, suggesting an exacerbation of pre-existing subclinical autoimmune thyroiditis.[129]

The incidence of thyroid dysfunction in patients treated with recombinant interleukin-2 is reportedly greater in females (30%) than males (7%).[130] Resolution of asymptomatic hypothyroidism within 9–10 months was reported in two patients who did not receive thyroid replacement therapy. Since thyroid replacement is routinely used for hypothyroid patients however, the time course of spontaneous resolution is not well defined.[129]

Recombinant interleukin-2 is associated with increased plasma levels of stress-related hormones.[43,47,131] Four hours after infusing recombinant interleukin-2 10^5 U/kg, Denicoff et al.[131] observed a 20-fold increase in the concentration of adrenocorticotropic hormone, a 10-fold increase in β-endorphin, and a 2-fold increase in cortisol above pretreatment values. Hormonal stimulation was more pronounced in the second course of therapy than in the first. The administration of LAK cells did not influence the magnitude of hormonal stimulation.

Dermatologic Effects

Macular erythema with burning and pruritus develops in 48–100% of patients receiving recombinant interleukin-2.[74,81,132] The onset of this rash is usually two to three days after the initiation of therapy. Usually the rash is confined to the head and neck; occasionally a generalized erythroderma occurs. Punch biopsies reveal nonspecific histological changes, including mild to moderate papillary edema, monocyte infiltration, spongiotic foci, and focal basal-cell degeneration. The blood vessels of the papillary dermis are surrounded by T cells, with fewer of these cells evident in the epidermis.[132]

Prophylactic administration of hydroxyzine 10–25 mg orally every four to six hours may be used to decrease the incidence and severity of rashes associated with recombinant interleukin-2.[84] It is important to avoid systemic corticosteroids, since these agents may interfere with the activity of recombinant interleukin-2.[123,133]

Recombinant interleukin-2 can exacerbate psoriasis.[134] Other dermatologic adverse effects, reported in 10% of patients or less, include multiple superficial punctate cutaneous erosions, telogen effluvium, and asymptomatic erosions in surgical scars.[132]

Gastrointestinal Effects

Treatment-related nausea, vomiting, and diarrhea are common during recombinant interleukin-2 therapy. Mild to moderate gastrointestinal symptoms have been reported in 80–100% of patients.[80,85,135] These adverse effects are treated symptomatically. Nausea and vomiting are generally controlled with standard doses of phenothiazine antiemetics, and standard doses of diphenoxylate and atropine are frequently used to control diarrhea.[74] Most patients are given ranitidine 50 mg intravenously every 8–12 hours or 150 mg orally once or twice daily as prophylaxis against gastrointestinal bleeding.[74,81]

Glossitis, which is manifested as erythema, edema, and tenderness of the tongue, occurs in up to 30% of patients.[132] Mucositis is reported to occur in fewer than 10% of patients[132]; a liquid diet is required in 3% of patients receiving recombinant interleukin-2.[80] Symptoms consistent with acute abdomen may be indicative of colonic perforation. This is reported infrequently (incidence, 1.3%) during therapy but must be considered when other etiologic factors are absent.[135]

Antibiotic Prophylaxis

Patients who are administered high-dose recombinant interleukin-2 with or without LAK cells or TIL routinely receive prophylaxis with antibiotics (oxacillin [as the sodium salt] 2 g intravenously every four hours) when a central venous catheter is inserted, even though central venous catheters used for the administration of adoptive immunotherapy are generally in place for only one to seven days.[136] In addition to the risk of sepsis from the placement of a central venous line, patients treated with recombinant interleukin-2 exhibit changes in neutrophil function that may increase their susceptibility to bacterial infection.[51] If sepsis does occur, its diagnosis may be delayed because the early signs and symptoms may be masked by the medications given as prophylaxis for the acute systemic adverse effects.[136]

Contraindications and Precautions

The use of recombinant interleukin-2 is contraindicated in patients with a history of hypersensitivity to this agent. Patient selection is critical to the outcome of therapy. Only patients whose performance status was good and who were in good health except for their malignant disease were enrolled in Phase I and Phase II trials.[74] An adverse drug reaction that is reversible in such a patient may not be as readily reversible in a patient whose health is more compromised. Recombinant interleukin-2 should be used with extreme caution in patients with pre-existing pathophysiological conditions that may be exacerbated during therapy. This includes patients with congestive heart failure, cardiac arrhythmias, pneumonia, and chronic obstructive pulmonary disease.

Recombinant interleukin-2 should also be used with caution in patients with impaired renal function. There is evidence that patients with compromised renal function are susceptible to more severe treatment-related renal toxicity.[113] Although renal function returns to normal after the discontinuation of recombinant interleukin-2 therapy in patients who undergo one or two treatment courses, the effect of repeated administration on renal function has not been determined.

The results of clinical trials evaluating the use of recombinant interleukin-2 in pediatric patients are not currently available. The teratogenic potential of recombinant interleukin-2 has not been investigated.

Recombinant interleukin-2 may worsen autoimmune thyroiditis.[129,130] Hypothyroidism may be a delayed effect of therapy. Therefore, thyroid function should be monitored routinely in patients receiving recombinant interleukin-2 and as a part of routine follow-up.

Drug–Drug Interactions

The administration of intravenous dexamethasone 4 mg every six hours to patients during therapy with recombinant interleukin-2 has been shown to decrease the incidence and severity of some adverse effects, including dyspnea, confusion, fever, elevation of serum creatinine, and elevation of serum bilirubin.[133] Other adverse effects associated with recombinant interleukin-2 treatment, such as anemia, eosinophilia, and thrombocytopenia, have not been diminished by the concurrent use of dexamethasone.[133] Despite evidence of their efficacy in the management of toxicity from recombinant interleukin-2 therapy, corticosteroids are generally not used clinically for this purpose, since there is concern that corticosteroids may reduce the efficacy of this lymphokine.[123]

To date, no other drug–drug interactions have been documented. Drugs that promote or exacerbate organ damage could increase the renal, hepatic, or cardiovascular toxicity associated with recombinant interleukin-2 therapy. Any drug that affects the cardiovascular system could have an exaggerated effect during therapy with recombinant interleukin-2. In addition, the ability of the body to compensate for the cardiovascular changes that occur during therapy with recombinant interleukin-2 could be compromised by the concomitant administration of negative inotropic agents, antihypertensives, or antiarrhythmics.

The pharmacokinetics of drugs administered concurrently during recombinant interleukin-2 therapy could be affected by the physiological changes that occur as adverse reactions to this immunotherapy. Extravascular partitioning alters the volume of distribution of many agents. In addition, the decreases in renal and hepatic function that occur during treatment with recombinant interleukin-2 could affect the clearance and safety profile of many drugs.

Dosage

The optimum dosage regimen for recombinant interleukin-2 has not been established. In the largest trials of recombinant interleukin-2 in adult patients with metastatic cancer, two dosage regimens have been used and maintained as tolerated: (1) 6×10^5 IU/kg administered as an intravenous bolus over 15 minutes every eight hours for four to five days, repeated in one week,[80] and (2) 1.8×10^7 IU/sq m/day administered as a continuous infusion for four to five days, repeated in one week.[87]

Availability, Cost, and Reconstitution

Recombinant interleukin-2 is undergoing Phase I and Phase II clinical trials. A product license application was submitted to the Food and Drug Administration in November 1988 for the approval of aldesleukin (Proleukin, Cetus) as a treatment for metastatic renal cell carcinoma.[b] As of this writing, aldesleukin has not been approved for use in the United States. Aldesleukin has been granted marketing approval for use in the treatment of metastatic renal cell cancer in Denmark, the Netherlands, Ireland, France, Spain, Italy, and West Germany.[c]

The wholesale cost of aldesleukin on the European market is approximately \$200 for a 2.16×10^7 IU (1.2-mg) vial.[d] The cost of one cycle of aldesleukin (6×10^5 IU/kg three times a day for 14 doses for a 70-kg patient) is \$6600. The cost of one cycle of aldesleukin when administered as a continuous infusion (1.8×10^7 IU/sq m/day for five doses for a patient with a body surface area of 1.8 sq m) is \$2000. Approval for LAK-cell or TIL therapy is not being sought in the United States.

If approved, aldesleukin (Proleukin) injection will be supplied in the United States as a lyophilized powder cake in packs of 10 individually boxed single-use vials. Each vial contains 2.16×10^7 IU (1.2 mg) of aldesleukin, 50 mg of mannitol, and 130 μg of sodium dodecyl sulfate per milligram of protein. The vials of lyophilized aldesleukin should be stored at 2–8 °C.[137] Teceleukin is currently formulated as a lyophilized powder cake in a single-use vial. Each vial contains 3.0×10^6 IU or 1.0×10^6 Nutley units of teceleukin, 5 mg of mannitol, and 25 mg of human albumin. Vials of lyophilized teceleukin should be stored at −20–8 °C. The manufacturer recommends that teceleukin be reconstituted with 1 mL of 0.9% sodium chloride injection.[e]

Reconstitution of a single vial of aldesleukin with 1.2 mL of sterile water for injection yields an aldesleukin concentration of 1.8×10^7 IU/mL (1 mg/mL). The vials are packaged under vacuum. Diluent should be aimed at the side wall of the vial to avoid foaming, and mixing should be accomplished with gentle swirling and slow inversion. Excessive agitation during dilution should be avoided. The reconstituted product is a clear, colorless solution that is stable for up to 48 hours when refrigerated (2 °C) or when stored at room temperature (30 °C). This product contains no preservative. The manufacturer recommends that the product not be filtered.[137]

Dilution of reconstituted aldesleukin with 5% dextrose injection containing 2% albumin maintains the biological activity of recombinant interleukin-2 signficantly better than when the agent is diluted with 5% dextrose injection that does not contain albumin.[138] The manufacturer recommends that the bolus dose of reconstituted aldesleukin be diluted with 50 mL of 5% Dextrose Injection, USP, containing 0.1% Human Albumin, USP, and infused over a 15-minute period. The total daily dose of reconstituted aldesleukin can be diluted with 500 mL of 5% Dextrose Injection, USP, containing 0.1% Human Albumin, USP[138,c] for infusion over a 24-hour period.

Aldesleukin is not compatible with bacteriostatic water for injection, 0.9% sodium chloride injection, or other solutions containing preservatives. Aldesleukin should not be admixed or infused with other drugs.[c]

Commentary

The importance of assessing the efficacy of therapy with recombinant interleukin-2 plus LAK cells in clinical trials was supported by animal data demonstrating the ability of LAK cells to mediate the regression of a variety of local and disseminated tumors.[116] The coadministration of intravenous recombinant interleukin-2 and LAK cells activated in vitro by incubation with the lymphokine was a logical first step in developing this immunotherapy for use in cancer patients. However, in vitro activation of LAK cells requires a large commitment of money, technical services, and space.[139] Furthermore, the ability of recombinant interleukin-2 to cause a response in cancer patients without the coadministration of exogenously activated LAK cells became evident during Phase I evaluation of recombinant interleukin-2 plus LAK cell therapy. Tumor responses were observed in patients who received recombinant interleukin-2 but were unable (usually because of toxicity) to receive LAK-cell infusions.[76] Consequently, it remains to be determined whether LAK cells will have an adjunctive role in recombinant interleukin-2 therapy.

Recombinant interleukin-2 costs $4,000–13,200 for one course (two cycles) of therapy, not including the cost of hospitalization. However, there is no other therapy for metastatic renal cell cancer that provides durable responses after one course. Traditional antineoplastic agents are ineffective against metastatic renal cell cancer, expose the patient to undue toxicity, and are inconvenient.[140] Interferon alfa costs approximately $125 for 1.8×10^7 U. Therefore, the cost to the hospital or clinic for a patient who receives interferon alfa 10^6 U/sq m every Monday, Wednesday, and Friday is also substantial—approximately $9750 for six months of therapy.

Conclusion

Recombinant interleukin-2 represents a tangible advance in immunotherapy, particularly in the treatment of metastatic renal cell cancer and malignant melanoma. Research is ongoing to evaluate the role of recombinant interleukin-2 in the treatment of patients with AIDS,[141] as an adjuvant to vaccines, and in the treatment of some infectious diseases.[142]

The overall treatment-related rate of mortality for patients who receive recombinant interleukin-2 therapy is low (1–1.5%).[74,80] However, because of the severe and frequent adverse effects, this treatment must be reserved for use in tertiary-care centers that have a sufficient number of trained personnel and adequate intensive-care facilities.

---

[a] Zeffren J, Hoffmann-La Roche Inc. Personal communication. 1990 Oct. 26.

[b] Cetus Corporation news release. Emeryville, CA; 1988 Dec 5.

[c] Cetus Corporation news release. Emeryville, CA; 1990 Mar 20.

[d] Quellhorst JK, EuroCetus. Personal communication. 1990 Oct 11.

[e] Hoffmann-La Roche Inc. Teceleukin package insert. Nutley, NJ.

References

1. Mizel SB. The interleukins. *FASEB J.* 1989; 3:2379–88.
2. Hansen LA. Immunotherapy of cancer. In: Koeller JM, Tami J, eds. Concepts in immunology and immunotherapeutics. Bethesda, MD: American Society of Hospital Pharmacists; 1990:335–6.
3. Matsushima K, Morishita K, Yoshimura T et al. Molecular cloning of a human monocyte-derived neutrophil chemotactic factor (MDNCF) and the induction of MDNCF mRNA by interleukin 1 and tumor necrosis factor. *J Exp Med.* 1988; 167:1883–93.
4. Samanta AK, Oppenheim JJ, Matsushima K. Interleukin 8 (monocyte-derived neutrophil chemotactic factor) dynamically regulates its own receptor expression on human neutrophils. *J Biol Chem.* 1990; 265:183–9.
5. Hoffmann-La Roche Inc. Recombinant interleukin-2 investigational drug brochure. Nutley, NJ; 1989 Jan.
6. Morgan DA, Ruscetti FW, Gallo RG. Selective in vitro growth of T lymphocytes from normal human bone marrows. *Science.* 1976; 193:1007–8.
7. Taniguchi T, Matsui H, Fujita T et al. Structure and expression of a cloned cDNA for human interleukin-2. *Nature.* 1983; 302:305–10.
8. Belldegrun A, Uppencamp I, Rosenberg SA. Anti-tumor reactivity of human lymphokine activated killer (LAK) cells against fresh and cultured preparations of renal cell cancer. *J Urol.* 1988; 139:150–5.
9. Carter CS, Leitman SF, Cullis H et al. Technical aspects of lymphokine-activated killer cell production. *J Clin Apheresis.* 1988; 4:113–7.
10. Grimm EA, Mazumder A, Zhang HA et al. Lymphokine-activated killer cell phenomenon. *J Exp Med.* 1982; 155:1823–41.
11. Belldegrun A, Muul LM, Rosenberg SA. Interleukin 2 expanded tumor-infiltrating lymphocytes in human renal cell cancer: isolation, characterization, and antitumor activity. *Cancer Res.* 1988; 48:206–14.
12. Muul LM, Speiss PJ, Director EP et al. Identification of specific cytolytic immune responses against autologous tumor in humans bearing malignant melanoma. *J Immunol.* 1987; 138:989–95.
13. Topalian SL, Solomon D. Rosenberg SA. Tumor-specific cytolysis by lymphocytes infiltrating human melanomas. *J Immunol.* 1989; 142:3714–25.
14. Lotze MT, Grimm EA, Mazumder A et al. In-vitro growth of cytotoxic human lymphocytes. IV. Lysis of fresh and cultured autologous tumor by lymphocytes cultured in T cell growth factor (TCGF). *Cancer Res.* 1981; 41:4420–5.
15. Fox BA, Rosenberg SA. Heterogeneous lymphokine-activated killer cell precursor populations. *Cancer Immunol Immunother.* 1989; 29:155–66.
16. Iwasaki K, Kikuchi H, Miyatake S et al. Infiltrative and cytolytic activities of lymphokine-activated killer cells against a human glioma spheroid model. *Cancer Res.* 1990; 50:2429–36.
17. Hook GR, Greenwood MA, Barba D et al. Morphology of interleukin-2-stimulated human peripheral blood mononuclear effector cells killing glioma-derived tumor cells in vitro. *J Natl Cancer Inst.* 1988; 80:171–7.
18. Haas GP, Solomon D, Rosenberg SA. Tumor-infiltrating lymphocytes from nonrenal urological malignancies. *Cancer Immunol Immunother.* 1990; 30:342–50.
19. Topalian SL, Solomon D, Avis FP et al. Immunotherapy of patients with advanced cancer using tumor-infiltrating lymphocytes and recombinant interleukin-2: a pilot study. *J Clin Oncol.* 1988; 6:839–53.
20. Rosenberg SA, Speiss P, Lafreniere R. A new approach to the adoptive immunotherapy of cancer with tumor-infiltrating lymphocytes. *Science.* 1986; 233:1318–21.
21. Fisher B, Packard BS, Read EJ et al. Tumor localization of adoptively transferred indium-111 labeled tumor infiltrating lymphocytes in patients with metastatic melanoma. *J Clin Oncol.* 1989; 7:250–61.
22. Griffith KD, Read EJ, Carrasquillo JA et al. In vivo distribution of adoptively transferred indium-111-labeled tumor

infiltrating lympocytes in patients with metastatic melanoma. *J Natl Cancer Inst.* 1989; 81:1709–17.
23. Ju G, Collins L, Kaffka KL et al. Structure-function analysis of human interleukin-2. Identification of amino acid residues for biological activity. *J Biol Chem.* 1987; 262:5723–31.
24. Fujita T, Takaoka C, Matsui H et al. Structure of the human interleukin 2 gene. *Proc Natl Acad Sci U S A.* 1983; 80:7437–41.
25. Holbrook NJ, Smith KA, Fornace AJ et al. T-cell growth factor: complete nucleotide sequences and organization of the gene in normal and malignant cells. *Proc Natl Acad Sci U S A.* 1984; 81:1634–8.
26. Robb RJ, Kutney RM, Chowdhry V. Purification and partial sequence analysis of human T-cell growth factor. *Proc Natl Acad Sci U S A.* 1983; 80:5990–4.
27. Devos R, Plaetinck G, Cheroutre H et al. Molecular cloning of human interleukin 2 cDNA and its expression in *E. coli. Nucleic Acids Res.* 1983; 11:4307–23.
28. Smith GE, Ju G, Ericson BL et al. Modification and secretion of human interleukin 2 produced in insect cells by baculovirus expression vector. *Proc Natl Acad Sci U S A.* 1985; 82:8404–8.
29. Rosenberg SA, Grimm EA, McGrogan M et al. Biological activity of recombinant human interleukin-2 produced in *Escherichia coli. Science.* 1984; 223:1412–5.
30. Konrad MW, Hemstreet G, Hersh EM et al. Pharmacokinetics of recombinant interleukin 2 in humans. *Cancer Res.* 1990; 50:2009–17.
31. Eberlein TJ, Schoof DD, Jung S-E et al. A new regimen of interleukin 2 and lymphokine-activated killer cells. Efficacy without significant toxicity. *Arch Intern Med.* 1988; 148:2571–6.
32. Doyle MV, Lee MT, Fong S. Comparison of biological activities of human recombinant interleukin-2(125) and native interleukin-2. *J Biol Response Mod.* 1985; 4:96–109.
33. Gearing AJ, Thorpe R. The international standard for human interleukin 2. Calibration by international collaborative study. *J Immunol Methods.* 1988; 114:3–9.
34. Robb RJ, Munck A, Smith KA. T-cell growth factor receptors. Quantitation, specificity, and biological relevance. *J Exp Med.* 1981; 154:1455–74.
35. Teshigawara K, Wang H-M, Kato K et al. Interleukin 2 high-affinity receptor expression requires two distinct binding proteins. *J Exp Med.* 1987; 165:223–38.
36. Weil-Hillman G, Voss SD, Fisch P et al. Natural killer cells activated by interleukin 2 treatment in vivo respond to interleukin 2 primarily through the p75 receptor and maintain the p55(TAC) negative phenotype. *Cancer Res.* 1990; 50:2683–91.
37. Rubin LA, Kurman CC, Biddison WE et al. A monoclonal antibody, 7G7/B6, binds to an epitope on the human interleukin-2 (IL-2) receptor that is distinct from that recognized by IL-2 or anti-Tac. *Hybridoma.* 1985; 4:91–102.
38. Tsudo M, Kozak RW, Goldman CK et al. Demonstration of a non-Tac peptide that binds interleukin 2: a potential participant in a multichain interleukin 2 receptor complex. *Proc Natl Acad Sci U S A.* 1986; 83:9694–8.
39. Wang H-M, Smith KA. The interleukin 2 receptor: functional consequences of its bimolecular structure. *J Exp Med.* 1987; 166:1055–69.
40. Smith KA. The interleukin 2 receptor. *Adv Immunol.* 1988; 42:165–79.
41. Robb RJ, Greene WC. Internalization of the interleukin 2 is mediated by the β chain of the high-affinity interleukin 2 receptor. *J Exp Med.* 1987; 165:1201–6.
42. Hank JA, Kohler PC, Weil-Hillman G et al. In vivo induction of the lymphokine-activated killer phenomenon: interleukin 2-dependent human non-major histocompatibility complex restricted cytotoxicity generated in vivo during administration of human recombinant interleukin 2. *Cancer Res.* 1988; 48:1965–71.
43. Lotze MT, Matory YL, Ettinghausen SE et al. In vivo administration of purified recombinant interleukin 2. II. Half life, immunologic effects, and expansion of peripheral lymphoid cells in vivo with recombinant IL 2. *J Immunol.* 1985; 135:2865–75.
44. Rosenthal NS, Hank JA, Kohler PC et al. The in vitro function of lymphocytes from 25 cancer patients receiving four to seven consecutive days of recombinant IL-2. *J Biol Response Mod.* 1988; 7:123–39.
45. Urba WJ, Steis RG, Longo DL et al. Immunomodulatory properties and toxicity of interleukin 2 in patients with cancer. *Cancer Res.* 1990; 50:185–92.
46. Thompson JA, Lee DJ, Lindgren CG et al. Influence of dose and duration of infusion of interleukin-2 on toxicity and immunomodulation. *J Clin Oncol.* 1988; 6:669–78.
47. Lotze MT, Frana LW, Sharrow SO et al. In vivo administration of purified human interleukin 2. I. Half life and immunologic effects of the Jurkat cell line-derived interleukin-2. *J Immunol.* 1985; 134:157–66.
48. Aronson FR, Libby P, Brandon EP et al. IL-2 rapidly induces natural killer cell adhesion to human endothelial cells. *J Immunol.* 1988; 141:158–63.
49. Wiebke EA, Rosenberg SA, Lotze MT. Acute immunological effects of interleukin-2 therapy in cancer patients: decreased delayed type hypersensitivity response and decreased proliferative response to soluble antigens. *J Clin Oncol.* 1988; 6:1440–9.
50. McMannis JD, Fisher RI, Creekmore SP et al. In vivo effects of recombinant IL-2. I. Isolation of circulating Leu-19+ lymphokine-activated killer effector cells from cancer patients receiving recombinant IL-2. *J Immunol.* 1988; 140: 1335–40.
51. Jablons D, Bolton E, Mertins S et al. IL-2-based immunotherapy alters circulating neutrophil Fc receptor expression and chemotaxis. *J Immunol.* 1990; 144:3630–6.
52. Jablons DM, Mule JJ, McIntosh JK et al. IL-6/IFN-beta-2 as a circulating hormone: induction by cytokine administration. *J Immunol.* 1989; 142:1542–7.
53. Gemlo BT, Palladino MA, Jaffe HS et al. Circulating cytokines in patients with metastatic cancer treated with interleukin 2 and lymphokine-activated killer cells. *Cancer Res.* 1988; 48:5864–7.
54. Cameron RB, McIntosh JK, Rosenberg SA. Synergistic antitumor effects of combination immunotherapy with recombinant interleukin-2 and recombinant hybrid α-interferon in the treatment of established murine hepatic metastases. *Cancer Res.* 1988; 48:5810–7.
55. McIntosh JK, Mule M, Krosnick JA et al. Combination cytokine immunotherapy with tumor necrosis factor-α, interleukin 2 and α-interferon and its synergistic antitumor effects in mice. *Cancer Res.* 1989; 49:1408–14.
56. Papa MZ, Yang JC, Vetto JT et al. Combined effects of chemotherapy and interleukin 2 in the therapy of mice with advanced pulmonary tumors. *Cancer Res.* 1988; 48:122–9.
57. Berd D, Maguire HC Jr, Mastrangelo MJ. Potentiation of human cell-mediated and humoral immunity by low-dose cyclophosphamide. *Cancer Res.* 1984; 44:5439–43.
58. Berd D, Maguire HC Jr, Mastrangelo MJ. Impairment of concanavalin A-induced suppressor activity following administration of cyclophosphamide to patients with advanced cancer. *Cancer Res.* 1984; 44:1275–80.
59. Cameron RB, Speiss PJ, Rosenberg SA. Synergistic antitumor activity of tumor-infiltrating lymphocytes, interleukin 2, and local tumor irradiation. Studies on the mechanism of action. *J Exp Med.* 1990; 171:249–63.
60. Allegretta M, Atkins MB, Dempsey RA et al. The development of anti-interleukin-2 antibodies in patients treated with recombinant interleukin-2 (IL-2). *J Clin Immunol.* 1986; 6:481–90.
61. Siegel JP, Lane HC, Stocks NI et al. Pharmacokinetics of lymphocyte-derived and recombinant DNA-derived interleukin-2 after intravenous administration to patients with the acquired immunodeficiency syndrome. *J Biol Re-*

sponse Mod. 1985; 4:596–601.

62. Lotze MT, Custer MC, Sharrow SO et al. In vivo administration of purified human interleukin 2 to patients with cancer: development of interleukin-2 receptor positive cells and circulating soluble interleukin-2 receptors following interleukin-2 administration. *Cancer Res.* 1987; 47:2188–95.
63. Rubin LA, Jay G, Nelson DL. The released interleukin 2 receptor binds interleukin 2 efficiently. *J Immunol.* 1986; 137: 3841–4.
64. Donohue JH, Rosenberg SA. The fate of interleukin-2 after in vivo administration. *J Immunol.* 1983; 130:2203–8.
65. Knauf MJ, Bell DP, Hirtzer P et al. Relationship of effective molecular size to systemic clearance in rats of recombinant interleukin-2 chemically modified with water-soluble polymers. *J Biol Chem.* 1988; 263:15064–70.
66. Shih Y, Konrad M, Warren K et al. Serum lymphokine profiles in cancer patients before and after administration of pegylated interleukin-2 (PEG IL-2). *Proc Am Soc Clin Oncol.* 1990; 9:184. Abstract.
67. Saris SC, Rosenberg SA, Friedman RB et al. Penetration of recombinant interleukin-2 across the blood–cerebrospinal fluid barrier. *J Neurosurg.* 1988; 69:29–34.
68. Lotze MT, Custer MC, Rosenberg SA. Intraperitoneal administration of interleukin-2 in patients with cancer. *Arch Surg.* 1986; 121:1373–9.
69. Cornaby A, Simpson MA, vann Rice R et al. Interleukin-2 production in plasma and urine, plasma interleukin-2 receptors, and urine cytology as a means of monitoring renal allograft recipients. *Transplant Proc.* 1988; 20:108–10.
70. Huang Y-P, Perrin LC, Miescher PA et al. Correlation of T and B cell activities in vitro and serum IL-2 levels in systemic lupus erythematosus. *J Immunol.* 1988; 141:827–33.
71. Trotter JL, Clifford DB, Anderson CB et al. Elevated serum interleukin-2 levels in chronic progressive multiple sclerosis. *N Engl J Med.* 1988; 318:1206. Letter.
72. Kozeny GA, Nicolas JD, Creekmore S et al. Effects of interleukin-2 immunotherapy on renal function. *J Clin Oncol.* 1988; 6:1170–6.
73. Lee RE, Lotze MT, Skibber JM et al. Cardiorespiratory effects of immunotherapy with interleukin-2. *J Clin Oncol.* 1989; 7:7–20.
74. Margolin KA, Raynor AA, Hawkins MJ et al. Interleukin-2 and lymphokine-activated killer cell therapy of solid tumors: analysis of toxicity and management guidelines. *J Clin Oncol.* 1989; 7:486–98.
75. Webb DE, Austin HA, Belldegrun A et al. Metabolic and renal effects of interleukin-2 immunotherapy for metastatic cancer. *Clin Nephrol.* 1988; 30:141–5.
76. Rosenberg SA, Lotze MT, Muul LM et al. A progress report on the treatment of 157 patients with advanced cancer using lymphokine-activated killer cells and interleukin-2 or high-dose interleukin-2 alone. *N Engl J Med.* 1987; 316:889–97.
77. Rosenberg SA, Lotze MT, Muul LM et al. New approaches to the immunotherapy of cancer using interleukin-2. *Ann Intern Med.* 1988; 10:853–64.
78. Aebersold P, Carter CS, Hyatt C et al. A simplified automated procedure for generation of human lymphokine-activated killer cells for use in clinical trials. *J Immunol Methods.* 1988; 112:1–7.
79. Hawkins MJ. IL-2/LAK: current status and possible future directions. In: DeVita VT, Hellman S, Rosenberg SA, eds. Principles and practice of oncology updates. Philadelphia: Lippincott; 1990:1–14.
80. Rosenberg SA, Lotze MT, Yang JC et al. Experience with the use of high-dose interleukin-2 in the treatment of 652 cancer patients. *Ann Surg.* 1989; 210:474–85.
81. Rosenberg SA, Lotze MT, Muul LM et al. Observations on the systemic administration of autologous lymphokine-activated killer cells and recombinant interleukin-2 to patients with metastatic cancer. *N Engl J Med.* 1985; 313:1485–92.
82. Fisher RI, Coltman CA, Doroshow JH et al. Metastatic renal cancer treated with interleukin-2 and lymphokine-activated killer cells. A Phase II clinical trial. *Ann Intern Med.* 1988; 108:518–23.
83. Dutcher JP, Creekmore S, Weiss GR et al. A Phase II study of interleukin-2 and lymphokine-activated killer cells in patients with metastatic malignant melanoma. *J Clin Oncol.* 1989; 7:477–85.
84. Rosenberg SA. Clinical immunotherapy studies in the surgery branch of the U.S. National Cancer Institute: brief review. *Cancer Treat Rev.* 1989; 16(Suppl A):115–21.
85. Lotze MT, Matory YL, Rayney AA et al. Clinical effects and toxicity of interleukin-2 in patients with cancer. *Cancer.* 1986; 58:2764–72.
86. Negrier S, Philip T, Stoter G et al. Interleukin-2 with or without LAK cells in metastatic renal cell carcinoma: a report of a European multicenter study. *Eur J Cancer Clin Oncol.* 1989; 25(Suppl):S21–8.
87. West WH, Tauer KW, Yannelli JR et al. Constant-infusion recombinant interleukin-2 in adoptive immunotherapy of advanced cancer. *N Engl J Med.* 1987; 316:898–905.
88. Rosenberg SA, Packard BS, Aebersold PM et al. Use of tumor-infiltrating lymphocytes and interleukin-2 in the immunotherapy of patients with metastatic melanoma: a preliminary report. *N Engl J Med.* 1988; 319:1676–80.
89. Stahel RA, Sculler JP, Jost LM et al. Tolerance and effectiveness of recombinant interleukin-2 (r-Met Hu IL-2 [Ala-125]) and lymphokine-activated killer cells in patients with metastatic solid tumors. *Eur J Cancer Clin Oncol.* 1989; 25:965–72.
90. Mitchell MS, Kempf RA, Harel W et al. Effectiveness and tolerability of low-dose cyclophosphamide and low-dose intravenous interleukin-2 in disseminated melanoma. *J Clin Oncol.* 1988; 6:409–24.
91. Budd GT, Osgood B, Barna B et al. Phase I clinical trial of interleukin 2 and α-interferon: toxicity and immunologic effects. *Cancer Res.* 1989; 49:6432–6.
92. Rosenberg SA, Lotze MT, Yang JC et al. Combination therapy with interleukin-2 and alpha-interferon for the treatment of patients with advanced cancer. *J Clin Oncol.* 1989; 7:1863–74.
93. Rosenberg SA, Schwarz SL, Speiss PJ. Combination immunotherapy for cancer: synergistic antitumor interactions of interleukin-2, alfa interferon, and tumor-infiltrating lymphocytes. *J Natl Cancer Inst.* 1988; 80:1393–7.
94. Linehan WM, Shipley WU, Longo DL. Cancer of the kidney and ureter. In: DeVita VT, Hellman S, Rosenberg SA, eds. Cancer: Principles and practice of oncology. 3rd ed. Philadelphia: Lippincott; 1989:993–8.
95. Horoszewicz JS, Murphy GP. An assessment of the current use of human interferons in therapy of urological cancers. *J Urol.* 1989; 142:1173–80.
96. Krigel RL, Padavic-Shaller KA, Rudolph AR et al. A Phase-I study of recombinant interleukin 2 plus recombinant β-interferon. *Cancer Res.* 1988; 48:3875–81.
97. Krigel RL, Padavic-Shaller KA, Rudolph AR et al. Renal cell carcinoma: treatment with recombinant interleukin-2 plus beta-interferon. *J Clin Oncol.* 1990; 8:460–7.
98. Ettinghausen SE, Lipford EH, Mule JJ et al. Systemic administration of recombinant interleukin 2 stimulates in vivo lymphoid cell proliferation in tissues. *J Immunol.* 1985; 135:1488–97.
99. Thatcher N, Dazzi H, Johnson RJ et al. Recombinant interleukin-2 (rIL-2) given intrasplenically and intravenously for advanced malignant melanoma. A Phase I and II study. *Br J Cancer.* 1989; 60:770–4.
100. Klasa RJ, Silver HKB, Kong S. In vivo induction of lymphokine-activated killer cells by interleukin-2 splenic artery perfusion in advanced malignancy. *Cancer Res.* 1990; 50:4906–10.
101. Jacobs SK, Wilson DJ, Kornblith PL et al. Interleukin-2 or autologous lymphokine-activated killer cell treatment of malignant glioma: Phase I trial. *Cancer Res.* 1986; 46:2101–4.

102. Ingram M, Jacques S, Freshwater DB et al. Salvage immunotherapy of malignant glioma. *Arch Surg*. 1987; 122:1483–6.
103. Merchant RE, Grant AJ, Merchant LH et al. Adoptive immunotherapy for recurrent glioblastoma multiforme using lymphokine activated killer cells and recombinant interleukin-2. *Cancer*. 1988; 62:665–71.
104. Barba D, Saris SC, Holder C et al. Intratumoral LAK cell and interleukin-2 therapy of human gliomas. *J Neurosurg*. 1989; 70:175–82.
105. Gottlieb DJ, Brenner MK, Heslop HE et al. A Phase I clinical trial of recombinant interleukin 2 following high dose chemo-radiotherapy for haematological malignancy: applicability to the elimination of minimal residual disease. *Br J Cancer*. 1989; 60:610–5.
106. Storb R. Current problems and future approaches. In: DeVita VT, Hellman S, Rosenberg SA., eds. Cancer: principles and practice of oncology. 3rd ed. Philadelphia: Lippincott; 1989:2485.
107. Sosman JA, Kohler PC, Hank JA et al. Repetitive weekly cycles of interleukin-2. II. Clinical and immunological effects of dose, schedule, and addition of indomethacin. *J Natl Cancer Inst U S A*. 1988; 80:1451–61.
108. Karp S, White D, Rosenberg SA. Dose tolerance in patients receiving interleukin-2 (IL-2). *Proc Am Soc Clin Oncol*. 1990; 9:195. Abstract.
109. Denicoff KD, Rubinow DR, Papa MZ et al. The neuropsychiatric effects of treatment with interleukin-2 and lymphokine-activated killer cells. *Ann Intern Med*. 1987; 107:293–300.
110. Fisher B, Keenan AM, Garra BS et al. Interleukin-2 induces profound reversible cholestasis: a detailed analysis in treated cancer patients. *J Clin Oncol*. 1989; 7:1852–62.
111. Gaynor ER, Vitek L, Sticklin L et al. The hemodynamic effects of treatment with interleukin-2 and lymphokine-activated killer cells. *Ann Intern Med*. 1988; 109:953–8.
112. Ognibene FP, Rosenberg SA, Lotze M et al. Interleukin-2 administration causes reversible hemodynamic changes and left ventricular dysfunction similar to those seen in septic shock. *Chest*. 1988; 94:750–4.
113. Belldegrun A, Webb DE, Austin HA III et al. Effects of interleukin-2 on renal function in patients receiving immunotherapy for advanced cancer. *Ann Intern Med*. 1987; 106:817–22.
114. McIntosh JK, Mule JJ, Merino MJ et al. Synergistic antitumor effects of immunotherapy with recombinant interleukin-2 and recombinant tumor necrosis factor-α. *Cancer Res*. 1988; 48:4011–7.
115. Redman BG, Flaherty L, Chou T-H et al. A Phase I trial of recombinant interleukin-2 combined with recombinant interferon-gamma in patients with cancer. *J Clin Oncol*. 1990; 8:1269–76.
116. Weisfuse IB, Graham DJ, Will M et al. An outbreak of hepatitis A among cancer patients treated with interleukin-2 and lymphokine-activated killer cells. *J Infect Dis*. 1990; 161:647–52.
117. Thatcher N, Dazzi H, Gosh A et al. Recombinant IL-2 given intrasplenically and intravenously in advanced malignant melanoma: a Phase I/II study. *Cancer Treat Rev*. 1989; 16(Suppl A):S49–52.
118. Parker MM, Parrillo JE. Septic shock: hemodynamics and pathogenesis. *JAMA*. 1983; 250:3324–7.
119. Rosenstein M, Ettinghausen SE, Rosenberg SA. Extravasation of intravascular fluid mediated by the systemic administration of recombinant interleukin 2. *J Immunol*. 1986; 137:1735–42.
120. Ettinghausen SE, Puri RK, Rosenberg SA. Increased vascular permeability in organs mediated by the systemic administration of lymphokine-activated killer cells and recombinant interleukin-2 in mice. *J Natl Cancer Inst*. 1988; 80:177–88.
121. Puri RK, Rosenberg SA. Combined effects of interferon α and interleukin 2 on the induction of a vascular leak syndrome in mice. *Cancer Immunol Immunother*. 1989; 28:267–74.
122. Cotran RS, Pober JS, Gimbrone MA et al. Endothelial activation during interleukin 2 immunotherapy. A possible mechanism for the vascular leak syndrome. *J Immunol*. 1988; 140:1883–8.
123. Papa MZ, Vetto JT, Ettinghausen SE et al. Effect of corticosteroid on the antitumor activity of lymphokine-activated killer cells and interleukin 2 in mice. *Cancer Res*. 1986; 46:5618–23.
124. Belldegrun A, Webb DE, Austin HA III et al. Renal toxicity of interleukin-2 administration in patients with metastatic renal cell cancer: effect of pre-therapy nephrectomy. *J Urol*. 1989; 141:499–503.
125. American Psychiatric Association. Diagnostic and statistical manual of mental disorders, third edition—revised (DSM-III-R). Washington, DC: American Psychiatric Press; 1987:103.
126. Saris SC, Patronas NJ, Rosenberg SA. The effect of intravenous interleukin-2 on brain water content. *J Neurosurg*. 1989; 71:169–74.
127. Wilson DE, Birchfield GR, Hejazi JS et al. Hypocholesterolemia in patients treated with recombinant interleukin-2: appearance of remnant-like lipoproteins. *J Clin Oncol*. 1989; 7:1573–7.
128. Ettinghausen SE, Moore JG, White DE et al. Hematological effects of immunotherapy with lymphokine-activated killer cells and recombinant interleukin-2 in cancer patients. *Blood*. 1987; 69:1654–60.
129. Atkins MB, Mier JW, Parkinson DR et al. Hypothyroidism after treatment with interleukin-2 and lymphokine-activated killer cells. *N Engl J Med*. 1988; 318:1557–63.
130. Atkins MB, Mier JW, Demchak P et al. Thyroid dysfunction following IL-2 therapy. *Proc Am Soc Clin Oncol*. 1990; 9:186. Abstract.
131. Denicoff KD, Durkin TM, Lotze MT et al. The neuroendocrine effects of interleukin-2 treatment. *J Clin Endocrinol Metab*. 1989; 69:402–10.
132. Gaspari AA, Lotze MT, Rosenberg SA et al. Dermatological changes associated with interleukin 2 administration. *JAMA*. 1987; 258: 1624–9.
133. Vetto JT, Papa MZ, Lotze MT et al. Reduction of toxicity of interleukin-2 and lymphocyte-activated killer cells in humans by the administration of corticosteroids. *J Clin Oncol*. 1987; 5:496–503.
134. Lee RE, Gaspari AA, Lotze MT et al. Interleukin 2 and psoriasis. *Arch Dermatol*. 1988; 124:1811–5.
135. Schwartzentruber D, Lotze MT, Rosenberg SA. Colonic perforation. An unusual complication of therapy with high-dose interleukin-2. *Cancer*. 1988; 62:2350–3.
136. Bock SN, Lee RE, Fisher B. A prospective randomized trial evaluating prophylactic antibiotics to prevent triple-lumen catheter-related sepsis in patients treated with immunotherapy. *J Clin Oncol*. 1990; 8:161–9.
137. Cetus Corporation. Proleukin package insert. Emeryville, CA; 1990 Mar.
138. Miles DW, Bird CR, Wadawa M et al. Reconstitution of interleukin 2 with albumin for infusion. *Lancet*. 1990; 335:1602–3. Letter.
139. Boldt DH, Mills BJ, Gemlo BT et al. Laboratory correlates of adoptive immunotherapy with recombinant interleukin-2 and lymphokine-activated killer cells in humans. *Cancer Res*. 1988; 48:4409–16.
140. Buzald A, Todd MB. Therapeutic options in renal cell carcinoma. *Semin Oncol*. 1989; 16:12–9.
141. Lane HC, Siegel JP, Rook AH et al. Use of interleukin-2 in patients with acquired immunodeficiency syndrome. *J Biol Response Mod*. 1984; 3:512–6.
142. Winkelhake JL, Gauny SS. Human recombinant interleukin-2 as an experimental therapeutic. *Pharmacol Rev*. 1990; 42:1–28.

Research Notes

Prospective evaluation of a vancomycin dosage guideline for neonates

MARIANE HARDENBROOK GABRIEL, CARL W. KILDOO III, JANE L. GENNRICH, HOUCHANG D. MODANLOU, AND SHELLY RAINFORTH COLLINS

Clin Pharm. 1991; 10:129–32

The emergence of methicillin-resistant strains of staphylococci that cause infection in neonatal intensive-care unit (NICU) patients has resulted in an increased use of vancomycin. Potential toxicity, particularly ototoxicity and nephrotoxicity, has prompted interest in the pharmacokinetics of vancomycin in term and preterm sick infants.[1–11] We previously described the pharmacokinetics of vancomycin in infants with a postconceptional age (PCA) of 26–44 weeks.[5] Vancomycin clearance appeared to be related to improvement in the serum creatinine concentration and increased PCA, particularly in patients with a PCA of 30–36 weeks. On the basis of these and other results,[1,3–6,8–11] we developed a vancomycin dosage guideline for neonates at Long Beach Memorial Medical Center. We report the results of a prospective evaluation of the guideline's effectiveness in achieving therapeutic serum vancomycin concentrations in NICU patients.

Table 1.
Vancomycin Dosage Guideline for Neonates

PCA[a] (Weeks)	Chronological Age (Days)	Serum Creatinine Concentration (mg/dL)[b]	Dosage (mg/kg)
<30	≤7	. . .[c]	15 q 24 hr
	>7	≤1.2	10 q 12 hr
30–36	≤14	. . .[c]	10 q 12 hr
	>14	≤0.6	10 q 8 hr
		0.7–1.2	10 q 12 hr
>36	≤7	. . .[c]	10 q 12 hr
	>7	≤0.6	10 q 8 hr
		0.7–1.2	10 q 12 hr

[a] PCA = postconceptional age (gestational age at birth plus chronological age).

[b] If the serum creatinine concentration is >1.2 mg/dL, use an initial dosage of 15 mg/kg q 24 hr and determine serum vancomycin concentrations within 24–48 hours of the start of therapy.

[c] Serum creatinine concentration is not used to determine the dosage for this type of patient because of its lack of reliability or because of lack of information.

Methods. All patients in the NICU who received vancomycin in accordance with the institution's vancomycin dosage guideline for neonates (Table 1) between November 1988 and August 1989 were entered into the study. The study met the ethical standards of the institution's committee on human experimentation and was performed as part of routine patient care. Patients were excluded if (1) vancomycin was discontinued before serum drug concentrations were determined; (2) renal function was severely impaired or unstable, as defined by a serum creatinine concentration of >1.3 mg/dL or a change in the serum creatinine concentration of >0.4 mg/dL; or (3) chronological age exceeded four months.

Vancomycin (as the hydrochloride salt) diluted to 5 mg/mL in 10% dextrose injection was administered intravenously over 60 minutes by syringe pump. A pediatric clinical pharmacist scheduled measurements of serum vancomycin concentration

MARIANE HARDENBROOK GABRIEL, PHARM.D., is Pharmacy Clinical Coordinator, Pediatric Infectious Disease, and Clinical Pharmacist, Pediatrics, Long Beach Memorial Medical Center (LBMMC), Long Beach CA, and Assistant Clinical Professor of Pharmacy, University of California (UC), San Francisco. CARL W. KILDOO III, PHARM.D., is Clinical Pharmacist, Pharmacokinetics Service, LBMMC, and Assistant Clinical Professor of Pharmacy, UC, San Francisco. JANE L. GENNRICH, PHARM.D., is Clinical Pharmacist, Pediatrics, LBMMC, and Assistant Clinical Professor of Pharmacy, UC, San Francisco. HOUCHANG D. MODANLOU, M.D., is Director, Neonatal–Perinatal Medicine, Miller Children's Hospital, LBMMC, and Associate Professor of Pediatrics, UC, Irvine. SHELLY RAINFORTH COLLINS, PHARM.D., is Assistant Director of Pharmacy, Mobile Infirmary, Mobile, AL.

Address reprint requests to Dr. Gabriel at the Department of Pharmacy, Long Beach Memorial Medical Center, P.O. Box 1428, Long Beach, CA 90801-1428.

The editorial assistance of Harris R. Stutman, M.D., and the technical assistance of Hugo L. Folli, Pharm.D., Jane H. Hodding, Pharm.D., and Lisa A. Veale, Pharm.D., are acknowledged.

for 36–72 hours after the initiation of vancomycin therapy. A venipuncture technician obtained the serum samples by heel capillary prick at the ordered times. Samples were analyzed daily by fluorescence polarization immunoassay (TDx, Abbott Diagnostics, Irving, Texas) by a medical technologist in the chemistry section of the pathology laboratory. It was later confirmed from the concentration data that all samples had been drawn after at least four times the half-life of the drug had elapsed.

Samples for peak vancomycin concentration determinations were obtained one hour after the end of a one-hour infusion to minimize the effect of incomplete distribution of the drug to the tissues. Samples for trough measurements were obtained one hour before the next dose was given. The extrapolated true peak concentrations at the end of the infusion and the extrapolated true trough concentrations just before the next dose were calculated by using pharmacokinetic equations (appendix).[12] Extrapolated concentrations were categorized as (1) peak concentration, 20–40 μg/mL and trough concentration, ≤10 μg/mL; (2) peak concentration, <20 μg/mL; and (3) peak concentration, >40 μg/mL or trough concentration, >10 μg/mL.

Results. A total of 66 patients received vancomycin during the study period. Thirty-seven of these patients were included in the study. One patient received two separate courses of vancomycin; thus, a total of 38 courses were evaluated. Of the 29 patients excluded, vancomycin was discontinued in 15 before the drug concentration determinations, 11 had impaired or unstable renal function, and three had a chronological age of more than four months. Table 2 summarizes the patient characteristics and drug concentration data for the patients studied.

Methicillin-resistant *Staphylococcus epidermidis* was isolated from blood cultures for 11 patients; the minimum inhibitory concentration (MIC) of vancomycin for these isolates was 1.0 μg/mL. All the patients were clinically improved at the end of their vancomycin therapy. Blood cultures were repeated for three patients and found to be negative. Repeat white blood cell counts were improved, and C-reactive protein determinations showed a decrease.

Thirty-five (92%) of the extrapolated peak serum vancomycin concentrations were 20–40 μg/mL, and 33 (87%) of the extrapolated trough concentrations were ≤10 μg/mL. Both peak and trough concentrations were within these ranges for 30 (79%) of the treatment courses. Three (8%) of the extrapolated peak concentrations were <20 μg/mL (range, 14–19 μg/mL). Five (13%) of the extrapolated trough concentrations were >10 μg/mL (range, 12–16 μg/mL). None of the extrapolated peak concentrations were >40 μg/mL.

Discussion. The pharmacokinetic profile of vancomycin is best described by a two- or three-compartment model. In our prior study,[5] data for five postinfusion serum samples were fitted to a two-compartment model to determine pharmacokinetic variables for vancomycin. The effect of the alpha distribution phase in determining vancomycin clearance did not appear to be important in these patients. Thus, as stated by Matzke,[13] a one-compartment model is adequate to describe the pharmacokinetics of vancomycin in the clinical setting, and such a model was used in this study. A one-compartment model has also been used in most recent studies of vancomycin pharmacokinetics in premature neonates.[1-4,6,8] Although some error is introduced by a one-compartment model, we believe that it is not clinically meaningful.

According to Schaad et al.,[10] therapeutic peak and trough serum vancomycin concentrations in pediatric patients are 25–40 and <12 μg/mL, respectively. In their study, the sample for the peak concentration determination was drawn immediately after a 60-minute infusion. This time for the peak level was also used in several other studies of

Table 2.
Extrapolated Peak and Trough Serum Vancomycin Concentrations and Patient Characteristics

PCA[a] (Weeks)	No. Treatment Courses[b]	No. (%) Treatment Courses Yielding Indicated Extrapolated Serum Vancomycin Concentration[c]							
		Peak Concentration (μg/mL)				Trough Concentration (μg/mL)			
		<20	20–30	>30–40	>40	<5	5–10	>10–15	>15
<30	10[d]	3 (30)	7 (70)	...	...	4 (40)	6 (60)	...	...
30–36	22[e]	...	21 (95)	1 (5)	...	1 (5)	18 (82)	1 (5)	2 (9)
>36	6[f]	...	5 (83)	1 (17)	...	1 (17)	3 (50)	2 (33)	...
Total	38	3 (8)	33 (87)	2 (5)	...	6 (16)	27 (71)	3 (8)	2 (5)

[a] PCA = postconceptional age (gestational age at birth plus chronological age).
[b] Each treatment course represents one patient, except for one patient who had two treatment courses.
[c] Calculated peak and trough concentrations at the end of the infusion and just before the next dose, respectively.
[d] Mean PCA, 29 weeks (range, 28–29.5); mean chronological age, 3.6 weeks (2.5–5.5); mean body weight, 770 g (550–1090).
[e] Mean PCA, 31.9 weeks (range, 30–36); mean chronological age, 4.5 weeks (1–8); mean body weight, 1030 g (580–2000).
[f] Mean PCA, 38.7 weeks (range, 37–42); mean chronological age, 4.3 weeks (3–7); mean body weight, 1990 g (1020–3050).

vancomycin pharmacokinetics in neonates.[5,6,8,9,11] In the present study, samples for peak concentration measurements were drawn one hour after the end of the 60-minute infusion to minimize the effect of incomplete drug distribution. To more closely match the timing of the sampling for peak determinations to that in the prior studies, we used pharmacokinetic calculations to extrapolate the true peak at the end of the infusion. The MIC of vancomycin for methicillin-resistant *Staph. epidermidis* was 1.0 μg/mL in the study patients. Thus, using a range of peak serum vancomycin concentrations of 20–40 μg/mL as the therapeutic goal would result in peak values greater than 20 times the MIC for the organism and should generate bactericidal titers in serum of at least the 1:8 value associated with efficacy. Samples for trough determinations were drawn one hour before the end of the dosage interval; therefore, the true trough concentration was extrapolated.

Our vancomycin dosage guideline for neonates was successful in facilitating the achievement of peak serum vancomycin concentrations of 20–40 μg/mL and trough concentrations of <10 μg/mL in the majority of patients. The dosage guideline was particularly successful for the patients with PCAs of 30–36 weeks, all of whom had extrapolated peak concentrations within the range of 20–40 μg/mL. The guideline was also successful for 70% of the patients with PCAs of <30 weeks and in 66.7% of the patients with PCAs of >36 weeks.

The three patients who had peak vancomycin concentrations of <20 μg/mL had a chronological age of greater than three weeks and a PCA of 28–29 weeks. In addition, they all had serum creatinine concentrations of <0.6 mg/dL. In the older PCA groups, this would have led to an increased dosage according to the guideline, and subtherapeutic values would be avoided. The guideline does not provide for dosage adjustment according to serum creatinine levels in patients with PCAs of <30 weeks because of insufficient data for this age category in our prior study.[5] The findings here may indicate that the serum creatinine concentration is a useful part of dosage adjustment for this age group also; further study is needed.

Leonard et al.[6] recommended a vancomycin dosage of 15 mg/kg every 24 hours for infants weighing <1000 g. In the present study, there were 12 patients with PCAs of 30–36 weeks and nine patients with PCAs of <30 weeks who weighed <1000 g at the time of therapy. A vancomycin dosage of 15 mg/kg every 24 hours would have resulted in subtherapeutic vancomycin concentrations during a large part of the dosage interval in these patients. Most of the infants weighing <1000 g received vancomycin 10 mg/kg every 12 hours, and three patients required 10 mg/kg every eight hours.

Reed et al.[9] recommended a vancomycin dosage of 10 mg/kg every 12 hours for infants with PCAs of ≤36 weeks. There were 32 such patients in this study; nine of them required 10 mg/kg every eight hours to achieve therapeutic peak and trough drug concentrations. Use of the additional factor of serum creatinine level in the dosage guideline predicted the increased clearance and thus the need for an increased daily dosage and shorter dosage interval for these patients. Therapeutic serum vancomycin concentrations are more likely to be achieved if PCA and serum creatinine concentration, as well as body weight, are used to determine the dosage.

Information on vancomycin-associated ototoxicity in infants and children is limited. One single-dose study in 16 infants and children showed peak concentrations of <40 μg/mL and trough concentrations of <12 μg/mL to be nontoxic.[10] Information on vancomycin ototoxicity and nephrotoxicity in adults is based on retrospective reviews. Vancomycin ototoxicity in adults is associated with peak concentrations of >50 μg/mL.[14] None of our patients had peak concentrations that would be considered potentially toxic according to these guidelines.

Vancomycin nephrotoxicity in the general adult population is associated with trough serum drug concentrations of >30 μg/mL.[14] A recent study in adult cancer patients associated vancomycin nephrotoxicity with trough concentrations of >10 μg/mL.[15] The sample was small (22 patients), and the incidence of vancomycin nephrotoxicity in cancer patients is higher than that in the general population, perhaps because cancer patients are frequently exposed to other nephrotoxic agents. Dean et al.[16] reported two cases of vancomycin nephrotoxicity in pediatric patients in whom the serum creatinine level returned to baseline when the vancomycin dosage was adjusted to produce peak serum vancomycin concentrations of 20–40 μg/mL and trough concentrations of 5–10 μg/mL. In our study, the extrapolated trough values for the five patients in the >10-μg/mL range were all <17 μg/mL. The dosage guideline includes a recommendation to determine serum drug concentrations if vancomycin therapy is to continue longer than 72 hours, so a dosage adjustment would have been made for these patients before further accumulation could occur.

Conclusion. Most patients (79%) whose vancomycin dosage was selected in accordance with the guideline had peak serum vancomycin concentrations of 20–40 μg/mL and trough concentrations of <10 μg/mL. Further study is needed in patients with postconceptional ages of <30 and >36 weeks because of the small number of patients in those groups in this study.

References

1. Alpert G, Campos JM, Harris MC et al. Vancomycin dosage

in pediatrics reconsidered. *Am J Dis Child*. 1984; 138:20–2.
2. Baumgart S, Hall SE, Campos JM et al. Sepsis with coagulase-negative staphylococci in critically ill newborns. *Am J Dis Child*. 1983; 137:461–3.
3. Gross JR, Kaplan SL, Kramer et al. Vancomycin pharmacokinetics in premature infants. *Pediatr Pharmacol*. 1985; 5:17–22.
4. James A, Koren G, Milliken J et al. Vancomycin pharmacokinetics and dose recommendations for preterm infants. *Antimicrob Agents Chemother*. 1987; 31:52–4.
5. Kildoo CW III, Lin L, Gabriel MH et al. Vancomycin pharmacokinetics in infants: relationship to post-conceptional age and serum creatinine. *Dev Pharmacol Ther*. 1990; 14:77–83.
6. Leonard MB, Koren G, Stevenson DK et al. Vancomycin pharmacokinetics in very low birth weight neonates. *Pediatr Infect Dis J*. 1989; 8:282–6.
7. Munson DP, Thompson TR, Johnson DE et al. Coagulase-negative staphylococcal septicemia: experience in a newborn intensive care unit. *J Pediatr*. 1982; 101:602–5.
8. Naqvi SH, Keenan WJ, Reichley RM et al. Vancomycin pharmacokinetics in small, seriously ill infants. *Am J Dis Child*. 1986; 140:107–10.
9. Reed MD, Kliegman RM, Weiner JS et al. The clinical pharmacology of vancomycin in seriously ill preterm infants. *Pediatr Res*. 1987; 22:360–3.
10. Schaad UB, McCracken GH, Nelson JD. Clinical pharmacology and efficacy of vancomycin in pediatric patients. *J Pediatr*. 1980; 96:119–26.
11. Schaible DH, Rocci ML, Alpert GA et al. Vancomycin pharmacokinetics in infants: relationships to indices of maturation. *Pediatr Infect Dis*. 1986; 5:304–8.
12. Gibaldi M, Perrier D. Pharmacokinetics. 2nd ed. New York: Dekker; 1982:27.
13. Matzke GR. Vancomycin. In: Evans WE, Schentag JJ, Jusko WJ, eds. Applied pharmacokinetics. 2nd ed. Spokane, WA: Applied Therapeutics; 1986:423–4.
14. Matzke GR, Zhanel GG, Guay DRP. Clinical pharmacokinetics of vancomycin. *Clin Pharmacokinet*. 1986; 11:257–82.
15. Cimino MA, Rotstein C, Slaughter RL et al. Relationship of serum antibiotic concentrations to nephrotoxicity in cancer patients receiving concurrent aminoglycoside and vancomycin therapy. *Am J Med*. 1987; 83:1091–7.
16. Dean RP, Wagner DJ, Tolpin MD. Vancomycin/aminoglycoside nephrotoxicity. *J Pediatr*. 1985; 106:861–2.

Appendix—Extrapolation of True Peak and Trough Serum Vancomycin Concentrations

True peak and trough serum vancomycin concentrations at steady state were extrapolated by using a one-compartment model. The elimination rate constant (k) was determined with equation 1:

$$k = -[\ln(C_{min}/C_{max})]/t_1 \quad (1)$$

where C_{min} is the measured trough value, C_{max} is the measured peak value, and t_1 is the time interval between C_{min} and C_{max}. The elimination half-life ($t_{1/2}$) was calculated with equation 2:

$$t_{1/2} = 0.693/k \quad (2)$$

The equation for determining the extrapolated true peak concentration at steady state ($C_{max_{ss}}$) is

$$C_{max_{ss}} = C_{max}e^{kt_2} \quad (3)$$

where t_2 is the time interval between the end of the infusion and the time of C_{max}.

The equation for determining the extrapolated true trough concentration at steady state ($C_{min_{ss}}$) is

$$C_{min_{ss}} = C_{min}e^{-kt_3} \quad (4)$$

where t_3 is the time interval between C_{min} and the end of the scheduled dosage interval.

Effect of ultrafiltration product and ultrafiltration–freezing sequence on free phenytoin determination

LEANNE B. SMITH, BRUCE D. ANDERSON, AND CAROL B. PUGH

Clin Pharm. 1991; 10:132–6

Phenytoin is a highly protein-bound drug for which there is generally a good correlation between total and free plasma concentrations.[1,2] When one suspects that protein binding is altered because of factors such as hypoalbuminemia,[3] uremia,[4] or concurrent administration of valproic acid[5] or aspirin,[6] it is advisable to monitor free phenytoin concentrations.[7]

Separation of free from albumin-bound phenytoin has been accomplished by equilibrium dialysis, ultracentrifugation, and ultrafiltration.[8] Although equilibrium dialysis, the oldest method, is considered by some to be the technique of choice, it is time consuming and not readily adaptable to the clinical setting. The commercially available ultrafiltration products use a fixed membrane (filter) to exclude high-molecular-weight substances such as albumin from the ultrafiltrate when centrifugal force is applied. Because of their low cost, reliability, and ease of use, these ultrafiltration products are popular in commercial and clinical research laboratories. The use of two ultrafiltration products—Centriflo membrane cones (Amicon, Danvers, MA)[9] and the Centrifree Micropartition System filter (Amicon)[10,11]—has been described, but the two have not been compared. We compared the Centriflo cones, the Centrifree filter, and the Uni-

LEANNE B. SMITH is a pharmacist in York, PA; at the time of this study, she was a Bachelor of Science in Pharmacy degree candidate, Philadelphia College of Pharmacy and Science (PCPS), Philadelphia, PA. BRUCE D. ANDERSON, PHARM.D., is Fellow in Clinical Toxicology, San Diego Regional Poison Center and University of California San Diego Medical Center, San Diego, CA; at the time of this study he was a Doctor of Pharmacy degree candidate, PCPS. CAROL B. PUGH, PHARM.D., is Decentral Clinical Coordinator, Department of Pharmacy, University of Virginia Health Sciences Center, Charlottesville, VA; at the time of this study she was Assistant Professor of Clinical Pharmacy, Department of Pharmacy Practice/Pharmacy Administration, PCPS, and Clinical Pharmacokinetics Consultant, Philadelphia Veterans Affairs Medical Center (PVAMC), Philadelphia, PA.

Address reprint requests to Dr. Pugh at the Department of Pharmacy, University of Virginia Health Sciences Center, Box 274-11, Charlottesville, VA 22908.

The assistance of Lorraine Lapetina and Alice Floyd of the PVAMC Toxicology Laboratory in performing the phenytoin assays is acknowledged.

Presented in part at the 24th Annual ASHP Midyear Clinical Meeting, Atlanta, GA, December 6, 1989.

sep Ultracent-30 filter (Bio-Rad, Richmond, CA), which is similar to the Centrifree system, to determine if they differed in the values produced for free phenytoin concentration and phenytoin free fraction.

Since it may take several weeks or months to collect the large number of plasma samples generally required in clinical investigations, researchers often freeze samples until a reasonably sized batch is accumulated for analysis. To our knowledge, investigators have not determined whether the timing of ultrafiltration, relative to freezing of samples, affects free plasma phenytoin concentration or free fraction. Thus, the second purpose of our study was to compare the values obtained from samples that had been frozen after ultrafiltration with those obtained from samples frozen before ultrafiltration.

Methods. We accumulated unfrozen plasma from the hospital's clinical laboratory. The laboratory had previously taken blood samples from hospitalized and nonhospitalized patients for routine determination of plasma phenytoin concentration; we were provided with the excess plasma from these samples. We used only plasma that the laboratory had determined to have a total phenytoin concentration of at least 5.0 mg/L. The plasma that we used came from patients whose albumin and serum creatinine concentrations were predominantly within normal limits. We created 23 pools of plasma; each pool contained approximately 10 mL of plasma and was derived from the blood of 4–10 patients.

All but 1 mL of each whole plasma pool was frozen at −20 °C for 11.6–19.3 weeks, defrosted, and divided into portions for (1) use with each filter product to create ultrafiltrate that would be assayed for free phenytoin concentration and (2) determination of total phenytoin concentration.

Comparison of Ultrafiltration Products. A defrosted 1-mL portion from each plasma pool was centrifuged with each filter type in a refrigerated, swing-head rotor centrifuge (Centra-7R, International Equipment Company, Needham Heights, MA) at 2000 *g* and 25 °C. The Centrifree (lot MU 0520 RAA; molecular weight cutoff, 50,000) and Unisep filters (lot BU 3-1040; molecular weight cutoff, 30,000) were left dry and centrifuged with their plasma-pool samples for 30 minutes. One set of Centriflo membrane cones (lot CA 13864; molecular weight cutoff, 50,000) was soaked in water for one hour and then centrifuged for 15 minutes; another set was handled identically but centrifuged for 45 minutes. Both sets of Centriflo membrane cones were then centrifuged with their plasma-pool samples for 30 minutes. We then measured total phenytoin concentration in each plasma pool and free phenytoin concentration in each portion of ultrafiltrate.

Comparison of Ultrafiltration–Freezing Sequence. The 1-mL portions of plasma that were removed from each pool before freezing were ultrafiltered with a Centrifree filter as described above, and the ultrafiltrate was then frozen at −20 °C for 11.6–19.3 weeks. The ultrafiltrates were defrosted at the same time as the whole plasma-pool samples and were assayed for free phenytoin concentration along with the ultrafiltrates obtained after freezing.

Assay Methods and Calculations. We used enzyme-multiplied immunoassay (EMIT, Syva, Palo Alto, CA) and a clinical chemistry analyzer (Monarch 2000, I. L. Fisher, Lexington, MA) to determine (1) total phenytoin concentration in plasma and (2) free phenytoin concentration in ultrafiltrate. EMIT standard and control solutions were diluted 1:10 with tromethamine (TRIS) buffer (0.055 M, pH 8.0) in class A volumetric glassware for the measurement of free phenytoin concentration. The sensitivities of the assays for total and free phenytoin were 2.5 and 0.25 mg/L, and the coefficients of variation were 6% and 8%, respectively. Samples were assayed in duplicate.

Means of duplicate determinations were used in calculations. The phenytoin free fraction in each pool was calculated by dividing the free by the total phenytoin concentration. For the study of ultrafiltration products, free concentration and free fraction results were compared by using one-way analysis of variance and the Duncan multiple-range test. Differences in free concentration and free fraction related to the timing and duration of freezing were analyzed with the two-tailed paired Student's *t* test. The level of significance was set at <0.05. All statistical analyses were performed with SPSS/PC+ (version 2.0).[12]

Results. *Comparison of Ultrafiltration Products.* The results are summarized in Table 1. Three plasma pools were too small to be used with all ultrafiltration products; thus, 20 pools were studied. Because of methodologic problems, we were unable to evaluate the free phenytoin concentration in two portions of ultrafiltrate created with the Unisep filter. The mean free phenytoin concentration and free fraction obtained with either set of the Centriflo membrane cones, whether centrifugation lasted 15 or 45 minutes, were significantly lower than the corresponding values obtained with the Centrifree and Unisep filters.

Comparison of Ultrafiltration–Freezing Sequences. The results are summarized in Table 2. The mean values for free phenytoin concentration and free fraction were significantly higher when ultrafiltration occurred before rather than after freezing of the samples. When ultrafiltration occurred before freezing, the free phenytoin concentration and the corresponding free fraction were higher in 18 of 23 plasma pools. The largest differences between portions ultrafiltered before freezing and those ultrafiltered after freezing occurred when

Table 1.
Comparison of Phenytoin Concentration Data from Three Ultrafiltration Products[a]

Ultrafiltration Product[b]	Free Phenytoin Conc. (mg/L)		Phenytoin Free Fraction	
	Mean ± S.D.	Range	Mean ± S.D.	Range
Centrifree	1.61 ± 0.50	0.79–2.90	0.094 ± 0.019	0.072–0.139
Unisep	1.61 ± 0.47	0.77–2.73	0.092 ± 0.017	0.072–0.130
Centriflo, 15 min	1.08 ± 0.44[c]	0.31–2.03	0.062 ± 0.020[c]	0.034–0.111
Centriflo, 45 min	1.25 ± 0.39[c]	0.54–2.04	0.073 ± 0.018[c]	0.050–0.110

[a] For each product, values were derived from the means of duplicate determinations of (1) free phenytoin concentration in 20 portions of ultrafiltrate (except for the Unisep product, for which evaluable results were available from 18 portions) and (2) total phenytoin concentration (mean ± S.D., 17.02 ± 3.75 mg/L; range, 9.00–23.45 mg/L) in the 20 corresponding pools of whole plasma.

[b] Plasma was centrifuged with each ultrafiltration product for 30 minutes; the Centriflo product, which must be soaked in water before use, was centrifuged for 15 or 45 minutes before ultrafiltration.

[c] Significantly different ($p < 0.05$, Duncan multiple-range test) from the corresponding values for the Centrifree and Unisep products.

Table 2.
Phenytoin Concentration Data Derived from Samples Ultrafiltered before or after Freezing[a]

Ultrafiltration–Freezing Sequence	Free Phenytoin Conc. (mg/L)		Phenytoin Free Fraction	
	Mean ± S.D.	Range	Mean ± S.D.	Range
Ultrafiltered first	1.89 ± 0.68	0.68–3.40	0.103 ± 0.021	0.076–0.162
Frozen first	1.72 ± 0.56[b]	0.79–2.90	0.095 ± 0.018[c]	0.072–0.139

[a] Values were derived from the means of duplicate determinations of (1) free phenytoin concentration in 23 portions of ultrafiltrate and (2) total phenytoin concentration (mean ± S.D., 17.97 ± 4.52 mg/L; range, 9.00–28.75 mg/L) in the 23 corresponding pools of whole plasma. Ultrafiltration was performed with the Centrifree product. Mean ± S.D. duration of freezing was 15.5 ± 2.9 weeks (range, 11.6–19.3 weeks).

[b] Significantly different ($p < 0.002$, two-tailed paired Student's t test) from the corresponding value for portions that were ultrafiltered first.

[c] Significantly different ($p < 0.005$) from the corresponding value for portions that were frozen first.

freezing duration was longest; the mean differences for free phenytoin and free fraction in samples that were frozen for more than 16 weeks were significantly greater than those in samples frozen for a shorter duration (Table 3).

Discussion. *Comparison of Ultrafiltration Products.* Variations in plasma albumin[3] and creatinine concentrations,[4] pH,[13] and temperature[14] may influence the degree of phenytoin protein binding. In our study, creatinine and albumin concentration and pH were not determined for each plasma pool. However, because each plasma pool was used with each ultrafiltration product, we do not believe that the comparative value of our study was compromised. We used a refrigerated centrifuge at 25 °C so that temperature would not be a variable. Although it may have been preferable to perform ultrafiltration at 37 °C, the only temperature-controlled centrifuge available to us that could accommodate the 30-mm diameter Centriflo collection tubes had a maximum temperature of 25 °C. We strove to make experimental conditions as uniform as possible by freezing each plasma pool after collection and by defrosting and ultrafiltering each pool at the same time.

Even though the molecular-weight cutoffs for the Centrifree (50,000) and Unisep filters (30,000) differ, there was no significant difference in the mean free phenytoin concentration or free fraction that resulted from use of these products. This is not surprising, since the molecular weight of phenytoin is 252.26 while that of albumin is 60,000.[15] It is reasonable to conclude that results from the use of the Centrifree and Unisep filters are directly comparable.

Table 3.
Association between Freezing Duration and Timing-Related Differences in Phenytoin Concentration Data[a]

Freezing Duration (wk)	No. Portions	Mean ± S.D. Difference in Free Phenytoin Conc. (mg/L)	Mean ± S.D. Difference in Phenytoin Free Fraction
18.4 or 19.3	8	0.33 ± 0.15[b]	0.016 ± 0.007[b]
14.1 or 15.6	7	0.16 ± 0.24	0.008 ± 0.014
11.6 or 13.3	8	0.00 ± 0.09	0.000 ± 0.007

[a] For each of the 23 portions, the timing-related difference in free phenytoin concentration and phenytoin free fraction was calculated by subtracting the value derived from the sample that was ultrafiltered after freezing from the value derived from sample that was ultrafiltered before freezing.

[b] Significantly different ($p < 0.001$, two-tailed paired Student's t test) from the corresponding values for the other durations.

We centrifuged the Centriflo membrane cones for 15 and 45 minutes before use. The shorter duration was used to simulate the condition, in which some water remains in the cones, that would result from following the manufacturer's directions; Booker and Darcey[9] estimated that 0.34 mL of water remains in a Centriflo membrane cone after preparation. The longer duration resulted in membrane cones from which no more water could be removed by centrifugation. We found that the free phenytoin concentration and free fraction obtained from use of "wet" Centriflo cones (centrifuged for 15 minutes before use) was about 30% lower than the values obtained from use of Centrifree and Unisep filters. This finding confirms the observations of Booker and Darcey[9] and is most likely a result of the water remaining in the Centriflo cones diluting the ultrafiltrate.

The significantly lower values that we obtained from "dry" Centriflo cones (centrifuged 45 minutes before use), compared with those obtained from Centrifree and Unisep filters, were unexpected. The difference could be due to the binding of phenytoin to the Centriflo cones. Phenytoin might also bind to wet cones, but the effect may not have been suspected until now because of the relatively large dilutional effect caused by water remaining in the cones. One way to determine if binding occurs would be to measure the amount of radiolabeled phenytoin remaining in the cones after centrifugation. There are no published data on the degree of phenytoin binding to Centriflo cones, but investigators have found that Centrifree filters bind less than 5% of free phenytoin.[16] Although there is no confirming evidence, the fact that Centrifree and Unisep filters yielded similar results in our study suggests that the degree of phenytoin binding in these filter types is similar.

The Centrifree product compares favorably with equilibrium dialysis in separating free from albumin-bound phenytoin.[11] Because Centrifree and Unisep filters produced similar results in our study, the Unisep product should also compare favorably with equilibrium dialysis. The Centrifree and Unisep products can easily be used in standard laboratory centrifuges. Both products can accommodate approximately 1 mL of plasma or serum, a volume that provides an amount of ultrafiltrate adequate for most clinical and many research applications. The Centriflo system can be used with as much as 7 mL of plasma or serum, but the membrane cones, in addition to presenting the dilutional problem described above, require the use of a centrifuge that can accommodate the large-diameter Centriflo collection tubes.

The Centrifree or Unisep product seems to be the best choice for separating free phenytoin in the clinical setting. If the ultrafiltrate is to be stored and assayed later, the Centrifree product, which provides caps for the reservoir cups, may be preferred. In comparing studies that present values for free phenytoin concentration or free fraction, readers should note which ultrafiltration methods were used.

Comparison of Ultrafiltration–Freezing Sequences. The temperature at the time of separation of free from albumin-bound phenytoin may influence the resultant free phenytoin concentration value,[14,17,18] but freezing and thawing of plasma have been reported to have no effect on the degree of phenytoin protein binding.[19] Allison and Comstock[18] separated free from albumin-bound phenytoin before freezing the samples for two weeks at −18 °C. They found that freezing and thawing did not affect phenytoin free concentration and free fraction. Some authors have interpreted that study as showing that freezing does not affect free phenytoin concentration regardless of whether separation occurs before or after freezing,[5,8] but we are not aware that this assumption has been proved.

We could not find reports describing the effect of long freezing duration on free phenytoin concentration. In addition, the time for which samples are frozen before being assayed has not consistently been reported in studies of phenytoin protein binding. We assumed at first that the duration of freezing would not be an important variable. However, a trend became apparent when the data were analyzed: Samples frozen for more than 16 weeks showed the largest differences related to the timing of ultrafiltration and freezing, and this timing had little effect when the freezing duration was shorter than 16 weeks. We expected that changes in albumin or creatinine concentration or pH, factors that influence phenytoin protein binding, would not occur during short-term freezing; although we did not measure these variables, the results for samples frozen for less than 16 weeks are consistent with this expectation. Further study, which should include the measurement of these influencing factors, should be conducted to determine why prolonged freezing causes the changes that we found.

In clinical practice, samples for the determination of free phenytoin concentration are not ordinarily frozen before assay. However, clinical researchers must often delay concentration analysis until enough samples have been generated for a batch or until all study samples have been collected. These researchers have the option of (1) ultrafiltering plasma immediately after collection and then freezing the ultrafiltrate or (2) freezing the plasma and performing ultrafiltration just before assay. Because of the decreases in free phenytoin concentration and free fraction described above, we recommend that ultrafiltration precede freezing if samples are to be frozen for more than 16 weeks.

Conclusion. The Centrifree and Unisep ultrafiltration products provide similar results for free phenytoin concentration and free fraction, but the Centriflo membrane cone produces significantly lower values. When the duration of freezing is more than 16 weeks, samples that are frozen before ultrafiltration yield free phenytoin concentration and free fraction values that are significantly lower than those from samples that are ultrafiltered before freezing.

References

1. Svensson CK, Woodruff MN, Baxter JG et al. Free drug

concentration monitoring in clinical practice: rationale and current status. *Clin Pharmacokinet*. 1986; 11:450–69.
2. Perucca E. Free level monitoring of antiepileptic drugs: clinical usefulness and case studies. *Clin Pharmacokinet*. 1984; 9(Suppl 1):71–8.
3. Bauer LA, Edwards WAD, Dellinger EP et al. Importance of unbound phenytoin serum levels in head trauma patients. *J Trauma*. 1983; 23:1058–60.
4. Liponi DF, Winter ME, Tozer TN. Renal function and therapeutic concentrations of phenytoin. *Neurology*. 1984; 34:395–7.
5. Miles MV, Snead OC III, Thorn MD. Predictability of unbound antiepileptic drug concentrations in children treated with valproic acid and phenytoin. *Clin Pharm*. 1988; 7:688–93.
6. Odar-Cederlof I, Borga O. Impaired plasma protein binding of phenytoin in uremia and displacement effect of salicylic acid. *Clin Pharm Ther*. 1976; 20:36–47.
7. Baird-Lambert J, Manglick MP, Wall M et al. Identifying patients who might benefit from free phenytoin monitoring. *Ther Drug Monit*. 1987; 9:134–8.
8. Porter RJ, Layzer RB. Plasma albumin concentration and diphenylhydantoin binding in man. *Arch Neurol*. 1975; 32:298–303.
9. Booker HE, Darcey B. Serum concentrations of free diphenylhydantoin and their relationship to clinical intoxication. *Epilepsia*. 1973; 14:177–84.
10. Argyle JC, Kinniburgh DW, Costa R et al. Evaluation of ultrafiltration–fluorescence polarization immunoassay for monitoring unbound phenytoin. *Ther Drug Monit*. 1984; 6:117–20.
11. Koike Y, Magnusson A, Steiner E et al. Ultrafiltration compared with equilibrium dialysis in the determination of unbound phenytoin in plasma. *Ther Drug Monit*. 1985; 7:461–5.
12. Norusis MJ, ed. SPSS/PC+ V2.0. Chicago, IL: SPSS Inc.; 1988.
13. Firemark H, Barlow CF, Roth LJ. The entry, accumulation and binding of diphenylhydantoin-2-C^{14} in the brain. *Neuropharmacol*. 1963; 2:25–38.
14. Lunde PKM, Rane A, Yaffe SJ et al. Plasma protein binding of diphenylhydantoin in man: interaction with other drugs and the effect of temperature and plasma dilution. *Clin Pharmacol Ther*. 1970; 11:846–55.
15. The Merck index. 10th ed. Windholz M, ed. Rahway, NJ: Merck and Co., Inc.; 1983: 33, 1054–5.
16. Zysset T, Zeugin T. Comparison of the Amicon Centrifree micropartition system with the Sartorius SM 13249E Centrisart I device to determine protein free phenytoin concentrations. *Ther Drug Monit*. 1986; 8:346–51.
17. Melten JW, Wittebrood AJ, Wimer J et al. On the modulating effects of temperature, albumin, pH, and calcium on the free fractions of phenobarbitone and phenytoin. *J Pharm Pharmacol*. 1986; 38:643–6.
18. Allison TB, Comstock TJ. Temperature dependence of phenytoin protein binding in serum: effects of uremia and hypoalbuminemia. *Ther Drug Monit*. 1988; 10:376–81.
19. Ehrnebo M, Agurell S, Jalling B et al. Age differences in drug binding by plasma proteins: studies on human foetuses, neonates, and adults. *Eur J Clin Pharmacol*. 1971; 3:189–93.

Hypoprothrombinemic effect of warfarin not influenced by ciprofloxacin

JOSEPH P. RINDONE, CATHERINE L. KEUEY, WILLIAM N. JONES, AND HARINDER S. GAREWAL

Clin Pharm. 1991; 10:136–8

Recent case reports have suggested that some fluoroquinolone antimicrobials may inhibit drug metabolism. For example, enoxacin and ciprofloxacin have been reported to decrease the clearance of theophylline, and norfloxacin and ciprofloxacin have been associated with enhancing the hypoprothrombinemic response to warfarin.[1–4] To date, researchers have not specifically examined the effect of ciprofloxacin on the pharmacodynamics of warfarin. The purpose of this study was to evaluate the effect of ciprofloxacin on the hypoprothrombinemic effect of long-term, low-intensity warfarin therapy.

Methods. Pharmacy clinic patients at the Veterans Affairs Medical Center, Tucson, who had stable prothrombin times (PTs) and who were receiving long-term, low-intensity anticoagulation therapy with warfarin (international normalized ratio [INR], 2–3) were eligible for participation in the study. A stable PT was defined as one that varied by less than 10% between measurements taken on two consecutive days at least seven days after a change in the dosage of warfarin. Patients were not recruited if any medication changes had been made two weeks before the study began. Other exclusion criteria were a history of hypersensitivity reactions to ciprofloxacin or another quinolone antimicrobial (e.g., nalidixic acid) and the use of antacids, sucralfate, or ferrous sulfate. The study was approved by the human subjects committee, and informed consent was obtained from all patients.

Eligible patients were instructed to take cipro-

JOSEPH P. RINDONE, PHARM.D., is Clinical Pharmacist, Veterans Affairs Medical Center (VAMC), Tucson, AZ, and Adjunct Assistant Professor, Department of Pharmacy Practice, College of Pharmacy, University of Arizona (UA), Tucson. CATHERINE L. KEUEY, PHARM.D., is Clinical Pharmacy Resident, VAMC. WILLIAM N. JONES, M.S., is Clinical Pharmacy Coordinator, VAMC, and Adjunct Assistant Professor, Department of Pharmacy Practice, College of Pharmacy, UA. HARINDER S. GAREWAL, M.D., is Staff Physician, Hematology-Oncology Section, VAMC, and Assistant Professor, Department of Internal Medicine, UA.

Address reprint requests to Dr. Rindone at the Veterans Affairs Medical Center (119), Tucson, AZ 85723.

Presented at the 10th Annual Western States Conference for Pharmacy Residents and Preceptors, Pacific Grove, CA, April 6, 1990.

floxacin (as the hydrochloride salt) 500 mg twice daily for seven days. A seven-day supply of ciprofloxacin was dispensed on the first day of treatment. The patients were asked about their ciprofloxacin intake at each clinic visit, and unused ciprofloxacin tablets were counted at the end of the study. Compliance was defined as a patient returning less than 10% of the ciprofloxacin doses dispensed. PT was measured approximately 24 hours after a warfarin dose on days 1, 3, and 7 of ciprofloxacin therapy.

PTs were determined by using a rabbit brain thromboplastin assay with an international sensitivity index (ISI) of 1.85. The ISI is a standardization value for thromboplastin reagents that allows comparison among them.[5] Variation for this test is ±1 second (S.D.) for PTs between 18.8 and 20.8 seconds. The PT ratio was calculated by using a control value of 12.2 seconds, which was obtained for 50 patients at the institution who were not receiving an anticoagulant. A PT ratio of 1.45 (17.7 seconds) to 1.80 (22 seconds) was necessary to attain an INR of 2 to 3 with the thromboplastin reagent used.

The maximum change in PT for each patient was calculated from the difference between the mean of the patient's baseline PTs on days −1 (two days before the first dose of ciprofloxacin) and 0 (one day before the first dose) and the highest or lowest PT during the period of ciprofloxacin therapy. Analysis of variance was used to compare the mean PTs before and during ciprofloxacin therapy. The level of significance was set at <0.05. Seven subjects were estimated to be needed to avoid a Type II error,[6] based on β set at 0.2, an S.D. for the control group of two seconds, and an estimate of three seconds for a clinically important change in PT.

Results. Nine men who had been receiving warfarin for three months to more than one year completed the study. The patients ranged in age from 45 to 75 years (mean ± S.D., 62 ± 12 years). The indications for warfarin therapy were atrial fibrillation (three patients), deep-vein thrombosis (two patients), congestive heart failure (one patient), pulmonary embolism (one patient), subclavian vein thrombosis (one patient), and amaurosis fugax (one patient). The patients were maintained on the same medication regimen before and during the study period. In all patients, warfarin dosages had not been changed for at least one month before the trial. Patients 1 and 5 received cimetidine before and during the study. Compliance for ciprofloxacin therapy was 93% to 100%.

There was no significant difference in mean ± S.D. PTs before and during ciprofloxacin treatment (Table 1). Maximum increases in PT of 13% and 22% occurred in patients 2 and 7, respectively, and a 12% maximum decrease occurred in patient 6. The PT ratio was never less than 1.3 or more than 2 during ciprofloxacin therapy.

Discussion. In a case report, ciprofloxacin 750 mg twice daily was apparently associated with a marked increase in PT in a patient with a prosthetic aortic valve who was receiving warfarin.[4] Ciprofloxacin may interfere with the microsomal metabolism of some drugs; it decreases antipyrine clearance.[7] Notwithstanding such findings, our study showed that ciprofloxacin does not alter the hypoprothrombinemic effect of warfarin, although the results could have been influenced by the dosage or duration of ciprofloxacin administration. Patients with prosthetic heart valves who receive intensive anticoagulation therapy may be at increased risk for a clinically meaningful interaction, in view of the 22% increase in PT in one of the patients we studied.

A dose-related interaction is possible. The dosage of ciprofloxacin selected for this study is the

Table 1.
Prothrombin Times (PTs) before and during Ciprofloxacin Administration

Patient	Warfarin Dosage (mg/wk)	PT in Seconds (PT Ratio) on Indicated Day of Study					Maximum Change in PT in Seconds (% Change)[b]
		−1	0	1[a]	3	7	
1	22.5	18.0 (1.48)	17.5 (1.43)	17.1 (1.40)	19.0 (1.56)	18.9 (1.55)	1.2 (7)
2	22.5	17.8 (1.46)	17.8 (1.46)	17.9 (1.47)	19.8 (1.62)	20.1 (1.65)	2.3 (13)
3	20	17.5 (1.43)	18.8 (1.54)	18.5 (1.52)	17.2 (1.41)	17.6 (1.44)	−1.0 (6)
4	30	19.9 (1.63)	19.0 (1.56)	17.9 (1.47)	18.6 (1.52)	18.3 (1.50)	−1.5 (8)
5	75	22.0 (1.80)	23.5 (1.93)	22.9 (1.88)	21.3 (1.75)	22.0 (1.80)	−1.5 (7)
6	12.5	21.6 (1.77)	22.4 (1.84)	21.2 (1.74)	19.3 (1.58)	21.0 (1.72)	−2.7 (12)
7	70	18.4 (1.51)	18.5 (1.52)	18.6 (1.52)	22.4 (1.84)	21.6 (1.77)	4.0 (22)
8	33.75	17.9 (1.47)	19.3 (1.58)	19.3 (1.58)	19.4 (1.59)	18.4 (1.51)	0.8 (4)
9	20	16.7 (1.37)	18.5 (1.52)	18.9 (1.55)	17.4 (1.43)	18.8 (1.54)	1.3 (7)
Mean		18.9 (1.55)	19.5 (1.60)	19.1 (1.57)	19.4 (1.59)	19.6 (1.61)	0.3 (2)
S.D.		1.9	2.1	1.8	1.7	1.6	2.1

[a] Day 1 of ciprofloxacin therapy. Subjects took ciprofloxacin (as the hydrochloride salt) 500 mg twice daily for seven days.
[b] Calculated for each patient as the difference between the mean of the baseline PTs (days −1 and 0) and the highest or lowest PT during the period of ciprofloxacin therapy.

recommended dosage for mild to moderate infections. A seven-day duration of ciprofloxacin therapy was chosen since it is a common duration of treatment for many infections. In patients requiring higher dosages or more prolonged treatment, an interaction might occur. Further investigations of various dosage regimens of ciprofloxacin, especially in patients receiving intensive anticoagulation therapy, are needed.

Conclusion. A seven-day course of ciprofloxacin (as the hydrochloride salt) 500 mg twice daily did not affect the prothrombin times of patients undergoing long-term, low-intensity warfarin therapy.

References

1. Wijnands WJA, Vree TB, Vanhervaarden CLA. Enoxacin decreases the clearance of theophylline in man. *Br J Clin Pharmacol.* 1986; 20:583–8.
2. Schartz J, Jauregue L, Lettieri J et al. Impact of ciprofloxacin on theophylline clearance and steady-state concentrations in serum. *Antimicrob Agents Chemother.* 1988; 32:75–7.
3. Linville T, Matanin D. Norfloxacin and warfarin. *Ann Intern Med.* 1989; 110:751–2.
4. Mott FE, Murphy S, Hunt V. Ciprofloxacin and warfarin. *Ann Intern Med.* 1989; 111:542–3.
5. Hirsh J, Poller L, Deykin D et al. Optimal therapeutic range for oral anticoagulants. *Chest.* 1989; 95:5s–11s.
6. Stolley PD, Strom BC. Sample size calculations for clinical pharmacology studies. *Clin Pharmacol Ther.* 1986; 39:489–90.
7. Ludwig E, Szekely E, Csiba A et al. The effect of ciprofloxacin on antipyrine metabolism. *J Antimicrob Chemother.* 1988; 22:61–7.

Acceptability of cholestyramine and colestipol formulations in three common vehicles

MATTHEW K. ITO and ANTHONY P. MORREALE

Clin Pharm. 1991; 10:138–40

The efficacy of bile acid sequestrants for the treatment of primary hypercholesterolemia type IIa has been well established, and in general the adverse effects, while common, are not considered severe.[1–3] However, a major concern with bile acid sequestrants is lack of patient compliance due to constipation and poor palatability. Constipation is normally managed by an increase in the intake of fluid, fruit, and vegetables and by the occasional use of stool softeners. Palatability remains an issue with bile acid sequestrants. In 1987 Shaefer et al.[4] compared the taste, texture, and smell of colestipol hydrochloride (Colestid, Upjohn) and cholestyramine (Questran, Bristol) in a variety of vehicles in a double-blind randomized trial in healthy volunteers. Testing was rated on a modified wine-tasting scale.[4,5] In all vehicles tested, Questran was rated significantly better than Colestid in all three categories.

Recently, Bristol Laboratories introduced a new cholestyramine product, Questran Light. Questran Light contains the same amount of dried cholestyramine resin (4 g) as the original product but only 5 g of powder, compared with 9 g in Questran. In addition, Questran Light contains NutraSweet (aspartame) instead of the sucrose found in the original product. The changes were designed to decrease powder volume, improve flavor, and decrease caloric content.

In 1990 Shaefer et al.[6] compared the acceptability of the two cholestyramine products in water and orange juice. Overall, Questran Light was preferred. Colestid was not tested in this trial, and the rating scale was different from that previously used, precluding direct comparisons.

In the study reported here, we assessed the overall acceptability of Questran Light, Questran, and Colestid when mixed with water, orange juice, or apple juice.

Methods. Healthy volunteers more than 18 years of age were considered for inclusion in the study. Health status was ascertained by questionnaire. Each volunteer gave written informed consent to participate, and the study protocol was approved by the institutional review board at the Department of Veterans Affairs Medical Center, San Diego.

This was a prospective, randomized, double-blind study. Each volunteer received samples of all of the following drug–vehicle mixtures in random order: (1) Questran 9 g in 120 mL of water, apple juice, or orange juice; (2) Questran Light 9 g in 120 mL of water, apple juice, or orange juice; and (3) Colestid 5 g in 120 mL of water, apple juice, or orange juice.

Subjects were excluded from the study for any of the following reasons: previous exposure to any of the study medications, hypersensitivity to any of the vehicles or medication components, any history of a disease causing taste impairment (e.g., diabetes mellitus), gastrointestinal conditions for which bile resins are contraindicated, tobacco smoking, any acute illness that might impair taste or smell, current use of medications known to alter or impair taste or smell (e.g., metronidazole, gris-

MATTHEW K. ITO, PHARM.D., is Assistant Professor of Clinical Pharmacy and Regional Coordinator, San Diego Program, School of Pharmacy, University of the Pacific, Stockton, CA. ANTHONY P. MORREALE, PHARM.D., is Assistant Chief of Pharmacy Service, Department of Veterans Affairs Medical Center, San Diego, CA.

Address reprint requests to Dr. Ito, Pharmacy Service (119), Department of Veterans Affairs Medical Center, 3350 La Jolla Village Drive, San Diego, CA 92161.

The technical assistance of Michele A. Dietrich, Pharm.D., and Adrienne T. St. George and the secretarial assistance of Marsha L. Towers are acknowledged.

eofulvin, angiotensin-converting-enzyme inhibitors, penicillamine, lithium, and rifampin), phenylketonuria, and current use of oral anticoagulants or cardiac glycosides.

All nine mixtures were prepared by a pharmacy technician the night before testing and refrigerated at 4 °C. All drug–vehicle combinations were allowed to return to room temperature before sampling in an effort to minimize temperature fluctuation throughout the study. The subjects were blindfolded, and the investigators did not know which product was involved in a given test. The subjects were asked to refrain from eating or drinking for at least four hours before testing began.

Each drug–vehicle combination was graded by the subjects on a 5-point modified wine-tasting scale (Table 1).[4,5] The investigators reviewed the rating scale with each subject before and throughout testing and recorded the subject's assessments of the taste, texture, and smell of each mixture. Each subject consumed a well-mixed 30-mL sample of each drug–vehicle combination at random and was then asked to rinse out the mouth with 30 mL of water, to eat a small bland cracker, and to rinse again with 30 mL of water. The subjects were asked to consume the entire 30-mL sample being tested before offering a response.

Differences in mean scores for taste, texture, and smell and in total mean scores for each drug–vehicle mixture were compared by analysis of variance. Post hoc analysis was performed with Duncan's range test to test for pairwise differences. The level of significance (α) and the power of the test ($1-\beta$) were set at 0.05 and 0.80, respectively, for a sample size of 44. All values are expressed as means ± S.D.

Results. Forty-five healthy volunteers (20 men and 25 women) 31.6 ± 3.2 years of age completed the study. Mean scores for taste, texture, and smell for each drug–vehicle combination are listed in Table 2. In terms of taste, Colestid in orange juice and in water and Questran Light in water scored lower than the other combinations. Questran in all the vehicles scored higher for texture than all other combinations except Questran Light in orange juice and Colestid in apple juice. Colestid in water was rated lower for smell than all other combinations.

Total mean preference scores for each drug–vehicle combination are listed in Table 3. Total scores for Questran Light in water, Colestid in orange juice, and Colestid in water were lower than total scores for the remaining combinations.

Discussion. In selecting an antihyperlipidemic agent, the clinician needs to consider several key issues: efficacy in reducing the incidence of coronary heart disease, long-term safety, and characteristics affecting patient acceptability and compliance, such as adverse-effect profile, convenience, and palatability. In general, the effectiveness of a medication can be influenced by noncompliance. The bile acid sequestrants have gained an unfavorable reputation because of their poor palatability.

Table 1.
Modified Wine-Tasting Scale Used To Grade the Drug–Vehicle Combinations[4,5]

Taste	Texture	Smell
1 = Vile	1 = Sandy	1 = Offensive
2 = Unpleasant	2 = Gritty	2 = Tolerable
3 = Neutral	3 = Coarse	3 = Neutral
4 = Acceptable	4 = Neutral	4 = Nice
5 = Delicious	5 = Smooth	5 = Very pleasant

Table 2.
Mean Preference Scores for Each Drug–Vehicle Combination

	Mean ± S.D. Score (95% Confidence Interval)		
Vehicle	Questran Light	Questran	Colestid
Taste			
Orange juice	3.36 ± 0.98[a] (3.06–3.65)	3.16 ± 0.93[a] (2.88–3.43)	2.40 ± 0.96 (2.11–2.69)
Apple juice	3.58 ± 0.92[a] (3.30–3.85)	3.69 ± 0.79[a] (3.45–3.93)	3.31 ± 1.02[a] (3.01–3.62)
Water	2.76 ± 0.96 (2.47–3.04)	3.16 ± 0.82[a] (2.91–3.40)	2.78 ± 0.85 (2.52–3.03)
Texture			
Orange juice	3.07 ± 1.50[b] (2.62–3.52)	2.73 ± 1.45[b] (2.30–3.17)	2.33 ± 1.13 (2.0–2.67)
Apple juice	2.24 ± 1.33 (1.84–2.65)	2.82 ± 1.59[b] (2.35–3.30)	2.76 ± 1.67[b] (2.25–3.26)
Water	2.00 ± 1.15 (1.66–2.34)	2.67 ± 1.46[b] (2.23–3.11)	1.76 ± 1.13 (1.42–2.10)
Smell			
Orange juice	3.80 ± 0.76[c] (3.57–4.03)	3.71 ± 0.87[c] (3.45–3.97)	3.67 ± 0.83[c] (3.42–3.91)
Apple juice	3.87 ± 0.87[c] (3.61–4.13)	3.98 ± 0.84[c] (3.73–4.23)	3.60 ± 0.91[c] (3.33–3.87)
Water	3.69 ± 0.82[c] (3.44–3.94)	3.53 ± 0.81[c] (3.29–3.78)	3.02 ± 0.40 (2.90–3.14)

[a] Significantly different from scores for Questran Light in water and Colestid in orange juice and in water ($p < 0.05$).
[b] Significantly different from scores for Questran Light in apple juice and in water and Colestid in orange juice and in water ($p < 0.05$).
[c] Significantly different from score for Colestid in water ($p < 0.05$).

Table 3.
Combined Mean Preference Scores for Each Drug–Vehicle Combination

	Mean ± S.D. Score (95% Confidence Interval)		
Vehicle	Questran Light	Questran	Colestid
Orange juice	10.22 ± 2.32[a] (9.52–10.92)	9.60 ± 1.94[a] (9.02–10.18)	8.40 ± 1.92 (7.82–8.98)
Apple juice	9.69 ± 2.10[a] (9.06–10.32)	10.49 ± 2.16[a] (9.84–11.14)	9.67 ± 2.50[a] (8.91–10.42)
Water	8.44 ± 1.91 (7.87 ± 9.02)	9.36 ± 2.17[a] (8.71–10.01)	7.56 ± 1.55 (7.09–8.02)

[a] Significantly different from scores for Questran Light in water and Colestid in orange juice and in water ($p < 0.05$).

Questran Light and Colestid appear to have a less desirable taste and texture than Questran. The combinations that were less preferred were Colestid mixed with orange juice or water and Questran Light in water. Apple juice appears to be an acceptable vehicle for all the drugs tested. Thus, in patients unable to tolerate the flavor of Colestid or Questran Light, the use of water as a vehicle should be limited to patients with caloric restrictions and to those unable to tolerate fruit juices.

Smell appears to be of limited importance in overall preference. Scores for smell were similar except for Colestid in water, which had a lower, neutral score (3.02 ± 0.40), probably because of the lack of a fruit flavoring in this drug product.

We limited our evaluation to the most commonly available nontextured vehicles. Textured vehicles were avoided not only because of limited availability in a variety of situations but to avoid overtly masking the texture of each drug product.

Total mean preference scores for Questran–vehicle combinations are similar between this study (10.49, 9.60, and 9.36 for Questran in apple juice, orange juice, or water, respectively) and the study by Shaefer et al.[4] (10.7, 10.5, and 9.9 for Questran in apple juice, orange juice, or water, respectively). In contrast, total mean preference scores for Colestid–vehicle combinations in our study (9.67, 8.40, and 7.56 for Colestid in apple juice, orange juice, or water, respectively) average 15% greater than those reported by Shaefer et al. (7.9, 7.6, and 6.3 for Colestid in apple juice, orange juice, or water, respectively). However, both studies disclose scores of increasing magnitude for both bile acid sequestrant products when mixed with water, orange juice, or apple juice in that order.

Both study groups were younger (mean age: 26.2 years, Shaefer et al.[4]; 31.6 years, this study) than the average patients who use these medications, and older patients may have slightly altered perceptions of taste, texture, and smell.

The cost and the caloric content of the juice vehicles were not evaluated in this study. Consideration of cost alone without regard to outcome factors (e.g., compliance, effectiveness, and quality of life) may not be valid. The cost of an 8-oz glass of orange juice or apple juice at a supermarket could range from $0.12 to $0.25 ($0.96 to $2.00 per 64 oz). Obviously, this expense adds to the total cost of therapy and could be an issue for certain patients. However, the cost of an inadequate response attributed to poor compliance also needs to be considered. In patients in whom caloric intake is clinically important, water, other noncaloric vehicles, or alternative lipid-lowering agents should be considered.

Conclusion. Apple juice appeared to be an acceptable vehicle for Questran Light, Questran, and Colestid. Vehicle choice had a greater effect on the acceptability of Questran Light or Colestid than Questran. The less preferred drug–vehicle combinations were Questran Light in water, Colestid in water, and Colestid in orange juice.

References

1. Gluck CJ, Ford, S, Scheel D et al. Colestipol and cholestyramine resin comparative effects in familial type II hyperlipoproteinemia. *JAMA*. 1972; 222:671–81.
2. Brensike JF, Levy RI, Kelsey, SF et al. Effects of therapy with cholestyramine on progression of coronary arteriosclerosis: results of the NHLBI type II coronary intervention study. *Circulation*. 1984; 69:313–24.
3. Anon. The lipid research clinic coronary primary prevention trial: (1) reduction in incidence of coronary heart disease; (2) the relationship of reduction in incidence of coronary heart disease to cholesterol lowering. *JAMA*. 1984; 251:351–74.
4. Shaefer MS, Jungnickel PW, Jacobs EW et al. Acceptability of cholestyramine or colestipol combinations with six vehicles. *Clin Pharm*. 1987; 6:51–4.
5. Brown RO, Hall NH, Elkordy M et al. Use of a wine-tasting scale to evaluate enteral nutritional supplements. *Nutr Support Serv*. 1985; 5:21–4.
6. Shaefer MS, Jungnickel PW, Miwa LJ et al. Sensory/mixability preference evaluation of cholestyramine powder formulations. *DICP*. 1990; 24:472–4.

“

Health Benefits of Smoking Cessation

On September 25, 1990, *The Health Benefits of Smoking Cessation: A Report of the Surgeon General, 1990,* was released. The major conclusions of the report are: 1) smoking cessation has major and immediate health benefits for persons of all ages and provides benefits for persons with and without smoking-related disease; 2) former smokers live longer than continuing smokers; 3) smoking cessation decreases the risk for lung and other cancers, heart attack, stroke, and chronic lung disease; 4) women who stop smoking before pregnancy or during the first 3 to 4 months of pregnancy reduce their risk for having a low-birth-weight infant to that of women who never smoked; and 5) the health benefits of smoking cessation substantially exceed any risks from the average 5-lb. (2.3-kg) weight gain or any adverse psychologic effects that may follow quitting.

—Anon. Health benefits of smoking cessation. *MMWR*. 1990; 39:653.

”

Editorial

Recombinant interleukin-2 and the quest for FDA approval

This issue of *CP* contains a comprehensive review of the biological response modifier, or cytokine, recombinant interleukin-2. The article focuses on the treatment of renal cell carcinoma, melanoma, and colorectal cancer with recombinant interleukin-2, often in combination with lymphokine-activated killer (LAK) cells. In fact, much of the data supporting the use of recombinant interleukin-2 in these disease states comes from National Cancer Institute and extramural studies in which recombinant interleukin-2 was used in combination with LAK cells.[1]

Members of Cetus Corporation met with the Food and Drug Administration (FDA) several months ago in a public forum seeking approval for the use of recombinant interleukin-2 as single-agent therapy in renal cell carcinoma. Unlike drugs, biological agents are being evaluated by the FDA's Center for Biologics Evaluation and Research. This arm of the agency is now responsible for the approval of biological response modifiers as well as many other recombinant DNA products, such as hematopoietic growth factors. The FDA is still inexperienced in this area and is adjusting to the flood of applications for approval of biotechnology products.

The FDA advisory panel that met with Cetus did not approve Cetus's petition. Some of the data presented to the panel had been given to the FDA only shortly before the meeting.[2] The advisory panel apparently believed that the information had to be reorganized and revised to better support an analysis of the benefits and risks of using recombinant interleukin-2 in the treatment of renal cell carcinoma.

One of the reasons for the denial may have been that much of the supporting data was based on the use of recombinant interleukin-2 in combination with other agents or cells, especially LAK cells. Cetus, however, was seeking approval of recombinant interleukin-2 as single-agent therapy. Perhaps the basis of Cetus's approach was the fact that in humans the addition of LAK cells has not substantially been shown to add anything to the clinical outcome. But the FDA sees recombinant interleukin-2 therapy and recombinant interleukin-2 plus LAK cell therapy as separate entities and furthermore believes that data from studies of recombinant interleukin-2 plus LAK cell therapy should not be extrapolated to recombinant interleukin-2 therapy alone.

One of the primary concerns over high-dose recombinant interleukin-2 therapy is toxicity, which carries a mortality rate of 1–2%. The decision not to approve the petition may have been affected by the fact that study patients were treated and monitored in intensive-care units in major university hospital settings. With approval of recombinant interleukin-2, the question might arise as to whether the toxicity or associated mortality rates would increase in settings that do not have such intensive observation and supportive care. Researchers are continuing to look at lower-dose regimens to see if they can decrease toxicity without detracting from efficacy.[3] There have been advances in this area, although much work remains. For patients, however, any advance in the treatment of these traditionally incurable diseases would be welcome. While AIDS activists have strongly petitioned for the right to experimental therapy and fast tracking of drugs, cancer patients have been less vocal.

In some patients, recombinant interleukin-2 therapy does work; some have durable complete or partial responses after only one or two courses of treatment. Maintenance therapy in these patients may not be required—in stark contrast to those given traditional antineoplastic therapy. It would be most useful to identify those subgroups of patients who are likely to respond.[4] This is easier said than done, however. Retrospective analysis of renal cell carcinoma patients treated with recombinant interleukin-2 suggests that those who have previously undergone nephrectomy, those without large tumors, and those who have only pulmonary metastases are more likely to gain beneficial results. Analysis of changes in peripheral blood cells has not yielded insights into patient selection.

Newer evidence suggests that the role of recombinant interleukin-2 as a biological response modulator via the stimulation of cytokine release may be a key to responsiveness. Researchers have correlated clinical response with the sustained production of tumor necrosis factor (TNF) after the cessation of recombinant interleukin-2 therapy.[5] Most studies of TNF as single-agent therapy in cancer patients have found it to be highly toxic. Stimulation of endogenous production of TNF via recombinant interleukin-2 may be a more physiologically sound approach. Other determinants correlating with response, such as human lymphocyte antigen (HLA) phenotype, tumor cell surface receptor expression, or presence of tumor-associated suppressive factors, may also need to be examined. The immunobiological effects of recombinant interleukin-2 on tumor cell cytolysis in vivo are still not clearly understood.

Elucidation of recombinant interleukin-2's mechanism of action could enable researchers and clinicians to identify those patients with the physiological characteristics necessary for a response. Large-scale studies in which patients are grouped by common tumor correlates could select out those who would respond. These correlates, as viewed by Parkinson,[6] could include phenotyping by immune response genes, HLA class I and II expression, and ability to induce expression of cytokines.

In summary, recombinant interleukin-2 reproducibly results in objective clinical responses in a small number of patients with renal cell carcinoma. The best dosage regimen is still open to question. The complexity of the disease state and the effects of recombinant interleukin-2 on the body make analysis of clinical trial results extremely difficult. Perhaps the bottom line is that we know it works; the greatest challenge now is to find out how and in whom so that we can select those patients most likely to respond and avoid subjecting others to the potential toxicities and cost of high-dose recombinant interleukin-2 therapy. With a shift toward addressing and answering those questions, FDA approval of recombinant interleukin-2 for the treatment of renal cell cancer and perhaps other malignancies may yet be hoped for.

1. Rosenberg SA. Adoptive immunotherapy for cancer. *Sci Am.* 1990; May:62–9.
2. Culliton BJ. Cetus's costly stumble on IL-2. *Science.* 1990; 250:20–1.
3. Clark JW, Smith JW II, Steis RG et al. Interleukin 2 and lymphokine-activated killer cell therapy: analysis of a bolus interleukin 2 and a continuous infusion interleukin 2 regimen. *Cancer Res.* 1990; 50:7343–50.
4. Parmiani G. An explanation of the variable clinical response to interleukin 2 and LAK cells. *Immunol Today.* 1990; 11:113–5.
5. Blay J-Y, Favrot MC, Negrier S et al. Correlation between clinical response to interleukin 2 therapy and sustained production of tumor necrosis factor. *Cancer Res.* 1990; 50:2371–4.
6. Parkinson DR. Interleukin-2: further progress through greater understanding. *J Natl Cancer Inst.* 1990; 82:1374–6. Editorial.

JOSEPH A. TAMI, PHARM.D.
Department of Medicine, Division of Hematology
The University of Texas Health Science Center at San Antonio
7703 Floyd Curl Drive
San Antonio, TX 78284-7880

"

When Is a Cancer Treatment Worthwhile?

There is no absolute measure of benefit that can be used to determine whether a particular treatment is worthwhile. The traditional end points in trials of cancer treatment are tumor response and duration of survival. Although the shrinkage of tumor (i.e., response) may give information about the biologic activity of the therapy, it does not necessarily mean benefit to the patient. Balancing small gains in survival against toxicity and cost has been particularly difficult, because they are fundamentally different considerations, like the proverbial apples and oranges. The more recent inclusion of quality of life as an end point in clinical trials of cancer therapy has provided a way to incorporate both positive outcomes (the relief of symptoms) and negative outcomes (the toxicity of treatment) into a measure of the overall value of a treatment. One thereby attempts to assess the quality of the apples and oranges, as well as count them. Indexes of the quality of life have now been developed and validated for use in patients with several types of cancer. They can be applied when the primary aim of treatment is to provide palliation or, in the setting of adjuvant chemotherapy, when the aim is to improve survival or delay relapse.

Complementary methods are being developed to estimate the differences in therapeutic outcome that patients (or their surrogates) regard as worthwhile. With trade-off methods, a patient is asked to choose between two potential outcomes. An example is the choice between a defined period of poor health due to treatment, followed by prolonged survival, and shorter survival with no immediate ill effects of treatment. The difference in survival (other end points can also be used) can then be varied until the patient reaches a point of indecision. Among patients with operable lung cancer, the method revealed that an appreciable number preferred radiation therapy to surgery (thus avoiding the risk of perioperative mortality), despite a lower probability of long-term survival. In contrast, among patients who have received chemotherapy for breast cancer, the method suggested that they would accept toxic treatment for rather small gains in survival.

—Tannock IF, Boyer M. When is a cancer treatment worthwhile? *N Engl J Med.* 1990; 323:989–90. Editorial.

"

DUE Criteria

The DUE Criteria *section of* Clinical Pharmacy *features model drug-use evaluation criteria that may be employed as a component of a comprehensive quality assurance program. The criteria sets are presented in the format used in the ASHP book* Criteria for Drug Use Evaluation. *Some of the criteria sets will have been originally published in that book; others will be presented here for the first time and published in future volumes of the ASHP book. The practitioners who developed a criteria set are acknowledged.*

In selecting drug products for coverage in DUE Criteria, *priority is given to products that have been recently marketed, those that are frequently prescribed, those that have high potential risk associated with their use, and those that are expensive. When feasible, a criteria set will be linked with a Drug Review that appears in the same issue.*

These criteria sets are a starting point for the development of DUE criteria for a specific practice setting. Readers are encouraged to modify the model criteria to fit their own circumstances.

Element	Standard 100%	Standard 0%	Exception[b] or Critical Preventive/ Responsive Measure[c]	Sources of Information
Justification for Use				
1. Anemia due to chronic renal failure (CRF) (hematocrit [Hct], <30%) in the following types of patients who had a nephrology consultation[1–6]: a. Hemodialysis patients b. Peritoneal dialysis patients c. Predialysis patients	X		1A. None	1. History and physical examination (H&P), laboratory reports, progress notes, nephrology consultation reports
or				
2. Anemia (Hct, <30%) in patient with AIDS undergoing zidovudine therapy (≤4200 mg/wk) and with endogenous serum erythropoietin concentration of ≤500 mU/mL[7,8]	X		2A. None	2. H&P, laboratory reports, progress notes
Critical (Process) Indicators				
<u>CRF and AIDS Patients</u>				
3. No history of allergy to mammalian cell-derived products, human albumin, or epoetin[3]	X		3A. None	3. H&P, allergy reports
<u>CRF Patients Only</u>				
4. Hct measured twice weekly for 6–8 weeks after initiation of epoetin therapy[3]	X		4A. None	4. Laboratory reports, progress notes, physician orders
5. Hct measured twice weekly for 6–8 weeks after dosage adjustment[3]	X		5A. None	5. Laboratory reports, progress notes, physician orders, medication administration records (MAR)
6. Complete blood count with differential and platelet count performed at least monthly during epoetin therapy[2,3]	X		6A. None	6. Laboratory reports, progress notes, physician orders

Prepared by Teresa A. Bennett, Pharm.D., Coordinator, Drug Usage Evaluation, Department of Pharmacy, University Medical Center, and Clinical Assistant Professor, College of Pharmacy, University of Florida Health Science Center/Jacksonville; Mark W. Todd; Pharm.D., Director, Drug Information and Research, Department of Pharmacy, University Medical Center, and Clinical Associate Professor, College of Pharmacy, University of Florida Health Science Center/Jacksonville; and Stephen Sandroni, M.D., Assistant Professor and Chief, Division of Nephrology, University of Florida Health Science Center/Jacksonville at University Medical Center.

Element	Standard 100%	Standard 0%	Exception[b] or Critical Preventive/ Responsive Measure[c]	Sources of Information
7. Serum chemistry, including concentrations of blood urea nitrogen, creatinine, phosphate, potassium, and uric acid, measured at least monthly during epoetin therapy[2,3]	X		7A. None	7. Laboratory reports, progress notes, physician orders
8. Adequate baseline iron stores, including transferrin saturation (serum iron/iron-binding capacity) of at least 20% and serum ferritin concentration of at least 100 ng/mL documented[1–3]	X		8A. None	8. H&P, laboratory reports, progress notes
9. Iron supplementation provided to patient with inadequate iron stores before initiation of epoetin therapy[1–3]	X		9A. None	9. Laboratory reports, progress notes, physician orders, MAR
10. Serum ferritin concentration measured monthly for first 3 months and then every 2–3 months[2]; transferrin saturation reassessed if response not maintained during extended epoetin therapy	X		10A. None	10. Laboratory reports, progress notes, physician orders
11. Pretreatment control of blood pressure achieved in hypertensive patient; blood pressure monitored closely during therapy[1–3]	X		11A. None	11. H&P, progress notes, nursing flow sheets, nursing notes
12. Patient counseled about importance of renal-failure dietary restrictions before and during epoetin therapy[2]	X		12A. None	12. Progress notes, nursing notes
13. Appropriate initial dosage: 50–100 units/kg 3 times a week i.v. in dialysis patient and i.v. or s.c. in nondialysis patient[3]	X		13A. Smaller doses (30–50 units/kg) given to patient in whom a slower rise in Hct is desired	13, 13A. Physician orders, progress notes, MAR
14. Dosage adjusted appropriately[3]: a. Dose reduced by 25 units/kg when Hct reaches 30–33% or when Hct increases by >4 percentage points in any 2-week period b. Dose increased by 25 units/kg if Hct does not increase by 5 or 6 percentage points after 8 weeks and remains below target range (30–33%)	X		14A. None	14. Physician orders, progress notes, laboratory reports, MAR
15. Appropriate maintenance dosage[3]: a. In dialysis and nondialysis patients, dose decreased by 25 units/kg if Hct is >33% or withheld if Hct is >36% and not resumed until Hct decreases to ≤33% b. In nondialysis patient, dosage decreased to 75–150 units/kg per week or lower, as tolerated, depending on response	X		15A. None	15. Physician orders, progress notes, laboratory reports, MAR
<u>AIDS Patients Only</u>				
16. Appropriate dosage[7,8]: a. Initial dosage of 100 units/kg i.v. or s.c. three times a week for 8 weeks (target Hct, 30–40% or decreased need for transfusions) b. If target Hct has not been achieved or need for transfusions has not decreased after 8 weeks, dose increased by 50–100 units/kg i.v. or s.c. and continued for 4–8 weeks c. Dose reduced or increased in increments of 50–100 units/kg s.c. or i.v. to maintain response. If patient has not responded to 300	X		16A. None	16. Physician orders, progress notes, MAR

Element	Standard 100%	Standard 0%	Exception[b] or Critical Preventive/ Responsive Measure[c]	Sources of Information
units/kg three times a week, response to a higher dosage unlikely d. If Hct is >40%, epoetin discontinued until Hct is ≤36%. Treatment then resumed at a dosage decreased by 25%				
17. Hct measured once a week until stable and periodically thereafter[8]	X		17A. None	17. Physician orders, progress notes
Complications				
18. Hypertension (CRF patients only)[1–9]		X	18A. Identify other drug and nondrug causes 18B. Stress compliance with antihypertensive medication 18C. Adjust antihypertensive medication dosage as needed. 18D. Reduce epoetin dosage or discontinue until blood pressure is controlled[3] 18E. Monitor blood pressure regularly	18. Progress notes, nursing flow sheets, nursing notes 18A. Physician orders, progress notes, nursing notes, MAR 18B. Physician orders, progress notes, nursing notes 18C, D. Physician orders, progress notes, MAR 18E. Physician orders, progress notes, nursing flow sheets, nursing notes
19. Decreased iron stores (transferrin saturation, <20%, and serum ferritin concentration, <100 ng/mL) (CRF and AIDS patients)[1–8]		X	19A. Identify other drug and nondrug causes 19B. Provide supplemental iron unless serum ferritin concentration is >500 ng/mL 19C. Monitor transferrin saturation and serum ferritin level regularly	19. Laboratory reports, progress notes 19A. Physician orders, progress notes, nursing notes, MAR 19B. Laboratory reports, physician orders, progress notes, MAR 19C. Laboratory reports, physician orders, progress notes
20. Premonitory neurological symptoms (aura and sensations of sinking and rising in epigastrium) or seizures during therapy when Hct is rising (CRF patients only)[1–3]		X	20A. Identify other drug and nondrug causes 20B. Provide symptomatic and supportive care if seizure occurs 20C. Monitor patient closely, especially during first 90 days of therapy[3] 20D. Counsel patient about early signs of seizure 20E. Counsel patient to avoid driving or operating machinery	20. Laboratory reports, progress notes, nursing notes 20A, B. Physician orders, progress notes, nursing notes, MAR 20C. Physician orders, nursing notes 20D, E. Physician orders, progress notes, nursing notes
21. Thrombotic events (CRF patients only)[3,9]		X	21A. Identify other drug and nondrug causes 21B. Closely monitor patient with pre-existing vascular disease 21C. Assess need for increased heparin during dialysis[2]	21. Progress notes, nursing notes 21A. Physician orders, progress notes, nursing notes, MAR 21B. H&P, progress notes, nursing notes 21C. Physician orders, dialysis reports
22. Hyperkalemia (CRF patients only)[1–3]		X	22A. Identify other drug and nondrug causes 22B. Monitor serum potassium level 22C. Stress compliance with renal-failure dietary restrictions 22D. Administer potassium-removing resin or increase dialysis time if needed	22. Laboratory reports, progress notes 22A. Physician orders, progress notes, nursing notes, MAR 22B. Laboratory reports, physician orders, progress notes 22C. Physician orders, progress notes, nursing notes 22D. Physician orders, progress notes, MAR, dialysis reports

Element	Standard 100%	Standard 0%	Exception[b] or Critical Preventive/ Responsive Measure[c]	Sources of Information
23. Allergic reaction (CRF and AIDS patients)[2]		X	23A. Identify other drug and nondrug causes 23B. If anaphylaxis occurs, discontinue epoetin immediately and provide symptomatic and supportive care 23C. Monitor for skin rash and urticaria (usually mild and transient)	23. Progress notes, nursing notes 23A, B. Physician orders, progress notes, nursing notes, MAR 23C. Progress notes, nursing notes
Outcome Measures				
24. Resolution of chronic anemia (Hct, 30–33% in CRF patient and 30–40% in AIDS patient)[1–7]	X		24A. Patient with osteodystrophy and documented aluminum deposition[1] 24B. Patient died 24C. Patient unable to tolerate epoetin 24D. Patient with untreated iron deficiency 24E. Patient with recent stress due to surgery, or transplantation patient taking corticosteroids	24. Laboratory reports 24A. Progress notes, bone biopsy reports 24B. Progress notes 24C. Progress notes, nursing notes 24D. Laboratory reports, progress notes 24E. Progress notes, MAR
or				
25. Decreased need for transfusions[1–7]	X		25A. Patient did not require transfusions at onset of epoetin therapy 25B. Patient died	25. Physician orders, progress notes 25A. H&P, physician orders, progress notes 25B. Progress notes
or				
26. Improved quality of life (improved exercise tolerance, appetite, and sense of well-being)[4,8,10]	X		26A. Patient died 26B. Patient unable to tolerate epoetin 26C. Patient unable to achieve Hct in target range	26, 26A, B. Progress notes, nursing notes 26C. Laboratory reports

[a] Criteria address justifications for use (indications), critical (process) indicators, complications of therapy, and patient outcome. Each criterion consists of an element, a standard, exceptions to the standard, and sources of information. The element is the minimum level of evidence needed to show that patient care was optimal. The standard defines the deviation from an element that is acceptable. If no deviation is acceptable, the standard is 100%. Exceptions are circumstances in which deviation is allowable. Sources of information listed are the most reliable sources. Sources pertaining to an element or exception are identified by the number assigned to the element or exception (e.g., 18, 18A).

[b] For justification for use and critical (process) indicators.

[c] For complications and outcome measures.

References

1. Flaharty KK, Grimm AM, Vlasses PH. Epoetin: human recombinant erythropoietin. *Clin Pharm.* 1989; 8:769–82.
2. Ad Hoc Committee for the National Kidney Foundation. Statement on the clinical use of recombinant erythropoietin in anemia of end stage renal disease (ESRD). New York: National Kidney Foundation; 1989.
3. Amgen Inc. Epogen package insert. Thousand Oaks, CA; 1989.
4. Lim VS, DeGowin RL, Zavala D et al. Recombinant human erythropoietin treatment in predialysis patients. *Ann Intern Med.* 1989; 110:108–14.
5. Eschbach JW, Egrie JC, Downing MR et al. Correction of the anemia of end-stage renal disease with recombinant erythropoietin. *N Engl J Med.* 1987; 316:73–8.
6. Eschbach JW, Kelly MR, Haley R et al. Treatment of the anemia of progressive renal failure with recombinant human erythropoietin. *N Engl J Med.* 1989; 321:158–63.
7. Fischl M, Galpin JE, Levine JD et al. Recombinant human erythropoietin for patients with AIDS treated with zidovudine. *N Engl J Med.* 1990; 322:1488–93.
8. Amgen Inc. Procrit package insert. 1990 Dec. Distributed by Ortho Biotech Division, Ortho Pharmaceutical, Raritan, NJ.
9. Watson AJ. Adverse effects of therapy for the correction of anemia in hemodialysis patients. *Semin Nephrol.* 1989; 9(Suppl 1):30–4.
10. Evans RW, Radar B, Manninem DL et al. The quality of life of hemodialysis recipients treated with recombinant human erythropoietin. *JAMA.* 1990; 263:825–30.

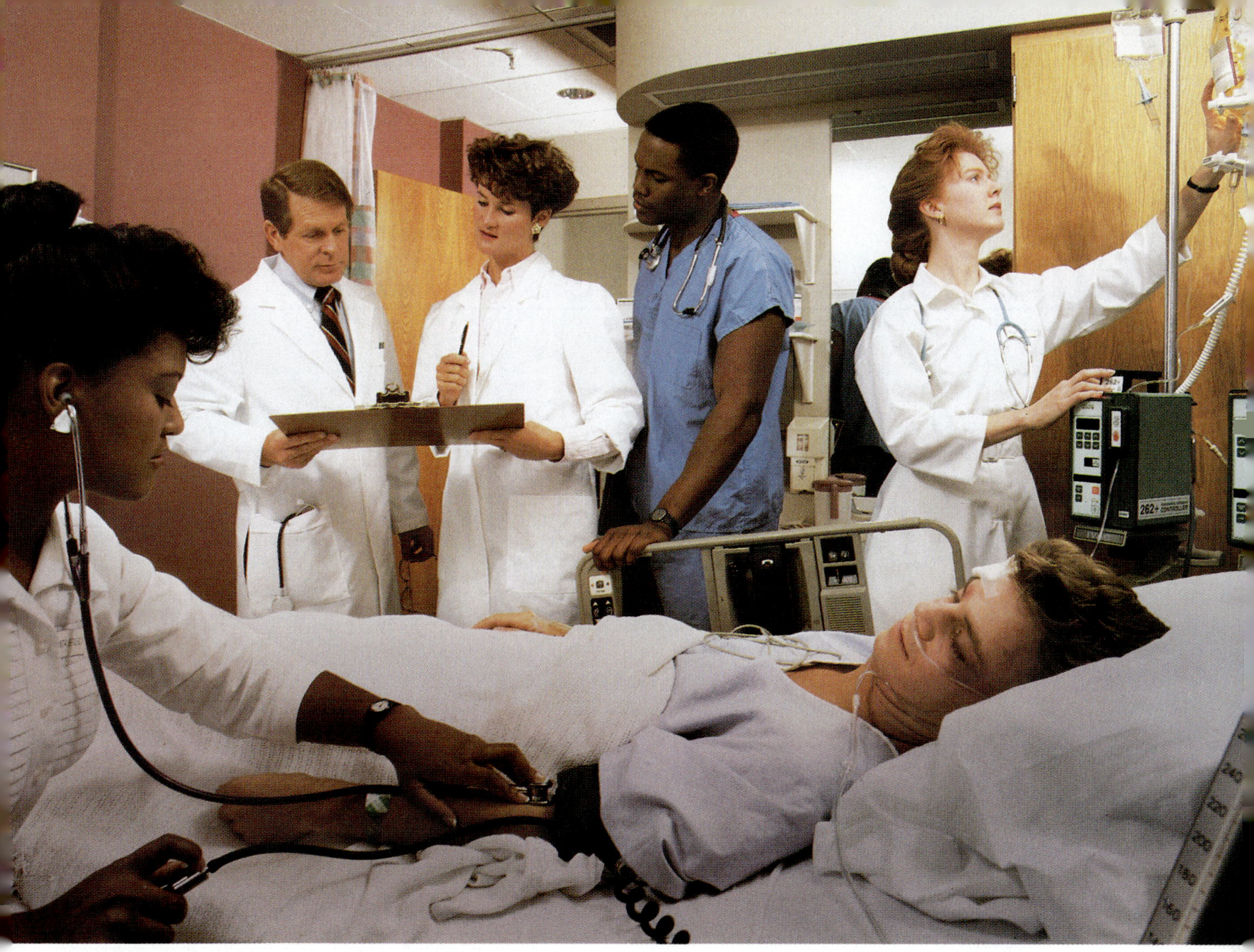

Current Literature

Drug Reaction Alerts 154

Book Review

Clinical Pharmacology of Psychotherapeutic Drugs, Third Edition 159
By Leo E. Hollister and John C. Csernansky
Reviewed by Timothy E. Welty

Drug Reaction Alerts

Drug Reaction Alerts focuses primarily on serious, unlabeled reactions to new chemical entities. The citations are compiled monthly from International Pharmaceutical Abstracts, *which covers over 800 pharmacy and health-related journals worldwide. An address for reprints (when available) follows the name of the corresponding author of each citation.*

Pharmacists may use the FDA Adverse Reaction Report form that appears in most issues of Clinical Pharmacy for submitting reports of adverse drug reactions directly to FDA.

Antifungals

Franklin IM, Elias E, Hirsch C (Department of Hematology, Queen Elizabeth Hospital, Birmingham B15 2TH, England). **Fluconazole**-induced jaundice. *Lancet*. 1990; 336:565. Case. (41-year-old man who was seropositive for human immunodeficiency virus; developed jaundice after several courses of fluconazole 50 mg/day for treatment of oral candidiasis; concomitant zidovudine, trimethoprim, and nystatin; previously diagnosed with chronic non-A, non-B hepatitis; withdrawal of fluconazole led to clinical improvement and decreases in serum bilirubin and aspartate aminotransferase concentrations)

Antituberculars

Mimouni A, Hodak E, Mimouni M (Department of Pediatrics B, Beilinson Medical Center, Petah Tiqva 49100, Israel). Fixed drug eruption following **rifampin** treatment. *DICP*. 1990; 24:947-8. Case. (24-year-old female physician who was exposed to patient with meningococcemia; received rifampin 600 mg every 12 hours for 48 hours; developed a fixed drug eruption 48 hours after completing therapy; two lesions on forearm resolved completely one week later; no residual hyperpigmentation)

Anxiolytics, Sedatives, and Hypnotics

Lurie Y, Gottesfeld F, Bass DD (Division of Gastroenterology, Kaplan Hospital, Rehovot, Israel). Benzodiazepines and fantasy. *Lancet*. 1990; 336:576. Case. (30-year-old man with epigastric pain; premedicated with **diazepam** 10 mg as slow i.v. injection before upper endoscopy; procedure was uneventful and showed no abnormalities; patient developed anterograde amnesia and asked when the endoscopy would occur; patient became abusive when told the endoscopy had been performed; second endoscopy was performed to calm patient; patient had complete amnesia of first endoscopy and subsequent incident)

Contraceptives, Oral

Leroy O, Beuscart C, Senneville E et al. (Beaucaire G, Intensive Care Unit, Center Hospital, 59208 Tourcoing, France). Deep venous thrombosis and antibodies to **cyproterone acetate**. *Lancet*. 1990; 336:509. Case. (19-year-old woman; received cyproterone acetate 2 mg in combination with ethinyl estradiol 35 µg as oral contraceptive for four months; developed thrombophlebitis; venogram showed thrombi in right iliac vein; patient was treated with streptokinase by i.v. injection for five days and heparin by i.v. injection for four weeks; positive test for circulating immune complexes; antibody testing showed antibody to cyproterone acetate but no antibodies to ethinyl estradiol or progesterone)

Drug Interactions

Baldwin CM, Safferman AZ (Department of Respiratory Medicine, Hillside Hospital, 75-59 263rd Avenue, Glen Oaks, NY 11004). Case of **lisinopril**-induced **lithium** toxicity. *DICP*. 1990; 24:946-7. Case. (49-year-old woman with bipolar depression and hypertension who received lithium carbonate 1500 mg/day and clonidine 0.1 mg/day as maintenance therapy; clonidine replaced with lisinopril 20 mg/day; three weeks later patient developed tremors, fatigue, nausea, diarrhea, slurred speech, and right bundle branch block; trough serum lithium concentration, 3.0 mM; withdrawal of all medications and three days of supportive therapy led to medical recovery and serum lithium concentration of 0.4 mM)

Blomley M, Teare EL, De Belder A et al. (Weston M, Chelmsford Public Health Laboratory, Chelmsford, Essex CM2 0YX, England). **Itraconazole** and anti-tuberculosis drugs. *Lancet*. 1990; 336:1255. Case. (53-year-old man with tuberculosis who received **rifampin** 600 mg/day, pyrazinamide 1.5 g/day, isoniazid 300 mg/day, ethambutol 1 g/day, and prednisolone 20 mg/day for eight weeks without improvement; received itraconazole 200 mg/day for treatment of pulmonary aspergillosis; itraconazole dose increased to 400 mg/day due to negligible serum levels; antitubercular treatment withdrawn due to possibility of interaction between itraconazole and rifampin; patient improved clinically and was discharged; improvement was not sustained and the patient died suddenly; cavitating lesions in both lungs with necrotizing granulomas found at autopsy; no evidence of mycobacterial or fungal infection)

Dyes

Nicolini U (Institute of Obstetrics and Gynecology, Royal Postgraduate Medical School, Queen Charlotte's and Chelsea Hospitals, London W6 0XG, England), Monni G. Intestinal obstruction in babies exposed in utero to **methylene blue**. *Lancet*. 1990; 336:1258-9. Cases. (seven infants born to mothers with twin pregnancies who had amniocentesis performed at 15-17 weeks gestation with methylene blue 10-30 mg; developed intestinal obstructions; four infants later required surgery for intestinal obstruction)

Gastrointestinal Drugs

Bourghol A, Rindone JP (Department of Pharmacy [119], Veterans Affairs Medical Center, Tucson, AZ 85723). **Cimetidine**-associated thrombocytopenia. *DICP*. 1990; 24:1007-8. Case. (76-year-old man with upper gastrointestinal bleeding; received cimetidine 300 mg every eight hours by i.v. injection for three doses; developed marked decrease in platelet count; withdrawal of cimetidine led to gradual rise in platelet count; platelet count was 227 x 10^9/L nine days after discontinuation of therapy)

Hypotensive Agents

Puppin D, Rybojad M, De La Chapelle C et al. (Morel P, Dermatology Clinic, Hopital St. Louis, 75475 Paris, France). Kaposi's sarcoma associated with **captopril**. *Lancet*. 1990; 336:1251-2. Case. (70-year-old man with hypertension; received captopril 75 mg/day and acebutolol hydrochloride 200 mg/day for six years; presented with two-month history of three nodular angiomatous lesions on left arm; clinical and histopathological findings were typical of Kaposi's sarcoma; withdrawal of captopril led to partial disappearance of lesions after one month; complete disappearance of lesions after three months; biopsy of arm showed residual features of Kaposi's sarcoma)

Immunotherapy

Farmer KL, Kurzrock R, Gutterman JU et al. (Duvic M, Department of Dermatology, University of Texas Medical School, 6431 Fannin, MSB 1.186, Houston, TX 77030). Necrotizing vasculitis at **granulocyte macrophage colony stimulating factor** injection sites. *Arch Dermatol*. 1990; 126:1243-4. Case. (59-year-old woman; received granulocyte–macrophage colony-stimulating factor 200 µg/day as s.c. injection for more than five days; developed necrotizing vasculitis at injection sites; concomitant clindamycin and ciprofloxacin; clindamycin and ciprofloxacin withdrawn after five days due to development of erythematous macular lesions; withdrawal of colony-stimulating factor and therapy with prednisone led to complete resolution of skin lesions and return of neutrophil levels to normal; negative rechallenge with ciprofloxacin)

Pediatrics

Jacqz-Aigrain E (Clinical Pharmacology, Nephrology and Immunohematology Service, Hopital Robert-Debre, 75019 Paris, France), Guillonneau M, Brun P et al. Toxic epidermal necrolysis due to pediatric **erythromycin/sulfisoxazole** combination. *Lancet*. 1990; 336:1010-1. Case. (4-year-old boy with otitis media; received erythromycin ethylsuccinate 1 g/day in combination with sulfisoxazole acetyl 3 g/day as Pediazole; experienced seizure and developed high fever associated with an erythematous rash on day 6 of therapy; withdrawal of Pediazole led to quick recovery; positive rechallenge)

Psychotherapeutic Agents

Skowron DM, Gutierrez MA (School of Pharmacy, University of Southern California, 1985 Zonal Avenue, Los Angeles, CA 90033), Epstein S. Precaution with titrating **nortriptyline** after the use of **fluoxetine**. *DICP*. 1990; 24:1008. Case. (56-year-old man with major depression; received fluoxetine up to 60 mg/day for 10 weeks but showed only a partial response; fluoxetine replaced with nortriptyline up to 150 mg/day over two days; experienced a hypotensive episode and fell after five days of therapy with nortriptyline; withdrawal of nortriptyline led to serum concentration of 200 ng/mL the following morning; experienced an apparent anticholinergic delirium one day later; resumed nortriptyline up to 100 mg/day nine days after withdrawal of fluoxetine; serum nortriptyline concentration was 133 ng/mL two months after withdrawal of fluoxetine)

Quinolones

Cain DB, O'Connor ME (Laboratory Medicine, Medicine Hat Regional Hospital, Medicine Hat, Alberta, Canada T1A 4H6). Pseudomembranous colitis associated with **ciprofloxacin**. *Lancet*. 1990; 336:946. Case. (79-year-old woman with recurrent cough, dyspnea, and wheezing; received ciprofloxacin 250 mg twice daily for 14 days; developed diarrhea; therapy with oral rehydration fluids and diphenoxylate unsuccessful; patient died two days later; previous therapy with sulfamethoxazole in combination with trimethoprim for two weeks; gross and microscopic changes characteristic of pseudomembranous colitis found at autopsy; cytotoxin-producing *Clostridium difficile* resistant to ciprofloxacin isolated from feces and colonic tissue)

Caumes E, Katlama C, Chapuis L et al. (Gentilini M, Department of Tropical Diseases, Hopital de la Salpetriere, 57013 Paris, France). Toxic reaction following treatment of typhoid fever with **pefloxacin**. *Lancet*. 1990; 336:252. Case. (25-year-old man with typhoid fever; received pefloxacin 250 mg twice daily by i.v. injection for five days followed by oral doses of 400 mg

Continued on page 159

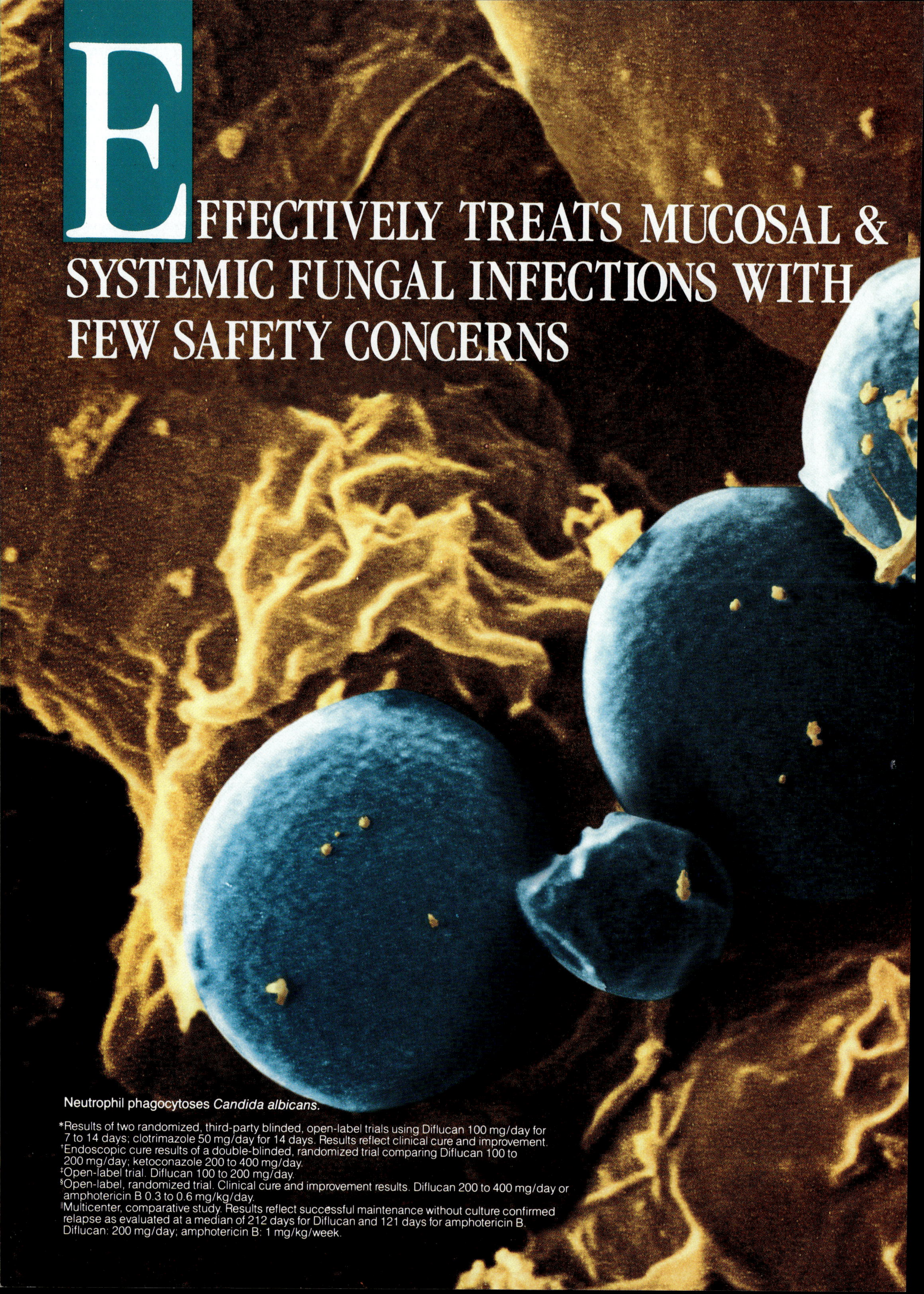

Neutrophil phagocytoses *Candida albicans.*

*Results of two randomized, third-party blinded, open-label trials using Diflucan 100 mg/day for 7 to 14 days; clotrimazole 50 mg/day for 14 days. Results reflect clinical cure and improvement.
†Endoscopic cure results of a double-blinded, randomized trial comparing Diflucan 100 to 200 mg/day; ketoconazole 200 to 400 mg/day.
‡Open-label trial. Diflucan 100 to 200 mg/day.
§Open-label, randomized trial. Clinical cure and improvement results. Diflucan 200 to 400 mg/day or amphotericin B 0.3 to 0.6 mg/kg/day.
||Multicenter, comparative study. Results reflect successful maintenance without culture confirmed relapse as evaluated at a median of 212 days for Diflucan and 121 days for amphotericin B. Diflucan: 200 mg/day; amphotericin B: 1 mg/kg/week.

Current Literature *Continued from page 155*

twice daily; experienced intense malaise, abdominal pain, vomiting, and decreased body temperature four hours after first oral dose; resumed i.v. therapy for two days; symptoms resolved; oral therapy resumed for 13 days without incident)

Sympathomimetic Agents

Shovlin CL, Tam FW (Respiratory Unit, Royal Postgraduate Medical School, Hammersmith Hospital, London W12 0NN, England). Salbutamol nebulizer and precipitation of critical cardiac ischemia. *Lancet*. 1990; 336:1258. Case. (60-year-old man with asthma; received **albuterol** 5 mg every four hours by nebulizer for five doses; experienced an acute myocardial infarction; patient recovered; concomitant oxygen therapy, high-dose corticosteroids, and oral aminophylline; received albuterol 200 μg four times daily by oral inhalation without incident)

Thrombolytic Agents

Rogers TK, Polacarz S, Channer KS et al. (Morice AH, Royal Hallamshire Hospital, Sheffield S10 2JF, England). Cardiac rupture and fibrinolytic therapy. *Lancet*. 1990; 336:259-60. Cases. (two women with myocardial infarction, aged 66 and 69 years; 66-year-old patient received **streptokinase** 1.5 million units; 69-year-old patient received streptokinase 1.5 million units and aspirin 300 mg; fibrinolytic therapy began before heart rupture was recognized; both patients died)

Book Review

Clinical Pharmacology of Psychotherapeutic Drugs, Third Edition

By Leo E. Hollister and John G. Csernansky.
Published by Churchill Livingstone Inc., 1560 Broadway, New York, NY 10036, 1990. ix + 194 p. Price $36.

Clinical Pharmacology of Psychotherapeutic Drugs could be categorized as an introductory textbook; the reader gains a rudimentary foundation in the subject but little depth or ability to apply the knowledge. To the beginner in psychotherapeutics, the book explains many of the basics of pharmaceutics, including brief sections in the introduction on the history of psychopharmacology; the testing, nomenclature, prescribing patterns, and risk-to-benefit ratios of psychotherapeutic drugs; and the definition of the ideal psychotherapeutic drug. The tone for the remainder of the book is set in the introductory chapter; each portion of this chapter summarizes the complexity of each concept but provides little depth for the reader.

The remainder of the book is divided into chapters that present each major category of psychotherapeutics: anxiolytics, hypnotics, antidepressants, antipsychotics, and mood-stabilizing drugs. Each category is discussed in terms of background of the disease, classification of the available agents, pharmacokinetics, clinical applications, investigational agents, and adverse reactions. However, these discussions are rather superficial and lack detail. Only the most important citations are referenced.

The book concludes with a rather unusual but important chapter on pediatric and adolescent psychother-

Continued on page 160

Continued from page 159

apeutics. The chapter not only presents the different pediatric therapeutic approaches to the standard adult disorders of depression, anxiety, and schizophrenia, but it also discusses special areas of pediatric practice: autism, mental retardation, attention-deficit disorder, hyperactivity disorder, and miscellaneous disorders (e.g., enuresis, appetite disorders, and narcolepsy). The authors emphasize the fact that children and adolescents cannot be managed as small adults but require unique approaches that are consistent with the physiological and psychological differences.

Because it is a general introduction to psychotherapeutics, *Clinical Pharmacology of Psychotherapeutic Drugs* does not belong on every pharmacist's shelf. The book would be more useful to the student who is embarking on a study of psychiatric pharmacotherapy. Most practicing pharmacists are probably already familiar with most of the information presented in the book. Therefore, the book would serve better as a textbook for an introductory course in psychotherapeutics.

Reviewed by Timothy E. Welty, Pharm.D., Department of Pharmaceutical Support Services, Methodist Hospital of Indiana, Inc., 1701 North Senate Boulevard, P.O. Box 1367, Indianapolis, IN 46206.

Advertising Index

Adria Laboratories
Idamycin, 160, inside back cover, outside back cover
American Society of Hospital Pharmacists
Clinical Pharmacy, 159
IV-Ease, 150
Safe Handling of Cytotoxic and Hazardous Drugs, 94
ASHP Research and Education Foundation
Institutional, 89
Burroughs Wellcome Company
Zovirax IV, 90-92
Charleston Area Medical Center
Position Available, 150
Department of Veterans Affairs (Richmond)
Positions Available, 83
Glaxo Inc.
Antiemetic, inside front cover
Kent General Hospital
Position Available, 94
Eli Lilly and Company
Hospital Division, 153
Lyphomed, Inc.
Amphotericin B, 84-86
Roerig, A Division of Pfizer Pharmaceuticals
Diflucan, 156-158
The Upjohn Company and Chugai-Upjohn, Inc.
Marogen, 87

News

Year-end review shows 23 new drugs approved, 14 important biologic licensing actions taken by FDA 167

New recommendations for prevention of bacterial endocarditis include amoxicillin use 168

Report assesses use of blood pressure monitoring devices for ambulatory patients 175

Upcoming Specialty Meetings 175

News Briefs 176

Year-end review shows 23 new drugs approved, 14 important biologic licensing actions taken by FDA

A total of 23 new drugs were approved for marketing in the United States during 1990. The average time from NDA filing to approval, at 27.7 months, was nearly five months less than the time required in 1989. Six of the 23 drugs were approved within 15 months of NDA submission. The 23 new drugs and their indications are as follows:

- Altretamine (Hexalen, U.S. Bioscience), for palliative treatment of persistent or recurrent ovarian cancer
- Bepridil hydrochloride (Vascor, McNeil, Wallace), for treatment of stable angina in patients who have not responded to or have not tolerated other therapies for angina
- Colfosceril palmitate, cetyl alcohol, and tyloxapol (Exosurf Neonatal, Burroughs Wellcome), a synthetic lung surfactant for treatment and prevention of neonatal respiratory distress syndrome
- Dapiprazole hydrochloride (Rev-Eyes, Angelini Pharmaceuticals), for reversal of pupillary dilatation induced by mydriatic agents used during ophthalmic examinations
- Doxazosin mesylate (Cardura, Pfizer), an α-receptor blocker used for treatment of hypertension
- Eflornithine hydrochloride (Ornidyl, Marion Merrell Dow), for treatment of the meningoencephalitic stage of African sleeping sickness
- Estazolam (ProSom, Abbott), for short-term management of insomnia
- Fluconazole (Diflucan, Pfizer), for treatment of oropharyngeal and esophageal candidiasis, cryptococcal meningitis, and serious systemic candidal infections
- Fluticasone propionate (Cutivate, Glaxo), a midpotency corticosteroid ointment for treatment of corticosteroid-responsive dermatoses
- Halobetasol propionate (Ultravate, Bristol-Myers Squibb), an ultrahigh potency corticosteroid for relief of inflammatory and pruritic manifestations of corticosteroid-responsive dermatoses
- Idarubicin hydrochloride (Idamycin, Adria), for use in combination therapy for acute myeloid leukemia in adults
- Isradipine (DynaCirc, Sandoz), a calcium-channel blocker for treatment of hypertension
- Levamisole hydrochloride (Ergamisol, Janssen), for adjuvant therapy with fluorouracil after surgical resection in patients with Dukes stage C colon cancer
- Moricizine hydrochloride (Ethmozine, Du Pont), for treatment of life-threatening ventricular arrhythmias
- Nafarelin acetate (Synarel, Syntex), a synthetic analogue of gonadotropin-releasing hormone for management of en-

dometriosis
- Ofloxacin (Floxin, McNeil, Ortho Johnson), a quinolone indicated for treatment of lower respiratory tract infections, infections of the skin and skin structures, infections of the prostate and urinary tract, and sexually transmitted diseases
- Olsalazine sodium (Dipentum, Pharmacia), for maintenance of remission of ulcerative colitis in patients who cannot tolerate sulfasalazine therapy
- Pegademase bovine (Adagen, Enzon), an enzyme replacement therapy for severe combined immunodeficiency disease associated with adenosine deaminase deficiency
- Pipecuronium bromide (Arduan, Organon), a neuromuscular blocking agent used as an adjunct to general anesthesia to provide skeletal muscle relaxation
- Sermorelin acetate (Geref, Serono), for evaluation of the ability of the pituitary gland to secrete growth hormone
- Technetium Tc 99m mertiatide (TechneScan MAG3, Mallinckrodt), a renal imaging agent
- Technetium Tc 99m sestamibi (Cardiolite, Du Pont Merck), a perfusion agent for evaluation of the myocardium in patients with suspected myocardial infarction
- Technetium Tc 99m teboroxime (CardioTec, Bristol-Myers Squibb), a perfusion agent for evaluation of the myocardium in patients with suspected coronary artery disease

Seven of these drugs received FDA's 1A rating for review, indicating that they represent significant therapeutic gains. These drugs are altretamine, colfosceril, eflornithine, fluconazole, levamisole, idarubicin, and pegademase.

Altogether 64 drug applications (excluding applications for generic drugs) were approved. In addition to the 23 new chemical entities were new combinations, chemical forms, and dosage forms of already marketed drugs. Notable among these approvals was an implantable contraceptive (Norplant, Wyeth-Ayerst).

Fourteen important biologic licensing actions were taken by FDA during 1990. These included three vaccines, four in vitro diagnostic agents, and seven therapeutic agents. Four of these actions involved new uses for existing products. The following biologic licensing applications were approved:

- Allergen patch test (Pharmacia AS), for use in diagnosing contact dermatitis
- BCG live, intravesical (TheraCys, Connaught), for treatment of carcinoma in situ of the urinary bladder
- BCG vaccine (Tice BCG, Organon), for treatment of carcinoma in situ of the urinary bladder
- CMV immune globulin intravenous (human) (Massachusetts Public Health Biologics Laboratory), for attenuation of primary cytomegalovirus disease associated with renal transplantation
- Coagulation factor IX, human (AlphaNine, Alpha Therapeutic), for prevention and control of bleeding in patients with factor IX deficiency due to hemophilia B
- Epoetin alfa (Amgen), for treatment of zidovudine-induced anemia in AIDS patients
- *Haemophilus* b conjugate vaccine (diphtheria CRM197 protein conjugate) (HibTITER, Lederle-Praxis), for immunization of infants two months of age
- *Haemophilus* b conjugate vaccine (meningococcal protein conjugate) (PedvaxHIB, Merck), for immunization of infants two months of age
- Hepatitis C virus encoded antigen (Abbott), a test for detection of hepatitis C virus
- Hepatitis C virus encoded antigen (Ortho Diagnostics), a test for detection of hepatitis C virus
- Human immunodeficiency virus type 1 (HIV-1) (Bio-Rad), a test for confirming the presence of antibodies to HIV-1
- Human immunodeficiency virus type 2 (HIV-2) (Genetic Systems), a test for detection of antibody to HIV-2
- Interferon gamma-1b (Actimmune, Genentech), for management of chronic granulomatous disease
- Poliovirus vaccine, inactivated (Ipol, Connaught), for immunization of infants, children, and adults

Included among these drug and biologic approvals were eight orphan products: altretamine, CMV immune globulin, coagulation factor IX, colfosceril, eflornithine, idarubicin, interferon gamma-1b, and pegademase.

New recommendations for prevention of bacterial endocarditis include amoxicillin use

The American Heart Association has updated its recommendations for prevention of bacterial endocarditis. The guidelines pertain to patients who have cardiac conditions that place them at risk for bacterial endocarditis after certain medical, dental, or surgical procedures that commonly cause transient bacteremia. The major revision is the recommendation for use of a different beta lactam, amoxicillin. Readers are referred to the full document for a complete discussion of indications and recommendations for prophylaxis and for advice on handling special situations.[1] Recommended regimens for antimicrobial prophylaxis are summarized below. Reprints of the statement may be obtained by writing to the Office of Scientific Affairs, American Heart Association, 7320 Greenville Avenue, Dallas, TX 75231.

Prophylactic Regimens for Dental, Oral, or Upper Respiratory Tract Procedures. The standard regimen for prophylaxis in patients at risk for bacterial endocarditis is amoxicillin 3 g (as the trihydrate) orally one hour before the procedure, followed by 1.5 g orally six hours after the first dose. For patients allergic to penicillin, erythromycin 800 mg (as the ethylsuccinate salt) or 1 g (as the stearate salt) should be given orally two hours before the procedure, followed six hours later by a dose one half the initial dose. If neither of these regimens can be tolerated, clindamycin 300 mg (as the hydrochloride salt) orally one hour before the procedure, followed by 150 mg six hours after the first dose, is recommended. Use of tetracyclines or sulfonamides is not recommended. For pediatric patients, initial doses are amoxicillin 50 mg/kg, erythromycin 20 mg/kg (ethylsuccinate or stearate), and clindamycin 10 mg/kg. Subsequent doses should be reduced by 50%, and the total dose should not exceed the total adult dose. The initial dose of amoxicillin may also be determined on the basis of the child's weight: <15 kg, 750 mg; 15–30 kg, 1500 mg; and >30 kg, 3000 mg.

If the patient cannot take medications orally, one of the following regimens is recommended:

- Ampicillin 2 g (as the sodium salt) i.m. or i.v. 30 minutes before the procedure, followed by ampicillin 1 g i.m. or i.v. or amoxicillin 1.5 g orally six hours after the first dose
- Clindamycin 300 mg (as the phosphate salt) i.v. 30 minutes before the procedure, followed by clindamycin 150 mg i.v. or orally six hours after the first dose (for patients with penicillin allergies)
- Ampicillin 2 g plus gentamicin 1.5 mg/kg (maximum dose, 80 mg) (as the sulfate salt) i.v. or i.m. 30 minutes before the

Continued on page 175

Continued from page 168

procedure, followed by (1) amoxicillin 1.5 g orally six hours after the first dose or (2) a second dose of ampicillin and gentamicin eight hours after the first dose (for patients considered to be at high risk and not considered to be candidates for the standard regimen)
- Vancomycin 1 g (as the hydrochloride salt) i.v. administered over one hour, starting one hour before the procedure (for penicillin-allergic patients considered to be at high risk)

Initial pediatric doses for the above regimens are ampicillin 50 mg/kg, clindamycin 10 mg/kg, gentamicin 2 mg/kg, and vancomycin 20 mg/kg. Subsequent doses should be reduced by 50%. The total dose should not exceed the total adult dose. No initial pediatric dose of amoxicillin is given; the recommended follow-up dose is 25 mg/kg.

Prophylactic Regimens for Genitourinary or Gastrointestinal Tract Procedures. The standard regimen for prophylaxis is ampicillin 2 g plus gentamicin 1.5 mg/kg (maximum dose, 80 mg) i.v. or i.m. 30 minutes before the procedure, followed by (1) amoxicillin 1.5 g orally six hours after the first dose or (2) a second dose of ampicillin and gentamicin eight hours after the first dose. Patients allergic to penicillin should receive vancomycin 1 g i.v. administered over one hour plus gentamicin 1.5 mg/kg (maximum dose, 80 mg) i.v. or i.m. one hour before the procedure; a second dose of vancomycin and gentamicin may be given eight hours after the first dose. An alternate regimen for low-risk patients is amoxicillin 3 g orally one hour before the procedure, followed by 1.5 g orally six hours after the first dose. For pediatric patients, initial doses are ampicillin 50 mg/kg, amoxicillin 50 mg/kg, gentamicin 2 mg/kg, and vancomycin 20 mg/kg. Subsequent doses should be reduced by 50%. The total dose should not exceed the total adult dose.

1. Dajani AS, Bisno AL, Chung KJ et al. Prevention of bacterial endocarditis: recommendations by the American Heart Association. *JAMA*. 1991; 264:2919-22.

Report assesses use of blood pressure monitoring devices for ambulatory patients

Indications for ambulatory blood pressure monitoring (ABPM) in the diagnosis and management of hypertension and the technical problems associated with the use of ABPM devices were assessed by the National High Blood Pressure Education Program (NHBPEP) Working Group on Ambulatory Blood Pressure Monitoring. The work was sponsored by the National Heart, Lung, and Blood Institute (NHLBI). Copies of the report are available from the Office of Prevention, Education, and Control, NHLBI, Bethesda, MD 20892 (301-496-0554).

ABPM devices make it possible to automatically obtain multiple blood pressure readings over one or more days. The devices, which must be carefully calibrated for each patient, use either oscillometric or auscultatory methods to obtain blood pressure readings. The data are then analyzed by using computer software. Patient diaries are often used in interpreting the results.

According to the report, ABPM is a useful research tool. Research applications have included the study of normal blood pressure patterns, target organ complications of hypertension, the prognosis of cardiovascular events and mortality, and the effects of antihypertensive drugs. Studies have shown that ABPM readings correlate better with target organ complications than do "casual" office or home measurements. ABPM is also a useful technique for excluding placebo responders from controlled clinical trials, thereby reducing the number of patients with mild hypertension who must be enrolled in the study in order to show drug efficacy.

The technique is not needed in the care of most patients with hypertension, concluded the working group. Indiscriminate use of the devices would increase costs but provide little benefit. ABPM was judged useful in the following clinical situations:

- Borderline hypertension with target organ damage,
- Resistant hypertension,
- Episodic hypertension,
- Hypotensive symptoms that occur during antihypertensive therapy,
- "Office" or "white-coat" hypertension,
- Blood pressure changes associated with nocturnal angina or pulmonary congestion,
- Autonomic dysfunction, and
- Carotid sinus syncope and pacemaker syndromes.

The working group concluded that more research is needed on the use of this technique in patients with transient "office" hypertension and normal self-measured blood pressure.

Some technical problems need to be resolved. The frequency of blood pressure measurements and methods of data analysis have not been standardized and may vary according to the indication for monitoring. Information on the accuracy and reliability of ABPM devices under conditions of use is needed, and auscultatory and oscillometric methods need to be compared to determine whether the two methods are interchangeable.

Upcoming Specialty Meetings

Recent Advances in the Prevention and Treatment of Ischemic Stroke. King of Prussia, PA, March 25–26. Contact IBC USA Conferences Inc., 8 Pleasant Street, Building D, South Natick, MA 01760; 508-650-4700, (fax) 508-653-1627.

Stereoisomerism in Pharmaceuticals: New Directions in Drug Discovery and Development. Atlanta, GA, March 26–27. Contact Technomic Publishing Company, Inc., Program Division, 851 New Holland Avenue, Box 3535, Lancaster, PA 17604; 800-233-9936, (fax) 717-295-4538.

Advantages in Emergency Medicine: Toxicology and Infectious Disease. Coronado, CA, April 5–6. Contact UCLA Extension, P.O. Box 24901, Los Angeles, CA 90024-0901; 213-825-9971 or 818-784-7006.

5th Annual Review and Update Course in Critical Care Medicine. Rockville, MD, April 17–21. Contact Svetlana Lisanti, Conference Administrator, Center for Bio-Medical Communication, Inc., 80 West Madison Avenue, Dumont, NJ 07268; 201-385-8080, (fax) 201-385-5650.

Continued on page 176

News *Continued from page 175*

AIDS Symposium: Pathogenesis of HIV Infection. Spokane, WA, April 30–May 1. Contact Conferences and Institutes, 208 Van Doren Hall, Washington State University, Pullman, WA 99164-5222; 509-335-2946.

23rd Meeting of the International Society of Paediatric Oncology. Isle of Rhodes, Greece, September 30–October 4. Contact Conference Secretariat, 23rd Meeting of the International Society of Paediatric Oncology, Bruistensingel 360, P.O. Box 3283, 5203 DG's-Hertogenbosch, the Netherlands; +31-73-429285, (fax) +31-73-414766.

News Briefs

- Schering–Plough has received approval to market **clotrimazole** (Gyne-Lotrimin) as a nonprescription product for the treatment of vaginal yeast infection.
- FDA has approved the start of clinical trials for a candidate **recombinant gp160 vaccine for AIDS** developed under an agreement between the National Institutes of Health and Immuno U.S., Inc.

Policies Regarding Personnel Advertising

Clinical Pharmacy

Personnel advertising is accepted in *Clinical Pharmacy* for Positions Open and Training Programs.

Only those employers who will not discriminate on the basis of race, sex, religion, age, color, or national origin should submit personnel advertising. Ads should include the statement "Equal Opportunity Employer." Employers are encouraged to specify salary range in their position advertising. Advertisers listing residency or fellowship positions are strongly encouraged to comply with the profession's consensus of definitions for these two types of training programs.

The deadline for receipt of final copy and for cancellations is the 1st of the month before the month of publication. The sizes available are: full page (7″ × 10″) at $1,175, half page (vertical = 3¼″ × 10″; horizontal = 7″ × 4¾″) at $790, and quarter page (3¼″ × 4⁹⁄₁₆″) at $520. There is a $35 charge for typesetting quarter- and half-page and $55 for full-page advertisements.

The address for insertions (which must be accompanied by payment, organizational purchase order, or advertising agency insertion order) is: Advertising Placement Manager, *Clinical Pharmacy*, 4630 Montgomery Avenue, Bethesda, MD 20814. The fax number is 301-657-1615.

For information regarding the Career Opportunities section of the *American Journal of Hospital Pharmacy*, please contact Advertising Placement Manager, 301-657-3000, ext. 288.

ASHP also offers the Personnel Placement Service, which consists of monthly listings of positions open and of brief résumés of individuals seeking positions. For more information, write to Personnel Placement Service, ASHP, 4630 Montgomery Avenue, Bethesda, MD 20814.

Letters

The Letters *column is a forum for rapid exchange of ideas among readers of* Clinical Pharmacy. *Liberal criteria are applied in the review of submissions to encourage contributions to this column.*

The Letters *column includes the following types of contributions: (1) comments, addenda, and minor updates on previously published work, (2) alerts on potential problems related to drug therapy or clinical research, (3) observations or comments on trends in drug therapy or clinical research, and (4) brief expressions of opinion about controversies in drug therapy or clinical research.*

Letters need not be submitted with the journal's manuscript checklist. The following conditions, however, must be adhered to: (1) the body of the letter must be no longer than two typewritten pages, (2) the use of references, tables, and illustrations should be minimized, (3) the authors' names, affiliations, and mailing addresses must be typed at the end of the letter in the format used by Clinical Pharmacy, *and (4) the entire letter (including references, tables, and authors' names) must be typed double-spaced on plain white paper (not letterhead). Following acceptance of a letter, the authors are required to sign an exclusive publication statement and a copyright-transferal form.*

Interferon for genital warts

The recommendations of the Centers for Disease Control (CDC) on the treatment of sexually transmitted diseases,[1] described in the January 1990 issue of *Clinical Pharmacy*,[2] contain a misleading statement. According to CDC, interferon therapy for genital warts is not recommended because of its toxicity, cost, and relatively poor efficacy.

Recombinant and natural interferon alfa has been given topically, intralesionally, and systemically for the treatment of genital human papilloma virus (HPV) infection. Several studies have shown intralesional interferon alfa to be effective and safe in the treatment of condylomata acuminata.[3-6] Some patients have had a reduction in the number of measurable lesions within days of the start of therapy. Although the degree of disease resolution varies among patients, 75–80% of patients treated with low doses of interferon for genital HPV disease show clear clinical benefit.[7] Intralesional interferon is associated with less frequent and less severe adverse effects than is systemic administration.

Friedman-Kien et al.[4] reported the results of a multicenter, randomized, double-blind, placebo-controlled trial that evaluated the efficacy of intralesional interferon alfa (Alferon N, Purdue Frederick) for the treatment of condylomata acuminata. Patients received a mean of 225,000 IU of interferon alfa or placebo into each wart twice weekly for up to eight weeks. Warts in 88% of patients had been recalcitrant or had recurred after previous therapy. Complete or partial resolution of warts occurred in 65 (80%) of 81 patients receiving interferon and in 33 (44%) of 75 patients receiving placebo ($p < 0.001$). Interferon reduced wart size and total wart volume per patient ($p < 0.001$). Among evaluable patients with previously recalcitrant warts, complete or partial resolution occurred in 58 (82%) of 71 of those receiving interferon and 29 (43%) of 67 of those receiving placebo ($p < 0.001$). The authors concluded that intralesional natural interferon alfa was effective and safe even in patients with recurrent or recalcitrant genital warts.

Interferon's therapeutic effect may be due to inhibition of viral replication, suppression of cell proliferation, or immunomodulation. Interferon is a welcome and valuable option for the eradication of external genital warts and should be included in CDC's recommendations for the treatment of sexually transmitted diseases.

1. Centers for Disease Control. 1989 sexually transmitted diseases treatment guidelines. *MMWR*. 1989; 38(S-8):1-43.
2. Anon. CDC updates recommendations on treatment of sexually transmitted diseases. *Clin Pharm*. 1990; 9:3,6,8-11. News.
3. Welander CE, Homesley HD, Smiles KA et al. Intralesional interferon alfa-2b for the treatment of genital warts. *Am J Obstet Gynecol*. 1990; 162:348-54.
4. Friedman-Kien AE, Eron LJ, Conant M et al. Natural interferon alfa for treatment of condylomata acuminata. *JAMA*. 1988; 259:533-8.
5. Gall SA, Hughes CE, Trofatter K. Interferon for the therapy of condyloma acuminatum. *Am J Obstet Gynecol*. 1985; 153:157-63.
6. Geffen JR, Klein RJ, Friedman-Kien AE. Intralesional administration of large doses of human leukocyte interferon for the treatment of condylomata acuminata. *J Infect Dis*. 1984; 150:612-5.
7. Weck PK, Buddin DA, Whismant JK. Interferons in the treatment of genital human papilloma virus infections. *Am J Med*. 1988; 85(Suppl 2A):159-64.

Celine M. Stahl-Bayliss, M.D., Assistant Medical Director
The Purdue Frederick Company
100 Connecticut Avenue
Norwalk, CT 06850-3590

Drug Reviews

Fluconazole: A new antifungal agent

STEVEN F. KOWALSKY AND DENNIS M. DIXON

Abstract: The chemistry, activity, pharmacokinetics, clinical efficacy, adverse effects, drug interactions, and administration of fluconazole are reviewed.

Fluconazole is a triazole antifungal agent labeled for use in the treatment of oropharyngeal and esophageal candidiasis and cryptococcal meningitis. Like the imidazoles, fluconazole inhibits the C-14 demethylation of lanosterol, but it has little or no effect on mammalian cytochrome P-450 enzymes. Fluconazole's activity in vitro does not reflect its effectiveness in vivo. Pharmacokinetic characteristics include water solubility and excellent bioavailability, low protein binding, extensive tissue distribution, and penetration into the cerebrospinal fluid. Fluconazole is eliminated primarily by the kidneys; dosage adjustments are necessary in patients with renal insufficiency. Studies have shown fluconazole to be effective in patients with cryptococcal meningitis and candidiasis, but the superiority of fluconazole over such agents as amphotericin B, ketoconazole, clotrimazole, and itraconazole remains to be proved. Fluconazole has shown varying degrees of success in the treatment of other systemic mycoses. The adverse effects of fluconazole are relatively infrequent and are primarily gastrointestinal. Tolbutamide, warfarin, rifampin, cyclosporine, and phenytoin interact with fluconazole. The drug is available in both oral and intravenous formulations.

Fluconazole is a broad-spectrum antifungal drug that appears to be similar in efficacy to other antifungals in the treatment of some systemic mycoses. More studies must be completed before fluconazole can be recommended as a first-line antifungal therapy.

Index terms: Antifungals; Drug interactions; Fluconazole; Pharmacokinetics; Toxicity
Clin Pharm. 1991; 10:179–94

Since its introduction in the late 1950s, amphotericin B has been the mainstay of therapy for deep-seated mycotic infections. Frequently used alone for the treatment of fungal infections, amphotericin B is occasionally used in combination with flucytosine for selected infections (e.g., cryptococcal meningitis). Despite amphotericin B's fungicidal activity and broad antifungal spectrum, the necessity of giving it as an intravenous infusion and the frequent occurrence of adverse effects (e.g., fever, chills, nausea, phlebitis, anemia, and renal insufficiency) remain important problems. Flucytosine has broad antifungal activity and is given orally, but rapid development of resistance and bone marrow toxicity make it a less than ideal agent.

Clotrimazole was the first oral imidazole studied. This drug induces its own metabolism, which markedly diminishes its systemic antifungal activity[1]; it is currently available only as an oral or topical formulation for the prevention and treatment of superficial fungal infections (e.g., thrush). Miconazole, unlike clotrimazole, is available for intravenous use, does not induce its own metabolism, and is effective against many systemic fungal diseases. Adverse effects such as phlebitis, pruritus, rash, fever, hyperlipidemia, and hepatotoxicity, coupled with the risk of cardiopulmonary arrest (attributable to the histamine-releasing properties of the polyoxyl 35 castor oil contained in the injection[2]), are limiting features of this derivative, and

STEVEN F. KOWALSKY, PHARM.D., is Professor of Pharmacy, Department of Pharmacy Practice, Albany College of Pharmacy and Adjunct Associate Professor of Medicine, Department of Medicine, Division of Infectious Diseases, Albany Medical College (AMC), Albany, NY. DENNIS M. DIXON, PH.D., is Director, Laboratories for Mycology, Wadsworth Center for Laboratories and Research, New York State Department of Health, Albany, and Adjunct Associate Professor, Department of Pathology and Laboratory Medicine, AMC.

Address reprint requests to Dr. Kowalsky at the Albany College of Pharmacy, 106 New Scotland Avenue, Albany, NY 12208.

This is **article 680-204-9106** in the **ASHP Continuing Education System;** it qualifies for 1.0 hour of continuing-education credit. See page **228** for learning objectives and test questions.

its use is primarily restricted to patients who do not respond to amphotericin B.

The introduction of ketoconazole provided the clinician with an orally active, broad-spectrum imidazole antifungal. Ketoconazole has a better adverse-reaction profile than miconazole; however, since its release, several endocrinologic adverse effects have been reported (e.g., gynecomastia, sexual impotence, azoospermia, oligospermia, and inhibition of steroid synthesis).[3] In addition, drug interactions with rifampin, histamine H_2-receptor antagonists, cyclosporine, warfarin, phenytoin, and theophylline have been described, and it has been reported that ketoconazole crosses the blood-brain barrier to only a limited extent in the presence of inflammation.[4]

The search for antifungal drugs with improved pharmacokinetic characteristics and safety has led to the development of a class of azole antifungals known as the triazoles.[5-7] Several triazole derivatives are under investigation; this review focuses on fluconazole.

Chemical Properties

The chemical name of fluconazole is 2,4-difluoro-α,α-bis(1*H*-1,2,4-triazol-1-ylmethyl)benzyl alcohol. The molecular formula is $C_{13}H_{12}F_2N_6O$, and the molecular weight is 306.3. Structural modifications of previously available imidazoles have led to the development of a number of triazole derivatives, including fluconazole.[8] Replacing the imidazole ring with a triazole ring, adding a second triazole ring, and substituting a difluorophenyl moiety for a dichlorophenyl moiety have provided fluconazole with more selective inhibition of fungal enzyme systems, greater metabolic stability (with higher concentrations in serum and lower protein binding), and enhanced solubility in water (10 mg/mL), respectively (Figure 1).[8]

Mechanism of Action

The mode of action of azole antifungal agents (both imidazoles [clotrimazole, miconazole, ketoconazole] and triazoles [fluconazole, itraconazole, SCH39304]) appears to be disturbance of fungal cell membrane permeability.[9-11] Unlike amphotericin B, which binds to ergosterol in fungal cell membranes, forming pores or channels that ultimately lead to leakage of vital intracellular constituents,[12] azoles specifically inhibit the C-14 demethylation step of lanosterol, which is necessary for ergosterol biosynthesis. This demethylation step is dependent on the cytochrome P-450 enzyme system. Inhibition of P-450 enzyme activity appears to be closely related to the affinity of azole binding to ferric P-450 at the sixth axial heme ligand position.[13] Binding occurs between the N-3 of imidazoles (or the N-4 of the triazoles) and the heme iron.[9,11] The N-substituted imidazoles are less selective than the triazole derivatives in their inhibition of the cytochrome P-450 enzyme system and in their inhibition of enzyme systems in several mammalian organs, including the testes,[14] ovaries,[15] adrenal glands,[16] kidneys,[17] and liver.[18,19] Another mechanism of antifungal activity proposed for the azole compounds is inhibition of cytochrome *c* oxidative and peroxidative enzymes, leading to increased production of intracellular peroxidase.[20-22]

Spectrum of Activity and Resistance

Evaluation of antifungal agents in vitro is complicated by several factors that affect the determination of antifungal activity. These include the size of the inoculum, the composition of the growth medium, the incubation time and temperature, and the endpoint chosen for the determination of the minimum inhibitory concentration (MIC). Furthermore, there is often difficulty in establishing a correlation between the in vitro activity of antifungal drugs and their activity in vivo.[23] Fluconazole represents one of the extremes in this regard, since it has been stated that the drug would never have been promoted on the basis of in vitro susceptibility data alone.[5] In many in vitro test systems, fluconazole appears to have little activity, yet it may become the drug of choice in some patients because of its activity in vivo. Because of the poor correlation, some have suggested that susceptibility testing is not justified for the triazole anti-

Figure 1. Structural components of ketoconazole and fluconazole. Compared with ketoconazole, fluconazole has two triazole rings and a difluorophenyl instead of dichlorophenyl structure.

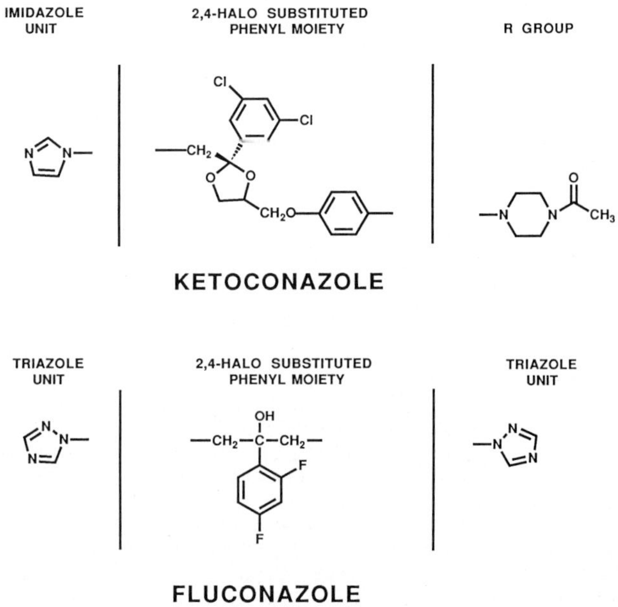

fungal agents.[24] Nonetheless, fluconazole MICs have been compiled for an array of medically important fungi. These data must be considered in the light of what is known about the agent's activity against these fungi in vivo.

Published MICs of fluconazole vary widely, not only for different fungal species but also for the same species tested under different conditions or in different laboratories (Table 1). For example, the MICs for *Candida albicans* vary by a factor of more than 1000. Some of the obfuscating variables can be eliminated by comparing the data for different species tested in a single laboratory by a single method. Gordon et al.[33] described an agar dilution method that gives clear endpoints without the "trailing" effect that is so problematic with the azoles and fungi. Trailing is said to occur when serial increases in drug concentration result in only partial inhibition of visible fungal growth. With the agar dilution method of Gordon et al., MICs are generally lower than other published values and, for many organisms, represent achievable serum concentrations. Furthermore, the method produces a range of MICs for multiple isolates of a given species. It is important that such a range of MICs be observed if one expects to correlate the data with in vivo outcomes, which usually comprise a range of responses.

Table 1.
Antifungal Activity of Fluconazole in Vitro

Organism	Reference	No. Strains	MIC[a] (μg/mL)	Test Conditions[b]
Aspergillus fumigatus	6	2	>40	A
	25	4	>100	B
	26	8	>100	C
Bipolaris spicifera	6	1	10	A
Candida albicans	6	8	0.625–2.0	A
	26	5	>100	C
	27	35	0.063–4.0	D
Candida guilliermondii	26	1	>100	C
Candida parapsilosis	6	1	2.5	A
Candida pseudotropicalis	26	1	>100	C
Candida tropicalis	6	1	1.25	A
Cryptococcus neoformans	6	6	1.25–10	A
	28	1	6.4, 12.8[c]	E
	28	1	>100	B
Dactylaria constricta var. *gallopava*	29	1	>100	B
Fonsecaea pedrosoi	6	1	20	A
Fusarium spp.	6	2	>40	A
Histoplasma capsulatum	6	1	2.5	A
	30	9	16–250	F
	31	1	3.3	B
Scedosporium apiospermum	6	2	20	A
Torulopsis glabrata	6	3	5.0–20	A
	26	1	>100	C
Trichosporon beigelii	6	1	2.5	A
	32	1	0.8	NS
Wangiella dermatitidis	29	1	55	B
Xylohypha bantiana	29	1	>100	B

[a] MIC = minimum inhibitory concentration.
[b] A = agar dilution with yeast nitrogen base (YNB), glucose, L-asparagine, and sodium phosphate buffer (pH 7); B = agar dilution with Casitone agar; C = agar dilution with YNB and glucose; D = broth dilution with synthetic amino acid medium fungal (SAAMF) and *N*-(2-hydroxyethyl)piperazine-*N*′-2-ethanesulfonic acid buffer (pH 7.4); E = broth dilution with SAAMF; F = broth dilution with YNB, glucose, and yeast extract; and NS = not specified.
[c] Values after 48 and 72 hours, respectively.

The emergence of resistance to the azole antifungals has been described for medically important yeasts. At least four isolates of *C. albicans* have been reported to have developed resistance to ketoconazole during prolonged therapy.[34] Studies indicate cross-resistance to fluconazole and all other triazole drugs tested. A 1988 report described the isolation of a strain of *Torulopsis glabrata* that became 10 times more resistant to fluconazole during therapy with fluconazole 400 mg once daily; the isolate was cross-resistant to other azoles, and urine cultures showed that it could not be cleared from the patient.[35] More recently, Redding et al.[36] suggested that in AIDS patients who are treated with fluconazole for thrush and then relapse, there is a substantial increase in MICs for the cultured fungi. Likewise, Fulton and Phillips[37] reported a case of possible fluconazole resistance after several months of suppressive therapy for oral and esophageal candidiasis. Prior therapy with azole antifungal agents was suggested as a possible reason for the inability of an AIDS patient with cryptococcal meningitis to respond to amphotericin B.[38] Alterations in fungal sterol metabolism after fluconazole therapy had resulted in a reduction in saponifiable sterols and consequent changes in susceptibility to amphotericin B.

Thus, while the incidence of resistance to fluconazole may be extremely low, it must remain a consideration and may affect susceptibility to other antifungal compounds.

Pharmacokinetics

Table 2 summarizes the pharmacokinetic data from selected clinical studies of oral and intravenous fluconazole. Among the azole antifungal agents, fluconazole has several unique pharmacokinetic characteristics.[5–7]

Absorption. Unlike ketoconazole and itraconazole, fluconazole is water-soluble and thus is readily absorbed from the gastrointestinal tract. Peak plasma concentrations in humans are reached two to four hours after oral administration and range from 1.4 μg/mL after a 50-mg dose to 2.82 μg/mL

Table 2.
Mean Pharmacokinetic Values for Fluconazole[a]

Reference	n	Dosage (mg) and Calculation Day[b]	C_{max} (μg/mL)	C_{24} (μg/mL)	$t_{1/2}$ (hr)	AUC (μg·hr/mL)[c]	V (L/kg)	CL (mL/min)	CL_R (mL/min)	fe (%)[d]
39	4	50 p.o. once	1.4	0.63	22	43	0.7	28	19	64
40	7	100 p.o. once	1.75	0.78	...	...	...	...	...	27
41	9	150 p.o. once	2.82	1.78	30	...	0.84	...[e]	...	...
42	10	50 i.v. daily for 7 days								
		Day 1	0.96	0.46	30	15	0.82	24	16	...
		Day 7	2.15	1.21	32	38	0.78	23	18	...
		100 i.v. daily for 7 days								
		Day 1	2.14	0.96	30	32	0.77	23	19	...
		Day 7	4.68	2.40	29	80	0.64	21	15	...
		100 i.v. once, then 50 i.v. daily for 6 days								
		Day 1	2.51	1.10	31	36	0.68	20	16	...
		Day 7	2.21	1.15	28	37	0.61	23	17	...

[a] C_{max} = peak serum concentration, C_{24} = serum concentration 24 hours after dose, $t_{1/2}$ = half-life, AUC = area under the serum concentration–time curve, V = volume of distribution, CL = total body clearance, CL_R = renal clearance, fe = fraction excreted unchanged.
[b] Values were calculated after a single dose in references 39 to 41 and after the first and seventh doses in reference 42.
[c] AUC represents the time from 0 hours to infinity in reference 39 and from 0 to 24 hours in reference 42.
[d] Fraction excreted unchanged in 72 and 24 hours in references 39 and 40, respectively.
[e] CL = 0.32 mL/min/kg.

after a 150-mg dose.[39–41] Seven bone marrow transplant recipients who received fluconazole 100 mg orally achieved peak serum concentrations that were not different from values in 12 healthy volunteers given a similar dose of fluconazole.[40] Houang et al.[41] studied the single-dose pharmacokinetics of fluconazole 150 mg (given orally as three 50-mg capsules) in patients being treated for vaginal candidiasis. Peak plasma concentrations were achieved two hours after the dose was given and ranged from 2.44 to 3.58 μg/mL.

From these studies, it appears that the amount of fluconazole absorbed is linearly proportional to the dose, while urinary excretion data indicate that the oral bioavailability of fluconazole is greater than 90%. This is in distinct contrast to older azole compounds, such as clotrimazole, miconazole, and econazole, which are characterized by poor oral bioavailability and low concentrations in plasma.[43–45] Unlike ketoconazole, which has limited solubility at high gastric pH, fluconazole, because of its greater water solubility, appears to be minimally affected by gastric pH. Drew et al.[46] reported excellent absorption of fluconazole in a patient with chronic mucocutaneous candidiasis and achlorhydria (intragastric pH, >8) who had previously failed to absorb ketoconazole. In addition, studies comparing peak concentrations and systemic exposure after the administration of oral fluconazole (capsules) to human volunteers indicate that food has little effect on fluconazole absorption.[47]

Distribution. Once absorbed, fluconazole has a volume of distribution of 0.6 to 0.8 L/kg.[39,41] Steady-state pharmacokinetic values were measured in 10 healthy male volunteers given a daily 30-minute intravenous infusion of fluconazole for seven days (Table 2).[42] A two-compartment analysis showed no substantial change in half-life, total body or renal clearance, or volume of distribution from day 1 to day 7. Terminal elimination half-life ranged from 28 to 32 hours, total body clearance ranged from 20 to 24 mL/min, renal clearance ranged from 15 to 19 mL/min, and volume of distribution ranged from 600 to 820 mL/kg. These data agree with the single-dose studies by Humphrey et al.[39] and Houang et al.[41]

Humphrey et al.,[39] using a dialysis technique for measuring plasma protein binding of fluconazole, found that approximately 11% of fluconazole was bound in humans and did not vary over a concentration range of 0.1 to 10 μg/mL. Fluconazole is a small molecule, is water-soluble, and has a low degree of protein binding—all characteristics that enhance the drug's ability to penetrate several tissue compartments, including the central nervous system (CNS). Many studies in animals[48–51] and humans[42,52,53] have demonstrated the ability of fluconazole to penetrate the CNS in the presence or absence of meningeal irritation. Investigators have also evaluated the distribution of fluconazole in tissues and fluids outside the CNS.[39,41,48,54–56] Table 3 summarizes the results of studies of fluconazole distribution in humans.

Elimination. The kidneys play a major role in the elimination of unchanged fluconazole. However, Milliken et al.[40] found the mean ± S.D. 24-hour urinary excretion of fluconazole to be significantly lower in bone marrow transplant patients (27.6 ± 8.6 mg) than in healthy controls (47 ± 16 mg) ($p < 0.05$). In the Humphrey et al.[39] study, three minor metabolites were detected in the urine of mice and dogs but accounted for less than 4% of the administered dose.

Table 3.
Fluconazole Concentrations in Fluids and Tissues

Fluid or Tissue	Reference	*n*	Fluconazole Dosage (mg)	Sampling Time (hr)[a]	Fluid Conc. (μg/mL) or Tissue Conc. (μg/g)[b]	Serum Conc. (μg/mL)[b]
Vaginal secretions	41	9	150 p.o. once	2	...	2.82
				8	2.42	...
				24	2.42	1.78
Sputum	54	11	150 p.o. once	4	3.71	3.54
				24	2.23	2.37
Cerebrospinal fluid	52	3	50/day i.v. × 6 doses	1	1.26	2.44
		3	100/day i.v. × 7 doses	1	2.74	4.44
		1	50/day p.o.	2	5.24	6.45
		1	200/day p.o.	4	2.57	4.49
		1	200/day intragastrically	22	4.44	7.46
Vaginal tissue	56	27	150 p.o. once	2	2.95	...
				72	0.61	...
Dialysate[c]	57	5	50 i.p. once	6	6.47	930
				144	0.47	220
		5	150 i.p. once	6	18.60	2160
				144	1.27	650
		5	100 p.o. once	6	2.47	1385
				144	0.96	460
Urine	40	6	100 p.o. once	24	13.20	0.78

[a] Time after dose at which fluid, tissue, or serum sample was collected.
[b] Reported as mean value if $n > 1$.
[c] Peritoneal dialysis solution containing fluconazole was instilled with a dwell time of six hours. Exchanges of peritoneal dialysis fluid were then performed every six hours with fluconazole-free solution.

Toon et al.[58] investigated the pharmacokinetics of fluconazole in three groups of patients with various degrees of renal function and found that while the volume of distribution was not affected by renal function, serum half-life and renal clearance were. The elimination half-life was 31 hours in subjects with normal renal function and 98 hours in subjects with creatinine clearance of <20 mL/min. Likewise, renal clearance was 1.04 L/hr in healthy volunteers and 0.19 L/hr in subjects with severe renal insufficiency. In addition, three hours of hemodialysis decreased plasma fluconazole levels by 48%. Debruyne et al.[57] studied the pharmacokinetics of fluconazole in patients undergoing continuous ambulatory peritoneal dialysis (CAPD). Fluconazole concentrations in serum and peritoneal dialysate fluid after intravenous or oral administration indicated that the drug readily and rapidly crossed the peritoneal membrane. The serum half-life and volume of distribution were 72 to 85 hours and 40 to 60 L, respectively. These studies suggest that dosage adjustments in patients with renal insufficiency might best be accomplished by extending the interval between doses rather than by reducing the dose.

Ahlmen et al.,[32] in treating a patient with CAPD-associated peritonitis caused by *Trichosporon beigelii*, measured dialysate fluconazole concentrations exceeding 2 μg/mL after five weeks of oral therapy (50 mg/day). The authors suggested that because of "slowly increasing concentrations in the overnight exchange dialysate...accumulation [of fluconazole] during CAPD [occurs]." Their recommendation was to decrease the daily dose of the drug after three weeks of therapy. Levine et al.[59] treated two patients with fungal peritonitis with oral fluconazole (a 200-mg loading dose followed by 100 mg/day) and found that the drug concentration in dialysate was at least 60% of that in serum.

Experimental Models

The lack of correlation between the in vitro susceptibility of fungi to triazole agents and the effectiveness of these agents in vivo has led to the use of animal models of fungal infections to investigate the antifungal activity of fluconazole. The experimental infections have included invasive aspergillosis,[60,61] coccidioidomycosis,[62–65] histoplasmosis,[30,31,66,67] candidiasis,[27,51,55,68–72] cryptococcosis,[28,51,60] blastomycosis,[73–75] systemic phaeohyphomycosis,[29] other *Candida* species infections,[76] and pityriasis versicolor.[77] The results of most of these studies have been summarized by Saag and Dismukes.[7] Fluconazole appeared to be more effective than ketoconazole against *Aspergillus flavus, C. albicans*, and *Blastomyces dermatitidis;* equal to ketoconazole against *Coccidioides immitis;* equal to itraconazole against *Cryptococcus neoformans;* and equal to amphotericin B against *Histoplasma capsulatum*. Fluconazole also had protective and life-prolonging effects in immunosuppressed mice infected with *H. capsulatum*. Amphotericin B was judged to be the better or best drug in experimental infections with

Aspergillus fumigatus, C. immitis, and *C. albicans.*

In life-threatening fungal infections in humans, amphotericin B alone or in combination with flucytosine remains the treatment of choice for most fungi and in most settings.[78,79] Exceptions could include systemic infection with *Pseudallescheria boydii,* amphotericin B-resistant strains of *Candida lusitaniae, C. albicans,* and refractory infections with *T. beigelii,* all of which pose significant treatment dilemmas. Other exceptions to the use of amphotericin B in mycoses include immunocompetent hosts with certain forms of histoplasmosis, blastomycosis, or paracoccidioidomycosis, for whom ketoconazole is replacing amphotericin B as the treatment of choice.[79]

Fluconazole has a place in the treatment of systemic fungal infections. The most promising results have come from studies in patients with cryptococcosis[80–102] and candidiasis[32,41,59,102–142] (Tables 4 and 5).

Efficacy against Cryptococcal Infections

Patients with AIDS. Because of its excellent penetration into cerebrospinal fluid, fluconazole is a logical candidate for use in the treatment of CNS

Table 4.
Fluconazole in the Treatment of Cryptococcal Infections[a]

Type of Infection	Reference	*n*	Dosage (mg)	Fraction (%) Cured[b]	Fraction (%) with Negative Cultures	Fraction (%) Relapsing
Meningitis						
Active	88	14	400/day p.o. × 10 days, then 200/day p.o. × 1 yr	6/14 (13)	6/14 (43)	2/4 (50)
		6	AmB 0.7/kg/day i.v. × 1 wk, then 3 times/wk × 9 wk + 5-FC 150/kg/day p.o. × 10 wk	6/6 (100)	6/6 (100)	1/6 (17)
	89	42	200–400/day p.o.	19/42 (45)	19/42 (45)	. . .
		23	AmB ≥15/kg i.v. (total)	11/23 (48)	11/23 (48)	. . .
	95	145	200 or 400/day p.o. or i.v.	36/59 (62)	25/38 (66)	2/35 (6)
	96	7	400 i.v. once, then 200/day i.v. × 2 wk, then 200/day p.o.	6/7 (86)	6/7 (86)	1/6 (17) 4/6 (67)[c]
	98	11	400 i.v. once, then 200/day i.v. × 2 wk, then 200/day p.o.	9/11 (82)[d]	2/11 (18)	6/11 (55)
		5	800 p.o. once, then 400/day p.o.	4/5 (80)	. . .	2/4 (50)
	100	1[e]	50 p.o. once	1/1 (100)	1/1 (100)	1/1 (100)
		1[e]	100 p.o. once, then 50/day p.o. × 10 wk, then 100/day p.o.	1/1 (100)	1/1 (100)	. . .
Inactive	87	19	50–200/day p.o.	9/19 (47)	9/19 (47)	2/19 (11)
	90	106	200/day p.o.	. . .	. . .	2/106 (2)
		77	AmB 1/kg/wk i.v.	. . .	. . .	13/77 (17)
	93	36	100/day p.o. × 12 wk	. . .	. . .	2/36 (6)
		47	200/day p.o.	. . .	. . .	. . .
Urinary tract	97	13	100–400/day p.o.	. . .	6/13 (46)	. . .
Cryptococcosis						
Active	85	7[f]	50–400/day p.o. × 8–64 wk	4/7 (57)	4/7 (57)	. . .
Inactive		15[g]	50–400/day p.o. × 8–64 wk	6/15 (40)	14/15 (93)	1/14 (7)
Disseminated	94	3	400 p.o. or i.v. once, then 200/day p.o. or i.v.	1/3 (33)	1/3 (33)	. . .
	99	18[h]	200–400/day (route unspecified)	. . .	10/10 (100)[i]	. . .
		11[h]	AmB 0.5/kg/day i.v. + 5-FC p.o. (dosage unspecified)	. . .	5/6 (83)[j]	. . .
Deep-seated	102	15[e]	Not reported	10/15 (67)	. . .	. . .

[a] Patients had AIDS and were treated with fluconazole unless otherwise noted. In some studies, some patients were not evaluated for cure, negative cultures, or relapse. AmB = amphotericin B, 5-FC = flucytosine.
[b] Includes patients who were cured and patients whose condition improved.
[c] Clinical relapse occurred in 17%, mycologic relapse in 67%.
[d] Result after 10 weeks of therapy. Fractions cured after 40 and 56 weeks were 4/11 (36%) and 2/4 (50%), respectively.
[e] The patient did not have AIDS.
[f] Of the seven patients, five had meningitis, two had cryptococcemia, and one had urinary tract infection.
[g] Of the 15 patients, 14 had meningitis and 1 had pneumonia.
[h] Of the total of 29 patients, 1 had pulmonary cryptococcosis.
[i] Value is for blood cultures. Cerebrospinal fluid cultures were negative in 7/11 (64%) of patients.
[j] Value is for blood cultures. Cerebrospinal fluid cultures were negative in 4/8 (50%) of patients.

Table 5.
Fluconazole in the Treatment of Noncryptococcal Infection[a]

Type of Infection	Reference	n	Dosage (mg)	Fraction (%) Cured	Fraction (%) with Negative Cultures	Fraction (%) Relapsing
Oropharyngeal esophageal candidiasis	103	18	50/day p.o. × 28 days	17/17 (100)	13/15 (87)	6/13 (46)
		28	KTZ 200/day p.o. × 28 days	12/16 (75)	9/13 (69)	1/9 (11)
	104	71	50/day p.o. × 5–20 days, then 50 q.o.d. × 6–49 days	42/42 (100)	30/71 (42)	(100)
	105	31	150 p.o. once	11/21 (52)	9/22 (41)	4/15 (27)
	108	28	50/day p.o. × 7 days	26/27 (96)	13/21 (62)	3/13 (23)
		28	150 p.o. once	21/24 (88)	6/17 (35)	5/13 (39)
	109	...	100/day p.o. × 14 days	(98)	(67)	(34)
		...	CLO 10 p.o. 5 times/day × 14 days	(97)	(54)	(43)
	111	45	150 p.o. once	16/43 (37)	...	...
	112	104	200 p.o. once, then 100/day p.o. × 3 wk	(90)	...	...
	113	...	50/day p.o. × 28 days	(96)	(44)	...
		...	KTZ 200 b.i.d. p.o. × 28 days	(92)	(42)	...
	115	36	200 p.o. once, then 100/day p.o. × 4 wk	33/33 (100)	33/33 (100)	2/33 (6)
	117	21	200 p.o. once/wk × 1 yr (preventive)	...	...	4/11 (36)
	120	17	100/day p.o. × 2 wk	16/16 (100)	12/16 (75)	9/15 (60)
		19	CLO 10 p.o. 5 times/day × 1 day	11/17 (65)	3/15 (20)	1/7 (14)
	125	15[b]	200 p.o. once, then 100/day p.o. × 13 days	...	11/15 (73)	13/14 (93)
	136	30[b]	50/day p.o. × 5–14 days	28/31 (90)[c]	16/31 (52)[c]	9/16 (56)
Vaginal candidiasis	121	180[b]	150 p.o. once	130/147 (88)	109/149 (73)	... (23)
	122	188[b]	150 p.o. once	141/152 (93)	115/160 (72)	...
		181[b]	CLO 200/day intravaginally × 3 days	113/135 (84)	90/145 (62)	...
	123	53[b]	150 p.o. once	38/47 (81)	27/47 (57)	...
		51[b]	ECZ 50/day intravaginally × 6 days	39/49 (80)	28/49 (57)	...
	124	92[b]	150 p.o. once	65/76 (86)	63/82 (71)	... (4–8)
		91[b]	KTZ 200 p.o. b.i.d. for 5 days	63/72 (88)	57/74 (77)	... (4–8)
Candidal UTI	126	7[b]	50/day p.o. or i.v. (duration unspecified)	6/7 (86)	6/7 (86)	...
Candidal ocular infection	128	3[b]	400 i.v. once, then 200/day × 18–21 days	3/3 (100)	...	...
CAPD-related peritonitis	32	1[b,d]	50 i.p. once, then 50/day p.o. × 5 wk	1/1 (100)	...	...
	59	2[b,e]	200 i.p. once, then 100/day p.o. × 6 wk	0/2 (0)	0/1 (0)	...
	129	1[b,f]	200 i.v. q.o.d. × 8 wk	1/1 (100)	1/1 (100)	0
Postoperative mycoses	130	26[b,g]	200–400 p.o. or i.v. × 8–26 days	22/26 (85)	(>50)	...
Deep candidal infection	132	6[b]	100–400/day i.v.	5/5 (100)	...	...
	102	47[b]	Unspecified	41/47 (87)	...	...
	133	17[b]	50/day or q.o.d. or 100/day p.o. × 8–194 days	10/11 (91)	8/11 (73)	...
Chronic mucocutaneous candidiasis	135	8[b]	50/day p.o. × 4 wk	8/8 (100)	8/8 (100)	3/8 (38)
Various candidal infections	119	24[h]	6–12/kg/day i.v. × 12 days	30/34 (88)	30/34 (88)	10/30 (30)
Antifungal prophylaxis	142	24[b]	400/day p.o.	...	...	2/24 (8)
		21[b]	AmB 0.5/kg i.v. 3 times/wk	...	...	3/21 (14)

[a] In some studies, not all patients were evaluated for cure, presence of negative cultures, or relapse. Evaluations were performed more than once in some studies; the latest results are provided here. In some reports, only percentage values were provided. KTZ = ketoconazole, CLO = clotrimazole, ECZ = econazole, UTI = urinary tract infection, CAPD = continuous ambulatory peritoneal dialysis, AmB = amphotericin B. Patients had AIDS or were seropositive for human immunodeficiency virus unless otherwise noted.

[b] The patients did not have AIDS.

[c] There were 31 episodes among 30 patients.

[d] The patient was infected with *Trichosporon beigelii.*

[e] One patient was infected with *Candida parapsilosis,* and the other was infected with *Candida albicans.*

[f] The patient was infected with *Torulopsis glabrata.*

[g] The patients were infected with *Candida* species or with *Aspergillus fumigatus.*

[h] The patients had oropharyngeal infection (17 patients), UTI (9), colonization (4), fungemia (2), otitis (1), and abscess (1).

mycoses. Cryptococcosis represents the most important mycosis in this category, and it is as a therapy for cryptococcosis that fluconazole has generated much excitement, especially with respect to patients with AIDS, who have a 10% incidence of cryptococcal meningitis. Although success also occurs with amphotericin B, both with and without flucytosine, as many as 50% of the patients who respond relapse within six months after completing therapy.[80] The efficacy of fluconazole, both as primary therapy for active cryptococcal meningitis, and as maintenance therapy, has been examined in many clinical trials.[81-96,98]

In a collaborative trial at several French centers in patients with AIDS and cryptococcal meningitis, fluconazole 400 mg/day was effective in converting cerebrospinal fluid cultures to negative and as maintenance therapy to prevent relapse.[81] Only a few trials in AIDS patients have compared fluconazole with amphotericin B (with or without flucytosine).[88-90] Fluconazole was not better than amphotericin B in terms of clinical or mycological outcomes. Relapse rates were lower with fluconazole in only one study.[90]

While fluconazole and amphotericin B do not appear to produce strikingly different outcomes, Larsen et al.[88] and Dismukes et al.[89] reported a slower conversion of cultures from positive to negative in patients with acute disease who were given fluconazole. In addition, treatment groups receiving fluconazole in the Dismukes et al. study were said to have experienced three times as many deaths during the first week of therapy.[143]

More studies are needed before fluconazole can be routinely substituted for amphotericin B as the drug of choice for treating acute cryptococcal meningitis. Several investigators have published their experiences with fluconazole in treating a limited number of patients with other types of cryptococcal infections.[85,94,97,99] In most cases, the clinical and mycological outcomes were excellent and occurred in patients previously unresponsive to or intolerant of traditional antifungal therapy.

Patients without AIDS. Only a few reports have appeared on the use of fluconazole to treat cryptococcal disease in patients who do not have AIDS.[100-102] These reports do not allow definitive statements to be made on differences in clinical or mycological outcomes or relapse rates between patients with and without AIDS.

Efficacy against Candidiasis

Patients with AIDS. The use of fluconazole for the treatment and prevention of candidal infections in patients with AIDS has been evaluated in a number of clinical trials. The majority of the investigators evaluated fluconazole alone, whereas others compared it with ketoconazole, clotrimazole, or itraconazole. Oropharyngeal or esophageal candidiasis or both were evaluated in all the trials. Viscoli et al.[119] evaluated the efficacy of fluconazole against oropharyngeal candidiasis, fungal abscess, urinary tract infection, fungemia, and fungal colonization in cancer patients; however, since patient response rates were pooled, the efficacy in AIDS patients only cannot be assessed.

The frequency of clinical cure (or improvement) and of conversion from positive to negative mycological cultures in the fluconazole-only studies ranged from 37% to 100% and from 35% to 100%, respectively. DeWit et al.[103] compared fluconazole and ketoconazole, but there is controversy over the interpretation of the clinical cure rates and the appropriateness of the ketoconazole dosage.[144-146] Nathwani et al.[106] compared fluconazole and itraconazole, but instead of providing objective data to substantiate clinical or mycological outcomes, reported that all patients were "successfully treated." An Italian study revealed a dramatic difference between the percentage of patients cured when treated with fluconazole (92%) and the percentage cured by ketoconazole (58%).[113] However, if patients with clinical outcomes graded as "improved" are combined with "cures," the difference becomes meaningless (96% versus 92%).

More recently, in a prospective, randomized trial comparing the efficacies of oral fluconazole once daily and clotrimazole troche five times daily, Koletar et al.[120] found a significantly better clinical outcome ($p = 0.018$) and mycological outcome ($p = 0.004$) with fluconazole on day 14. By day 28 after therapy, fluconazole-treated patients were significantly ($p = 0.014$) more likely to be disease free than patients in the clotrimazole group who initially responded. Despite poor compliance in the clotrimazole-treated patients, fluconazole appeared to lead to superior clinical and mycological outcomes in these human immunodeficiency virus-infected patients with documented oral candidiasis.

At least three studies have evaluated fluconazole alone in immunocompromised patients with and without HIV positivity[104,119] or AIDS.[107] In only one of these studies were outcomes specifically reported for both AIDS and non-AIDS immunosuppressed patients.[107] While the mycological outcomes were not stated, 63% of the patients with AIDS were clinically cured or improved, compared with 75% and 71% of leukemic and transplant patients, respectively. Although the number of patients evaluated in this trial was small, it appears that fluconazole may be effective against serious candidal infections in immunocompromised patients. The other two trials did not separate the clinical and mycological outcomes on the basis of patient type.

Because of the limited number of studies comparing fluconazole with other antifungal regimens in AIDS patients with candidal infections, definitive conclusions about the superiority of any agent must wait.

Patients without AIDS. In general, investigators who have evaluated the efficacy of fluconazole against vaginal candidiasis used a single 150-mg oral dose and reported that *C. albicans* was the only fungal pathogen isolated from most patients or cultured at baseline. Trials comparing fluconazole with clotrimazole vaginal tablets, econazole topical treatment,[122-124] or oral ketoconazole have shown fluconazole to be superior ($p < 0.02$) in producing a favorable long-term clinical outcome.[122] In addition, patients treated with fluconazole had more rapid resolution of their symptoms than those treated with intravaginal clotrimazole ($p < 0.001$).[122] Herzog and Ansmann[123] found no significant differences in clinical outcomes between groups treated wth fluconazole or econazole, but rectal smears produced negative mycological findings more commonly in fluconazole-treated women ($p < 0.1$). Kutzer et al.[124] conducted a randomized, double-blind, placebo-controlled multicenter trial comparing single-dose fluconazole with five days of oral ketoconazole in vaginal candidiasis. There were no significant differences in clinical or mycological outcomes, but fluconazole did have the advantage of being equally effective at a single dose.

Hendel et al.[125] found that in patients with esophageal candidiasis and progressive systemic sclerosis, the frequency of negative mycological cultures was approximately 70% after two weeks of fluconazole therapy. However, the recurrence rate was quite high (>90% within three months). Clinical outcomes were not reported, since all patients had relief of symptoms (heartburn) after the institution of antireflux therapy.

Because of its renal clearance, fluconazole would be a logical candidate for use in treating fungal infections of the urinary tract. Nito[126] described excellent results (both clinically and mycologically) of treating fungal urinary tract infection in seven patients with a variety of underlying urinary tract disorders (bladder tumors [three patients], neurogenic bladder [three patients], and hydronephrosis [one patient]). Dave et al.[127] described renal candidiasis (*C. albicans*) in a patient with renal papillary necrosis and obstruction. Despite effective treatment with fluconazole, the patient relapsed and was retreated (successfully) and maintained on fluconazole therapy.

Van't Wouk et al.[133] used fluconazole in 17 nonneutropenic patients with deep-seated fungal infections. Eleven of the patients were infected by *Candida* species, and fluconazole appeared to be effective in these patients. Three patients were infected by *T. glabrata*; of these, one failed to improve.

Cohen[134] treated five profoundly immunosuppressed patients who had culture-proved deep-seated infection with *C. albicans* and *Candida parapsilosis*. Four of the patients had successful clinical and mycological outcomes.

Anaissie et al.[142] found that both fluconazole and amphotericin B were 100% effective in preventing oral candidiasis (thrush) in leukemic patients. However, two patients in the fluconazole group developed disseminated infection (one with *T. glabrata* and one with *Aspergillus terreus*), as did three in the amphotericin B group (one with *C. albicans* and two with *Aspergillus* species). Although the number of patients evaluated in this study was small, fluconazole might have an advantage over amphotericin B in terms of a more convenient dosage form and less toxicity.

Case descriptions of fluconazole treatment for candidal endocarditis,[137] peritonitis,[32,59,129] ocular infections,[128] mediastinitis,[138] invasive infection,[139] colonization,[140] and disseminated disease[141] have also appeared.

Efficacy against Other Fungal Infections

Although not labeled for such use, fluconazole has been used in the treatment of aspergillosis and coccidioidomycosis. Unlike the other important mycoses in this category, cryptococcosis and candidiasis, invasive aspergillosis does not appear to be particularly responsive to fluconazole in the immunocompromised host. This contrasts with findings for another triazole antifungal agent, itraconazole, which has been used as an effective alternative to amphotericin B in invasive aspergillosis.[147] Of particular importance in recovery from this disease is restoration of the host's neutrophils; unless this occurs, no antifungal agent can be said to be effective. In less invasive forms of aspergillosis, such as chronic pulmonary disease and aspergilloma, clinical responses to fluconazole have been documented.[102,148-151] However, some investigators have found the drug to be ineffective.[130,152]

Fluconazole has also been used to treat coccidioidal meningitis.[53,153,154] Tucker et al.[153] updated (as of August 1988) the results of a multicenter investigation evaluating the use of fluconazole for the treatment of patients ($n = 18$, including one patient with AIDS) with coccidioidal meningitis. The initial dosage of fluconazole was 50 mg/day; once safety was established, up to 400 mg/day was given. Nine of the 18 patients received concomitant therapy with amphotericin B or miconazole. Of 15 assessable patients, 10 responded to therapy and 4 did not.

In another study, two patients with meningitis caused by *C. immitis* initially responded to intravenous and intrathecal amphotericin B but developed problems related to the intrathecal administration route.[154] One of these patients deteriorated while receiving ketoconazole therapy (up to 1200 mg/day) and was treated successfully with fluconazole 50 to 150 mg/day. The second patient was also considered to have responded to fluconazole before dying of causes apparently unrelated to the drug.

Catanzaro et al.[155] evaluated the efficacy of oral fluconazole in cases of persistent pulmonary or disseminated coccidioidomycosis. Fourteen patients were treated with fluconazole 50 mg/day initially, followed by 100 mg/day if there was no satisfactory response. The average duration of treatment was 13 months. A favorable clinical response was achieved in 12 (86%) of 14 patients. Follow-up cultures were established for five of the responders; all were negative. Six (55%) of 11 surviving responders relapsed between nine days and 15 months after treatment. Higher dosages of fluconazole need to be evaluated in the treatment of coccidioidomycosis.

Phaeohyphomycoses include a spectrum of fungal diseases characterized histologically by the appearance of dematiaceous (darkly pigmented) filamentous or yeastlike cells. Therapy ranges from simple surgical excision to administration of intravenous amphotericin B. Fluconazole was effective in treating a foot lesion caused by an unidentified dematiaceous fungus[156] but was ineffective in treating a subcutaneous leg abscess caused by *Phialophora parasitica*.[157] Fluconazole also failed to produce a response in a case of *Exophiala* species tenosynovitis.[133] If the results of experimental infections in animals are borne out in clinical experience, then the activity of fluconazole may depend on the fungal species involved.[29]

The disseminated histoplasmosis of a 33-year-old HIV-seropositive patient receiving zidovudine 1200 mg/day was reported to be successfully treated with intravenous fluconazole 200 mg/day for two months.[158] A follow-up examination at 10 months revealed no signs of relapse or other opportunistic infections.

Adverse Effects

The adverse-effect profiles of amphotericin B, flucytosine, ketoconazole, and miconazole have been reviewed elsewhere.[159] Toxicological studies in animals indicate that fluconazole has little toxicity in relation to its potency as an antifungal agent.[160] Fluconazole has not been shown to be teratogenic or mutagenic.

In the experimental and clinical trials reported to date, fluconazole appears to be a well-tolerated antifungal agent. Approximately 16% of patients treated with fluconazole 50 to 400 mg/day for at least one week experienced an adverse effect considered to be "possibly related" to the drug.[161] The gastrointestinal tract was most frequently involved (7% of patients), followed by the CNS (3%) and the skin (3%). Specific adverse effects reported were nausea (3.8%), abdominal pain (2%), headache (1.9%), rash (1.7%), diarrhea (1.6%), vomiting (1.6%), and flatulence (0.9%). The occurrence of these reactions does not appear to be related to either the dosage or the duration of fluconazole administration.

Adverse effects have been considered severe enough to require discontinuation of therapy in 1.6% of patients.[161] Abdominal pain, nausea, and vomiting were the most frequent reasons for discontinuing therapy. Severe life-threatening skin rashes have been reported, including Stevens-Johnson syndrome (three patients) and toxic epidermal necrolysis (one patient); each of these patients had a diagnosis of AIDS and was receiving other medications concomitantly.

Two cases of hepatic necrosis and death in association with fluconazole therapy have been reported (Shaw GL, Pfizer Central Research. Personal communication. 1989 Dec 6). One patient was receiving fluconazole 50 mg/day for intertriginous candidiasis, and the second was being given 200 mg/day because a bronchial lavage specimen was positive for *C. albicans*. Shortly after the start of fluconazole treatment, both patients died. Autopsy results for the first patient revealed "ischemic injury" to the liver. In the second patient, a needle biopsy of the liver revealed hepatic necrosis consistent with "toxic injury."

Liver aminotransferase levels have been clinically abnormal (more than three times the upper limit of normal) in approximately 3% of patients given fluconazole. Kidd et al.[162] reported three cases of hypokalemia associated with low-dose (50 mg/day) fluconazole therapy. In each case, serum potassium returned to pretreatment levels after the discontinuation of therapy.

Schulman et al.[163] found the intravitreal use of fluconazole 5, 10, 20, 50, or 100 μg/0.1 mL to be without corneal, lenticular, or retinal toxicity in rabbits.

Drug Interactions

Drug interactions involving fluconazole have been investigated extensively,[164–167] and case reports are beginning to appear in the literature.[137,139,168–172] Much of the research has centered on the enzyme-inhibiting capability of fluconazole and its predecessor, ketoconazole. Since its approval, ketoconazole has been shown to have inhibitory effects on cytochrome P-450 isoenzymes,[173] which result in alterations in steroid biosynthesis.[14–17] Evaluation of fluconazole's effect on drug-metabolizing enzymes[174–176] and on steroidogenesis[177] indicates that it could be considered intermediate in enzyme-inducing ability when compared with ketoconazole and itraconazole and to be without substantial effect on circulating testosterone concentrations. Extensive studies have shown clinically significant interactions of drugs with fluconazole to be limited to tolbutamide,[164] warfarin,[164] rifampin,[164] cyclosporine,[166] and phenytoin.[167] The dosages of fluconazole used in these studies have ranged from 50 to 200 mg/day, and the duration of treatment has ranged from a single dose to two weeks.

Coadministration of fluconazole and tolbutamide resulted in a significant increase in the maximum serum concentration and the area under the serum drug concentration–time curve (AUC) for tolbutamide.[164] A similar result was obtained when glipizide and glyburide were evaluated for potential interactions with fluconazole.[178] Not all patients became clinically hypoglycemic or required medical treatment; however, patients receiving these agents along with fluconazole may need to be carefully monitored for hypoglycemic episodes.

In a crossover study assessing the effects of fluconazole 200 mg/day on the pharmacodynamics of warfarin in healthy volunteers, a 7% increase in the area under the prothrombin activity curve was detected.[164] While the clinical importance of this observation is unknown, anecdotal reports suggest the need for caution in patients receiving fluconazole and warfarin.[137]

Rifampin administration has caused a significant reduction in the AUC and half-life of fluconazole.[164] While this interaction raises some interesting questions about the liver metabolism and first-pass effect of fluconazole, it may be necessary to administer increased doses of fluconazole if it is given with rifampin.

Graves et al.[166] studied 16 renal transplant patients receiving long-term cyclosporine therapy to evaluate the effect of fluconazole 200 mg/day on the AUC and minimum plasma concentration (C_{min}) of cyclosporine. A significant ($p < 0.05$) increase in cyclosporine AUC and C_{min} occurred when fluconazole was given. Therefore, patients receiving cyclosporine might be at increased risk of toxicity when that agent is given with fluconazole.

An investigation of the effect of fluconazole on the disposition of phenytoin showed a 75% increase in the phenytoin AUC from 0 to 24 hours.[167] In the same study, the C_{min} of phenytoin increased 128% between day 4 (phenytoin only) and day 21 (phenytoin administered with fluconazole).

Availability, Dosage, and Administration

Fluconazole (Diflucan, Roerig Division of Pfizer Pharmaceuticals) is available in pink trapezoidal tablets containing 50, 100, or 200 mg of fluconazole for oral administration. Fluconazole is also available in a sterile solution (100- or 200-mL volume) containing fluconazole 2 mg/mL for intravenous administration.[179] The following dosages (oral or intravenous single daily doses) are recommended for patients with normal renal function: for oropharyngeal candidiasis, 200 mg on day 1, followed by 100 mg/day thereafter; for esophageal candidiasis, 200 mg on day 1, followed by 100 to 400 mg/day; for systemic candidiasis, 400 mg on day 1, followed by 200 mg/day; and for acute cryptococcal meningitis, 400 mg on day 1, followed by 200 to 400 mg/day. High-dose fluconazole (800 mg/day) was given without adverse effect by Ansari et al.[180] for the treatment of recurrent oropharyngeal candidiasis in a patient with AIDS. The use of higher dosages has yet to be described.

Intravenous fluconazole should be infused at a rate not higher than 200 mg/hr. Adjustments of fluconazole dosages are necessary in patients with impaired renal function and should follow suggested guidelines based on creatinine clearance (CL_{cr}): If CL_{cr} is >50 mL/min, give 100% of the recommended daily dose; if CL_{cr} is 21 to 50 mL/min, give 50% of the recommended daily dose; if CL_{cr} is 11 to 20 mL/min, give 25% of the recommended daily dose; and if the patient is receiving regular hemodialysis, give the regularly recommended dose after each dialysis procedure.[179]

Cost

Table 6 gives the costs (based on average wholesale prices) of 14 days of therapy with fluconazole and other antifungal agents.[181] Preparation, administration, and laboratory-monitoring costs are not included.

FDA-Approved Labeling

Indications in FDA-approved labeling for fluconazole are the treatment of oropharyngeal and

Table 6.
Drug Acquisition Costs for 14 Days of Antifungal Therapy

Drug Product	Dosage	Average Wholesale Cost ($)[a]
Fluconazole (Diflucan)		
Tablets	200 mg once, then 100 mg/day	84.72
	400 mg once, then 200 mg/day	142.09
Injection	200 mg once, then 100 mg/day	513.08
	400 mg once, then 200 mg/day	999.32
Amphotericin B (Fungizone) injection	50 mg/day	480.90[b]
Ketoconazole (Nizoral) tablets	200 mg twice daily	46.32
Nystatin (Mycostatin) oral suspension	500,000 units q.i.d.	31.77
Clotrimazole (Mycelex) oral lozenges[c]	10 mg five times daily	38.96

[a] Based on *American Druggist Blue Book.*[181] Costs do not include associated expenses such as those of diluent, i.v. sets, or premedications.

[b] Cost of maintenance dosage only; cost of upward adjustment of dosage not included.

[c] Cost of treatment of vulvovaginal candidiasis is $13.06 (Mycelex-G vaginal tablet 100 mg/day for seven days) or $10.90 (Mycelex-G vaginal tablet 500 mg once).

esophageal candidiasis and cryptococcal meningitis.

Formulary Recommendation

Fluconazole is a broad-spectrum antifungal agent whose properties in vitro do not accurately reflect its potential therapeutic value. Experimental and clinical data have established the effectiveness and safety of fluconazole in vivo and have identified a number of unique pharmacokinetic features. Although labeled indications include only the treatment of oropharyngeal and esophageal candidiasis and cryptococcal meningitis, fluconazole may prove useful in the treatment of other systemic mycoses.

Fluconazole provides the clinician with an effective alternative drug that can be safely used in patients unable to tolerate the adverse effects associated with amphotericin B. In addition, because fluconazole does not interact with P-450 enzyme systems, it may have fewer interactions with drugs or endogenous substances metabolized by this pathway and consequently may be safer then ketoconazole.

Given these advantages, the use of fluconazole is likely to expand even in the absence of clinical data demonstrating superior efficacy. The threshold for beginning antifungal chemotherapy or prophylaxis is likely to drop, and concomitant regimens of antibacterial and antifungal agents may become more commonplace. Therefore, it might be appropriate to restrict or otherwise focus the use of fluconazole until additional findings support its routine use as first-line antifungal therapy. Studies support fluconazole as being more appropriate for maintenance (rather than initial) therapy of cryptococcal meningitis. Although information on the use of fluconazole for prophylaxis is limited, the drug is likely to be frequently used (e.g., in the febrile, granulocytopenic patient unresponsive to a 7- to 10-day course of antibacterials). The possibility that fungi may develop resistance to fluconazole or cross-resistance to other antifungal agents should discourage routine use of fluconazole for this indication. As familiarity with fluconazole increases and as higher dosages and more extended treatment regimens are studied, clinicians will need to re-evaluate therapies and be alert to potential adverse effects and drug interactions not yet described.

Conclusion

Fluconazole is a broad-spectrum antifungal drug that appears comparable in efficacy to other antifungal agents in the treatment of some systemic mycoses and that offers unique pharmacokinetic properties, relative safety, and convenience. More studies must be completed before fluconazole can be recommended as a first-line antifungal therapy.

References

1. Holt RJ, Newman RL. Laboratory assessment of the antimycotic drug clotrimazole. *J Clin Pathol*. 1972; 25:1089–97.
2. Heel RC, Brogden RN, Pakes GE et al. Miconazole: a preliminary review of its therapeutic efficacy in systemic fungal infections. *Drugs*. 1980; 19:7–30.
3. Sonino N. The use of ketoconazole as an inhibitor of steroid production. *N Engl J Med*. 1987; 317:812–8.
4. Daneshmend TK, Warnock DW. Clinical pharmacokinetics of ketoconazole. *Clin Pharmacokinet*. 1988; 14:13–34.
5. Graybill JR. New antifungal agents. *Eur J Clin Microbiol Infect Dis*. 1989; 8:402–12.
6. Fromtling RA. Overview of medically important antifungal azole derivatives. *Clin Microbiol Rev*. 1988; 1:187–217.
7. Saag MS, Dismukes WE. Azole antifungal agents: emphasis on new triazoles. *Antimicrob Agents Chemother*. 1988; 32:1–8.
8. Richardson K, Cooper K, Marriott MS et al. Design and evaluation of a systemically active agent, fluconazole. *Ann NY Acad Sci*. 1988; 544:4–11.
9. Vanden Bossche H. Biochemical targets for antifungal azole-derivatives. Hypothesis of the mode of action. *Curr Top Med Mycol*. 1985; 1:313–51.
10. Vanden Bossche H, Willemsens G, Cools W et al. In vitro and in vivo effects of the antimycotic drug ketoconazole on sterol synthesis. *Antimicrob Agents Chemother*. 1980; 17:922–8.
11. Vanden Bossche H, Willemsens G, Cools W et al. Hypothesis on the molecular basis of the antifungal activation of N-substituted imidazoles and triazoles. *Biochem Soc Trans*. 1983; 11:665–7.
12. Brajtburg J, Powderly WG, Kobayashi GS et al. Amphotericin B: current understanding of mechanisms of action. *Antimicrob Agents Chemother*. 1990; 34:183–8.
13. Murray M. Mechanisms of the inhibition of cytochrome P-450-mediated drug oxidation by therapeutic agents. *Drug Metab Rev*. 1987; 18:55–81.
14. Pont A, Williams PL, Azhar S et al. Ketoconazole blocks testosterone synthesis. *Arch Intern Med*. 1982; 142:2137–40.
15. Malozowski S, Merico V, Cassoria F. Effects of ketoconazole on rat ovarian steroidogenic enzymatic activities. *Res Commun Chem Pathol Pharmacol*. 1986; 52:403–6.
16. Pont A, Williams PL, Loose DS et al. Ketoconazole blocks adrenal steroid synthesis. *Ann Intern Med*. 1982; 97:370–2.
17. Loose DS, Kna PB, Hirst MA et al. Ketoconazole blocks adrenal steroidogenesis by inhibiting cytochrome P450-dependent enzymes. *J Clin Invest*. 1983; 71:1495–9.
18. Mosca P, Bonazzi P, Novelli G et al. In vivo and in vitro inhibition of hepatic microsomal drug metabolism by ketoconazole. *Br J Exp Pathol*. 1985; 66:737–42.
19. Sheets JJ, Mason JL. Ketoconazole: a potent inhibitor of cytochrome P-450-dependent drug metabolism in rat liver. *Drug Metab Dispos*. 1984; 12:603–6.
20. Denollin S, Vanbelle H, Goossens F et al. Cytochemical and biochemical studies of yeasts after in vitro exposure to miconazole. *Antimicrob Agents Chemother*. 1977; 11:500–13.
21. Shigematsu ML, Uno J, Arai T. Effect of ketoconazole on isolated mitochondria from *Candida albicans*. *Antimicrob Agents Chemother*. 1982; 21:919–24.
22. Uno J, Shigematsu ML, Arai T. Primary site of action of ketoconazole on *Candida albicans*. *Antimicrob Agents Chemother*. 1982; 21:912–8.
23. Polak A, Dixon DM. In vitro/in vivo correlation of antifungal susceptibility testing using 5-fluorocytosine and ketoconazole as examples of two extremes. In: Fromtling RA, ed. Recent trends in the discovery, development and evaluation of antifungal agents. Barcelona, Spain: Prous; 1987:45–59.
24. Kobayashi GS, Spitzer ED. Testing of organisms for susceptibility to triazoles: is it justified? *Eur J Clin Microbiol Infect Dis*. 1989; 8:387–9.

25. Polak A. Combination therapy of experimental candidiasis, cryptococcosis, aspergillosis and wangiellosis in mice. *Chemotherapy.* 1987; 33:381–95.
26. Odds FC, Chessman SL, Abbott AB. Antifungal effects of fluconazole (UK 49858), a new triazole. *J Antimicrob Chemother.* 1986; 18:473–8.
27. Roger TE, Galgiani JN. Activity of fluconazole (UK 49,858) and ketoconazole against *Candida albicans* in vitro and in vivo. *Antimicrob Agents Chemother.* 1986; 30:418–22.
28. Palou de Fernandez E, Patino MM, Graybill JR et al. Treatment of cryptococcal meningitis in mice with fluconazole. *J Antimicrob Chemother.* 1986; 18; 261–70.
29. Dixon DM, Polak A. In vitro and in vivo drug studies with three agents of central nervous system phaeohyphomycosis. *Chemotherapy.* 1987; 33:129–40.
30. Kobayashi GS, Travis SJ, Medoff G. Comparison of fluconazole and amphotericin B in treating histoplasmosis in immunosuppressed mice. *Antimicrob Agents Chemother.* 1987; 31:2005–6.
31. Polak A, Dixon DM. Fungistatic and fungicidal effects of amphotericin B, ketoconazole and fluconazole (UK-49,858) against *Histoplasma capsulatum* in vitro and in vivo. *Mykosen.* 1987; 30;186–94.
32. Ahlmen J, Edebo L, Eriksson C et al. Fluconazole therapy for fungal peritonitis in continuous ambulatory peritoneal dialysis (CAPD). A case report. *Peritoneal Dial Int.* 1989; 9:79–80.
33. Gordon MA, Lapa EW, Passero PG. Improved method for azole antifungal susceptibility testing. *J Clin Microbiol.* 1988; 26:1874–7.
34. Smith KJ, Warnock DW, Kennedy CT et'al. Azole resistance in *Candida albicans. J Med Vet Mycol.* 1986; 24:133–44.
35. Warnock DW, Burke J, Cope NJ et al. Fluconazole resistance in *Candida glabrata. Lancet.* 1988; 2:1310.
36. Redding SW, Smith JA, Rinaldi MG et al. In vitro susceptibility patterns in AIDS patients receiving fluconazole for thrush. Paper presented at 30th Interscience Conference on Antimicrobial Agents and Chemotherapy. Atlanta, GA: 1990 Oct 24.
37. Fulton P, Phillips P. Fluconazole resistance during suppressive therapy of AIDS-related thrush and esophagitis caused by *Candida albicans.* Paper presented at Sixth International Conference on AIDS. San Francisco, CA: 1990 Jun 21.
38. Powderly WG, Keath EJ, Little JR et al. Resistant *Cryptococcus neoformans* in a patient with AIDS. Paper presented at 30th Interscience Conference on Antimicrobial Agents and Chemotherapy. Atlanta, GA: 1990 Oct 24.
39. Humphrey MJ, Jevons S, Tarbit MH. Pharmacokinetic evaluation of UK-49,858, a metabolically stable triazole antifungal drug, in animals and humans. *Antimicrob Agents Chemother.* 1985; 28:648–53.
40. Milliken S, Powles R, Jones A et al. Pharmacokinetics of oral fluconazole in autologous bone marrow transplantation recipients given TBI and high-dose melphalan. *Transplant Proc.* 1989; 21:3067.
41. Houang ET, Chappatte O, Byrne O et al. Fluconazole levels in plasma and vaginal secretions of patients after a 150-milligram single oral dose and rate of eradication of infection in vaginal candidiasis. *Antimicrob Agents Chemother.* 1990; 34:909–10.
42. Foulds G, Wajszczuk C, Weidler DJ et al. Steady state parenteral kinetics of fluconazole in man. *Ann NY Acad Sci.* 1988; 544:427–30.
43. Brugman J, VanCusten J, Heykants J et al. Systemic antifungal potential, safety and transport of miconazole nitrate. *Eur J Clin Pharmacol.* 1972; 5:93–9.
44. Duhm B, Maul W, Medenwald H et al. The pharmacokinetics of clotrimazole-^{14}C. *Postgrad Med J.* 1974; 50(Suppl 1):13–6.
45. Heel RC, Brogden RN, Speight TM et al. Econazole: a review of its antifungal activity and therapeutic efficacy. *Drugs.* 1978; 16:177–201.
46. Drew RH, Perfect JR, Gallis HA. Use of fluconazole in a patient with documented malabsorption of ketoconazole. *Clin Pharm.* 1988; 7:622–3.
47. Brammer KW, Tarbit MH. A review of the pharmacokinetics of fluconazole (UK-49,858) in laboratory animals and man. In: Fromtling RA, ed. Recent trends in the discovery, development and evaluation of antifungal agents. Barcelona, Spain: Prous; 1987:141–9.
48. Walsh TJ, Foulds G, Pizzo PA. Pharmacokinetics and tissue penetration of fluconazole in rabbits. *Antimicrob Agents Chemother.* 1989; 33:467–9.
49. Perfect JR, Durack DT. Penetration of imidazoles and triazoles into cerebrospinal fluid of rabbits. *J Antimicrob Chemother.* 1985; 16:81–6.
50. Arndt CAS, Walsh TJ, McCully CL et al. Fluconazole penetration into cerebrospinal fluid: implications for treating fungal infections of the central nervous system. *J Infect Dis.* 1988; 157:178–80.
51. Perfect JR, Savari DV, Durack DT. Comparison on itraconazole and fluconazole in treatment of cryptococcal meningitis and *Candida* pyelonephritis in rabbits. *Antimicrob Agents Chemother.* 1986; 29:579–83.
52. Foulds G, Brennan DR, Wajszczuk C et al. Fluconazole penetration into cerebrospinal fluid in humans. *J Clin Pharmacol.* 1988; 28:363–6.
53. Tucker RM, Williams PL, Arathoon EG et al. Pharmacokinetics of fluconazole in cerebrospinal fluid and serum in human coccidioidal meningitis. *Antimicrob Agents Chemother.* 1988; 32:369–73.
54. Ebden P, Neill P, Farrow PR. Sputum levels of fluconazole in humans. *Antimicrob Agents Chemother.* 1989; 33:963–4.
55. Savani DV, Perfect JR, Cobo LM et al. Penetration of new azole compounds into the eye and efficacy in experimental *Candida* endophthalmitis. *Antimicrob Agents Chemother.* 1987; 31:6–10.
56. Dellenbach P. Penetration of fluconazole into vaginal tissue and secretions. *R Soc Med Int Congr Symp Ser.* 1989; 160:19–22.
57. Debruyne D, Ryckelynck J-P, Moulin M et al. Pharmacokinetics of fluconazole in patients undergoing continuous ambulatory peritoneal dialysis. *Clin Pharmacokinet.* 1990; 18:491–8.
58. Toon S, Ross CE, Gokal R et al. Effects of impaired renal function on the oral pharmacokinetics of fluconazole. Paper presented at 10th International Congress of the Society for Human and Animal Mycology. Barcelona, Spain: 1988 Jun 27–Jul 1.
59. Levine J, Bernard DB, Idelson BA et al. Fungal peritonitis complicating continuous ambulatory peritoneal dialysis: successful treatment with fluconazole, a new orally active antifungal agent. *Am J Med.* 1989; 86:825–7.
60. Troke PF, Andrews RJ, Marriott MS et al. Efficacy of fluconazole (UK-49,858) against experimental aspergillosis and cryptococcosis in mice. *J Antimicrob Chemother.* 1987; 19:663–70.
61. Patterson TF, Miniter P, Andriole VT. Efficacy of fluconazole in experimental invasive aspergillosis. *Rev Infect Dis.* 1990; 12(Suppl 3):S281–5.
62. Graybill JR, Sun SH, Ahrens J. Treatment of murine coccidioidal meningitis with fluconazole (UK49,858). *J Med Vet Mycol.* 1986; 24:113–9.
63. Graybill JR, Griffith L, Sun SH. Fluconazole therapy for coccidioidomycosis in Japanese macaques. *Rev Infect Dis.* 1990; 12(Suppl 3):S286–90.
64. Levine HB. Fluconazole in murine coccidioidomycosis. Paper presented at 26th Interscience Conference on Antimicrobial Agents and Chemotherapy. New Orleans, LA: 1986 Sep 30.
65. Clemons KV, Hanson LH, Perlman AM et al. Efficacy of SCH39304 and fluconazole in a murine model of disseminated coccidioidomycosis. *Antimicrob Agents Chemother.* 1990; 34:928–30.
66. Kobayashi GS, Travis S, Medoff G. Comparison of the in

vitro and in vivo activity of the bis-triazole derivative UK 49,858 with that of amphotericin B against *Histoplasma capsulatum*. *Antimicrob Agents Chemother*. 1986; 29:660–2.
67. Graybill JR, Palou E, Ahrens J. Treatment of murine histoplasmosis with UK 49,858 (fluconazole). *Am Rev Respir Dis*. 1986; 134; 768–70.
68. Richardson K, Brammer KW, Marriott MS et al. Activity of UK-49,858, a bis-triazole derivative, against experimental infections with *Candida albicans* and *Trichophyton mentagrophytes*. *Antimicrob Agents Chemother*. 1985; 27:832–5.
69. Troke PF, Andrews RJ, Brammer KW et al. Efficacy of UK-49,858 (fluconazole) against *Candida albicans* experimental infections in mice. *Antimicrob Agents Chemother*. 1985; 825–8.
70. Hughes CE, Bennett RL, Tuna IC et al. Activities of fluconazole (UK 49,858) and ketoconazole against ketoconazole-susceptible and -resistant *Candida albicans*. *Antimicrob Agents Chemother*. 1988; 32:209–12.
71. Fisher MA, Lee PG, Tarry WF. Fluconazole (UK-49,858) treatment of candidiasis in normal and diabetic rats. *Antimicrob Agents Chemother*. 1989; 33:1042–5.
72. Martin MV. A comparison of fluconazole and ketoconazole in the treatment of rat palatal candidosis. *J Med Vet Mycol*. 1989; 27:63–70.
73. Lyman CA, Sugar AM, Diamond RD. Comparative activities of UK-49,858 and amphotericin B against *Blastomyces dermatitidis* infections in mice. *Antimicrob Agents Chemother*. 1986; 29:161–1.
74. Sugar AM, Picard M, Noble L. Comparison of SCH 39304, fluconazole, and amphotericin B in the treatment of murine pulmonary blastomycosis. Paper presented at 29th Interscience Conference on Antimicrobial Agents and Chemotherapy. Houston, TX: 1989 Sep 19.
75. Stevens DA, Brummer E, McEwen JG et al. Comparison of fluconazole and ketoconazole in experimental murine blastomycosis. *Rev Infect Dis*. 1990; 12(Suppl 3):S304–6.
76. Fisher MA, Shen SH, Haddad J et al. Comparison of in vivo activity of fluconazole with that of amphotericin B against *Candida tropicalis*, *Candida glabrata*, and *Candida krusei*. *Antimicrob Agents Chemother*. 1989; 33:1443–6.
77. Faergemann J. Activity of triazole derivatives against *Pityrosporum orbiculare* in vitro and in vivo. *Ann NY Acad Sci*. 1988; 544;348–53.
78. Dixon DM, Walsh TJ. Antifungal agents. In: Barron S, ed. Medical microbiology. 3rd ed. New York: Churchill Livingstone; in press.
79. Walsh TJ. Recent advances in the treatment of fungal infections. *Methods Find Exp Clin Pharmacol*. 1987; 9:769–78.
80. Zuger A, Louis E, Holzman RS et al. Cryptococcal disease in patients with the acquired immunodeficiency syndrome. Diagnostic features and outcome of treatment. *Ann Intern Med*. 1986; 104:234–40.
81. Dupont B. Traitement d'attaque et d'entretien des meningoencephalites cryptococciques ali cours du sida. *Med Mal Infect*. 1988; 18:737–41.
82. Dupont B, Drouhet E. Cryptococcal meningitis and fluconazole. *Ann Intern Med*. 1987; 106:778.
83. Byrne WR, Wajszczuk CP. Cryptococcal meningitis in the acquired immunodeficiency syndrome (AIDS): successful treatment with fluconazole after failure of amphotericin B. *Ann Intern Med*. 1988; 108; 384–5.
84. Esposito R, Foppa CU, Antinori S. Fluconazole for cryptococcal meningitis. *Ann Intern Med*. 1989; 110:170. Letter.
85. Stern JJ, Hartman BJ, Sharkey P et al. Oral fluconazole therapy for patients with acquired immunodeficiency syndrome and cryptococcosis: experience with 22 patients. *Am J Med*. 1988; 85:477–80.
86. Tozzi V, Bordi E, Galgani S et al. Fluconazole treatment of cryptococcosis in patients with acquired immunodeficiency syndrome. *Am J Med*. 1989; 87:353.
87. Sugar AM, Saunders C. Oral fluconazole as suppressive therapy of disseminated cryptococcosis in patients with acquired immunodeficiency syndrome. *Am J Med*. 1988; 85:481–9.
88. Larsen RA, Leal MAE, Chan LS. Fluconazole compared with amphotericin B plus flucytosine for cryptococcal meningitis in AIDS. *Ann Intern Med*. 1990; 113:183–7.
89. Dismukes W, Cloud G, Thompson S et al. Fluconazole versus amphotericin B therapy of acute cryptococcal meningitis. Paper presented at 29th Interscience Conference on Antimicrobial Agents and Chemotherapy. Houston, TX: 1989 Sep 20.
90. Powderly W, Saag M, Cloud G et al. Fluconazole versus amphotericin B as maintenance therapy for prevention of relapse of AIDS-associated cryptococcal meningitis. Paper presented at 30th Interscience Conference on Antimicrobial Agents and Chemotherapy. Atlanta, GA: 1990 Oct 24.
91. Squires K, Rowland V, Gassyuk E et al. Fluconazole as therapy for acute cryptococcal meningitis. Paper presented at 30th Interscience Conference on Antimicrobial Agents and Chemotherapy. Atlanta, GA: 1990 Oct 23.
92. Pietroski N, Buckley RM, Braffman MN et al. Intravenous and oral fluconazole in treatment of acute cryptococcal meningitis in AIDS. Paper presented at 30th Interscience Conference on Antimicrobial Agents and Chemotherapy. Atlanta, GA: 1990 Oct 23.
93. Bozzette SA, Larsen R, Chiu J et al. Successful secondary prophylaxis of cryptococcal meningitis with fluconazole: a placebo-controlled trial. Paper presented at 30th Interscience Conference on Antimicrobial Agents and Chemotherapy. Atlanta, GA: 1990 Oct 24.
94. Gritti MF, Raise E, Vannini V et al. Fluconazole treatment for fungal infections in ARC and AIDS. Paper presented at Fifth International Conference on AIDS. Montreal, Que.: 1989 Jun 5.
95. Rubin R, Robinson PA, Knirsch AK et al. Fluconazole therapy of patients with AIDS and cryptococcal meningitis and failed conventional antifungal therapy. Paper presented at Fifth International Conference on AIDS. Montreal, Que.: 1989 Jun 7.
96. Sanjana V, Davidson M, Mullen M et al. Intravenous and oral fluconazole for the treatment of acute cryptococcal meningitis. Paper presented at Fifth International Conference on AIDS. Montreal, Que.: 1989 Jun 7.
97. Bozzette SA, Larsen RA, Chiu J et al. Fluconazole treatment of persistent urinary cryptococcosis after cryptococcal meningitis. Paper presented at Fifth International Conference on AIDS. Montreal, Que.: 1989 Jun 7.
98. Sanjana V, Davidson M, Mullen M et al. Intravenous and oral fluconazole in the treatment of acute cryptococcal meningitis. Paper presented at Sixth International Conference on AIDS. San Francisco, CA: 1990 Jun 21.
99. Marchou B, Pascal C, Carles M et al. Fluconazole: a first-line drug for cryptococcosis in AIDS. Paper presented at Sixth International Conference on AIDS. San Francisco, CA: 1990 Jun 21.
100. Van't Wout JW, deGraeff-Meeder ER, Paul LC et al. Treatment of two cases of cryptococcal meningitis with fluconazole. *Scand J Infect Dis*. 1988; 20:193–8.
101. Shuttleworth D, Philpot CM, Knight AG. Cutaneous cryptococcosis: treatment with oral fluconazole. *Br J Dermatol*. 1989; 120:683–7.
102. Ikemoto H, Watanabe K, More T et al. Clinical study of fluconazole on deep seated fungal infections. *Jpn J Antibiot*. 1989; 42:63–116.
103. DeWit S, Goossens H, Weerts D et al. Comparison of fluconazole and ketoconazole for oropharyngeal candidiasis in AIDS. *Lancet*. 1989; 1:746–7.
104. Dupont B, Drouhet E. Fluconazole for the treatment of fungal diseases in immunosuppressed patients. *J Med Vet Mycol*. 1986; 26:67–71.
105. Chave JP, Cajot A, Bille J et al. Single-dose therapy for oral candidiasis with fluconazole in HIV-infected adults: A pilot study. *J Infect Dis*. 1989; 19:806–7.
106. Nathwani D, Green ST, McGuire W et al. New triazole antifungal agents (fluconazole and itraconazole) in the

treatment of HIV-related gastrointestinal candidiasis. *Scand J Infect Dis*. 1989; 21:355–6.
107. Rubin RH, Debruin MF, Knirsch AK. Fluconazole therapy for patients with serious *Candida* infections who have failed standard therapy. Paper presented at 29th Interscience Conference on Antimicrobial Agents and Chemotherapy. Houston, TX: 1989 Sep 18.
108. DeWit S, Rahir F, Weerts D et al. Single dose versus 7 days fluconazole for treatment of oral candidiasis in HIV infected patients: a prospective randomized study. Paper presented at 30th Interscience Conference on Antimicrobial Agents and Chemotherapy. Atlanta, GA: 1990 Oct 24.
109. Pons VG, Greenspan D, Koletar SL et al. Comparative study of fluconazole and clotrimazole troches for the treatment of oral thrush in AIDS. Paper presented at 30th Interscience Conference on Antimicrobial Agents and Chemotherapy. Atlanta, GA: 1990 Oct 24.
110. Chave JP, Vernazza P, Margalith D et al. Single-dose therapy for esophageal candidiasis with fluconazole: a pilot study. Paper presented at Fifth International Conference on AIDS. Montreal, Que.: 1989 Jun 8.
111. Cajot A. Single dose therapy for oral candidiasis with fluconazole in HIV-infected adults. Paper presented at Fifth International Conference on AIDS. Montreal, Que.: 1989 Jun 8.
112. Just G, Schnellbach M, Bottinger C et al. Fluconazole in the treatment of oropharyngeal candidiasis in HIV-positive patients. Paper presented at Fifth International Conference on AIDS. Montreal, Que.: 1989 Jun 8.
113. Espositio R, Uberti CF, Cernuschi M. Treatment of HIV+ patients with oropharyngeal and/or oesophageal candidiasis: the results of A.D.B. study. Paper presented at Fifth International Conference on AIDS. Montreal, Que.: 1989 Jun 8.
114. Lim SG, Hales M, Lee CA et al. Fluconazole for oropharyngeal candidiasis in anti-HIV positive haemophiliacs. Paper presented at Fifth International Conference on AIDS. Montreal, Que.: 1989 Jun 8.
115. Gil A, Lavilla P, Gonzalez A et al. Fluconazole treatment of esophageal candidiasis in AIDS patients. Paper presented at Fifth International Conference on AIDS. Montreal, Que.: 1989 Jun 5.
116. Tschechne B, Brunkhorst U, Schedel I et al. Treatment of therapy-resistent oro-pharyngeal candidiasis with fluconazole in HIV-1-infected patients. Paper presented at Fifth International Conference on AIDS. Montreal, Que.: 1989 Jun 5.
117. Lavilla P, Gil A, Valencia ME et al. Fluconazole preventive therapy for *Candida* esophagitis in AIDS. Paper presented at Sixth International Conference on AIDS. San Francisco, CA: 1990 Jun 21.
118. DeWit S, Rahir F, Urbain D et al. Treatment of esophageal candidiasis with fluconazole: a prospective study. Paper presented at Sixth International Conference on AIDS. San Francisco, CA: 1990 Jun 21.
119. Viscoli C, Castagnola E, Barigione D et al. Fluconazole in the treatment of candidiasis in compromised children. Paper presented at 30th Interscience Conference on Antimicrobial Agents and Chemotherapy. Atlanta, GA: 1990 Oct 23.
120. Koletar SL, Russell JA, Fass RJ et al. Comparison of oral fluconazole and clotrimazole troches as treatment for oral candidiasis in patients infected with human immunodeficiency virus. *Antimicrob Agents Chemother*. 1990; 34:2267–8.
121. Lebech PE, Nielsen NC, Lundvall F et al. Treatment of vaginal candidiasis with a single oral dose of fluconazole. *Eur J Microbiol Infect Dis*. 1988; 7:364–7.
122. Anderson GM, Barrat J, Bergan T et al. A comparison of single-dose oral fluconazole with 3-day intravaginal clotrimazole in the treatment of vaginal candidiasis. Report of an international multicentre trial. *Br J Obstet Gynaecol*. 1989; 96:226–32.
123. Herzog RE, Ansmann EB. Treatment of vaginal candidosis with fluconazole. *Mycoses*. 1989; 32:204–8.
124. Kutzer E, Oittner R, Leodolter S et al. A comparison of fluconazole and ketoconazole in the oral treatment of vaginal candidiasis: report of a double-blind multicentre trial. *Eur J Obstet Gynecol Reprod Biol*. 1988; 29:305–13.
125. Hendel L, Svejgaard E, Walsoe I et al. Esophageal candidosis in progressive systemic sclerosis: occurrence, significance and treatment with fluconazole. *Scand J Gastroenterol*. 1988; 23:1182–6.
126. Nito H. Clinical efficacy of fluconazole in urinary tract fungal infections. *Jpn J Antibiot*. 1989; 42:171–8.
127. Dave J, Hickey MM, Wilkins EGL. Fluconazole in renal candidosis. *Lancet*. 1989; 1:163–4.
128. Cruciani M, DiPerri G, Concia E et al. Fluconazole and fungal ocular infection. *J Antimicrob Chemother*. 1990; 25:718–20.
129. Thomas MG, Ellis-Pegler RB. Fluconazole treatment of *Candida glabrata* peritonitis. *J Antimicrob Chemother*. 1989; 24:94–6.
130. Kujath P, Lerch K. Secondary mycosis in surgery: treatment with fluconazole. *Infection*. 1989; 17:111–7.
131. Bunin IS, Camitta B. Oral fluconazole for treatment of disseminated fungal infection. *Pediatr Infect Dis J*. 1989; 8:62. Letter.
132. Maruta A, Matsuzaki M, Fukawa H et al. Clinical evaluation of fluconazole in the case of deep mycosis associated with leukemia. *Jpn J Antibiot*. 1989; 42:117–26.
133. Van't Wouk JW, Mattie H, vanFurth R. A prospective study of the efficacy of fluconazole (UK-49,858) against deep-seated fungal infections. *J Antimicrob Chemother*. 1988; 21:665–72.
134. Cohen J. Treatment of systemic yeast infection with fluconazole. *J Antimicrob Chemother*. 1989; 23:294–5.
135. Hay RJ, Clayton YM. Fluconazole in the management of patients with chronic mucocutaneous candidiasis. *Br J Dermatol*. 1988; 119:683–5.
136. Meunier F, Gerain J, Snoeck R et al. Fluconazole therapy of oropharyngeal candidiasis in cancer patients. In: Fromtling RA, ed. Recent trends in the discovery, development and evaluation of antifungal agents. Barcelona, Spain: Prous; 1987:169–74.
137. Isalska BJ, Stanbridge TN. Fluconazole in the treatment of candidal prosthetic valve endocarditis. *Br Med J*. 1988; 297:178–9.
138. Kirk AJB, Gould FK, Freeman R et al. Fluconazole and candidosis. *Lancet*. 1989; 1:339. Letter.
139. Conti DJ, Tolkoff-Rubin NE, Baker GP et al. Successful treatment of invasive fungal infection with fluconazole in organ transplant recipients. *Transplantation*. 1989; 48: 692–5.
140. Viscoli C, Castagnola E, Corsini M et al. Fluconazole therapy in an underweight infant. *Eur J Microbiol Infect Dis*. 1989; 8:925–6.
141. Jakab K, Kelemen E, Prinz G et al. Amphotericin-resistant invasive hepatosplenic candidiasis controlled by fluconazole. *Lancet*. 1990; 335:473–4.
142. Anaissie E, Reuben A, Cunningham K et al. Randomized trial of fluconazole versus intravenous amphotericin B for antifungal prophylaxis in neutropenic patients with leukemia. Paper presented at 30th Interscience Conference on Antimicrobial Agents and Chemotherapy. Atlanta, GA: 1990 Oct 23.
143. Galgiani JN. Fluconazole, a new antifungal agent. *Ann Intern Med*. 1990; 113:177–9.
144. Kibbler CC, Odds FC. Fluconazole versus ketoconazole in oropharyngeal candidiasis in AIDS. *Lancet*. 1989; 1:1130. Letter.
145. Cauwenbergh G. Fluconazole versus ketoconazole in oropharyngeal candidiasis in AIDS. *Lancet*. 1989; 1:1130. Letter.
146. Smith DE, Gazzard BG. Fluconazole versus ketoconazole in oropharyngeal candidiasis in AIDS. *Lancet*. 1989; 1:1131. Letter.

147. Vivani MA, Tortorano AM, Woenstenborgs R et al. Experience with itraconazole in deep mycosis in northern Italy. *Mykosen*. 1987; 30:233–44.
148. Lee Y, Ikeda S, Katsura A et al. Clinical efficacy of fluconazole in the patient with pulmonary mycosis. *Jpn J Antibiot*. 1989; 42:138–43.
149. Yoneda R. A clinical study of fluconazole in pulmonary aspergillosis. *Jpn J Antibiot*. 1989; 42:40–6.
150. Matsushima T, Ikeda H, Tomizawa S et al. Clinical evaluation of fluconazole in patients with mycotic infection. *Jpn J Antibiot*. 1989; 42:153–63.
151. Lee Y, Shiota T, Ikeda S et al. Clinical efficacy of fluconazole in the patient with pulmonary mycosis. *Jpn J Antibiot*. 1989; 42:138–43.
152. Nakashima M. The clinical study of fluconazole against pulmonary cryptococcosis and aspergillosis. *Jpn J Antibiot*. 1989; 42:127–37.
153. Tucker RM, Galgianni JN, Denning DW et al. Treatment of coccidioidal meningitis with fluconazole. *Rev Infect Dis*. 1990; 12(Suppl 3):S380–9.
154. Classen DC, Burke JP, Smith CB. Treatment of coccidioidal meningitis with fluconazole. *J Infect Dis*. 1988; 158:903–4.
155. Catanzaro A, Fierer J, Fiedman PJ. Fluconazole in the treatment of persistent coccidioidomycosis. *Chest*. 1990; 97: 666–9.
156. Noel SB, Greer DL, Abadie SM et al. Primary cutaneous phaeohyphomycosis. Report of three cases. *J Am Acad Dermatol*. 1988; 18:1023–30.
157. Fincher RME, Fisher JF, Padhye AA et al. Subcutaneous phaeohyphomycotic abscess caused by *Phialophora parasitica* in a renal allograft recipient. *J Med Vet Mycol*. 1988; 26:311–4.
158. Smith E, Franzmann M, Mathiesen LR. Disseminated histoplasmosis in a Danish patient with AIDS. *Scand J Infect Dis*. 1989; 21:573–7.
159. Benson JM, Nahata MC. Clinical use of systemic antifungal agents. *Clin Pharm*. 1988; 7:424–38.
160. Tachibana M, Noguchi Y, Monro AM. Toxicology of fluconazole in experimental animals. In: Fromtling RA, ed. Recent trends in the discovery, development and evaluation of antifungal agents. Barcelona, Spain: Prous; 1987: 93–102.
161. Anon. Investigator's brochure. Fluconazole (UK-49,858). Groton, CT: Pfizer Central Research; 1989:25.
162. Kidd D, Ranaghan EA, Morris TCM. Hypokalemia in patients with acute myeloid leukemia after treatment wih fluconazole. *Lancet*. 1989; 1:1017. Letter.
163. Schulman JA, Peyman G, Fiscella B et al. Toxicity of intravitreal injection of fluconazole in the rabbit. *Can J Ophthalmol*. 1987; 22:304–6.
164. Lazar JD, Wilmer KD. Drug interactions with fluconazole. *Rev Infect Dis*. 1990; 12(Suppl 3):S327–33.
165. Thrope JE, Baker N, Bromet-Petit M. Effect of oral antacid administration on the pharmacokinetics of oral fluconazole. *Antimicrob Agents Chemother*. 1990; 34:2032–3.
166. Graves NM, Matas AJ, Hilligoss DM et al. Fluconazole/cyclosporine interaction. *Clin Pharmcol Ther*. 1990; 47:208. Abstract.
167. Blum RA, Wilton JH, Hilligoss DM et al. Effect of fluconazole on the disposition of phenytoin. *Clin Pharmacol Ther*. 1990; 47:182. Abstract.
168. Kruger HU, Schuler U, Zimmerman R et al. No severe drug interaction of fluconazole, a triazole antifungal, with cyclosporin. *Bone Marrow Transplant*. 1988; 3:271.
169. Ehlninger G, Jaschonek K, Schuler U et al. Interaction of fluconazole with cyclosporin. *Lancet*. 1989; 2:104–5. Letter.
170. Collignon P, Hurley B, Mitchell D. Interaction of fluconazole with cyclosporin. *Lancet*. 1989; 1:1262. Letter.
171. Sugar AM, Saunders C, Idelson BA et al. Interaction of fluconazole and cyclosporine. *Ann Intern Med*. 1987; 110:844. Letter.
172. Mitchell AS, Holland JT. Fluconazole and phenytoin: a predictable interaction. *Br Med J*. 1989; 298:1315. Letter.
173. Higashi Y, Omura M, Suzuki K et al. Ketoconazole as a possible universal inhibitor of cytochrome P-450 dependent enzymes: its mode of inhibition. *Endocrinol Jpn*. 1987; 34:105–15.
174. Lavrijsen KLM, VanHoudt JMG, VanDyck DMJ et al. Induction potential of fluconazole toward drug-metabolizing enzymes in rats. *Antimicrob Agents Chemother*. 1990; 34:402–8.
175. Houston JB, Humphrey MJ, Matthew DE et al. Comparison of two azole antifungal drugs, ketoconazole and fluconazole, as modifiers of rat hepatic monooxygenase activity. *Biochem Pharmacol*. 1988; 37:401–8.
176. Shaw JTB, Tarbit MH, Troke PF. Cytochrome P-450 mediated sterol synthesis and metabolism: differences in sensitivity to fluconazole and other azoles. In: Fromtling RA, ed. Recent trends in the discovery, development and evaluation of antifungal agents. Barcelona, Spain: Prous; 1987:125–39.
177. Hanger DP, Jevons S, Shaw JTB. Fluconazole and testosterone: in vivo and in vitro studies. *Antimicrob Agents Chemother*. 1988; 32:646–8.
178. Lazar JD, Wilner KD. Key drug interaction studies with fluconazole. Paper presented at Major Developments in the Management of Bacterial and Fungal Infections: A Look to the Future. Vancouver, B.C.: 1989 Aug 20.
179. Pfizer, Inc. Diflucan package insert. New York; 1990 Jan.
180. Ansari AM, Gould IM, Douglas JG. High dose oral fluconazole for oropharyngeal candidosis in AIDS. *J Antimicrob Chemother*. 1990; 25:720–1.
181. American Druggist blue book. Lee FH, ed. Oradell, NJ: Hearst; 1989.

Therapy Reviews

Evaluation and treatment of ventricular arrhythmias: an update

PATRICK L. MCCOLLAM AND ROBERT B. PARKER

Abstract: An overall approach to evaluating and treating ventricular arrhythmias based on objective monitoring criteria is described.

A clinically useful system classifies patients based on whether their ventricular arrhythmias are benign, potentially lethal, or lethal. Some clinicians believe that antiarrhythmic drug therapy improves survival in patients with potentially lethal arrhythmias. However, disappointing results from the Cardiac Arrhythmia Suppression Trial have led to a greater awareness of the potential adverse effects of antiarrhythmics.

Various risk factors for arrhythmia-related death have been identified, such as the presence of frequent and complex ventricular ectopy, abnormal signal-averaged electrocardiography (SAECG) tracings, and poor left ventricular ejection fraction (LVEF). Antiarrhythmic drugs remain the primary mode of therapy for patients with recurrent symptomatic tachycardias. Antiarrhythmic drug efficacy has been evaluated by methods including symptom assessment, continuous ambulatory electrocardiographic monitoring (Holter monitoring), exercise testing, and invasive electrophysiologic testing. There may be an extremely wide range of effective serum concentrations for the class IA agents. Individual target concentrations of antiarrhythmic agents may be determined for individual patients and should assist the clinician in optimizing long-term antiarrhythmic drug therapy.

The risk-to-benefit ratio of treatment should be weighed before antiarrhythmic drug therapy is begun, and careful, objective monitoring of drug efficacy should be performed. When pharmacologic treatment of ventricular arrhythmias is considered, treatment algorithms that incorporate LVEF measurements, Holter monitor recordings, and SAECG may aid the clinician.

Index terms: Arrhythmia; Blood levels; Cardiac drugs; Methodology; Protocols; Rational therapy; Toxicity
Clin Pharm. 1991; 10:195–205

Since the publication of an earlier review in *Clinical Pharmacy*,[1] two factors have led to a great deal of uncertainty and confusion regarding the proper approach to the evaluation and treatment of ventricular arrhythmias. First, the introduction of new antiarrhythmic drugs such as encainide, flecainide, and amiodarone has complicated the selection of appropriate antiarrhythmic drug therapy. Second, the results of the Cardiac Arrhythmia Suppression Trial (CAST) indicated that antiarrhythmic drug therapy with flecainide or encainide in post-myocardial-infarction patients increased mortality compared with that observed in a control group receiving placebo.[2] In addition, several other factors warrant this update on therapy, including additional insight into patient evaluation that has been gained by considering cardiac risk factors, wider use of complex antiarrhythmic agents such as amiodarone, and more appropriate use of serum antiarrhythmic drug concentration determinations. This review will suggest an approach to therapy that is based on objective monitoring criteria. Specific antiarrhythmic therapies will not be the main focus of this review; rather, we will discuss an

PATRICK L. MCCOLLAM, PHARM.D., is Assistant Professor of Pharmacy, Department of Hospital Pharmacy Practice and Administration, College of Pharmacy, Medical University of South Carolina, Charleston. ROBERT B. PARKER, PHARM.D., is Assistant Professor of Pharmacy, College of Pharmacy, University of Georgia, Athens, and Clinical Assistant Professor of Medicine, Medical College of Georgia, Augusta.

Address reprint requests to Dr. McCollam at the Department of Hospital Pharmacy Practice and Administration, 171 Ashley Avenue, Medical University of South Carolina, Charleston, SC 29425.

This is **article 680-204-9107** in the **ASHP Continuing-Education System;** it qualifies for 1.0 hour of continuing-education credit. See page 229 for learning objectives and test questions.

overall approach to evaluating and treating the patient with ventricular arrhythmias. Ventricular arrhythmias occurring in the acute stages of myocardial infarction (MI) will not be specifically addressed in this review.

Classification of Ventricular Arrhythmias

Before classification systems for ventricular arrhythmias are discussed, several terms must first be defined. Unless stated to the contrary in this review, sustained ventricular tachycardia (VT) is defined as a ventricular tachyarrhythmia of >100 beats/min lasting ≥30 seconds. Sustained VT may also last <30 seconds if therapeutic intervention is required to restore hemodynamic stability. Nonsustained VT (NSVT) is less than 30 seconds or 15 beats in duration and terminates spontaneously. Usually, patients with NSVT are asymptomatic or mildly symptomatic (e.g., palpitations, dizziness). When used to describe ventricular ectopy, "frequent" is defined as >10 premature ventricular contractions (PVCs) per hour, and "complex" is defined as anything other than a unifocal PVC (i.e., couplets, multifocal PVCs).

A number of classification systems have been developed to help evaluate patients with ventricular arrhythmias. The Lown grading scale for classifying PVCs has historically been used in evaluating patients with ventricular ectopy after acute MI.[3] This system uses the frequency of ventricular ectopic activity and the PVC morphology to form a hierarchy of mutually exclusive grades. The underlying assumption of this system is that higher grades of ectopic activity indicate a poorer prognosis. Although this hierarchic system may be useful in descriptive reports, it does not provide the clinician with useful information such as whether ischemic heart disease is present, the prognostic significance of the tachycardia, or symptoms the patient may be experiencing. Further, this system does not take into account the spontaneous variability of PVC frequency that has been noted by other investigators.[4,5] Finally, considerable controversy exists about Lown's assignment of the R-on-T phenomenon as the highest grade of PVC.[6]

Myerburg et al.[7] suggested a second PVC classification system that allows simultaneous assignment of PVCs to parallel hierarchies of frequency and form. Using this system, clinicians and investigators can more uniformly describe both PVC frequency and morphology. However, this classification scheme is also limited by several factors. First, this system provides no information about the presence or absence of underlying heart disease, a factor known to affect prognosis of patients with ventricular ectopy.[8] Second, neither patient symptoms nor the degree of impairment caused by the symptoms is taken into account by this system. Finally, the prognostic significance of a reduction in the classification of PVC frequency or form from a more advanced grade to a less advanced grade after therapeutic intervention is unknown.

A broader, more clinically useful classification system that provides the clinician with information about prognosis has been suggested by Bigger[9] and Morganroth.[10] This system classifies patients with ventricular arrhythmias based on whether the arrhythmias are (1) benign, (2) prognostically significant (potentially lethal), or (3) lethal. Also, this system takes into account the presence of underlying heart disease. Patients with PVCs and no underlying heart disease are classified as having benign arrhythmias. Epidemiologic data suggest that these patients are at no increased risk of sudden cardiac death.[8] Drug treatment is indicated only if the patient's symptoms are sufficiently bothersome that the benefits of treatment would outweigh the risk of adverse reactions to antiarrhythmic drugs (e.g., proarrhythmia). At the opposite end of the classification system are the patients who have underlying heart disease (usually prior MI) with lethal arrhythmias, such as sustained VT producing hemodynamic instability or ventricular fibrillation (VF), that are not associated with the acute phase of MI. Aggressive treatment has been assumed to be necessary because of the high one-year recurrence rate (30–40%) of these malignant tachycardias.[11,12] Patients with organic heart disease and ventricular ectopy characterized by frequent or complex PVCs or NSVT who are asymptomatic or mildly symptomatic (e.g., dizziness, palpitations) are assigned to the potentially lethal category.

Patients assigned to the potentially lethal category are the most problematic with regard to treatment. Epidemiologic studies indicate that these patients are at increased risk of sudden cardiac death.[13–17] The assumption among some clinicians has been that suppression of ventricular ectopy with antiarrhythmic drugs would improve survival in these patients. However, CAST has demonstrated that, although flecainide and encainide suppressed ventricular ectopy in patients after MI, they increased total mortality and sudden cardiac death rates compared with placebo.[2] Although not proved, this increase in mortality is generally attributed to the proarrhythmic effects of these two drugs. Therefore, two major questions raised by CAST are the applicability of these results to other antiarrhythmic drugs when used in post-MI patients and how best to manage these patients, who are at increased risk of sudden cardiac death.

Evaluation and Prognostic Importance of Ventricular Arrhythmias

Historical Perspective. With respect to the determination of drug efficacy, a marked evolution has occurred over time. Early efficacy studies often used subjective methods of assessment. One example is an often-cited study of procainamide efficacy.[18] In this study, the physician was usually blinded to procainamide concentrations and determined drug efficacy by clinical assessment of the patient. No continuous electrocardiographic monitoring or electrophysiologic (EP) testing methods were used. Other studies of disopyramide[19] and quinidine[20] also used periodic electrocardiograms (ECGs) and frequent clinical observations in determining drug efficacy. Indeed, many clinicians now believe that the correlation between symptomatology and the occurrence of arrhythmias is rather poor. Perhaps because of this perception, objective monitoring by continuous electrocardiography (telemetry or Holter monitoring) became the standard for determining efficacy. However, subjective assessment may be appropriate in patients without organic heart disease who have benign but symptomatic arrhythmias.

Many antiarrhythmic drugs have been assessed by evaluating their effectiveness against chronic ventricular ectopy because the number of PVCs over time was a measurable endpoint. One of the earliest studies to use this technique evaluated lidocaine for the treatment of ventricular tachyarrhythmias. This study used telemetry and Holter monitoring to determine efficacy, empirically defined as a 50% reduction in PVC frequency.[21] Many other drug efficacy trials also used a simple statistical difference in PVC frequency to determine drug efficacy. Only later did Morganroth et al.[4] show that a 50% reduction or a simple statistical difference in PVC frequency between control and drug treatment groups was not necessarily an adequate measure of drug efficacy. In this study,[4] the authors determined that a 65% reduction in PVC frequency over two 72-hour monitoring periods, or an 83% reduction over two 24-hour periods, was needed to conclude that an observed change was due to drug therapy rather than simple spontaneous variability. A pertinent example of this variability was found in the study by Winkle,[5] who demonstrated that simple spontaneous variability in PVC frequency could mimic antiarrhythmic drug efficacy; therefore, spontaneous variability in PVC frequency must be differentiated from drug response in patients evaluated by continuous electrocardiographic monitoring. In addition, recent data indicate a need for periodic assessment of PVC frequency over time to rule out long-term spontaneous variability.[22]

Holter Monitoring. Ambulatory electrocardiographic monitoring (Holter monitoring) is a frequently used noninvasive technique for detecting ventricular ectopy and for evaluating drug therapy. Over the last 15 years, Holter monitoring has provided clinicians with valuable data about the prognostic importance of ventricular ectopy. Holter monitoring for 24–48 hours has shown that ventricular ectopy occurs in 40–75% of persons without underlying heart disease and that the incidence and frequency of ventricular ectopy increase with age.[23–27] However, those individuals without underlying heart disease do not appear to be at increased risk of sudden cardiac death.[8]

One of the most useful contributions of Holter monitoring is the identification of patients at risk for increased mortality after MI.[13,17] The Multicenter Postinfarction Research Group assessed left ventricular function by radionuclide ventriculography and performed 24-hour Holter monitoring before hospital discharge in 866 patients with acute MI.[14] After adjustment for left ventricular dysfunction, patients with more than 10 PVCs/hour detected by Holter monitoring were at increased risk for cardiac mortality in the first two years after an MI. Similar results were described by Mukharji et al.,[15] reporting for the Multicenter Investigation of the Limitation of Infarct Size study group. These investigators noted an increased incidence of sudden cardiac death after acute MI in 533 patients with more than 10 PVCs/hour detected by a 24-hour Holter recording performed before hospital discharge. Meinertz et al.[16] reported a similar increased risk of sudden cardiac death in patients with idiopathic dilated cardiomyopathy and ventricular ectopy.

The Holter monitor has also confirmed ventricular tachyarrhythmias as the cause of sudden cardiac death in ambulatory patients. Bayes de Luna et al.[28] recently compiled the results of a number of case reports of sudden cardiac death that occurred in patients wearing Holter monitors. Of 157 cases of sudden cardiac death compiled, 131 (83%) were found to be due to ventricular tachyarrhythmias. Only 20 of these cases were due to torsade de pointes. The majority of the cases of ventricular tachyarrhythmias were sudden onset of VF (13 cases) or sustained VT that degenerated into VF (98 cases). Ninety-three percent of patients without torsade de pointes had ischemic heart disease. Therefore, these data confirm the previously assumed role of ventricular tachyarrhythmias as the mechanism of sudden cardiac death in patients with ischemic heart disease.

Holter monitoring is indicated in a number of situations for the management of patients with ventricular arrhythmias. First, Holter monitoring can be used to correlate patient symptoms with recorded arrhythmias. Second, both the frequency and morphology of ventricular ectopy can be recorded with the Holter monitor. Third, proarrhythmic responses to antiarrhythmic drugs, such as an increase in the frequency of ventricular ectopy or drug-induced changes in cardiac conduction, can be detected. Fourth, the Holter monitor can be used before hospital discharge in patients with acute MI to identify individuals at increased risk for sudden cardiac death. However, after the results of CAST,[2] in which encainide and flecainide increased mortality despite an 80% decrease in PVC frequency detected by Holter monitoring, the use of this popular method of monitoring antiarrhythmic drug therapy must be questioned.

Signal-Averaged Electrocardiography. In recent years, the use of signal-averaged electrocardiography (SAECG) has provided important prognostic information about patients at risk for spontaneous or inducible sustained VT (during EP testing) or sudden cardiac death after MI.[29-34] Signal averaging amplifies the recording of a repetitive waveform from the surface ECG, usually the QRS complex, while simultaneously decreasing the random noise (such as skeletal muscle activity) recorded from the body surface (Figure 1). After amplification of the QRS complex, low-amplitude late potentials that occur in the terminal portion of the QRS complex can be detected. These late potentials are thought to be due to areas of slow and fragmented conduction through damaged ventricular tissue.[35] These areas of slow and fragmented conduction are believed to provide the necessary environment for initiation and perpetuation of reentrant tachycardias.

The prognostic importance of late potentials in post-MI patients has been described by several investigators. In an early study by Simson,[29] the results of SAECG in 39 post-MI patients with inducible VT during EP testing were compared with the results in a control group of 27 post-MI patients with <200 PVCs and no complex ectopy on a 24-hour Holter recording. Late potentials were found in 92% of the patients with inducible sustained VT, whereas only 7% of the patients without VT had late potentials. Also, the filtered QRS duration was longer ($p < 0.0001$) in patients with VT (mean ± S.D., 139 ± 26 msec) than in patients without VT (95 ± 10 msec).

More recent studies involving larger numbers of patients have provided additional data demonstrating the prognostic value of SAECG in post-MI patients. Kuchar et al.[30] performed SAECG in 165 survivors of acute MI. Eleven of 65 patients (17%) with an abnormal SAECG tracing had an arrhythmic event (sudden cardiac death or sustained VT), whereas only 1 of 92 patients (1%) with a normal SAECG tracing had an arrhythmic event ($p <$ 0.001). Gomes et al.[34] prospectively performed SAECG, 24-hour Holter recordings, and radionuclide ventriculography in 102 patients after acute MI. Twenty-nine percent of patients with an abnormal SAECG tracing had an arrhythmic event (sustained VT, sudden cardiac death, or both) compared with 3.5% of patients with a normal SAECG tracing (p = 0.003) during follow-up of 12 ± 6 months (mean ± S.D.). Patients at highest risk for an arrhythmic event had an abnormal SAECG tracing, a left ventricular ejection fraction (LVEF) of <40%, and frequent or complex ectopy on Holter recordings. Fifty percent of these patients experienced an arrhythmic event during follow-up. These investigators also determined that SAECG provided prognostic information that was inde-

Figure 1. Portions of normal (left) and abnormal (right) signal-averaged electrocardiograms. The vertical axis is voltage, and the horizontal axis is time. The large complex in the center of each tracing is the filtered QRS complex. The normal tracing, from a patient without ventricular tachycardia, has a filtered-QRS-complex duration of 85 msec (normal, <114 msec) and no ventricular late potentials. The abnormal tracing, from a patient with ventricular tachycardia, has a prolonged filtered-QRS-complex duration of 154 msec and ventricular late potentials (indicated by braces).

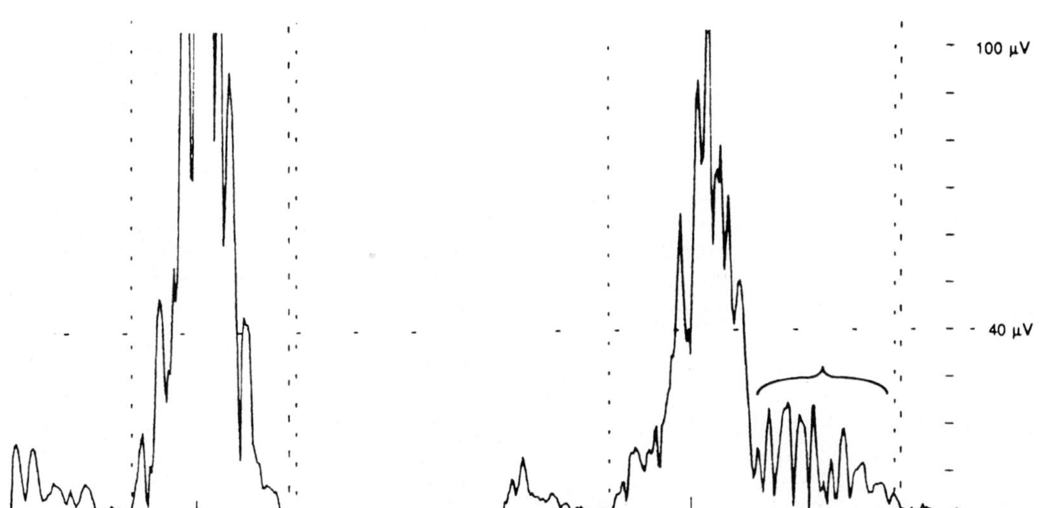

pendent of LVEF or ventricular ectopy. Similar results have been reported by other investigators.[31,33,36] Unfortunately, the most effective treatment for those individuals at high risk for recurrent arrhythmic events is unknown. Interestingly, recent data suggest that thrombolytic therapy with recombinant tissue plasminogen activator can decrease the incidence of late potentials in patients with acute MI.[37]

Although SAECG provides valuable prognostic information in patients after acute MI, the SAECG tracing does not appear useful as an endpoint for monitoring antiarrhythmic drug therapy. Early data collected by Simson et al.[38] in 23 patients with VT treated with either class I antiarrhythmic drugs or amiodarone suggested that antiarrhythmic drugs did not abolish late potentials, even in patients whose arrhythmias were rendered noninducible during EP testing. Also, these class I antiarrhythmic drugs prolonged the filtered QRS duration measured by SAECG.[38] In a similar report, neither class I nor class II antiarrhythmic drugs had an effect on late potentials even when inducible VT was suppressed.[39] In fact, oral loading therapy with amiodarone (1400 mg/day for seven days) followed by a maintenance dose of 400 mg/day increased the duration of late potentials. Of four patients who had no late potentials on a baseline SAECG tracing, three exhibited late potentials within 10 days of initiation of amiodarone treatment.[40] Thus, it appears that SAECG is not useful in providing an endpoint for monitoring antiarrhythmic drug therapy because drugs can control VT without abolishing late potentials.

Exercise Testing. Exercise testing can also be useful in the evaluation of ventricular arrhythmias. Some arrhythmias may be provoked by exercise through a combination of increased sympathetic stimulation or decreased vagal tone.[41] During exercise testing unifocal PVCs occur in 60–70% and complex ectopy occurs in 20% of patients with ischemic heart disease. Velebit et al.[42] reported that a number of cases of antiarrhythmic-induced proarrhythmia were uncovered during exercise testing. Another study of exercise-induced antiarrhythmic drug effects was performed by Ranger et al.[43] These investigators found that when patients receiving flecainide (an agent that primarily slows ventricular conduction) underwent exercise testing, the mean ± S.D. QRS duration increased from 94 ± 22 to 116 ± 25 msec ($p < 0.001$), compared with the increase observed in a control group not receiving flecainide (79 ± 10 to 80 ± 10 msec; not significant). The authors postulated that this drug-induced effect could facilitate a reentrant tachycardia, which occurred in one patient in this study. Exercise testing may be helpful in evaluating those patients whose arrhythmias are controlled by drug therapy at rest but who either develop their typical arrhythmia during exercise or develop new symptoms (i.e., possible proarrhythmia) during exercise.

Electrophysiologic Testing. EP testing (or programmed electrical stimulation) has several important indications in the evaluation of ventricular arrhythmias. For the purposes of this review we will limit the discussion of EP testing to the clinical indications, use in serial drug testing, and potential prognostic value in patients with ventricular arrhythmias.

In simplest terms, an EP study for ventricular arrhythmias is performed in a specialized cardiac catheterization laboratory by venous insertion of electrode catheters into the right side of the heart. By using these catheters, the electrical activity of the heart can be recorded and programmed stimulation can be performed in an attempt to induce the patient's problematic tachycardia (the "clinical arrhythmia").[44,45] Unfortunately, there are several different stimulation protocols that use various modes of stimulation, which makes precise study comparisons difficult. Also, because these stimulation procedures use rapid pacing and insertion of extra beats at critically timed intervals, reentrant tachycardias are the main types of ventricular arrhythmias initiated by EP testing; arrhythmias arising from other mechanisms (e.g., enhanced automaticity, triggered activity, or delayed afterdepolarizations) may not be elicited as readily.

The typically desired endpoint of the control EP study is induction of VF or sustained monomorphic VT of >15 beats' or >30 seconds' duration. Although some investigators use NSVT as an endpoint,[46] NSVT and polymorphic VT must be recognized as possible artifacts of the stimulation protocol in some cases.[47] The induced tachycardia is then terminated by rapid pacing or direct-current cardioversion. Obviously, one of the most important problems with EP testing is found in the patient whose clinical arrhythmia is noninducible at baseline but who has previously experienced an episode of VF or sustained VT. In these patients, the workup then shifts back to Holter monitoring and exercise testing to define the type of arrhythmia and test therapeutic agents. Another potential problem is daily reproducibility of the study, which some investigators suggest may vary considerably.[48]

The most recent guidelines (December 1989) for EP testing from the American College of Cardiology and the American Heart Association have categorized the indications for the procedure into three classes according to the risk-to-benefit ratio and the potential for the study to yield useful information for patient management.[49] In the report, a class I recommendation is given for a generally agreed indication. Class I recommendations include (1) testing survivors of cardiac arrest who lack evidence of an acute MI, (2) testing patients who have had cardiac arrest ≥48 hours after acute MI, and (3) conducting serial drug testing in patients with VF or sustained VT. Additional class I recommendations are given in the report for other specific arrhythmias. Importantly, in patients with only PVCs or ventricular couplets there are no class I recommendations.[49] We emphasize this point because it highlights the questionable rationale for treating asymptomatic PVCs.

Several reviews have described the use of serial drug testing for serious ventricular arrhythmias.[44,45] Briefly, patients undergo a baseline EP study to characterize the tachycardia and then usually receive one of the class IA antiarrhythmic drugs.[50,51] After drug administration (and presumed steady-state conditions with oral agents), the stimulation protocol is repeated. However, clinicians should be aware that EP testing may not account for the contribution of active metabolites (e.g., *N*-acetylprocainamide) when a parent drug is administered in the EP laboratory. A positive response is commonly defined as (1) failure to induce VF or sustained VT or (2) induction of a brief, self-terminating asymptomatic episode of <15 beats. When baseline studies induce NSVT, a positive response after drug administration would be noninduction of tachycardia. Drug testing may then continue with other class IA, IB, or IC agents.

Other authors have suggested an analysis of clinical variables to identify those patients who have the best possibility for a positive EP study. Swerdlow et al.[52] analyzed clinical variables to categorize patients as low-yield or high-yield candidates for EP testing. This study determined three variables that were strong predictors of drug response during EP testing: less diffuse coronary artery disease, female gender, and fewer numbers of arrhythmic episodes.

In a separate study, Swerdlow et al.[53] described EP testing as one means of predicting long-term survival in patients with VF or sustained VT. Patients for whom effective antiarrhythmic drugs were found during serial drug testing and who received long-term therapy with an effective agent had a higher survival rate (less cardiac death) than those patients whose arrhythmia remained inducible during drug testing ($p < 0.0001$). An important question is whether EP testing or Holter monitoring is the better method for predicting efficacy of antiarrhythmic drugs. Although this issue is controversial, some studies have shown EP testing to be more accurate than Holter monitoring in predicting effective therapy for the prevention of recurrent VT.[54,55] A more definitive answer to this question will be available when the multicenter, randomized Electrophysiologic Study Versus Electrocardiographic Monitoring trial is completed.[56]

Finally, EP testing may be of prognostic value. For example, what is the prognosis for the patient with an inducible tachycardia if he or she has survived MI or out-of-hospital cardiac arrest? Although their study was not randomized, Gomes et al.[57] provided some interesting data on the likelihood of cardiac death using EP testing as the evaluation method. EP testing was performed in 73 patients with Lown grade III and IV PVCs (multiformed PVCs and at least two consecutive PVCs, respectively) during Holter monitoring. Patients were then grouped and followed according to whether a sustained tachycardia was inducible (group I, $n = 20$) or noninducible (group II, $n = 53$). The patients in group I had significantly worse underlying heart disease, and 17 of 20 were prescribed long-term therapy with an antiarrhythmic agent found effective during EP testing. The one-year mortality rate in group I was higher than that in group II (32% versus 2%; $p < 0.001$) regardless of antiarrhythmic therapy. The authors concluded that patients with inducible tachycardia and an LVEF of <40% had a less favorable prognosis. In a similar study in 40 patients with underlying NSVT, EP testing identified those at subsequent risk for developing sustained arrhythmias.[58] In 22 patients with inducible arrhythmias, nine cases of sudden death or spontaneous sustained arrhythmia occurred, although patients whose therapy was determined by EP testing had fewer episodes ($p < 0.01$). Of the 18 patients without inducible tachycardias, none experienced a clinical arrhythmic episode or died during follow-up (1–57 months; mean, 14 months) regardless of therapy.

Another important patient group comprises survivors of out-of-hospital cardiac arrest (sudden cardiac death) not related to acute MI. Wilber et al.[12] studied the prognostic implications of EP testing in 166 survivors of out-of-hospital cardiac arrest. In this study, the authors used VT of <100 beats that terminated spontaneously as the definition of NSVT (which is considerably different from other studies). Of these patients, 61 (37%) of 166 had inducible sustained VT, 25 (15%) had inducible polymorphic VT that degenerated into VF, 45 (27%) had inducible NSVT (mean duration of 15 beats), and tachycardia was not inducible in 35 (21%). Patients then underwent serial drug testing, which identified an effective antiarrhythmic agent in 72% of patients with inducible tachycardias. After a mean follow-up period of 21 months, three patients were not evaluable, and cardiac arrest had recurred in 11 of 91 (12%) who had effective therapy determined at baseline, in 12 of 36 (33%) who had a continually inducible tachycardia, and in 6 of 35 (17%) who did not have inducible tachycardias at baseline. Multivariate analysis revealed that patients whose tachycardias remained inducible during drug therapy were at higher risk for recurrent cardiac arrest ($p = 0.0006$). Similarly, Skale et al.[55] found that a noninducible tachycardia during drug therapy predicted a better outcome in sudden-death survivors.

Finally, Cripps et al.[59] performed a trial to determine the value of EP testing, Holter monitoring,

SAECG, and clinical variables for predicting the occurrence of ventricular arrhythmias in post-MI patients. This study is of particular interest in that no patients received long-term prophylaxis with antiarrhythmic agents. Of 75 patients studied, 23 (32%) had inducible NSVT, 8 (11%) had inducible sustained VT, and 14 (19%) had inducible polymorphic VT or VF during EP testing. During follow-up (6–30 months; mean, 16 months) six patients had documented serious arrhythmic events; all of these patients had inducible sustained monomorphic VT at baseline. Multivariate analysis of these data revealed that factor to be the most highly significant variable that is predictive of arrhythmia occurrence ($p < 0.002$).

EP testing is an established method for evaluating ventricular arrhythmias and guiding drug therapy. The ability of antiarrhythmic agents to suppress inducible tachyarrhythmias during EP testing indicates a decreased risk for sudden cardiac death.[53] EP testing also appears to possess prognostic value in that it identifies some patient groups that are at increased risk of experiencing arrhythmic events or sudden cardiac death.

Antiarrhythmic Class Responses. Serial drug testing during an EP study could become quite expensive and time consuming if one were to test all of the available IA, IB, and IC drugs. Because i.v. procainamide is usually the first drug to be tested, the obvious question is whether a positive (or negative) response to procainamide typifies the response to other IA drugs. Kuchar et al.[60] analyzed data obtained during the initial EP test in 106 patients with inducible sustained ventricular tachyarrhythmias. When i.v. procainamide was used as the first agent for serial drug testing, two variables were identified that were predictive of a positive response to subsequent oral therapy. They were a noninducible tachycardia and an LVEF of ≥40%. However, the long-term efficacy of the oral agents was not described in this study. In a broader study, Waxman et al.[61] found that, in patients with a tachycardia that became noninducible after i.v. procainamide administration, this response was a positive predictor of response to other agents ($p < 0.001$). Unfortunately, many antiarrhythmic agents were grouped in this "other" category, and relationships among individual drugs were not discussed.

Swiryn et al.[62] reviewed the response to IA agents in patients undergoing serial drug testing who had inducible sustained ventricular tachyarrhythmias at baseline. A concordant response rate was found between procainamide and quinidine (83%; $p < 0.025$) but not between either procainamide or quinidine and disopyramide. However, other studies have failed to show concordance between procainamide and other IA drugs.[63,64] Oseran et al.[63] found a concordance rate of 75% (15 of 20 patients) between oral and i.v. procainamide and between oral procainamide and oral quinidine. Only 10 of 20 patients had concordant responses to i.v. procainamide and oral quinidine. Wyse et al.[64] evaluated the concordance among disopyramide, procainamide, and quinidine after acute i.v. administration of the drugs in a nonrandomized study. The authors found only a 45% concordance rate between any two drugs and only 36% when all three drugs were considered. However, a 75% concordance rate was shown among all three drugs when continued inducibility was the variable. The lack of concordance among procainamide, disopyramide, and quinidine may be explained in part by the differences in these agents' metabolite profiles and protein binding. In summary, conflicting data exist regarding concordance among the class IA drugs, and unfortunately, little information is available regarding concordance among other classes of antiarrhythmic drugs.

As discussed earlier, noninducibility during drug therapy is an indicator of a decreased risk for recurrent arrhythmias. However, failure of amiodarone to prevent arrhythmia induction is not necessarily associated with a poor response to long-term amiodarone therapy. In a small study, Hamer et al.[65] followed nine patients receiving chronic amiodarone therapy after drug efficacy was assessed by repeat EP testing. Eight of nine patients had inducible tachycardias during the control EP study, and seven of nine patients continued to have inducible tachycardias after a mean of 11 weeks of amiodarone therapy. All patients remained free from spontaneous arrhythmias during a mean follow-up of 15 months (range, 10–24 months). Interestingly, the tachyarrhythmias that were induced while patients were receiving amiodarone were generally slower and had a prolonged QRS duration. A more recent study by Bauman et al.[66] reviewed patients receiving chronic amiodarone therapy to determine any electrophysiologic variables that would predict long-term efficacy. Sustained tachycardias were still inducible in 27 (75%) of 36 patients who underwent repeat EP testing after three weeks of amiodarone therapy. Data analysis revealed that the mode of arrhythmia induction was the only significant predictor of long-term efficacy ($p < 0.025$). Patients with a tachycardia that was more difficult to induce had a better chance for successful chronic therapy than patients whose tachycardias were more easily induced during amiodarone therapy. Therefore, long-term efficacy may still occur in some patients who have continually inducible tachycardias while receiving amiodarone therapy.

Use of Serum Drug Concentration Data. Therapeutic serum concentration ranges have been proposed for most of the available antiarrhythmic drugs.[18,20,67,68] However, these therapeutic ranges were determined by a variety of methods in patients with various types of arrhythmias. A recent study found an extremely wide range of effective concentrations for the class IA agents (e.g., procainamide 2.9–22.2 μg/mL and quinidine 1.0–9.1 μg/mL) when these concentrations were determined during EP serial drug testing.[51] These data, coupled with the previous studies, suggest that there may be a specific threshold or "target" concentration at which efficacy may occur for each individual patient. If this hypothesis were true, then a target concentration could be used to develop a more effective long-term antiarrhythmic drug regimen.

Recently, we described the use of this concept.[69] Nineteen patients were reviewed to determine whether recurrence of their tachycardia was related to their target concentration as determined during EP testing. All patients had a symptomatic recurrent tachycardia that was inducible during a control EP study and responded to at least one class IA antiarrhythmic drug. When a positive response occurred, the patient's serum concentration was determined in the electrophysiology laboratory for use as the target serum concentration. Acute response was defined as the inability to induce the tachycardia or induction of a brief (<15 beats), spontaneously terminating asymptomatic episode. During follow-up (1–65 months; mean ± S.D., 23 ± 23 months) 7 patients had a documented arrhythmia recurrence and 12 patients had no recurrence. However, all seven patients with a recurrence had antiarrhythmic concentrations at the time that were below the initial target value; this was a significant finding ($p < 0.05$). Clearly, an antiarrhythmic drug serum concentration that simply lies within a predetermined therapeutic range should not be viewed as a therapeutic endpoint.[51] When the target method described above is used, antiarrhythmic drug dosage during long-term therapy is adjusted to achieve a trough serum concentration above the target. Although this method will not define the minimally effective serum concentration, it should assist the clinician in optimizing long-term antiarrhythmic drug therapy.

Recommendations

The results of CAST have once again pointed out that the treatment of arrhythmias with drugs possessing a low therapeutic ratio can be quite hazardous. As many authors have observed, clinicians must first optimize their patients' overall cardiovascular drug regimen before setting out a course of therapy with antiarrhythmic drugs. For example, in patients with ischemic heart disease (especially post-MI patients) β-adrenergic blockers are clearly indicated because these are the only drugs that have been shown to reduce cardiovascular mortality.[70] The use of aspirin in appropriate patients should also be recommended.[70] In patients with congestive heart failure, one should examine the use of angiotensin-converting-enzyme inhibitors because they have been shown to reduce mortality in these patients.[71] Finally, serum electrolytes (particularly potassium and magnesium) should be routinely monitored to avoid imbalances that are reversible causes of arrhythmias.

When considering antiarrhythmic treatment, one might stratify patients into three groups based on the type of arrhythmias: benign, potentially lethal, and lethal. The first group includes those patients with benign arrhythmias and no underlying heart disease; these patients have no increased risk of sudden cardiac death. Treatment is indicated in these individuals only if the benefits of alleviating a patient's symptoms outweigh the risk of antiarrhythmic drug treatment. Also, there is a general consensus among clinicians that patients with lethal arrhythmias, because they are at high risk for recurrent arrhythmic events, should undergo EP testing followed by serial drug testing even though an effective agent can be identified in fewer than 50% of patients. Although the optimum order for serial drug testing is unknown, the usual clinical practice is to administer a class IA agent initially (usually i.v. procainamide in the EP laboratory). If the tachycardia remains inducible, an oral class IB agent such as mexiletine is typically administered (until steady state is achieved) before the next attempt to reinduce the patient's tachycardia. If the tachycardia is still inducible, some clinicians suggest combining a class IA agent with a class IB agent. However, others would suggest (1) a class IC drug, (2) amiodarone, or (3) an automatic implantable cardiac defibrillator. If an effective drug is identified, then the drug's serum concentration should be determined at the time when efficacy is demonstrated and it should be used as the target concentration for long-term therapy.

Which patients with potentially lethal arrhythmias should be treated is more controversial. The ultimate goal of treatment in these patients is decreasing the risk of sudden cardiac death. Before CAST, many believed that suppression of ventricular ectopy in post-MI patients would decrease the risk of sudden cardiac death. However, the results of CAST certainly call into question the benefits of using a reduction in PVC frequency as an endpoint for antiarrhythmic drug therapy. A number of studies performed in post-MI patients have consistently identified an LVEF of <40%, abnormal SAECG tracings, and >10 PVCs/hour on a 24-hour Holter recording as independent risk factors for subsequent sustained VT or sudden cardiac death. The presence of more than one of these risk factors in an individual patient places the patient at even higher risk for a serious arrhythmic event (sustained VT or sudden cardiac death).

We recommend stratifying these patients into those who are at high risk for developing serious arrhythmias (candidates for EP testing) and those who should have close clinical follow-up by (1) evaluating the LVEF, (2) obtaining a 24-hour Holter recording, and (3) performing SAECG. If a patient has an LVEF of <40%, frequent or complex ventricular ectopy, and an abnormal SAECG tracing, EP testing should be strongly considered because these patients are at higher risk for subsequent arrhythmic events. Patients with any two risk factors are also at higher risk for an arrhythmic event and should undergo EP testing.

Should patients with only one risk factor undergo EP testing? Currently, more data are needed to definitively answer this question, although some general conclusions can be made. Patients with only frequent or complex ventricular ectopy probably do not require EP testing because ventricular ectopy is not as powerful a predictor of subsequent events as an LVEF of <40% or an abnormal SAECG tracing.[35] Further, the sheer number of patients with frequent or complex ventricular ectopy and organic heart disease would preclude EP testing for all of these patients. However, EP testing should be considered in patients with either an abnormal SAECG tracing or an LVEF of <40%. If patients with potentially lethal arrhythmias have no tachycardia induced during EP testing, the risk of subsequent sustained VT or VF appears to be low and antiarrhythmic drug therapy is warranted only to relieve symptoms. If a sustained tachyarrhythmia is induced, then repeat EP studies with serial drug testing are indicated. Although this approach seems reasonable based on current data, there are no studies on the use of the combination of LVEF evaluation, 24-hour Holter monitoring, and SAECG to predict which patients will have inducible tachycardias during EP testing. Further prospective studies will be required to assess the utility of these prognostic factors in identifying patients for EP testing and the subsequent effects on cardiovascular morbidity and mortality.

Conclusion

Various risk factors for arrhythmia-related death have been identified, including frequent and complex ventricular ectopy, an abnormal SAECG tracing, and a poor LVEF. CAST reinforces the need to (1) carefully weigh the risk-to-benefit ratio of treatment in any patient before antiarrhythmic drug therapy is begun and (2) perform careful, objective monitoring of drug efficacy. When pharmacologic treatment of ventricular arrhythmias is considered, treatment algorithms that incorporate LVEF measurements, Holter monitor recordings, and SAECG may aid the clinician.

References

1. Batenhorst RL, Bottorff MB, Kuo CS. Mechanisms and control of ventricular tachyarrhythmias. *Clin Pharm.* 1983; 2:320–9.
2. The Cardiac Arrhythmia Suppression Trial (CAST) Investigators. Preliminary report: effect of encainide and flecainide on mortality in a randomized trial of arrhythmia suppression after myocardial infarction. *N Engl J Med.* 1989; 321:406–12.
3. Lown B, Wolf M. Approaches to sudden death from coronary heart disease. *Circulation.* 1971; 44:130–42.
4. Morganroth J, Michelson EL, Horowitz LN et al. Limitations of routine long term electrocardiographic monitoring to assess ventricular ectopic frequency. *Circulation.* 1978; 58:408–14.
5. Winkle RA. Antiarrhythmic drug effect mimicked by spontaneous variability of ventricular ectopy. *Circulation.* 1978; 57:1116–21.
6. Surawicz B. R on T phenomenon: dangerous and harmless. *J Appl Cardiol.* 1986; 1:39–61.
7. Myerburg RJ, Kessler KM, Luceri RM et al. Classification of ventricular arrhythmias based on parallel hierarchies of frequency and form. *Am J Cardiol.* 1984; 54:1355–8.
8. Kennedy HL, Whitlock JA, Sprague MK et al. Long-term follow up of asymptomatic healthy subjects with frequent and complex ventricular ectopy. *N Engl J Med.* 1985; 312:193–7.
9. Bigger JT. Definition of benign versus malignant ventricular arrhythmias: targets for treatment. *Am J Cardiol.* 1983; 52:47C–54C.
10. Morganroth J. Premature ventricular complexes. Diagnosis and indications for therapy. *JAMA.* 1984; 252:673–6.
11. Surawicz B. Prognosis of ventricular arrhythmias in relation to sudden cardiac death: therapeutic implications. *J Am Coll Cardiol.* 1987; 10:435–7.
12. Wilber DJ, Garan H, Finkelstein D et al. Out-of-hospital cardiac arrest: use of electrophysiologic testing in the prediction of long-term outcome. *N Engl J Med.* 1988; 318:19–24.
13. Ruberman W, Weinblatt E, Goldberg JD et al. Ventricular premature beats and mortality after MI. *N Engl J Med.* 1977; 297:750–7.
14. The Multicenter Postinfarction Research Group. Risk stratification and survival after MI. *N Engl J Med.* 1983; 309:331–6.
15. Mukharji J, Rude RE, Poole WK et al. Risk factors for sudden death after acute MI: two year follow up. *Am J Cardiol.* 1984; 54:31–6.
16. Meinertz T, Hofmann T, Kasper W et al. Significance of ventricular arrhythmias in idiopathic dilated cardiomyopathy. *Am J Cardiol.* 1984; 53:902–7.
17. Bigger JT, Fleiss JL, Kleiger R et al. The relationships among ventricular arrhythmias, left ventricular dysfunction, and mortality in the 2 years after MI. *Circulation.* 1984; 69:250–8.
18. Koch-Weser J, Klein SW. Procainamide dosage schedules, plasma concentrations, and clinical effects. *JAMA.* 1971; 215:1454–60.
19. Niarchos AP. Disopyramide: serum level and arrhythmia conversion. *Am Heart J.* 1976; 92:57–64.
20. Sokolow M, Edgar AL. Blood quinidine concentrations as a guide in the treatment of cardiac arrhythmias. *Circulation.* 1950; 1:576–92.
21. Gianelly R, Von der Groeben JO, Spivack AP et al. Effect of lidocaine on ventricular arrhythmias in patients with coronary heart disease. *N Engl J Med.* 1967; 277:1215–9.
22. Anastasiou-Nana MI, Menlove RL, Nanas JN et al. Changes in spontaneous variability of ventricular ectopic activity as a function of time in patients with chronic arrhythmias. *Circulation.* 1988; 78:286–95.
23. Brodsky M, Wu D, Denes P et al. Arrhythmias documented by 24 hour continuous electrocardiographic monitoring in 50 male medical students without apparent heart disease. *Am J Cardiol.* 1977; 39:390–5.
24. Sobotka PA, Mayer JH, Bauernfeind RA et al. Arrhythmias documented by 24-hour continuous ambulatory electrocardiographic monitoring in young women without apparent heart disease. *Am Heart J.* 1981; 101:753–9.
25. Bjerregaard P. Premature beats in healthy subjects 40–79 years of age. *Eur Heart J.* 1982; 3:493–503.

26. Fleg JL, Kennedy HL. Cardiac arrhythmias in a healthy elderly population: detection by 24-hour ambulatory electrocardiography. *Chest*. 1982; 81:302–7.
27. Kostis JB, McCrone K, Moreya AE et al. Premature ventricular complexes in the absence of identifiable heart disease. *Circulation*. 1981; 63:1351–6.
28. Bayes de Luna A, Coumel P, Leclercq JF. Ambulatory sudden cardiac death: mechanisms of production of fatal arrhythmia on the basis of data from 157 cases. *Am Heart J*. 1989; 117:151–9.
29. Simson MB. Use of signals in the terminal QRS complex to identify patients with ventricular tachycardia after myocardial infarction. *Circulation*. 1981; 64:235–42.
30. Kuchar DL, Thorburn CW, Sammel NL. Late potentials detected after myocardial infarction: natural history and prognostic significance. *Circulation*. 1986; 74:1280–9.
31. Nalos PC, Gang ES, Mandel WJ et al. The signal-averaged electrocardiogram as a screening test for inducibility of sustained ventricular tachycardia in high risk patients: a prospective study. *J Am Coll Cardiol*. 1987; 9:539–48.
32. Gomes JA, Mehra R, Barreca P et al. Quantitative analysis of the high frequency components of the signal-averaged QRS complex in patients with acute myocardial infarction: a prospective study. *Circulation*. 1985; 72:105–11.
33. Denniss AR, Richards DA, Cody DV et al. Prognostic significance of ventricular tachycardia and fibrillation induced at programmed stimulation and delayed potentials detected on the signal-averaged electrocardiograms of survivors of acute myocardial infarction. *Circulation*. 1986; 74:731–45.
34. Gomes JA, Winters SL, Stewart D et al. A new noninvasive index to predict sustained ventricular tachycardia and sudden death in the first year after myocardial infarction: based on signal-averaged electrocardiogram, radionuclide ejection fraction and Holter monitoring. *J Am Coll Cardiol*. 1987; 10:349–57.
35. Simson MB, Untereker WJ, Spielman SR et al. Relation between late potentials on the body surface and directly recorded fragmented electrograms in patients with ventricular tachycardia. *Am J Cardiol*. 1983; 51:105–12.
36. Lindsay BD, Ambos HD, Schechtman KB et al. Improved selection of patients for programmed ventricular stimulation by frequency analysis of signal-averaged electrocardiograms. *Circulation*. 1986; 73:675–83.
37. Gang ES, Lew AS, Hong M et al. Decreased incidence of ventricular late potentials after successful thrombolytic therapy for acute myocardial infarction. *N Engl J Med*. 1989; 321:712–6.
38. Simson MB, Spielman SR, Horowitz LN et al. Effects of antiarrhythmic drugs on body surface late potentials in patients with ventricular tachycardia. *Am J Cardiol*. 1982; 49:1030. Abstract.
39. Denniss AR, Ross DL, Richards DA et al. Effects of antiarrhythmic therapy on delayed potentials detected by the signal-averaged electrocardiogram in patients with ventricular tachycardia after acute myocardial infarction. *Am J Cardiol*. 1986; 58:261–5.
40. Borbola J, Denes P. Oral amiodarone loading therapy: I. The effect on serial signal-averaged electrocardiographic recordings and the QT_c in patients with ventricular tachyarrhythmias. *Am Heart J*. 1988; 115:1202–8.
41. Podrid PJ, Graboys TB. Exercise stress testing in the management of cardiac rhythm disorders. *Med Clin North Am*. 1984; 68:1139–52.
42. Velebit V, Podrid P, Lown B et al. Aggravation and provocation of ventricular arrhythmias by antiarrhythmic drugs. *Circulation*. 1982; 65:886–94.
43. Ranger S, Talajic M, Lemery R et al. Amplification of flecainide-induced ventricular conduction slowing by exercise. *Circulation*. 1989; 79:1000–6.
44. Hammill SC, Sugrue DD, Gersh BJ et al. Clinical intracardiac electrophysiologic testing: technique, diagnostic indications, and therapeutic uses. *Mayo Clin Proc*. 1986; 61:478–503.
45. Cameron J, Isner JM, Salem DM et al. Cardiac electrophysiologic testing: its role in the selection of antiarrhythmic drug regimens for supraventricular and ventricular arrhythmias. *Pharmacotherapy*. 1985; 5:95–108.
46. Podrid PJ, Schoeneberger A, Lown B et al. Use of nonsustained ventricular tachycardia as a guide to antiarrhythmic drug therapy in patients with malignant ventricular arrhythmia. *Am Heart J*. 1983; 105:181–188.
47. Freedman RA, Anderson KP, Mason JW. Electrophysiologic studies in patients with ventricular tachycardia. *Annu Rev Med*. 1986; 37:1–12.
48. Lombardi F, Stein J, Podrid PJ et al. Daily reproducibility of electrophysiologic test results in malignant ventricular arrhythmia. *Am J Cardiol*. 1986; 57:96–101.
49. Zipes DP, Akhtar M, Denes P et al. Guidelines for clinical intracardiac electrophysiologic studies. *Circulation*. 1989; 80:1925–39.
50. Horowitz LN, Josephson ME, Farshidi A et al. Recurrent sustained ventricular tachycardia. 3. Role of the electrophysiologic study in selection of antiarrhythmic regimens. *Circulation*. 1978; 58:986–97.
51. Berry NS, Bauman JL, Gallastegui JL et al. Analysis of antiarrhythmic drug concentrations determined during electrophysiologic drug testing in patients with inducible tachycardias. *Am J Cardiol*. 1988; 61:922–4.
52. Swerdlow CD, Gong G, Echt DS et al. Clinical factors predicting successful electrophysiologic-pharmacologic study in patients with ventricular tachycardia. *J Am Coll Cardiol*. 1983; 1:409–16.
53. Swerdlow CD, Winkle RA, Mason JW. Determinants of survival in patients with ventricular tachyarrhythmias. *N Engl J Med*. 1983; 308:1436–42.
54. Mitchell LB, Duff HJ, Manyari DE et al. A randomized clinical trial of the noninvasive and invasive approaches to drug therapy of ventricular tachycardia. *N Engl J Med*. 1987; 317:1681–7.
55. Skale BT, Miles WM, Heger JJ et al. Survivors of cardiac arrest: prevention of recurrence by drug therapy as predicted by electrophysiologic testing or electrocardiographic monitoring. *Am J Cardiol*. 1986; 57:113–9.
56. The ESVEM Investigators. The ESVEM trial: electrophysiologic study versus electrocardiographic monitoring for selection of antiarrhythmic therapy of ventricular tachyarrhythmias. *Circulation*. 1989; 79:1354–60.
57. Gomes JAC, Hariman RI, Kang PS et al. Programmed electrical stimulation in patients with high-grade ventricular ectopy: electrophysiologic findings and prognosis for survival. *Circulation*. 1984; 1:43–51.
58. Klein RC, Machell C. Use of electrophysiologic testing in patents with nonsustained ventricular tachycardia: prognostic and therapeutic implications. *J Am Coll Cardiol*. 1989; 14:155–61.
59. Cripps T, Bennett D, Camm AJ et al. Inducibility of sustained monomorphic ventricular tachycardia as a prognostic indicator in survivors of recent myocardial infarction: a prospective evaluation in relation to other prognostic variables. *J Am Coll Cardiol*. 1989; 14:289–96.
60. Kuchar DL, Rottman J, Berger E et al. Prediction of successful suppression of sustained ventricular tachyarrhythmias by serial drug testing from data derived at the initial electrophysiologic study. *J Am Coll Cardiol*. 1988; 12:982–8.
61. Waxman HL, Buxton AE, Sadowski LM et al. The response to procainamide during electrophysiologic study for sustained ventricular tachyarrhythmias predicts response to other medications. *Circulation*. 1983; 67:30–7.
62. Swiryn S, Bauernfeind RA, Strasberg B et al. Prediction of response to class I antiarrhythmic drugs during electrophysiologic study of ventricular tachycardia. *Am Heart J*. 1982; 104:43–50.
63. Oseran DS, Gang ES, Rosenthal ME et al. Electropharmacologic testing in sustained ventricular tachycardia associated with coronary heart disease: value of the response to intravenous procainamide in predicting the response to oral

procainamide and oral quinidine treatment. *Am J Cardiol.* 1985; 56:883–6.
64. Wyse DG, Mitchell LB, Duff HJ. Procainamide, disopyramide and quinidine: discordant antiarrhythmic effects during crossover comparison in patients with inducible ventricular tachycardia. *J Am Coll Cardiol.* 1987; 9:882–9.
65. Hamer AW, Finerman WB, Peter T et al. Disparity between the clinical and electrophysiologic effects of amiodarone in the treatment of recurrent ventricular tachyarrhythmias. *Am Heart J.* 1981; 102:992–1000.
66. Bauman JL, Berk SI, Hariman RJ et al. Amiodarone for sustained ventricular tachycardia: efficacy, safety, and factors influencing long-term outcome. *Am Heart J.* 1987; 114:1436–44.
67. Kessler KM, Lowenthal DT, Warner H et al. Quinidine elimination in patients with congestive heart failure or poor renal function. *N Engl J Med.* 1974; 290:706–9.
68. Anderson JL, Stewart JR, Perry BA et al. Oral flecainide acetate for the treatment of ventricular arrhythmias. *N Engl J Med.* 1981; 305:473–7.
69. McCollam PL, Bauman JL, Beckman KJ et al. A simple method of monitoring antiarrhythmic drugs during short- and long-term therapy. *Am J Cardiol.* 1989; 63:1273–5.
70. Yusuf S, Wittes J, Friedman L. Overview of results of randomized clinical trials in heart disease: I. Treatments following myocardial infarction. *JAMA.* 1988; 260:2088–93.
71. The CONSENSUS Trial Study Group. Effects of enalapril on mortality in severe congestive heart failure. *N Engl J Med.* 1987; 316:1429–35.

“

Reassessment of Benefit–Risk Ratio and Treatment Algorithms for Antiarrhythmic Drug Therapy

The Cardiac Arrhythmia Suppression Trial (CAST) has led to serious reconsideration of both the benefit–risk ratio of antiarrhythmic drug therapy and the appropriate therapeutic approach to various cardiac arrhythmias. Class IC drugs, such as encainide and flecainide, should not be used to treat asymptomatic postinfarction arrhythmias. Furthermore, because the CAST raises serious questions about the concept of treating asymptomatic but "potentially malignant" (prognostically important) arrhythmias guided by ambulatory monitoring, the prophylactic use of any of the antiarrhythmic agents (except beta blockers) must be considered inappropriate and potentially harmful until otherwise established by specific clinical trials.

For prophylaxis of malignant ventricular arrhythmias (sustained ventricular tachycardia or ventricular fibrillation), treatment may still begin with standard agents in classes IA, IB, or both, preferably guided by electrophysiologic testing alone or in combination with noninvasive testing. Class IC therapy may be most useful in those patients in this group who do not have such high-risk characteristics for proarrhythmia as a history of multiple myocardial infarctions (MIs), congestive heart failure, or low ejection fraction. Amiodarone is moderately effective for treating these arrhythmias but is reserved as second- or third-line therapy because of its potential organ toxicity. Sotalol, a beta blocker with class III activity, is often effective and relatively well tolerated in these patients and may become a preferred drug when approved.

For symptomatic but nonmalignant ventricular arrhythmias, a more conservative approach is more appropriate than in the past, with therapy reserved for those with debilitating symptoms. An initial trial of beta blockade is often appropriate before class I agents are considered. Class IC therapy should be avoided in patients with a history of MI (especially recent or multiple MIs), and probably in other patients with symptomatic coronary artery disease (e.g., angina, heart failure). The CAST emphasizes the need for further experimental and clinical trials and the development of new agents based on a better understanding of the overall benefit–risk ratio. As this occurs, treatment algorithms will continue to evolve.

—Anderson JL. Reassessment of benefit–risk ratio and treatment algorithms for antiarrhythmic drug therapy after the Cardiac Arrhythmia Suppression Trial. *J Clin Pharmacol.* 1990; 30:981–9. Abstract.

”

Research

Comparison of MS-DOS and Macintosh pharmacokinetic analysis programs using a two-compartment, two-infusion dosing scheme

EDWARD M. HAMPTON, KYLE HRDLICKA, AND DAVID W. A. BOURNE

Abstract: Pharmacokinetic values derived by three nonlinear least-squares regression computer programs for sets of serum drug concentration data were compared.

The three programs selected for comparison were the MS-DOS-based programs PCNONLIN and ADAPT and the Macintosh program BOOMER. Data on serum recainam hydrochloride concentration in 10 patients given an i.v. loading dose followed by a maintenance infusion were fitted by the appropriate models in each program. Samples had been subjected to reverse-phase isocratic high-performance liquid chromatography with ultraviolet light detection; intraday and interday coefficients of variation were less than 8% over the range of concentrations measured. A two-compartment model was used for all regressions. Each program was given identical initial estimates, and the simplex minimization algorithm of each program was used to fit the model to the data. An identical weighting scheme was used for all three programs.

The mean pharmacokinetic values estimated by each program for the 10 data sets were essentially identical. Slightly larger rate constants and smaller volume terms were derived by BOOMER. BOOMER yielded the lowest weighted sum of squares and the highest correlation coefficient. A mean concentration–time plot showed that the programs all produced values that described the data very well.

The three computer programs used in this analysis derived essentially the same pharmacokinetic values to describe sets of serum drug concentration data. The BOOMER program provides an acceptable alternative to MS-DOS-based programs for pharmacokinetic analysis.

Index terms: Blood levels; Cardiac drugs; Computers; Methodology; Models; Pharmacokinetics; Recainam hydrochloride
Clin Pharm. 1991; 10:206–9

Compartmental analysis of pharmacokinetic data requires relatively large, sophisticated computer programs. Two of the earlier programs used extensively for pharmacokinetic analysis were the SAAM program of Berman and Weiss[1] developed at the National Institutes of Health and NONLIN of Metzler et al.[2] Both programs were widely used for data analysis and modeling, especially pharmacokinetic analysis. At the time of their development, a mainframe computer was necessary to provide the capacity and computational power needed. Since then, microcomputers and desktop computers have become more affordable and much more powerful.[3,4] Two MS-DOS programs for pharmacokinetic analysis, PCNONLIN[5] and ADAPT PC COLLECTION[6] (ADAPT) have enjoyed widespread use.

Since 1984, the 68000-based family of Macintosh computers has become popular among educators, researchers, and practitioners. Academics and clinicians have used these machines to solve complex pharmacokinetic and pharmacodynamic problems.

EDWARD M. HAMPTON, PHARM.D., is Clinical Specialist in Pharmacokinetics, Pharmacy Service, Department of Veterans Affairs Medical Center, Oklahoma City, and Clinical Assistant Professor, Section of Pharmacy Practice, College of Pharmacy, University of Oklahoma Health Sciences Center, Oklahoma City. KYLE HRDLICKA is a student at the College of Osteopathic Medicine, Oklahoma State University, Oklahoma City. DAVID W. A. BOURNE, PH.D., is Associate Professor, Pharmaceutics Section, College of Pharmacy, University of Oklahoma Health Sciences Center.

Address reprint requests to Dr. Hampton at the Pharmacy Service, Department of Veterans Affairs Medical Center, 921 NE 13th Street, Oklahoma City, OK 73104.

The assistance of Patricia Lurvey, Ph.D., University of Oklahoma Health Sciences Center, is acknowledged.

Presented at the 24th Annual ASHP Midyear Clinical Meeting, Atlanta, GA, December 6, 1989.

Until recently, however, no comparable program was available for the Apple Macintosh computer, even though many high-level language compilers had been available for some time. Translation and extension of the BASIC program MULTI[7] resulted in the general-purpose nonlinear regression program BOOMER[8] for the Macintosh. Since BOOMER was written for a new operating system and was compiled from a variety of source codes, an evaluation of the program's performance relative to the two commonly used programs, with real data, was desired.

The objective of this study was to compare the pharmacokinetic values estimated by three programs—PCNONLIN, ADAPT, and BOOMER—for given sets of serum drug concentration data.

Methods

PCNONLIN[a] and ADAPT[b] evaluations were performed on an IBM-XT computer equipped with 640K of random-access memory (RAM) and an 8087 math coprocessor. BOOMER[c] evaluations were performed on a standard Macintosh Plus computer with 1 megabyte of RAM.

Ten sets of serum drug concentration data collected during a previous investigation were fitted by models described in each program.[9] The data were for 10 subjects who had been treated with the class 1C antiarrhythmic recainam hydrochloride. An i.v. loading dose of 3 mg/kg was given over 40 minutes, followed by a maintenance infusion of 0.9 mg/kg/hr for 23 hours 20 minutes. A total of 15 blood samples from each subject were collected in heparin-containing tubes at frequent intervals and frozen at −20 °C until analysis.

The samples had been subjected to reverse-phase isocratic high-performance liquid chromatography with ultraviolet light detection at 214 nm. A Partisil ODS III (10-μm) column (Alltech Applied Sciences Laboratories, State College, PA) was used. The mobile phase consisted of 8.5% acetonitrile and 91.5% 0.1 M monobasic sodium phosphate buffer (pH 4.0). An analogue of recainam was used as an internal standard, with good resolution, and calculations were performed by using the peak height ratio of the two compounds. Intraday and interday coefficients of variation were less than 8% over the range of concentrations measured.[9]

The data had been well described by a two-compartment model[9]; therefore this model was used for all regressions with the three programs. Each program was given identical initial estimates, and the simplex minimization algorithm of each program was used to fit the model to the data. The identical weighting scheme of $1/y_{\text{observed}}$ was used for all three programs. Each set of data was run a single time on each program for standardization.

Since the implied hypothesis suggests that there is no significant difference in the estimates by the programs, multiple discriminant analysis[d] was used to detect any factor or variable that might discriminate among the programs. Multiple discriminant analysis allows analysis of a nonmetric dependent variable (the computer programs) and continuous independent variables (the pharmacokinetic variables). This statistical method allows for both univariate and multivariate analysis in an attempt to detect and distinguish discriminating factors. For all analyses, the a priori level of significance was set at ≤ 0.05.

Figure 1 illustrates the model used for all analyses and identifies those variables used to build the model in the BOOMER program. The model has two timed events or infusions (load and maintenance), two corresponding time interrupts (1 and 2), three rate constants to describe drug flow, and a single reciprocal volume term to describe the volume of distribution of the central compartment.

The appropriate variables were chosen from the variable menu to build the model in BOOMER. For ADAPT, the closed form solution provided in the ID3 module was used with one input and three dosing events (start and stop times for each infusion). To ensure that equal weights were used by all three programs, the generalized weighting option was selected so that the weights could be individually entered. For PCNONLIN, the integrated equation 1 was used as a function input. The equation contains a pre-exponential term that is multiplied by an exponential term describing the accumulation of the drug during infusion and a second exponential term describing the decay after infusion:

$$C = (R/V_c)[(k_{21} - \alpha)/(\beta - \alpha)][1 - e^{-\alpha(D)}][e^{-\alpha(t-D)}] + (R/V_c)[(k_{21} - \beta)/(\alpha - \beta)][1 - e^{-\beta(D)}][e^{-\beta(t-D)}] \quad (1)$$

Figure 1. Two-compartment, two-infusion model. $dC_1/dt = k_{21}C_2 - (k_{12} + k_{10})C_1$, where k_{12}, k_{21}, and k_{10} are distribution rate constants from the central compartment to the peripheral compartment, the peripheral compartment to the central compartment, and the central compartment to the external compartment, respectively; V_c is the volume of the central compartment; and C_1, C_2, and C_0 are apparent drug concentrations in the central, peripheral, and external compartments, respectively.

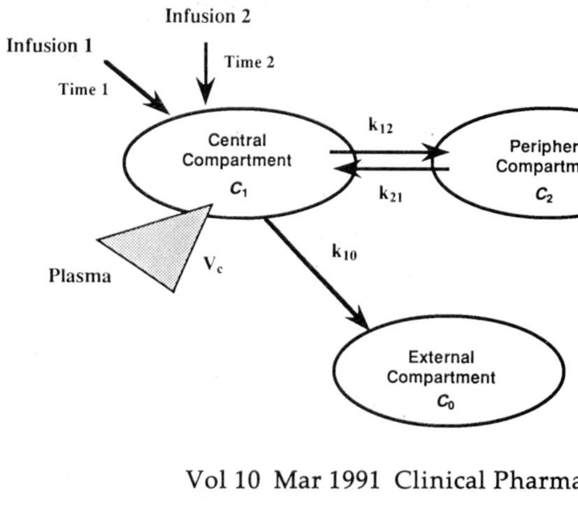

where C = drug concentration, R = rate of infusion, V_c = volume of central compartment, k_{21} = the distribution rate constant from the peripheral compartment to the central compartment, α = rate constant associated with distribution phase of concentration–time curve, and β = rate constant associated with terminal phase of concentration–time curve. Time functions were calculated as follows: when $t < T$ then $D = t$, and when $t > T$ then $D = T$, where T = time of infusion and t = elapsed time.

A separate equation (equations 2 and 3) was necessary for each infusion, and the function (F) was equal to the sum of the concentrations predicted from each equation ($C_1 + C_2$):

$$C_1 = A*(DEXP(-ALPHA*T) - DEXP(-ALPHA*TSTAR)) + B*(DEXP(-BETA*T) - DEXP(-BETA*TSTAR)) \quad (2)$$

$$C_2 = X1*A*(DEXP(-ALPHA*(T-TI)) - DEXP(-ALPHA*TSTAR2)) + B*(DEXP(-BETA*(T-TI)) - DEXP(-BETA*TSTAR2)) \quad (3)$$

A third data point was used to toggle in C_2 when the second infusion began. A logic statement was also required to allow the program to determine which time to use in each of the exponential terms.

Results

The mean pharmacokinetic values estimated by each of the three programs for the 10 data sets are listed in Table 1. The calculated values were essentially identical; slightly larger rate constants and smaller volume terms were derived by BOOMER. BOOMER yielded the lowest weighted sum of squares and the highest correlation coefficient of the three programs.

A mean concentration–time plot showed that PCNONLIN, ADAPT, and BOOMER all produced values that described the data very well. When superimposed, the three plots were almost indistinguishable (Figure 2).

A plot of each program's weighted residuals versus observed concentrations for a representative patient (Figure 3) revealed random scatter about zero, suggesting that the weighting scheme used was appropriate. Despite minimization of the y-axis to accentuate distances between points, the residuals calculated with the three programs were indistinguishable.

Visual examination of the data suggested that the programs produced identical pharmacokinetic values. The univariate component of the statistical analysis confirmed that there was no difference

Table 1.
Pharmacokinetic Values, Weighted Sums of Squares, and Correlation Coefficients for the Three Programs Evaluated[a]

Variable	PCNONLIN	ADAPT	BOOMER
V(L)	23.4 ± 3.2	23.5 ± 3.3	22.8 ± 2.9
k_{10} (hr^{-1})	0.921 ± 0.171	0.926 ± 0.186	0.948 ± 0.187
k_{12} (hr^{-1})	1.59 ± 0.5	1.60 ± 0.5	1.72 ± 0.4
k_{21} (hr^{-1})	0.486 ± 0.386	0.494 ± 0.105	0.519 ± 0.108
WSS	0.452 ± 0.386[b]	0.276 ± 0.186	0.260 ± 0.196
CC	0.967 ± 0.250	0.967 ± 0.200	0.983 ± 0.013

[a] Reported as mean ± S.D. of results for 10 patients. V = volume of distribution; k_{10}, k_{12}, and k_{21} = distribution rate constants from the central compartment to the external compartment, the central compartment to the peripheral compartment, and the peripheral compartment to the central compartment, respectively; WSS = weighted sum of squares; CC = correlation coefficient.

[b] PCNONLIN calculations of WSS involve a weighting scheme normalized for the number of data points.

Figure 2. Estimated (superimposed continuous and dashed lines) and observed (▲) mean concentration-versus-time plot for ADAPT, BOOMER, and PCNONLIN.

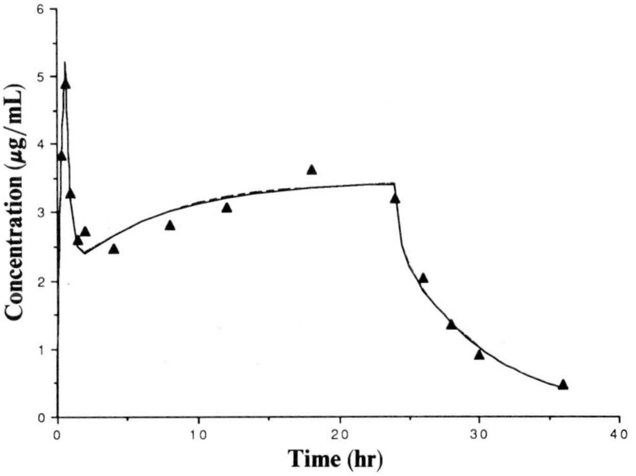

Figure 3. Plot of weighted residuals versus observed concentration for ADAPT (O), BOOMER (△), and PCNONLIN (□) for patient 1. (The values for PCNONLIN were calculated by hand by using standard methods.[8])

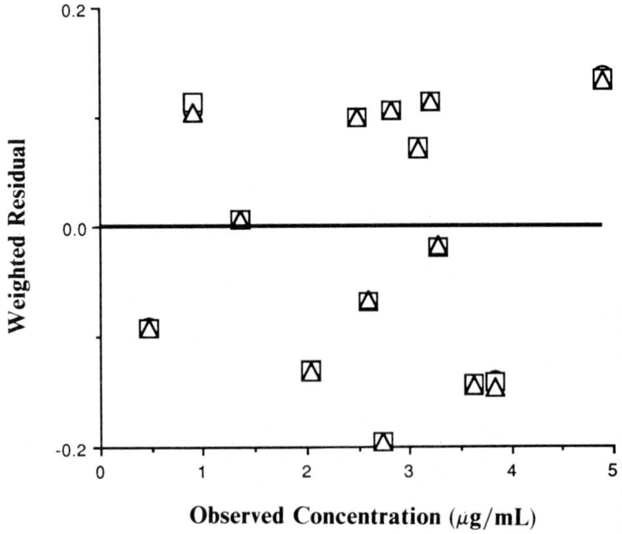

between the programs with respect to value estimation (minimum $p = 0.789$). Multivariate analysis further indicated that the programs did not have any distinguishing variables with respect to performance (minimum $p = 0.99$).

The results of the discriminant analysis can be illustrated by examining a discriminant function plot (Figure 4) in which the data points represent program performance for each of the data sets plotted against the two discriminant functions derived from the statistical operation. The considerable overlap in these data points suggests that the programs possessed no discriminating variables. Had the programs truly performed differently, the discriminant functions would have produced more disparate clusters.

Discussion

The minor differences in the estimates by the three programs are practically and statistically insignificant. The differences are less than 1 standard deviation of any of the estimates and probably reflect differences in each program's estimates of initial value sets for the simplex algorithm. The detailed output of all three programs varied, but each provided information and plots useful for evaluating goodness of fit. For the particular model in question, the version of PCNONLIN evaluated required a user-generated subroutine to create the model. Both ADAPT and BOOMER were capable of analyzing the data without the need for subroutines. Although this investigation did not subjectively evaluate speed—it varies with hardware configuration—the ADAPT program ran several orders of magnitude faster than PCNONLIN on the same system. BOOMER was slightly slower than ADAPT but considerably faster than PCNONLIN at convergence.

Figure 4. Multivariate analysis discriminatory function plot for ADAPT (○), BOOMER (△), and PCNONLIN (□).

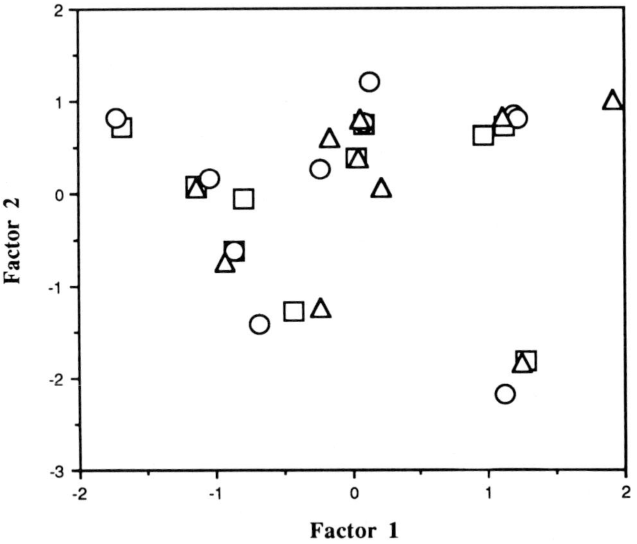

Since the time of this analysis, all three programs have been upgraded. The changes enhance the ease of use and speed of the programs but have little to no influence on output performance. All three programs are extremely useful, and although each has unique attributes, all perform similarly. Detailed information about the programs is available elsewhere.[5,6,8]

Conclusion

Three computer programs used in pharmacokinetic analysis—PCNONLIN, ADAPT, and BOOMER—derived essentially the same pharmacokinetic values to describe sets of serum drug concentration data. The study failed to reject the null hypothesis that the programs are indistinguishable. The primary differences between the programs are the hardware requirements and how the models are described and entered. Since it appears that the three programs provide equivalent results, the primary considerations in choosing one for pharmacokinetic analysis are hardware preference, ease of use, flexibility, and speed.

---

[a] Version 2.0C, Statistical Consultants, Inc., Lexington, KY 40508.

[b] Version written in June 1987, Laboratory of Applied Pharmacokinetics, School of Medicine, University of Southern California, Los Angeles, CA 90033.

[c] From David W. A. Bourne, College of Pharmacy, University of Oklahoma Health Sciences Center, Oklahoma City, OK 73190.

[d] Systat, Inc., Evanston, IL 60201.

References

1. Berman M, Weiss MF. Users manual for SAAM. Bethesda, MD: National Institute for Arthritis and Metabolic Disease; 1968.
2. Metzler CM, Elfring GK, McEwen AJ. A package of computer programs for pharmacokinetic modeling. *Biometrics.* 1974; 30:562–3.
3. Peck CC, Barrett BB. Nonlinear least-squares regression programs for microcomputers. *J Pharmacokinet Biopharm.* 1979; 7:537–41.
4. Peck CC. Computer-assisted clinical pharmacokinetics. In: Benet LZ, Massoud N, Gambertoglio JG, eds. Pharmacokinetic basis for drug treatment. New York: Raven; 1984:349–56.
5. Weiner DL. NONLIN84/PCNONLIN: software for the statistical analysis of nonlinear models. *Methods Find Exp Clin Pharmacol.* 1986; 8:625–8.
6. Jelliffe RW. User's manual for the PC programs from the USC Laboratory of Applied Pharmacokinetics. Los Angeles, CA: University of Southern California School of Medicine; 1987.
7. Yamaoka K, Tanigawara Y, Nakagawa T et al. A pharmacokinetic analysis program (MULTI) for microcomputer. *J Pharmacobiodyn.* 1981; 4:879–85.
8. Bourne DWA. BOOMER, a simulation and modeling program for pharmacokinetic and pharmacodynamic data analysis. *Comput Programs Biomed.* 1989; 29:191–5.
9. Hampton EM, Anastasiou-Nana MI, Nanas JN et al. The disposition of recainam hydrochloride during and after intravenous loading and maintenance infusion in cardiac patients. *J Clin Pharmacol.* 1987; 27:951–6.

Editorials

Trials and tribulations of evaluating ventricular arrhythmias

In this issue McCollam and Parker (pages 195-205) outline a number of ways of evaluating the patient who has a ventricular arrhythmia. One can assess the patient on the basis of clinical findings or his or her report of symptoms. As the authors point out, however, these methods correlate poorly with actual episodes of ventricular arrhythmias. Continuous ambulatory electrocardiographic recordings (Holter monitoring) can be used to measure the frequency and type of rhythm abnormality. In addition, some Holter monitors can assess the ST segment of the electrocardiogram and count the ischemic episodes, which may (or may not) relate to the arrhythmia in question. Cardiologists may also evaluate the patient under conditions of stress (exercise testing) in hopes of unmasking an arrhythmia that may not be present under normal conditions. Additional tools are signal-averaged electrocardiography and the electrophysiologic study (EPS).

A major question in the utilization of these various means of evaluating arrhythmias is how well they predict long-term prognosis, drug efficacy, and the efficacy of nonpharmacologic methods of controlling or abolishing ventricular arrhythmias. The evaluation and management of ventricular arrhythmias are complex and confusing and have become more so since results of the Cardiac Arrhythmia Suppression Trial (CAST) became available.[1] Although the risks associated with antiarrhythmics, especially proarrhythmia, have been recognized for years, CAST proved that encainide and flecainide, drugs that were shown by Holter monitoring to suppress ventricular ectopy, actually shortened survival. By conventional wisdom, one would have suspected that patients who had significant suppression of premature ventricular contractions (PVCs) would have fared better than those without such suppression. This theory is still being tested as CAST continues with the use of moricizine. CAST raises other questions: Is Holter monitoring really useful in evaluating ventricular arrhythmias or drug efficacy? Is ventricular ectopy a marker of poor clinical outcome but not necessarily the cause of death? The latter is an interesting question since β-adrenergic blockade has improved survival after myocardial infarction, yet β-blockers are not particularly effective in suppressing ventricular ectopy.

McCollam and Parker cite a number of studies in which some arrhythmias that were inducible during EPS became noninducible after antiarrhythmics were administered. Clinical outcome was better in patients whose arrhythmias became noninducible than in patients whose arrhythmias remained inducible. Does EPS predict drug efficacy or merely identify those patients (whose arrhythmias are easily rendered noninducible) who have a better prognosis due to some unrecognized factor?

In contrast to the study by Wilber and colleagues,[2] which McCollam and Parker describe, is one by Poole et al.,[3] in which 241 survivors of out-of-hospital ventricular fibrillation (VF) were evaluated. Patients whose initially inducible arrhythmias (sustained ventricular tachycardia [VT] or VF) were subsequently rendered noninducible as determined by EPS-guided drug therapy did *not* have improved survival when compared with patients whose tachyarrhythmia could not be rendered noninducible by drug therapy. Clearly, one must use caution when evaluating these complex studies. They may differ in their definition of positive response or in the stimulation protocol employed. Long-term outcomes may also be difficult to compare because of differences in long-term therapy. Frequently, patients whose arrhythmia becomes noninducible in response to drug therapy are treated with type I antiarrhythmics, while those whose arrhythmia remains inducible are treated with amiodarone. The use of automatic implantable defibrillators further complicates the picture.

McCollam and Parker suggest that there is a consensus among clinicians (cardiologists) that patients with lethal arrhythmias should undergo EPS. This is not surprising when one considers the financial remuneration for such a procedure. As of yet, it has not been clearly shown that EPS is superior to Holter monitoring in predicting drug efficacy. As mentioned by McCollam and Parker, this possibility is being investigated in a large prospective randomized multicenter trial funded by the National Institutes of Health. The Electrophysiologic Study Versus Electrocardiographic Monitoring (ESVEM) trial is comparing the usefulness of serial EPS and serial Holter monitoring in predicting drug efficacy in patients with lethal arrhythmias.[4] To be enrolled in ESVEM, patients must have survived an episode of sudden cardiac death or have documented sustained ventricular tachycardia. To be randomized for one of the methods of evaluation, all patients must have inducible sustained VT and >10 PVCs per hour. A similar trial has been completed[5] but has been criticized because of its small number of patients (57), the unusually small number of arrhythmia recurrences in the EPS group, and the resultant low statistical power (approximately 0.50).[6] The ESVEM study plans to follow almost 300 patients discharged on "effective" drug therapy as determined by either Holter monitoring or EPS.

The accuracy of using EPS in predicting drug efficacy may vary substantially depending on the nature of the underlying disease. EPS may be more useful in patients with sustained VT who have coronary artery disease than in patients with sustained VT who have idiopathic cardiomyopathy or other cardiac conditions in which coronary artery disease is not present. In addition, other factors outlined by McCollam and Parker may affect long-term prognosis.

As pharmacists, we are interested in how to best monitor our patients. Are the drugs that patients are receiving efficacious? What is the therapeutic outcome? In the case of the patient with a lethal or potentially lethal arrhythmia, we are faced with a dilemma. The drugs used to treat these disorders have a narrow therapeutic range and cause proarrhythmia in 10% to 15% of patients. We should become familiar with the advantages and disadvantages of each of the methods available for evaluating arrhythmias and antiarrhythmic agents.

1. The Cardiac Arrhythmia Suppression Trial (CAST) Investigators. Preliminary report: effect of encainide and flecainide on mortality in a randomized trial of arrhythmia suppression after myocardial infarction. *N Engl J Med.* 1989; 321:406-12.
2. Wilber DJ, Garan H, Finkelstein D et al. Out-of-hospital cardiac arrest: use of electrophysiologic testing in the prediction of long-term outcome. *N Engl J Med.* 1988; 318:19-24.
3. Poole JE, Mathisen TL, Kudenchuk PJ et al. Long-term outcome in patients who survive out of hospital ventricular fibrillation and undergo electrophysiologic studies: evaluation by electrophysiologic subgroups. *J Am Coll Cardiol.* 1990; 16:657-65.
4. ESVEM Investigators. The ESVEM trial: electrophysiologic study versus electrocardiographic monitoring for selection of antiarrhythmic therapy of ventricular tachyarrhythmias. *Circulation.* 1989; 79:1354-60.
5. Mitchell LB, Duff HJ, Mayari DE et al. A randomized clinical trial of the noninvasive and invasive approaches to drug therapy of ventricular tachycardias. *N Engl J Med.* 1987; 317:1681-7.
6. Mason JW, Moon TE. Treatment of ventricular tachycardia. *N Engl J Med.* 1988; 318:1693-4. Letter.

Jean Nappi, Pharm.D., Professor of Clinical Pharmacy
College of Pharmacy
Texas Medical Center
University of Houston
Houston, TX 77030

Antiarrhythmic monitoring: Misplaced emphasis

There is something intellectually appealing about using the achievement of a predetermined serum antiarrhythmic drug concentration as a therapeutic endpoint. This alternative to trial-and-error dosing correctly assumes that antiarrhythmic response is often more closely related to serum concentration than dosage and that patients differ in the amount of drug needed to attain a target concentration. McCollam and Parker, however, warn in this issue that the attainment of a preestablished drug concentration should not generally be the sole endpoint; other authors have expressed a similar opinion.[1,2] Nevertheless, many physicians and pharmacists continue to use concentration data as if cardiac rhythm disturbances in all patients were caused by the same imaginary microbe that always succumbed to a "therapeutic level" of a drug. Practitioners too often base their description of an antiarrhythmic concentration—as "subtherapeutic," "therapeutic," or "toxic"—on the value itself rather than the patient's clinical response.

The proper use of antiarrhythmic concentration data is anything but simple. Familiar pharmacokinetic considerations (e.g., the degree of protein binding, the presence of active metabolites, and drug interactions) complicate the monitoring of concentrations. In addition, a predetermined therapeutic range is often irrelevant for a patient because that range was determined for another arrhythmia; derived from patients with a different type, chronicity, or severity of illness; or established using an obsolete definition of success.

Why, then, do health-care professionals continue to rely on predetermined therapeutic concentration ranges? Many practitioners are not taught to do otherwise. Educators might argue that there simply is not enough time to cover all important aspects of antiarrhythmic therapy. Indeed, the number of drugs now available and our expanding knowledge of arrhythmias and their treatment make adequate coverage of the topic seemingly impossible. In many pharmacy schools, the antiarrhythmics section (if there is one) of the therapeutics course emphasizes information that is easily found in reference books (e.g., dosages, pharmacokinetic values, and adverse effects) rather than the harder-to-explain evaluation of efficacy. Many pharmacy students never get a chance to learn the finer points of antiarrhythmic therapy during clinical clerkships.

Even if they were taught about the evaluation of antiarrhythmic efficacy, students might still overemphasize the importance of concentration ranges. Pharmacy students are conditioned to approach problems numerically. When students are not calculating the dosage associated with a given drug concentration (or vice versa), they are observing their faculty mentors measuring drug concentrations in some body fluid. Thus, students might easily suppose that drug concentration is practically synonymous with drug efficacy.

It is easy—and some might say medicolegally prudent—to pay at least as much attention to laboratory values as to patients, and patients with heart disease are already likely to be described in terms of quantifiable variables such as blood pressure and cardiac index. Practitioners often give no more thought to forcing an antiarrhythmic concentration into the "normal" or "therapeutic" range indicated on a laboratory report than they do to manipulating heparin or potassium dosages to attain the same goal. Pharmacists, anxious to demonstrate their skill in pharmacokinetics, may also focus too much on the adjustment of antiarrhythmic dosage and not enough on the meaning of the concentration values. Finally, because predetermined therapeutic ranges are employed with other commonly used drugs (e.g., aminoglycosides, theophylline, and anticonvulsants), it is natural to assume that such ranges should also be applicable for antiarrhythmics.

To be sure, monitoring antiarrhythmic concentrations has valuable applications. One of the most important, as

 0278-2677/91/0301-0211$00.50.

McCollam and Parker suggest, is the determination of a patient's own therapeutic threshold. Other valid applications include the investigation of drug interactions, unexpected clinical outcomes, toxicity, and compliance in individual patients. Attainment of a pre-established concentration range may be appropriate when the use of other endpoints is not practical. For example, if an arrhythmia is not inducible during programmed electrical stimulation and occurs so rarely that its suppression cannot be convincingly demonstrated by electrocardiographic monitoring, a concentration range may serve as a sensible, but not ideal, dosage guideline.

The quantitative approach to medicine provides invaluable insight into the pathogenesis of disease and the properties of drugs. In fact, for many patients the response to antiarrhythmics may be most appropriately expressed in quantitative terms, such as the duration of arrhythmia during programmed electrical stimulation and the frequency of ectopy during electrocardiographic monitoring. Health-care providers, however, should know that appropriate drug therapy, whether it involves antiarrhythmics or not, is rarely a matter of simply attaining a pre-established drug concentration. Pharmacists, in particular, should realize that they need more than a calculator to contribute optimally to antiarrhythmic therapy.

1. Kates RE. Plasma level monitoring of antiarrhythmic drugs. *Am J Cardiol.* 1983; 52:8C-13C.
2. Kupersmith J. Monitoring of antiarrhythmic drug levels: values and pitfalls. *Ann N Y Acad Sci.* 1984; 432:138-54.

GUY R. HASEGAWA

Grand Rounds

Elemental mercury poisoning

MAURO J. FLORENTINE AND DOMINIC J. SANFILIPPO II

Abstract: Three siblings with inhaled elemental mercury toxicity are described, and the signs and symptoms of mercury toxicity, interpretation of mercury concentrations, and management of elemental mercury exposure are reviewed.

A 4-year-old girl was admitted to the hospital with a history of fever and increasing irritability, fatigue, malaise, insomnia, headache, anorexia, and ataxia. She was discharged two days later with a diagnosis of acute cerebellar ataxia. During the following 18 days, the child's condition worsened, and she was rehospitalized. Meanwhile her 11-year-old sister was hospitalized for evaluation of fatigue, weakness, lower back pain, and ataxia. The older girl's blood mercury concentration, at 5.5 µg/dL, was in the toxic range. Twenty-four-hour urine mercury screening confirmed mercury intoxication in both children. Questioning revealed that the girls' brother had recently spilled 0.5–l oz of elemental mercury in the house. All family members underwent blood and urine mercury testing. The brother underwent a dimercaprol challenge to determine his tissue mercury burden, which was found to be >2.4 µg/dL. The sisters underwent two courses of chelation therapy with dimercaprol. Symptoms persisted in all three children, and they underwent five 10-day cycles of *N*-acetyl-D,L-penicillamine (NAP) therapy; the youngest underwent a third dimercaprol regimen. All siblings continued NAP chelation therapy because of extensive tissue mercury burden until the results of repeated urine mercury concentration determinations were normal.

The cases presented illustrate several challenges in diagnosing and managing mercury toxicity: lack of agreement upon toxic versus normal levels of blood and urine mercury, lack of correlation between symptomatology and blood and urine test results, and the absence of endpoints for initiation and cessation of chelation therapy. Treatment options include dimercaprol, penicillamine, and the investigational agents NAP and 2,3-dimercaptosuccinic acid (DMSA).

DMSA may be the most effective agent available for mercury chelation therapy; however, further study is needed to determine toxic levels of blood and urine mercury and endpoints for initiation and cessation of therapy.

Index terms: *N*-Acetyl-D,L-penicillamine; Antidotes; Blood levels; Dimercaprol; Heavy-metal antagonists; Mercury; Metals; Pediatrics; Poisoning; Tissue levels; Toxicity; Toxicity, environmental; Urine levels

Clin Pharm. 1991; 10:213-21

Mercury is one of the oldest industrial poisons. Its toxic properties have been documented for centuries; its most famous victim was perhaps the Mad Hatter of *Alice in Wonderland*.[1] Despite improvements in working conditions, mercury is second only to lead as a cause of heavy-metal poisonings today. One reason for this is the widespread use of mercury in many branches of manufacturing, including the chemical, pharmaceutical, and electrochemical industries, as well as in the production of measuring apparatus and dental amalgams. Organic mercury intoxication has historically been associated with a more severe acute or subacute disorder than has elemental mercury inhalation. Recently, however, the inhalation of elemental mercury has been shown to cause many of the signs and symptoms attributed to organic mercury poisoning.[2-5] The following cases illustrate the myriad medical, psychological, scientific, and financial problems associated with inhalational elemental mercury poisoning.

MAURO J. FLORENTINE is Clinical Coordinator, Pharmacy Department, Butterworth Hospital (BH), Grand Rapids, MI. DOMINIC J. SANFILIPPO II, M.D., is Assistant Professor of Pediatrics, Michigan State University College of Human Medicine, Lansing, and Director, Pediatric Intensive Care, BH.

Address reprint requests to Mr. Florentine at Mail Code 1, Butterworth Hospital, 100 Michigan NE, Grand Rapids, MI 49503.

The editorial assistance of Jim Cwengros and Lyn Florentine and the secretarial assistance of Arlene Sprengelmeyer and Shirley Bergin are acknowledged.

This is **article 680-204-9108** in the **ASHP Continuing Education System**; it qualifies for 1.0 hour of CE credit. See page 230 for learning objectives and test questions.

Papers in the Grand Rounds *section are patient case reports and literature review combined in a way that gives them high educational value. The papers lead off with a well-documented case report of an unusual drug experience (e.g., adverse drug reaction or other unexpected drug response, experimental use of a drug). The case generally deals with a difficult therapeutic problem or dilemma that is commonly encountered but may be overlooked or misunderstood. (Esoteric or rare occurences of minor impportance do not make good* Grand Rounds *material.) A literature review puts the case in perspective with previously reported similar cases and alternative treatments. The review is integrated with related discussion of the case being reported.*

CP *readers are encouraged to use* Grand Rounds *for educational group discussions. For this purpose, discussion questions are printed at the end of* Grand Rounds *papers.*

Case Reports

A four-year-old girl was admitted to the hospital on August 21, 1989, with ataxia. Her illness had first received medical attention approximately two weeks earlier, when she was evaluated by her pediatrician for nausea, diarrhea, and an erythematous, macular rash of the extremities. These symptoms were attributed to gastroenteritis and seemed to respond to clear liquids and Donnagel (A. H. Robins Co., Inc., Richmond, VA). Approximately five days before admission, the mother reported that the child was febrile and developed increasing irritability, fatigue, malaise, insomnia, headache, ataxia, anorexia, and a 2–3 kg weight loss.

On the day of admission, her temperature was 37.2 °C rectally, blood pressure was 133/78 mm Hg, respiratory rate was 32 breaths/min, and heart rate was 128 beats/min. The physical examination also revealed irritability, fatigue, a decrease in overall muscle tone, decreased deep-tendon reflexes, a wide-based ataxic gait, and truncal ataxia.

Laboratory analysis revealed that complete blood count (CBC), serum electrolytes, and urinalysis were within normal limits. A lumbar puncture revealed no white blood cells, a cerebrospinal fluid (CSF) protein concentration of 125 mg/dL, and a glucose concentration of 79 mg/dL. A nonenhanced computed-tomography (CT) scan of the head was normal. Results of Epstein-Barr viral studies were negative. She was discharged on August 23 with a diagnosis of acute cerebellar ataxia that was thought to be caused by a postinfectious radiculocerebellar syndrome.

The patient was home for 18 days, during which time she became progressively weaker. Ataxia progressed to the point where she was no longer able to walk. Her irritability, insomnia, and fatigue persisted, and she became encephalopathic, exhibiting inappropriate behavior and experiencing hallucinations. The frequency and severity of her headaches increased. The skin of her hands and feet was erythematous; it had begun to peel and was extremely itchy. She was evaluated at this time by her pediatrician. Results of laboratory analyses, including CBC, serum chemistry, and erythrocyte sedimentation rate (ESR), were within normal limits. Because of her encephalopathic behavior and progressive weakness, she was readmitted to the hospital on September 11. Her vital signs included a blood pressure of 140/90 mm Hg and a heart rate of 125 beats/min. Physical examination revealed a weak, irritable child who was unable to walk. Deep-tendon reflexes were absent. A lumbar puncture revealed a CSF protein concentration of 262 mg/dL; all other CSF values were within normal limits. Results of tests for oligoclonal banding and myelin basic proteins were normal. Lyme titers and antinuclear antibody test results were negative. Results of magnetic-resonance imaging (MRI) studies were within normal limits and did not reveal any demyelinization. She was diagnosed as having benign essential hypertension and a postviral encephaloradiculopathy or a Guillain-Barré-like syndrome. She was started on a course of prednisone 1.5 mg/kg/day, chloral hydrate (for irritability), and propranolol (for hypertension). Despite this treatment, she showed no improvement and suffered a seizure on September 19. At the time of her seizure, her serum sodium concentration was 120 meq/L, which was thought to be attributable to a syndrome of inappropriate secretion of antidiuretic hormone. The seizure responded well to diazepam and infusion of 3% sodium chloride solution. Urinalysis revealed proteinuria with a urine sodium concentration of 60 meq/L. Serum sodium and osmolality returned to normal within 24 hours after therapy, and no further seizures were observed. In retrospect, this hyponatremia was likely due to renal tubular dysfunction with salt loss secondary to mercury intoxication.

During this time, the child's 11-year-old sister also was hospitalized for evaluation of generalized fatigue, weakness, severe lower back pain, and ataxia. The older girl's blood pressure was 141/97 mm Hg, heart rate was 90–100 beats/min, and temperature was 37.7 °C. A neurologic examination revealed bilateral thigh and calf pain, toe and finger numbness, and decreased response to pinprick in all four extremities. She exhibited no personality changes or irritability. CSF examination revealed a protein concentration of 376 mg/dL. All other CSF values were normal, as were serum electrolytes and CBC.

Because the two sisters had such similar symptoms and the likelihood of a postviral polyradiculopathy occurring in two family members at the same time was low, investigation for heavy-metal intoxication was pursued. Whole-blood mercury concentration determinations were performed on both sisters. Results (Table 1) were interpreted as within normal limits by house staff physicians and consultants as well as by the toxicology laboratory that performed the test. On September 20, the older girl underwent an MRI and an electromyogram study. The MRI results were normal; results of the electromyogram study were interpreted as consistent with a mild demyelinating neuropathy.

While reviewing the sisters' case histories, a pediatric intensive-care specialist recognized that the older girl's blood mercury concentration of 5.5 mg/dL, originally interpreted as normal, was indicative of toxicity. Twenty-four-hour urine mercury determinations confirmed mercury intoxication in both sisters (Table 1). Interrogation of family members revealed that the sisters' 10-year-old brother had accidentally spilled approximately 0.5–1 oz of elemental mercury, discovered in the garage among his father's tools, on his bedroom carpet. All the children occasionally slept in the boy's bedroom during the summer, and the younger girl frequently slept on the area of the floor closest to the contaminated site.

The Michigan Department of Public Health (MDPH) was contacted to determine the extent of household contamination. Blood and urine mercury determinations were subsequently ordered for the boy and both parents.

The sisters began chelation therapy with dimercaprol (BAL) on September 26, receiving a total of two 30-dose i.m. courses (3.75 mg/kg every four hours) with a three-day rest period between treatments. They received i.v. fluids containing sodium bicarbonate, which were infused at a rate that maintained a urinary pH >7.0 during chelation therapy. Aspartate aminotransferase (AST), alanine aminotransferase (ALT), lactate dehydrogenase (LDH), blood urea nitrogen (BUN), serum creatinine, and 24-hour urine mercury levels (Table 2) were closely monitored throughout therapy.

The major adverse reactions encountered during dimercaprol therapy were pain at the injection site, nausea, and vomiting. Hypertension was well controlled with propranolol. Both sisters were discharged on October 10. At the time of discharge, the younger girl remained emotionally labile, ataxic, and areflexic in all extremities; she was transferred to a rehabilitation hospital for two weeks of inpatient physiotherapy. Her sister still experienced fatigue, lower extremity weakness, and pain; she received physical therapy on an outpatient basis. Although the boy remained asymptomatic, he was admitted on October 4 for a total of six dimercaprol injections (dimercaprol challenge) to determine his mercury burden. The reported blood mercury concentration was >2.4 mg/dL. The parents' blood and urine mercury levels were within normal limits.

Because of their continued symptomatology and the good results with dimercaprol chelation, all three children received five 10-day cycles of *N*-acetyl-D,L-penicillamine (NAP) (30 mg/kg/day) on an outpatient basis between October 20 and November 15. The patients' laboratory results were within normal limits during each NAP course. Their urine mercury levels were monitored during each NAP regimen (Figure 1).

The younger girl was readmitted on November 13 for a third dimercaprol regimen because of the questionable effectiveness of NAP chelation therapy as well as persistent irritability, difficulty in ambulation, and diminished deep-tendon reflexes. She was discharged after completion of dimercaprol therapy and resumed outpatient chelation therapy with NAP.

After the mercury intoxication was discovered, the

Figure 1. Urine mercury concentrations in 4-year-old girl, 11-year-old girl, and 10-year-old boy (from top to bottom).

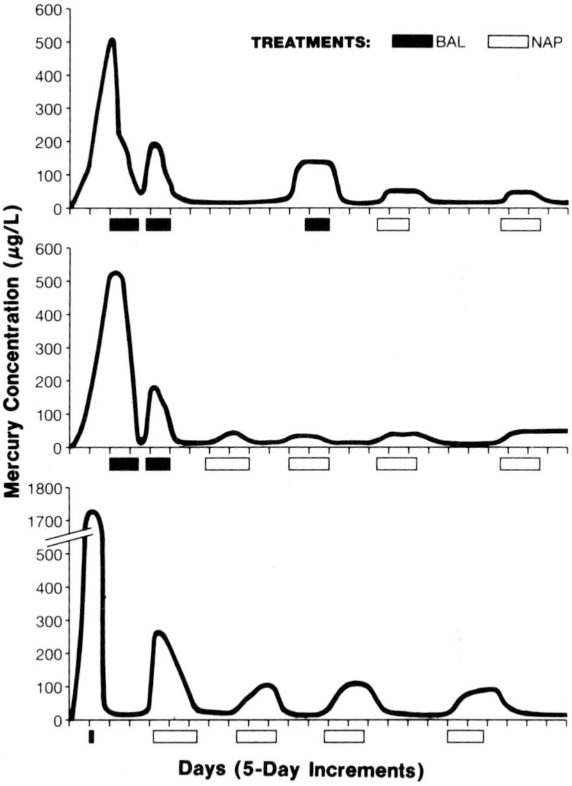

Table 1.
Results of Heavy-Metal Screening

Metal	Patient Value: 4-Year-Old Girl	Patient Value: 11-Year-Old Girl	Normal Value
Blood			
Arsenic (µg/dL)	1.0	<1.0	<7.0
Cadmium (µg/dL)	0.3	<0.10	<0.5
Lead (µg/dL)	<5	<5	<25
Mercury (µg/dL)	<1.0	5.5	<6.0
Urine			
Arsenic (µg/24 hr)	<5	<5	<25
Lead (µg/24 hr)	<5	<5	<80
Mercury (µg/24 hr)	120	58	<20

Table 2.
Laboratory Values during Three Courses of Dimercaprol Therapy[a]

Laboratory Value[b]	Course 1: 4-Year-Old Girl	Course 1: 11-Year-Old Girl	Course 2: 4-Year-Old Girl	Course 2: 11-Year-Old Girl	Course 3: 4-Year-Old Girl	Course 3: 11-Year-Old Girl
AST (mU/mL)	37–60	59–121	40	43–45	38–41	20–27
ALT (mU/mL)	20–34	38–80	23–40	40–64	23	17–19
LDH (mU/mL)	190–281	120–197	...	...	...	...
BUN (mg/dL)	7–13	9–14	8–12	6–13	7–10	7–12
Serum creatinine (mg/dL)	0.2–0.3	0.5–0.6	0.2–0.3	0.4–0.5	0.3	0.4–0.5

[a] Course 1 was from September 26 to October 2, course 2 from October 5 to October 11, and course 3 from November 14 to November 17.
[b] AST = aspartate aminotransferase, ALT = alanine aminotransferase, LDH = lactate dehydrogenase.

Table 3.
Residential Mercury Concentrations[a]

Area	9/28/89	10/4/89	10/20/89	1/11/90
Family room	0.041	0.48	0.002	0.005
Basement game room	0.069	0.114	0.003	0.002
Older girl's bedroom	0.015	0.008	0.002	0.000
Younger girl's bedroom	0.018	0.005	0.008	0.001
Boy's bedroom	0.070–>1.0	0.231	0.200	0.001
Old vacuum cleaner (bag and housing)	0.4	. . .	. . .	. . .
New vacuum cleaner (inside)				1.125

[a] Reported as milligrams per cubic meter. Acceptable industrial concentration = <0.05 mg/cu m.

MDPH evaluated the mercury-vapor levels throughout the house. Elevated mercury levels were found in various areas of the house (Table 3). The family evacuated the premises from September 28 to October 19, and numerous household items were discarded. Eradication of all remaining mercury was attempted.

Both girls have completed their physical therapy. The younger one now walks without difficulty and no longer exhibits abnormal behavior. Two years after diagnosis some visual field defects remain. The three children continued chelation therapy with NAP until the results of repeated urine mercury concentration determinations were normal.

Mercury Poisoning

Mercury compounds are divided into three chemical classes: elemental ("quicksilver," "liquid"), inorganic (elemental mercury is often included in this class), and organic (e.g., phenyl, alkyl, methyl).[6-11] Elemental mercury is a component in dental amalgams and laboratory mounting and preserving solutions. It is also used in the photoengraving industry and in the manufacture of medical and electrical instruments (thermometers, barometers). Inorganic salts (mercurous and mercuric) are used in disinfectants, antiseptics, diuretics, pigments, dry batteries, and explosives. Organic compounds are used in diuretics, antiseptics, insecticides, and fungicides as well as in the processing of wood, paper, and plastics.[6-11] Elemental mercury exists in the nonionized form, is highly lipid soluble, and is the most volatile of all mercury compounds. It is the only metal known that remains a liquid at 0 °C.[11]

Pharmacokinetics of Mercury. Unlike organic compounds, elemental mercury is poorly absorbed from the intact gastrointestinal (GI) tract.[12-13] Substantial mercury absorption can occur in individuals with decreased GI motility or large areas of intestinal stasis or inflammation. In contrast, inhaled mercury is almost completely absorbed (74–86%) through the alveolar membrane.[12-16] Because of its high lipid solubility, elemental mercury easily crosses the blood–brain barrier and accumulates in the cerebral cortex and cerebellum. Elemental mercury and organic and inorganic salts can all be absorbed through the skin.[4,6] The toxicity associated with dermal exposures via broken thermometers (elemental), diaper powders or rinses (mercuric chloride), teething lotions, and antiseptic ointments (organic) has been well documented.[4,6,7]

Studies with radioactively labeled mercury have shown that immediately after inhalational exposure, the majority of the whole-blood mercury content is concentrated in the red blood cell (RBC).[16] The amount in plasma is initially very low and rises to a maximum value approximately 20 hours after the initial exposure. Thereafter, the plasma and RBC concentrations equilibrate to a final ratio of 2:1 (RBC:plasma). The plasma half-life of mercury ranges from two to five days.[15,16] Mercury is well distributed to the brain, liver, and kidney in both its elemental and oxidized forms. The tissue half-life has been estimated to range from three months to one year.[15,16] It is commonly thought that mercury avidly binds to and is sequestered in tissue protein complexes. Many authors, however, suggest that an exchangeable pool of oxidized and nonoxidized mercury exists in most body tissues.[11-16]

Most absorbed mercury is quickly oxidized to divalent or mercuric ions via a hydrogen peroxide catalase pathway present in plasma, RBCs, and tissue.[11,15,16]

Mercury can be excreted via the lungs and feces, but only during the brief period immediately after an acute inhalational exposure.[15,16] The major excretory pathway for chronic and subacute inorganic and elemental mercury exposures is the kidney. Organic mercury is excreted mainly in the bile.

Mechanism of Toxicity. Oxidized mercury strongly binds to sulfhydryl radicals on various protein molecules. The protein–mercury complex leads to the inhibition of many enzyme systems and the denaturation and precipitation of structural proteins. These cellular changes are manifested in the neurologic and metabolic toxicities commonly associated with mercury poisoning.

Signs and Symptoms of Toxicity. *Ingestion.* Organic mercury (ethyl, methyl, phenyl) ingestion produces a severe acute or subacute disorder manifested by paresthesias, sensory loss, tunnel vision, ataxia, dysarthria, memory loss, and dementia.[7-10] Many epidemics have resulted from the ingestion of grain treated with mercury-containing fungicides or pesticides.[6-11] Recent epidemics have been reported in Japan (Minimata Bay Disease, 1975) and among North-

Table 4.
Published Urine and Blood Mercury Concentrations

Reference	Yr	Urine		Blood	
		Toxic	Normal	Toxic	Normal
9	1980	>300 μg/L (symptomatic); >100 μg/L (asymptomatic)	<50 μ/L	. . .	. . .
6	1982	>20 μg/L	. . .	>2–4 μg/dL	. . .
7	1989	>100–300 μg/L	. . .	3 μg/dL	. . .
8	1983	>100–300 μg/L	. . .	3 μg/L	. . .
11	1986	>100–300 μg/L	. . .	3 μg/dL	. . .
19	1987	>150 μg/L	. . .	>3.5 μg/dL[a]	. . .
10	1987	>0.1 ppm	. . .	>0.1 ppm	. . .
20	1980, 1984	>100 μg/L[b]	. . .	>10 μg/dL	. . .
17	1990	. . .	<15 μg/L	. . .	<1.5 μg/dL

[a] Reported in reference 19 as 35 ng/mL.
[b] Reported in reference 20 as 10 μg/dL.

ern American Indian tribes who subsist on fish and game whose food chain has been contaminated by organic mercury compounds.[6] The ingestion of inorganic mercury salts can be rapidly fatal. Symptoms include stomatitis, nausea, vomiting, diarrhea, cardiovascular collapse, acute tubular necrosis, and psychological disturbances.

Inhalation. The signs and symptoms of acute inhalational mercury exposure include salivation, a burning sensation of the oropharynx, cough, dyspnea, tachypnea, bronchitis, interstitial pneumonitis, nausea, vomiting, and chest pain.[6-11] The manifestations of chronic inhalational mercury exposure, by contrast, have a more insidious onset and involve primarily the central nervous system, kidneys, and liver.[6-11,16] Common symptoms include oral-cavity disorders (gingivitis, stomatitis), tremor (hand, foot), psychological disturbances (anxiety, irritability, depression), renal compromise (proteinuria, tubular necrosis), anorexia, and weight loss. Pruritus and sometimes-painful scaling or peeling of the skin of the hands and feet have historically been associated with infantile acrodynia (pink disease); they are also common in adults. Both girls exhibited many of the classic symptoms of both acute and chronic inhalational mercury intoxication.

Interpretation of Mercury Concentrations

Since the mercuric ion is excreted primarily through the kidney, many authors believe that poisoning from elemental, inorganic, and some long-chain organic compounds can best be assessed by measuring urine mercury concentrations.[6-11,17-21] Blood mercury levels may be reliable indicators of acute exposure; however, they are less useful than urine levels in assessing chronic exposure.[6-11] Of note, however, are the discrepancies in the published literature regarding the assignment of normal versus toxic blood and urine mercury levels.[6-11,17-21] Table 4 compares the guidelines for toxic and normal urine and blood mercury levels that appear in commonly used texts. It is apparent that clinicians and toxicology laboratories may be easily misled by the varied toxic and normal ranges (or lack thereof) as well as by the various units reported. Moreover, such values have been derived entirely from data obtained in adults exposed to mercury in the work place; the data do not include children. Teleologically, no mercury should be found in the blood or urine of any symptomatic, "nonexposed" child or adult. Any mercury found in a child's blood or urine should be cause for investigation.

A further dilemma is that urine or blood mercury concentrations may often be nondiagnostic in persons with chronic exposure, who have gradually developed an extensive and relatively unexchangeable tissue mercury burden.[6-11,22] Thus, while the finding of any mercury in the blood or urine can confirm exposure, it may often correlate poorly with the manifestation of symptoms.

Mercury levels in hair (scalp, pubic) correlate well with symptoms of organic (short-chain) intoxications. Hair concentrations of 50–125 μg/g denote mild toxicity. Although most authors agree that monitoring hair mercury levels has little value in detecting chronic exposures, Sikorski et al.[23] have recently shown this measurement to be a reliable indicator of metabolic and reproductive toxicity caused by chronic mercury inhalation in female dental workers.

Management Pitfalls and Guidelines

There are many pitfalls in the management of elemental mercury poisoning. The three patients presented illustrate how the aforementioned discrepancies in the literature can lead to delays in diagnosis and treatment. The lack of correlation between symptomatology and mercury levels in both blood and urine is well illustrated by the fact that the younger girl had the lowest initial blood concentration (<l μg/dL) but exhibited the most serious symptoms. The other children had much higher blood and urine levels but had relatively milder symptoms. The urine

mercury levels collected from all three patients during chelation therapy were reported by the toxicology laboratory in units of micrograms per 24 hours. These values should have been corrected to micrograms per liter, a unit that accurately compensates for the amount of urine voided during the 24-hour collection period.

According to a consensus of toxicology experts, the following approach should be taken to diagnose mercury intoxication in children. The patient should be observed closely for characteristic signs and symptoms. Clinicians should maintain a high index of suspicion, as there may be no history of exposure until the diagnosis is made. Nerve-conduction studies should be performed. A definitive diagnosis can be made by a 24-hour urine collection for mercury (normal = 0). Whole-blood mercury levels, while sometimes helpful, may not correlate well with symptomatology or with extensive tissue mercury burden (i.e., chronic exposures). In asymptomatic patients such as the boy described in this report, existing literature supports the use of chelation challenge as a means of determining the chelatable mercury pool.

Pharmacotherapy of Inhalational Mercury Exposure

The efficacy of chelation therapy for chronic inhalational exposure has been questioned by many authors because of the perceived inability of the available agents to effectively mobilize oxidized mercury from relatively unexchangeable tissue stores.[7-10] Regardless of the acute or chronic nature of the exposure, it is recommended that all individuals who are symptomatic or have toxic blood or urine mercury concentrations (blood, >0–1.5 μg/dL; urine, >25–50 μg/L) undergo chelation therapy.[11-17] The most effective mercury-chelating agents currently available in the United States are dimercaprol and penicillamine (both commercially available) and the investigational agents NAP and 2,3-dimercaptosuccinic acid (DMSA).

Dimercaprol. Dimercaprol (British Anti-Lewisite [BAL], 2,3-dimercapto-1-propanol) was developed as a means of counteracting Lewisite, an arsinedichloride gas employed during World War II. The dimercaprol molecule contains two sulfhydryl groups that are available to complex with mercury, thus preventing or reversing its binding to tissue (enzymatic and structural proteins) sulfhydryl groups. Dimercaprol forms a 2:1 or 1:1 chelate with mercury that is reversible, especially at a low urine pH.

Pharmacokinetics. Peak plasma dimercaprol concentrations are achieved within 30 to 60 minutes after a deep i.m. injection.[18] Free dimercaprol is rapidly converted in the liver to inactive metabolites. Dimercaprol metabolites, the dimercaprol–mercury complex, and other divalent and trivalent cations (i.e., zinc and iron) are mainly excreted via the kidney (approximately 50%), and to a lesser extent in the bile and feces. Elimination is usually complete within four hours after administration. This rapid clearance necessitates frequent administration to ensure that an excess of free dimercaprol is present in body fluids.[17-21]

Monitoring Therapy. Although most references recommend monitoring urine mercury levels in order to assess the efficacy of chelation, appropriate therapeutic endpoints are either ambiguous or not addressed. Acceptable mercury concentrations (blood and urine) upon which the drug may be discontinued are also lacking. Thus, a clinician who bases therapy on one of the commonly used reference texts may undertreat the patient, either by prescribing too low a dosage or by underestimating the length of time that the drug is needed. Illustrating this treatment dilemma, both girls remained symptomatic during their first dimercaprol regimen, even though the drug proved to be an effective chelating agent during all treatment regimens (Figure 1). Some authors believe that chelation therapy has minimal benefit in treating chronic mercury exposures, presumably because of a relatively unexchangeable tissue mercury complex. Dimercaprol therapy has been reported to transiently increase brain mercury levels in patients with organic poisonings.[3-5,19-21] Many authors, however, have found dimercaprol chelation therapy to be of great benefit in reducing the total body mercury burden in patients with elemental and inorganic poisonings. Aronow et al.[24] and Eastman[25] recommend that patients be chelated until all clinical symptoms abate and the urine mercury concentration is <10–20 μg/L. They also recommend five-day treatment periods interspersed with 7- to 10-day rest periods until the therapeutic endpoints are reached. Unfortunately, the extreme discomfort of frequent deep i.m. injections is a major limiting factor associated with prolonged dimercaprol treatments; both girls experienced such a reaction. In cases such as these, an oral chelating agent may be necessary.

Adverse Effects. Approximately 50% of patients treated with dimercaprol experience an adverse drug reaction (ADR).[17-21] Doses exceeding 5 mg/kg may precipitate vomiting, seizures, stupor, and coma. These reactions can appear 30 minutes after the injection and last from one to six hours.[18] An increase in systolic or diastolic blood pressure is the most frequent ADR; this may be accompanied by tachycardia. Hypertension, tachycardia, or both, usually appear 15–30 minutes after the injection and are dose related.[17,18] Less-frequent ADRs include urticaria (responsive to diphenhydramine); nausea; vomiting; unpleasant taste; burning sensation of the lips, mouth, throat, and eyes; headache; conjunctivitis; blepharospasm; myalgias; arthralgias; and paresthesias. Children may exhibit febrile reactions that can persist until the drug is discontinued. Transient elevations of hepatic enzymes may occur during therapy. Hemolytic anemia has also been reported in individuals with glucose 6-phosphate dehydrogenase deficiency. Dimercaprol is potentially nephrotoxic. The dosage interval should be lengthened in patients with renal failure.

The most bothersome ADRs experienced by both girls were pain at the injection site, burning of the lips and mouth, unpleasant taste, nausea, and vomiting. Their AST and ALT levels were transiently elevated during therapy; however, renal function remained normal (Table 2).

Dosing. The preferred dimercaprol regimen is that recommended in Poisindex, *Toxicologic Emergencies*, and *AHFS Drug Information*: 3–5 mg/kg i.m. every four hours on days 1 and 2, 2.5–3 mg/kg i.m. every six hours on days 3 and 4, and 2.5–3 mg/kg every 12 hours for one week thereafter.[11,17,18] *Harrison's Principles of Internal Medicine* recommends only that the total daily dimercaprol dosage not exceed 24 mg/kg and that the length of therapy not exceed five days (therapy may be reinstituted after a "suitable" rest period).[19] Most references also state or imply that dimercaprol therapy is ineffective unless initiated within three hours after a mercury exposure.[17-21]

Penicillamine. The chelating properties of penicillamine (D-penicillamine) were first documented in 1956, when Walshe observed that it increased the urinary excretion of copper in patients treated for Wilson's disease.[26] This observation led to its eventual use by Aposhian in 1958 in the treatment of heavy-metal poisonings.[26]

Penicillamine is well absorbed orally (on an empty stomach), undergoes minimal metabolism, and is renally excreted. The pediatric dosage is 100 mg/kg/day (maximum 1 g/day) administered in four doses; the adult dosage is 250–500 mg four times daily.

The more serious ADRs include anorexia, nausea, vomiting, nephrotoxicity, optic neuritis, and systemic lupus erythematosus; these reactions, however, have been reported only in patients receiving prolonged (one- to two-year) penicillamine therapy for rheumatoid arthritis or Wilson's disease. The ADRs associated with the short (one- to four-month) courses of therapy used for mercury intoxication have been limited to hypersensitivity reactions (fever, rash, leukopenia, eosinophilia, and thrombocytopenia), which usually appear early in the course of therapy. The incidence of an allergic reaction in a penicillin-sensitive individual is approximately 2.5–10%.

Urine mercury levels should be closely monitored during therapy with penicillamine to assess the efficacy of chelation. The practitioner should be aware that penicillamine can deplete copper, zinc, and iron stores.

***N*-Acetyl-D,L-penicillamine.** In 1959, Aposhian et al.[24] reported that of the penicillamine analogues, *N*-acetyl-D,L-penicillamine (NAP) was the most effective oral agent (it was equally efficacious to i.m. dimercaprol) in a study involving rats poisoned with mercurous chloride. Numerous authors have more recently reported successful chelation therapy with NAP in approximately 88% of persons with inhalational mercury exposures.[24,25,27-29]

NAP is well absorbed orally (on an empty stomach), undergoes minimal metabolism, and is renally excreted. The pediatric dosage is 30 mg/kg/day (maximum of 1 g/day) administered in four divided doses; the adult dosage is 250–500 mg four times daily. Since NAP is still considered a chemical, an investigational new drug number must be obtained from the Food and Drug Administration. NAP is produced by the Aldrich Chemical Company (414-273-3850).

There was a noticeable difference in the amount of mercury excreted during dimercaprol versus NAP chelation therapy in all three children (Figure 1). These differences could be attributed to claims that NAP is less effective than dimercaprol.[30-32] An alternative explanation is that the patients' exchangeable mercury burdens were lowered during the dimercaprol treatment regimens, and any remaining mercury was sequestered in relatively unexchangeable tissue complexes. In the cases reported here, chelation therapy with NAP was continued, because all three patients remained symptomatic, had urinary mercury concentrations of >25–50 μg/L, or both.

2,3-Dimercaptosuccinic Acid (DMSA). DMSA is a water-soluble analogue of dimercaprol. Extensive laboratory and clinical research on DMSA and related compounds was done between 1956 and 1975 in China, Japan, and the Soviet Union.[30,31] These agents, however, received little attention in the United States and Western Europe until 1975, when Friedheim et al.[32] reported good results with the use of DMSA in treating inhalational mercury intoxications. DMSA has consistently been shown to be of equal or superior efficacy to dimercaprol, penicillamine, and NAP in comparative studies conducted in Europe, Japan, and China.[30-32] In the United States, Campbell et al. and Fornier et al. have used DMSA successfully to treat symptomatic patients exposed to elemental mercury vapor through industrial accidents.[17] Heath et al.[33] have recently shown that DMSA was more effective and less toxic than NAP in treating 35 symptomatic adults exposed to mercury vapors as a result of industrial accidents.

The dosage of DMSA is 30 mg/kg/day administered orally every four to six hours. DMSA is primarily renally excreted (80–85%); biliary and fecal excretion are minimal. Common ADRs include nausea, vomiting, and abdominal bloating. Allergic reactions are rare. DMSA is available in the United States for compassionate use only from the Johnson & Johnson Company.

Environmental Decontamination

Current occupational standards for allowable mercury-vapor concentrations are referred to as the TWA (time-weighted average) and STEL (short-term exposure limit).[17] The TWA is "the time-weighted average concentration for a normal 8-hour working day or a 40-hour week to which a healthy worker may be repeatedly exposed, day after day, without adverse effect."[34] Although the established TWA for mercury vapor is 0.05 mg/cu m, the standard recommends that "all efforts should be made to control the mercury concentration within the working environment to at most one-quarter of this value (0.0125 mg/cu m)."[34]

The MDPH determined the mercury vapor levels in the family's home on three occasions. The results are presented in Table 3. Certain areas of the home (the boy's bedroom carpet, the garage, the basement game and family rooms), as well as the vacuum cleaner, contained mercury vapors well in excess of industrial levels established as minimally safe. The MDPH supervised the following clean-up procedure. On September 28, the home was closed (except for the window in the boy's bedroom). On October 4, the carpeting and pad, as well as any visible mercury beads, were removed from his bedroom, the game room, and the garage. The vacuum cleaner and children's sleeping bags were discarded, and several pieces of linen and clothing were dry-cleaned. On October 20, all of the carpeting was removed from the home, with the exception of that in the living room, the master bedroom, and the sisters' bedrooms. The wooden floor and subfloor were removed from the boy's bedroom on October 21. The house was evacuated between September 28 and October 19 and aired out (all windows opened) regularly. The family's plight, as well as the lack of direction and regulations experienced by the MDPH, is summarized in the following observations of a supervising sanitarian: "No established procedures are available for the clean-up of the home. Proper disposal of the contaminated materials continues to pose a problem. Mercury standards for residential structures do not exist; therefore, safe standards for reoccupancy do not exist. Apparently homeowners' insurance will not compensate for clean-up costs or other losses. It should also be indicated that the homeowner has experienced severe frustration because of the lack of residential standards and, therefore, positive directions for dealing with this situation."

Conclusion

These case reports illustrate the controversies and ambiguities that were encountered in detecting and treating inhalational mercury poisonings. Clinicians and toxicology laboratories should be aware of the inconsistencies in established blood and urine mercury levels. Hospital laboratories receiving results from an independent toxicology laboratory should verify that the reported value and its units correlate with those that are established by general toxicological consensus. Definitive therapeutic endpoints for the initiation and cessation of chelation therapy need to be established. DMSA may be the ideal chelating agent because of the documented efficacy, low incidence of ADRs, and extensive experience reported with this drug. State and local health departments should establish guidelines regarding reimbursement and the clean-up procedures necessary for mercury contamination.

Discussion Questions

1. Explain the pathophysiology of inhalational mercury intoxication.
2. Discuss the pharmacokinetics of inhaled mercury vapor.
3. What are the most commonly recognized normal and toxic blood and urine values for mercury intoxication? How well do they correlate with the patient's symptomatology? How useful are they in diagnosing acute versus chronic intoxication?
4. List six factors that are most important in diagnosing chronic inhalational mercury intoxication in children.
5. What chelation regimen(s) should be recommended for a symptomatic child with detectable blood and urine mercury levels? Include recommendations for drug, dosage, route of administration, duration of therapy, and patient and laboratory monitoring.

References

1. Hunter D. The diseases of the occupations. Boston: Little Brown; 1955.
2. Kark PR, Poskanzer DC, Bullock JD et al. Mercury poisoning and its treatment with *N*-acetyl-D,L-penicillamine. *N Engl J Med*. 1971; 285:10-6.
3. Vroom FQ, Greer M. Mercury vapour intoxication. *Brain*. 1972; 95:305-18.
4. Nakayma H, Niki F, Shono M et al. Mercury exanthem. *Contact Dermatitis*. 1983; 9:411-7.
5. McFarland RB, Reigel H. Chronic mercury poisoning from a single brief exposure. *J Occup Med*. 1978; 20:532-4.
6. Aronow R. Mercury. In: Haddad LM, Winchester JF, eds. Clinical management of poisoning and drug overdose. Philadelphia: Saunders; 1983:637-43.
7. Bryson PD, ed. Comprehensive review in toxicology. 2nd ed. Rockville, MD: Aspen; 1989.
8. Arena JM, ed. Poisoning: toxicology, symptoms, treatments. 5th ed. Springfield, IL: Thomas; 1986.
9. Kaye S, ed. Handbook of emergency toxicology: a guide for the identification, diagnosis and treatment of poisoning. 4th ed. Springfield, IL: Thomas; 1980.
10. Driesbach RH, ed. Handbook of poisoning: prevention, diagnosis and treatment. Norwalk, CT: Appleton-Lange; 1987.
11. Goldfrank LR, Bresnitz EA, Howland MA et al. Mercury. In: Goldfrank LR, Flomenbaum NE, Lewin NA et al., eds. Toxicologic emergencies. 3rd ed. Norwalk, CT: Appleton-Century-Crofts; 1986:645-9.
12. Moutinho ME, Tomkins AL, Rowland TW et al. Acute mercury vapor poisoning (fatality in an infant). *Am J Dis Child*. 1981; 135:42-4.
13. McNeil NI, Olver RE, Issler HC et al. Domestic metallic mercury poisoning. *Lancet*. 1984; 1:269-71.
14. Hallee TJ. Diffuse lung disease caused by inhalation of mercury vapor. *Am Rev Respir Dis*. 1969; 99:430-6.
15. Lien DC, Todoruk DN, Hasmukhal RR et al. Accidental inhalation of mercury vapour: respiratory and toxicologic consequences. *Can Med Assoc J*. 1983; 129:591-5.
16. Cherian MG, Hursh JB, Clarkson TW et al. Radioactive mercury distribution in biological fluids and excretion in human subjects after inhalation of mercury vapor. *Arch Environ Health*. 1978; 33:109-14.
17. Poisindex. Toxicologic managment of mercury poisoning. Denver, CO: Micromedex; 1989: 64.
18. AHFS drug information 90. McEvoy GK, ed. Dimercaprol. Bethesda, MD: American Society of Hospital Pharmacists; 1990:1711-3.
19. Graef JW, Lovejoy FH. Heavy metal poisoning. In: Braunwald E, Isselbacher KJ, Petersdorf RG et al., eds. Harrison's principles of internal medicine. 11th ed. New York: McGraw-Hill;

1987:853-4.
20. Gosselin RE, Hodge HC, Smith RP et al., eds. Clinical toxicology of commercial products. 5th ed. Baltimore: Williams & Wilkins; 1984.
21. Meyboom RHB. Metal antagonists. In: Dukes MNG, ed. Meyler's side effects of drugs. 9th ed. Amsterdam, the Netherlands: Excerpta Medica; 1980:383-9.
22. Roels H, Gennart JP, Lauwerys R et al. Surveillance of workers exposed to mercury vapour: validation of a previously proposed biological threshold limit value for mercury concentration in urine. *Am J Indust Med.* 1985; 7:45-71.
23. Sikorski R, Juszkiewicz T, Paszkowski T et al. Women in dental surgeries: reproductive hazards in occupational exposure to metallic mercury. *Int Arch Occup Environ Health.* 1987; 59:551-7.
24. Aronow R, Fleischman LE. Mercury poisoning in children. *Clin Pediatr.* 1976; 15:936-45.
25. Eastmond CJ, Holt S. A case of acute mercury vapour poisoning. *Postgrad Med J.* 1975; 51:428-30.
26. Klaassen CD. Heavy metals and heavy metal antagonists. In: Gilman AG, Goodman LS, Rall TW et al., eds. Goodman and Gilman's the pharmacological basis of therapeutics. 7th ed. New York: Macmillan; 1985:1605-27.
27. Hirschman SZ, Feingold M, Boylen G. Mercury in house paint as a cause of acrodynia. *N Engl J Med.* 1963; 269:889-92.
28. Markowitz L, Schaumburg HH. Successful treatment of inorganic mercury neurotoxicity with *N*-acetyl-penicillamine despite an adverse reaction. *Neurology.* 1980; 30:1000-1.
29. Smith AD, Miller JW. Treatment of inorganic mercury poisoning with *N*-acetyl-D,L-penicillamine. *Lancet.* 1961; 280:640-2.
30. Aaseth J. Recent advances in the therapy of metal poisonings with chelating agents. *Human Toxicol.* 1983; 2:257-72.
31. Aposhian HV. DMSA and DMPS—water-soluble antidotes for heavy metal poisoning. *Ann Rev Pharmacol Toxicol.* 1983; 23:193-215.
32. Freidheim E. MESO-dimercaptosuccinic acid, a chelating agent for the treatment of mercury poisoning. *J Pharm Pharmacol.* 1975; 27:624-6.
33. Heath A, Bluhm R. 2,3-Dimercaptosuccinic acid (DMSA) vs. *N*-acetyl-penicillamine (NAP) for the treatment of elemental mercury toxicity. Paper presented at the 1989 American Academy of Toxicologists, American Association of Poison Control Centers, and Canadian Association of Poison Control Centers Annual Scientific Meeting. Atlanta, GA: 1989 Oct 12–15.
34. Gelbier S, Ingram J. Possible foetotoxic effects of mercury vapour: a case report. *Public Health.* 1989; 103:35-40.

DUE Criteria

The DUE Criteria *section of* Clinical Pharmacy *features model drug-use evaluation criteria that may be employed as a component of a comprehensive quality assurance program. The criteria sets are presented in the format used in the ASHP book* Criteria for Drug Use Evaluation. *Some of the criteria sets will have been originally published in that book; others will be presented here for the first time and published in future volumes of the ASHP book. The practitioners who developed a criteria set are acknowledged.*

In selecting drug products for coverage in DUE Criteria, *priority is given to products that have been recently marketed, those that are frequently prescribed, those that have high potential risk associated with their use, and those that are expensive. When feasible, a criteria set will be linked with a Drug Review that appears in the same issue.*

These criteria sets are a starting point for the development of DUE criteria for a specific practice setting. Readers are encouraged to modify the model criteria to fit their own circumstances.

Criteria for use of fluconazole in adult and pediatric inpatients and outpatients[a]

Element	Standard 100%	Standard 0%	Exception[b] or Critical Preventive/ Responsive Measure[c]	Sources of Information
Justification for Use				
1. Suppressive maintenance therapy of culture-documented cryptococcal meningitis[1–10]	X		1A. None	1. History and physical (H&P), laboratory reports, progress notes, physician orders, infectious disease (ID) consultation report
or				
2. Therapy of suspected or culture-documented acute cryptococcal meningitis in patient unable to take amphotericin B because of allergy, intolerance, or underlying renal disease (serum creatinine [SCr] concentration, >2.5 mg/dL) or failing to respond to amphotericin B therapy[1–7,9,11,12]	X		2A. None	2. H&P, laboratory reports, progress notes, physician orders, ID consultation report
or				
3. Suspected or culture-documented esophageal candidiasis in patient unable to take ketoconazole because of hypochlorhydria or concomitant therapy with drug that interacts significantly with ketoconazole (e.g., histamine H_2-receptor antagonist or antacid)[1–4,6,11–15]	X		3A. None	3. H&P, laboratory reports, progress notes, physician orders, ID consultation report
or				
4. Suspected or culture-documented oropharyngeal candidiasis in patient	X		4A. None	4. H&P, laboratory reports, progress notes, physician

Prepared by Kimberly M. Bourne, Pharm.D., Pharmacy Resident, Department of Pharmacy, and S. Diane Goodwin, Pharm.D., Clinical Research Pharmacist, Division of Infectious Diseases, Department of Medicine, Duke University Medical Center, Durham, NC.

Review of these criteria by John R. Perfect, M.D., is acknowledged.

Element	Standard 100%	Standard 0%	Exception[b] or Critical Preventive/ Responsive Measure[c]	Sources of Information
not responsive to local treatment or unable to take ketoconazole because of hypochlorhydria or concomitant therapy with drug that interacts significantly with ketoconazole (e.g., histamine H_2-receptor antagonist or antacid)[1,2,4,6,13,15–18] or				orders, ID consultation report
5. Suspected or culture-documented systemic candidiasis in patient unable to take amphotericin B because of allergy, intolerance, or underlying renal disease (SCr concentration, >2.5 mg/dL) or failing to respond to amphotericin B therapy[1–4,6,11,14,19]	X		5A. None	5. H&P, laboratory reports, progress notes, physician orders, ID consultation report
Critical (Process) Indicators				
6. No history of hypersensitivity to fluconazole	X		6A. None	6. H&P, allergies
7. Fluconazole not used in pregnant or lactating woman[10]	X		7A. Fluconazole used when benefit outweighs risk	7, 7A. H&P, laboratory reports, progress notes
8. Fungal cultures obtained from suspected body sites (e.g., cerebrospinal fluid, blood, and urine) within 48 hr before initiation of fluconazole therapy	X		8A. Empirical therapy with fluconazole begun after previously given antifungal agent failed or was not tolerated 8B. Suspected oropharyngeal candidiasis	8, 8A. H&P, laboratory reports, progress notes, physician orders 8B. H&P, progress notes
9. Baseline laboratory test results obtained within 48 hr before initiation of fluconazole therapy: a. Liver function tests: serum aspartate aminotranferase, alanine aminotransferase, alkaline phosphatase, and total bilirubin b. Complete blood count (CBC) with differential c. Platelet count d. SCr level	X		9A. None	9. Laboratory reports, progress notes, physician orders
10. Lumbar puncture performed within 48 hr before initiation of fluconazole therapy	X		10A. Suspected or culture-documented esophageal candidiasis, oropharyngeal candidiasis, or systemic candidiasis	10, 10A. H&P, laboratory reports, progress notes, physician orders
11. Cryptococcal antigen titer in cerebrospinal fluid and serum determined within 48 hr before initiation of fluconazole therapy	X		11A. Suspected or culture-documented esophageal candidiasis, oropharyngeal candidiasis, or systemic candidiasis	11, 11A. H&P, laboratory reports, progress notes, physician orders
12. Endoscopy performed within 48 hr before initiation of fluconazole therapy	X		12A. Suspected or culture-documented oropharyngeal candidiasis or cryptococcal meningitis or suppression of cryptococcal meningitis	12, 12A. H&P, laboratory reports, progress notes, physician orders, endoscopy reports
13. Urinalysis performed within 24 hr before initiation of fluconazole therapy	X		13A. Suspected or culture-documented oropharyngeal candidiasis, esophageal candidiasis, or cryptococcal meningitis or suppression of cryptococcal meningitis	13, 13A. H&P, laboratory reports, progress notes, physician orders
14. Chest roentgenogram obtained within 48 hr before initiation of fluconazole therapy	X		14A. Suspected or culture-documented esophageal candidiasis, oropharyngeal candidiasis, systemic candidiasis other than pneumonia, or suppression of cryptococcal meningitis	14, 14A. H&P, progress notes, physician orders, roentgenographic reports
15. Fluconazole administered i.v. to patient with nothing-by-mouth orders or severe cryptococcal meningitis, esophageal candidiasis, or systemic candidiasis[1–4,6]	X		15A. None	15. Progress notes, physician orders, nursing notes, medication administration record (MAR)

Element	Standard 100%	Standard 0%	Exception[b] or Critical Preventive/ Responsive Measure[c]	Sources of Information
16. Appropriate adult dosage in suppressive therapy for cryptococcal meningitis: 200 mg once daily[3, 10]	X		16A. Patient without AIDS may not require maintenance therapy 16B. Patient with renal disease (CL_{cr}, <50 mL/min) (see element 22) 16C. ID consultation recommendation for alternative dosage regimen	16, 16A. H&P, progress notes, physician orders, MAR 16B. Laboratory reports, progress notes 16C. ID consultation report, physician orders
17. Appropriate adult dosage in acute cryptococcal meningitis: 400 mg on first day, then 200 mg once daily for 10–12 weeks after cerebrospinal fluid culture is negative[3, 10]	X		17A. In severe disease (cryptococcal antigen titer, >1:1024), dosage may be increased to 400 mg/day 17B. Patient with renal disease (CL_{cr}, <50 mL/min) (see element 22) 17C. ID consultation recommendation for alternative dosage regimen or length of treatment	17. H&P, progress notes, physician orders, MAR 17A, B. Laboratory reports, progress notes 17C. ID consultation report, physician orders
18. Appropriate adult dosage in oropharyngeal candidiasis: 200 mg on first day, then 100 mg once daily for 14 days[3, 10]	X		18A. Patient with renal disease (CL_{cr}, <50 mL/min) (see element 22) 18B. ID consultation recommendation for alternative dosage regimen or length of treatment	18. H&P, progress notes, physician orders, MAR 18A. Laboratory reports, progress notes 18B. ID consultation report, physician orders
19. Appropriate adult dosage in esophageal candidiasis: 200 mg on first day, then 100 mg once daily for 21 days (with ≥2 weeks of therapy after symptoms resolve)[3, 10]	X		19A. Dosage may be increased to 200 mg/day for patient failing to respond after 1 week 19B. Patient with renal disease (CL_{cr}, <50 mL/min) (see element 22) 19C. ID consultation recommendation for alternative dosage regimen or length of treatment	19, 19A. H&P, progress notes, physician orders, MAR 19B. Laboratory reports, progress notes 19C. ID consultation report, physician orders
20. Appropriate adult dosage in systemic candidiasis: 400 mg on first day, then 200 mg once daily for 28 days[3, 10]	X		20A. Patient with renal disease (CL_{cr}, <50 mL/min) (see element 22) 20B. ID consultation recommendation for alternative dosage regimen or length of treatment	20. H&P, progress notes, physician orders, MAR 20A. Laboratory reports, progress notes 20B. ID consultation report, physician orders
21. Appropriate dosage for children 3–13 years of age: 3–6 mg/kg once daily[3]	X		21A. Patient with renal disease (CL_{cr}, <50 mL/min) (see element 22)	21. Progress notes, physician orders, MAR 21A. Laboratory reports, progress notes
22. Dosage adjusted for renal impairment based on CL_{cr} estimated by the Cockcroft-Gault method[10,20]: If CL_{cr} is >50 mL/min, give 100% of dose; if 21–50 mL/min, 75%; and if 11–20, 25%. Loading dose of 50–400 mg given on first day[10]	X		22A. Full dose given after each hemodialysis session[10]	22. Laboratory reports, progress notes, physician orders, MAR 22A. Physician orders, MAR, dialysis reports
23. Fluconazole dosage increased in patient receiving rifampin concomitantly[3,21]	X		23A. None	23. Progress notes, physician orders, MAR
24. Serum chemistry (SCr concentration and liver function) monitored weekly during fluconazole therapy	X		24A. Monitoring performed monthly if patient receiving suppressive maintenance therapy, unless clinical condition changes 24B. Monitoring performed more frequently in patient with rapidly changing renal function	24, 24A, B. Laboratory reports, progress notes, physician orders
25. Temperature and other vital signs monitored once daily during first 2 weeks of therapy	X		25A. Therapy conducted on outpatient basis	25. Progress notes, physician orders, nursing notes, nursing flow sheets 25A. Progress notes

Element	Standard 100%	Standard 0%	Exception[b] or Critical Preventive/ Responsive Measure[c]	Sources of Information
26. Chest roentgenogram obtained monthly during fluconazole therapy	X		26A. Suspected or culture-documented cryptococcal meningitis, esophageal candidiasis, oropharyngeal candidiasis, systemic candidiasis other than pneumonia, or suppression of cryptococcal meningitis 26B. Chest roentgenography performed more frequently in patient with poor response to fluconazole	26, 26A, B. H&P, roentgenographic reports, progress notes, physician orders
27. CBC with differential and platelet count performed after 1 week of fluconazole therapy and then every 2 weeks	X		27A. Monitoring performed monthly if patient receiving suppressive maintenance therapy	27, 27A. Laboratory reports, progress notes, physician orders
28. Lumbar puncture performed after 2 weeks of therapy, at end of therapy, and at follow-up visit	X		28A. Lumbar puncture not performed initially 28B. Monitoring more frequent in patient with poor response to fluconazole 28C. If cerebrospinal fluid culture positive after 2 weeks of therapy, lumbar puncture performed after another 2–4 weeks	28, 28A–C. Laboratory reports, progress notes, physician orders
29. Urinalysis performed during first week of therapy, at end of therapy, and at follow-up visit	X		29A. Pretreatment urine culture negative 29B. If urine culture positive after 1 week of therapy, urine cultured at least weekly until negative	29, 29A, B. Laboratory reports, progress notes, physician orders
30. For patient undergoing anticoagulant (e.g., warfarin) therapy, prothrombin time (PT) measured before and weekly during fluconazole therapy; anticoagulant dosage adjusted until PT stable[3,10,21]	X		30A. None	30. H&P, laboratory reports, progress notes, physician orders, MAR
31. For patient receiving cyclosporine, baseline serum cyclosporine concentration measured, serum cyclosporine and SCr concentrations monitored every 1–2 weeks until stable, and cyclosporine dosage adjusted as needed[3,10,21,22]	X		31A. None	31. Laboratory reports, progress notes, physician orders, MAR
32. For patients taking phenytoin, serum phenytoin concentration determined initially and every 1–2 weeks until stable, patient monitored for signs of phenytoin toxicity (e.g., nystagmus and ataxia), and phenytoin dosage adjusted to achieve desired serum concentration[3,10,21,23]	X		32A. None	32. Laboratory reports, progress notes, physician orders, MAR
33. For patient receiving oral hypoglycemic, serum glucose concentration measured initially and every week until stable, patient monitored for signs of hypoglycemia, and oral hypoglycemic dosage adjusted to maintain desired glucose concentration[3,10,21]	X		33A. None	33. Laboratory reports, progress notes, physician orders, MAR
Complications				
34. Anaphylaxis: difficulty breathing, hypotension, and cardiac arrest[3,10]		X	34A. Identify other drug and nondrug causes 34B. Discontinue fluconazole 34C. Provide symptomatic and supportive care, including airway re-establishment and cardiopulmonary resuscitation	34. Progress notes, nursing notes 34A–C. Progress notes, physician orders, nursing notes, MAR

Element	Standard 100%	Standard 0%	Exception[b] or Critical Preventive/ Responsive Measure[c]	Sources of Information
35. Rash or other dermatologic manifestation[3,7,10,22]		X	35A. Identify other drug and nondrug causes 35B. Treat mild reaction symptomatically with antihistamines or topical or systemic anti-inflammatory agents 35C. If severe reaction, discontinue fluconazole and institute alternative antifungal therapy	35. Progress notes, nursing notes 35A–C. Progress notes, physician orders, nursing notes, MAR
36. Gastrointestinal effects: nausea, vomiting, diarrhea, abdominal pain, and anorexia[3,7,8,10]		X	36A. Identify other drug and nondrug causes 36B. Provide symptomatic and supportive care 36C. If patient unable to tolerate fluconazole, discontinue it and institute alternative antifungal therapy	36. Progress notes, nursing notes 36A–C. Progress notes, physician orders, nursing notes, MAR
37. Elevations in liver function test results from baseline or signs and symptoms of hepatotoxicity[3,7,8,10]		X	37A. Identify other drug and nondrug causes 37B. Provide symptomatic and supportive care 37C. Discontinue fluconazole and institute alternative antifungal therapy if liver functon test results more than three times baseline values or if patient has signs and symptoms of hepatitis 37D. Peform follow-up tests until values return to baseline	37. Laboratory reports, progress notes, nursing notes 37A, B. Progress notes, physician orders, nursing notes, MAR 37C, D. Laboratory reports, physician orders, progress notes
38. Local effects of i.v. therapy: phlebitis, pain, and inflammation		X	38A. Provide symptomatic and supportive care 38B. Reduce infusion rate 38C. Alternate i.v. sites	38. Progress notes, nursing notes 38A–C. Progress notes, physician orders, nursing notes, MAR
Outcome Measures				
39. Normalization of body temperature within 5 days of start of fluconazole therapy	X		39A. Initial temperature not obtained or within normal limits 39B. New source of infection suspected or identified 39C. Patient died	39, 39A. Progress notes, nursing flow sheets, nursing notes 39B. Laboratory reports, progress notes, nursing notes 39C. Progress notes
40. Resolution of chest roentgenographic abnormalities	X		40A. Initial chest roentgenogram not obtained or within normal limits 40B. New source of infection suspected or identified 40C. Patient failed to return for follow-up 40D. Patient died	40, 40A. Progress notes, roentgenographic reports 40B. Laboratory reports, progress notes, nursing notes 40C, D. Progress notes
41. Normalization of leukocyte count by end of fluconazole therapy	X		41A. Initial leukocyte count not obtained or within normal limits 41B. Altered leukocyte count due to underlying disease state (e.g., AIDS or cancer) 41C. New source of infection suspected or documented 41D. Patient failed to return for follow-up 41E. Patient died	41, 41A. Laboratory reports, progress notes 41B. Laboratory reports, progress notes, H&P 41C. Laboratory reports, progress notes, nursing notes 41D, E. Progress notes
42. Fungal cultures negative at end of therapy	X		42A. Initial culture not performed or results within normal limits 42B. New source of infection suspected or documented 42C. Patient with relapse at follow-up visit 42D. Patient failed to return for follow-up	42, 42A. Laboratory reports, progress notes 42B. Laboratory reports, progress notes, nursing notes 42C. Laboratory reports, progress notes 42D, E. Progress notes

Element	Standard 100%	Standard 0%	Exception[b] or Critical Preventive/ Responsive Measure[c]	Sources of Information
			42E. Patient died	
43. Lumbar puncture: cerebrospinal fluid glucose concentration within normal limits at end of therapy	X		43A. Initial values not obtained or within normal limits	43, 43A. Laboratory reports, progress notes
			43B. New source of infection suspected or documented	43B. Progress notes, nursing notes, laboratory reports
			43C. Patient failed to return for follow-up	43C, D. Progress notes
			43D. Patient died	
44. Improvement in or resolution of clinical signs and symptoms of infection	X		44A. No signs or symptoms present initially	44, 44A. Progress notes, nursing notes, nursing flow sheets
			44B. Patient failed to return for follow-up	44B, C. Progress notes
			44C. Patient died	
45. Patient alive at end of therapy			45A. Patient failed to return for follow-up	45, 45A. Progress notes

[a] Criteria address justification for use (indications), critical (process) indicators, complications of therapy, and patient outcome. Each criterion consists of an element, a standard, exceptions to the standard, and sources of information. The element is the minimum level of evidence needed to show that patient care was optimal. The standard defines the deviation from an element that is acceptable. If no deviation is acceptable, the standard is 100%. Exceptions are circumstances in which deviation is allowable. Sources of information listed are the most reliable sources. Sources pertaining to an element or exception are identified by the number assigned to the element or exception (e.g., 14, 14A).

[b] For justification for use and critical (process) indicators.

[c] For complications and outcome measures.

References

1. Crowe HM. Focus on fluconazole: a potent antifungal agent. *Hosp Formul.* 1990; 25:611–6.
2. Galgiani JN. Fluconazole, a new antifungal agent. *Ann Intern Med.* 1990; 113:177–9.
3. Grant SM, Clissold SP. Fluconazole: a review of its pharmacodynamic and pharmacokinetic properties, and therapeutic potential in superficial and systemic mycoses. *Drugs.* 1990; 36:877–916.
4. Pasko MT, Piscitelli SC, Van Slooten AD. Fluconazole: a new triazole antifungal agent. *DICP.* 1990; 24:860–7.
5. Larsen RA, Leal ME, Chan LS. Fluconazole compared with amphotericin B plus flucytosine for cryptococcal meningitis in AIDS. *Ann Intern Med.* 1990; 113:183–7.
6. Robinson PA, Knirsch AK, Joseph JA. Fluconazole for life-threatening fungal infections in patients who cannot be treated with conventional antifungal agents. *Rev Infect Dis.* 1990; 12(Suppl 3):S349–63.
7. Stern JJ, Hartman BJ, Sharkey P et al. Oral fluconazole therapy with acquired immunodeficiency syndrome and cryptococcosis: experience with 22 patients. *Am J Med.* 1988; 85:477–80.
8. Sugar AM, Saunders C. Oral fluconazole as suppressive therapy of disseminated cryptococcosis in patients with acquired immunodeficiency syndrome. *Am J Med.* 1988; 85: 481–9.
9. Sugar AM, Stern JJ, Dupont B. Overview: treatment of cryptococcal meningitis. *Rev Infect Dis.* 1990; 12(Suppl 3):S338–48.
10. Roerig. Diflucan package insert. New York; 1990 Jan.
11. Thomas MG. Fluconazole for fungal disease. *N Z Med J.* 1990; 103:108.
12. Van't Wout JU, De Graeff-Meeder ER, Paul LC et al. Treatment of two cases of cryptococcal meningitis with fluconazole. *Scand J Infect Dis.* 1988; 20:193–8.
13. Benson JM, Nahata MC. Clinical use of systemic antifungal agents. *Clin Pharm.* 1988; 7:424–38.
14. Cleary JD, Taylor JW, Chapman SW. Imidazoles and triazoles in antifungal therapy. *DICP.* 1990; 24:148–52.
15. Lake-Bakaar G, Tom W, Lake-Bakaar D et al. Gastropathy and ketoconazole malabsoprtion in the acquired immunodeficiency syndrome (AIDS). *Ann Intern Med.* 1988; 109:471–3.
16. Hay RJ. Overview of studies of fluconazole in oropharyngeal candidiasis. *Rev Infect Dis.* 1990; 12(Suppl 3):S334–7.
17. Meunier F, Aoun M, Gerard M. Therapy for oropharyngeal candidiasis in the immunocompromised host: a randomized double-blind study of fluconazole vs. ketoconazole. *Rev Infect Dis.* 1990; 12(Suppl 3):S364–8.
18. Warnock DW. Itraconazole and fluconazole: new drugs for deep fungal infection. *J Antimicrob Chemother.* 1989; 24:275–6.
19. Bunin N, Camitta B. Oral fluconazole for treatment of disseminated fungal infection. *Pediatr Infect Dis J.* 1989; 8:62.
20. Cockcroft DW, Gault HM. Prediction of creatinine clearance from serum creatinine. *Nephron.* 1976; 16:31–41.
21. Lazar JD, Wilner KD. Drug interactions with fluconazole. *Rev Infect Dis.* 1990; 12(Suppl 3):S327–33.
22. Collignon P, Hurley B, Mitchell D. Interaction of fluconazole with cyclosporin. *Lancet.* 1989; 1:1262.
23. Mitchell AS, Holland JT. Fluconazole and phenytoin: a predictable interaction. *Br Med J.* 1989; 298:1315.

CP Continuing Education

The ASHP Continuing-Education System gives readers a self-assessment mechanism for selected articles in Clinical Pharmacy *and* AJHP. *It allows readers to obtain continuing-education credit for these articles.*

For the purpose of CE-credit enrollment, a blank answer sheet is published at the end of each installment of the column for the CE articles in that issue. An enrollee accumulates these answer sheets until the enrollment is submitted, using the form that is published in the June and December issues of Clinical Pharmacy *and in the June and December issues of* AJHP. *Any combination of tests within an 18-month period, from both* Clinical Pharmacy *and* AJHP, *may be included in an enrollment. More complete details about enrollment in the system appear in the semiannual enrollment form.*

Article 680-204-9106 (see page 179)
Qualifies for 1.0 hour of CE credit

Fluconazole: A new antifungal agent

Learning Objectives

After studying this article, the reader should be able to

1. Describe how fluconazole exerts antifungal effects.
2. Name two pharmacokinetic advantages of fluconazole over other antifungal agents.
3. List three infections for which fluconazole may be clinically useful.
4. List the three organ systems most commonly involved in fluconazole-associated adverse effects.

Self-assessment Questions

For each question there is only one best answer.

1. Fluconazole is

   a. Able to cross the blood–brain barrier readily.
   b. Extensively metabolized and cleared by the liver.
   c. Less specific than ketoconazole for fungal cytochrome P-450 enzymes.
   d. None of the above alternatives is correct.

2. Fluconazole exerts its antifungal activity by

   a. Binding to ergosterol in the fungal cell membrane.
   b. Incorporating itself into fungal DNA and causing misreading of the genetic code.
   c. Inhibiting the demethylation of lanosterol.
   d. Interfering with fungal DNA synthesis and arresting cell division.

3. Fungal resistance to fluconazole in vivo

   a. Is generally predicted accurately by in vitro tests.
   b. Has occurred during fluconazole therapy.
   c. Is not associated with cross-resistance to other antifungal agents.
   d. None of the above alternatives is correct.

4. The pharmacokinetic properties of fluconazole include

   a. A low (<50%) degree of oral bioavailability.
   b. A marked (>80%) degree of protein binding.
   c. Primary excretion by the kidneys.
   d. pH-dependent gastric absorption.

5. Inhibition by azole antifungal agents of the cytochrome P-450 enzyme system is closely related to the drugs'

   a. Lipid solubility.
   b. Degree of protein binding.
   c. Affinity for ferric P-450.
   d. Degree of first-pass metabolism.

6. Compared with values observed in patients with normal renal function, the (1) volume of distribution and (2) renal clearance of fluconazole in patients with renal dysfunction are

   a. Comparable and lower, respectively.
   b. Higher and lower, respectively.
   d. Lower and higher, respectively.
   d. Higher and comparable, respectively.

7. Compared with amphotericin B, fluconazole

   a. Is clearly more efficacious for the treatment of cryptococcal meningitis.
   b. Causes important adverse effects more frequently.
   c. Has a much lower daily cost (average wholesale price) when given by injection at typical dosages.
   d. None of the above alternatives is correct.

8. The adverse effects of fluconazole most commonly involve the

   a. Kidneys.
   b. Gastrointestinal tract.
   c. Central nervous system.
   d. Cardiovascular system.

9. Studies suggest that clinically important interactions may occur between fluconazole and
   a. Cyclosporine or phenytoin.
   b. Cimetidine or antacids.
   c. Oral contraceptives.
   d. All of the above alternatives are correct.
10. FDA-approved labeling for fluconazole includes indications for
    a. Coccidioidomycosis and cryptococcal meningitis.
    b. Cryptococcal meningitis and esophageal candidiasis.
    c. Oropharyngeal candidiasis and aspergillosis.
    d. Aspergillosis, coccidioidomycosis, and candidiasis.

Article 680-204-9107 (see page 195)
Qualifies for 1.0 hour of CE credit

Evaluation and treatment of ventricular arrhythmias: An update

Learning Objectives

After studying this article, the reader should be able to

1. List three criteria that have been used to classify ventricular arrhythmias.
2. List four methods of evaluating ventricular arrhythmias.
3. Compare the benefits and limitations of electrocardiographic monitoring and electrophysiologic testing in the evaluation of antiarrhythmic efficacy.
4. Construct a basic plan for evaluating and managing a patient with ventricular arrhythmias.

Self-assessment Questions

For each question there is only one best answer.

1. Ventricular arrhythmias have been classified according to their
   a. Frequency.
   b. Electrocardiographic morphology.
   c. Lethality.
   d. All of the above alternatives are correct.
2. Continuous electrocardiographic monitoring has shown that
   a. Up to 75% of persons without heart disease have ventricular arrhythmia.
   b. The incidence and frequency of ventricular arrhythmia decreases with age.
   c. A 50% decrease in arrhythmia frequency during a 24-hour monitoring period is sufficient proof of drug efficacy.
   d. None of the above alternatives is correct.
3. Flecainide and encainide have been shown to
   a. Suppress ventricular ectopy.
   b. Increase mortality in patients who have had myocardial infarction.
   c. Possess proarrhythmic effects.
   d. All of the above alternatives are correct.
4. The signal-averaged electrocardiogram is useful in
   a. Correlating symptoms with recorded arrhythmias.
   b. Providing an objective endpoint for antiarrhythmic therapy.
   c. Identifying patients at risk of developing lethal arrhythmias.
   d. Identifying patients whose arrhythmias are provoked by stimulation of the sympathetic nervous system.
5. Electrophysiologic testing provides
   a. Uniform results regardless of the protocol employed.
   b. An objective method of testing drugs serially for efficacy.
   c. A simple, noninvasive means of evaluation than can be conducted in a physician's office.
   d. All of the above alternatives are correct.
6. Electrophysiologic testing is likely to be most useful in patients with
   a. Cardiac arrest within the first day after acute myocardial infarction.
   b. Asymptomatic premature ventricular contractions that occur less frequently than 10 times per hour.
   c. Recurrent sustained ventricular tachycardia.
   d. Paired premature ventricular contractions (couplets).
7. A positive response to one antiarrhythmic agent predicts with >90% certainty a positive response to another antiarrhythmic agent if both drugs are in class
   a. IA.
   b. IB.
   c. IC.
   d. None of the above alternative is correct.
8. Electrophysiologic testing has shown that amiodarone
   a. Exhibits long-term efficacy only if it prevents arrhythmia induction.
   b. May slow the rate of induced arrhythmias.
   c. Shortens the QRS duration of induced arrhythmias.
   d. Alternatives a and b only are correct.
9. The effective serum concentration of an antiarrhythmic agent
   a. Consistently lies within the same narrow range for the vast majority of patients.
   b. Is independent of the arrhythmia being treated.
   c. May vary widely depending on the patient and the arrhythmia.
   d. Alternatives a and b only are correct.
10. Appropriate management of the patient with arrhythmia includes
    a. Estimating the risk of sudden cardiac death.

b. Initiating drug therapy to suppress all arrhythmia.
c. Discontinuing treatment with other cardiovascular drugs.
d. All of the above alternatives are correct.

Article 680-204-9108 (see page 213)
Qualifies for 1.0 hour of CE credit.

Elemental mercury poisoning

Learning Objectives

After studying this article, the reader should be able to

1. List the physiologic (toxic) effect of inhaled elemental mercury vapors.
2. State two potential problems in the interpretation of blood or urine mercury concentrations in cases of acute or chronic mercury exposure.
3. State the indications for chelation therapy for elemental mercury exposure.
4. Recommend loading and maintenance regimens of dimercaprol, *N*-acetyl-D,L-penicillamine (NAP), penicillamine, and 2,3-dimercaptosuccinic acid (DMSA). Include dose, route of administration, and appropriate patient and laboratory monitoring.
5. Identify the decontamination measures that should be attempted after an elemental mercury exposure in a residential setting.

Self-assessment Questions

For each question there is only one best answer.

1. Which of the following statements is inconsistent with the pharmacokinetics of inhaled elemental mercury vapor?

 a. Inhaled mercury vapor is almost completely absorbed through the alveolar membrane.
 b. Mercury accumulates in the cerebral cortex and cerebellum.
 c. The tissue half-life of mercury is <2 hours.
 d. Absorbed mercury is rapidly oxidized to mercuric ions in plasma, red blood cells, and tissues.

2. Which of the following signs and symptoms are not indicative of chronic inhalational mercury exposure?

 a. Irritability, anxiety, depression, and hallucinations.
 b. Hunger, weight gain, and edema.
 c. Tremor (hand, foot), ataxia, and paresthesias.
 d. Proteinuria and tubular necrosis.

3. Symptoms of acute exposure to mercury vapors include all of the following except

 a. Salivation.
 b. Mucosal bleeding.
 c. Cough.
 d. Chest pain.

4. Which of the following statements best describes the problems associated with interpretation of blood and urine mercury levels?

 a. The published values have been derived entirely from the pediatric population.
 b. Urinary or blood mercury concentrations may be nondiagnostic in chronic exposures.
 c. The correlation between clinical symptomatology and blood or urine mercury levels associated with acute exposures is poor.
 d. Hair mercury concentrations are frequently used in determining the chronicity of an exposure.

5. The laboratory assessment of a child with suspected mercury poisoning should include

 a. A 24-hour urine mercury determination.
 b. A blood mercury concentration.
 c. Nerve-conduction studies.
 d. All of the above alternatives are correct.

6. Which of the following patient populations should receive chelation therapy?

 a. Any symptomatic patient.
 b. An asymptomatic patient with a blood mercury concentration >0–1.5 μg/dL.
 c. An asymptomatic patient with a urine mercury concentration >25–50 μg/L.
 d. All of the above alternatives are correct.

7. When dimercaprol is used for treatment of chronic exposure to mercury,

 a. An appropriate therapeutic endpoint is an asymptomatic patient with a urine mercury concentration <10–20 μg/L.
 b. The efficacy of chelation therapy should not be assessed by frequent monitoring of blood mercury levels.
 c. Five-day treatment courses followed by 7- to 10-day rest periods should be employed until the desired therapeutic endpoint is reached.
 d. All of the above alternatives are correct.

8. Which of the following adverse reactions are not associated with dimercaprol therapy?

 a. Hypertension with or without tachycardia.
 b. Unpleasant taste, nausea, and vomiting.
 c. Fever.
 d. Irreversible hepatic enzyme elevation.

9. Which of the following statements best describes chelation therapy with NAP, penicillamine, or DMSA?

 a. DMSA has demonstrated equal or superior efficacy when compared with dimercaprol, penicillamine, and NAP.
 b. Serious adverse drug reactions associated with penicillamine (nephrotoxicity, systemic lupus erythematosus, optic neuritis) are frequently encountered with regimens commonly used for chelation therapy.
 c. NAP has been reported to be as efficacious as dimercaprol in treating mildly symptomatic or asymptomatic patients.
 d. Routine monitoring of urine mercury levels is not necessary if penicillamine is selected as the chelating agent.

10. Measures that should be employed in residential decontamination should include
    a. Evacuate and "air out" the premises until measured mercury-vapor levels are within an acceptably safe range.
    b. Do not use a household vacuum to remove elemental mercury droplets.
    c. Mercury spills onto carpeted surfaces may necessitate removal of the carpet and subfloor.
    d. All of the above alternatives are correct.

Answer Sheet

February 1991 *Clinical Pharmacy*

Note: An enrollment form for the ASHP Continuing-Education System appears in the June and December issues. Please accumulate all the answer sheets you wish to use in one enrollment and submit them at one time with a completed enrollment form.

The American Society of Hospital Pharmacists is approved by the American Council on Pharmaceutical Education as a provider of continuing pharmaceutical education.

ACPE®

Place an X in the box(es) at the top of the column(s) corresponding to the test(s) you are taking. Darken the boxes corresponding to the correct answers.

	☐ ACPE 680-204-9106 1.0 C.E.U.	☐ ACPE 680-204-9107 1.0 C.E.U.	☐ ACPE 680-204-9108 1.0 C.E.U.
	a b c d	a b c d	a b c d
1.	☐☐☐☐	☐☐☐☐	☐☐☐☐
2.	☐☐☐☐	☐☐☐☐	☐☐☐☐
3.	☐☐☐☐	☐☐☐☐	☐☐☐☐
4.	☐☐☐☐	☐☐☐☐	☐☐☐☐
5.	☐☐☐☐	☐☐☐☐	☐☐☐☐
6.	☐☐☐☐	☐☐☐☐	☐☐☐☐
7.	☐☐☐☐	☐☐☐☐	☐☐☐☐
8.	☐☐☐☐	☐☐☐☐	☐☐☐☐
9.	☐☐☐☐	☐☐☐☐	☐☐☐☐
10.	☐☐☐☐	☐☐☐☐	☐☐☐☐

ASHP Use Only
(1.0)9106 ________ (3)
(1.0)9107 ________ (3)
(1.0)9108 ________ (3)

Current Literature

Drug Reaction Alerts 235

Book Reviews

Cancer Chemotherapy by Infusion, Second Edition 239
Edited by Jacob J. Lokich
Reviewed by James H. Keller

Poisoning and Drug Overdose 243
Edited by Kent R. Olson, Charles E. Becker, Neal L. Benowitz et al.
Reviewed by James J. Kresel

Books Received 246

Drug Reaction Alerts

Drug Reaction Alerts focuses primarily on serious, unlabeled reactions to new chemical entities. The citations are compiled monthly from International Pharmaceutical Abstracts, *which covers over 800 pharmacy and health-related journals worldwide. An address for reprints (when available) follows the name of the corresponding author of each citation.*

Pharmacists may use the FDA Adverse Reaction Report form that appears in most issues of Clinical Pharmacy for submitting reports of adverse drug reactions directly to FDA.

Abortifacients

Brandenburg H, Jahoda MG, Wladimiroff JW et al. (Lindhout D, Department of Obstetrics and Gynecology and Clinical Genetics, Academy Hospital Dijkzigt, Erasmus University, 3015GD Rotterdam, the Netherlands). Convulsions in epileptic women after administration of prostaglandin E2 derivative. *Lancet*. 1990; 336:1138. Cases. (four pregnant women with epilepsy who were stabilized on valproic acid before conception, aged 24–29 years; spina bifida detected in fetuses; women received **sulprostone** 500 μg every four hours by i.m. injection for elective termination of pregnancies; three patients developed convulsions)

Anti-infective Agents

Fisch A, Prazuck T, Malkin JE et al. (Lafaix C, University Hospital, Villeneuve St. George, 94190 France). Diabetes mellitus in a patient with AIDS after treatment with **pentamidine** aerosol. *Br Med J*. 1990; 301:875. Case. (56-year-old patient with acquired immunodeficiency syndrome; received pentamidine isethionate 300 mg monthly by aerosol inhalation for treatment of *Pneumocystis carinii* pneumonia; developed asthenia, polyuria, and polydipsia eight days after third inhalation; fasting serum glucose concentration, 25.3 mM; symptoms resolved after therapy with regular insulin 35 units for 10 days; pentamidine replaced with dapsone)

Anti-inflammatory Agents

Helfgott SM, Sandberg-Cook J, Zakim D et al. (Nestler J, 85 Seymour Street, Hartford, CT 06106). **Diclofenac**-associated hepatotoxicity. *JAMA*. 1990; 264:2660-2. Cases. (six women and one man with rheumatoid arthritis, osteoarthritis, or fibromyalgia, aged 45–69 years; six patients received diclofenac sodium 75 mg twice daily and oldest patient received 25 mg three times daily; developed signs and symptoms of hepatitis within

Continued on page 237

several weeks of initiation of diclofenac; withdrawal of diclofenac led to general resolution of signs and symptoms within four to six weeks; 46-year-old patient rechallenged and developed recurrence of hepatic abnormalities; 65-year-old patient developed fatal fulminant hepatitis despite early withdrawal of diclofenac)

Antilipemic Agents

Pizarro S, Bargay J, D'Agosto P (Primary Care Center, Son Servera, La Vileta, Palma de Mallorca, Majorca, Spain). **Gemfibrozil**-induced impotence. *Lancet*. 1990; 336:1135. Case. (48-year-old man with hypertension, coronary heart disease, and hyperlipoproteinemia; received gemfibrozil 600 mg twice daily for two weeks; patient noted impotence; concomitant propranolol; withdrawal of gemfibrozil led to resumption of sexual activity in a few days; positive rechallenge)

Antineoplastic Agents

Cervantes F, Salgado C, Montserrat E et al. (Rozman C, Postgraduate School of Hematology "Farreras Valenti," Hospital Clinic, 08037, Barcelona, Spain). **Fludarabine** for prolymphocytic leukemia and risk of interstitial pneumonitis. *Lancet*. 1990; 336:1130. Case. (40-year-old man with prolymphocytic leukemia unresponsive to conventional chemotherapy; received fludarabine phosphate 20 mg/sq m/day for five days every four weeks for three cycles; developed productive cough, fever with dyspnea, hypoxemia, and diffuse interstitial pneumonia; white blood cell count fell rapidly from 5.9×10^{11}/L to 4.6×10^{10}/L with 84% mature lymphocytes and 7% prolymphocytes; negative microbiological studies; therapy with antibiotics and prednisone 1 mg/kg/day led to resolution of clinical symptoms; respiratory symptoms reappeared two weeks later during fourth cycle of fludarabine; clinical symptoms resolved again after treatment with antibiotics and prednisone; fludarabine discontinued; patient died from disease progression)

Carbonic Anhydrase Inhibitors

McMurdo ME, Hutchison GL, Lindsay G (Department of Medicine and Anesthetics, and Pharmacy, Ninewells Hospital and Medical School, Dundee DD1 9SY, Scotland). Taste disturbance with **acetazolamide**. *Lancet*. 1990; 336:1190-1. Cases. (three patients; received acetazolamide 500 mg/day for five days as prophylaxis for altitude sickness while touring Andes mountains; developed peripheral paresthesia; two patients developed taste disturbance six hours after first dose; resolution of taste disturbance 24 hours after final dose)

Drug Interactions

Figge J (Division of Endocrinology and Metabolism, Albany Medical College, A44, 47 New Scotland Avenue, Albany, NY 12208), Dluhy RG. Amiodarone-induced elevation of thyroid stimulating hormone in patients receiving **levothyroxine** for primary hypothyroidism. *Ann Intern Med*. 1990; 113:553-5. Cases. (two patients with primary hypothyroidism who were stabilized on levothyroxine, aged 73 and 83 years; one patient received levothyroxine sodium 0.075 mg/day and other received 0.1 mg/day; received amiodarone hydrochloride for treatment of tachycardia; developed elevation of serum thyroid stimulating hormone concentration; resolution of symptoms of hypothyroidism and normal serum thyroid stimulating hormone concentration after levothyroxine increased from 0.075 up to 0.112 mg/day in one patient; other remained clinically euthyroid without change to levothyroxine dose)

Monahan BP, Ferguson CL, Killeavy ES et al. (Cantilena LR, Division of Clinical Pharmacology, Uniformed Services University

Continued on page 238

Current Literature *Continued from page 237*

of the Health Sciences, 4301 Jones Bridge Road, Bethesda, MD 20814-4799). Torsades de pointes occurring in association with **terfenadine** use. *JAMA.* 1990; 264:2788-90. Case. (39-year-old woman; received terfenadine 60 mg twice daily for 10 days and **ketoconazole** 200 mg twice daily during last two days; developed symptoms of cardiac arrhythmia; withdrawal of terfenadine and ketoconazole led to resolution of tachycardia as shown by electrocardiographic and symptomatic evidence; serum terfenadine concentration excessive and serum concentration of main metabolite reduced proportionately)

Gastrointestinal Drugs

La Vecchia C (Instituto di Ricerche Farmacologiche Mario Negri, Via Eritrea 62, 20157 Milan, Italy), Negri E, D'Avanzo B et al. Histamine-2-receptor antagonists and gastric cancer risk. *Lancet.* 1990; 336:355-7. Study. (nonrandomized retrospective study; 2064 patients; 563 patients with recently diagnosed gastric cancer and 1501 controls without neoplastic or gastrointestinal disorders; 6.3% of case patients and 3.3% of control patients received **cimetidine** or **ranitidine** before study began; relative risk for development of gastric cancer by patients who used either drug was 1.8; increased risk restricted to patients who began treatment with H_2-receptor antagonists within five years of diagnosis of gastric cancer)

Hemostatics

McLeod BC (Department of Medicine, Rush-Presbyterian-St. Luke's Medical Center, Chicago, IL 60612). Myocardial infarction in a blood donor after administration of **desmopressin**. *Lancet.* 1990; 336:1137-8. Case. (47-year-old man who was a regular blood donor and previously received desmopressin stimulation for 88 of 143 donations; received desmopressin 0.3 μg/kg as i.v. infusion over 30 minutes; developed chest pain; electrocardiogram showed subtle ST segment changes in the inferior leads; serum creatine kinase concentration initially was 103 IU/L but was 549 IU/L with 14% in the MB fraction six hours later; recovery upon dechallenge)

Immunosuppressive Agents

DeJong DJ, Sayler DJ (Department of Pharmacy, Methodist Medical Center, 301 W. Colorado, Dallas, TX 75208). Possible **cyclosporine**-associated thrombocytopenia. *DICP.* 1990; 24:1007. Case. (70-year-old man with renal transplant; received cyclosporine 150 mg twice daily; developed thrombocytopenia; platelet count, 2.1×10^{10}/L; withdrawal of cyclosporine led to slow increase of platelet count; therapy with immune globulin 30 g/day for four days led to resolution of thrombocytopenia)

Quinolones

Bates CJ (Department of Bacteriology, Royal Hallamshire Hospital, Sheffield S10 2JF, England), Wilcox MH, Spencer RC et al. **Ciprofloxacin** and *Clostridium difficile* infection. *Lancet.* 1990; 336:1193. Cases. (two patients with symptomatic enteric salmonellosis; received ciprofloxacin 500 mg twice daily for seven days; resolution of symptoms; fecal samples obtained on day 7 contained *Clostridium difficile* toxin, which was not present initially; withdrawal of ciprofloxacin led to absence of toxin in fecal samples)

Mumford CJ, Ginsberg L (Addenbrooke's Hospital, Cambridge CB2 2QQ, England). **Ciprofloxacin** and myasthenia gravis. *Br Med J.* 1990; 301:818. Case. (73-year-old man with subclinical myasthenia gravis; received ciprofloxacin 250 mg twice daily for less than 48 hours; developed severe dysphagia, dysarthria, and blepharoptosis on left side that varied with fatigue; withdrawal of ciprofloxacin led to resolution of severe bulbar symptoms but blepharoptosis persisted; therapy with i.v. injection of edrophonium and oral pyridostigmine led to resolution of blepharoptosis)

Skin and Mucous Membrane Preparations

Brenner S, Wolf R, Landau M (Department of Dermatology, Sackler Facility of Medicine, Tel Aviv University, Ichilov Hospital, Tel Aviv Sourasky Medical Center, 64239, Tel Aviv, Israel). Ectropion: adverse effect of **etretinate** therapy for psoriasis. *DICP*. 1990; 24:1007. Case. (75-year-old man with psoriasis; received etretinate 75 mg/day for six weeks; developed bilateral ectropion; symptoms remain two years after end of treatment for psoriasis)

Vaccines

Gutierrez K, Abzug MJ (Department of Infectious Diseases, Children's Hospital, 1056 E. 19th Avenue, Denver, CO 80218). Vaccine-associated poliovirus meningitis in children with ventriculoperitoneal shunts. *J Pediatr*. 1990; 117:424-7. Cases. (two infants with ventriculoperitoneal shunts; one infant received **poliovirus live oral vaccine** at five months of age and other received vaccine at two months; developed aseptic meningitis; poliovirus isolated from cerebrospinal fluid; five-month-old infant treated with i.v. injections of ampicillin and nafcillin; other treated with i.v. injections of vancomycin and ceftriaxone)

Vasodilating Agents

Chassagne P, Mejjad O, Noblet C et al. (Deshayes P, Hopital de Boisguillaume, BP 100, 76233 Boisguillaume Cedex, France). Pseudopolymyalgia rheumatica with **dipyridamole**. *Br Med J*. 1990; 301:875. Case. (59-year-old patient with cardiac problems; received dipyridamole 225 mg/day; developed severe muscular pain in all limbs; muscle pain increased sharply 20 minutes after each dose of dipyridamole and then slowly decreased but did not disappear completely before next dose; substitution of another brand of dipyridamole did not reduce symptoms; therapy with aspirin 1.5 g/day did not reduce symptoms; withdrawal of dipyridamole by patient led to complete resolution of symptoms)

Vitamins

Mehta JB, Singhal SB, Mehta BC (Blood Respiratory Center, 400058 Bombay, India). **Ascorbic acid**-induced hemolysis in G-6-PD deficiency. *Lancet*. 1990; 336:944. Cases. (two boys with glucose 6-phosphate dehydrogenase deficiency; drank 8–10 servings of an orange-flavored drink and 2–3 glasses of a lemon-flavored soft drink over four to six hours; developed severe hemolysis; one boy was treated twice with packed cells, 3 units per treatment; other did not receive transfusion)

Book Reviews

Cancer Chemotherapy by Infusion, Second Edition

Edited by Jacob J. Lokich.
Published by Precept Press, Inc., 160 East Illinois Street, Chicago, IL 60611, 1990. xxiv + 659. Price $129.

During the last 10 years, the discovery of novel antineoplastic agents has slowed dramatically. With fewer new drugs available for cancer chemotherapy, investigators are increasing their efforts to optimize the effectiveness and safety of existing drugs. The prolonged infusion of antineoplastic agents is one of these efforts.

The editor of *Cancer Chemotherapy by Infusion*, physician Jacob Lokich, has been a long-time leader and innovator in the field of infusion techniques. For this book he compiled chapters that explain the rationale behind the use of specific drugs for specific disease categories.

Continued on page 243

Continued from page 239

The first five chapters thoroughly present the basic and technical aspects of infusion therapy. However, little of the information is new but would be useful to the practitioner who is not familiar with this type of therapy.

Chapter 4 is extremely important to any pharmacist who prepares antineoplastic agents for prolonged infusions; it is fairly complete in its discussion of stability and compatibility issues for infusion therapy—probably the most complete single reference for this information. In addition to the practical information, the chapter provides pharmaceutic principles for practitioners interested in pursuing further evaluations of drug stability and compatibility.

The second section of the book explains the pharmacology of several different antineoplastic agents. In general, the chapters in this section provide thorough discussions of the pharmacologic bases for the individual compounds or classes of compounds that can be used in infusion therapy. The information is current and provides a good reference for pharmacists who want to obtain information beyond the basic technical information provided in the first section of the book. For example, important clinical studies that support the continuous infusion of a class of drugs are included. Section 2 also contains limited information on infusion techniques with biological response modifiers (e.g., interleukins, interferons, colony-stimulating factors, and monoclonal antibodies). Lokich wrote the chapter that explains infusion schedules for investigational agents; the information is somewhat limited, but Lokich provides some impetus for examining infusion techniques at an early stage in drug development.

The third section of the text is devoted to disease-oriented information and discusses infusion techniques for specific tumor sites. These chapters are good reviews of clinical studies that involve infusion techniques alone or infusion techniques as part of combined modality treatments.

The last section contains chapters that pertain to unique categories of infusion chemotherapy; these chapters explain topics such as chemotherapy combined with radiation therapy, intraperitoneal chemotherapy, local or regional perfusion with antineoplastic agents, and the monitoring of serum concentrations. The data are fairly current and provide background information for pharmacists involved in settings where chemotherapy is administered by various infusion techniques. Like the preceding chapters, these chapters may not provide the specific details of preparation and administration that would be useful to the practicing pharmacist.

The last chapter discusses therapeutic drug monitoring, which is in its infancy. The author provides a foundation for further growth and development in this area. Although relatively short, the chapter may provide an area of research for pharmacists in the academic or research setting.

Cancer Chemotherapy by Infusion provides a compilation of important information about infusion techniques for cytotoxic agents, biological response modifiers, and drugs involved in combined modality treatments. It presents an overview of drug preparation, administration techniques, compatibilities, stabilities, and other pharmacy-related topics but does not always explain the details. The book would be a good reference book in a drug information center that receives questions about the infusion of cancer chemotherapy.

Reviewed by James H. Keller, Pharm.D., Itasca Medical Center, 126 First Avenue Southeast, Grand Rapids, MN 55744.

Poisoning and Drug Overdose

Edited by Kent R. Olson, Charles E. Becker, Neal L. Benowitz et al.

Published by Appleton & Lange, 25 Van Zant Street, East Norwalk, CT 06855, 1990. ix + 575 p. Price $24.50.

The editors of this book assembled a vast quantity of information on poisoning and drug overdose and turned it into a compact, yet comprehensive, manual that is separated logically into four distinct sections. This first edition is a very appropriate manual for pharmacists who have a general understanding of toxicologic principles; it distills many of the facts contained in the large literature base into a format that is easy to read and understand. However, *Poisoning and Drug Overdose* is not a substitute for the vast, often overwhelming, body of information that is available on the computer databases found in virtually all poison information centers and in many hospitals.

Section I is a review of the principles and techniques used to evaluate the poisoned patient; the section partially resembles a check list. For the pharmacist, this section either provides a review of these techniques or offers an introduction to the area. As an introduction, this section provides a clear description of the initial approach to dealing with the poisoned patient. The section also offers the pharmacist a valuable opportunity to expand his or her knowledge base and reviews how toxicologic principles may be integrated into clinical decision making.

Section II focuses on chemicals and drug products that are associated often with poisonings and describes the mechanisms of toxicity and toxic dose and the clinical presentation of the poisoned patient. The section explains the often subtle distinction between toxicologic and pharmacologic attributes of a drug and groups the drugs by pharmacologic class, then presents the class as a whole (e.g., hypoglycemics and diuretics).

Section III describes drugs and pharmacologic classes of drugs that have antidotal potential. A clear, concise monograph of each agent is presented including a brief review of the drug's pharmacology, indications, dosage, and method of administration.

The fourth section of this manual presents environmental and occupational toxicology. This final section contains a reasonably extensive listing of chemicals that may be encountered in the work place. The reader not familiar with the lexicon of occupational health can find good descriptions of relevant terms such as threshold limit value (TLV) and permissible exposure limit (PEL). This fourth section offers general information that can be useful to pharmacists, especially those who are involved in evaluating a work site within the hospital. Also, this section contains a list of chemicals known or suspected to have carcinogenic potential.

Poisoning and Drug Overdose is an easy-to-use review manual. As with any book that reviews a broad subject, this manual does not replace existing encyclopedic

Continued on page 246

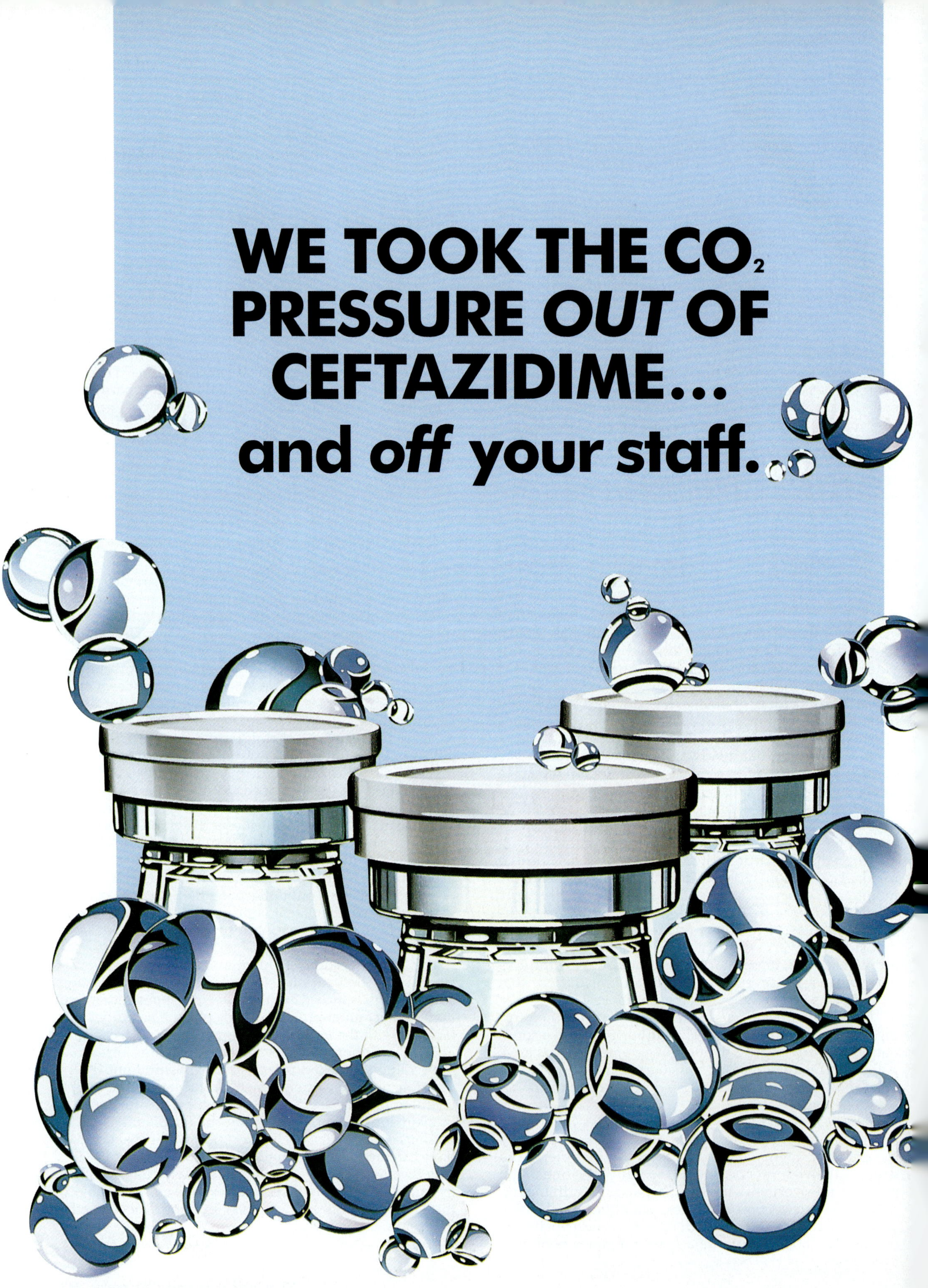
WE TOOK THE CO_2
PRESSURE *OUT* OF
CEFTAZIDIME...
and *off* your staff...

Current Literature *Continued from page 243*

sources, either printed or electronic. For the reader with a background in pharmacology and toxicology, this manual augments that background and provides rapid, concise information.

Reviewed by James J. Kresel, Ph.D., Mary Hitchcock Memorial Hospital, 2 Maynard Street, Hanover, NH 03756.

Books Received

Books are listed as soon as received; selected books may be reviewed in Book Reviews in subsequent issues.

Drug Safety in Pregnancy, edited by Peter I. Folb and M. N. Graham Dukes. Published by Elsevier Science Publishers B.V., P.O. Box 211, 1000 AE Amsterdam, the Netherlands, 1990. xxi + 520 p. Price $243.

The Essentials of Homeopathic Therapeutics, by Jacques Jouanny. Published by Boiron Laboratories, 20, rue de la Libération, 69110 Ste-Foy-lés-Lyon, France, 1985. 417 p. Price $40.

Handbook of Psychiatric Emergencies, by William R. Dubin and Kenneth J. Weiss. Published by Springhouse Corporation, 1111 Bethlehem Pike, Springhouse PA 19477, 1991. x + 294 p. Price $22.95.

Advertising Index

American Society of Hospital Pharmacists
AHFS Drug Information 91, 239
Aseptic Preparation of Parenteral Products, 238
ASHP Membership, 212
Clinical Pharmacy, 221
Handbook on Injectable Drugs, 6th Edition, 232
International Pharmaceutical Abstracts, 231
Medication Teaching Manual, Fourth Edition, 178
Pocket Guide to Injectable Drugs, 1991 Edition, 236
Burroughs Wellcome Company
Zovirax I.V., 240-242
Department of Veterans Affairs (Richmond)
Positions Available, 163
Eisenhower Medical Center
Position Available, 237
Glaxo Inc.
Ceptaz, 244-246
Zofran, 169-174
Eli Lilly and Company
Hospital Division, inside front cover
Lyphomed, Inc.
Amphotericin B, 164-166
SmithKline Beecham
Tagamet, inside back cover, outside back cover
Wyeth-Ayerst Laboratories, Inc.
Position Available, 176

News

Ondansetron granted marketing approval 249

Rubella prevention guidelines updated by CDC 249

Two reports on hypertension available from National Heart, Lung, and Blood Institute 253

News Briefs 253

Ondansetron granted marketing approval

Ondansetron hydrochloride injection (Zofran, Glaxo), a selective antagonist of serotonin type 3 receptors, was approved by FDA in January for the prevention of nausea and vomiting associated with emetogenic cancer chemotherapy, including high-dose cisplatin therapy. (Ondansetron will be reviewed in an upcoming issue of *Clinical Pharmacy*.)

Serotonin type 3 receptors are found peripherally on vagus nerve terminals and centrally in the chemoreceptor trigger zone. The exact mechanism of ondansetron's antiemetic activity is uncertain. Effects could be mediated at central or peripheral receptors, or both. However, cytotoxic agents appear to release serotonin from the enterochromaffin cells of the small intestine. Released serotonin may initiate the vomiting reflex by stimulating serotonin receptors on the vagus nerve.

Ondansetron is extensively metabolized; about 5% of a dose is recovered as unchanged drug in the urine. The elimination half-life in adult cancer patients is about four hours. The half-life is longer (about 5.5 hours) in healthy volunteers older than 75 years and shorter (2.4 hours) in patients 4–14 years. Because ondansetron is metabolized by cytochrome P-450 enzymes, drugs that induce or inhibit the activity of these enzymes could affect the clearance of ondansetron; however, no dosage adjustment is currently recommended for patients treated with these drugs.

Headache and diarrhea were the most frequently reported adverse events in premarketing comparative clinical trials; these events were reported by 16% and 22% of patients, respectively.

A series of three intravenous 0.15-mg/kg doses is recommended. The first dose should be infused over 15 minutes beginning 30 minutes before the start of cytotoxic therapy. Additional doses should be given four and eight hours after the initial dose. The same dosage schedule is recommended for elderly persons and children 4 to 18 years of age.

Zofran is supplied as a 2-mg/mL solution in 20-mL multidose vials.

Rubella prevention guidelines updated by CDC

Recommendations for the prevention of rubella have been updated by the Immunization Practices Advisory

Continued on page 253

Continued from page 249

Committee of the Centers for Disease Control (CDC).[1] The goal of rubella immunization programs is prevention of fetal infection and subsequent congenital anomalies. The guidelines reflect the new two-dose schedule for measles–mumps–rubella vaccine that has been recommended to achieve better control of measles. Included in the statement are general recommendations for rubella vaccine use, recommendations for vaccinating women of child-bearing age, and special considerations involving immunocompromised patients and patients receiving immune globulin therapy. Also included is information about vaccine efficacy and adverse effects; contraindications to vaccine administration; the simultaneous administration of rubella vaccine and other widely used vaccines; strategies for eliminating congenital rubella syndrome (CRS); and surveillance of rubella and CRS.

1. Immunization Practices Advisory Committee. Rubella prevention. *MMWR*. 1990; 39(RR-15):1–18.

Two reports on hypertension available from National Heart, Lung, and Blood Institute

Two reports from working groups of the National High Blood Pressure Education Program and the National Cholesterol Education Program are available from the National Heart, Lung, and Blood Institute (NHLBI). They can be ordered from the Office of Prevention, Education, and Control, NHLBI, Bethesda, MD 20892 (301-496-0554).

"Hypertension and Chronic Renal Failure" describes the pathology and pathophysiology of hypertension and chronic renal insufficiency, reviews the effects of various classes of antihypertensive agents on renal hemodynamics, and provides recommendations for treatment that help to protect the kidneys.

"Hypertension and High Blood Cholesterol" provides an integrated approach to the management of patients who have multiple risk factors for cardiovascular disease. Sections of the report review epidemiologic data, the effects of hypertension and high blood cholesterol on atherosclerosis, and results of intervention trials; provide guidelines for the treatment of patients with hypertension and high blood cholesterol; cover special considerations, such as smoking, hormonal therapy, the patient's age, cost barriers, and the presence of diabetes mellitus, peripheral or carotid artery disease, coronary artery disease, cardiac or renal transplantation, and renal, cardiovascular, or cerebrovascular disease; and provide information on developing educational messages for patients.

News Briefs

- **Two videotapes about clinical trials** are available at no cost to health professionals from the Office of Cancer Communications, National Cancer Institute, Building 31, Room 4B43, National Institutes of Health, Bethesda, MD 20892. One videotape is intended for viewing by patients; the other is being promoted to physicians and other health professionals involved in cancer treatment studies.
- **"Alcohol, Tobacco, and Other Drugs May Harm the Unborn Child,"** an 80-page booklet from the U.S. Department of Health and Human Services, is intended for use by health professionals who work with women of childbearing age. The booklet (stock no. 017-024-01422-2) is available for $2.50 from the Superintendent of Documents, Department 36-IV, U.S. Government Printing Office, Washington, DC 20402-9325 (202-783-3238).
- Alcon Laboratories has marketed ciprofloxacin hydrochloride as an **ophthalmic solution containing 0.3% ciprofloxacin.**

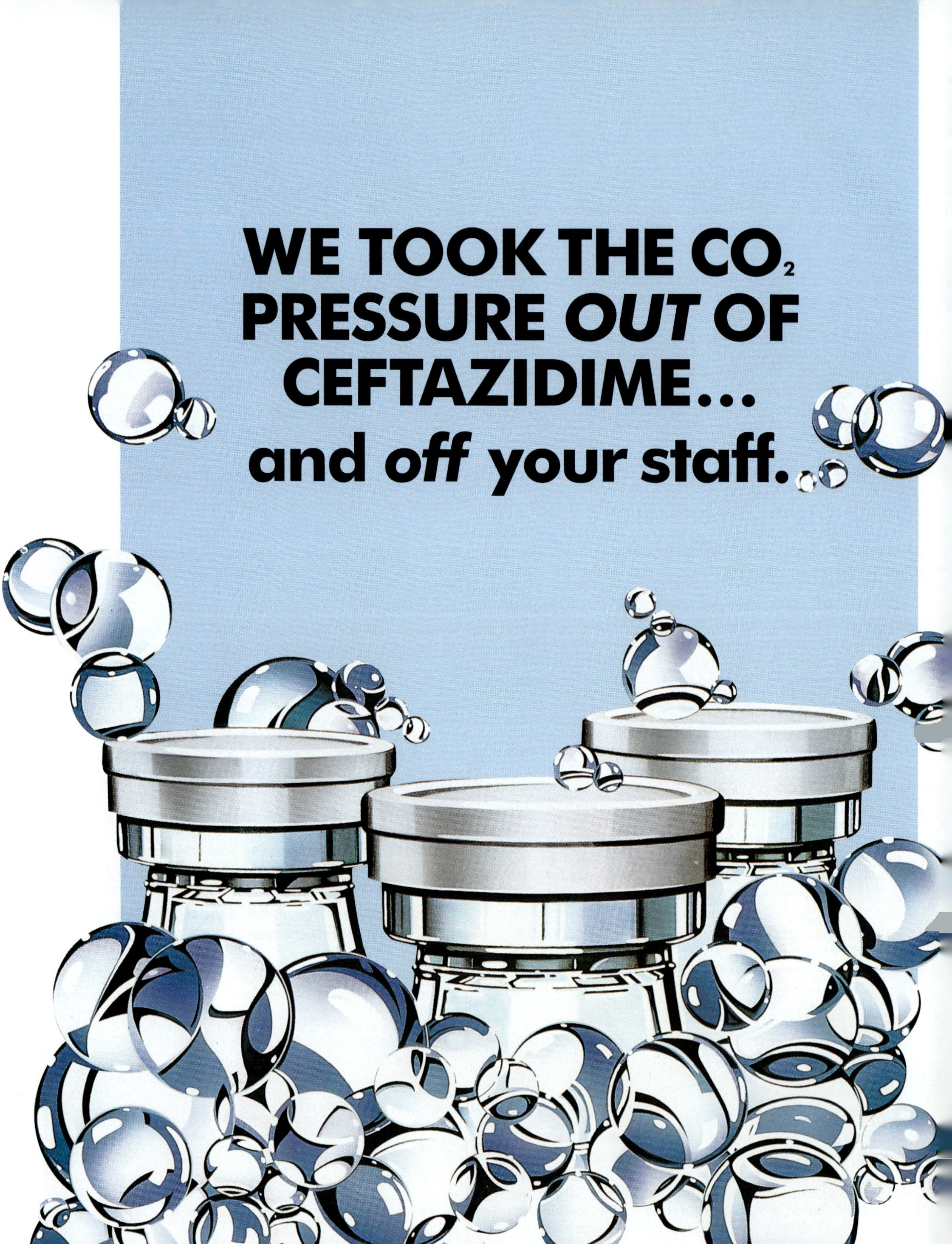
WE TOOK THE CO_2
PRESSURE *OUT* OF
CEFTAZIDIME...
and *off* your staff.

Letters

Pentamidine-induced facial numbness 257
Anne Y. F. Lin and Candace Smith

Corrections 261

The Letters *column is a forum for rapid exchange of ideas among readers of* Clinical Pharmacy. *Liberal criteria are applied in the review of submissions to encourage contributions to this column.*

The Letters *column includes the following types of contributions: (1) comments, addenda, and minor updates on previously published work, (2) alerts on potential problems related to drug therapy or clinical research, (3) observations or comments on trends in drug therapy or clinical research, and (4) brief expressions of opinion about controversies in drug therapy or clinical research.*

Letters need not be submitted with the journal's manuscript checklist. The following conditions, however, must be adhered to: (1) the body of the letter must be no longer than two typewritten pages, (2) the use of references, tables, and illustrations should be minimized, (3) the authors' names, affiliations, and mailing addresses must be typed at the end of the letter in the format used by Clinical Pharmacy, *and (4) the entire letter (including references, tables, and authors' names) must be typed double-spaced on plain white paper (not letterhead). Following acceptance of a letter, the authors are required to sign an exclusive publication statement and a copyright-transferal form.*

Pentamidine-induced facial numbness

The use of pentamidine has increased dramatically over the past few years as a result of the increasing number of cases of *Pneumocystis carinii* pneumonia (PCP) in patients with AIDS. Information on pentamidine-associated adverse reactions has been accumulating. We report here a case of pentamidine-associated facial numbness. The causal relationship was evaluated by using the Jones nomogram.[1]

A 21-year-old man (170 cm, 64 kg) was admitted to the hospital for the treatment of presumed PCP. He had hemophilia (factor VIII deficiency) and no known allergies. His vital signs on physical examination were temperature, 39.2 °C; pulse, 120 beats/min; respiration, 32/min; and blood pressure, 120/70 mm Hg. Serum electrolyte concentrations were within normal limits. Diffuse bilateral infiltration consistent with PCP was noted on chest roentgenography. An HIV antibody test result available on the day of discharge was positive.

On admission, the patient was given trimethoprim 250 mg–sulfamethoxazole 1.3 g i.v. every six hours for presumed PCP and erythromycin 500 mg p.o. every six hours for possible infection by *Mycoplasma pneumoniae.* On hospital day 4, a bronchoalveolar lavage specimen was positive for *P. carinii,* and erythromycin administration was discontinued. On hospital day 10 the patient remained febrile and developed a diffuse maculopapular rash; trimethoprim–sulfamethoxazole was discontinued and daily treatment with pentamidine isethionate 300 mg i.v. (over 60 minutes) was started. Other medications included acetaminophen 650 mg p.o. on day 10 and diphenhydramine hydrochloride 25 mg p.o. every six hours as needed.

Within minutes of the start of the first pentamidine infusion, the patient complained of dizziness (which he described as "the same feeling as when you come off a roller coaster") and bilateral numbness of the face ("not feeling anything even if you tap your finger on my face"). The reaction resolved within 15 minutes after the end of the infusion. The patient was not hypotensive during this reaction (blood pressure, 124/70 mm Hg). He described similar reactions while receiving pentamidine over the next six days. On four of these occasions when blood pressure was measured, the patient was not hypotensive (range, 100/70 to 124/70 mm Hg), and on three occasions blood glucose concentrations determined with the Chemstrip bG were 120, 140, and

Continued on page 261

Letters *Continued from page 257*

210 mg/dL. Ninety minutes after receiving the eighth dose, the patient experienced diaphoresis and orthostasis (seated blood pressure, 104/60 mm Hg; supine blood pressure, 160/110 mm Hg). Blood pressure readings were 108/60 and 110/60 mm Hg during the infusion and approximately one-half hour after the infusion, respectively. The blood glucose concentration was 84 mg/dL. The patient was not hypocalcemic during treatment with pentamidine (serum calcium concentration, 9.1 mg/dL).

Finally, the patient could no longer tolerate these adverse effects and requested that treatment with pentamidine be discontinued. However, because clinical improvement had been noted since the pentamidine therapy began, it was decided to change the method of administration to inhalation rather than to use other agents. The patient remained afebrile and was discharged on hospital day 19. The patient has not reported any similar reactions after being treated with aerosolized pentamidine for one and a half years.

Common pentamidine-associated adverse effects include rash, hypoglycemia, dizziness without hypotension, hypotension, nausea and vomiting, hematologic disturbances, and elevations of liver enzyme levels.[2,3]

A literature search did not reveal any reports of pentamidine-associated facial numbness. One report of lip numbness in a patient receiving aerosolized pentamidine was made by Leoung et al.[4] Although hypesthesia is mentioned in the NebuPent package insert,[5] the patient described here has not reported any such adverse reaction. To our knowledge, this is the first case report of facial numbness possibly due to i.v. pentamidine.

1. Jones JK. Adverse drug reactions in the community health setting: approaches to recognizing, counseling, and reporting. *Fam Community Health.* 1982; 5(Aug):58-67.
2. Sands M, Kron MA, Brown RB. Pentamidine: a review. *Rev Infect Dis.* 1985; 7:625-33.
3. Lyphomed, Inc. Pentam 300 package insert. Rosemont, IL; 1987 Apr.
4. Leoung GS, Feigal DW, Montgomery AB et al. Aerosolized pentamidine for prophylaxis against *Pneumocystis carinii* pneumonia. *N Engl J Med.* 1990; 323:769-75.
5. Lyphomed, Inc. NebuPent package insert. Rosemont, IL; 1989 Jun.

ANNE Y. F. LIN, PHARM.D., Assistant Clinical Professor
CANDACE SMITH, PHARM.D., Assistant Clinical Professor

College of Pharmacy and Allied Health Professions
St. John's University
Grand Central and Utopia Parkways
Jamaica, NY 11439

Corrections

Attention-deficit hyperactivity disorder (August 1990, Therapy Review). On page 639, the dosage of clonidine hydrochloride in references 61 and 62 was 0.005 mg/kg/day, not 0.05 mg/kg/day.

Olsalazine approved for use in ulcerative colitis (December 1990, News). On page 908, the labeled indication for olsalazine is maintenance of remission of ulcerative colitis in patients who cannot tolerate sulfasalazine therapy.

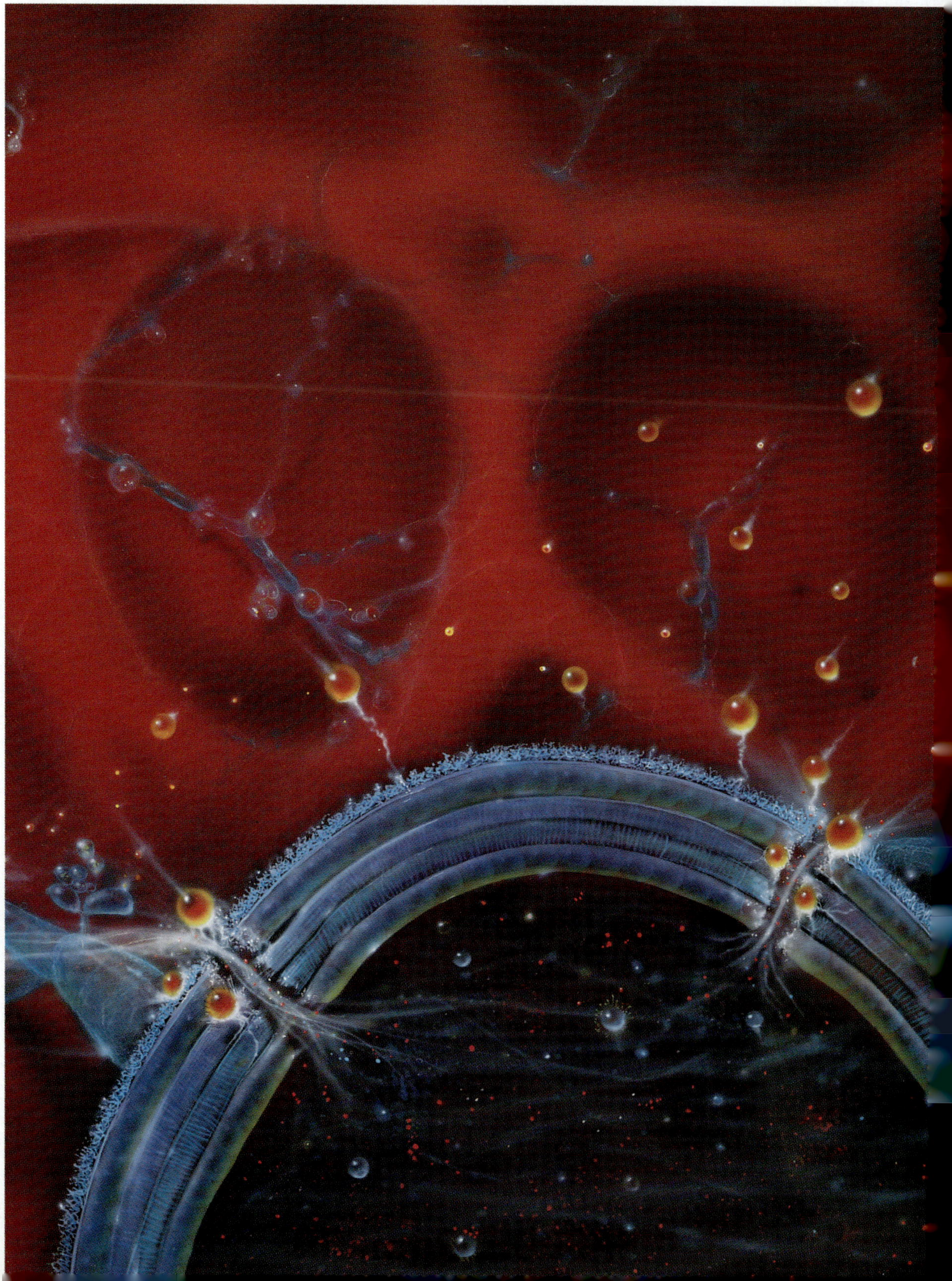

Guard against harmful drug interactions with

Rx Triage™

Software support for drug interaction decisions

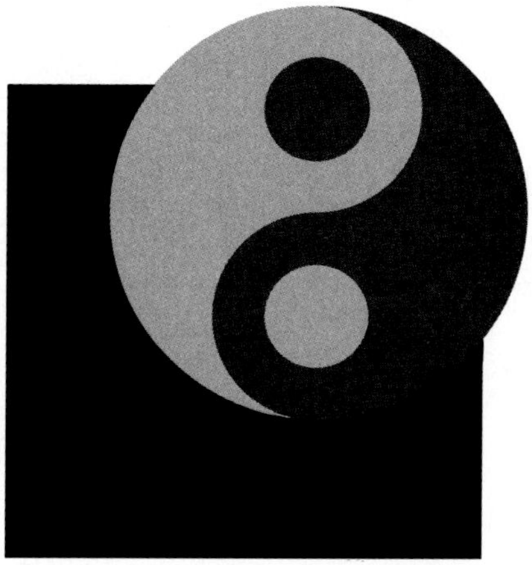

Order today - or try our demo package first!

Many of the patients you see are taking more than one drug to treat any number of medical conditions. How can you ensure that potentially harmful drug interactions are avoided?

ASHP, in cooperation with First DataBank, can help make this task easier and more reliable, with Rx Triage software. The clinical drug information in Rx Triage has been used for over 10 years by thousands of health care professionals - and it's updated quarterly by a panel of drug interaction experts from around the country.

Program Features:

- ❑ **Drug Interaction Screening** - drug interaction monographs for virtually every product available in the U.S.
- ❑ **Drug-to-Food Interaction Data** - important information about potential drug-food problems.
- ❑ **Decision Support and Risk Management** - clinical information tables to help you select the optimum method of drug therapy.
- ❑ **Patient Education Leaflets** - for printing take-home monographs in easy-to-understand language.

System Requirements:

- ❑ DOS 2.0 or higher
- ❑ 512K random access memory
- ❑ one 3½" or 5¼" floppy disk drive
- ❑ hard drive (with 3.5 megabytes of disk space)
- ❑ monochrome or color monitor
- ❑ dot matrix printer

Order Form

❑ Please send me______ copies of Rx Triage software (P327) at:

❑ $480 ASHP Members (please provide ASHP Member ID #, below)

❑ $530 Nonmembers

❑ Please send me______ copies of the demo package (P327-DEMO) at:

❑ $25 ASHP Members

❑ $31 Nonmembers

❑ Enclosed is my check for $__________, made payable to ASHP. (Checks must be drawn on a U.S. bank.)

❑ Enclosed is our purchase order #__________; please issue an invoice and add postage and handling charges.

❑ Charge $__________ to my: ❑ VISA ❑ MasterCard

Account#__________________ Exp. date__________ month/year

Signature__________________________

Name__________________________

Institution__________________________

Address__________________________

City______________ State______ Zip______

ASHP Member ID #____________________
(must include to receive member price)

Send to: ASHP Customer Service Dept.
4630 Montgomery Avenue
Bethesda, MD 20814
FAX: 301-657-1251

ASHP

To order by phone, call ASHP Customer Service at 301-657-4383. Please have your VISA, MasterCard, or purchase order number ready.

Payments to ASHP are not deductible as charitable contributions for Federal Income Tax purposes. However, they may be deductible under other provisions of the Internal Revenue Code.

Neutropenia in patients infected with human immunodeficiency virus

DEB S. ISRAEL AND KAREN I. PLAISANCE

Abstract: The possible mechanisms of neutropenia associated with both human immunodeficiency virus (HIV) infection and drug treatment in adults are examined, and the current and investigational strategies for managing neutropenia are reviewed.

Neutropenia associated with HIV arises from diverse mechanisms, including cellular immune dysfunction, direct effects on progenitor cells, humoral immune dysfunction, and vitamin deficiencies. Drug-induced neutropenia may be related to direct cytotoxic effects, immunologic mediators, and the effects of vitamin depletion on the bone marrow. Bone marrow toxicity in patients receiving zidovudine appears to be more frequent in those patients with advanced disease, low CD4 cell counts, a pretreatment anemia, low serum vitamin B_{12} levels, and low or low normal serum folic acid levels. Patients with AIDS also are at increased risk for adverse events associated with folate antagonists and sulfonamides compared with other patient populations.

Lithium therapy has improved neutrophil counts in patients receiving zidovudine; however, the toxicities associated with use of lithium, combined with the lower dosages of zidovudine now recommended, may obviate its use. The use of colony-stimulating factors appears promising for increasing the number and function of circulating neutrophils. Although concomitant use of interferon alfa and zidovudine may result in a strong synergistic anti-HIV effect, dose-limiting neutropenia has been reported in patients receiving the combination. There are currently no controlled data assessing the effectiveness of intravenous immune globulin in the treatment of HIV-related or drug-related neutropenia.

In evaluating neutropenia, the clinician must attempt to discern whether the neutropenia is more likely related to disease state(s) or drug therapies. Potential management strategies include modulation of the disease state, discontinuation or dose reduction of the offending agent, or administration of exogenous immune enhancer.

Index terms: Antimanic agents; Antivirals; Colony-stimulating factors; Globulin immune; HIV infections; Immunotherapy; Lithium; Neutropenia; Toxicity; Zidovudine
Clin Pharm. 1991; 10:268-79

Drug therapies have prolonged the life span of patients who are infected with the human immunodeficiency virus (HIV), including those with the acquired immunodeficiency syndrome (AIDS).[1,2] This benefit, however, is not without cost. It has become clear that patients with AIDS are at increased risk of developing adverse drug reactions, such as neutropenia, compared with patients who do not have AIDS.[3-5]

Neutrophils play an integral role in the proper functioning of the immune system and are responsible for chemotaxis, phagocytosis, and digestion of microorganisms. Leukopenia can be defined as a leukocyte count of less than 3000 cells/cu mm; neutropenia is an absolute neutrophil count of less than 1000 cells/cu mm, although definitions range from less than 500 to 1500 cells/cu mm.[6-9] The susceptibility of immunocompromised cancer patients to bacterial infections increases significantly when their absolute neutrophil count falls below 500 cells/cu mm.[10] Although the risk of bacterial sepsis in neutropenic patients infected

DEB S. ISRAEL, PHARM.D., is Infectious Diseases Pharmacotherapy Fellow, Medical College of Virginia, Richmond, VA; at the time this manuscript was prepared, she was a Doctor of Pharmacy student, School of Pharmacy, University of Maryland, Baltimore. KAREN I. PLAISANCE, PHARM.D., is Associate Professor, School of Pharmacy, University of Maryland.

Address reprint requests to Dr. Plaisance at the School of Pharmacy, University of Maryland, 20 North Pine Street, Baltimore, MD 21201.

This is **article 680-204-9109** in the **ASHP Continuing-Education System;** it qualifies for 1.0 hour of continuing-education credit. See page 308 for learning objectives and test questions.

with HIV may not be as high as that in granulocytopenic cancer patients, neutropenia in patients with AIDS further compromises their already deficient host defenses.[8,11] The prevalence of neutropenia has been reported to range from 20% to 25% in patients with symptomatic HIV illness.[12,13]

Most drug therapies directed at patients infected with HIV are limited by their adverse effects. It is increasingly important that pharmacists be able to manipulate drug therapies to minimize toxicity and maximize efficacy. This article will examine the possible mechanisms of neutropenia associated with both HIV infection and drug treatments in adults. Current and investigational strategies to manage neutropenia will be reviewed. Anemia and thrombocytopenia may also be present in HIV-infected patients. Although this paper will deal specifically with neutropenia, these other cytopenias should also be considered when evaluating and suggesting modifications in drug therapies.

HIV-Associated Neutropenia

Infection with HIV is a progressive illness with a wide spectrum of manifestations. After seroconversion, the HIV-infected individual often remains clinically well for a long period of time. The worsening immune defects, however, ultimately result in symptoms and secondary illnesses that define AIDS.[14,15] Neutropenia associated with HIV arises from diverse mechanisms, including cellular immune dysfunction, direct effects on progenitor cells, humoral immune dysfunction, and vitamin deficiencies.

Cellular Immune Dysfunction. One of the more striking effects on the immune system caused by HIV is the selective depletion of CD4 (helper–inducer) cells and the resultant inversion of the CD4:CD8 (suppressor:cytotoxic) ratio. This leads to cellular immune dysfunction, which eventually is manifested by the development of neoplasms and opportunistic infections such as *Pneumocystis carinii* pneumonia (PCP) and cryptococcal meningitis.[16-18] A deficiency in systemic glutathione may contribute to the cellular immune defects of HIV infection. Glutathione is found in virtually all mammalian cells and is a storage and transport form of cysteine, which is present in most tissues at much lower concentrations than those of glutathione.[19,20] Glutathione functions in the synthesis of deoxyribonucleotide precursors of DNA, in the reduction of protein disulfide linkages, and as an antioxidant, protecting cells against free radicals and toxic compounds of endogenous and exogenous origin. In addition, glutathione has a role in the transport of amino acids and serves as a coenzyme for several enzyme systems. Glutathione is also believed to be involved in the initiation and progression of lymphocyte activation by mitogens and promotes lymphocyte-mediated cytotoxicity.[19,21]

Buhl et al.[19] examined whether systemic glutathione depletion contributes to immunodeficiency in asymptomatic patients infected with HIV. Venous plasma and bronchoalveolar lavage (BAL) fluid were obtained from 14 HIV-positive patients and 19 healthy HIV-seronegative control subjects and assayed for glutathione. Mean plasma total and reduced glutathione concentrations in the HIV-seropositive group were about one third of those in the healthy group. Similarly, the total and reduced glutathione concentrations in the BAL fluid of the HIV-seropositive individuals were 60% of those in the BAL fluid of the healthy volunteers. These authors concluded that a relative glutathione deficiency was a generalized process occurring in both blood and lung compartments.

The precise role of glutathione as one of the factors responsible for the immune deficiency in patients infected with HIV is not known. Intracellular glutathione deficiency inhibits the action of lymphocytes, thus suppressing cell-mediated cytotoxic functions, whereas administration of glutathione has been shown to enhance the activation of cytotoxic T cells in vitro.[22] Because glutathione protects cells by acting as a free-radical scavenger, glutathione depletion may also contribute to the high incidence of adverse drug reactions seen in patients infected with HIV.[23,24] Much remains to be understood about the role of glutathione depletion in the development of neutropenia. Whether administration of systemic glutathione will enhance the depressed immune functions or modulate drug toxicity in patients who are infected with HIV remains to be investigated.

Progenitor Cells. An understanding of the effects of HIV on hematopoietic progenitor cells is also evolving. Leiderman et al.[25] investigated the mechanism of HIV-associated neutropenia by studying the proliferative capacity of granulocyte–macrophage colony-forming units (progenitor cells). Examination of the bone marrow of 18 patients with AIDS and concurrent leukopenia revealed that the mean number of granulocyte–macrophage colony-forming units per 2×10^5 cells was 13.8 ± 2.3 in patients with AIDS compared with 29 ± 1.3 in healthy individuals. When the bone marrow from the patients with AIDS was cocultured with normal peripheral blood mononuclear cells, significant inhibition of colony formation was observed. Inhibition was observed whether the patient-derived cells were in direct contact with or were physically separated from the normal cells. This study suggested that bone marrow cells derived from patients with AIDS release a soluble factor that inhibits normal granulopoietic progenitor cells. It remains to be clarified whether this soluble factor is present in nonleukopenic patients with AIDS.

Humoral Immune Dysfunction. Patients infected with HIV also develop defects in humoral immunity, including polyclonal B-cell activation and hypergammaglobulinemia. The development of autoantibodies, resulting in peripheral destruction of cells, may contribute to the evolution of cytopenias.[16,18] Antibodies to cellular antigens have been detected in patients infected with herpesviruses, in whom B-cell activation resulted in hypergammaglobulinemia.[26] Autoantibodies against CD4 lymphocytes, platelets, red blood cells, and neutrophils have all been observed in patients with AIDS.[26]

Murphy et al.[12] investigated the incidence and mechanism of neutropenia and thrombocytopenia in 105 HIV-infected patients. The incidence of neutropenia was 20–25% in patients with symptomatic disease (persistent generalized lymphadenopathy and AIDS), and neutropenia was absent in 26 asymptomatic HIV-positive patients. The serum of 34 of these patients was analyzed for the presence of antibodies to platelets and granulocytes and circulating immune complexes. Serologic examination revealed that 10 (29%) had developed antigranulocyte antibodies, 5 (15%) had antibodies to platelets, and 14 (41%) had increased levels of circulating immune complexes. There was no apparent correlation between elevated immune complexes and presence of antibodies. The relationship between antibodies and corresponding neutropenia and thrombocytopenia did not reach statistical significance, perhaps because of the small number of patients studied. However, these investigators suggest that the presence of autoantibodies contributes to the development of cytopenias in patients infected with HIV.

The bone marrow of 49 patients with AIDS was examined by Castella et al.[27] Twenty-one of these patients were neutropenic, although at least 6 of the 21 were receiving trimethoprim–sulfamethoxazole or pentamidine. The majority of neutropenic patients (15 of 21) had normocellular marrow with normal or increased myeloid:erythroid ratios, suggesting peripheral destruction of neutrophils. Interestingly, acid-fast bacilli were identified in five of the nine patients with hypocellular marrow, six of whom were neutropenic. The authors also noted that peripheral cytopenias were, in some instances, associated with trimethoprim–sulfamethoxazole or pentamidine use; however, the data were not provided. Although hypergammaglobulinemia was frequently observed in this series, whether peripheral destruction was caused by formation of autoantibodies was unclear.

Vitamin Deficiencies. Ganser[16] observed leukopenia in 10% of patients with AIDS-related complex (ARC) and 35% of patients with AIDS. This investigator suggests that deficiencies in vitamin B_{12} and folate may contribute to the cytopenias observed in these patients. The major impact of folic acid deficiency is on the hematopoietic system. Because folic acid is an essential vitamin in humans, it must be provided from an outside source. Folate deficiencies may result from malabsorption, increased requirements, inadequate folate intake, and interference with folate metabolism by drugs.[28] Vitamin deficiencies may contribute to the increased hematopoietic sensitivity to antimetabolite drug therapy that patients with AIDS experience. In addition, it is possible that the hematopoietic progenitor cells of patients with AIDS are more sensitive to deficiencies in folate and vitamin B_{12}, resulting in leukopenia.[25]

Concomitant Illnesses

Even in the absence of HIV illness, neutropenia may occur as a manifestation of other infections. Neutropenia is frequently associated with salmonellosis, brucellosis, and pertussis and with some viral, rickettsial, and protozoal infections.[29] In addition, patients with bone marrow invasion by *Mycobacterium avium* complex may develop anemia, thrombocytopenia, and leukopenia.[30] Because patients with AIDS are susceptible to opportunistic infections, including some of those listed above, concomitant illnesses occurring in this setting complicate evaluation of neutropenia.

Drug-Induced Neutropenia

Many of the drugs used in the management of patients infected with HIV may cause neutropenia. Because these patients often receive multiple drug therapies, the ability to manipulate the regimens in an effort to minimize toxicity while retaining efficacy becomes imperative. The risks associated with either discontinuing therapy with a drug or decreasing the dose (and potentially the effectiveness) must be weighed against the risks associated with neutropenia.

Once neutropenia develops, it is often difficult to definitively establish the causative agent(s), especially because the development of the neutropenia may also be a result of disease progression. This dilemma emphasizes the importance of frequent hematologic monitoring in patients with AIDS to attempt to define temporal relationships. Various algorithms to assess the likelihood of a drug-induced reaction have been evaluated and judged to be clinically useful.[31,32]

Several mechanisms of drug action are thought to contribute to the development of bone marrow suppression. These include direct bone marrow suppression (cytotoxic effects), immunologic effects, and adverse reactions thought to be related to vitamin depletion. Idiosyncratic neutropenia is outside the scope of this paper. This should not be construed as minimizing the importance of drugs that cause idiosyncratic neutropenia. The clinician must also consider the need for altering therapy with these agents to manage neutropenia.

Zidovudine. Zidovudine is a nucleoside analogue that is ultimately phosphorylated to zidovudine triphosphate. Zidovudine triphosphate competes with cellular deoxynucleoside 5'-triphosphate, essential in the formation of viral DNA through reverse transcriptase, and acts as a chain terminator in the synthesis of viral DNA.[33,34] The experience with zidovudine in patients at various stages of HIV infection is summarized in Table 1.

The most frequent dose-limiting adverse effect of zidovudine is hematologic toxicity, with anemia, leu-

Table 1.
Efficacy of Zidovudine

Population (Reference)	No. Patients	Regimen	Follow-up (months)	Outcome
Advanced AIDS or ARC (36)	145	1500 mg/day p.o.	4[b]	1 death[a]
	137	Placebo		19 deaths
AIDS (35)	262	1500 mg/day p.o.	26[b]	188 deaths
	262	1200 mg/day p.o. for 4 weeks, then 600 mg/day p.o.		169 deaths[a]
Mild symptoms (37)				
200–500 CD4+ cells cu/mm	260	1200 mg/day p.o.	11[b]	12 deaths in patients with AIDS or ARC[a]
	253	Placebo		34 deaths in patients with AIDS or ARC
500–799 CD4+ cells cu/mm	100	1200 mg/day p.o.	11[b]	3 deaths in patients with AIDS or ARC
	98	Placebo		2 deaths in patients with AIDS or ARC
Asymptomatic with <500 CD4+ cells cu/mm (38)	457	1500 mg/day p.o.	13[c]	14 progressions to AIDS[a]
	453	500 mg/day p.o.	14[c]	11 progressions to AIDS[a]
	428	Placebo	15[c]	33 progressions to AIDS

[a] $p \leq 0.05$ compared with placebo or standard regimen.
[b] Approximate median value.
[c] Approximate mean value.

kopenia, granulocytopenia, thrombocytopenia, and thrombocytosis being reported.[33,34,39] Both the macrocytic anemia and neutropenia appear to be dose dependent. Bone marrow toxicity appears to be more frequent in those patients with AIDS, low CD4 cell counts, pretreatment anemia, low serum vitamin B_{12} levels, and low or low normal serum folic acid levels.[33,34] A placebo-controlled, double-blind study assessed the toxicity of zidovudine in 282 patients with AIDS or advanced ARC.[36,39] Differences in neutrophil count between the placebo and zidovudine recipients were apparent by week 4, and by week 12, 24% of the people receiving zidovudine had neutrophil counts lower than 1000 cells/cu mm and 7% had counts lower than 500 cells/cu mm. Furthermore, neutropenia was most marked in the zidovudine recipients with AIDS and low pretreatment CD4 cell counts (<100 cells/cu mm).[39] Fischl et al.[1] evaluated 229 patients with AIDS or ARC receiving zidovudine therapy for a mean of 21 months. During this time, 58% of all subjects had granulocytopenia (<750 cells/cu mm) with 45% having a first granulocytopenic episode within the first four months of zidovudine therapy and 57% having a first episode within the first six months. Granulocytopenia was reversed in most cases after the zidovudine therapy either was discontinued or the dosage was lowered.

Previously, the bone marrow toxicity of zidovudine was thought to be a consequence of a nonspecific effect on cellular DNA polymerase.[40] However, recent in vitro data suggest that the mechanism of this toxicity is related to effects on bone marrow hematopoietic progenitor cells. Zidovudine has been shown to inhibit colony formation of the pluripotent hematopoietic progenitor cells derived from the bone marrow of healthy persons and patients with AIDS. This inhibition occurred at concentrations of zidovudine (0.13–1.9 μM) lower than the concentration necessary to inhibit the cytopathic effect of HIV on T-cell lines (1 μM). Because patients with HIV infection may already have defective hematopoietic progenitor cells, it is difficult to distinguish between the actions of zidovudine on the bone marrow and the bone marrow suppressive effects of HIV itself.[41,42]

Concomitant drugs may increase the risk of marrow toxicity. It is clear that drugs known to cause hematologic adverse effects, such as ganciclovir, interferon alfa, and trimethoprim–sulfamethoxazole, may have additive suppressive effects on marrow when combined with zidovudine.[34,43-45] In these cases, when neutropenia develops, the benefits of combination therapy must be weighed against the risks of reduced drug doses, single-agent therapy, or no therapy at all. Other drugs, such as probenecid, may enhance zidovudine toxicity by inhibition of hepatic glucuronidation and renal secretion.[46] Richman et al.[39] observed an increase in marrow suppression in patients receiving concomitant zidovudine and acetaminophen. However, on further analysis, Burroughs Wellcome concluded that a greater prevalence of neutropenia was present in acetaminophen users before zidovudine exposure, perhaps reflecting progressive HIV illness. Additionally, recent pharmacokinetic studies suggest that the metabolism and clearance of zidovudine are not inhibited by acetaminophen.[33,47] It appears that the concerns regarding occasional concomitant administration of acetaminophen and zidovudine may have been overstated and should be re-evaluated.

The neutropenia associated with zidovudine is usually reversible.[1,2] The management of zidovudine-induced neutropenia has relied on dose reduction or discontinuation of therapy until the cell counts rise. The optimal dose and schedule for zidovudine have not been determined. Based on a serum half-life of 1.1 hours and the results of a dose-finding study,[48] a dosage interval of every four hours was chosen for Phase II testing of the drug. However, the intracellular half-life of the active moiety, zidovudine triphosphate, is approximately 3 hours—suggesting the possibility that anti-HIV activity may be maintained with dosage intervals as long as 8–12 hours.[34]

Until recently, the adult dosage of zidovudine was 200 mg orally every four hours in patients with CD4 lymphocyte counts of fewer than 200 cells/cu mm. Modifications in the dosage (100 mg orally every four hours) were recommended when granulocyte counts fell to below 750 cells/cu mm. However, patients with AIDS and ARC appeared to receive no greater benefit from zidovudine at 1000–1200 mg/day than they did when their dosage was reduced to 600 mg/day because of intolerance.[49,50]

This dose-related bone marrow suppression prompted the evaluation of reduced dosages of zidovudine in patients with symptomatic and asymptomatic HIV disease (Table 1). A randomized, double-blind trial assessing the efficacy of zidovudine in adults with asymptomatic HIV infection was recently reported.[38] After a mean follow-up of 55 weeks, neutropenia (absolute neutrophil count of <750 cells/cu mm) developed in 7 (1.6%) patients in the placebo group, 8 (1.8%) patients in the group receiving zidovudine 500 mg/day, and 29 (6.3%) patients in the group receiving zidovudine 1500 mg/day. Both zidovudine groups had lower rates of progression to AIDS and ARC compared with the placebo group. These authors concluded that therapy with zidovudine 500 mg/day delayed the onset of AIDS and was associated with less hematologic toxicity than therapy with zidovudine 1500 mg/day. Whether zidovudine use at these lower dosages will ultimately affect survival remains to be determined.

Reduced dosages of zidovudine also appear to be effective and better tolerated in patients with AIDS. After a median follow-up of approximately two years, a significantly better survival rate (72% versus 65% mortality) was noted in the group receiving zidovudine 600 mg/day compared with the patients receiving "standard" therapy. No significant differences in occurrences of opportunistic infections, times to next infection, declines in CD4 cell counts, or p24 antigen levels or changes from baseline were noted. However, serious anemia and neutropenia occurred earlier and more frequently in those receiving standard dosages.[35]

The incidence of neutropenia associated with zidovudine appears to be greater in patients with more advanced disease. In a placebo-controlled trial of the efficacy of zidovudine in mildly symptomatic patients, the incidence of serious neutropenia in placebo and zidovudine recipients was 1% and 4%, respectively.[37] This is similar to the 6% incidence observed in asymptomatic individuals receiving zidovudine 1500 mg/day but markedly lower than the incidence observed in patients with advanced disease (37–44%).

Table 2.
In Vitro Antiretroviral Activity and Bone Marrow Toxicity of Dideoxynucleoside Analogues[a]

Dideoxynucleoside	Median Effective Dose (μmol/L) ATH8[b]	MT4[b]	Median Bone Marrow Inhibitory Dose (μmol/L)
Zidovudine	2.4	0.006	1.0
2′,3′-Dideoxyadenosine and didanosine	2.7	2.5	100.0
2′,3′-Dideoxycytidine	0.2	0.046–0.06	10.0
2′,3′-Didehydro-2′,3′-dideoxythymidine	4.1	0.01	100.0
Azidodeoxyuridine	0.4	0.36	21.0

[a] Adapted from reference 52.
[b] ATH8 and MT4 are human T-lymphocyte cell lines.

The currently recommended zidovudine dosages reflect the outcomes of these trials.[35,37,38] For adults with symptomatic HIV infection, including AIDS, a starting dosage of 200 mg orally every four hours (1200 mg/day) for one month, followed by 100 mg orally every four hours (600 mg/day), is recommended. For persons with asymptomatic HIV infection and a CD4 cell count of ≤500 cells/cu mm, the recommended dosage is 100 mg orally every four hours while awake (500 mg/day).[51] It is anticipated that these lower dosage regimens will decrease the adverse effects of the drug while maintaining efficacy.

Other Dideoxynucleosides. Other dideoxynucleosides under evaluation for the treatment of HIV infection are listed in Table 2.[52] Human cells phosphorylate these compounds at different rates, resulting in the variation in antiretroviral activity. In vitro and limited clinical data suggest that, unlike zidovudine, these compounds have little marrow toxicity.[34]

The antiretroviral activity of 2',3'-dideoxycytidine (ddC) is more potent than that of didanosine (2',3'-dideoxyinosine, ddI); however, its use is associated with a severe peripheral neuropathy that limits its clinical application. In HIV-infected cell culture, Spector et al.[53] demonstrated that a three-day alternating regimen of zidovudine and ddC produced antiviral inhibition superior to that achieved with zidovudine alone. This type of alternating regimen might not only decrease the toxicities of both drugs but also prove to be more efficacious than zidovudine alone. A Phase I study examined the use of ddC as a single agent and alternating with zidovudine in patients with severe HIV infection. Neutropenia did not occur with ddC alone, even with escalating doses (maximum dosage, 0.09 mg/kg every four hours).[54]

Both didanosine and 2',3'-dideoxyadenosine (ddA) undergo cleavage in acid environments to form a purine base and dideoxyribose. Although the free base of didanosine, hypoxanthine, is relatively nontoxic, the free base of ddA, adenine, has been reported to cause renal damage.[34] Yarchoan et al.[55] examined eight dosage regimens of didanosine for periods extending to 42 weeks in 26 patients with AIDS or ARC, 10 of whom could not tolerate zidovudine. These authors found no bone marrow suppression at any of the dosage schedules (maximum dosage, 3.2 mg/kg every eight hours intravenously). Thus far, the major adverse effects associated with this drug have been peripheral neuropathy and pancreatitis.[56,57] Clinical trials with didanosine are currently under way. Additionally, didanosine has been made available outside formal clinical trials to patients with AIDS or advanced ARC who cannot take zidovudine.

Table 2 summarizes the differential antiretroviral activity and bone marrow suppressive effects of these nucleoside analogues. These drugs, used alone, in combination, or in alternating regimens with zidovudine, may ultimately yield efficacy and toxicity profiles superior to those achieved with zidovudine.

Acyclovir and Ganciclovir. In vitro, acyclovir has been shown to have little effect on human bone marrow,[58] and there have been only a few case reports of acyclovir-associated neutropenia.[59,60] In contrast, neutropenia has been reported to develop in 25% to 68% of patients receiving ganciclovir therapy.[61] Although the neutropenia is generally reversible on discontinuation of ganciclovir therapy, there have been several reports of irreversible leukopenia.[62] Acyclovir and ganciclovir are prodrugs requiring phosphorylation by kinases to the active triphosphate moiety. Initial phosphorylation of acyclovir requires a viral-specific thymidine kinase. Although the precise phosphorylation pathways for ganciclovir are unclear, cytomegalovirus (CMV) cellular kinases may act to phosphorylate ganciclovir from the monophosphate form to the active triphosphate.[7,62] Thus, acyclovir is selectively toxic to virus-infected cells, whereas the toxicity from ganciclovir is less specific.

Studies have shown that neutropenia is the result of a direct, dose-dependent inhibition of progenitor cells. The time course for the development of neutropenia is varied. Although neutropenia is usually observed early during induction therapy, it may also develop during maintenance therapy.[61,62] Dosage reductions are recommended when the absolute neutrophil count falls below 1000 cells/cu mm, and ganciclovir therapy should be discontinued if the absolute neutrophil count drops below 500 cells/cu mm. Treatment may be reinstituted when the absolute neutrophil count rises above 750 cells/cu mm.[7,63]

Ganciclovir must be used cautiously with other drugs that also cause bone marrow suppression, such as trimethoprim–sulfamethoxazole, flucytosine, dapsone, and pentamidine. The manufacturer cautions against the concomitant use of ganciclovir and zidovudine because severe granulocytopenia may result.[43,63] This myelosuppression may be the result of an additive or synergistic effect on the bone marrow.[43,44] Severe or life-threatening hematologic toxicity occurred in 90% and 82% of patients with AIDS-related CMV disease receiving ganciclovir and zidovudine orally at 1200 mg/day and 600 mg/day, respectively.[44] Without maintenance therapy, patients with CMV retinitis will relapse,[7] so again, one must weigh the comparative benefits of maintaining one essential therapy at the expense of therapy with another agent. Investigational strategies, such as foscarnet for CMV disease and other dideoxynucleosides for HIV infection, may alleviate this dilemma in the future.

Flucytosine. Flucytosine has been used in combination with amphotericin B to treat serious fungal infections. In patients with AIDS, the use of this combination is problematic because of the serious hematologic toxicity that may result.[64] The antifungal activity of flucytosine results from the ability of the fungal cell to selectively deaminate flucytosine to form fluorouracil. However, in the colon, small amounts of flucytosine may be deaminated by intestinal bacteria and then reabsorbed as fluorouracil. This conversion to fluorouracil may account for the hematologic effects of the drug.[65]

Both leukopenia and gastrointestinal disturbances are among the adverse effects associated with flucytosine use. High serum concentrations of flucytosine (100–150 μg/mL) are thought to correlate with an increase in bone marrow toxicity.[65] If the combination of flucytosine and amphotericin B is used, monitoring of serum flucytosine concentrations is essential. Alternatives to the flucytosine–amphotericin B combination are being developed. Recently, a new oral triazole antifungal agent, fluconazole, gained FDA approval for the treatment of cryptococcal meningitis in patients with AIDS. However, its role in the acute management of this disease is controversial.

Sulfonamides. As mentioned previously, patients with AIDS have a higher incidence of adverse drug reactions to sulfonamides. The major toxicities associated with sulfonamides include hypersensitivity reactions and hematologic adverse effects, both of which may be dose limiting and life threatening. Hematologic reactions are complex because these patients generally receive sulfonamides and folate antagonists concomitantly.

Sulfonamides may mediate toxicity either through the formation of haptens and immunologic reactions or through direct cytotoxicity, perhaps by the formation of reactive metabolites. As mentioned earlier, glutathione stores are depleted in patients with AIDS.

Work by Rieder and associates[66] in patients without AIDS demonstrated pre-existing glutathione depletion in patients with severe reactions to sulfonamides. Their work has shown that depressed glutathione levels lead to defective detoxification of the oxidative metabolites of sulfonamides, thus predisposing these patients to adverse reactions to sulfonamides. The contribution of glutathione depletion to the frequency of adverse drug reactions in patients with AIDS is a potentially intriguing avenue of investigation.

Dihydrofolate Reductase Inhibitors. Folate antagonists, including trimetrexate, pyrimethamine, and trimethoprim, act as inhibitors of the enzyme dihydrofolate reductase (DHFR). This enzyme catalyzes the reduction of folic acid (dihydrofolic acid) to folinic acid (tetrahydrofolic acid). Folate inhibitors have a much greater affinity for bacterial and protozoal DHFRs than for the mammalian enzyme.[67-69] Despite the selective binding of these compounds to microbial enzymes, folate antagonists also interfere with normal hematopoiesis, especially at high doses. In vitro studies of human bone marrow have shown that there was little or no effect on folate metabolism when trimethoprim concentrations did not exceed those attained with normal doses. Abnormalities did occur when there was a 10-fold increase in trimethoprim concentrations. The abnormalities were completely corrected by folinic acid but only partially corrected by folic acid.[70]

Folinic acid enters mammalian cells via a specific carrier-mediated transport system and is itself a functional folate coenzyme. Therefore, folinic acid is not dependent on the action of DHFR to be active.[28] Folinic acid will not interfere with the antibacterial or antiprotozoal action of folic acid antagonists. Bacteria and protozoa do not possess the active transport pathways necessary to use preformed dihydrofolates and tetrahydrofolates.[68,70,71]

Patients with pre-existing folate and vitamin B_{12} deficiencies, those with renal insufficiency, and those receiving immunosuppressants or other drugs associated with hematologic adverse effects (such as sulfonamides) are predisposed to the development of hematologic toxicities.[68] Compared with other patient populations, patients with AIDS are at increased risk for adverse events associated with folate antagonists and sulfonamides.[3,4] The hematologic effects of folate antagonists are reversible on discontinuation of therapy with the offending drug.[68,72] Although most authorities recommend that leucovorin (folinic acid) accompany regimens containing pyrimethamine or trimetrexate, its use to treat or prevent hematologic reactions associated with trimethoprim remains controversial.

Combination Therapies. Sulfonamides such as sulfamethoxazole and sulfadiazine are commonly prescribed in combination with DHFR inhibitors to treat or prevent a variety of infections in patients who are infected with HIV or whose illness has progressed to AIDS. Minimal data are available correlating drug concentrations of trimethoprim and sulfamethoxazole with the development of blood dyscrasias. Details of these studies are summarized in Table 3.

Trimethoprim and sulfamethoxazole concentrations were reported in seven patients with AIDS and confirmed PCP.[73] Toxicities requiring a change in therapy were observed in all seven patients. During the first 10 days of therapy, average serum trimethoprim concentrations ranged from 8.7 to 9.4 μg/mL (usual range, 4–10 μg/mL), and average serum sulfamethoxazole concentrations ranged from 274.2 to 342.5 μg/mL (usual range, 80–120 μg/mL). Elevated concentrations of sulfamethoxazole may have contributed to the toxicities that developed. Fong[74] examined 38 patients with AIDS who were being treated for 40 episodes of PCP. Eight of 20 patients (40%) with serum sulfamethoxazole concentrations of >200 μg/mL developed leukopenia compared with only 2 of 20 patients (10%) with serum sulfamethoxazole concentrations of <200 μg/mL. Four patients, all with elevated sulfamethoxazole concentrations, developed severe leukopenia. Fong suggests that the incidence of leukopenia may be lessened by maintaining serum sulfamethoxazole concentrations at <200 μg/mL. Finally, Sattler et al.[75] evaluated the use of trimethoprim–sulfamethoxazole and pentamidine in patients with AIDS. These investigators adjusted dosages of trimethoprim–sulfamethoxazole to maintain serum trimethoprim concentrations at 5–8 μg/mL, resulting in a mean trimethoprim dosage of approximately 12 mg/kg/day. Sattler et al. concluded that, with pharmacokinetic monitoring of trimethoprim–sulfamethoxazole concentrations, the severe myelosuppression associated with the drug can at least be partially avoided.

The relationships between the serum concentrations and toxicities associated with trimethoprim, sulfamethoxazole, or both are not well defined. Additional studies are needed to fully understand the potential concentration dependence of this toxicity.

The prophylactic use of leucovorin in patients being treated for PCP with high doses of trimethoprim–sulfamethoxazole or in patients receiving tri-

Table 3.
Trimethoprim–Sulfamethoxazole (TMP–SMX) Concentrations and Incidence of Leukopenia

Reference	No. Patients	Dosage (mg/kg/day)		Time between Dose and Conc. Determination (hr)	Concentration (μg/mL)		No. Patients with Leukopenia	
		TMP	SMX		TMP	SMX	Any	Severe
73	7	20	100	1.5 (p.o. or i.v.)	4.7–11.9	241–536	NS[a,b]	NS[a,b]
74	38[c]	NS	NS	2 (p.o.)	NS	>200	8/20	4/20
				0.5 (i.v.)	NS	<200	2/20	0/20
75	36	12 ± 3.4	NS	1.5 (i.v.)	5–8	NS	26/36	0/36

[a] NS = not stated.
[b] Although incidence of leukopenia was not stated, all seven patients required discontinuation of TMP–SMX because of adverse reactions.
[c] Data reported for 38 patients with 40 episodes of *Pneumocystis carinii* pneumonia.

methoprim–sulfamethoxazole who have pre-existing borderline folate deficiency is controversial. Various authors have suggested that patients may benefit from 400 μg to 15 mg of leucovorin daily while receiving trimethoprim–sulfamethoxazole.[68,76,77] Bygbjerg et al.[78] examined the effects of folic acid and leucovorin in 12 patients with AIDS or ARC being treated for PCP with trimethoprim–sulfamethoxazole. Patients were randomized to receive either folic acid (5 mg daily) or leucovorin (as the calcium salt) (7.5 mg every other day) orally for 3.5 to 4 months. Patients concurrently received trimethoprim–sulfamethoxazole 320 mg/1600 mg orally four times a day for 10 to 20 days, followed by low-dose trimethoprim–sulfamethoxazole therapy (160 mg/800 mg twice daily). These patients were not receiving any other drugs that were known to affect hematologic values, and no patient had folate deficiency before or during the study. The results of this small study suggested that leucovorin was no better than folic acid in preventing cytopenias. Because patients with AIDS may develop folate deficiency secondary to recurrent infections and because that folate deficiency may play a role in the neurologic complications of AIDS, these authors recommend that patients with AIDS routinely receive folic acid 5 mg/day.

Lack of response to leucovorin in AIDS patients receiving trimethoprim–sulfamethoxazole for PCP has been reported by several authors.[3,72] Granulocytopenia rarely responds to leucovorin administration, but lowering the dosage of trimethoprim–sulfamethoxazole may reduce adverse reactions while maintaining efficacy. The lack of response to leucovorin may indicate that alternative mechanisms are responsible for the bone marrow suppression. It should be emphasized that the routine use of leucovorin to prevent hematologic reactions from trimethoprim–sulfamethoxazole is not supported by controlled evaluations.

Other combinations of DHFR inhibitors and sulfonamides are frequently prescribed for patients with AIDS. Specifically, pyrimethamine and sulfadiazine are generally prescribed for the treatment of *Toxoplasma gondii* encephalitis. Several dosage regimens are recommended, and because pyrimethamine is a potent DHFR inhibitor, proponents of these regimens advocate the use of leucovorin throughout the therapy. Dosage recommendations for leucovorin (as the calcium salt) vary from 10 mg to 50 mg per day, depending on the aggressiveness of the regimen and the degree of hematologic toxicity that develops.[79,80] Alternatives to this combination regimen for the treatment of *T. gondii* are being evaluated, and one promising therapy is the combination of pyrimethamine and clindamycin.[81,82]

Pentamidine. Leukopenia was rarely associated with pentamidine therapy before AIDS became prevalent. Early reports of leukopenia in patients with AIDS stimulated the Centers for Disease Control to evaluate retrospectively the occurrence of leukopenia in patients with AIDS who had received pentamidine. Over 20 months, leukopenia was reported in 26 (14.5%) of 179 patients who had received pentamidine. In 12 cases, the physician discontinued pentamidine therapy because of leukopenia.[83] Prospective studies report leukopenia occurring in 30–50% of AIDS patients receiving pentamidine.[75,84]

Neither the precise mechanism of the drug's activity against *P. carinii* nor the mechanism for the development of leukopenia is known. However, one report of the development of folate deficiency in a patient suggests that antagonism of folate metabolism may contribute to pentamidine's effects.[85] Additionally, in one assay system, pentamidine, as well as sulfonamides, inhibits metabolism of *p*-aminobenzoic acid labeled with tritium, suggesting that folate antagonism may be important to pentamidine's effects on *P. carinii*.[71] It may be speculated that the leukopenia associated with pentamidine results from folate antagonism. However, there are no data on the ability of exogenous folate to reverse this effect. Finally, it is also noteworthy that pentamidine appears to adversely affect the function of neutrophilic granulocytes in vitro.[86-88] The clinical importance of this effect is unknown.

Potential Therapies for Neutropenia

Lithium. As early as 1973, lithium carbonate was shown to induce prolonged leukocytosis and neutrophilia in patients receiving lithium for psychiatric disorders. Lapierre and Stewart[89] examined 35 patients who were receiving lithium for psychiatric illness and found that the leukocytosis observed in these patients was drug related but neither dose nor concentration related. Lithium has also been used to partially reverse neutropenia in patients who have received myelosuppressive therapy. Herbert et al.[90] observed that lithium could stimulate production of CD4 lymphocytes in AIDS patients. The mechanism of this action is not well defined; however, lithium has been shown to enhance the activity of colony-stimulating factors in vitro.

The effect of lithium was evaluated in five patients with zidovudine-associated neutropenia, all of whom had required discontinuation of zidovudine therapy because of neutropenia. The mean total neutrophil count was 674 cells/cu mm in the two weeks before treatment. Lithium dosages were gradually adjusted to achieve serum lithium concentrations of 0.6 to 1.2 meq/L. Zidovudine therapy was reinstituted once the absolute neutrophil count was greater than 750 cells/cu mm. Three of the five patients were able to tolerate at least 1000 mg/day of zidovudine.[91]

Lithium, with its narrow therapeutic index, requires close monitoring of serum lithium and electrolyte levels. Toxic reactions to lithium may occur more frequently in AIDS patients because they are often anorectic and are prone to diarrhea and gastroenteritis, factors that can affect electrolyte balance and the pharmacokinetics of lithium.[92] It may also be difficult to differentiate confusion, slurred speech, and tremors associated with lithium from the neurologic complications of HIV. Although these reactions usually are associated with serum lithium concentrations of 1.5 to 2.0 meq/L, some patients may experience these effects at lithium concentrations lower than 1.5 meq/L. Leukopenia has also been observed in association with high serum lithium concentrations observed with lithium overdosages.[93] Finally, there is some suggestion that lithium-associated improvement in leukopenia is a transient phenomenon.[94]

The toxicities associated with lithium therapy preclude its widespread use until placebo-controlled trials demonstrate its usefulness. However, the lower dosages of zidovudine now recommennded and the availability of alternative therapies probably obviate the need for lithium and, consequently, these trials.

Immunomodulators. Whether the neutropenia occurring in patients with AIDS is drug induced or related to these patients' disease state, immunomodulators may play a role in modulating either the occurrence or the severity of the neutropenia.

Colony-Stimulating Factors. Colony-stimulating factors stimulate bone marrow progenitor cells to differentiate into erythrocytes, monocytes, basophils, eosinophils, and neutrophils. Colony-stimulating factors not only function in the proliferation of these cells but also play a role in maintaining host defense by influencing even the fully mature cells. Four colony-stimulating factors have been identified, and they are available as cloned gene products. Several of these factors stimulate the production of neutrophils, including granulocyte colony-stimulating factor (G-CSF), granulocyte–macrophage colony-stimulating factor (GM-CSF), and interleukin-3. Mature neutrophils have receptors for G-CSF and GM-CSF only. Studies show that GM-CSF primes neutrophils for enhanced biologic functions, increases macrophage tumoricidal activity, and, with G-CSF, increases neutrophil cytotoxicity.[95]

Recent reports have evaluated the use of colony-stimulating factors to treat or minimize neutropenia induced by cancer chemotherapy.[96,97] Success in this setting led to the evaluation of colony-stimulating factors to modulate neutropenia in patients with AIDS. Baldwin et al.[98] examined the use of GM-CSF and G-CSF to stimulate the cytotoxic function of the neutrophils toward HIV-infected cells. These authors concluded that both GM-CSF and G-CSF enhance neutrophil numbers and cytotoxicity toward HIV-infected T lymphocytes in vitro.

The ability of colony-stimulating factors to modulate the bone marrow toxicity of zidovudine has been investigated. Bhalla and coworkers[99] examined the effects of recombinant human granulocyte–macrophage colony-stimulating factor (rGM-CSF) on zidovudine-induced cytotoxic effects on normal myeloid progenitor cells in vitro. Coadministration of rGM-CSF reduced intracellular concentrations of zidovudine triphosphate while partially restoring the intracellular pools of thymidine and deoxycytidine triphosphates. In addition to partially correcting these zidovudine-induced biochemical changes, rGM-CSF reduced the cytotoxicity of zidovudine on normal progenitor cells. It appears that the reduction of zidovudine toxicity may be due to the ability of rGM-CSF to expand intracellular pools of deoxycytidine triphosphate and thymidine triphosphate. Thus, intracellular concentrations of zidovudine triphosphate and its subsequent incorporation into DNA would be reduced, resulting in reduced zidovudine cytotoxicity to normal human granulocyte–macrophage colony-forming units. Whether these reduced concentrations might also result in reduced antiviral effect is unclear. The activity of GM-CSF and zidovudine was further examined in the monocyte–macrophage system.[100] Cells were exposed to various concentrations of GM-CSF and zidovudine, separately and in combination, for 14 to 17 days. Nearly all combinations of GM-CSF and zidovudine synergistically inhibited HIV replication.

Finally, Groopman et al.[101] conducted a Phase I–II study to assess the effects of GM-CSF in neutropenic patients with AIDS. Patients were ineligible for the study if they had received myelosuppressive or cytotoxic drugs within six weeks of the study. Doses of rGM-CSF ranged from 0.5 to 8 μg/kg. Sixteen patients initially received a single intravenous bolus followed after 48 hours by a 14-day continuous infusion. After the bolus injection, circulating leukocytes increased transiently but returned to baseline before the continuous infusion began. After discontinuation of the infusion, leukocyte counts returned to baseline within three to nine days in all the patients. While receiving rGM-CSF, however, all patients were reported to have at least a twofold increase in blood leukocyte counts. No life-threatening toxic effects occurred, and the authors concluded that use of rGM-CSF was relatively nontoxic yet efficacious in stimulating granulocyte counts in this patient population.

The potential for colony-stimulating factors to actually increase HIV replication has caused concern. Because colony-stimulating factors enhance the number of circulating immune cells (e.g., neutrophils, macrophages), it is not clear whether there will be a corresponding increase in cells that are also HIV infected.[102] This concern will need to be addressed for colony-stimulating factors to become rational adjunctive therapy.

The use of colony-stimulating factors appears promising for increasing the number and function of circulating neutrophils, thus augmenting the host defense system. However, the inability to maintain an increased and sustained leukocyte count after discontinuation of rGM-CSF therapy remains a limitation on the use of these agents.

Interferon Alfa. Interferon alfa has been shown to have substantial antitumor activity in the treatment of Kaposi's sarcoma in patients with AIDS. As with zidovudine, the dose-limiting effects of interferon alfa include anemia and leukopenia. Berman et al.[103] examined the synergistic cytotoxic effect of zidovudine and interferon alfa on normal human bone marrow progenitor cells. Their results suggest that lower doses of a combination of zidovudine and interferon alfa may maintain a strong synergistic anti-HIV effect while avoiding hematologic toxicity. It was anticipated that this combination might exert synergistic antitumor and antiviral effects at dosages low enough to spare the bone marrow. Results of Phase I trials of interferon alfa combined with zidovudine were recently reported.[45] Dose-limiting toxicity included constitutional symptoms and hematologic toxicity. Neutropenia was the most frequent reason for dosage reduction. Maximum tolerated dosages were 18 million units/day i.m. of interferon alfa with zidovudine 600 mg/day orally. Neutropenia occurred in one of six patients at this dosage. In addition to antitumor effects, both immunologic and virologic improvement were observed.

Immune Globulins. Immune globulins have been used since 1952 to treat immune deficiency disease. Currently, immune globulin is used in the management of transplant patients at risk for CMV disease and patients with idiopathic thrombocytopenic purpura or Kawaski disease. Idiopathic thrombocytopenic purpura is an immune-mediated disease wherein antibody-coated platelets are destroyed. Intravenous immune globulin appears to be effective in treating both the acute and chronic forms of this disease. Intravenous immune globulin may increase platelet counts by blocking splenic phagocytosis of antibody-coated platelets, although the precise mechanism of action is not completely understood. It has been suggested that some patients with AIDS and immune-mediated thrombocytopenia, granulocytopenia, or anemia, or a combination of these disorders may benefit from exogenous immune globulin in a manner similar to patients with idiopathic thrombocytopenic purpura.[104] There are currently no controlled data assessing the effectiveness of intravenous immune globulin in the treatment of HIV-related or drug-related neutropenia. Clinical trials will be needed to evaluate the role of immune globulins in this patient population.

Conclusion

The development of neutropenia in patients infected with HIV requires a careful assessment of the potential etiologies of this condition. In evaluating neutropenia, the clinician must attempt to discern whether the neutropenia is more likely related to disease state(s) or drug therapies. Potential management strategies include modulation of the disease state, discontinuation or dose reduction of the offending agent, or administration of exogenous immune enhancer. Decisions to change drug therapy must be made on an individual basis.

References

1. Fischl MA, Richman DD, Causey DM et al. Prolonged zidovudine therapy in patients with AIDS and advanced AIDS-related complex. *JAMA*. 1989; 262:2405-10.
2. Masur H. Therapy for AIDS. In: Mandell GL, Douglas RG, Bennett J, eds. Principles and practice of infectious diseases. New York: John Wiley; 1990:1102-11.
3. Kovacs JA, Hiemenz JW, Macher AM et al. *Pneumocystis carinii* pneumonia: a comparison between patients with the acquired immunodeficiency syndrome and patients with other immunodeficiencies. *Ann Intern Med*. 1984; 100:663-71.
4. Gordin FM, Simon GL, Wofsy CB et al. Adverse reactions to trimethoprim-sulfamethoxazole in patients with the acquired immunodeficiency syndrome. *Ann Intern Med*. 1984; 100:495-9.
5. Purdy B, Plaisance K, Furth P. Adverse reactions to antibiotics in AIDS patients. *Clin Pharmacol Ther*. 1988; 43:144. Abstract.
6. Gallin JI. Disorders of phagocytic cells. In: Braunwald E, Isselbacher KJ, Petersdorf RG et al., eds. Harrison's principles of internal medicine. 11th ed. New York: McGraw-Hill; 1987:278-83.
7. Drew WL, Buhles W, Erlich KS. Herpesvirus infections (caused by cytomegalovirus, herpes simplex virus, varicella zoster virus): how to use ganciclovir (DHPG) and acyclovir. In: Sande MA, Volberding PA, eds. The medical management of AIDS. Philadelphia: Saunders; 1988:271-90.
8. Shaunak S, Bartlett JA. Zidovudine-induced neutropenia: are we too cautious? *Lancet*. 1989; 2:91-2.
9. Lehrer RI, moderator. Neutrophils and host defense. *Ann Intern Med*. 1988; 109:127-42.
10. Schimpff SS. Overview of empiric antibiotic therapy for the febrile neutropenic patient. *Rev Infect Dis*. 1985; 7:S734-40.
11. Chaisson RE. Infections due to encapsulated bacteria, salmonella, shigella and campylobacter. In: Sande MA, Volberding PA, eds. The medical management of AIDS. Philadelphia: Saunders; 1988:247-58.
12. Murphy MF, Metcalfe P, Waters AH et al. Incidence and mechanism of neutropenia and thrombocytopenia in patients with human immunodeficiency virus infection. *Br J Haematol*. 1987; 66:337-40.
13. Clement M. General approach to the human immunodeficiency virus-infected patient. In: Leoung G, Mills G, eds. Opportunistic infections in patients with the acquired immunodeficiency syndrome. New York: Marcel Dekker; 1989:88-101.
14. Baltimore D, Feinberg MB. HIV revealed: toward a natural history of the infection. *N Engl J Med*. 1989; 321:1673-5. Editorial.
15. Purdy BD, Plaisance KI. Infection with the human immunodeficiency virus: epidemiology, pathogenesis, transmission, diagnosis, and manifestations. *Am J Hosp Pharm*. 1989; 46:1185-1209.
16. Ganser A. Abnormalities of hematopoiesis in the acquired immunodeficiency syndrome. *Blut*. 1988; 56:49-53.
17. Fauci AS, moderator. Acquired immunodeficiency syndrome: epidemiologic, clinical, immunologic and therapeutic considerations. *Ann Intern Med*. 1984; 100:92-106.
18. Bowen DL, Lane HC, Fauci AS. Immunologic abnormalities in the acquired immunodeficiency syndrome. *Prog Allergy*. 1986; 37:207-23.
19. Buhl R, Jaffe HA, Holroud KJ et al. Systemic glutathione deficiency in symptom-free HIV-seropositive individuals. *Lancet*. 1989; 2:1294-8.
20. Meister A. New developments in glutathione metabolism and their potential application in therapy. *Hepatology*. 1984; 4:739-42.
21. Hamilos DL, Wedner HJ. The role of glutathione in lymphocyte activation: I. Comparison of inhibitory effects of buthionine sulfoximine and 2-cyclohexene-1-one by nuclear size transformation. *J Immunol*. 1985; 135:2740-7.
22. Dröge W, Pottmeyer-Gerber C, Schmidt H et al. Glutathione augments the activation of cytotoxic T lymphocytes in vivo. *Immunobiology*. 1986; 172:151-6.

23. Rieder MJ, Uetrecht J, Shear NH et al. Synthesis and in vitro toxicity of hydroxylamine metabolites of sulfonamides. *J Pharmacol Exp Ther*. 1988; 244:724-8.
24. Leeder JS, Cannon M, Nakhooda A et al. Drug metabolite toxicity assessed in human lymphocytes with a purified reconstituted, cytochrome P-450 system. *J Pharmacol Exp Ther*. 1988; 245:956-62.
25. Leiderman IZ, Greenberg ML, Adelsberg BR et al. Defective myelopoiesis in acquired immunodeficiency syndrome (AIDS). In: Gottlieb MS, Groopman JE, eds. Acquired immunodeficiency syndrome. New York: Alan R Liss; 1984:281-9.
26. Levy JA. The human immunodeficiency virus and its pathogenesis. In: Sande MA, Volberding PA, eds. The medical management of AIDS. Philadelphia: Saunders; 1988:3-18.
27. Castella A, Croxson TS, Mildvan D et al. The bone marrow in AIDS. A histologic, hematologic and microbiologic study. *Am J Clin Pathol*. 1985; 84:425-32.
28. Hillman RS. Vitamin B12, folic acid and the treatment of megaloblastic anemia. In: Goodman and Gilman's the pharmacological basis of therapeutics. 7th ed. Gilman AG, Goodman LS, Rall TW et al., eds. New York: Macmillan; 1985:323-7.
29. Hoeprich PD, O'Grady LF. Manifestations of infectious diseases. In: Hoeprich PD, Jordan MC, eds. Infectious diseases. 4th ed. Philadelphia: Lippincott; 1989:83-94.
30. Schecter GF. Mycobacteria diseases. In: Leoung G, Mills J, eds. Opportunistic infections in patients with the acquired immunodeficiency syndrome. New York: Marcel Dekker; 1989:253-64.
31. Michel DJ, Knodel LC. Comparison of three algorithms used to evaluate adverse drug reactions. *Am J Hosp Pharm*. 1986; 43:1709-14.
32. Jones JK. Adverse drug reactions in the community health setting: approaches to recognizing, counseling, and reporting. *Fam Community Health*. 1982; 5:58-67.
33. Yarchoan R, Mitsuya H, Broder S. Clinical and basic advances in the antiretroviral therapy of human immunodeficiency virus infection. *Am J Med*. 1989; 87:191-200.
34. Yarchoan R, Mitsuya H, Myers C et al. Clinical pharmacology of 3'-azido-2',3'-dideoxythymidine (zidovudine) and related dideoxynucleosides. *N Engl J Med*. 1989; 321:726-38.
35. Fischl MA, Parker CB, Pettinelli C et al. A randomized controlled trial of a reduced daily dose of zidovudine in patients with the acquired immunodeficiency syndrome. *N Engl J Med*. 1990; 323:1009-14.
36. Fischl MA, Richman DD, Grieco MH et al. The efficacy of azidothymidine (AZT) in the treatment of patients with AIDS and AIDS-related complex. A double-blind, placebo-controlled trial. *N Engl J Med*. 1987; 317:185-91.
37. Fischl MA, Richman DD, Hansen N et al. The safety and efficacy of zidovudine (AZT) in the treatment of subjects with mildly symptomatic human immunodeficiency virus type 1 (HIV) infection: a double-blind, placebo-controlled trial. *Ann Intern Med*. 1990; 112:727-37.
38. Volberding PA, Lagakos SW, Koch MA et al. Zidovudine in asymptomatic human immunodeficiency virus infection. A controlled trial in persons with fewer than 500 CD4-positive cells per cubic milliter. *N Engl J Med*. 1990; 322:941-9.
39. Richman DD, Fischl MA, Grieco MH et al. The toxicity of azidothymidine (AZT) in the treatment of patients with AIDS and AIDS-related complex. A double-blind, placebo-controlled trial. *N Engl J Med*. 1987; 317:192-7.
40. Anon. Zidovudine (AZT). *Lancet*. 1987; 1:957-8.
41. Ganser A, Greher J, Volkers B et al. Inhibitory effect of azidothymidine, 2'-3'-dideoxyadenosine, and 2'-3'-dideoxycytidine on in vitro growth of hematopoietic progenitor cells from normal persons and from patients with AIDS. *Exp Hematol*. 1989; 17:321-5.
42. Gogu SR, Beckman BS, Agrawal KC. Anti-HIV drugs: comparative toxicities in murine fetal liver and bone marrow erythroid progenitor cells. *Life Sci*. 1989; 45:3-7.
43. Jacobson MA, De Miranda P, Gordon SM et al. Prolonged pancytopenia due to combined ganciclovir and zidovudine therapy. *J Infect Dis*. 1988; 158:489-90.
44. Hochster H, Dieterich D, Bozzette S et al. Toxicity of combined ganciclovir and zidovudine for cytomegalovirus disease associated with AIDS: an AIDS clinical trials group study. *Ann Intern Med*. 1990; 113:111-7.
45. Krown SE, Gold JWM, Niedzwiecki D et al. Interferon-alfa with zidovudine: safety, tolerance, and clinical and virologic effects in patients with Kaposi sarcoma associated with the acquired immunodeficiency syndrome (AIDS). *Ann Intern Med*. 1990; 112:812-21.
46. Hedaya MA, Elmquist WF, Sawchuck RJ. Probenecid inhibits the metabolic and renal clearances of zidovudine (AZT) in human volunteers. *Pharm Res*. 1990; 7:411-7.
47. Steffe EM, King JH, Inciardi JF et al. The effect of acetaminophen on zidovudine metabolism in HIV-infected patients. *J AIDS*. 1990; 3:691-4.
48. Yarchoan R, Klecker RW, Weinhold KJ et al. Administration of 3'-azido-3'-deoxythymidine, an inhibitor of HTLV-III/LAV replication, to patients with AIDS or AIDS-related complex. *Lancet*. 1986; 1:575-80.
49. Dournon E, Matheron S, Rozenbaum W et al. Effects of zidovudine in 365 consecutive patients with AIDS or AIDS-related complex. *Lancet*. 1988; 2:1297-1302.
50. Sette P, Narciso P, Tozzi V et al. Low-dose zidovudine for AIDS. *Lancet*. 1989; 1:1136-7. Letter.
51. Burroughs Wellcome. Retrovir package insert. Research Triangle Park, NC; 1990 May.
52. Myers MW. New antiretroviral agents in the clinic. *Rev Infect Dis*. 1990; 12:944-50.
53. Spector SA, Ripley D, Hsia K. Human immunodeficiency virus inhibition is prolonged by 3'-azido-3'-deoxythymidine alternating with 2',3'-dideoxycytidine compared with 3'-azido-3'-deoxythymidine alone. *Antimicrob Agents Chemother*. 1989; 33:920-3.
54. Yarchoan R, Perno CF, Thomas RV et al. Phase I studies of 2',3'-dideoxycytidine in severe human immunodeficiency virus infection as a single agent and alternating with zidovudine (AZT). *Lancet*. 1988; 1:76-81.
55. Yarchoan R, Mitsuya H, Thomas RV et al. In vivo activity against HIV and favorable toxicity profile of 2',3'-dideoxyinosine. *Science*. 1989; 245:412-5.
56. Lambert JS, Seidlin M, Reichman RC et al. 2',3'-Dideoxyinosine (ddI) in patients with the acquired immunodeficiency syndrome or AIDS-related complex. A phase I trial. *N Engl J Med*. 1990; 322:1333-40.
57. Cooley TP, Kunches LM, Saunders CA et al. Once daily administration of 2',3'-dideoxyinosine (ddI) in patients with the acquired immunodeficiency syndrome or AIDS-related complex. Results of a phase I trial. *N Engl J Med*. 1990; 322:1340-5.
58. Kucers A, Bennett NM. The use of antibiotics. 4th ed. Philadelphia: Lippincott; 1987:1551-77.
59. McPherson MC, Plaisance KI. Neutropenia associated with oral acyclovir and multiple antibacterial agents in a patient with acquired immunodeficiency syndrome. *Clin Pharm*. 1988; 7:398-401.
60. Bean B, Fletcher C. Neutropenia in immunocompromised patients receiving intravenous acyclovir. In: Program and abstracts of the 25th Interscience Conference on Antimicrobial Agents and Chemotherapy. Washington, DC: American Society for Microbiology; 1985:237. Abstract 786.
61. Jacobson MA, Mills J. Serious cytomegalovirus diseases in the acquired immunodeficiency syndrome (AIDS). Clinical findings, diagnosis and treatment. *Ann Intern Med*. 1988; 108:585-94.
62. Drew WL. Cytomegalovirus infection in patients with AIDS. *J Infect Dis*. 1988; 158:449-56.
63. Syntex Laboratories. Ganciclovir package insert. Palo Alto, CA; 1989 Jun.
64. Chuck SL, Sande MA. Infections with *Cryptococcus neoformans* in the acquired immunodeficiency syndrome. *N Engl J Med*. 1989; 321:794-9.
65. Kucers A, Bennett NM. The use of antibiotics. 4th ed. Phila-

delphia: Lippincott; 1987:1534-50.
66. Rieder MJ, Uetrecht J, Shear NH et al. Diagnosis of sulfonamide hypersensitivity reactions by in vitro "rechallenge" with hydroxylamine metabolites. *Ann Intern Med.* 1989; 110:286-9.
67. Jewkes RF, Edwards MS, Grant BJB. Haematological changes in a patient on long-term treatment with a trimethoprim-sulphonamide combination. *Postgrad Med J.* 1970; 46:723-6.
68. Kahn SB, Fein SA, Brodsky I. Effects of trimethoprim on folate metabolism in man. *Clin Pharmacol Ther.* 1968; 9:550-60.
69. Allegra CJ, Chabner BA, Tuazon CU et al. Trimetrexate for the treatment of *Pneumocystis carinii* pneumonia in patients with the acquired immunodeficiency syndrome. *N Engl J Med.* 1987; 317:978-85.
70. Kucers A, Bennett NM. The use of antibiotics. 4th ed. Philadelphia: Lippincott; 1987:1118-1202.
71. Masur H, Lane HC, Kovacs JA et al. Pneumocystis pneumonia: from bench to clinic. *Ann Intern Med.* 1989; 111:813-26.
72. Jaffe HS, Abrams DI, Ammann AJ. Complications of cotrimoxazole in treatment of AIDS-associated *Pneumocystis carinii* pneumonia in homosexual men. *Lancet.* 1983; 2:1109-11.
73. Bowden FH, Harman PJ, Lucas CR. Serum trimethoprim and sulphamethoxazole levels in AIDS. *Lancet.* 1986; 1:853. Letter.
74. Fong IW. Correlation of side effects of trimethoprim/sulfamethoxazole with blood levels in AIDS patients treated for *Pneumocystis carinii* pneumonia. In: Program and abstracts of the 28th Interscience Conference on Antimicrobial Agents and Chemotherapy. Washington, DC: American Society for Microbiology; 1988:328. Abstract 1226.
75. Sattler FR, Cowan R, Nielson D et al. Trimethoprim-sulfamethoxazole compared with pentamidine for treatment of *Pneumocystis carinii* pneumonia in the acquired immunodeficiency syndrome. *Ann Intern Med.* 1988; 109:280-7.
76. Kinzie BJ, Taylor JW. Trimethoprim and folinic acid. *Ann Intern Med.* 1984; 101:565. Letter.
77. Stock C. Trimethoprim-sulfamethoxazole and folinic acid. *Ann Intern Med.* 1985; 102:277. Letter.
78. Bygbjerg IC, Lund JT, Hørding M. Effect of folic and folinic acid on cytopenia occurring during co-trimoxazole treatment of *Pneumocystis carinii* pneumonia. *Scand J Infect Dis.* 1988; 20:685-6.
79. Leport C, Raffi F, Matheron S et al. Treatment of central nervous system toxoplasmosis with pyrimethamine/sulfadiazine combination in 35 patients with the acquired immunodeficiency syndrome. Efficacy of long-term continuous therapy. *Am J Med.* 1988; 84:94-100.
80. Israelski DM, Remington JS. Toxoplasmic encephalitis in patients with AIDS. In: Sande MA, Volberding PA, eds. The medical management of AIDS. Philadelphia: Saunders; 1985:193-212.
81. Rolston KVI, Hoy J. Role of clindamycin in the treatment of central nervous system toxoplasmosis. *Am J Med.* 1987; 83:551-4.
82. Leport C, Bastuji-Garin S, Perronne C et al. An open study of the pyrimethamine-clindamycin combination in AIDS patients with brain toxoplasmosis. *J Infect Dis.* 1989; 160:557-8. Letter.
83. Centers for Disease Control. Severe neutropenia during pentamidine treatment of *Pneumocystis carinii* pneumonia in patients with acquired immunodeficiency syndrome—New York City. *MMWR.* 1984; 33:65-7.
84. Wharton JM, Coleman DL, Wofsy CB et al. Trimethoprim–sulfamethoxazole or pentamidine for *Pneumocystis carinii* pneumonia in the acquired immunodeficiency syndrom: a prospective randomized trial. *Ann Intern Med.* 1986; 105:37-44.
85. Robbins JB, Miller RH, Arean VM et al. Successful treatment of *Pneumocystis carinii* pneumonitis in a patient with congenital hypogammaglobulinaemia. *N Engl J Med.* 1965; 272:708-13.
86. Arnott MA, Hay J. The effect of pentamidine salts on the in-vitro responses of neutrophilic granulocytes. *J Antimicrob Chemother.* 1989; 23:557-64.
87. Arnott MA, Hay J. The effect of pentamidine salts on the respiratory burst of human neutrophilic granulocytes. *J Antimicrob Chemother.* 1989; 24:339-45.
88. Arnott MA, Hay J. The effect of pentamidine salts on the NADPH-dependent oxidase of stimulated neutrophilic granulocytes. *J Antimicrob Chemother.* 1990; 25:247-53.
89. Lapierre G, Stewart RB. Lithium carbonate and leukocytosis. *Am J Hosp Pharm.* 1980; 37:1525-8.
90. Herbert V, Jacobson J, Shevchuck O et al. Lithium in AIDS. *Clin Res.* 1988; 36:620A. Abstract.
91. Roberts DE, Berman SM, Nakasato S et al. Effect of lithium carbonate on zidovudine-associated neutropenia in the acquired immunodeficiency syndrome. *Am J Med.* 1988; 85:428-31.
92. Nathwani D, Green ST. Lithium for zidovudine-induced neutropenia in AIDS. *JAMA.* 1989; 262:775-6. Letter.
93. Klutman NE. Lithium carbonate therapy for zidovudine-associated neutropenia in patients with the acquired immunodeficiency syndrome. *Am J Med.* 1989; 87:362-3. Letter.
94. Worthington M. Lack of effect of lithium carbonate on zidovudine-associated neutropenia in patients with AIDS. *J Infect Dis.* 1990; 162:777-8.
95. Weisbart RH, moderator. Colony-stimulating factors and host defense. *Ann Intern Med.* 1989; 110:297-303.
96. Antman KS, Griffin JD, Elias A et al. Effect of recombinant human granulocyte-macrophage colony-stimulating factor on chemotherapy-induced myelosuppression. *N Engl J Med.* 1988; 319:593-8.
97. Glaspy JA, Baldwin GC, Robertson PA et al. Therapy for neutropenia in hairy cell leukemia with recombinant human granulocyte colony-stimulating factor. *Ann Intern Med.* 1988; 109:789-95.
98. Baldwin GC, Fuller ND, Roberts RL et al. Granulocyte and granulocyte-macrophage colony-stimulating factors enhance neutrophil cytotoxicity toward HIV-infected cells. *Blood.* 1989; 74:1673-7.
99. Bhalla K, Birkhofer M, Grant S et al. The effect of recombinant human granulocyte-macrophage colony-stimulating factor (rGM-CSF) on 3'-azido-3'-deoxythymidine (AZT) mediated biochemical and cytotoxic effects on normal human myeloid progenitor cells. *Exp Hematol.* 1989; 17:17-20.
100. Hammer SM, Gillis JM. Synergistic activity of granulocyte-macrophage colony stimulating factor and 3'-azido-3'-deoxythymidine against human immunodeficiency virus in vitro. *Antimicrob Agents Chemother.* 1987; 31:1046-50.
101. Groopman JE, Mitsuyasu RT, DeLeo MJ et al. Effect of recombinant human granulocyte-macrophage stimulating factor on myelopoiesis in the acquired immunodeficiency syndrome. *N Engl J Med.* 1987; 317:593-8.
102. Merigan TC. A personal view of the efforts in the treatment of human immunodeficiency virus infection in 1988. *J Infect Dis.* 1989; 159:390-9.
103. Berman E, Duigou-Osterndorf R, Krown SE et al. Synergistic cytotoxic effect of azidothymidine and recombinant interferon alpha on normal human bone marrow progenitor cells. *Blood.* 1989; 74:1281-6.
104. Berkman SA, Lee ML, Gale RP. Clincial uses of intravenous immunoglobulins. *Ann Intern Med.* 1990; 112:278-92.

Current and investigational therapies for AIDS-associated *Mycobacterium avium* complex disease

R. Chris Rathbun, Emory S. Martin III, Virginia E. Eaton, and Earl B. Matthew

Abstract: The epidemiology, pathogenesis, clinical manifestations, and treatment of *Mycobacterium avium* complex (MAC) infection are reviewed.

MAC infection is one of the most common infections in AIDS patients. Its pathogenesis is poorly understood, but it is believed to develop by gastrointestinal colonization followed by systemic invasion. The relatively poor response to treatment may be partly accounted for by the tremendous mycobacterial load present by the time patients develop systemic symptoms. Clinically, MAC infection is difficult to differentiate from the signs and symptoms of AIDS or from other opportunistic infections. Signs and symptoms include fever, malaise, anorexia, night sweats, and weight loss; diarrhea and abdominal pain may also be present.

There is no established therapy for MAC infection, although combinations of three to five antimicrobial agents are typically used. There has been consistently poor correlation between in vitro results and in vivo outcomes in the treatment of MAC infection. Currently, the role of treatment is mainly to suppress the progression of infection and to relieve symptoms. Recent in vitro studies and animal studies have revealed possible alternative agents and combinations of agents (e.g., macrolide antibiotics, quinolones, amikacin, cytokines) that may influence therapy of MAC infection.

No known therapy for MAC has been shown to prolong survival in AIDS patients, possibly because of the high organism load that exists once patients become symptomatic. Research is needed to find improved methods for earlier detection of MAC infection, determine optimal dosage regimens of current antimycobacterial agents, develop better antimycobacterial drug-delivery systems (e.g., liposomes), and discover new antimicrobials with better activity against MAC and methods of immune modulation that will overcome immune system defects.

Index terms: Acquired immunodeficiency syndrome; Amikacin; Aminoglycosides; Anti-infective agents; Antibiotics; Cytokines; *Mycobacterium avium* complex; Quinolones
Clin Pharm. 1991; 10:280-91

The *Mycobacterium avium* complex (MAC), also termed *Mycobacterium avium–intracellulare*, is a group of slow-growing, nonchromogenic mycobacteria consisting of *Mycobacterium avium* and *Mycobacterium intracellulare*.[1,2] With the widespread use of prophylaxis for *Pneumocystis carinii* pneumonia, MAC is now believed to be one of the most common infections found in patients with the acquired immunodeficiency syndrome (AIDS). It is observed clinically in 4.2% of human immunodeficiency virus (HIV)-infected patients at the time AIDS is diagnosed[3] and is found in up to 50% of AIDS patients at the time of autopsy.[4-6] Before the 1980s and the AIDS epidemic, MAC infection was uncommon, being seen primarily as a slowly progressive pneumonitis in elderly patients with chronic pulmonary disorders. Very rarely, disseminated MAC infection was found in immunocompromised leukemic patients.[1] With the onset of the AIDS epidemic, the incidence of MAC infection, predominantly disseminated disease, has increased dramatically.[2,7,8]

Compared with tuberculosis (a more common mycobacterial disease in non-AIDS patients), AIDS-associated disseminated MAC infection is much more resistant to drug therapy.[9] Response to therapy is often poor, and clinical improvements are frequently short-lived despite continued treatment. Currently, there is no standardized treatment for MAC infection, and because of the high incidence of adverse effects associated with multiple drug therapy, many AIDS patients are not treated for their MAC disease. A review of MAC infection and its treatment, as well as other opportunistic infections in patients with AIDS, was presented in this journal in 1985.[10] The purpose of this article is to review the results of recent investigations that provide new information regarding antimycobacterial therapy and describe future directions in managing MAC disease.

Epidemiology

Both *M. avium* and *M. intracellulare* are ubiquitous in the environment, being found in water, dust, and soil, and are common causes of disease in animals.[1,11] The two organisms resemble one another so closely that on routine laboratory examination they cannot be distinguished; however, serotyping has been performed in

R. Chris Rathbun, Pharm.D., is Clinical Science Fellow in Infectious Disease, and Emory S. Martin III, Pharm.D., is Clinical Assistant Professor, College of Pharmacy, University of Texas at Austin, TX. Virginia E. Eaton, Pharm.D., is Pharmacy Resident in Clinical Oncology, University of Texas M. D. Anderson Cancer Center, Houston. Earl B. Matthew, M.D., is Infectious Disease Specialist and Director of Medical Service and Education, Central Texas Medical Foundation, Austin.

Address reprint requests to Dr. Martin at the Clinical Division, College of Pharmacy, University of Texas at Austin, Austin, TX 78712.

an attempt to classify the two species. Colony appearance has been correlated with virulence, and particular serotypes of MAC may also have increased virulence.[1] However, the relationship between serotype and virulence is not firmly established.[2,12]

It is clear that the immunocompromised state of AIDS patients is an important predisposing factor in the development of MAC infection. Evidence in AIDS patients of impaired gamma interferon production and inadequate proliferation of T cells in response to mycobacterial antigens may explain the propensity for disseminated disease in these patients.[13] However, some evidence indicates that the particular strains of MAC that cause disease in AIDS patients have certain unique characteristics that may relate to increased virulence and contribute to patients' poor clinical response to antimycobacterial therapy.[2,5,9,12,14,15] The majority of isolates from AIDS patients have been found to be *M. avium*,[16] which may indicate that this species is more pathogenic than *M. intracellulare* for AIDS patients. In addition, virtually all MAC isolates from AIDS patients contain plasmids, compared with only one third of the isolates from the environment.[17] The higher incidence of plasmids in AIDS patients may confer a greater degree of resistance to drug therapy or allow the organism to elude cellular defense mechanisms.[18] The predominance of *M. avium* and prevalence of plasmids in isolates from AIDS patients may also suggest that there is a common route of infection or source of exposure in these patients.

Pathogenesis of Infection

Several hypotheses have been proposed to explain the preponderance of disseminated MAC disease with gastrointestinal involvement in persons with AIDS. According to an early theory, disseminated MAC infection in AIDS patients was merely an extension of initial respiratory MAC infection or colonization, acquired by inhalation of aerosolized organisms from the environment. However, this theory of pathogenesis was questioned when it was shown that MAC is rarely isolated from lung tissue of AIDS patients at autopsy.[6] An alternate theory of pathogenesis in AIDS patients is that the gastrointestinal tract may serve as the portal of entry for MAC.[4-6,19,20] This theory is supported by the large bacterial load present in gut biopsy specimens of some patients with disseminated disease and the associated malabsorption or wasting syndrome frequently seen in these patients.[2] Affinity of the MAC organisms for specific receptors on the intestinal mucosal surface may facilitate the organisms' attachment and allow for a point of entry into the gut-associated lymphoid tissue.[21] The incidence of MAC disease in patients who contracted AIDS through sexual contact is similar to that in patients who contracted AIDS through needle sharing; therefore, the risk of acquiring MAC disease may not correlate with any particular type of behavior. Rather, this similarity seems to indicate that a more universal source is responsible for exposure, such as water or food contaminated with the mycobacteria.[22]

It has been hypothesized that MAC colonization of the gut leads to localized infection of the gut mucosa.[6,19] As the number of mycobacterial colony-forming units (CFUs) steadily increases, the disease is manifested clinically as diarrhea and malabsorption.[14] Pathologically, these patients may have evidence of diffuse granulomas with large, foamy-appearing macrophages and enlarged mesenteric lymph nodes.[6] The clinical features are similar to those of Whipple's disease but can be distinguished by a relative nonresponsiveness to broad-spectrum antimicrobials.[14,23] Once localized infection has become established, MAC organisms then presumedly invade the blood stream and spread hematogenously to distant body sites.[19] The presence of hepatic lesions and the involvement of the mesenteric lymph nodes seem to indicate that dissemination from the bowel proceeds through the lymphatics and portal circulation.[23] Once the organisms enter the systemic circulation, the mycobacterial load steadily increases as the organisms continue to multiply in tissues throughout the body. The time course from initial colonization of the gut to the development of systemic infection and symptomatic illness is not known, but it may be a period of months.[24] Patients may remain relatively asymptomatic despite large numbers of CFUs/mL of blood, with no apparent signs of systemic involvement. This may be due to the lack of an inflammatory response to the infection.[6] The inability of macrophages to kill MAC intracellularly promotes continued, uninhibited replication of the organisms. The relatively poor response to treatment may be accounted for, in part, by the tremendous mycobacterial load present by the time patients develop systemic symptoms, making resolution of infection unlikely.[2,6]

Clinical Manifestations

The nonspecific nature of symptoms makes it difficult to distinguish MAC from other AIDS-related infections. Symptomatic MAC infection commonly occurs late in the course of HIV disease when patients have usually had several episodes of *Pneumocystis carinii* pneumonia as well as other opportunistic infections.[4,6,7,25] Despite favorable responses to treatment, patients' overall clinical condition may continue to deteriorate.[2] Signs and symptoms include fever, malaise, anorexia, night sweats, and weight loss; diarrhea and abdominal pain may also be present.[4,6,8,25] Laboratory findings usually show abnormal liver function tests with evidence of anemia, hypergammaglobulinemia, and either leukocytosis or leukopenia[6,8]; CD4 lymphocyte counts are typically low as well (<50 cells/cu mm).[26,27] On physical examination, patients may appear cachectic and have hepatosplenomegaly and lymphadenopathy.[28] Computed-tomography scans may show intra-abdominal lymphadenopathy,[29] and chest roentgenograms may or may not show infiltration.[28] Blood culture is the most efficient and reliable method of documenting infection; however, bone marrow biopsy and stool cultures can also be useful.[2,5,14,30] Because organisms may be sequestered within leukocytes, processing of blood cultures should include lysis centrifugation[29] to increase the yield.[5] Additionally, analysis of the whole blood buffy coat may also increase the recovery of organisms.[30,31] The presence of acid-fast bacilli in stool and biopsy specimens may provide evidence of infection before blood cultures become positive, allowing for earlier treatment. The presence of MAC in the stool alone, though, does not necessarily indicate dissemination and currently is not an indication for treatment. Like *M. tuberculosis, M. avium* and *M. intracellulare* are very slow growing organisms, making rapid detection desirable to distinguish between tuberculosis and MAC infection because of the different approaches to treatment. Radiometric testing, which measures cellular respiration, provides the quickest way of detecting growth, typically with results within 7 to 14 days and as early as 4 days.[30] Within hours, genetic probes can then be used to identify the culture as MAC or *M. tuberculosis*.[32]

Current Therapy

An effective short course of antimicrobial monotherapy for MAC disease would be desirable, but hopes for finding such a regimen may be unrealistic. Finding a lifelong, multiple-drug regimen capable of merely suppressing the infection and its symptoms would be a great advance in therapy. Traditionally, combinations of four to six drugs have been used with varying degrees of success to treat MAC infection. An overview of these agents is found in Table 1. Based on clinical research findings, many recently published recommendations for the therapy of MAC infection correctly state that there is no standard treatment approach to the disease and that investigational drug therapy to date has not reliably changed the outcome of the disease. In a position paper on the treatment of mycobacterial diseases in 1987, the Centers for Disease Control (CDC) reported that no therapy had been found that consistently decreased the level of bacteremia or had an influence on mortality, but that a regimen consisting of rifabutin (Adria), isoniazid, ethambutol, and clofazimine was being used by some clinicians.[46] In a separate report that year,[47] the CDC recommended that patients who were empirically started on a three-drug regimen (rifampin, isoniazid, and ethambutol or pyrazinamide) for presumed *M. tuberculosis* infection who were found to have MAC infection should continue to receive the same therapy or be switched to rifabutin, isoniazid, ethambutol, and clofazimine. At the National Consensus Conference for Tuberculosis in 1985, the Committee on *M. intracellulare* Disease recommended a five-drug regimen for adult patients with disseminated MAC infection who were immunocompromised. This regimen included rifampin (600 mg/day) or rifabutin (150–300 mg/day), depending on results of susceptibility tests, clofazimine (100 mg t.i.d.), ethambutol hydrochloride (25 mg/kg/day for 6 weeks, then 15 mg/kg/day), ethionamide (250 mg b.i.d.–q.i.d.), and streptomycin (as the sulfate salt) (15 mg/kg/day i.m. for 60 days, then a reduced dosage for six months). Other agents could be added or substituted as needed based on

Table 1.
Current Agents for Treatment of *Mycobacterium avium* Complex Infection

Drug	Dosing Regimen[4,33,41–45]	Dose-Limiting Adverse Effects[33–40]
Rifabutin	150–600 mg p.o. daily	Hematologic (leukopenia, thrombocytopenia, hemolytic anemia), hepatitis[a]
Clofazimine	100–300 mg p.o. divided every 8–24 hr	Discoloration of tissues and body fluids (especially skin, 80%; cornea or conjunctiva, 10–38%), severe GI intolerance (abdominal pain or diarrhea, 40–50%; malabsorption or constipation, <1%)
Cycloserine	500–1000 mg p.o. daily, divided every 12 hr	Central nervous system (dizziness, 22%; insomnia, 15%; nervousness, 10%; disorientation, 9%; loss of memory, 7%; depression, 5%; tremor, 3.5%; vertigo, 3%; paresthesia, <3.5%; seizures or coma[a]), dysarthria[a]
Ethionamide	500–1000 mg p.o. daily, divided every 6–24 hr	GI intolerance (vomiting, 66%; abdominal pain, 26%; nausea, 22%), nervous system, 13% (depression, peripheral neuritis, seizures, hallucinations, optic and olfactory disturbances[a]), hepatitis[a]
Isoniazid	300 mg p.o. daily	Nervous system (peripheral neuritis, 0.2%; seizures, optic neuritis, dizziness, ataxia, paresthesia, toxic encephalopathy, psychosis[a]), hepatitis, 0.3–2.3%
Ethambutol hydrochloride	15–25 mg/kg p.o. daily	Nervous system (optic neuritis, 1–5%; peripheral neuritis, 1.5%; dizziness, disorientation, hallucinations[a])
Ciprofloxacin (as the hydrochloride salt)	1500 mg p.o. daily, divided every 12 hr	Central nervous system (headache, 1.2%; dizziness, restlessness, nightmares, ataxia, seizures, or hallucinations, <1%)
Amikacin (as the sulfate salt)	15 mg/kg i.v. daily, divided every 8–12 hr	Ototoxicity[b] (auditory and vestibular, 0.5–3%), nephrotoxicity (tubular necrosis or nonoliguric azotemia, 2–10%), neuromuscular blockade[a]

[a] Incidence not known.
[b] Defined as clinically important.

susceptibility test results (except for ethambutol and ethionamide) or lack of patient tolerance. The recommendation was to continue this regimen for 12 months and then change to clofazimine, ethambutol, and rifampin or rifabutin for an additional year.[48]

Clinical studies by Masur et al.[41] and Hawkins et al.[4] exemplify the poor response of this infection to drug therapy despite the long-term use of regimens combining multiple antimicrobial agents; these studies are the basis of the prevailing attitude that therapy is futile. Masur and colleagues found that a two-drug regimen of rifabutin 150 or 300 mg and clofazimine 100 mg daily resulted in a sustained clearing of mycobacteremia in only 4 of 13 patients, despite long-term therapy. Hawkins et al. found that treatment of mycobacteremia with a three-drug regimen of rifabutin, clofazimine, and ethionamide or ethambutol was successful in only 2 of 26 patients.

In the face of such discouraging results, it is not surprising that clinicians and persons with AIDS often make no attempt to treat or be treated for MAC disease once a diagnosis is made. But case reports that drug therapy may relieve the symptoms of MAC infection in certain patients have provided some support for aggressive treatment of the disease.[49] Several recently published clinical reports provide some promising evidence of potentially effective therapy for advanced MAC disease.

In a small retrospective review, Agins et al.[42] summarized the response of seven AIDS patients with recently diagnosed mycobacteremia to long-term therapy with rifabutin (150 mg/day), clofazimine (100 mg/day), isoniazid (300 mg/day), and ethambutol hydrochloride (15 mg/kg/day). In six of the seven patients, mycobacteremia was cleared and symptoms of MAC disease were reduced. There was no evidence that these treated patients had improved survival over untreated patients, however.

Hoy et al.[43] treated a larger group of patients ($n = 25$) with a drug regimen consisting of rifabutin (300–600 mg/day), clofazimine (100 mg/day), isoniazid (300 mg/day), and ethambutol hydrochloride (15 mg/kg/day, up to 1 g), which was continued indefinitely. The patients were HIV antibody-positive with culture-proven mycobacteremia, and they had symptoms consistent with MAC disease (most notably, night sweats, fever, lethargy). All had CD4 cell counts below 200 cells/μL, and 18 had counts of <100 cells/μL. Only patients who completed at least one month of anti-MAC therapy were included in the report. The duration of MAC disease before therapy was begun was not reported. Patients completed an average of 38 weeks of therapy (range, 6–74 weeks). With this four-drug regimen, mycobacteremia was cleared in 22 of 25 patients with AIDS. Of the three patients whose mycobacteremias were not initially cleared, one had cryptosporidial diarrhea that may have compromised drug absorption and contributed to the failure. All patients who responded microbiologically had some symptomatic relief, and 18 patients had an early remission of all their symptoms of MAC disease. These findings are somewhat offset by the fact that 6 of the 22 patients eventually had recurrence of mycobacteremia, but compliance with the four-drug regimen was reportedly compromised in half of these patients. Recurrence occurred most often in the group of patients receiving rifabutin 300 mg daily. Symptoms recurred in five patients, with most having simultaneous recurrence of mycobacteremia. Coadministration of zidovudine did not appear to affect the rate of response or relapse. The study's positive clinical results were observed notwithstanding the finding that two thirds of the isolates were resistant to rifabutin (minimum inhibitory concentration [MIC] of >2 μg/mL), and all were resistant to clofazamine (MIC of >8 μg/mL), isoniazid (MIC of >4 μg/mL), and ethambutol (MIC of >4 μg/mL) using in vitro testing standards for *M. tuberculosis*. It may be noteworthy that the isolates from the three patients whose mycobacteremias were not initially cleared were rifabutin resistant. Despite MAC therapy, there was greater than 50% mortality in the study due to a variety of AIDS-related diseases, yet there was little evidence of MAC disease at autopsy in the patients whose mycobacteremias were cleared.

As one reviews this report of success in permanent clearing of mycobacteremia in almost two thirds of patients (with particular success in those receiving >300 mg of rifabutin per day) and the accompanying relief of MAC disease symptoms in many patients, several points must be recognized, namely, the small sample, the lack of a control group, the lack of blinding, and the sustained high mortality associated with other AIDS-associated diseases. But the authors present some encouraging data that may provide the basis for therapy of MAC infection and future clinical investigations. It is important to note that many AIDS patients are currently receiving rifabutin through the CDC as part of a compassionate-use protocol. The CDC has stopped enrolling patients in this protocol because the manufacturer of rifabutin has begun formal MAC treatment studies.

Preliminary results of a clinical study involving a four-drug regimen consisting of rifampin (600 mg/day), ethambutol hydrochloride (15 mg/kg/day), clofazimine (100–200 mg/day), and ciprofloxacin (as the hydrochloride salt) (750 mg b.i.d.) for 12 weeks have recently been reported. Six of the 40 patients entered also received amikacin during a portion of the study period. Of the patients who were evaluable, clinical signs and symptoms improved in most, and the improvement appeared to correspond to decreases in CFUs.[44] An overview of this study and other clinical studies performed to date is presented in Table 2.

Limitations of In Vitro Testing

It is well recognized that there has been poor correlation between in vitro results and in vivo outcomes in the treatment of MAC infection.[48] One of the major obstacles has been the lack of a standardized method for susceptibility testing of MAC organisms against various agents.[2,52] Methods used to determine the degree of susceptibility of *M. tuberculosis* strains and to assign cutoffs (e.g., susceptible, moderately susceptible, resistant) cannot be used to evaluate the susceptibility of MAC organisms because of their widespread resistance to antitubercular drugs. Many agents, when tested alone, may have little if any activity against MAC but are capable of producing a therapeutic response when combined with other agents.[53] Thus, poor in vitro activity does not always indicate an unsatisfactory in vivo response. The absence of a systematic approach has made it difficult to determine the relevance of in vitro findings to treatment and whether or not they should influence drug selection and therapy. Another limitation of susceptibility test-

Table 2.
Clinical Studies of Treatment for Disseminated *Mycobacterium avium* Complex (MAC) Infection

Reference	Study Design,[a] *n*	Drug Regimen[b]	No. Patients	% Susceptible (μg/mL)	Duration of Therapy	Comments
4	R, 29	Rifabutin 150–300 mg/day	21	100 (2)	4–30 weeks (mean, 6 weeks)	29 patients were treated with two or more drugs; all 29 patients had positive cultures indicating persistent infection (e.g., blood, bone marrow, liver, lymph nodes) despite treatment; 24 of 26 patients had persistent MAC bacteremia; 7 patients received <1 month of therapy (6 died, 1 dropped from study)
		Clofazimine 300 mg/day	20	100 (1)		
		Ethionamide 750 mg/day	14[c]	92 (15)		
		Ethambutol hydrochloride 15 mg/kg/day		81 (15)		
		(Rifampin)[d]	9	42 (10)		
		(Isoniazid)[d]	6	22 (5)		
		(Amikacin)[d]	4	NR[e]		
		(Pyrazinamide)[d]	3	NR		
		(Cycloserine)[d]	1	100 (60)		
41	P, 13	Rifabutin 150–300 mg/day	13	NR	33–530 days	6 patients had consecutive sets of negative blood cultures; 2 patients relapsed while receiving therapy; only one MAC isolate developed resistance (to rifabutin)
		Clofazimine 100 mg/day	13	NR		
		Amikacin 7.5 mg/kg i.v. b.i.d.	10	9 (12)		
		(Ceftizoxime + ciprofloxacin)	1	NR		
		(Isoniazid + cycloserine)	1	0 (5)/16 (30)		
		(Ethambutol)	1	76 (10)		
45	P, 4	(Amikacin)	4	50 (20)	3 weeks–5 months	All 4 patients had clinical improvement (decreased fever, malaise; increased well-being); 3 patients developed negative blood cultures on follow-up[f] (no cultures were available for the fourth patient); in the one autopsy that was performed, there was no sign of MAC infection in the spleen, liver, or brain
		(Ethambutol)	4	50 (10)		
		(Rifampin)	4	50 (8)		
42	R, 7	Rifabutin 150 mg/day	7	97 (2)	4–23 months	Only one patient remained bacteremic on therapy; 6 patients had clinical signs of improvement (decreased fever, night sweats; increase in weight); treatment did not prolong survival
		Clofazimine 100 mg/day	7	86 (1)		
		Isoniazid 300 mg/day	7	0 (5)		
		Ethambutol hydrochloride 15 mg/kg/day	7	47 (10)		
43	P, 25	Rifabutin 300–600 mg/day	25	33 (2)	6–74 weeks (mean, 38.4 weeks)	22 patients developed consecutive negative blood cultures; 6 patients relapsed; 2 later redeveloped negative blood cultures
		Clofazimine 100 mg/day	25	0 (8)		
		Isoniazid 300 mg/day	25	0 (4)		
		Ethambutol hydrochloride 15 mg/kg/day	25	0 (4)		
50	R, 8	(Rifampin)	4	8 (NR)	NR	4 patients receiving rifampin, isoniazid, ethambutol, and pyrazinamide had no response; 2 patients treated with rifabutin, isoniazid, and pyrazinamide had clinical improvement (undefined); 2 patients who also received amikacin had clinical improvement (undefined); other medications were not specified
		(Isoniazid)	6	0 (NR)		
		(Ethambutol)	4	0 (NR)		
		(Pyrazinamide)	6	NR		
		(Rifabutin)	2	78 (NR)		
		(Amikacin)	2	40 (NR)		
51	P, 15	Rifampin 600 mg/day	15	50 (NR)	4–35 weeks	3 of 10 patients who completed 12 weeks of therapy developed negative blood cultures; mean colony count (CFUs/mL) in the blood declined 30-fold during treatment
		Amikacin 7.5 mg/kg/day[g]	15	100[h]		
		Ethambutol hydrochloride 15 mg/kg/day	15	88 (NR)		
		Ciprofloxacin 750 mg b.i.d.	15	38 (NR)		

Continued on next page

Table 2 *(continued)*

Reference	Study Design,[a] *n*	Drug Regimen[b]	No. Patients	% Susceptible (μg/mL)	Duration of Therapy	Comments
						and was associated with an improvement in clinical signs (fever, night sweats)
44	P, 31	Rifampin 600 mg/day	31	NR	12 weeks (mean, 9.8 weeks)	Clinical signs improved in the majority of patients (fevers improved in 25 of 28, night sweats in 24 of 27, diarrhea in 9 of 14); the mean colony count in the blood of the study population declined by 2 logarithms within 4 weeks; 4 patients developed negative blood cultures after 4 weeks of therapy
		Ethambutol hydrochloride 15 mg/kg/day	31	NR		
		Clofazimine 100–200 mg/day	31	NR		
		Ciprofloxacin 750 mg b.i.d.	31	NR		
		(Amikacin)	6[i]	NR		

[a] R = retrospective, P = prospective.
[b] For drugs listed in parentheses, authors did not state dosage.
[c] Twelve patients received clofazimine with either ethambutol or ethionamide; two patients received all three.
[d] Combined with one or more of the following drugs: rifabutin, clofazimine, ethionamide, and ethambutol.
[e] NR = not reported.
[f] Two patients had two consecutive sets of negative blood cultures; one patient had only one set of blood cultures drawn, which were negative.
[g] Amikacin was given for only the first four weeks of therapy.
[h] If 99% of isolates had a minimum inhibitory concentration that was less than the peak concentration (not reported), the isolate was considered susceptible.
[i] Six of the 40 patients originally entered received amikacin during weeks 5–8 of the study.

ing is that many techniques currently used allow for the determination of inhibitory activity (MIC) but provide no information regarding the antimicrobial concentration necessary to produce killing.[54] Often, minimum bactericidal concentrations (MBCs) of agents are many times higher (e.g., 32 times for rifabutin and clofazimine) than concentrations that are capable of inhibiting growth, resulting in continued growth once the antimicrobial concentration drops below the MIC. To optimize therapeutic strategies, studies are needed to determine which agents can achieve concentrations in serum that are capable of producing killing without producing intolerable adverse effects.

Another matter that complicates the interpretation of in vitro data is that different strains of MAC exhibit highly variable susceptibility to a given antimicrobial,[55] a factor that greatly limits the ability to predict how a particular strain will respond to therapy. To make the approach to treatment more rational, quantitative in vitro procedures must be developed and the activity of antitubercular agents must be re-evaluated so that standard concentrations for testing can be established.[56]

Future Therapies

Several preliminary clinical studies suggest possible future approaches to treatment of MAC disease. Also, drug therapy trials in animal models of MAC infection have provided information on possible treatments. The beige mouse model has been developed to evaluate the efficacy of different combinations of agents under in vivo conditions.[57,58] The beige mouse model uses mice that have the murine equivalent of Chédiak–Higashi syndrome,[59] a disease in humans in which neutrophils and monocytes have an impaired response to infection and that is characterized by abnormally slow rates of bacterial killing. Although the model does not portray the full extent of disease in patients with AIDS, it does mimic the defective response to infection and allows MAC to be studied as an acute infection, an advantage over previous models in which MAC was able to subsist as a chronic infection but was not capable of inducing death in the animal.[57] Other model systems, such as human and murine macrophages, are also being used to test new agents and various combinations in an in vitro environment. These new systems make it possible to observe how intracellular organisms such as MAC are processed at a cellular level and how antimicrobial therapy influences the response to infection. The only major disadvantage is that many of the studies using this methodology include macrophages from healthy human donors or from normal mice. This methodology does not accurately portray the immune status in patients with AIDS.

Macrolide Antimicrobials. Clarithromycin (Abbott) and azithromycin (Pfizer) are investigational macrolide antimicrobials noted for achieving high tissue concentrations with oral therapy, and they are active in vitro against many strains of MAC. Some experimental data suggest that clarithromycin has in vivo efficacy as a single agent.[60] In one study examining MICs against 12 strains of MAC, clarithromycin had MICs that were 8 to 32 times lower than those of erythromycin. In the beige mouse model, clarithromycin was significantly more effective than all other single-agent treatments in reducing CFUs in the spleen. Clarithromycin maintained concentrations in the spleen and serum longer than erythromycin.[61] In a separate study, azithromycin significantly reduced mortality and colony counts in beige mice compared with those in untreated controls.[62] Other investigational macrolides are currently being studied to determine their activity against MAC.[63]

In recent clinical studies, the efficacy of clarithromycin as a single agent and in combination therapy has been evaluated. In one study,[64] 23 AIDS patients with disseminated MAC infection were randomized to receive clarithromycin 1000 mg orally b.i.d. or placebo for six weeks (phase 1). Of the 23 patients entered, 15 were evaluable. Although the severity of MAC disease (blood CFUs) in the two groups appeared similar at the initiation of this phase, the groups appeared quite different at the end of six weeks. All eight patients treated with clarithromycin had a dramatic decrease in the number of CFUs in the blood, whereas the seven patients who received placebo had continuously elevated CFUs, had an increase in the absolute number of CFUs, or died. Ten patients went on to phase 2 of the study. Seven patients who originally received clarithromycin were assigned to receive a four-drug regimen consisting of rifampin (10 mg/kg), isoniazid (5 mg/kg), ethambutol hydrochloride (20 mg/kg), and clofazimine (100 mg) daily for six weeks. These patients began this phase with low or negative blood CFUs. Counts continued to remain low in four patients after six weeks, whereas two patients had elevations in the number of CFUs; the remaining patient withdrew. Three patients who originally received placebo were assigned to receive the same four-drug regimen plus clarithromycin. These patients began this phase with high blood CFUs. After six weeks, however, counts substantially decreased in all three patients. The authors concluded that these results validated the efficacy of clarithromycin against MAC but that an optimal dose and combination drug regimen for treatment needed further study. In a similar study,[65] 11 patients were treated with either clarithromycin 1000 mg orally b.i.d. or placebo for six weeks. All seven patients receiving clarithromycin had decreases in CFUs in the blood, whereas the patients receiving placebo showed little change or a progressive increase in the number of blood CFUs. Two patients receiving clarithromycin had an impressive 2-logarithm reduction in the number of CFUs after two weeks, suggesting that clarithromycin has substantial activity against MAC.

Quinolones. The quinolones have been tested for activity against mycobacteria, and several have been found to have good in vitro activity against *M. tuberculosis* and variable activity against strains of MAC.[66,67] The quinolone that currently appears to have the most potential is ciprofloxacin; 20–38% of MAC strains are estimated to be susceptible (≤2 μg/mL).[68,69] In spite of its marginal activity at concentrations achievable in serum, ciprofloxacin has been observed to penetrate macrophages, producing levels two to three times higher than those in serum,[70] and reportedly has low MBC:MIC ratios for many strains of MAC.[53] When ciprofloxacin is combined with other agents (particularly with an aminoglycoside), bactericidal activity against MAC isolates from AIDS patients has been observed.[68] Several investigators have tested ciprofloxacin for synergy with other antimicrobial agents. Hoffner et al.[71] were able to show synergism between ciprofloxacin and ethambutol against 70 strains of MAC based on a growth index grading system. A possible explanation for the synergism is that cellular penetration of the quinolone is enhanced by ethambutol. In another study, Yajko et al.,[72] using MAC strains isolated from AIDS patients, assessed combination therapies in mouse macrophages. This study found combination therapy to be more effective than single-drug therapy. The combination of ciprofloxacin, ethambutol, and either rifabutin or rifampin resulted in a kill rate of 91% compared with 70% when two-drug combinations were used. In more recent studies, the investigational quinolones temafloxacin (Abbott), PD-117,558 (Parke-Davis), Win 57273 (Sterling), and sparfloxacin (Parke-Davis) have also been reported to have in vitro activity comparable to that of ciprofloxacin against MAC isolates from AIDS and cancer patients.[73,74] In a beige mouse model, Win 57273 and sparfloxacin were found to reduce mortality in disseminated MAC infection when given as single-agent therapy and are being evaluated further in combination drug regimens in mice. Further studies are needed to determine the role of these agents in therapy.

Amikacin. The utility of amikacin in combination therapy for MAC disease has been examined in several studies with beige mice. In a study by Gangadharam et al.,[75] amikacin alone or in combination with clofazimine or rifabutin, or both, was tested for a period of six weeks as a treatment of early and established MAC infection. All combinations tested were found to be significantly better than no treatment. Amikacin alone was similar to the combination of amikacin and clofazimine in its ability to reduce CFUs in the spleen and liver after six weeks of treatment of early infection. Combination therapy with amikacin and clofazimine produced the greatest drop in CFUs at two weeks and the most rapid reduction in CFUs in patients with either early or established infection. The authors concluded that regimens containing amikacin should be considered for future studies.

Another study by Inderlied et al.[76] examined the effectiveness of four weeks of therapy with amikacin, ciprofloxacin, and imipenem in beige mice. Amikacin alone and in combination with ciprofloxacin and imipenem significantly reduced the number of CFUs in the blood, liver, and spleen. Despite improvement during therapy, the combination of amikacin, ciprofloxacin, and imipenem was less effective than amikacin alone with respect to mortality and reduction in the degree of tissue infection. This trend was observed for monotherapy with ciprofloxacin or imipenem as well. Mice treated with either ciprofloxacin or imipenem alone had a greater degree of mortality than untreated controls. There was little or no difference between controls and mice treated with ciprofloxacin or imipenem with respect to reduction of CFUs in liver and spleen. Despite these poor results, the combination of amikacin, ciprofloxacin, and imipenem was significantly more effective in clearing mycobacteremia than all other treatments, including amikacin monotherapy. The authors did not speculate as to why the combination of amikacin, ciprofloxacin, and imipenem appeared to result in greater mortality than amikacin monotherapy or state whether this difference was significant.

A liposomal preparation of amikacin has also been used to treat experimental MAC infection in beige mice, with more favorable results than with nonliposomal preparations.[77-79] Liposomal delivery may be favorable because of its preferential drug distribution to reticuloendothelial tissues such as the liver, spleen, and bone marrow and its ability to incorporate drug into macrophages, thereby making it attractive for treatment of intracellular pathogens such as MAC.

Preliminary results of a clinical study using amikacin in patients with disseminated MAC infection suggest that amikacin may be effective in suppressing MAC infection.[80] Twenty patients with disseminated MAC infection were treated with a combination of amikacin (as the sulfate salt) (15 mg/kg/day) i.v. and rifampin (600 mg/day), clofazimine (150–300 mg/day), ethambutol hydrochloride (15 mg/kg/day), and ciprofloxacin (as the hydrochloride salt) (750 mg b.i.d.) orally. Of 20 patients, 19 had what the investigators termed a "favorable clinical/microbiological response." One patient who did not receive amikacin remained bacteremic, whereas two patients developed bacteremia when amikacin therapy was discontinued on day 14 and day 30. Another patient receiving oral therapy remained bacteremic until amikacin therapy was started. Therapy with amikacin was continued for a mean of 45.3 ± 28.8 days. Severe ototoxicity (not defined) was reported in three patients after 60 days of therapy. The authors concluded that a prospective trial with a regimen containing amikacin was warranted.

Other Antimicrobials. A variety of mouse and human macrophage studies using rifamycin antimicrobials such as rifabutin,[81] rifapentine (Merrell Dow),[79] and liposomal rifampin[82] have also been done. These agents may prove to be useful in combination drug regimens. Clinical trials with rifabutin in the treatment of MAC infection may soon be under way.

Dapsone is an antileprosy drug, with little anti-MAC activity of its own. However, when dapsone is combined with other antifolate drugs such as sulfamethazine, synergistic in vitro activity against MAC infection has been observed.[63] The mechanism of this synergism and its relevance to therapy, though, remain to be determined.

Immunomodulators. Another approach to therapy includes the use of immunomodulators to enhance the immune response to MAC infection. It is believed that the secretion of certain cytokines such as tumor necrosis factor, gamma interferon, and interleukin-2 is impaired in patients with AIDS or in patients with disseminated MAC infection and may contribute to their lack of response to antimycobacterial therapy for MAC disease.[13,83,84] In studies using mouse-derived and human-derived macrophages under in vitro and in vivo conditions, enhanced killing has been demonstrated when therapy was supplemented with cytokines. Bermudez et al.[85] evaluated the effectiveness of recombinant tumor necrosis factor (rTNF), recombinant interferon gamma (rINF-γ), and recombinant interleukin-2 (rIL-2) in stimulating mouse and human macrophages before MAC infection and after infection had developed using two separate strains of MAC. In addition, the activity of macrophages activated in vivo by previous MAC infection was examined. Compared with controls, significant killing was achieved by macrophages that had been activated in vivo by a prior MAC infection and harvested from mice. To evaluate whether macrophages could be stimulated with cytokines before infection, rINF-γ, rIL-2, and rTNF were given singly or in combination to macrophages that were subsequently infected. Of the cytokines used alone, only rTNF was observed to effectively stimulate macrophages, producing significant killing of both MAC strains compared with controls. The combination of rIL-2 followed by rTNF (10^4 units/mL) was similarly effective in stimulating macrophages and producing killing. rTNF at a lower dose (10 units/mL) followed by rIL-2 was also very effective. The combination of rIFN-γ and rTNF was not found to be any more effective than rTNF alone.[85]

To determine whether immunotherapy would be beneficial after infection had already occurred, rTNF was added to macrophages 24 or 48 hours after their exposure to organisms, followed by incubation. It appeared that rTNF continued to kill MAC organisms for four days. Lower doses given on a daily basis for four days after infection also produced significant killing at all concentrations compared with controls. Despite the lack of efficacy of rINF-γ when given before MAC infection, macrophages given rINF-γ doses for two to seven days after infection were found to produce more intracellular killing than controls. However, it is believed that rINF-γ's mechanism of killing may be stimulation of the release of endogenous tumor necrosis factor by macrophages.[85]

To further test their results in vivo, Bermudez et al.[84] examined rIL-2 and rTNF in mice that had been infected with MAC. After infection was established, mice were treated daily with rIL-2, rTNF, or rIL-2 plus rTNF at half doses for 14 days. Because tumor necrosis factor is associated with hypotension and cachexia,[86] mice treated with rTNF were given a drug holiday every fourth day in an attempt to decrease toxicity. Both rTNF and rIL-2, alone and in combination, decreased CFUs in the blood. However, only rIL-2 plus rTNF decreased CFUs below those present before therapy was initiated. Similarly, reductions in CFUs in the liver and spleen were noted with each of the treatments. Although rTNF toxicity was difficult to assess, the authors stated that about 60% of the mice were unable to eat or had changes in their fur that indicated rTNF toxicity. Given that there was no mortality, however, the researchers believed that the dose of rTNF (25 μg/kg) given daily for three days, followed by a one-day drug holiday, was effective in alleviating rTNF toxicity.

Using human macrophages in vitro, Bermudez et al.[87] have also reported on the use of rTNF alone and in combination with antimicrobials. The anti-MAC activity of amikacin, roxithromycin (Hoechst-Roussel) and azithromycin (two investigational macrolides), and rTNF, alone and in combination, was compared with that of untreated controls in three separate experiments. In the first series, amikacin, azithromycin, roxithromycin, and rTNF were added to separate groups of infected macrophages immediately after infection and then washed out after 24 hours. Amikacin, roxithromycin, and azithromycin alone were initially inhibitory to MAC compared with untreated controls; however, regrowth of MAC was evident after 48 hours with all three drugs. rTNF, on the other hand, produced killing of the organisms that was continuous throughout the study period. When each of the agents was added on a daily basis, all were found to produce killing. When rTNF was combined with amikacin, roxithromycin, or azithromycin, significantly more killing was observed than with antimicrobial therapy alone in all cases. The three-drug combination of amikacin–roxithromycin–rTNF appeared to be most effective, with 91% killing.[87] In a separate study, rTNF combined with amikacin was given to beige mice and found to be more effective in reducing colony counts in blood and tissue than single-agent therapy, with greater bactericidal activity.[88]

Squires et al.[89] reported on the use of both natural and recombinant INF-γ in human monocytes and macrophages and beige mice with disappointing findings consistent with those of Bermudez et al.[84] In contrast to these findings, Squires et al. did report that two AIDS patients who had been treated for more than six months with at least three antimycobacterials and continued to have persistent mycobacteremia and positive bone marrow cultures were treated with rIFN-γ for four weeks in addition to their antimycobacterial therapy. Although bone marrow cultures remained positive in both patients after four weeks, mycobacteremia decreased within two weeks of treatment in one patient and continued to decline until therapy was discontinued. The second patient's mycobacteremia appeared to plateau with no progressive increases during the treatment period. Both patients had subsequent rises in mycobacteremia one month after rIFN-γ therapy was stopped. The authors remarked that exacerbation of disease by rIFN-γ could not be ruled out because of the increase in CFUs after therapy was stopped, but that in light of these findings and the poor response to conventional therapy, they were initiating a pilot study to define the role of rIFN-γ in the treatment of MAC infection.[89]

Such preliminary results make it difficult to draw conclusions regarding the place of immunomodulators in therapy. In theory, immunotherapy appears to be a logical approach to overcoming the immune defect in AIDS. Despite reports that some cytokines may actually be elevated in AIDS patients,[90] in vitro and in vivo results seem to indicate that supplementation with cytokines can influence the response to infection and that cytokines may enhance the effectiveness of antimicrobials. However, the toxicity of these agents when used for treatment remains undefined, and their true potential in overcoming immune system deficits in patients with AIDS is unclear. The majority of studies evaluating immunomodulators in MAC infection have used relatively immunocompetent models (e.g., human macrophages harvested from healthy donors) that may not be representative of the immune response in AIDS; however, other studies suggest that infection with HIV does not influence the ability of cells to be activated by cytokines.[83,91,92] Continued research in this area will help to clarify the role of these agents.

As evidenced by these and other results, many avenues of antimycobacterial therapy that have not been fully evaluated may hold promise. Both new and old agents are being identified that may have a place in therapy. Unless a method of overcoming the immune deficiency in AIDS is discovered, continued efforts to evaluate new combinations of antimycobacterial agents that are minimally toxic and more effective are essential to solving this treatment dilemma.

Conclusion

Definitive treatment for disseminated MAC infection has been a perplexing issue. The fact that no known therapy for MAC infection has been shown to prolong survival in AIDS patients is discouraging but may be more related to the point at which MAC disease is identified in patients. The poor clinical responses reported in many of the published studies on treatment of MAC infection in AIDS patients may be due to the low drug dosages used and the high organism load that exists once patients become symptomatic. Earlier recognition of infection or the prevention of colonization may be effective in decreasing the number of CFUs present in the body because it would allow therapy to be initiated before the mycobacterial burden becomes overwhelming. Current therapy may be successful in suppressing the infection in some patients. The decision to treat a patient should be based on the assessment of whether treatment would improve the patient's quality of life. In the HIV-infected population, antimicrobial prophylaxis may be justifiable to prevent colonization of the gut with MAC or to control pre-existing colonization or localized infection. Studies to examine the impact of prophylaxis are under way.

Research is needed to find improved methods for earlier detection of MAC infection, determine optimal dosage regimens of current antimycobacterial agents, develop antimycobacterial drug-delivery systems to enhance intracellular killing of mycobacteria (e.g., liposomes), and discover new antimicrobials with greater intrinsic activity against MAC and methods of immune modulation that will overcome immune system defects. Advances in these areas may make treatment of MAC disease more successful in the future.

References

1. Wolinski E. Nontuberculous mycobacteria and associated diseases. *Am Rev Respir Dis*. 1979; 119:107-59.
2. Young LS, Inderlied CB, Berlin OG et al. Mycobacterial infections in AIDS patients, with an emphasis on the *Mycobacterium avium* complex. *Rev Infect Dis*. 1986; 8:1024-33.
3. Selik RM, Starcher ET, Curran JW. Opportunistic diseases reported in AIDS patients: frequencies, associations, and trends. *AIDS*. 1987; 1:175-82.
4. Hawkins CC, Gold JWM, Whimbey E et al. *Mycobacterium avium* complex in patients with the acquired immunodeficiency syndrome. *Ann Intern Med*. 1986; 105:184-8.
5. Kiehn TE, Edwards FF, Brannon P et al. Infections caused by *Mycobacterium avium* complex in immunocompromised patients: diagnosis by blood culture and fecal examination, antimicrobial susceptibility tests, and morphological and seroagglutination characteristics. *J Clin Microbiol*. 1985; 21:168-73.
6. Wallace JM, Hannah JB. *Mycobacterium avium* complex infection in patients with the acquired immunodeficiency syndrome: a clinicopathologic study. *Chest*. 1988; 93:926-31.
7. Zakowski P, Fligiel S, Berlin OGW et al. Disseminated *Mycobacterium avium-intracellulare* infection in homosexual men dying of acquired immunodeficiency. *JAMA*. 1982; 248:2980-2.
8. Horsburgh CR, Mason UG III, Farhi DC et al. Disseminated infection with *Mycobacterium avium-intracellulare*: a report of 13 cases and a review of the literature. *Medicine*. 1985; 64:36-48.
9. Horsburgh CR, Cohn DL, Roberts RB et al. *Mycobacterium avium-M. intracellulare* isolates from patients with or without acquired immunodeficiency syndrome. *Antimicrob Agents Chemother*. 1986; 30:955-7.
10. Furio MM, Wordell CJ. Treatment of infectious complications of acquired immunodeficiency syndrome. *Clin Pharm*. 1985; 4:539-54.
11. Centers for Disease Control. Isolation of nontuberculous mycobacteria in the United States, 1980. *J Infect Dis*. 1982; 146:829-33.
12. Hampson SJ, Thompson J, Moss MT et al. DNA probes demonstrate a single highly conserved strain of *Mycobacterium avium* infecting AIDS patients. *Lancet*. 1989; 1:65-8.
13. Murray HW, Scavuzzo DA, Chaparas SD et al. T lymphocyte responses to mycobacterial antigen in AIDS patients with disseminated *Mycobacterium avium-Mycobacterium intracellulare* infection. *Chest*. 1988; 93:922-5.
14. Armstrong D, Gold JWM, Dryjanski J et al. Treatment of infections in patients with the acquired immunodeficiency syndrome. *Ann Intern Med*. 1985; 103:738-43.
15. Inderlied CB, Young LS, Yamada JK. Determination of in vitro susceptibility of *Mycobacterium avium* complex isolates to antimycobacterial agents by various methods. *Antimicrob Agents Chemother*. 1987; 31:1697-1702.
16. Guthertz LS, Damsker B, Bottone EJ et al. *Mycobacterium avium* and *Mycobacterium intracellulare* infections in patients with and without AIDS. *J Infect Dis*. 1989; 160:1037-41.
17. Crawford JT, Bates JH. Analysis of plasmids in *Mycobacterium avium-intracellulare* isolates from persons with acquired immunodeficiency syndrome. *Am Rev Respir Dis*. 1986; 134:659-61.
18. Gangadharam PRJ, Perumal VK, Crawford JT et al. Association of plasmids and virulence of *Mycobacterium avium* complex. *Am Rev Respir Dis*. 1988; 137:212-4.
19. Damsker B, Bottone EJ. *Mycobacterium avium-Mycobacterium intracellulare* from the intestinal tracts of patients with the acquired immunodeficiency syndrome: concepts regarding acquisition and pathogenesis. *J Infect Dis*. 1985; 151:179-81.
20. Stacey AR. Isolation of *Mycobacterium avium-intracellulare-scrofulaceum* complex from faeces of patients with AIDS. *Br Med J*. 1986; 293:1194.
21. Collins FM. Mycobacterial disease, immunosuppression, and acquired immunodeficiency syndrome. *Clin Microbiol Rev*. 1989; 2:360-77.
22. Horsburgh CR, Selik RM. The epidemiology of disseminated nontuberculous mycobacterial infection in the acquired immunodeficiency syndrome (AIDS). *Am Rev Respir Dis*. 1989; 139:4-7.
23. Roth RI, Owen RL, Keren DF et al. Intestinal infection with *Mycobacterium avium* in acquired immune deficiency syndrome (AIDS): histological and clinical comparison with Whipple's disease. *Dig Dis Sci*. 1985; 30:497-504.
24. Bessesen MT, Berry CD, Johnson MA et al. Site of origin of disseminated MAC infection in AIDS. Proceedings of the 30th Interscience Conference on Antimicrobial Agents and Chemotherapy. Atlanta, GA: 1990 Oct 21–24. Abstract 1268.
25. Young LS. AIDS commentary. *J Infect Dis*. 1988; 157:863-7.
26. Masur H, Ognibene FP, Yarchoan R et al. CD4 counts as predictors of opportunistic pneumonias in human immunodeficiency virus (HIV) infection. *Ann Intern Med*. 1989; 111:223-31.
27. Havlik JA, Horsburgh CR, Metchock B et al. Clinical risk factors for disseminated *Mycobacterium avium* complex infection (DMAC) in persons with HIV infection. Sixth International Conference on AIDS final program and abstracts. San Francisco, CA: 1990 Jun 20–24. Abstract Th.B. 515
28. Pitchenik AE, Fertel D, Bloch AB. Mycobacterial disease: epidemiology, diagnosis, treatment, and prevention. *Clin Chest Med*. 1988; 9:425-41.
29. Nyberg DA, Federle MP, Jeffrey RB et al. Abdominal CT findings of disseminated *Mycobacterium avium-intracellulare* in AIDS. *AJR*. 1985; 145:297-9.
30. Wong B, Edwards FF, Kiehn TE et al. Continuous high-grade *Mycobacterium avium-intracellulare* bacteremia in patients with the acquired immune deficiency syndrome. *Am J Med*. 1985; 78:35-40.
31. Damsker B, Bottone EJ. Mycobacteria and cryptococci cultured from the buffy coat of AIDS patients prior to symptomatology: a rationale for early therapy. *AIDS Res*. 1986; 2:343-8.
32. Drake TA, Hindler JA, Berlin OGW et al. Rapid identification of *Mycobacterium avium* complex in culture using DNA probes. *J Clin Microbiol*. 1987; 25:1442-5.
33. AHFS drug information 90. McEvoy GK, ed. Bethesda, MD: American Society of Hospital Pharmacists; 1990:56-7,340-8,403-13,442-6.
34. Mandell GL, Sande MA. Antimicrobial agents: drugs used in the chemotherapy of tuberculosis and leprosy. In: Goodman and Gilman's the pharmacological basis of therapeutics. 7th ed. Gilman AG, Goodman LS, Rall TW et al., eds. New York: Macmillan; 1985:1199-1218.
35. Baroni V, Foddai G, Lukinovich N et al. Clinical evaluation of intolerance to cycloserine. *Scand J Respir Dis [Suppl]*. 1970; 71:217-9.
36. Stephanopoulos C, Zoumbouloglou H. Clinical tolerance to cycloserine. *Scand J Respir Dis [Suppl]*. 1970; 71:235-8.
37. Tala E, Tevola K. Side effects and toxicity of ethionamide and prothionamide. *Ann Clin Res*. 1969; 1:32-5.
38. Wilson TM. Clinical experience with ethambutol. *Antibiot Chemother*. 1970; 16:222-9.
39. Miles Laboratories. Ciprofloxacin package insert. West Haven, CT; 1987 Oct.

40. Zaske DE, Shikuma LR, Tholl DA. Aminoglycosides. In: Taylor WJ, Diers Caviness MH, eds. A textbook for the clinical application of therapeutic drug monitoring. Irving, CA: Abbott Laboratories; 1986:285-320.
41. Masur H, Tuazon C, Gill V et al. Effect of combined clofazimine and ansamycin therapy on *Mycobacterium avium-Mycobacterium intracellulare* bacteremia in patients with AIDS. *J Infect Dis*. 1987; 155:127-9.
42. Agins BD, Berman DS, Spicehandler D et al. Effect of combined therapy with ansamycin, clofazimine, ethambutol, and isoniazid for *Mycobacterium avium* infection in patients with AIDS. *J Infect Dis*. 1989; 159:784-7.
43. Hoy J, Mijch A, Sandland M et al. Quadruple-drug therapy for *Mycobacterium avium-intracellulare* bacteremia in AIDS patients. *J Infect Dis*. 1990; 161:801-5.
44. Kemper CA, Chiu J, Meng TC et al. Microbiologic and clinical response of patients with AIDS and MAC bacteremia to a four oral drug regimen. Proceedings of the 30th Interscience Conference on Antimicrobial Agents and Chemotherapy. Atlanta, GA: 1990 Oct 21–24. Abstract 1267.
45. Baron EJ, Young LS. Amikacin, ethambutol, and rifampin for treatment of disseminated *Mycobacterium avium-intracellulare* infections in patients with acquired immune deficiency syndrome. *Diagn Microbiol Infect Dis*. 1986; 5:215-20.
46. American Thoracic Society. Mycobacterioses and the acquired immunodeficiency syndrome. *Am Rev Respir Dis*. 1987; 136:492-6.
47. Centers for Disease Control. Diagnosis and management of mycobacterial infection and disease in persons with human immunodeficiency virus infection. *Ann Intern Med*. 1987; 106:254-6.
48. National Consensus Conference on Tuberculosis. Disease due to *Mycobacterium avium-intracellulare*. *Chest*. 1985; 87(Suppl):139S-49S.
49. Bach MC. Treating disseminated *Mycobacterium avium-intracellulare* infection. *Ann Intern Med*. 1989; 110:169-70. Letter.
50. Helbert M, Robinson D, Buchanan D et al. Mycobacterial infection in patients infected with the human immunodeficiency virus. *Thorax*. 1990; 45:45-8.
51. Chiu J, Nussbaum J, Bozette S et al. Treatment of disseminated *Mycobacterium avium* complex infection in AIDS with amikacin, ethambutol, rifampin, and ciprofloxacin. *Ann Intern Med*. 1990; 113:358-61.
52. Inderlied CB, Young LS, Yamada JK. Determination of in vitro susceptibility of *Mycobacterium avium* complex isolates to antimycobacterial agents by various methods. *Antimicrob Agents Chemother*. 1987; 31:1697-1702.
53. Hoffner SE, Svenson SB, Kallenius G. Synergistic effects of antimycobacterial drug combinations on *Mycobacterium avium* complex determined radiometrically in liquid medium. *Eur J Clin Microbiol*. 1987; 6:530-5.
54. Yajko DM, Nassos PS, Hadley WK. Therapeutic implications of inhibition versus killing of *Mycobacterium avium* complex by antimicrobial agents. *Antimicrob Agents Chemother*. 1987; 31:117-20.
55. Ozenne G, Morel A, Menard JF et al. Susceptibility of *Mycobacterium avium* complex to various two-drug combinations of antituberculosis agents. *Am Rev Respir Dis*. 1988; 138:878-81.
56. Heifets LB, Iseman MD, Lindholm-Levy PJ. Determination of MIC's of conventional and experimental drugs in liquid medium by the radiometric method against *Mycobacterium avium* complex. *Drugs Exp Clin Res*. 1987; 9:529-38.
57. Gangadharam PR, Edwards CK III, Murthy PS et al. An acute infection model for *Mycobacterium intracellulare* disease using beige mice: preliminary results. *Am Rev Respir Dis*. 1983; 127:648-9.
58. Bertram MA, Inderlied CB, Yadegar S et al. Confirmation of the beige mouse model for study of disseminated infection with *Mycobacterium avium* complex. *J Infect Dis*. 1986; 154:194-5.
59. Gallin JI. Disorders of phagocytic cells. In: Harrison's principles of internal medicine. 11th ed. Braunwald E, Isselbacher KJ, eds. New York: McGraw-Hill, 1987:278-83.
60. Fernandes PB, Hardy DJ, McDaniel D et al. In vitro and in vivo activities of clarithromycin against *Mycobacterium avium*. *Antimicrob Agents Chemother*. 1989; 33:1531-4.
61. Naik S, Ruck R. In vitro activities of several new macrolide antibiotics against *Mycobacterium avium* complex. *Antimicrob Agents Chemother*. 1989; 33:1614-6.
62. Inderlied CB, Kolonoski PT, Wu M et al. In vitro and in vivo activity of azithromycin (CP 62,993) against the *Mycobacterium avium* complex. *J Infect Dis*. 1989; 159:994-7.
63. Gonzalez AH, Berlin OGW, Bruckner DA. In-vitro activity of dapsone and two potentiators against *Mycobacterium avium* complex. *Antimicrob Agents Chemother*. 1989; 24:19-22.
64. Dautzenberg B, Legris S, Truffot C, Mehoyas MC et al. Clarithromycin clears *Mycobacterium avium-intracellulare* (MAIC) from blood of AIDS patients. A randomized trial. Proceedings of the 30th Interscience Conference on Antimicrobial Agents and Chemotherapy. Atlanta, GA: 1990 Oct 21–24. Abstract 1264.
65. Prokocimer P, Dellerson M, Craft C et al. Effect of clarithromycin on blood cultures positive for *Mycobacterium avium* complex (MAC) in HIV+ patients. Proceedings of the 30th Interscience Conference on Antimicrobial Agents and Chemotherapy. Atlanta, GA: 1990 Oct 21–24. Abstract 634.
66. Fenlon CH, Cynamon MH. Comparative in vitro activities of ciprofloxacin and other 4-quinolones against *Mycobacterium tuberculosis* and *Mycobacterium intracellulare*. *Antimicrob Agents Chemother*. 1986; 29:386-8.
67. Heifets LB, Lindholm-Levy PJ. Bacteriostatic and bactericidal activity of ciprofloxacin and ofloxacin against *Mycobacterium tuberculosis* and *Mycobacterium avium* complex. *Tubercle*. 1987; 68:267-76.
68. Young LS, Berlin OGW, Inderlied CB. Activity of ciprofloxacin and other fluorinated quinolones against mycobacteria. *Am J Med*. 1987; 82(Suppl 4A):S23-6.
69. Johnson SM, Roberts GD. In vitro activity of ciprofloxacin and ofloxacin against the *Mycobacterium avium-intracellulare* complex. *Diagn Microbiol Infect Dis*. 1987; 7:89-91.
70. Easmon CSF, Crane JP. Uptake of ciprofloxacin by macrophages. *J Clin Pathol*. 1985; 35:442-4.
71. Hoffner SE, Kratz M, Olsson-Liljequist B et al. In-vitro synergistic activity between ethambutol and fluorinated quinolones against *Mycobacterim avium* complex. *Antimicrob Agents Chemother*. 1989; 24:317-24.
72. Yajko DM, Nassos PS, Sanders CA et al. Killing by antimycobacterial agents of AIDS-derived strains of *Mycobacterium avium* complex inside cells of the mouse macrophage cell line J774. *Am Rev Respir Dis*. 1989; 140:1198-203.
73. Khardori H, Rolston K, Tosenbaum B et al. In vitro activity of quinolones against *Mycobacterium avium-Mycobacterium intracellulare*. *Rev Infect Dis*. 1989; 2(Suppl 5):S987-8.
74. Kolonoski PT, Wu M, Inderlied CB et al. Therapeutic efficacy of WIN 57273 and sparfloxacin for disseminated *Mycobacterium avium* complex (MAC) infection in beige mice. Proceedings of the 30th Interscience Conference on Antimicrobial Agents and Chemotherapy. Atlanta, GA: 1990 Oct 21–24. Abstract 1247.
75. Gangadharam PR, Perumal VK, Podapati PNR et al. In vivo activity of amikacin alone or in combination with clofazimine or rifabutin or both against acute experimental *Mycobacterium avium* complex infections in beige mice. *Antimicrob Agents Chemother*. 1988; 32:1400-3.
76. Inderlied CB, Kolonoski PT, Wu M et al. Amikacin, ciprofloxacin, and imipenem treatment for disseminated *Mycobacterium avium* complex infection of beige mice. *Antimicrob Agents Chemother*. 1989; 33:176-80.
77. Cynamon MH, Swenson CE, Palmer GS et al. Liposome-encapsulated amikacin therapy of *Mycobacterium avium* complex infection in beige mice. *Antimicrob Agents Chemother*. 1989; 33:1179-83.
78. Bermudez LE, Yau-Young AO, Lin JP et al. Treatment of disseminated *Mycobacterium avium* complex infection of beige mice with liposome-encapsulated aminoglycosides. *J Infect*

Dis. 1990; 161:1262-8.
79. Bermudez LEM, Wu M, Young LS. Intracellular killing of *Mycobacterium avium* complex by rifapentine and liposome-encapsulated amikacin. *J Infect Dis*. 1987; 156:510-3.
80. Benson C, Pottage J, Kessler H. Treatment of AIDS-related disseminated *Mycobacterium avium* complex disease (D-MAC) with a multiple drug regimen including amikacin. Sixth International Conference on AIDS final program and abstracts. San Francisco, CA: 1990 Jun 20–24. Abstract. Th.B 517.
81. Saito H, Sato K. Activity of rifabutin alone and in combination with clofazimine, kanamycin and ethambutol against *Mycobacterium intracellulare* infections in mice. *Tubercle*. 1989; 70:201-5.
82. Saito H, Tomioka H. Therapeutic efficacy of liposome-entrapped rifampin against *Mycobacterium avium* complex infection induced in mice. *Antimicrob Agents Chemother*. 1989; 33:429-33.
83. Murray HW, Rubin BY, Masur H et al. Impaired production of lymphokines and immune (gamma) interferon in the acquired immunodeficiency syndrome. *N Engl J Med*. 1984; 310:883-9.
84. Bermudez LEM, Stevens P, Kolonoski P et al. Treatment of experimental disseminated *Mycobacterium avium* complex infection in mice with recombinant IL-2 and tumor necrosis factor. *J Immunol*. 1989; 143:2996-3000.
85. Bermudez LEM, Young LS. Tumor necrosis factor, alone or in combination with IL-2, but not INF-γ, is associated with macrophage killing of *Mycobacterium avium* complex. *J Immunol*. 1988; 140:3006-13.
86. Oliff A. The role of tumor necrosis factor (cachectin) in cachexia. *Cell*. 1988; 54:141-2.
87. Bermudez LEM, Young LS. Activities of amikacin, roxithromycin, and azithromycin alone or in combination with tumor necrosis factor against *Mycobacterium avium* complex. *Antimicrob Agents Chemother*. 1988; 32:1149-53.
88. Bermudez LE, Petrofsky M, Kolonoski P et al. Amikacin plus tumor necrosis factor (TNF) for treatment of *Mycobacterium avium* complex (MAC) infection in beige mice. Proceedings of the 30th Interscience Conference on Antimicrobial Agents and Chemotherapy. Atlanta, GA: 1990 Oct 21–24. Abstract 1266.
89. Squires KE, Murphy WF, Madoff LC et al. Interferon-γ and *Mycobacterium avium-intracellulare* infection. *J Infect Dis*. 1989; 159:599-600.
90. Lahdevirta J, Maury CPJ, Teppo AJ et al. Elevated levels of circulating cachectin/tumor necrosis factor in patients with acquired immunodeficiency syndrome. *Am J Med*. 1988; 85:289-91.
91. Murray HW, Gellene RA, Libby DM et al. Activation of tissue macrophages from AIDS patients: in vitro response of AIDS alveolar macrophages to lymphokines and interferon-γ. *J Immunol*. 1985; 135:2374-7.
92. Murray HW, Scavuzzo D, Jacobs JL et al. In vitro and in vivo activation of human mononuclear phagocytes by interferon-γ. *J Immunol*. 1987; 138:2457-62.

Drug Experience

Straightforward reports of unusual drug experiences are included in this section. These may be confirmations of previously reported drug experiences or brief apparent first reports. While selected references may be cited, the purpose of a Drug Experience *report is not to present an extensive review of the literature.*

A related section, Grand Rounds, *includes papers that are well-documented patient case reports with a thorough review of the important literature to help put the case in perspective.*

Continuous subcutaneous infusion of terbutaline for suppression of preterm labor

JANET R. FISCHER AND BRIAN L. KAATZ

Clin Pharm. 1991; 10:292-6

Prematurity continues to be a major cause of morbidity and mortality in the newborn. The incidence of preterm delivery (generally defined as birth before 37 weeks of gestation) has remained fairly stable over the past 35 years, despite improvements in screening techniques, diagnosis, and treatment.[1] Currently, 10% of births in the United States are premature.[2] There is evidence that prematurity, in addition to frequently necessitating expensive stays in the intensive-care nursery (ICN), contributes to mental retardation and other neurological deficits.[3]

Several causes of preterm delivery have been identified, but 25–50% of such births are due to preterm labor alone.[4] For the past 15 years, various drugs have been safely and effectively used to prevent preterm labor, including magnesium sulfate and the β-sympathomimetic agents ritodrine hydrochloride and terbutaline sulfate.[5,6] Ritodrine is currently the only agent with FDA-approved labeling for use in the treatment of preterm labor, but many practitioners use terbutaline because of its lower cost and documented efficacy.[7-9] Indomethacin and nifedipine have also been used to treat preterm labor but are considered second-line agents because of their potential adverse effects and need for further evaluation in clinical trials.[6,10,11] Several oral magnesium salts have also been administered, but results are preliminary; their use is considered experimental.[12]

Currently, β-sympathomimetic agents are considered the drugs of choice for the treatment and prevention of preterm labor.[6] However, their use has been complicated by troubling adverse effects and problems with long-term effectiveness.[6-9,13] Studies addressing the issue of tocolytic efficacy have shown that 25–50% of patients maintained with long-term oral terbutaline sulfate have a recurrence of preterm labor and that 30% of preterm deliveries in women receiving prenatal care are a result of failure of attempted tocolytic therapy.[8,13,14]

Because of these limitations of standard tocolytic therapy, researchers and clinicians are investigating alternative treatment modalities. A new and promising therapy is continuous subcutaneous infusion of low-dose terbutaline sulfate. Two studies have shown terbutaline infusion-pump therapy to be significantly more effective than oral terbutaline, with improved prolongation of pregnancy, decreased recurrence of preterm labor, and reduced ICN admissions.[14,15]

This paper describes our experiences in using continuous subcutaneous terbutaline infusion to treat cases of preterm labor at a private community hospital.

Patient Eligibility. Candidates for the study were between weeks 20 and 35 of pregnancy and had an established diagnosis of preterm labor based on the presence of uterine contractions (two in a 10-minute period or more than four in one hour) and one of the following findings: progressive effacement or dilation of the internal os, cervical dilation of 2 cm, and 75% effacement. Candidates also had to have intact uterine membranes, cervical dilation of less than 4 cm, and stabilization of contraction patterns before the start of terbutaline infusion. Contraindications to terbutaline treatment included a nonreassuring fetal heart rate pattern, significant maternal electrocardiographic changes due to therapy with intravenous β-sympa-

JANET R. FISCHER, PHARM.D., is Assistant Professor, Department of Clinical Pharmacy, College of Pharmacy, South Dakota State University (SDSU), Brookings, and Clinical Pharmacist, Sioux Valley Hospital, Sioux Falls, SD. BRIAN L. KAATZ, PHARM.D., is Associate Professor and Head, Department of Clinical Pharmacy, College of Pharmacy, SDSU.

Address reprint requests to Dr. Fischer at the Department of Pharmaceutical Services, Sioux Valley Hospital, 1100 S. Euclid Avenue, Sioux Falls, SD 57117-5039.

The assistance of Teresa Buell, M.S.N.; Cindy Schuttler; and the physicians of the Department of Obstetrics and Gynecology, Sioux Valley Hospital, is acknowledged.

Presented at the 24th Annual ASHP Midyear Clinical Meeting, Atlanta, GA, December 7, 1989.

thomimetic drugs, abruptio placentae, and progressive pre-eclampsia. The decision to use the terbutaline pump rather than other forms of tocolytic therapy was made by the attending physicians. Patients with preterm labor that was judged to be more progressive based on the degree of cervical dilation, the frequency of contractions, and the lack of a response to previously used β-sympathomimetic agents were stabilized with intravenous magnesium sulfate before terbutaline infusion-pump therapy began. Patients who were judged by their physicians to have less severe preterm labor began terbutaline therapy directly.

Infusion Method. The continuous subcutaneous administration of terbutaline was accomplished with portable infusion pumps (model 404-S, MiniMed Technologies, Sylmar, CA). This pump allows a continuous basal rate of infusion to be programmed, as well as scheduled bolus doses. In addition, it permits nonscheduled bolus doses to be given as needed for sudden changes in contraction patterns. The pump was used with specially adapted 3-mL Luer-Lok syringes (3 mg of terbutaline sulfate per 3 mL) prepared by the pharmacy department. The terbutaline was administered through a bent needle placed subcutaneously in the abdomen or thigh. The tubing between the pump and the needle was long enough to enable the patient to carry the pump in a pocket.

Inpatient Therapy. Therapy was started in the hospital with a continuous subcutaneous infusion of terbutaline sulfate, usually at the rate of 0.05 mg/hr, to maintain general relaxation in the tone of the uterine wall. A bolus dose of 0.25 mg was given over 10 minutes at the beginning of the infusion to promote a rapid therapeutic effect. The infusion rate had to be increased in a few patients to control basal uterine activity. Regularly scheduled bolus doses of 0.25 mg were used in some patients, depending on uterine contraction patterns. Additional nonscheduled bolus doses were given as needed if a patient experienced two contractions in a 10-minute period or more than four contractions in 60 minutes. If a patient was receiving intravenous magnesium sulfate, it was tapered off during the first hour of terbutaline pump therapy. Contraction patterns, fetal heart rates, and maternal heart rates were monitored during the first 48 hours of terbutaline therapy and as needed thereafter. Maternal heart rates were also checked when any nonscheduled bolus doses were given. Terbutaline syringes were changed daily, usually in the evening to ensure an adequate supply of drug overnight. Injection sites were varied every three or four days. Standard nonpharmacologic measures, such as bed rest, were part of the therapeutic regimen.

Home Therapy. Once the terbutaline infusion-pump therapy was established, the patients were given extensive instructions on how to program the pump, change the batteries, load the syringes, change the tubing, and care for and change the injection sites. The potential adverse effects of terbutaline were reviewed, and each patient was instructed to evaluate her heart rate when giving additional bolus doses. Uterine self-palpation was taught as a method for detecting contractions. Twice a day the patients palpated the abdomen with both hands for an hour at a time to try to detect uterine tightening. Self-palpation was also done for an hour whenever the patients felt contractions. While the patients practiced this technique, nurses used a uterine monitor to evaluate their success. Once the contractions had been adequately controlled with the pump and training was complete, the patients were discharged from the hospital. Most of the patients were hospitalized for three to five days before going home with the pump. Follow-up care included weekly appointments with physicians, daily telephone calls from a perinatal nurse clinician, and home visits as needed. The patients were instructed to telephone their physicians if they noted a persistently increased contraction rate or a heart rate above 110 beats/min.

Goals of Therapy. The goals of the continuous subcutaneous terbutaline therapy were to stop labor, suppress contractions, and prolong gestation to term. Because of the nature of preterm labor, success was determined on an individual basis. In general, treatment was considered successful if contractions were suppressed and delivery was delayed by at least one week, ideally to 36 weeks. However, any prolongation of pregnancy judged by the attending physician to allow for substantially improved neonatal viability was also considered to represent a successful outcome.

Results. During a 12-month period, continuous subcutaneous infusions of terbutaline were given to 19 patients, two of whom bore twins. Details on the individual cases are reported in Table 1.

Prolongation of Pregnancy. In 14 (74%) of the 19 patients, the terbutaline pump therapy successfully terminated labor and prolonged pregnancy. Eleven patients delivered infants with gestational ages of more than 36 weeks. (In one of these women [patient 3], terbutaline therapy was stopped after one day because of adverse effects. Although her pregnancy was prolonged by other means for 25 days [gestational age at delivery, 36.9 weeks], the outcome was not considered a terbutaline-associated success.) Four patients (nos. 1, 10, 12, and 14) who gave birth between weeks 34 and 36 were also judged by their physicians to have responded successfully.

In the successful cases, pregnancy was prolonged by a mean ± S.D. of 43 ± 27 days, the mean ± S.D. gestational age of infants at delivery was 36.9 ± 1.3 weeks, and the mean birth weight was 2.96 ± 0.55 kg. The modes of Apgar scores in successful cases were 8 and 9 (out of a possible maximum score of 10) at one and five minutes, respectively.

Of the 15 babies delivered in the successful cases (including one set of twins), 6 required admission to the ICN. Four were admitted because of respiratory distress, one because of sepsis and meningitis, and one for observation because the mother was diabetic.

Table 1.
Efficacy of Continuous Subcutaneous Infusion of Terbutaline Sulfate in Patients in Preterm Labor[a]

Patient	Maternal Age (yr)	Final Dosage (mg/hr)	Duration of Infusion (days)	Gestational Age at Start of Infusion (wk)	Gestational Age at Delivery (wk)	Weight of Infant (kg)	Apgar Scores (1 min/5 min)[b]
1	25	0.05[c]	16	33 1/7	35 3/7	2.64	8/9[d]
2	32	0.05[c]	19	34 4/7	37 6/7	2.92	8/9
3	21	0.05[c]	1	33 2/7	36 6/7	3.15	9/9[d]
4	26	0.05[c]	71	26 6/7	37 1/7	3.54	9/9
5	22	0.05	24	30	38 5/7	3.32	8/9
6	37	0.07	4	31 6/7	32 3/7	1.91	1/7[d]
7	29	0.05[c]	32	32 1/7	36 6/7	3.80	8/9
8	27	0.09[c,e]	6	30 1/7	31	1.58	8/9[d]
						1.35	6/7[d]
9	23	0.05[c]	72	26 1/7	36 3/7	2.27	8/10
10	31	0.01[c,f]	78	24 5/7	35 5/7	1.94	8/9[d]
						2.07	8/9[d]
11	36	0.05	1	32 1/7	32 3/7	1.73	8/8[d]
12	34	0.12[c]	18	33 1/7	35 5/7	2.82	8/9[d]
13	25	0.05	19	32 2/7	37 5/7	2.38	8/8
14	32	0.08[c]	91	21	34	2.64	8/9[d]
15	22	0.08[c,g]	5	23	23 5/7	0.60	3/6[d]
16	20	0.05[c]	17	34 3/7	37	3.01	7/8[d]
17	31	0.06[c]	39	33	38 4/7	3.35	8/9
18	31	0.09[c]	22	34	37 3/7	3.09	9/9
19	33	0.07[c,e]	13	34 5/7	36 4/7	3.66	7/8
Mean ± S.D.	28 ± 5	0.07 ± 0.02	29 ± 28	30.6 ± 4.1	35.6 ± 3.6	2.56 ± 0.84	

[a] All the patients received an initial bolus dose of terbutaline sulfate 0.25 mg. For all but three patients, the initial basal rate of terbutaline sulfate infusion was 0.05 mg/hr.
[b] Apgar scores are usually determined one and five minutes after birth. The highest score, representing the best status, is 10.
[c] Patient received scheduled or as-needed bolus doses of terbutaline sulfate 0.25 mg.
[d] Infant admitted to intensive-care nursery.
[e] Initial basal rate of terbutaline sulfate infusion was 0.07 mg/hr.
[f] Patient received terbutaline sulfate at the rate of 0.05 mg/hr for 41 days, 0.09 mg/hr for 27 days, and 0.1 mg/hr for 10 days.
[g] Initial basal rate of terbutaline sulfate infusion was 0.08 mg/hr.

None of the babies required assisted ventilation, and their mean length of stay in the ICN was 10 days.

In six patients, contraction patterns had to be stabilized with intravenous magnesium sulfate before terbutaline infusion-pump therapy could begin. Three of these women had not responded to previous attempts at tocolysis with intravenous ritodrine, oral terbutaline, and oral magnesium oxide. Five patients began infusion-pump therapy after failing to respond to one or more other tocolytic modalities, including intravenous magnesium sulfate, oral magnesium oxide, intermittent subcutaneous terbutaline, and oral terbutaline. Three patients began using the terbutaline pump without receiving any prior treatment.

The highest dosage delivered in the short term was terbutaline sulfate 3.16 mg/day for two days in a patient (no. 7) who was having breakthrough contractions. The pump therapy was subsequently discontinued for 24 hours, and intravenous terbutaline was used to control the contractions. Therapy with the pump was then resumed, and the patient was well controlled with 2.2 mg/day. The patient had not received intravenous magnesium sulfate before pump therapy began, which probably contributed to the initial difficulty in controlling her contractions.

The highest dosage that was used on a sustained basis was 2.88 mg/day for 14 days in a patient (no. 12) who also had gestational diabetes. In this case, the physician chose to increase the basal infusion rate (rather than give bolus doses) so that the dosage of insulin needed to manage the hyperglycemic effect of the terbutaline could be more easily adjusted.

Two patients (nos. 10 and 18) developed breakthrough contractions that necessitated a short course of treatment with intravenous magnesium sulfate. Suspending terbutaline pump therapy for 24 hours and administering magnesium sulfate allowed both patients to resume pump therapy, which then provided good control of contractions.

Four patients received a short course of indomethacin while using the terbutaline pump. In two of these patients (nos. 2 and 7), the indomethacin was given at the beginning of pump therapy to help control the contraction pattern. In the other two patients (nos. 10 and 12), the indomethacin was used during pump therapy to help avoid increasing the terbutaline dosage.

Home Infusion. Of the 14 patients in whom continuous subcutaneous terbutaline therapy was eventually successful, 11 were discharged and continued to use the pump at home until delivery. Two patients (nos. 14 and 18) were kept in the hospital for the remainder of their pregnancy because of the precariousness of their condition. One of these had experienced premature rupture of the uterine membranes, and the other had a very incompetent cervix. A third patient (no. 16) remained hospitalized, awaiting a decision on whether Medicaid would pay for use of the pump at home. Payment was refused, and an attempt was made to switch the patient to oral terbutaline therapy. The patient was noncompliant with the therapy, however, and gave birth the day after pump therapy was discontinued.

Unsuccessful Outcomes. Five (26%) of the 19 women did not respond or had an inadequate response to continuous subcutaneous infusion of terbutaline. Three of these patients had had acute vaginal bleeding and therefore were poor candidates for any form of tocolysis. In two of the five patients (nos. 8 and 11), including one insulin-dependent diabetic, contractions persisted despite the use of both intravenous magnesium sulfate and intermittent subcutaneous terbutaline. One of these women was also given intravenous terbutaline, without success. The failure of intravenous agents in these cases makes it unlikely that the lack of efficacy of the terbutaline pump was due to the subcutaneous route of administration. Two patients (nos. 6 and 15), both of whom had vaginal bleeding, required emergency cesarean sections due to abruptio placentae and acute cord prolapse. Patient 3 had troublesome adverse effects, including heart palpitations, diaphoresis, and hypertension, necessitating stopping the terbutaline pump. The babies born to all five of these patients were admitted to the ICN.

Adverse Effects. Other than patient 3, whose adverse effects are described above, two patients reported adverse effects while receiving the infusion. One patient reported a single episode of chest pain, believed to have been due either to the drug or to anxiety. Her dosage was not altered, and she had no further problems. A second patient reported lightheadedness and flushing after her first bolus dose of terbutaline at the beginning of therapy. She had no further symptoms, however, despite receiving additional bolus doses and having a relatively high basal rate of terbutaline infusion. In addition, this patient had gestational diabetes, and her insulin requirements increased as her basal rate of terbutaline infusion was increased. Her blood glucose level was maintained within an acceptable range by avoiding bolus doses as much as possible.

Discussion. One of the main difficulties with current methods of treating preterm labor is the maintenance of prolonged contraction-free periods after the initial cessation of labor. Numerous studies have documented the efficacy of ritodrine and terbutaline in halting labor, but few demonstrate long-term suppression, typically regarded as the attainment of 36 or 37 weeks of gestation.[5]

A leading theory to explain the lack of long-term effectiveness of tocolytic therapy with β-sympathomimetics is desensitization of the β-adrenergic receptors in the myometrium. Several studies in animals and humans have documented the development of tolerance to the metabolic and cardiovascular effects of β-receptor agonists.[16,17] Such tolerance also occurs in myometrial tissue and may be due to decreased density of β-receptors or increased activity of phosphodiesterase.[18,19] Myometrial tolerance develops most rapidly with the continuous intravenous infusion of β sympathomimetics or with intermittent administration of long-acting β-agonists such as ritodrine. In contrast, intermittent administration of the short-acting agent isoproterenol prevents desensitization.[20,21] Thus it seems that tolerance is influenced by both the duration and the extent of exposure of the β-receptors to the β-agonist.

Adverse effects are another problem commonly seen with β-sympathomimetics. A wide variety of metabolic and cardiovascular effects have been reported in both mother and baby.[5] Common reactions are maternal hyperglycemia, tachycardia, hypotension, tremor, palpitations, nervousness, and headache. Fetal tachycardia is also frequently noted. Adverse-effect incidences as high as 65% have been reported for intravenous β-agonist tocolytics.[7,9] The incidence of adverse effects associated with oral therapy has not been well documented, but dosages are usually two to eight times higher than those used for bronchospasm and so are also likely to cause reactions that may interfere with compliance.

The dilemma is thus one of finding a way of using these highly effective tocolytic agents such that efficacy and ease of administration are maintained while adverse effects and tolerance are minimized. Continuous low-dose subcutaneous terbutaline seems to answer all these needs.

Two studies have been done to compare the long-term tocolytic efficacy of oral terbutaline with that of continuously infused subcutaneous terbutaline. In one study, 68 patients in preterm labor were randomly assigned to receive oral terbutaline or terbutaline infusion-pump therapy.[14] Pump therapy prolonged pregnancy 8.6 weeks on average, and premature labor recurred in less than 20% of the women. Oral terbutaline prolonged pregnancy for an average of only 2.4 weeks, and the rate of recurrence was 90%. Overall, 93% of the patients reached the goal of 36 weeks of pregnancy, compared with 34% given oral therapy. In the second study, which involved 1556 patients, use of the terbutaline pump in patients with recurrent preterm labor reduced the overall frequency of preterm delivery from 5.18% to 2.69%.[15] In addition, pump therapy reduced ICN admissions by 40%. Thus it appears that terbutaline given by continuous subcutaneous infusion is more effective than oral terbutaline for long-term management of preterm labor.

Several theories have been proposed to explain the effectiveness of terbutaline pump therapy. One theory involves the type of uterine activity seen in patients in preterm labor. Most patients not only have full, organized, high-amplitude contractions of labor but also high-frequency, low-amplitude waves of uterine irritability that may be precursors to full uterine contractions.[22] Studies of terbutaline pump therapy have shown that the low-dose continuous basal infusion suppresses this uterine irritability and that bolus doses interrupt most breakthrough high-amplitude uterine contractions that do occur.[23,24] Thus the combination of a low basal infusion rate and bolus doses effectively suppresses labor with very small total daily doses.

A closely related theory is based on the low dosage delivered by the pump. Since the total daily dose rarely exceeds 3 mg, it is believed that there should be fewer problems with down-regulation of β-receptors.[24] Indeed, this may be true, since less breakthrough labor has occurred with pump therapy. Also, the relatively low incidence of adverse effects seen with such low doses may produce better compliance than that seen with oral terbutaline.

Finally, terbutaline infusion-pump therapy may be superior because it allows greater individualization of therapy.[23] Most patients with preterm labor have regular, predictable times during the day when uterine activity is increased. Most of the increased activity occurs in the evening, but the timing can vary from patient to patient. By charting a patient's uterine contractions, the times of heightened activity can be identified and bolus doses can be scheduled to suppress these contractions. Thus the amount of drug administered matches the patient's changing needs.

Our findings confirm that continuous subcutaneous infusion of terbutaline can successfully treat preterm labor and that home therapy is feasible. Patient acceptance of the infusion pump has been excellent, and our success rate in achieving delivery beyond 34 weeks of gestation has been more than 70%.

Conclusion. Continuous subcutaneous infusion of terbutaline appears to be safe and effective in the treatment of preterm labor and can be self-administered at home.

References

1. Main DM. The epidemiology of preterm birth. *Clin Obstet Gynecol.* 1988; 31:521-32.
2. National Center for Health Statistics. Advance report of final natality statistics, 1987. Hyattsville, MD: National Center for Health Statistics, 1989; PHS publication no. 89-1120.
3. Behrman RE. The field of neonatal–perinatal medicine and neonatal risk. In: Fanaroff AA, Martin RJ, eds. Neonatal–perinatal medicine. 4th ed. St. Louis: Mosby; 1987:1-7.
4. Meis PJ, MacErnest J, Moore ML. Causes of low birthweight births in public and private patients. *Am J Obstet Gynecol.* 1987; 156:1165-8.
5. Souney PF, Kaul AF, Osathanondh R. Pharmacotherapy of preterm labor. *Clin Pharm.* 1983; 2:29-44.
6. Caritis SN, Darby MJ, Chan L. Pharmacologic treatment of preterm labor. *Clin Obstet Gynecol.* 1988; 31:635-51.
7. Beall MH, Edgar BW, Paul RH et al. A comparison of ritodrine, terbutaline, and magnesium sulfate for the suppression of preterm labor. *Am J Obstet Gynecol.* 1985; 153:854-9.
8. Brown SM, Tejani NA. Terbutaline sulfate in the prevention of recurrence of premature labor. *Obstet Gynecol.* 1981; 57:22-5.
9. Caritis SN, Toig G, Heddinger LA et al. A double blind study comparing ritodrine and terbutaline in the treatment of preterm labor. *Am J Obstet Gynecol.* 1984; 150:7-14.
10. Gerson A, Abbasi S, Johnson A et al. Safety and efficacy of long term tocolysis with indomethacin. *Am J Perinatol.* 1990; 7:71-4.
11. Read MD, Welby DE. The use of a calcium antagonist (nifedipine) to suppress preterm labour. *Br J Obstet Gynaecol.* 1986; 93:933-9.
12. Martin RW, Gaddy DK, Martin JN et al. Tocolysis with oral magnesium. *Am J Obstet Gynecol.* 1987; 156:433-4.
13. Main DM, Gabbe SG, Richardson D et al. Can preterm deliveries be prevented? *Am J Obstet Gynecol.* 1985; 151:892-8.
14. Lam F, Gill PJ, Smith M et al. Comparison of portable subcutaneous terbutaline pump and oral terbutaline treatment for long term tocolysis: a randomized clinical trial. Paper presented at Eighth Annual Meeting of the Society of Perinatal Obstetricians. Las Vegas, NV: 1988 Feb 5.
15. Lam F, Graves WK, Peacock WG et al. The impact of portable tocodynamometry and subcutaneous terbutaline pump therapy on preterm birth in a private obstetrical practice. Paper presented at American College of Obstetricians and Gynecologists Districts VIII and IX Meeting. Las Vegas, NV: 1987 Sep 2.
16. Harden TK. Agonist-induced desensitization of the β-adrenergic receptor-linked adenylate cyclase. *Pharmacol Rev.* 1983; 35:5-32.
17. Fredholm BB, Lunell NO, Persson B et al. Development of tolerance to the metabolic actions of β_2-adrenoceptor stimulating drugs. *Acta Obstet Gynecol Scand Suppl.* 1982; 108:53-9.
18. Berg G, Andersson RG, Ryden G. β-Adrenergic receptors in human myometrium during pregnancy: changes in the number of receptors after β-mimetic treatment. *Am J Obstet Gynecol.* 1985; 151:392-6.
19. Ryden G, Andersson RG, Berg G. Is the relaxing effect of β-adrenergic agonists on the human myometrium only transitory? *Acta Obstet Gynecol Scand Suppl.* 1982; 108:47-51.
20. Casper RF, Lye SJ. Myometrial desensitization to continuous but not to intermittent β-adrenergic agonist infusion in the sheep. *Am J Obstet Gynecol.* 1986; 154:301-5.
21. Ke R, Vohra M, Casper R. Prolonged inhibition of human myometrial contractility by intermittent isoproterenol. *Am J Obstet Gynecol.* 1984; 149:841-4.
22. Creasy RK. Preterm labor and delivery. In: Creasy RK, Resnik R, eds. Maternal–fetal medicine: principles and practice. Philadelphia: Saunders; 1989: 477-504.
23. Lam F, Gill P, Smith M et al. Use of the subcutaneous terbutaline pump for long term tocolysis. *Obstet Gynecol.* 1988; 72:810-3.
24. Sala DJ, Moise KJ. The treatment of preterm labor using a portable subcutaneous terbutaline pump. *J Obstet Gynecol Neonatal Nurs.* 1990; 19:108-15.

Vancomycin half-life in a patient with hepatic and renal dysfunction

ROBERT E. PACHOREK AND FREDERICK WOOD

Clin Pharm. 1991; 10:297-300

Recent studies in both healthy and seriously ill humans indicate that the renal component of vancomycin clearance is in the range of 70–94%.[1-3] The correlation of vancomycin clearance with creatinine clearance is sufficient to justify basing initial empirical dosage guidelines on estimated or measured creatinine clearance and body weight.[4-6]

Equations involving the patient's age, serum creatinine concentration, sex, and weight as variables have been useful in estimating creatinine clearance in many patients.[7-9] However, in patients with certain conditions (e.g., liver dysfunction, obesity, and malnutrition), estimates of creatinine clearance may be unreliable.[8-12] In some patients with severe liver disease, even the measured 24-hour creatinine clearance may provide an inaccurate estimate of the glomerular filtration rate (GFR).[13,14]

Empirical adjustment of vancomycin dosage because of hepatic disease is generally not deemed necessary.[2,4,15] Few reports suggest that hepatic clearance accounts for a substantial portion of the nonrenal clearance of vancomycin.[16,17]

The following case report describes a patient with acute bacterial endocarditis, liver dysfunction, and renal dysfunction whose vancomycin clearance was disproportionately low relative to estimated and measured creatinine clearances.

Case Report. A 77-year-old man with a history of mitral and aortic stenosis, chronic atrial fibrillation, bacterial endocarditis, and cirrhosis was admitted to the hospital in May 1988 after the sudden onset of fever, chills, and confusion. He had developed acute bacterial endocarditis, which involved the mitral valve, in 1986 after a dental procedure. The cause of his cirrhosis was unknown, but it was unrelated to infectious hepatitis, alcoholism, or known exposure to drugs. He had been treated for hepatic encephalopathy with lactulose and spironolactone, and he had been maintained on warfarin anticoagulation because of his atrial fibrillation.

He was initially taken to another hospital and there found to have a temperature of 39.4 °C. Intravenous cefazolin was started. On admission to our hospital he was cachectic and confused, with a blood pressure of 100/60 mm Hg, an irregular pulse rate of 88 beats/min, and a temperature of 38.1 °C. There was no evidence of peripheral embolization, lymph nodes were not enlarged, and his chest was clear on auscultation and percussion. On cardiac examination, an irregularly irregular rhythm was noted, and a grade III/VI systolic crescendo murmur along the left sternal border was heard. There were no thrills, rubs, or gallops. Abdominal examination showed a slightly enlarged liver palpable 3 cm below the costal margin, with minimal ascites. Moderate (2+) ankle edema was noted. Laboratory values were as follows: hemoglobin concentration, 8.5 g/dL; hematocrit, 25.3%; platelet count, 78,000/cu mm; leukocyte count, 4,500/cu mm; prothrombin time, 25.1 seconds; blood urea nitrogen concentration, 23 mg/dL; serum creatinine concentration, 1.5 mg/dL; aspartate aminotransferase concentration, 29 units/L; alkaline phosphatase concentration, 38 units/L; total bilirubin concentration, 1.2 mg/dL; serum protein concentration, 4.3 g/dL; and serum albumin concentration, 1.8 g/dL. Urinalysis showed three to five leukocytes, a few bacteria, and 10–12 hyaline casts per field at low magnification. A chest roentgenogram was unremarkable.

Antimicrobial treatment was begun with cefazolin (as the sodium salt) 1 g i.v. every eight hours and tobramycin (as the sulfate salt) 60 mg i.v. every eight hours. Other medications included digoxin, furosemide, spironolactone, potassium chloride, and warfarin. Initially, the patient defervesced and improved. Blood cultures were positive for *Staphylococcus aureus*, however. On day 8 of hospitalization, the patient developed a temperature of 38.3 °C; cefazolin and tobramycin were discontinued, and therapy with vancomycin (as the hydrochloride salt) 1 g i.v. every 12 hours was started at 1200. The patient's serum creatinine concentration fell to 1.2 mg/dL after rehydration. On day 11 he became hypotensive and was transferred to the medical intensive-care unit for the treatment of presumed sepsis. His serum creatinine concentration had risen to 2.7 mg/dL. Vancomycin was discontinued after the dose at 0600; a total of six doses had been given. All other medications were also discontinued. Vancomycin concentration data and renal function test results for days 8–25 are summarized in Table 1.

On day 12 at 0500 the serum vancomycin concentration was 40.3 μg/mL (TDx, Abbott Laboratories, Chicago, IL 60064). The serum creatinine concentration increased to 3.1 mg/dL, and the total serum bilirubin concentration rose to 2.4 mg/dL. Blood pressure was maintained with intravenous pressors. On day 13 at 0500 the vancomycin concentration was 36.7 μg/mL, and the serum creatinine concentration increased to 3.4 mg/dL. A chest roentgenogram showed diffuse in-

ROBERT E. PACHOREK, PHARM.D., is Clinical Pharmacist and Pharmacokinetic Service Coordinator, Department of Pharmacy, Mercy Hospital and Medical Center, San Diego, and Assistant Clinical Professor of Pharmacy, University of Southern California, Los Angeles, CA. FREDERICK WOOD, M.D., is Chief Medical Resident, Department of Medical Education, Mercy Hospital and Medical Center, and Clinical Instructor, School of Medicine, University of California, San Diego.

Address reprint requests to Dr. Pachorek at the Department of Pharmacy, Mercy Hospital and Medical Center, San Diego, CA 92103.

Table 1.
Vancomycin Administration Times, Serum Vancomycin Concentrations, and Renal Function Test Results

Variable	Time or Value on Indicated Hospital Day																	
	8	9	10	11	12	13	14	15	16	17	18	19	20	21	22	23	24	25
Vancomycin[a] administration times	1200	0000, 1800	0600, 1800	0600	...	...	...	...	...	...	...	...	...	...	...	...	...	...
Serum vancomycin concentration (μg/mL)	...	...	...	...	40.3	36.7	...	29.8	...	...	...	24.7	...	...	...	...	...	16.1
Serum creatinine concentration (mg/dL)	1.2	...	...	2.7	3.1	3.4	3.6	4.0	4.1	4.1	3.7	3.6	3.2	3.0	2.9	2.9	2.8	2.8
Urine output (mL/24 hr)	...	...	...	...	901	912	667	417	592	924	1224	1265	556	721	737	549	391	298
Measured creatinine clearance (mL/min)	...	...	...	...	...	...	...	...	...	...	...	14	...	...	...	...	...	18

[a] Vancomycin (as the hydrochloride salt) 1 g i.v.

filtration, suggesting pneumonia or pulmonary edema. By the next day the serum creatinine concentration had increased to 3.6 mg/dL. Furosemide 160 mg i.v. and mannitol 25 g i.v. were given to induce diuresis. On day 15 the patient's cough yielded purulent sputum, and empirical treatment with cefoperazone (as the sodium salt) 2 g i.v. followed by 1 g i.v. every 12 hours was started; sputum cultures subsequently grew *Pseudomonas aeruginosa, Enterobacter cloacae, Citrobacter freundii,* and *Klebsiella pneumoniae.* At 0500 the serum vancomycin concentration was 29.8 μg/mL, and the serum creatinine concentration had risen to 4.0 mg/dL.

On day 19 at 0530 the serum vancomycin concentration was 24.7 μg/mL. The serum creatinine concentration had decreased to 3.6 mg/dL, and the creatinine clearance, measured from a 24-hour urine collection, was 14.0 mL/min. Aggressive diuresis was continued to maintain a urine output of 500–1200 mL/day. By day 23 the serum creatinine concentration had fallen to 2.9 mg/dL. Chest roentgenography showed persistent infiltration despite the use of antimicrobials, and urine cultures grew yeast. The patient became unresponsive to painful stimuli, and serum ammonia concentrations were found to exceed 80 μmol/L.

On day 25, because of declining respiratory function, the patient was placed on mechanical ventilation. At 0500 the vancomycin concentration was 16.1 μg/mL and the serum creatinine concentration was 2.8 mg/dL. The measured creatinine clearance, determined from a 24-hour urine collection, was 18 mL/min. The patient became progressively more oliguric, despite diuretic therapy.

On day 27 continuous arteriovenous hemofiltration with hemodialysis (CAVH/D) was initiated. The serum creatinine concentration had climbed to 3.1 mg/dL. Later in the day the patient developed ecchymoses and bled from his mucous membranes, i.v.-line sites, and gastrointestinal tract secondary to disseminated intravascular coagulation (confirmed by coagulation and hematologic studies). The patient's mental status progressively deteriorated, despite treatment with lactulose.

The patient remained oliguric on CAVH/D; on day 33 the serum creatinine concentration was 2.6 mg/dL. Despite continued intensive management, the patient's condition continued to deteriorate, progressing to multiple-organ-system failure. On day 34 CAVH/D was stopped, pressors were withdrawn, and the patient died.

Discussion. The terminal elimination half-life of vancomycin in this patient, calculated from the concentration data for days 12–25 by using nonlinear least-squares regression analysis (USC PC Pack, Laboratory of Applied Pharmacokinetics, University of Southern California, Los Angeles, CA 90033), was 244 hours, or approximately 10 days. The elimination phase is illustrated in Figure 1. The correlation coefficient relating the serum vancomycin concentration data to the model estimates is 0.992.

We were unable to accurately estimate the patient's apparent steady-state volume of distribution because of the change in his renal function during the period of vancomycin therapy and the fact that the concentration data were obtained after the last dose. Between days 12 and 25 the patient's weight ranged from 66.6 to 73.0 kg and the serum creatinine concentration from 3.1 to 4.1 mg/dL. The measured 24-hour creatinine clearances on days 19 and 25 were 14.0 and 18.0 mL/min, respectively, and the estimated creatinine clearances (determined by the method of Cockcroft and Gault[7]) for those days were 15.9 and 20.5 mL/min, respectively. The average measured 24-hour creatinine clearance (16 mL/min) was used in calculating the population-based clearance: 3.66 + (0.689 × CL_{cr}).[1,18] The volume of distribution was estimated from the average ranges reported for adults with renal dysfunction (0.39–0.92 L/kg).[4] Based on these esti-

Figure 1. Serum vancomycin concentration versus time. Time zero was the time of the last dose of vancomycin, 0600 on day 11. The terminal elimination half-life was 244 hours.

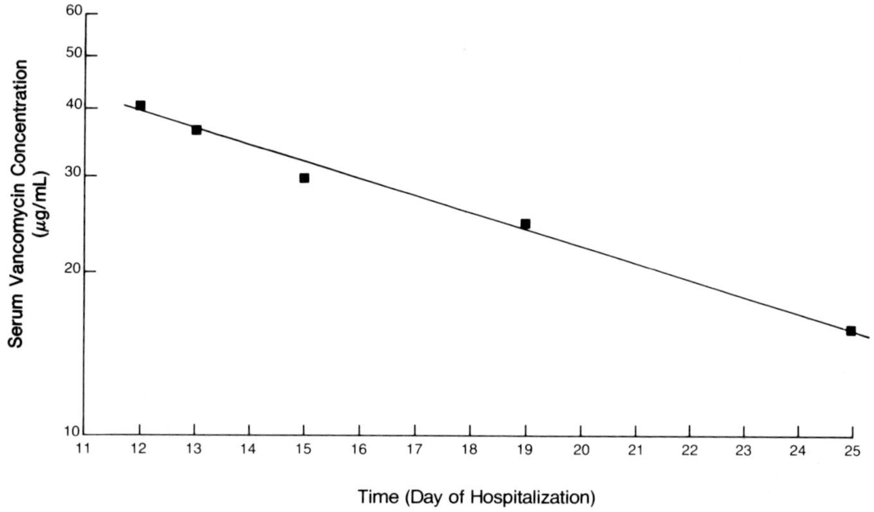

mates of vancomycin clearance and volume of distribution, the estimated half-life in this patient on days 12–25 ranged from 20.4 to 52.8 hours.

Reported terminal elimination half-lives of vancomycin in patients with very poor renal function and patients undergoing hemodialysis are 130–190 hours; few patients have vancomycin half-lives greater than 240 hours.[1,4] If one were to have estimated a dosage regimen for this patient on the basis of creatinine clearance, the prediction would have been grossly in error.[2,18]

Possible explanations for the discrepancy in the actual and estimated vancomycin half-lives include (1) inaccurate assessment of GFR from the measured 24-hour creatinine clearance because of the presence of liver disease, (2) greatly reduced nonrenal clearance of vancomycin because of liver dysfunction, (3) interference with the creatinine assay by some substance in the patient's serum, and (4) interference with the vancomycin assay by some interfering substance, such as a metabolite or a vancomycin-like immunoreactive substance.

In patients with low GFRs, even the measured 24-hour creatinine clearance can substantially exceed the inulin clearance (inulin clearance is a more accurate measure of GFR).[19] This overestimation could account for the difficulty in accurately estimating vancomycin dosages in patients with creatinine clearances of less than 25 mL/min. With some estimates, an incremental decrease in the creatinine clearance of only 9 mL/min would indicate a change in the recommended dosage interval from 3 days to 6 days.[18]

Overestimation of GFRs by using measured 24-hour creatinine clearances was reported in cirrhotic patients by Papadakis and Arieff.[14] In that study, some cirrhotic patients had a markedly decreased GFR (measured from inulin clearance) despite an apparently normal serum creatinine concentration and normal measured 24-hour creatinine clearance. The 13 cirrhotic patients with the lowest GFRs (measured from inulin clearance) had measured 24-hour creatinine clearances that overestimated the GFR by 96%. A better correlation of vancomycin clearance and renal function might be found by estimating the GFR more accurately, although this might not improve the accuracy of dosage estimates for patients with renal and hepatic impairment.

Another explanation for the very low vancomycin clearance in this patient may be that nonrenal clearance was reduced secondary to his liver dysfunction. Decreases in vancomycin clearance in patients with liver dysfunction have been reported, but the association remains speculative.[4] Golper et al.,[3] by measuring the clearances of vancomycin, creatinine, inulin, and aminohippurate sodium simultaneously, found that the renal clearance of vancomycin in healthy adults represented only 70% of total vancomycin clearance. They also found that nonrenal clearance of vancomycin was concentration dependent (i.e., as serum vancomycin concentration increased, nonrenal clearance increased). The authors did not hypothesize where this 30% nonrenal elimination occurred anatomically but speculated that the very reduced vancomycin clearances reported for patients with severe renal impairment may occur because uremia itself greatly reduces nonrenal elimination.

We were unable to determine the nonrenal clearance of vancomycin in this patient. Nor were we able to determine whether the patient's liver dysfunction actually affected nonrenal vancomycin clearance, but with his apparently very low vancomycin clearance, the patient can be considered to have been functionally anephric despite having an average measured 24-hour creatinine clearance of 16 mL/min. It is also possible that uremia in combination with liver disease could have contributed to his very long vancomycin half-life.

The serum and urinary creatinine determinations

for this patient were assayed by using an automated system incorporating a modification of the Jaffe reaction designed to create less susceptibility than conventional methods to interference from non-creatinine-containing, Jaffe-positive compounds (Dimension, Du Pont, Wilmington, DE 19898). Our patient was not receiving any drugs known to interfere with the assay, nor did he have substantially elevated levels of any other known interfering substance. His slightly elevated total bilirubin concentration, 1.2 mg/dL, was much less than the 20 mg/dL reported by the manufacturer to depress the creatinine result by 0.7 mg/dL.

There may be a vancomycin-like immunoreactive substance in patients with renal disease that interferes with the commonly used TDx fluorescence polarization immunoassay (FPIA) for vancomycin.[20,21] The substance, possibly a degradation product or, less likely, a metabolite, appears to interfere with polyclonal antibody-based immunoassays (e.g., the radioimmunoassay [RIA] and FPIA for vancomycin) but not with high-performance liquid chromatography.

Interference with the vancomycin assay could have occurred in our patient, especially if his GFR was actually less than that estimated from creatinine clearance. In one study of nine patients undergoing continuous ambulatory peritoneal dialysis, the overestimation of the peak vancomycin concentration after three weeks of weekly treatment averaged 39.6%.[20] Indeed, the vancomycin RIA or FPIA used in earlier studies of patients with renal disease may also have measured a vancomycin-like immunoreactive substance[1,2,16,17] The results of studies in which these vancomycin assays have been used for patients with renal dysfunction should be interpreted with great caution.

Conclusion. In a patient with renal and hepatic dysfunction, estimated and measured creatinine clearances were inconsistent with the vancomycin elimination half-life, which was very long. Serum vancomycin concentrations should be monitored closely in patients with renal and hepatic impairment.

References

1. Matzke GR, McGory RW, Halstenson CE et al. Pharmacokinetics of vancomycin in patients with various degrees of renal function. *Antimicrob Agents Chemother*. 1984; 25:433-7.
2. Rodvold KA, Blum RA, Fischer JH et al. Vancomycin pharmacokinetics in patients with various degrees of renal function. *Antimicrob Agents Chemother*. 1988; 32:848-52.
3. Golper TA, Noonan HM, Elzinga L et al. Vancomycin pharmacokinetics, renal handling, and nonrenal clearances in normal human subjects. *Clin Pharmacol Ther*. 1988; 43:565-70.
4. Matzke GR, Zhanel GG, Guay DRP. Clinical pharmacokinetics of vancomycin. *Clin Pharmacokinet*. 1986; 11:257-82.
5. Rybak MJ, Boike SC. Individualized adjustment of vancomycin dosage: comparison with two dosage nomograms. *Drug Intell Clin Pharm*. 1986; 20:64-8.
6. Zokufa HZ, Rodvold KA, Blum RA et al. Simulation of vancomycin peak and trough concentrations using five dosing methods in 37 patients. *Pharmacotherapy*. 1989; 9:10-6.
7. Cockcroft DW, Gault MH. Prediction of creatinine clearance from serum creatinine. *Nephron*. 1976; 16:31-41.
8. Lott RS, Hayton WL. Estimation of creatinine clearance from serum creatinine concentration—a review. *Drug Intell Clin Pharm*. 1978; 12:140-50.
9. Hull JH, Hak LJ, Koch GG et al. Influence of range of renal function and liver disease on predictability of creatinine clearance. *Clin Pharmacol Ther*. 1981; 29:516-21.
10. Echizen H, Ishizaki T. Superiority of disease-specific over conventional formula in predicting creatinine clearance from serum creatinine in patients with liver cirrhosis. *Ther Drug Monit*. 1988; 10:369-75.
11. Cocchetto DM, Tschanz C, Bjornsson TD. Decreased rate of creatinine production in patients with hepatic disease: implications for estimation of creatinine clearance. *Ther Drug Monit*. 1983; 5:161-8.
12. Boyce EG, Dickerson RN, Cooney GF et al. Creatinine clearance estimation in protein-malnourished patients. *Clin Pharm*. 1989; 8:721-6.
13. Takabatake T, Ohta H, Ishida Y et al. Low serum creatinine levels in severe hepatic disease. *Arch Intern Med*. 1988; 148:1313-5.
14. Papadakis MA, Arieff AI. Unpredictability of clinical evaluation of renal function in cirrhosis. *Am J Med*. 1987; 82:945-52.
15. Matzke GR. Vancomycin. In: Evans WE, Schentag JJ, Jusko WJ, eds. Applied pharmacokinetics: principles of therapeutic drug monitoring. Spokane, WA: Applied Therapeutics; 1986:399-436.
16. Rotschafer JC, Crossley K, Zaske DE et al. Pharmacokinetics of vancomycin: observations in 28 patients and dosage recommendations. *Antimicrob Agents Chemother*. 1982; 22:391-4.
17. Brown N, Ho DHW, Fong KL et al. Effects of hepatic function on vancomycin clinical pharmacology. *Antimicrob Agents Chemother*. 1983; 23:603-9.
18. Brown DL, Mauro LS. Vancomycin dosing chart for use in patients with renal impairment. *Am J Kidney Dis*. 1988; 11:15-9.
19. Bauer JH, Brooks CS, Burch RN. Clinical appraisal of creatinine clearance as a measurement of glomerular filtration rate. *Am J Kidney Dis*. 1982; 2:337-46.
20. Morse GD, Nairn DK, Bertino JS et al. Overestimation of vancomycin concentrations utilizing fluorescence polarization immunoassay in patients on peritoneal dialysis. *Ther Drug Monit*. 1987; 9:212-5.
21. Anne L, Hu M, Chan K et al. Potential problem with fluorescence polarization immunoassay cross-reactivity to vancomycin degradation product cdp-1: its detection in sera of renally impaired patients. *Ther Drug Monit*. 1989; 11:585-91.

Preventing recurrent varicella and herpes zoster with oral acyclovir in HIV-seropositive patients

PIERRE DELLAMONICA, MICHEL CARLES, FRANÇOIS LOKIEC, VÉRONIQUE MONDAIN, EVELYNE BERNARD, AND FRANCK JOHANSON

Clin Pharm. 1991; 10:301-2

Recurrent manifestations of varicella-zoster virus (VZV) infection, such as herpes zoster, occur in approximately 16% of immunocompromised patients.[1] Thus, therapy to prevent such recurrence is desirable. We used oral acyclovir in two patients who were seropositive for human immunodeficiency virus (HIV) in an attempt to prevent recurrent varicella or herpes zoster.

Case Reports. *Patient 1.* Patient 1 was a 38-year-old, 66-kg homosexual man who was in group IV C-1 according to the system (since revised) used by the Centers for Disease Control (CDC) for classifying persons infected with HIV.[2] This category included patients with at least one of the infectious diseases used in the CDC definition of acquired immunodeficiency syndrome. The patient had been receiving weekly treatment with aerosolized pentamidine for *Pneumocystis carinii* pneumonia. He was also receiving zidovudine 200 mg orally every four hours.

The patient developed disseminated varicella. Over a five-day period, he developed an oral temperature of 38.5 °C and a generalized macular rash that evolved into vesicles filled with cloudy fluid and then into black crusts. There were lesions in the buccal mucosa as well, but no bullae or ecchymoses were observed. Acyclovir sodium 10 mg/kg i.v. was given over 30 minutes every eight hours for 10 days. Defervescence and drying of the lesions occurred within four days of the initiation of acyclovir therapy. Oral acyclovir 200 mg five times daily was prescribed in an effort to prevent recurrence of disease. Serum acyclovir concentrations were measured after at least three days of therapy for both routes of administration (Table 1).

One month later, the patient was hospitalized with varicella. I.V. acyclovir therapy was repeated at the same dosage, and the varicella resolved as before. Oral acyclovir was prescribed at a dosage of 400 mg five times daily. The patient had no sign of recurrence of varicella after three months. Renal function remained normal throughout the episodes, and the patient had no adverse reactions to acyclovir.

Patient 2. Patient 2 was a 36-year-old, 70-kg homosexual man, also classified in CDC group IV C-1, whose anti-HIV therapy consisted of oral zidovudine 200 mg every four hours. He developed intercostal herpes zoster in the left T5–T6 dermatome, with painful, necrotic vesicles. Acyclovir sodium 10 mg/kg i.v. was given over 30 minutes every eight hours for 10 days. Serum acyclovir concentrations were measured (Table 1). Clinical improvement, manifested by drying of the lesions, occurred within eight days of the initiation of acyclovir treatment, but scars remained. The patient was discharged from the hospital without maintenance acyclovir therapy.

One month later, the patient was readmitted with the identical presentation of herpes zoster. He was treated, and he recovered as before and was discharged taking oral acyclovir 200 mg five times daily; serum acyclovir concentrations were measured again. A third episode of herpes zoster occurred 15 days later and resolved after i.v. acyclovir treatment was repeated at the same dosage. The patient was given maintenance therapy with oral acyclovir 400 mg five times daily and had no further recurrence after two months. No adverse effects of acyclovir were noted, and the patient's renal function was normal throughout the episodes.

Discussion. Viral resistance is a possible explanation for the failure of drug treatment to prevent recurrent varicella or herpes zoster. Resistance of VZV to acyclovir is due primarily to the virus's lack of thymidine kinase.[3,4] The satisfactory response of both pa-

Table 1.
Acyclovir Concentrations in Two Patients Seropositive for Human Immunodeficiency Virus[a]

Route of Administration and Time after Dose (hr)	Serum Acyclovir Concentration (μmol/L)	
	Patient 1	Patient 2
Oral		
0	2.60	0.40
1	3.15	1.58
2	2.37	1.74
4	1.50	0.73
5	1.27	0.83
I.V.		
0	2.88	1.67
0.25	19.35	21.50
0.50	18.70	95.40

[a] Blood samples collected during i.v. therapy were taken from the arm contralateral to the arm receiving the infusion. Samples were collected after at least three days of oral or i.v. therapy. Acyclovir concentration was measured by radioimmunoassay. The i.v. dosage of acyclovir sodium was 10 mg/kg given over 30 minutes every eight hours. The oral dosage of acyclovir was 200 mg five times daily.

PIERRE DELLAMONICA, M.D., is Professor of Infectious Diseases and MICHEL CARLES, M.D., is Assistant Physician, Infectious Diseases, Archet Hospital, Nice, France. FRANÇOIS LOKIEC, M.D., is Hospital Pharmacist, Pharmacology, René Huguenin Center, St. Cloud, France. VÉRONIQUE MONDAIN, M.D., EVELYNE BERNARD, M.D., and FRANCK JOHANSON, M.D., are Assistant Physicians, Infectious Diseases, Archet Hospital.

Address reprint requests to Dr. Dellamonica at Infectious Diseases, Archet Hospital, Route St-Antoine-de-Ginestière, B.P. 689, 06012 Nice Cedex, France.

tients to i.v. acyclovir, however, suggests that viral resistance was unlikely. In addition, VZV in patient 1 was isolated and found to have thymidine kinase; thus, this mechanism of resistance was ruled out.

The initial oral dosage of acyclovir was probably not sufficient to prevent recurrence of varicella or herpes zoster. In both patients, i.v. acyclovir produced drug concentrations many times higher than did oral administration. Balfour[5] measured serum acyclovir concentrations in HIV-seronegative patients who were receiving the same oral and i.v. dosages as our patients and obtained mean peak and trough concentrations of 2.5 and 1.3 µmol/L, respectively, during oral administration and 73.1 and 7.0 µmol/L during i.v. administration. Because these concentrations are similar to the ones we measured, we cannot conclude that HIV seropositivity is associated with decreased gastrointestinal absorption of acyclovir.

The differences between concentrations measured after i.v. and oral acyclovir administration demonstrate the need for an adequate oral dosage. Although the minimum serum acyclovir concentration necessary to prevent recurrence of varicella or herpes zoster in HIV-seropositive patients is unknown, we found that disseminated varicella and herpes zoster resolved when relatively high drug concentrations were present. In prescribing therapy to prevent recurrence, then, it might be useful to give patients enough oral acyclovir to produce concentrations similar to those achieved by the i.v. route.

The initial oral dosage of acyclovir may have failed to prevent recurrence of varicella or herpes zoster for other reasons. Acyclovir may diffuse poorly at the site of infection in HIV-seropositive patients, or VZV in such patients may be relatively resistant to the drug. Whether the presence of zidovudine interferes with acyclovir activity is not known.

Conclusion. Oral acyclovir 200 mg five times a day failed to prevent recurrent varicella or herpes zoster in two HIV-seropositive patients, but 400 mg five times daily was apparently effective.

References

1. Meyer JD. Treatment of varicella-zoster virus infection in immunocompromised patients. *Res Clin Forums.* 1987; 9:65-74.
2. Centers for Disease Control. Classification system for human T-lymphotropic virus type III/lymphadenopathy-associated virus infections. *Ann Intern Med.* 1986; 105:234-7.
3. Larder BA, Darby G. Virus drug-resistance: mechanisms and consequences. *Antiviral Res.* 1984; 4(Apr):1-42.
4. Biron KK, Fyfe JA, Noblin JE et al. Selection and preliminary characterization of acyclovir-resistant mutants of varicella zoster virus. *Am J Med.* 1982; 73(Suppl 1A):383-6.
5. Balfour HH Jr. Aciclovir. *Antimicrob Agents Annu 2.* 1987; 32:315-29.

DUE Criteria

The DUE Criteria *section of* Clinical Pharmacy *features model drug-use evaluation criteria that may be employed as a component of a comprehensive quality assurance program. The criteria sets are presented in the format used in the ASHP book* Criteria for Drug Use Evaluation. *Some of the criteria sets will have been originally published in that book; others will be presented here for the first time and published in future volumes of the ASHP book. The practitioners who developed a criteria set are acknowledged.*

In selecting drug products for coverage in DUE Criteria, *priority is given to products that have been recently marketed, those that are frequently prescribed, those that have high potential risk associated with their use, and those that are expensive. When feasible, a criteria set will be linked with a Drug Review that appears in the same issue.*

These criteria sets are a starting point for the development of DUE criteria for a specific practice setting. Readers are encouraged to modify the model criteria to fit their own circumstances.

Criteria for use of epoetin[a]

Element	Standard 100%	Standard 0%	Exception[b] or Critical Preventive/ Responsive Measure[c]	Sources of Information
Justification for Use				
1. Anemia due to chronic renal failure (CRF) (hematocrit [Hct], <30%) in the following types of patients who had a nephrology consultation[1–6]: a. Hemodialysis patients b. Peritoneal dialysis patients c. Predialysis patients or	X		1A. None	1. History and physical examination (H&P), laboratory reports, progress notes, nephrology consultation reports
2. Anemia (Hct, <30%) in patient with AIDS undergoing zidovudine therapy (≤4200 mg/wk) and with endogenous serum erythropoietin concentration of ≤500 mU/mL[7,8]	X		2A. None	2. H&P, laboratory reports, progress notes
Critical (Process) Indicators				
CRF and AIDS Patients				
3. No history of allergy to mammalian cell-derived products, human albumin, or epoetin[3]	X		3A. None	3. H&P, allergy reports
CRF Patients Only				
4. Hct measured twice weekly for 6–8 weeks after initiation of epoetin therapy[3]	X		4A. None	4. Laboratory reports, progress notes, physician orders
5. Hct measured twice weekly for 6–8 weeks after dosage adjustment[3]	X		5A. None	5. Laboratory reports, progress notes, physician orders, medication administration records (MAR)
6. Complete blood count with differential and platelet count performed at least monthly during epoetin therapy[2,3]	X		6A. None	6. Laboratory reports, progress notes, physician orders

Prepared by Teresa A. Bennett, Pharm.D., Coordinator, Drug Usage Evaluation, Department of Pharmacy, University Medical Center, and Clinical Assistant Professor, College of Pharmacy, University of Florida Health Science Center/Jacksonville; Mark W. Todd; Pharm.D., Director, Drug Information and Research, Department of Pharmacy, University Medical Center, and Clinical Associate Professor, College of Pharmacy, University of Florida Health Science Center/Jacksonville; and Stephen Sandroni, M.D., Assistant Professor and Chief, Division of Nephrology, University of Florida Health Science Center/Jacksonville at University Medical Center.

The criteria are being reprinted in this issue because we failed to include a title with their earlier printing in the February issue.

Element	Standard 100%	Standard 0%	Exception[b] or Critical Preventive/ Responsive Measure[c]	Sources of Information
7. Serum chemistry, including concentrations of blood urea nitrogen, creatinine, phosphate, potassium, and uric acid, measured at least monthly during epoetin therapy[2,3]	X		7A. None	7. Laboratory reports, progress notes, physician orders
8. Adequate baseline iron stores, including transferrin saturation (serum iron/iron-binding capacity) of at least 20% and serum ferritin concentration of at least 100 ng/mL documented[1–3]	X		8A. None	8. H&P, laboratory reports, progress notes
9. Iron supplementation provided to patient with inadequate iron stores before initiation of epoetin therapy[1–3]	X		9A. None	9. Laboratory reports, progress notes, physician orders, MAR
10. Serum ferritin concentration measured monthly for first 3 months and then every 2–3 months[2]; transferrin saturation reassessed if response not maintained during extended epoetin therapy	X		10A. None	10. Laboratory reports, progress notes, physician orders
11. Pretreatment control of blood pressure achieved in hypertensive patient; blood pressure monitored closely during therapy[1–3]	X		11A. None	11. H&P, progress notes, nursing flow sheets, nursing notes
12. Patient counseled about importance of renal-failure dietary restrictions before and during epoetin therapy[2]	X		12A. None	12. Progress notes, nursing notes
13. Appropriate initial dosage: 50–100 units/kg 3 times a week i.v. in dialysis patient and i.v. or s.c. in nondialysis patient[3]	X		13A. Smaller doses (30–50 units/kg) given to patient in whom a slower rise in Hct is desired	13, 13A. Physician orders, progress notes, MAR
14. Dosage adjusted appropriately[3]: a. Dose reduced by 25 units/kg when Hct reaches 30–33% or when Hct increases by >4 percentage points in any 2-week period b. Dose increased by 25 units/kg if Hct does not increase by 5 or 6 percentage points after 8 weeks and remains below target range (30–33%)	X		14A. None	14. Physician orders, progress notes, laboratory reports, MAR
15. Appropriate maintenance dosage[3]: a. In dialysis and nondialysis patients, dose decreased by 25 units/kg if Hct is >33% or withheld if Hct is >36% and not resumed until Hct decreases to ≤33% b. In nondialysis patient, dosage decreased to 75–150 units/kg per week or lower, as tolerated, depending on response	X		15A. None	15. Physician orders, progress notes, laboratory reports, MAR
<u>AIDS Patients Only</u>				
16. Appropriate dosage[7,8]: a. Initial dosage of 100 units/kg i.v. or s.c. three times a week for 8 weeks (target Hct, 30–40% or decreased need for transfusions) b. If target Hct has not been achieved or need for transfusions has not decreased after 8 weeks, dose increased by 50–100 units/kg i.v. or s.c. and continued for 4–8 weeks c. Dose reduced or increased in increments of 50–100 units/kg s.c. or i.v. to maintain response. If patient has not responded to 300	X		16A. None	16. Physician orders, progress notes, MAR

Element	Standard 100%	Standard 0%	Exception[b] or Critical Preventive/ Responsive Measure[c]	Sources of Information
units/kg three times a week, response to a higher dosage unlikely d. If Hct is >40%, epoetin discontinued until Hct is ≤36%. Treatment then resumed at a dosage decreased by 25%				
17. Hct measured once a week until stable and periodically thereafter[8]	X		17A. None	17. Physician orders, progress notes
Complications				
18. Hypertension (CRF patients only)[1–9]		X	18A. Identify other drug and non-drug causes 18B. Stress compliance with antihypertensive medication 18C. Adjust antihypertensive medication dosage as needed. 18D. Reduce epoetin dosage or discontinue until blood pressure is controlled[3] 18E. Monitor blood pressure regularly	18. Progress notes, nursing flow sheets, nursing notes 18A. Physician orders, progress notes, nursing notes, MAR 18B. Physician orders, progress notes, nursing notes 18C, D. Physician orders, progress notes, MAR 18E. Physician orders, progress notes, nursing flow sheets, nursing notes
19. Decreased iron stores (transferrin saturation, <20%, and serum ferritin concentration, <100 ng/mL) (CRF and AIDS patients)[1–8]		X	19A. Identify other drug and non-drug causes 19B. Provide supplemental iron unless serum ferritin concentration is >500 ng/mL 19C. Monitor transferrin saturation and serum ferritin level regularly	19. Laboratory reports, progress notes 19A. Physician orders, progress notes, nursing notes, MAR 19B. Laboratory reports, physician orders, progress notes, MAR 19C. Laboratory reports, physician orders, progress notes
20. Premonitory neurological symptoms (aura and sensations of sinking and rising in epigastrium) or seizures during therapy when Hct is rising (CRF patients only)[1–3]		X	20A. Identify other drug and non-drug causes 20B. Provide symptomatic and supportive care if seizure occurs 20C. Monitor patient closely, especially during first 90 days of therapy[3] 20D. Counsel patient about early signs of seizure 20E. Counsel patient to avoid driving or operating machinery	20. Laboratory reports, progress notes, nursing notes 20A, B. Physician orders, progress notes, nursing notes, MAR 20C. Physician orders, nursing notes 20D, E. Physician orders, progress notes, nursing notes
21. Thrombotic events (CRF patients only)[3,9]		X	21A. Identify other drug and non-drug causes 21B. Closely monitor patient with pre-existing vascular disease 21C. Assess need for increased heparin during dialysis[2]	21. Progress notes, nursing notes 21A. Physician orders, progress notes, nursing notes, MAR 21B. H&P, progress notes, nursing notes 21C. Physician orders, dialysis reports
22. Hyperkalemia (CRF patients only)[1–3]		X	22A. Identify other drug and non-drug causes 22B. Monitor serum potassium level 22C. Stress compliance with renal-failure dietary restrictions 22D. Administer potassium-removing resin or increase dialysis time if needed	22. Laboratory reports, progress notes 22A. Physician orders, progress notes, nursing notes, MAR 22B. Laboratory reports, physician orders, progress notes 22C. Physician orders, progress notes, nursing notes 22D. Physician orders, progress notes, MAR, dialysis reports

Element	Standard 100%	Standard 0%	Exception[b] or Critical Preventive/ Responsive Measure[c]	Sources of Information
23. Allergic reaction (CRF and AIDS patients)[2]		X	23A. Identify other drug and nondrug causes 23B. If anaphylaxis occurs, discontinue epoetin immediately and provide symptomatic and supportive care 23C. Monitor for skin rash and urticaria (usually mild and transient)	23. Progress notes, nursing notes 23A, B. Physician orders, progress notes, nursing notes, MAR 23C. Progress notes, nursing notes
Outcome Measures				
24. Resolution of chronic anemia (Hct, 30–33% in CRF patient and 30–40% in AIDS patient)[1–7]	X		24A. Patient with osteodystrophy and documented aluminum deposition[1] 24B. Patient died 24C. Patient unable to tolerate epoetin 24D. Patient with untreated iron deficiency 24E. Patient with recent stress due to surgery, or transplantation patient taking corticosteroids	24. Laboratory reports 24A. Progress notes, bone biopsy reports 24B. Progress notes 24C. Progress notes, nursing notes 24D. Laboratory reports, progress notes 24E. Progress notes, MAR
or				
25. Decreased need for transfusions[1–7]	X		25A. Patient did not require transfusions at onset of epoetin therapy 25B. Patient died	25. Physician orders, progress notes 25A. H&P, physician orders, progress notes 25B. Progress notes
or				
26. Improved quality of life (improved exercise tolerance, appetite, and sense of well-being)[4,8,10]	X		26A. Patient died 26B. Patient unable to tolerate epoetin 26C. Patient unable to achieve Hct in target range	26, 26A, B. Progress notes, nursing notes 26C. Laboratory reports

[a] Criteria address justifications for use (indications), critical (process) indicators, complications of therapy, and patient outcome. Each criterion consists of an element, a standard, exceptions to the standard, and sources of information. The element is the minimum level of evidence needed to show that patient care was optimal. The standard defines the deviation from an element that is acceptable. If no deviation is acceptable, the standard is 100%. Exceptions are circumstances in which deviation is allowable. Sources of information listed are the most reliable sources. Sources pertaining to an element or exception are identified by the number assigned to the element or exception (e.g., 18, 18A).

[b] For justification for use and critical (process) indicators.

[c] For complications and outcome measures.

References

1. Flaharty KK, Grimm AM, Vlasses PH. Epoetin: human recombinant erythropoietin. *Clin Pharm*. 1989; 8:769–82.
2. Ad Hoc Committee for the National Kidney Foundation. Statement on the clinical use of recombinant erythropoietin in anemia of end stage renal disease (ESRD). New York: National Kidney Foundation; 1989.
3. Amgen Inc. Epogen package insert. Thousand Oaks, CA; 1989.
4. Lim VS, DeGowin RL, Zavala D et al. Recombinant human erythropoietin treatment in predialysis patients. *Ann Intern Med*. 1989; 110:108–14.
5. Eschbach JW, Egrie JC, Downing MR et al. Correction of the anemia of end-stage renal disease with recombinant erythropoietin. *N Engl J Med*. 1987; 316:73–8.
6. Eschbach JW, Kelly MR, Haley R et al. Treatment of the anemia of progressive renal failure with recombinant human erythropoietin. *N Engl J Med*. 1989; 321:158–63.
7. Fischl M, Galpin JE, Levine JD et al. Recombinant human erythropoietin for patients with AIDS treated with zidovudine. *N Engl J Med*. 1990; 322:1488–93.
8. Amgen Inc. Procrit package insert. 1990 Dec. Distributed by Ortho Biotech Division, Ortho Pharmaceutical, Raritan, NJ.
9. Watson AJ. Adverse effects of therapy for the correction of anemia in hemodialysis patients. *Semin Nephrol*. 1989; 9(Suppl 1):30–4.
10. Evans RW, Radar B, Manninem DL et al. The quality of life of hemodialysis recipients treated with recombinant human erythropoietin. *JAMA*. 1990; 263:825–30.

Criteria for use of misoprostol[a]

Element	Standard 100%	Standard 0%	Exception[b] or Critical Preventive/ Responsive Measure[c]	Sources of Information
Justification for Use				
1. Combined with nonsteroidal anti-inflammatory drug (NSAID), including aspirin, to decrease gastric ulcer development in high-risk adult patient[1–10] who meets one or more of the following criteria: a. Is >60 years of age[11–13] b. Has history of gastric ulcer or bleeding[1,8,13–15] c. Has history of melena[14] d. Is cigarette smoker[13,14] e. Has rheumatoid arthritis[13,15] f. Has severe concomitant disease[1,8]	X		1A. None (product information for misoprostol (Cytotec) and FDA's Gastrointestinal Drugs Advisory Committee state that severe concomitant disease places patient at high risk, but "severe" has not been defined with objective criteria in the literature)	1. History and physical (H&P), physician orders, progress notes, medication administration record (MAR)
Critical (Process) Indicators				
2. Misoprostol not used in pregnant woman[1,5,8]	X		2A. None	2. H&P, progress notes, nursing notes
3. Misoprostol not used in woman of childbearing potential[1,5,8]	X		3A. Patient provided with oral and written warnings of hazards of misoprostol[8] and 3B. Negative serum pregnancy test performed within 2 weeks of initial misoprostol therapy[8] and 3C. Misoprostol therapy started only on 2nd or 3rd day of next normal menstrual period[8] and 3D. Patient compliant with effective birth control method[8]	3. H&P 3A. Progress notes, nursing notes 3B. Laboratory reports 3C. Progress notes, nursing notes, physician orders 3D. H&P, progress notes, nursing notes, physician orders
4. Appropriate dosage: 200 μg four times daily, after meals and at bedtime with food[1,2,5,8]	X		4A. If intolerance develops, dosage decreased to 100 μg four times daily, after meals and at bedtime with food[5,8]	4. Physician orders, MAR 4A. Progress notes, nursing notes, physician orders, MAR
5. Misoprostol discontinued once NSAID (or aspirin) therapy is stopped or if intolerance develops[1,4,5,8]	X		5A. None	5. Physician orders, MAR, progress notes
6. Patient provided with oral and written information about misoprostol[8]: a. Indication b. Administration instructions c. Warning not to give drug to another person d. Adverse effects, especially likelihood of diarrhea e. Pregnancy contraindication	X		6A. None	6. Progress notes, nursing notes, physician orders
Complications				
7. Pregnancy during misoprostol therapy		X	7A. Discontinue misoprostol[1,4,5,8,10] 7B. Inform patient of potential risks to fetus[8]	7,7A, B. Progress notes, physician orders, nursing notes
8. Diarrhea[1–10]		X	8A. Provide supportive care 8B. If possible, discontinue magnesium-containing antacids[5,8] 8C. Identify other drug and nondrug causes	8. Progress notes, nursing notes 8A. Progress notes, nursing notes, physician orders 8B. Physician orders

Prepared by Mark W. Todd, Pharm.D., Director, Drug Information and Research, Department of Pharmacy, University Medical Center, and Clinical Associate Professor, College of Pharmacy, University of Florida Health Science Center/Jacksonville.

Element	Standard 100%	Standard 0%	Exception[b] or Critical Preventive/ Responsive Measure[c]	Sources of Information
			8D. If mild to moderate reaction, decrease misoprostol dosage to 100 μg four times daily[4,5,8,10] 8E. If severe reaction, discontinue misoprostol	8C. Progress notes, physician orders 8D, E. Physician orders, progress notes, MAR
9. Other gastrointestinal effects (abdominal pain, nausea, vomiting, flatulence, dyspepsia, and constipation) or headache[2–10]		X	9A. Identify other drug and nondrug causes 9B. Provide supportive care 9C. If mild to moderate reaction, decrease misoprostol dosage to 100 μg four times daily[8] 9D. If severe reaction, discontinue misoprostol	9. Progress notes, nursing notes 9A. Progress notes, MAR 9B–D. Progress notes, physician orders, nursing notes
10. Gynecological disorders: spotting, cramps, hypermenorrhea, menstrual disorders, and dysmenorrhea[1–10]		X	10A. Identify other drug and nondrug causes 10B. Provide supportive care 10C. If condition persists, discontinue misoprostol	10, 10A. Progress notes, nursing notes 10B. Progress notes, nursing notes, physician orders 10C. Progress notes, physician orders
Outcome Measures				
11. No interruption in NSAID therapy because of gastric bleeding or ulceration	X		11A. None	11. Physician orders, MAR

[a] Criteria address justification for use (indications), critical (process) indicators, complications of therapy, and patient outcome. Each criterion consists of an element, a standard, exceptions to the standard, and sources of information. The element is the minimum level of evidence needed to show that patient care was optimal. The standard defines the deviation from an element that is acceptable. If no deviation is acceptable, the standard is 100%. Exceptions are circumstances in which deviation is allowable. Sources of information listed are the most reliable sources. Sources pertaining to an element or exception are identified by the number assigned to the element or exception (e.g., 4, 4A).

[b] For justification for use and critical (process) indicators.

[c] For complications and outcome measures.

References

1. Stern WR. Summary of the 33rd Meeting of the Food and Drug Administration's Gastrointestinal Drugs Advisory Committee. *Am J Gastroenterol.* 1989; 84:351–4.
2. Graham DY, Agrawal NM, Roth SH. Prevention of NSAID-induced gastric ulcer with misoprostol: multicentre double-blind placebo-controlled trial. *Lancet.* 1988; 2:1277–80.
3. Knodel LC. Preventing NSAID-induced gastric ulcers: the role of misoprostol. *Hosp Formul.* 1989; 24:27–30.
4. Misoprostol. *Med Lett Drugs Ther.* 1989; 31:21–2.
5. Garris RE, Kirkwood CF. Misoprostol: a prostaglandin E_1 analogue. *Clin Pharm.* 1989; 8:627–44.
6. Lanza F, Peace K, Gustitus L et al. A blinded endoscopic comparative study of misoprostol versus sucralfate and placebo in the prevention of aspirin-induced gastric and duodenal ulceration. *Am J Gastroenterol.* 1988; 83:143–6.
7. Silverstein FE, Kimmey MD, Saunders DR. Gastric protection by misoprostol against 1300 mg of aspirin. An endoscopic dose-response study. *Am J Med.* 1987; 83(Suppl 1A):32–6.
8. G. D. Searle & Co. Cytotec package insert. Chicago, IL; 1988 Dec.
9. Jiranek GC, Kimmey MD, Saunders DR et al. Misoprostol reduces gastroduodenal injury from one week of aspirin: an endoscopic study. *Gastroenterology.* 1989; 96:656–61.
10. Jones JB, Baily RT. Misoprostol: a prostaglandin E_1 analog with antisecretory and cytoprotective properties. *DICP.* 1989; 23:276–82.
11. Langman MJ. Antiinflammatory drug intake and the risk of ulcer complication. *Med Toxicol.* 1986; 1(Suppl 1):34–8.
12. Jick SS, Perera DR, Walker AM et al. Non-steroidal anti-inflammatory drugs and hospital admission for perforated peptic ulcer. *Lancet.* 1987; 2:380–2.
13. Fries JF, Miller SR, Spitz PW et al. Toward an epidemiology of gastropathy associated with nonsteroidal antiinflammatory drug use. *Gastroenterology.* 1989; 96:647–55.
14. Roth SH, Bennett RI. NSAID and gastropathy. A rheumatologist's review. *J Rheumatol.* 1988; 15:912–8.
15. Grahm DY. Prevention of gastroduodenal injury induced by chronic nonsteroidal antiinflammatory drug therapy. *Gastroenterology.* 1989; 96:675–81.

Current Literature

Drug Reaction Alerts 313

Book Reviews

Drugs in Pregnancy and Lactation, Third Edition 316
Gerald G. Briggs, Roger K. Freeman, and Sumner J. Yaffe
Reviewed by Don R. Porter

Goodman and Gilman's The Pharmacological Basis of Therapeutics, 8th edition 317
Edited by Alfred Goodman Gilman, Theodore W. Rall, Alan S. Nies et al.
Reviewed by Burgunda W. Volger

Books Received 318

Drug Reaction Alerts

Drug Reaction Alerts focuses primarily on serious, unlabeled reactions to new chemical entities. The citations are compiled monthly from International Pharmaceutical Abstracts, *which covers over 800 pharmacy and health-related journals worldwide. An address for reprints (when available) follows the name of the corresponding author of each citation.*

Pharmacists may use the FDA Adverse Reaction Report form that appears in most issues of Clinical Pharmacy for submitting reports of adverse drug reactions directly to FDA.

Analgesics and Antipyretics

Sgro C (Center of Pharmacovigilance, CHRU Dijon, France), Escousse A, Tennenbaum D et al. Perinatal adverse effects of **nalbuphine** given during labor. *Lancet.* 1990; 336:1070. Case. (30-year-old primigravid woman at full term; received nalbuphine hydrochloride 7 mg by i.v. injection after five hours of labor; delivery of 2.75-kg infant one hour later; infant cyanotic and hypotonic; Apgar score, 9, 10, 10; infant treated with oxygen therapy; bradycardia and bradypnea resolved within 24 hours)

Anthelmintics

Cork MJ, Cooke NJ, Mellor E (Leeds General Infirmary, Leeds LS1 3EX, England). Pruritus ani, **piperazine** and thrombocytopenia. *Br Med J.* 1990; 301:1398. Case. (61-year-old man with self-diagnosed threadworm infestation; self-medicated with piperazine hydrate 2.25 g/day for two one-week courses and piperazine phosphate 4 g as a single dose three and seven weeks later; developed hemoptysis and epistaxis five days after last dose; platelet count was 2.6×10^{10}/L four days after hemoptysis resolved; platelet count increased to 1.7×10^{11}/L three weeks later; previous exposure to piperazine)

Anticoagulants

Gruel Y (Hematology Laboratory and Cardiology Department, Centre Hôspitalier and Universitaire Trousseau, 37044 Tours Cedex, France), Lang M, Darnige L et al. Fatal effect of re-exposure to **heparin** after previous heparin-associated thrombocytopenia and thrombosis. *Lancet.* 1990; 336:1077-8. Case. (71-year-old woman with history of heparin-associated thrombocytopenia and thrombosis; received unfractionated heparin 30,000 IU/day by s.c. injection and alteplase by i.v. injection for treatment of severe venous thromboembolism; developed thrombocytopenia and low fibrinogen concentrations by day 15 of heparin therapy; developed thrombi in abdominal aorta and pulmonary embolism during subsequent days; heparin discontinued; patient died on day 21 after recurrence of arterial thrombosis)

Antivirals

Bouvet E, Casalino E, Prevost MH et al. (Vachon F, Clinic de Reamination des Maladies Infections, Hopital Bichat, 75018

Paris, France). Fatal case of **2',3'-dideoxyinosine**-associated pancreatitis. *Lancet.* 1990; 336:1515. Case. (30-year-old woman with acquired immunodeficiency syndrome; received 2',3'-dideoxyinosine 250 mg twice daily for three months; developed relapse of cytomegalovirus retinitis; blood glucose concentration, 16.9 mM; elevated hepatic enzyme concentrations; retreated with ganciclovir; 2',3'-dideoxyinosine discontinued; one day later patient experienced severe abdominal pain that continued for six days; diagnosed with pancreatitis; serum amylase, 172 IU/mL; concomitant valproic acid, folinic acid, pyrimethamine, clindamycin, fluconazole, and pentamidine by aerosolization; patient died)

Cathartics and Laxatives

Lantner RR (Allergy Section, Loyola University Medical Center, 21605 First Ave., Building 117, Room 15, Maywood, IL 60153), Espiritu BR, Zumerchik P et al. Anaphylaxis following ingestion of a **psyllium**-containing cereal. *JAMA.* 1990; 264:2534-6. Case. (60-year-old female nurse; consumed one bowl of plantago seed-containing cereal with milk; developed anaphylactic reaction without hypotension 30 to 60 minutes after exposure; therapy with oral diphenhydramine led to resolution of symptoms; previous external exposure to psyllium-containing bulk laxative)

Drug Administration

Khan SA, Pace JE, Cox ML (Watford General Hospital, Watford, Hertfordshire WD1 8HB, England). Respiratory distress secondary to **naftidrofuryl**. *Br Med J.* 1990; 301:1219. Case. (93-year-old man with peripheral vascular disease; received nafronyl for several years; accidentally chewed one capsule; developed shortness of breath after drinking milk to relieve burning sensation in throat; concomitant pilocarpine ophthalmic solution; therapy with oxygen, sympathomimetic agents by nebulization, and corticosteroids by i.v. injection led to resolution of symptoms)

Folk Medicine

Koren G, Randor S, Martin S et al. (Danneman D, The Motherisk Program, Hospital for Sick Children, Toronto, Ontario, Canada). Maternal **ginseng** use associated with neonatal androgenization. *JAMA.* 1990; 264:2866. Case. (2-week-old male infant whose mother self-medicated with ginseng 1300 mg/day throughout pregnancy and during first two weeks of lactation for irritability and mood swings; infant developed pubic and head hair growth and enlarged testes; discontinuation of breast feeding after two weeks led to slow resolution of excess hair growth; infant demonstrated increased growth and weight gain during first seven weeks of life; mother experienced increased hair growth during ginseng use)

Immunotherapy

Janssen HL, Berk L, Vermeulen M et al. (Schalm SW, Department of Internal Medicine II and Neurology, University Hospital Dijkzigt, 3015GD Rotterdam, the Netherlands). Seizures associated with low-dose **α-interferon**. *Lancet.* 1990; 336:1580. Cases. (three men, aged 24–49 years, with chronic hepatitis B; 24- and 49-year-old patients received interferon alfa 1.5–5 million units daily; 28-year-old patient received interferon alfa 3 million units three times weekly; all patients developed seizures within 10 weeks; therapy with phenytoin or diazepam led to resolution of seizures; interferon therapy discontinued in 28-year-old patient)

Thrombolytic Agents

Dickinson RJ, Rosser A (Hinchingbrooke Hospital, Huntingdon PE18 8NT, England). Low back pain associated with **streptokinase**: 1. *Br Med J.* 1991; 302:111-2. Cases. (two patients, aged 73 and 74 years, with myocardial infarction; 73-year-old patient received streptokinase 200,000 units by i.v. infusion; 74-year-old patient received streptokinase 150,000 units by i.v. infusion; within 10 minutes both patients developed severe low back pain; withdrawal of streptokinase led to rapid resolution of pain; one patient received diacetylmorphine 5 mg by i.v. injection for pain relief; 73-year-old patient developed petechial rash 10 days later)

Partanen HJ, Nieminen MS (First Department of Medicine, University Central Hospital, SF-00290 Helsinki, Finland). Intracerebellar fatal hemorrhage after thrombolytic therapy of suspected non-Q-wave myocardial infarction. *Lancet.* 1990; 336:883. Case. (50-year-old man with suspected non-Q-wave myocardial infarction; received **streptokinase** 600,000 units by i.v. infusion over 10 minutes followed by 1.2 million units over 30 minutes; patient died; occlusion of left common carotid and left vertebral arteries due to thrombosis found at autopsy; right cerebellar hemorrhagic infarction with cerebral edema noted; no evidence of intracoronary thrombosis or myocardial infarction)

Porter NJ, Nikoletatos K (Royal Newcastle Hospital, Newcastle, NSW 2300, Australia). Low back pain associated with **streptokinase**: 2. *Br Med J.* 1991; 302:112. Case. (50-year-old woman with ventricular myocardial infarction; received streptokinase 1.5 million units by i.v. infusion over 60 minutes; after 20 minutes patient developed severe low back pain that radiated bilaterally down back of legs; discontinuation of streptokinase and therapy with morphine 5 mg by i.v. injection led to complete resolution of pain within five minutes; reinstitution of streptokinase without further incident)

Shah M, Taylor RT (Kidderminster General Hospital, Kidderminster, England). Low back pain associated with **streptokinase**. *Br Med J.* 1990; 301:1219. Cases. (three men, aged 35–64 years, with presumed myocardial infarction; 54-year-old patient with hypertension and asthma received aspirin and streptokinase 350,000 units; 35-year-old patient with diabetes mellitus received aspirin and streptokinase 300,000 units; 64-year-old patient with angina received streptokinase 255,000 units; all patients developed severe, acute low back pain; withdrawal of streptokinase led to resolution of pain; 64-year-old patient treated with hydrocortisone 100 mg and chlorpheniramine 10 mg by i.v. injections before continuation of streptokinase infusion)

Topical Preparations

Pavlovitch JH (CNRS URA 583, Hopital des Enfants Malades, 75743 Paris, France), Hubert H, Leibovitch J. Angiogenesis and **minoxidil**. *Lancet.* 1990; 336:889. Cases. (two patients, aged 26 and 27 years, with alopecia; applied minoxidil solution to scalp; after three months 26-year-old patient, who was seropositive for human immunodeficiency virus and had Kaposi's sarcoma on legs and trunk, developed two hemorrhagic lesions with features of Kaposi's sarcoma at site of minoxidil applications; after two months 27-year-old patient developed angioma of scalp, which was similar to a childhood lesion that spontaneously resolved)

Toxicity

Spearing RL (Department of Hematology, Christchurch Hospital, Private Bag, Christchurch, New Zealand), Hickton CM, Sizeland P et al. **Quinine**-induced disseminated intravascular coagulation. *Lancet.* 336:1535-7. Cases. (three women, aged 18–74 years, with leg cramps; self-medicated with quinine sulfate 200–300 mg; developed disseminated intravascular coagulation with high concentrations of circulating quinine-dependent antiplatelet antibodies; 18-year-old patient developed thrombotic microangiopathic hemolytic anemia, renal failure, and acute respiratory distress; 33-year-old patient developed rhabdomyolysis, severe hypoglycemia, and quinine-associated

Continued on page 316

Continued from page 314

red-cell hemolysis and died; 74-year-old patient developed less severe systemic symptoms and coagulopathy that spontaneously resolved)

Book Reviews

Drugs in Pregnancy and Lactation, Third Edition

By Gerald G. Briggs, Roger K. Freeman, and Sumner J. Yaffe.

Published by Williams & Wilkins, 428 East Preston Street, Baltimore, MD 21202, 1990. xx + 732 p. Price $59.95.

Health-care professionals are constantly asked about the effects of drugs on a fetus or nursing infant. We have a responsibility to be as well informed as allowed by current studies and available literature. *Drugs in Pregnancy and Lactation* summarizes this information and presents it in an easy-to-assess format; knowledge-based, prompt decisions can be made about maternal drug therapy and its effects.

The authors organized this book to resemble an encyclopedia; entries can be found easily and there are extensive appendixes and an index with cross-references. The introduction discusses some basics about the interactions between drugs, placenta, and fetus and emphasizes the importance of remembering horrendous past experiences such as the thalidomide and diethylstilbestrol catastrophies. The point is well made that drugs in maternal circulation, with few exceptions, will be transferred to breast milk.

The main text of the book is organized alphabetically by generic drug name and includes monographs on more than 500 drugs. Within each listing in the main text, the pharmacologic class is identified immediately below the generic drug name; this serves as a helpful refresher for seldom-used medications. The "Risk Factor" section of each monograph is very useful for hurried practitioners. The definitions of risk that are used by the authors are the same as those used by the Food and Drug Administration: A, B, C, D, and X are based on the level of risk posed to the fetus. The authors assigned most of the risk factors; when the assignment of risk factor matches the drug manufacturer's assignment, a subscript "M" appears alongside. When the authors and manufacturer differ in their assignment of risk, an asterisk appears, to indicate that the manufacturer's assignment is shown elsewhere in the monograph.

The bulk of the information on each drug is contained in the "Fetal Risk Summary" section, where a review of the literature concerning the drug is presented. In some cases the amount of information can be considerable, such as the seven pages devoted to ethanol. This approach allows the reader to digest the available information and make a knowledgeable recommendation about the drug in question. The summaries in this section are well referenced, which is useful to readers who want to study the issue in more detail.

The final part of each drug monograph is the "Breast Feeding Summary." Pay close attention to the distinction between the amount of drug excreted into breast milk and the effect of the drug on the infant.

When insufficient data are available, references are

made to other drugs in the same class (e.g., cloxacillin, see Penicillin G). The appendix lists drugs and their assigned risk factors by therapeutic class. This allows the clinician, at a glance, to assess the risks within that class of drugs and choose the least toxic alternative. The extensive index at the end lists drugs by both trade and generic names and includes many foreign names.

This easy-to-use reference book would be a helpful addition to any clinical library. I plan to use it on a regular basis.

Reviewed by Don R. Porter, Carteret General Hospital, 3500 Arendell Street, Morehead City, NC 28557.

Goodman and Gilman's The Pharmacological Basis of Therapeutics, 8th edition

Edited by Alfred Goodman Gilman, Theodore W. Rall, Alan S. Nies et al.

Published by Pergamon Press, Inc., Maxwell House, Fairview Park, Elmsford, NY 10523, 1990. xvi + 1811 p. Price $79.50.

Though this is the eighth edition of *Goodman and Gilman's The Pharmacological Basis of Therapeutics*, the three objectives of the first edition remain intact: to correlate pharmacology with related medical sciences; to reinterpret the actions and uses of drugs from the viewpoint of important advances in medicine; and to place emphasis on the applications of pharmacodynamics to therapeutics. The list of individuals who were involved in publication of the eighth edition includes several new contributing authors and two new editors.

The basic format of *Goodman and Gilman's The Pharmacological Basis of Therapeutics* has not changed. This edition is divided into 18 different sections and subdivided into chapters of related topics. Reorganization of the seventh edition created three new sections: "Drugs Affecting Gastrointestinal Function," "Drugs Used for Immunosuppression," and "Dermatology." Newly organized sections include chapters on renin, angiotensin, and angiotensin-converting enzyme inhibitors; antiviral agents; antifungal agents; hematopoietic agents; and sedative and hypnotic agents. In addition, many sections have been revised extensively. The section "General Principles" now includes a chapter on the principles of toxicology. There is new information about the structures and functions of several receptors and descriptions of more than 50 new drugs that were marketed in the past five years, including drugs produced by DNA technology, and many investigational agents. The book continues to convey the importance of the interplay between pharmacodynamics and pharmacokinetics.

Clinicians may find the two appendixes particularly useful. The first is a complete review of principles of prescription order writing and instructions for increasing patient compliance. The second is entitled "Design and Optimization of Dosage Regimen; Pharmacokinetic Data"; this table has been expanded to include pharmacokinetic parameters for 243 drug entries. The appendix that listed drug interactions, which appeared in the seventh edition, was deleted.

Goodman and Gilman's The Pharmacological Basis of Therapeutics continues to be a useful and informative ref-

Continued on page 318

Continued from page 317

erence book for the health-care practitioner. The revisions make the book current and include the rapid advances being made in health care. This book is a valuable reference not only to the hospital practitioner but also to those clinicians practicing in the community setting.

Reviewed by Burgunda W. Volger, Pharm.D., Drug Information and Investigational Drug Services, The University of Michigan Hospitals, 1500 E. Medical Center Drive, Ann Arbor, MI 48109-0008.

Books Received

Books are listed as soon as received; selected books may be reviewed in Book Reviews in subsequent issues.

Clinical Laboratory Tests: Values and Implications, edited by Helen Klusek Hamilton. Published by Springhouse Publishing Company, 1111 Bethlehem Pike, Springhouse, PA 19477, 1991. xii + 724 p. Price $24.95.

Infections in Intravenous Drug Abusers, edited by Donald P. Levine and Jack D. Sobel. Published by Oxford University Press, 200 Madison Avenue, New York, NY 10016, 1991. x + 395 p. Price $75.

Pharmacological Treatment of Endocrinopathies: Bone Disease, Kidney Stones and Related Disorders, by Charles Y. C. Pak. Published by S. Karger AG, P.O. Box CH-4009 Basel, Switzerland, 1991. viii + 141 p. Price $116; Sw.fr.145; DM174; £63.10.

Advertising Index

Adria Laboratories
Idamycin, 318, inside back cover, outside back cover
American Society of Hospital Pharmacists
CiteSearch, 256
Clinical Pharmacy, 291
Concepts in Clinical Pharmacokinetics, 317
Criteria for Drug Use Evaluation, Volumes 1 & 2, 261
European Drug Index, 315
Handbook on Injectable Drugs, Sixth Edition, 302
Medication Teaching Manual, Fourth Edition, 266
Rx Triage, 267
Safe Handling of Cytotoxic and Hazardous Drugs, 253
Burroughs Wellcome Company
Zovirax I.V., 258-260
Department of Veterans Affairs (Richmond)
Positions Available, 265
Glaxo Inc.
Ceptaz, 254-256
Lyphomed, Inc.
Amphotericin B, 262-264
Roerig, A Division of Pfizer Pharmaceuticals
Diflucan, 250-252
St. Jude Children's Research Hospital
Institutional, 310
The Upjohn Company and Chugai-Upjohn, Inc.
Marogen, inside front cover

News

Marketing of recombinant granulocyte–macrophage colony-stimulating factor approved by FDA	411
Etodolac approved for marketing in United States	416
Anabolic steroids reclassified as Schedule III controlled substances	417
Latex in medical devices may cause severe reactions; extra care advised	417
CDC revises mefloquine dosage recommendations	417
News Briefs	417

Marketing of recombinant granulocyte–macrophage colony-stimulating factor approved by FDA

In March, FDA approved marketing of sargramostim (Leukine, Immunex; Prokine, Hoechst–Roussel), a recombinant human granulocyte–macrophage colony-stimulating factor (GM-CSF), for use in accelerating myeloid recovery in patients with Hodgkin's disease, non-Hodgkin's lymphoma, or acute lymphoblastic leukemia (ALL) who are undergoing autologous bone marrow transplantation.

GM-CSF promotes division and differentiation of partially committed hematopoietic progenitor cells in the granulocyte–macrophage pathways. It also activates mature granulocytes and macrophages. Along with other factors, GM-CSF promotes proliferation of megakaryocytic and erythroid progenitor cells.

Sargramostim has been found to speed myeloid engraftment, reduce the duration of antimicrobial therapy and infectious episodes, and shorten the duration of hospitalization in patients with Hodgkin's disease, non-Hodgkin's lymphoma, or ALL who are undergoing bone marrow transplantation.

Sargramostim therapy is contraindicated in patients with excessive leukemic myeloid blast cells in the bone marrow or peripheral blood (≥10%) and in those with known hypersensitivity to GM-CSF, yeast-derived products, or any component of the product. Therapy with sargramostim is generally well tolerated; adverse events occurred at similar frequencies in the placebo and sargramostim groups in controlled clinical trials.

The recommended dosage of sargramostim is 250 μg/sq m as a two-hour intravenous infusion given daily for 21 days. Therapy should begin two to four hours after the bone marrow infusion and not less than 24 hours after the last dose of antineoplastic agents or 12 hours after the last dose of radiotherapy. Treatment should be discontinued if blast cells appear or the underlying disease progresses. Treatment should also be discontinued if the absolute neutrophil count exceeds 20,000/cu mm.

Leukine is available as a lyophilized powder in vials containing 250 or 500 μg of sargramostim. Immunex has set the price at $85 per 250-μg vial and $160 per 500-μg vial. The vials are packaged individually or in cartons of 10. Prokine is supplied in individually packaged 500-μg vials.

Continued on page 416

Gammagard®

Immune Globulin Intravenous (Human)

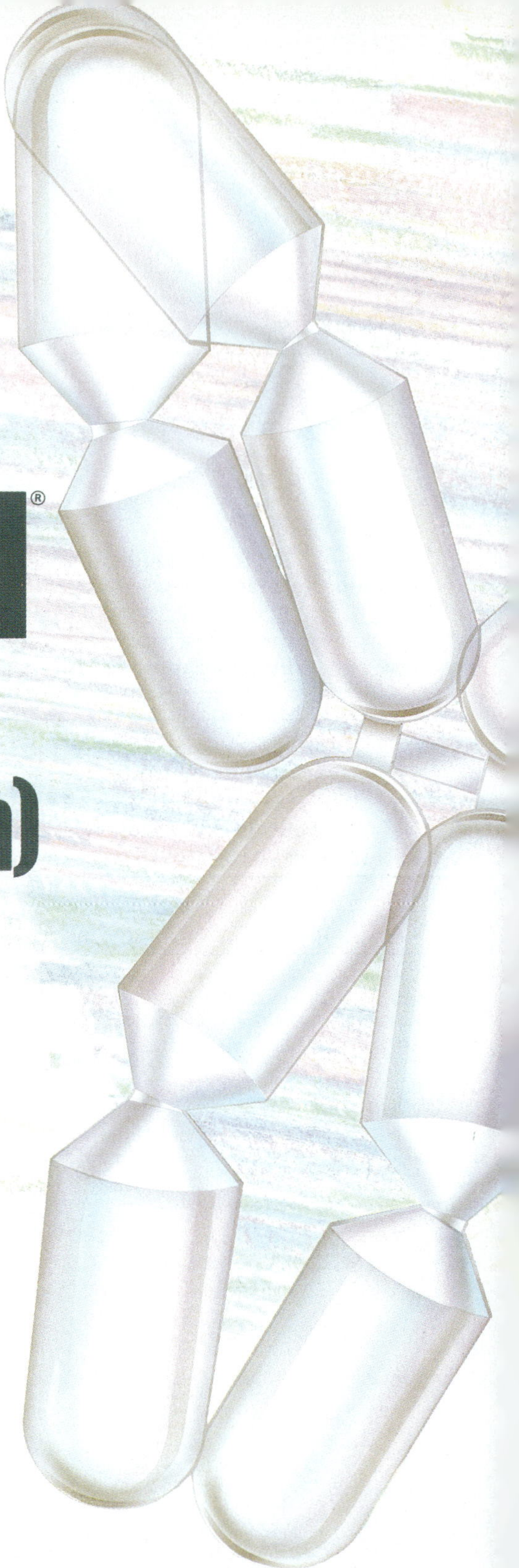

persons weighing 60 kg or less).

Lodine is available as 200- and 300-mg capsules in bottles and unit dose packages of 100.

Anabolic steroids reclassified as Schedule III controlled substances

Consistent with the requirements of the Anabolic Steroids Act of 1990, the Drug Enforcement Agency has reclassified all anabolic steroids as Schedule III controlled substances. Prescriptions for anabolic steroids issued on or before February 27, 1991, may be refilled up to five times before August 27, 1991, if refills were initially authorized. The only exceptions to the regulations are certain anabolic steroid implants intended for veterinary use. All salts, esters, and isomers of the following drugs are covered by the regulations: boldenone, chlorotestosterone, clostebol, dehydrochloromethyltestosterone, dihydrotestosterone, drostanolone, ethylestrenol, fluoxymesterone, formebolone, mesterolone, methandienone, methandranone, methandriol, methandrostenolone, methenolone, methyltestosterone, mibolerone, nandrolone, norethandrolone, oxandrolone, oxymesterone, oxymetholone, stanolone, stanozolol, testolactone, testosterone, and trenbolone.

Latex in medical devices may cause severe reactions; extra care advised

Reports of severe allergic reactions to medical devices containing latex have prompted FDA to advise health-care professionals to identify patients sensitive to latex and to be prepared to treat allergic reactions promptly. Reported reactions have ranged from contact urticaria to systemic anaphylaxis. An estimated 6–7% of surgical personnel and 18–40% of spina bifida patients are sensitive to latex. Recommendations to health-care professionals are as follows:

- Ask questions about latex sensitivity when taking general histories from all patients. This recommendation is especially important for surgical and radiology patients, spina bifida patients, and health-care workers. Questions about itching, rash, or wheezing after wearing latex gloves or inflating toy balloons may be useful. If the history suggests latex sensitivity, the patient's chart should be flagged.
- If latex sensitivity is suspected, consider using devices made with alternative materials, such as plastic. For example, a health-care professional could wear a nonlatex glove over a latex glove if the patient is sensitive. If both the health-care professional and the patient are sensitive, a latex middle glove could be used. Latex gloves labeled "hypoallergenic" may not always prevent adverse reactions.
- Be alert to the possibility of an allergic reaction whenever latex-containing medical devices are used, especially when the latex comes in contact with mucous membranes.
- If an allergic reaction does occur and latex is the suspected cause, advise the patient of a possible latex sensitivity and consider an immunologic evaluation.
- Advise patients to tell health-care professionals and emergency personnel about any known latex sensitivity before they undergo medical procedures. Consider advising patients with severe latex sensitivity to wear a medical identification bracelet.

Reports of adverse reactions to latex or other materials used in medical devices should be reported to the Medical Device and Laboratory Product Problem Reporting Program operated by the U.S. Pharmacopeia (800-638-6725 or 301-881-0256 [call collect] in Maryland).

CDC revises mefloquine dosage recommendations

The Centers for Disease Control (CDC) has changed its dosage recommendations for mefloquine for malaria prevention.[1] Travelers to areas with drug-resistant *Plasmodium falciparum* should take the first dose of mefloquine one week before travel. Therapy should be continued with doses given once weekly throughout the stay in areas with endemic malaria and for four weeks after departure. Previous recommendations called for doses to be given weekly for four weeks followed by one dose every other week.

1. Centers for Disease Control. Change of dosing regimen for malaria prophylaxis with mefloquine. *MMWR*. 1991; 40:72-3.

News Briefs

• In March an FDA advisory committee recommended against approving **tacrine** (Cognex, Warner–Lambert) without additional studies documenting the effectiveness of the drug in patients with Alzheimer's disease.

• Copies of a **cumulative list of orphan drugs and biologics** (docket number 84N-0102) can be obtained from the Dockets Management Branch (HFA-305), FDA, Room 4-62, 5600 Fishers Lane, Rockville, MD 20857, or from the National Information Center for Orphan Drugs and Rare Diseases, P.O. Box 1133, Washington, DC 20013.

• FDA plans to revise the labeling of corticosteroid products to strengthen the **warning about risks associated with varicella or herpes infection in patients taking corticosteroids.** This plan was prompted by a report describing the development of fatal disseminated varicella in an asthmatic child during a single course of corticosteroid therapy (October 1990 issue of the *Pediatric Infectious Disease Journal*) and several other case reports submitted to FDA.

• Miles Inc. has introduced an **injectable formulation of ciprofloxacin** (Cipro I.V.). The product is supplied in 200- and 400-mg strengths in vials (10 mg/mL) and flexible containers (0.2% ciprofloxacin in 5% dextrose injection).

• **Miconazole nitrate vaginal cream and suppositories** (Monistat 7, Ortho Pharmaceutical Corporation) are now available without a prescription.

• **Glutethimide** has been transferred from Schedule III to Schedule II of the Controlled Substances Act.

Therapy Consultation

The Therapy Consultation *section provides brief advice, in question-and-answer format, on how to handle specific drug-therapy problems. Readers are invited to submit questions, which will be referred to a consultant for an answer. The problems should not be highly specialized or unusual, nor should they be mundane. Questions are answered briefly, based largely on the judgment and personal experience of the consultant, although selected references may be cited to substantiate the consultant's advice.*

Assistance in identifying Therapy Consultation *topics is provided by the drug information centers at Medical College of Virginia Hospitals, Richmond; University of California Medical Center, San Diego; and University of Michigan Medical Center, Ann Arbor.*

Treatment of nocturnal leg cramps and restless leg syndrome

Question: Not all of our patients with nocturnal leg cramps obtain relief from using quinine sulfate. Are alternative treatments available? Should the patients be evaluated for restless leg syndrome, or would the treatment be the same?

Answer: The symptomatology, etiology, and treatment of idiopathic nocturnal leg cramps and restless leg syndrome are different, and proper diagnosis is necessary for successful treatment. Idiopathic nocturnal leg cramps are involuntary, painful contractions of muscles; cramps are usually confined to the calf but may affect other muscle groups. They usually occur during the first few hours of sleep and may disrupt sleep patterns. Nocturnal leg cramps frequently afflict persons middle-aged or older, pregnant women, and persons with vascular disease. The mechanism of nocturnal cramps is unknown. One hypothesis states that cramps may be caused by pathologic changes in the motor neuron cell body that cause abnormal neuron firing. Cramps usually do not follow a predictable pattern of onset, frequency, or duration. Cramping may occur regularly for a few days or weeks before resolving, but in some instances cramping may occur nightly for several years.

Restless leg syndrome (RLS) often goes unrecognized but is believed to be the fourth leading cause of insomnia. Patients with RLS have disturbing sensations of creeping or restlessness in their legs, usually bilaterally, that are worse at night. These patients also experience periodic movements of sleep that usually affect the legs predominantly and consist of flexion movements that occur at regular 20- to 40-second intervals during non-rapid-eye-movement sleep. Some evidence implicates central dopamine, as well as norepinephrine, in the pathophysiology of RLS.

A variety of home remedies have been used for preventing or treating nocturnal leg cramps. Among these treatments are soaking the affected leg in extremely hot water, massaging the affected area, elevating the foot of the bed, wrapping the legs tightly with cloth, and emptying the bladder immediately before going to bed. One novel idea involved placing a horseshoe magnet under the affected limb, between the sheet and the mattress.

The mainstay of therapy for the past 50 years has been quinine, but its use in recent years has become controversial. Most of the data concerning the use of quinine come from two studies: a noncontrolled study in 15 elderly subjects, published in 1940, that showed quinine to be effective in treating nocturnal leg cramps[1] and a double-blind study in nine patients, published in 1983.[2] More recently, Warburton et al.[3] conducted a double-blind, placebo-controlled, crossover trial in 22 elderly patients (mean ± S.D. age, 74 ± 8 years) with leg cramps at rest. A standard nightly dose of quinine bisulfate (300 mg at bedtime for three weeks) did not reduce the number or severity of cramps. Other controlled studies have also found quinine to be ineffective in the treatment of nocturnal leg cramps.[4,5] Quinine is not without potential adverse effects, which range from cinchonism (headache, tinnitus, unsteady gait, nausea, and visual disturbances) to blindness, thrombocytopenia, convulsions, coma, cardiac arrhythmias, and hypotension.

Several other treatments have been evaluated. Unfortunately all these studies had methodological flaws and none included statistical analyses. Ayres and Mihan[6] performed an unblinded, noncontrolled study of vitamin E in 125 subjects with nocturnal leg cramps. Approximately 82% of the subjects reported complete or almost complete relief at dosages of 300–400 IU/day. No adverse effects were noted. Carisoprodol 350 mg four times daily was compared with placebo in a double-blind study.[7] Of the 26 subjects, 81% showed improvement with carisoprodol. Adverse effects of carisoprodol in the general population include dizziness, drowsiness, vertigo, ataxia, and insomnia. In a double-blind, placebo-controlled study, chloroquine phosphate 250 mg/day relieved cramping.[8] However, since long-term chloroquine use is associated with retinal degeneration, its use for treatment of nocturnal leg cramps cannot be recommended. Seven of eight patients in an eight-week noncontrolled study had cessation of leg cramps while receiving verapamil hydrochloride 120 mg at bedtime.[9] An effect was usually noted in six days. Although verapamil was effective in treating nocturnal leg cramps, another calcium-channel blocker, nifedipine, has been implicated in precipitating leg cramps.[10]

The drugs reported to be successful in amelioration of RLS fall into three broad categories: anticonvulsants, dopaminergic agents, and drugs that inhibit noradrenergic or opiate activity. Carbamazepine 100–300 mg daily (median dose, 236 mg) was found in a randomized double-blind study to be more effective than placebo in decreasing both the number and severity of attacks.[11] Placebo produced a statistically significant therapeutic effect. Thirty-four of 84 subjects receiving carbamazepine and 20 of 88 subjects receiving placebo experienced unwanted effects, none serious. In several noncontrolled studies clonazepam was reported to be effective in the treatment of RLS. Dosages usually ranged from 0.5 to 2 mg daily given in divided doses. At higher dosages, somnolence was noted.

Bromocriptine (as the mesylate salt)[12] and levodopa/benserazide[13] have both been found effective at dosages of 7.5 mg at bedtime and 100 mg/25 mg at bedtime, respectively. Both significantly improved subjective complaints and decreased periodic movements during sleep. Many of the responders had been previously treated unsuccessfully with clonazepam. Transient nasal stuffiness and lightheadedness were reported. Handwerker and Palmer[14] reported that clonidine hydrochloride, at dosages of 0.1–0.3 mg daily, was effective therapy for RLS in three patients. RLS developed in one of these patients after the combination of oxycodone and aspirin was discontinued. Phenoxybenzamine, an α-adrenergic-receptor blocker, was reported to improve sleep disturbances and sleep-related myoclonus in one patient.[15] Although the patient was able to sleep without difficulty, his other symptoms of RLS remained.

Iatrogenic causes of RLS should not be overlooked. Both initiation and withdrawal of tricyclic antidepressant therapy have been implicated in the development of RLS. Because tricyclic antidepressants are frequently prescribed for geriatric patients, this may be an important cause of RLS in the elderly. In one patient, propranolol hydrochloride 40 mg three times daily relieved the severe tonic–clonic leg jerking that occurred after the dosage of imipramine hydrochloride was reduced from 75 mg at bedtime to less than 50 mg at bedtime.[16] Trimipramine and imipramine were found to increase sleep-related myoclonic events in those subjects who experienced these disturbances during a placebo period.[17] Myoclonic events decreased over the course of 44 days, suggesting a change in receptor sensitivity.

The treatment of nocturnal leg cramps and RLS can be problematic. The first step is to exclude potential iatrogenic causes. On the basis of our experience and review of the available data, we believe that the best method of relieving and preventing most nocturnal leg cramps is stretching of the affected limbs before sleep and during cramping episodes. If this is ineffective, some evidence suggests that vitamin E, carisoprodol, or verapamil may be effective and cause minimal adverse effects. The preferred treatment for RLS is much less clear. The dopaminergic agents, particularly bromocriptine, and carbamazepine appear to be preferred treatments.

1. Moss HK, Herrmann LG. Use of quinine for relief of "night cramps" in the extremities. *JAMA.* 1940; 115:1358.
2. Jones K, Castleden CM. A double-blind comparison of quinine sulphate and placebo in muscle cramps. *Age Ageing.* 1983; 12:155-8.
3. Warburton A, Royston JP, O'Neill CJ et al. A quinine a day keeps the leg cramps away? *Br J Clin Pharmacol.* 1987; 23:459-65.
4. Whitley AM. Cramps, stiffness and restless legs. *Practitioner.* 1982; 226:1085-7.
5. Lim SH. Randomized double-blind trial of quinine sulphate for nocturnal leg cramp. *Br J Clin Pract.* 1986; 40:462.
6. Ayres S Jr, Mihan R. Nocturnal leg cramps (systremma): a progress report on response to vitamin E. *South Med J.* 1974; 67:1308-12.
7. Chesrow EJ, Kaplitz SE, Breme JT et al. Use of carisoprodol for treatment of leg cramps associated with vascular, neurologic or arthritic disease. *J Am Geriatr Soc.* 1963; 11:1014-6.
8. Parrow A, Samuelsson SM. Use of chloroquine phosphate: a new treatment for spontaneous leg cramps. *Acta Med Scand.* 1967; 181:237-44.
9. Baltodano N, Gallo BV, Weidler DJ. Verapamil vs quinine in recumbent nocturnal leg cramps in the elderly. *Arch Intern Med.* 1988; 148:1969-70.
10. Keidar S, Binenboim C, Palant A. Muscle cramps during treatment with nifedipine. *Br Med J (Clin Res).* 1982; 285:1241-2.
11. Telstad W, Sørensen Ø, Larsen S et al. Treatment of the restless legs syndrome with carbamazepine: a double blind study. *Br Med J.* 1984; 288:444-6.
12. Walters AS, Hening WA, Kavey N et al. A double-blind randomized crossover trial of bromocriptine and placebo in restless legs syndrome. *Ann Neurol.* 1988; 24:455-8.
13. Brodeur C, Montplaisir J, Godbout R et al. Treatment of restless legs syndrome and periodic movements during sleep with L-dopa: a double-blind controlled study. *Neurology.* 1988; 38:1845-8.
14. Handwerker JV, Palmer RF. Clonidine in the treatment of restless leg syndrome. *N Engl J Med.* 1985; 313:1228-9. Letter.
15. Ware JC, Pittard JT, Blumoff RL. Treatment of sleep related myoclonus with an alpha-receptor blocker. *Sleep Res.* 1981; 10:242.
16. Ginsberg HN. Propranolol in the treatment of restless legs syndrome induced by imipramine withdrawal. *Am J Psychiatry.* 1986; 143:938. Letter.
17. Ware JC, Brown FW, Moorad PJ et al. Nocturnal myoclonus and tricyclic antidepressants. *Sleep Res.* 1984; 13:72.

TED WALTON, Pharm.D. Degree Candidate
School of Pharmacy, Medical College of Virginia/Virginia Commonwealth University (MCV/VCU)

KENNETH W. KOLB, PHARM.D.
Assistant Professor, School of Pharmacy, MCV/VCU
Chief, Pharmacotherapy Section, McGuire Veterans Affairs Medical Center

Richmond, VA 23298

Letters

The Letters *column is a forum for rapid exchange of ideas among readers of* Clinical Pharmacy. *Liberal criteria are applied in the review of submissions to encourage contributions to this column.*

The Letters *column includes the following types of contributions: (1) comments, addenda, and minor updates on previously published work, (2) alerts on potential problems related to drug therapy or clinical research, (3) observations or comments on trends in drug therapy or clinical research, and (4) brief expressions of opinion about controversies in drug therapy or clinical research.*

Letters need not be submitted with the journal's manuscript checklist. The following conditions, however, must be adhered to: (1) the body of the letter must be no longer than two typewritten pages, (2) the use of references, tables, and illustrations should be minimized, (3) the authors' names, affiliations, and mailing addresses must be typed at the end of the letter in the format used by Clinical Pharmacy, *and (4) the entire letter (including references, tables, and authors' names) must be typed double-spaced on plain white paper (not letterhead). Following acceptance of a letter, the authors are required to*

Cryoprecipitate for uremic bleeding

Couch and Stumpf[1] suggested in the November 1990 issue of *CP* that the use of cryoprecipitate may be an effective alternative to transfusion and dialysis in the management of uremic bleeding. However, the evidence for cryoprecipitate's efficacy in this clinical situation should be carefully examined. Although the initial reports of this product's value in uremia were positive, there have been few recent studies.

The experience in our blood bank is that cryoprecipitate often does not control uremic bleeding. This impression was confirmed by Triulzi and Blumberg,[2] who described five patients with uremia and prolonged bleeding times. Three patients did not respond to cryoprecipitate; one of these received multiple infusions of the product. One patient subsequently responded to desmopressin. A reason for the lack of reports similar to Triulzi and Blumberg's could be that clinicians are more likely to report treatment successes than failures.

Because treatment with cryoprecipitate carries risks, including the transmission of infectious diseases, its use in the treatment of uremic bleeding should be carefully deliberated.

1. Couch P, Stumpf JL. Management of uremic bleeding. *Clin Pharm.* 1990; 9:673-81.
2. Triulzi DJ, Blumberg N. Variability in response to cryoprecipitate treatment for hemostatic defects in uremia. *Yale J Biol Med.* 1990; 63(Jan-Feb):1-7.

Robertson Davenport, M.D., Associate Medical Director
Blood Bank and Transfusion Service
University of Michigan Hospitals, 2G332/0054
1500 East Medical Center Drive
Ann Arbor, MI 48109-0054

In the paper cited by Dr. Davenport, Triulzi and Blumberg reviewed the records of 82 patients who had received cryoprecipitate. Three of five evaluable patients with end-stage renal disease failed to respond to cyroprecipitate. Because bleeding times after cryoprecipitate administration were not determined for many of the remaining 77 patients, efficacy in these patients was not evaluated further. As mentioned by Dr. Davenport, other (earlier) reports of the use of cryoprecipitate in uremic bleeding have been predominantly positive.

Controlled studies of cryoprecipitate in large numbers of uremic patients are necessary to definitely establish the product's efficacy. The risk of disease transmission and the variable response to cryoprecipitate are indeed good reasons to carefully deliberate the product's use in uremic patients. In light of these considerations, desmopressin may be the preferred alternative to transfusion and dialysis in the management of uremic bleeding.

Patricia Couch, Pharm.D., Pediatric Pharmacy Resident
Department of Pharmacy
University of Michigan Medical Center
1500 East Medical Center Drive
Ann Arbor, MI 48109-0008

Correction

Hypoprothrombinemic effect of warfarin not influenced by ciprofloxacin (February 1991, Research Notes). On page 136, the second author's name is Catherine L. Kelley, not Catherine L. Keuey.

Drug Review

Ondansetron—the first of a new class of antiemetic agents

Betty J. Chaffee and Roberta M. Tankanow

Abstract: The chemistry, pharmacokinetics, adverse effects, stability, compatibility, and dosage of ondansetron hydrochloride are described, and clinical studies of the use of ondansetron for the prophylaxis of nausea and vomiting induced by antineoplastic therapy are reviewed.

Ondansetron hydrochloride is a specific antagonist of serotonin type 3 (5-HT_3) receptors, both in the chemoreceptor trigger zone and in the GI tract. Peak plasma concentrations of ondansetron occur approximately one hour after an oral dose and 6 to 20 minutes after an i.v. dose. The mean elimination half-life is approximately 3.5 hours in healthy volunteers, but it is extended in elderly patients (mean of 7.9 hours).

In clinical trials, ondansetron has been shown to provide excellent control of nausea and vomiting in patients treated with cisplatin. Comparisons of ondansetron with metoclopramide in patients treated with various types of chemotherapy have shown better response rates with ondansetron. Ondansetron has also been shown to be effective in controlling nausea and vomiting in patients receiving cyclophosphamide with an anthracycline and in patients receiving combination therapy with cyclophosphamide, methotrexate, and fluorouracil. Adverse effects appear to be mild and include headache, constipation, diarrhea and transient abnormalities in liver function tests. The dose of ondansetron (as the hydrochloride salt) for the prophylaxis of chemotherapy-induced nausea and vomiting in adults is 0.15 mg/kg i.v. every four hours for three doses, beginning 30 minutes before antineoplastic therapy.

The efficacy of ondansetron is comparable to that of metoclopramide, and the adverse-effect profile is much less problematic. The cost of ondansetron is much higher than that of metoclopramide; thus its use should be limited to patients at high risk for metoclopramide-induced adverse effects and patients in whom metoclopramide is ineffective.

Index terms: Antiemetics; Antineoplastic agents; Clinical studies; Dosage; Incompatibilities; Ondansetron hydrochloride; Pharmacokinetics; Stability; Toxicity
Clin Pharm. 1991; 10:430-46

Ondansetron hydrochloride dihydrate (Zofran, Glaxo) is one of a new class of antiemetic agents known as serotonin type 3 (5-hydroxytryptamine type 3; 5-HT_3)-receptor antagonists. Since 1986, ondansetron has been studied for the prophylaxis of nausea and vomiting induced by antineoplastic drugs. Ondansetron was approved by the FDA in January 1991 and was marketed in February 1991.

Nausea and Vomiting Induced by Antineoplastic Drugs

The importance of nausea and vomiting as serious adverse effects of antineoplastic drugs is evidenced by the rapid proliferation of literature on this subject in recent years.[1-4] Nausea and vomiting are the most feared symptoms related to therapy with antineoplastic drugs,[5] and when severe, they can lead to dehydration, esophageal rupture, or refusal of potentially curative treatment.[4] Additionally, recent work documents the detrimental effect of antineoplastic-drug-induced nausea and vomiting on the quality of life of cancer patients.[6]

The 1981 discovery that high-dose metoclopramide was effective for the prevention of cisplatin-induced emesis[7] was a major breakthrough in the management

Betty J. Chaffee, Pharm.D., is Clinical Pharmacist, Hematology/Oncology, and Clinical Assistant Professor, University of Michigan Medical Center and College of Pharmacy, Ann Arbor. Roberta M. Tankanow, M.S., is Clinical Pharmacist, Investigational Drug Service, University of Michigan Medical Center.

Address reprint requests to Dr. Chaffee at the Department of Pharmacy Services, UH-B2D301, Box 0008, University of Michigan Medical Center, 1500 East Medical Center Drive, Ann Arbor, MI 48109.

This is **article 680-204-9113** in the **ASHP Continuing Education System.** It qualifies for 1.0 hour of continuing-education credit. See page 474 for learning objectives and test questions.

of nausea and vomiting induced by antineoplastic drugs. Since that time, high-dose metoclopramide has been considered the most effective single-agent antiemetic,[4] with up to 65% of patients remaining relatively free of emesis during the 24 hours after receiving high-dose cisplatin.[8] Although this success rate is far better than that seen with placebo or prochlorperazine for the prevention of cisplatin-induced emesis,[7] approximately 35% of patients still experience severe nausea and vomiting after receiving high-dose cisplatin therapy. In addition, successful prophylaxis of nausea and vomiting on the day that an antineoplastic drug is administered does not guarantee that a patient will be free from nausea and vomiting on the days after drug therapy or during the next course.[9,10] It has also been shown that patients who suffer nausea and vomiting during one course of therapy with antineoplastic drugs are at an even higher risk of suffering severe nausea and vomiting with subsequent courses.[11] Finally, dose-limiting adverse effects of metoclopramide, such as acute dystonic reactions, akathisia, and diarrhea,[7,8,12-14] cause some patients to refuse further treatment with this effective antiemetic, resulting in even more difficult control of nausea and vomiting.

The problems described above have led researchers to look for alternative methods of preventing nausea and vomiting induced by antineoplastic therapy. The 5-HT_3-receptor antagonists are the newest class of agents found to be effective. Ondansetron, the first of these agents to come to market, will be the focus of this paper.

Chemistry and Pharmacology

The chemical formula of ondansetron is 1,2,3,9-tetrahydro-9-methyl-3[(2-methyl-1*H*-imidazol-1-yl)methyl]-4*H*-carbazol-one. Its structure is shown in Figure 1. Ondansetron is soluble in water (3.2% w/v) and in 0.9% sodium chloride (0.8% w/v).[15] Doses of the drug are expressed as milligrams of ondansetron, although ondansetron is formulated as the hydrochloride salt. It is a potent, selective, reversible 5-HT_3-receptor antagonist. This has been shown by its antagonism of 5-HT-induced depolarization in the vagus nerve and superior cervical ganglion of the rat.[16] Ondansetron is selective for the 5-HT_3 receptor, as compared with the 5-HT_1 or 5-HT_2 receptors. This selectivity has been proven by its lack of effect against 5-HT-induced contractions in the rabbit aorta (5-HT_2 receptors) and the dog saphenous vein (5-HT_1 receptors). Additionally, it had no activity against the 5-HT-induced relaxed cat saphenous vein.[17] Low concentrations of ondansetron antagonized the positive chronotropic effect of 5-HT and 2-methyl-5-HT on the isolated heart of the rabbit.[16] Ondansetron has been shown to have negligible agonist or antagonist activity at the α_1, α_2, β_1, or β_2 adrenoreceptors, as well as the histamine H_1 and H_2 receptors. Ondansetron has no antagonist activity at the muscarinic and central or

Figure 1. Structure of ondansetron.

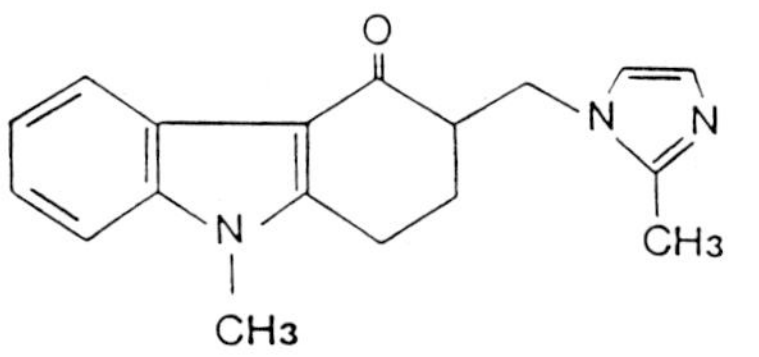

peripheral dopaminergic receptor sites. This drug does not seem to possess any extrapyramidal reactions that have been associated with dopamine antagonist activity.[16-18]

The specific central 5-HT_3 receptor-binding site of action for ondansetron appears to be in the area postrema, the medullary structure that contains the chemoreceptor trigger zone.[19] This has been demonstrated by the fact that cisplatin-induced emesis was inhibited by discrete injections of ondansetron into the area postrema of the ferret brain. The peripheral site of action is possibly the upper GI tract because 5-HT is abundant in the enterochromaffin cells near the afferent pathway. It is postulated that the area postrema acts as a relay between activated visceral afferents in the GI tract and the vomiting center in the medulla to cause the muscular movements of the abdomen and diaphragm.[20]

Antineoplastic drugs and radiation therapy have been shown to induce the release of serotonin from the enterochromaffin cells of the GI tract, where most of the body's serotonin stores are located.[20,21] 5-HT_3 receptors are found in the sympathetic and parasympathetic postganglionic neurons, sensory neurons, neurons in the GI tract, and vagal afferents in the CNS.[22] Serotonin, a neurotransmitter, stimulates the afferent fibers of the peripheral nerves in mammals. The serotoninergic neurons and the 5-HT_3 receptors of the central and peripheral nervous system play a role in the emetogenic pathways. Serotonin mediates the neural reflex arc of emesis.[21,23,24]

Cubeddu et al.[21] studied the effect of cisplatin on endogenous serotonin kinetics in patients who were enrolled in a double-blind, placebo-controlled study of ondansetron. All patients received a cisplastin dose of at least 50 mg/sq m. Urinary excretion of the primary metabolite of serotonin, 5-hydroxyindoleacetic acid (5-HIAA), was measured for a 10-hour period beginning 2 hours before cisplatin therapy in 28 patients (14 patients received ondansetron and 14 received placebo). The relationship of urinary 5-HIAA excretion to nausea and vomiting was an important finding in this study. Six healthy volunteers who received only hydration and mannitol without cisplatin showed no changes in the urinary excretion of 5-HIAA during the study period. Conversely, all 28 patients treated with cisplatin showed a significantly increased urinary excretion of the metabolite from a mean of 490 μg/hr during the two hours before cisplatin therapy to a mean of 1242 μg/hr during the four- to six-hour period after cisplatin therapy. There was no difference between the placebo- and ondansetron-treated groups in the magnitude of the change. A positive correlation existed between the concentrations of urinary 5-HIAA and the number of emetic episodes in patients treated with cisplatin. The increase in urinary 5-HIAA points to the mechanism of cisplatin-induced emesis (i.e., increased release of serotonin from enterochromaffin cells in the gut) and explains the high efficacy of ondansetron in these patients.

The ferret model has been used to demonstrate antiemetic efficacy. In the ferret, the initial response to noxious compounds is initiated in the gut. This response is in contrast to the response of the rat and other animals that do not vomit as easily. The ferret displays an acute emetic response to apomorphine, suggesting that this animal has an emetic chemoreceptor trigger zone. [19,25-28]

The antiemetic activity of ondansetron has been demonstrated in the ferret. Intravenous doses of ondansetron 0.01–1 mg/kg were compared with metoclopramide 2–4 mg/kg in animals receiving cisplatin 10 mg/kg. Ondansetron was shown to be 200 times more potent than metoclopramide in reducing or abolishing the emetic response, as well as increasing the latency period to the onset of emesis.[29] A further study by Stables et al.[30] has shown the effect of ondansetron against retching and vomiting induced by cyclophosphamide, x-ray radiation, or cisplatin in the ferret. In the animals receiving cisplatin, there was a significant increase in ileal mucosal levels of 5-HT and its principal metabolite, 5-HIAA. Andrews et al.[25] further substantiated these results by inducing emesis in ferrets with cyclophosphamide or radiation. Ondansetron (0.5 mg/kg) abolished the retching and vomiting responses. Because abdominal vagotomy and ondansetron have similar effects on the emetic response to these two treatments, it is thought that ondansetron acts by blocking $5\text{-}HT_3$ receptors on the vagal afferent input pathways to the emetic coordinating centers in the brain stem.[25]

Other Pharmacologic Actions. Costall et al.[31] studied the action of ondansetron on scopolamine-induced cognitive deficits in rats. Treatment with ondansetron and three other $5\text{-}HT_3$-receptor antagonists inhibited the impaired mental performance produced by scopolamine (a muscarinic-receptor antagonist). This discovery may indicate a role for future studies in patients with cognitive deficits linked with a cholinergic dysfunction. Other $5\text{-}HT_3$ receptors have been shown to be located in brain areas such as the entorhinal cortex, amygdala, and nucleus accumbens. The actions of ondansetron on these areas indicate potential usefulness of this agent in the treatment of schizophrenia, obsessive–compulsive disorders, anxiety, and substance abuse.[18,32] No clinical trials of ondansetron in patients with these disease states have yet been published. Ondansetron has shown no effect in motion sickness.[33]

The effect of ondansetron on gastric emptying has been studied in a double-blind, placebo-controlled, crossover trial involving 12 patients with persistent nausea and gastric stasis syndrome. After administration of ondansetron 16 mg or placebo three times daily for two days, solid and liquid gastric emptying tests were performed. There was no significant difference between patients who received ondansetron or placebo with respect to gastric emptying rate of the solid or liquid phases.[34] In controlled studies with human volunteers, single i.v. doses of ondansetron also did not seem to have an effect on gastric emptying compared with placebo. It is possible that ondansetron does not affect a normal basal emptying rate.[35] However, further controlled trials using large patient populations are needed to better assess this potential action, especially to determine if it could be useful in certain subgroups of patients with diabetic gastroparesis.[33] Ondansetron has been shown to have an effect on colonic transit. In healthy volunteers, ondansetron 16 mg three times daily slowed left colon transit but caused no change in the right colon or small intestine.[35,36] This action of ondansetron is likely to be the cause of constipation in patients treated with this drug.

Pharmacokinetics

The distribution of ondansetron has been studied after single and multiple oral and i.v. dosing in healthy volunteers, in patients (children and adults), and in the elderly. Absolute oral bioavailability in healthy volunteers has been shown to be about 50–60%. Ondansetron is approximately 70–76% protein bound and has a large volume of distribution of about 163 L.[33] Ondansetron is extensively metabolized, with less than 10% of the parent compound recovered unchanged in the urine. The metabolites are mainly formed by hydroxylation, glucuronidation, and *N* demethylation.[37] Kinetic studies were done by Priestman et al.[38] in eight elderly patients (≥65 years of age) undergoing either antineoplastic drug therapy or radiation therapy. Ondansetron 8 mg was administered every eight hours for four days. The median maximum plasma drug concentration (C_{max}) was 107.5 ng/mL, with a time to reach maximum concentration (T_{max}) of one hour. The median elimination half-life ($t_{1/2}$) was increased to 7.9 hours, as opposed to 3.5 hours in younger healthy volunteers.[38,39] Another trial[40] comparing age groups of healthy volunteers reported similar trends. Systemic clearance of ondansetron tended to be lower in the elderly (>75 years of age) than in the younger volunteers (20–40 years of age). Additionally, females cleared the drug slightly more slowly than males.

Colthup et al.[41] reported results to kinetic studies of ondansetron in 18 healthy male volunteers. Single and repeated oral and i.v. doses were tested. After a single i.v. dose of 8 mg, C_{max} ranged from a median of 80 to 95.6 ng/mL; after a single oral dose of 8 mg, the median C_{max} was about 32 ng/mL. The steady state serum drug concentration (C_{ss}) after an infusion of 1 mg/hr for 24 hours ranged from 20 to 30 ng/mL. T_{max} ranged from 0.1 to 0.3 hours after an 8-mg i.v. infusion and was approximately 1 hour after a single 8-mg oral dose.[33,39,41] The renal clearance of ondansetron from plasma (CL_R) after oral and i.v. doses was 17.5 mL/min and 10 mL/min, respectively. The median total body clearance of drug from plasma (CL) after single and continuous infusion was 578 mL/min and 602 mL/min, respectively.[33] The pharmacokinetic profile of ondansetron is nonlinear, suggesting a saturation of first-pass metabolism.[39]

Lazarus et al.[42] studied the pharmacokinetics of ondansetron in 12 patients before autologous bone marrow transplantation and before cisplatin therapy (40 mg/sq m daily for five days). The dose of ondansetron was 0.15 mg/kg i.v. every two hours three times daily for five days. On day 1, after doses 1 and 3, the mean C_{max} was 119 and 244 ng/mL, respectively. Based on data compiled from day 1, mean T_{max} was 0.25 hours, mean $t_{½}$ was 3.9 hours, and mean systemic CL was 398.3 mL/min. Compared with healthy volunteers, these patients had the same $t_{½}$ but a higher C_{max}. The clearance also seemed to be lower in these patients.

The pharmacokinetics of ondansetron in children has not been studied extensively. Blumer et al.[43] studied the kinetics of this drug in nine children aged 8 to 18 years who were naive to antineoplastic drugs. The children received ondansetron 0.15 mg/kg every four hours for three doses; $t_{½}$ ranged from 1.8 to 5.1 hours. Volume of distribution and clearances of drug from plasma were generally within the ranges reported for adults.

Serum concentrations are not correlated with antiemetic efficacy, and there does appear to be accumulation after multiple dosing.[26,33,44] It is not known yet whether renal failure or hepatic failure would alter the pharmacokinetics and hence the dose of ondansetron. Because of its extensive hepatic metabolism, ondansetron should be used with caution in patients with known or suspected severe liver dysfunction. Like the antagonists of the H_2 receptor that are known inhibitors of cytochrome P-450, ondansetron contains an imidazole ring. Although drug interactions with ondansetron have not been reported in the literature, the potential for drug interactions will become clear only after many patients have been exposed to this agent.

Clinical Efficacy

Methodological Considerations and Definition of Terms. Efficacy studies of antiemetics for the prevention of antineoplastic-drug-induced nausea and vomiting are difficult to design and often to interpret. Study design and patient population variables can substantially influence the results of a study. Unblinded and nonrandomized study designs present the problem of investigator or patient bias, or both, toward one treatment or another. The crossover design, commonly used in antiemetic studies, can introduce a less obvious source of bias. It is well known that patients who have been previously exposed to antineoplastic drugs are more likely to suffer nausea and vomiting.[11,45] Patients who serve as their own controls may be naive to antineoplastic drugs during the first treatment period; however, by the second treatment period they will have been previously exposed to antineoplastic drugs and may not have the same underlying potential for nausea and vomiting. This type of bias is known as a "treatment-by-period interaction."[46] To consider the results of a crossover study valid, the investigators must test for this type of interaction.

In addition to study design, patient variables may also substantially influence study results. Because antineoplastic drugs differ in the mechanism, incidence, and severity of nausea and vomiting they evoke, studies that include patients receiving a wide variety of drugs may be difficult to interpret (Table 1).[11] Factors such as age, gender, alcohol use,[47,48] previous exposure to antineoplastic drugs, and the dose and duration of administration of the antineoplastic drug have been shown to significantly influence the responses of patients to antiemetics.[11,45,49,50]

Recently, antiemetic studies have become somewhat more uniform in design, allowing for easier comparison of trials. Ideally, antiemetic trials should study parallel groups of patients who are naive to antineoplastic drugs and who all receive the same emetic stimulus. Studies that employ a crossover design must test for a treatment-by-period interaction and statistically compare the results of only the first treatment period if necessary. The dose and duration of infusion of the antineoplastic drug(s) should be reported to the reader. Strict inclusion and exclusion criteria, randomization, and double-blinding procedures should be used.

The efficacy of antiemetic agents is reported in a similar way in most recently published studies. The following definitions will be used in this paper: "complete response" will refer to complete absence of emesis; "major reponse" will refer to zero, one, or two emetic episodes during the study period; and "failure" will refer to more than two emetic episodes. The term "emetic episode" will refer not only to episodes of vomiting but will include episodes of retching not productive of liquid. Nausea, most often measured on a 100-mm visual analogue scale that denotes 0 mm as "no nausea" and 100 mm as "worst nausea," will be reported in millimeters. Deviations from these definitions will be specifically described.

Doses of ondansetron hydrochloride and metoclopramide hydrochloride are expressed as milligrams of ondansetron and metoclopramide, respectively.

Cisplatin-Containing Antineoplastic Therapy. Cisplatin is generally considered one of the most potent and predictable emetic stimuli among antineoplastic drugs, producing emesis in nearly 100% of patients to whom it is administered without antiemetic prophylaxis.[7,21] Emesis after a single high dose of cisplatin

Table 1.
Relative Emetic Potential of Antineoplastic Drugs[a]

High (>90%)	Moderately High (60–90%)	Moderate (30–60%)	Moderately Low (10–30%)	Low (<10%)
Cisplatin	Semustine	Fluorouracil	Bleomycin	Busulfan
Dacarbazine	Carmustine	Doxorubicin	Hydroxyurea	Chlorambucil
Mechlorethamine	Lomustine	Daunorubicin	Melphalan	Thioguanine
Streptozocin	Cyclophosphamide	Asparaginase	Etoposide	Vincristine
Cytarabine[b]	Dactinomycin	Mitomycin	Teniposide	Estrogens
	Plicamycin	Azacitidine	Cytarabine[d]	Progestins
	Procarbazine	Hexamethylmelamine	Mercaptopurine	Corticosteroids
	Methotrexate[c]		Methotrexate[e]	Androgens
			Thiotepa	
			Vinblastine	

[a] Originally published in: Craig JB, Powell B. Review: the management of nausea and vomiting in clinical oncology. *Am J Med Sci.* 1987; 29:34–44. Reprinted with permission.
[b] Only with high-dose therapy (>500 mg/sq m).
[c] Doses >200 mg/sq m.
[d] Standard doses.
[e] Low dose.

(≥100 mg/sq m by short i.v. infusion) has an onset of between three and six hours after the dose and is usually most severe during that time.[13,21,51] Additionally, nausea and vomiting severe enough to affect daily activities commonly occur between 48 and 72 hours after cisplatin is administered, even in patients who experienced little or no nausea and vomiting on the day of antineoplastic therapy.[2] Because of the widespread use of cisplatin and the high incidence and severity of cisplatin-induced nausea and vomiting, many trials of ondansetron have been conducted in patients receiving cisplatin.

Noncomparative Trials. Pilot studies showed that ondansetron was safe and effective for the prophylaxis of nausea and vomiting in patients treated with a variety of antineoplastic drugs.[52-55] Investigators then proceeded to conduct dose-ranging studies of ondansetron for the prophylaxis of cisplatin-induced nausea and vomiting (Table 2).

The first study to be published included 13 patients scheduled to receive cisplatin 70 to 120 mg/sq m over four hours.[10] All patients were initially naive to antineoplastic drugs; five patients were studied twice. Overall, complete antiemetic response was achieved in 45% of the treatment courses, whereas major response was achieved in 72% of the courses. A dose–response relationship was not found. Median nausea scores were 7 mm in the complete responders, 53 mm in the major responders, and 39.5 mm in the patients who failed to respond. Adverse effects included mild sedation (six patients), flushing (five patients), and headache (two patients).

An open, dose-ranging study was performed in 45 patients (38 of whom were naive to antineoplastic drugs) scheduled to receive cisplatin 60 to 120 mg/sq m over two hours.[56] Eight dose levels of ondansetron were studied on an every-four-hour schedule. Ondansetron 0.18 mg/kg was also studied on an every-six-hour schedule. The degree of nausea was measured in hours instead of by severity. The overall complete antiemetic response rate in the 43 evaluable patients was 44%, with 81% of the patients achieving a major response. In addition, 44% of the patients suffered two or fewer hours of nausea. Dose–response relationships included a somewhat higher failure rate at the 0.01-mg/kg dose and a significantly higher rate of complete response in patients who received high-dose cisplatin (≥100 mg/sq m) when ondansetron was given in doses of at least 0.3 mg/kg. Adverse effects included dose-related headache in 40% of patients (more severe at the 0.48-mg/kg dose), lightheadedness in 21%, asymptomatic elevations of serum aminotransferases in 19%, and one apparent anaphylactic reaction that responded to standard treatment. The authors concluded that ondansetron lacked efficacy at 0.01 mg/kg and that the adverse effects were more intense at 0.48 mg/kg; they recommended that further studies be performed with 0.36 mg/kg as the maximum dose. However, the small patient population and lack of randomization brings into question the validity of the dose comparisons made.

Kris et al.[57] reported a series of trials using ondansetron in patients receiving cisplatin. One of these trials included eight patients who were naive to antineoplastic drugs. Ondansetron 0.04 mg/kg failed to prevent nausea and vomiting in seven of the eight patients studied. The researchers concluded that ondansetron in the doses used is not effective for the prevention of cisplatin-induced nausea and vomiting.

An open-label, controlled, randomized, dose-finding study was initiated to confirm the lack of effectiveness of lower doses of ondansetron.[23] Thirty-six patients who were naive to antineoplastic drugs and scheduled to receive high-dose cisplatin were studied. Complete antiemetic response was achieved in 41% of the patients receiving the higher dose of ondansetron and in only 5% of the patients receiving the lower dose ($p < 0.02$). Nausea scores were slightly lower in the

Table 2.
Noncomparative Trials of Ondansetron in Cisplatin-Treated Patients

Reference	No. Patients	Cisplatin Regimen	Ondansetron Regimen	% Response[a] MR	CR
10	13	70–120 mg/sq m over 4 hours	4 mg i.v. before cisplatin, then 2 mg Q6h × 2 (6 patients)	72	45[b]
			8 mg i.v. before cisplatin, then 4 mg Q6h × 2 (7 patients)		
56	45	60–120 mg/sq m over 2 hours	0.01–0.48 mg/kg Q4h × 3; one dose infused before cisplatin	81	44
57	28	≥100 mg/sq m over 20 min	0.04 mg/kg Q2h × 3; one dose infused before cisplatin (8 patients)	12	0
			0.18 mg/kg Q2h × 3 (10 patients)	50	30
			0.18 mg/kg Q4h × 3 (10 patients)	60	40
23	36	≥100 mg/sq m over 60 min	0.01 mg/kg Q4h × 6; one dose infused before cisplatin	26	5
			0.18 mg/kg Q4h × 6; one dose infused before cisplatin	65	41
58	85	≥75 mg/sq m over 5 min to 8 hours	0.18 mg/kg Q6h × 3; one dose infused before cisplatin (42 patients)	83	59
			0.18 mg/kg Q8h × 3; one dose infused before cisplatin (43 patients)	72	50
59	28	70–120 mg/sq m over 1 hour	8 mg i.v. before cisplatin, immediately followed by 1 mg/hr × 24 hours	69	46
60	23	100–120 mg/sq m over 12 hours	8 mg i.v. before cisplatin, immediately followed by 1 mg/hr × 24 hours (7 patients)	28	28
			10 mg i.v. before cisplatin, immediately followed by 2 mg/hr × 24 hours (6 patients)	50	33
			12 mg i.v. before cisplatin, immediately followed by 4 mg/hr × 24 hours (10 patients)	30	20
61	45	70–120 mg/sq m over an unspecified time period	8 mg i.v., immediately followed by 1 mg/hr × 24 hours	63	37[b]
			10 mg i.v., immediately followed by 2 mg/hr × 24 hours		
			12 mg i.v., immediately followed by 4 mg/hr × 24 hours		

[a] MR = major response, CR = complete response. All patients were monitored for 24 hours.
[b] Response rates include patients from all the treatment groups in the trial.

higher-dose group (42 mm versus 57 mm); this difference was not statistically significant. Interestingly, the time to onset of emesis was much shorter in the lower-dose group: in the six hours after cisplatin administration, 89% of the lower-dose group had vomited compared with only 6% of the higher-dose group. Adverse effects were not dose related and included headache in three patients, diarrhea in one patient, and elevated serum aminotransferases in six patients. Ondansetron was shown to be ineffective when given in a dose of 0.01 mg/kg, confirming the results seen by others.[57]

Kris et al.[57] also studied ondansetron in different dosing schedules. Twenty patients who were naive to antineoplastic drugs and scheduled to be treated with high-dose cisplatin were randomized to receive the same dose of ondansetron every two hours or every four hours for three doses. Complete response was achieved in 35% of the 20 patients, whereas major responses were achieved in 55% of them. The visual analogue scale scores for nausea were 36 mm in the every-two-hour group and 6 mm in the every-four-hour group. No significant difference was found between the two schedules; unfortunately, the statistical power of the study may have been too low to detect a clinically important difference.

A multi-institutional dose-finding study was conducted in 85 patients who were naive to antineoplastic drugs and scheduled to receive high-dose cisplatin.[58] Patients were randomized to receive ondansetron for three doses given every six hours or every eight hours. The groups were relatively comparable with respect to gender, age, and history of ethanol consumption; comparability of groups with respect to dose and duration of cisplatin infusion was not reported. No statistically significant difference was found between the groups for complete response rate or major response rate. Nausea scores were not significantly different between the two groups. Analysis of data with respect to alcohol intake showed that patients with a prior or current history of heavy ethanol use (one or more drinks daily) had a 74% complete response rate, compared with a 33% complete response rate in those without such a history. Adverse effects included transient elevation of serum aminotransferases in 17% of patients, mild

Table 3.
Comparative Trials of Ondansetron in Cisplatin-Treated Patients

Reference	No. Patients	Cisplatin Regimen	Antiemetic Regimen: Ondansetron	Antiemetic Regimen: Control	% Response[a] Ondansetron MR	Ondansetron CR	Control MR	Control CR	Monitoring Period
21	28	≥50 mg/sq m over 1 hour	0.15 mg/kg Q4h × 3; one dose infused before cisplatin	Placebo	79	14	0	0	24 hours
66	97	80–100 mg/sq m over 1 hour	8 mg i.v. before cisplatin, immediately followed by 1 mg/hr × 24 hours	Metoclopramide 3 mg/kg i.v. before cisplatin, immediately followed by 0.5 mg/kg/hr × 8 hours, and then placebo i.v. × 16 hours	75	46	42	16	24 hours, then diary cards for days 2–6
51	121	50–100 mg/sq m over 3–4 hours	8 mg i.v. before cisplatin, immediately followed by 1 mg/hr × 24 hours	Metoclopramide 3 mg/kg i.v. before cisplatin, immediately followed by 0.5 mg/kg/hr × 8 hours, and then placebo i.v. × 16 hours	72	NR	41	NR	24 hours, then diary cards for days 2–6
67	307	≥100 mg/sq m over ≤3 hours	0.15 mg/kg Q4h × 3; one dose infused before cisplatin	Metoclopramide 2 mg/kg Q2h × 3, then Q3h × 3; one dose infused before cisplatin	65	40	51	30	24 hours

[a] MR = major response, CR = complete response, NR = not reported.

headache in 11%, diarrhea in 7%, dizziness in 5%, and drowsiness in 5%. Constipation was reported in one patient. Ondansetron 0.18 mg/kg for three doses was shown to be effective for the prevention of cisplatin-induced nausea and vomiting; the six-hour and eight-hour dosing intervals were equally effective. However, the variable doses and infusion times of cisplatin may have biased the results if the two groups were not comparable in this regard.

The efficacy of ondansetron given as a continuous i.v. infusion has also been studied.[59-61] The first published trial[59] was uncontrolled and unblinded and included patients who were naive to antineoplastic drugs and previously treated patients; some were given other emetogenic antineoplastic drugs in addition to cisplatin during the trial. The complete and major response rates were 46% and 69%, respectively. In those patients with complete response, the median nausea score was 0 mm (range, 0–25 mm); in those patients with major response it was 27 mm (range, 1–52 mm). As expected, patients who were naive to antineoplastic drugs and received relatively lower doses of cisplatin (≤100 mg/sq m) responded more favorably than previously exposed patients treated with higher doses of cisplatin (major responses of 100% versus 30%, respectively). Adverse effects included sedation in five patients, headache in four, diarrhea in four, and asymptomatic, transient increases in serum aminotransferases in three.

Another uncontrolled, unblinded trial[60] of continuous i.v. infusion ondansetron included 23 patients; 10 were previously treated and considered refractory to standard antiemetics. Three dose schedules were used. Patient characteristics within each group were not described. The higher doses of ondansetron had no significant advantage over the lower doses. The overall major response rate of 35% is comparable to that observed in the study by Marty et al.[59] (in which previously treated patients receiving high doses of cisplatin achieved a 30% major response) and is not particularly impressive. However, the uncontrolled nature of the trial may have led to the relative lack of success compared with other trials involving patients who were naive to antineoplastic drugs. The only adverse effect reported was headache in 22% of patients.

The third trial[61] of continuous-infusion ondansetron was uncontrolled and involved patients who were naive to antineoplastic drugs and patients who had been previously treated. Ondansetron was given in three doses. Forty-three of the 45 enrolled patients were evaluable; of these, 37% achieved a complete antiemetic response and 63% achieved a major response. No dose–response relationship was noted. The visual analogue scale score for nausea was ≤10 mm in 40% of patients.

The results of these dose-finding studies seem to indicate that a wide range of ondansetron doses are safe and effective for the prophylaxis of cisplatin-induced nausea and vomiting. In addition, the optimal dose interval appears to range from two to eight hours. Continuous i.v. infusion of ondansetron appears to be effective for the prophylaxis of cisplatin-induced nausea and vomiting, but the comparative efficacy of continuous infusion and intermittent dosing has not yet been studied.

Comparative Trials. Several comparative trials of ondansetron in cisplatin-treated patients have been conducted (Table 3). Among them was a placebo-controlled trial of ondansetron for the prophylaxis of cisplatin-induced nausea and vomiting.[21] Many ethical questions have been raised about this trial,[62-65] as it has been shown that without antiemetics nearly all patients treated with cisplatin suffer severe nausea and vomiting.[7] Twenty-eight patients who were naive to antineoplastic drugs were randomized to receive placebo or ondansetron. Patients were given rescue antiemetic treatment if they suffered intense or frequent vomiting (three or more episodes in one hour). As expected, there was a significant difference between the patients receiving placebo and the patients receiving ondansetron with respect to the need for antiemetic rescue ($p < 0.001$), median number of emetic episodes in 24 hours (5.5 versus 1.5; $p < 0.001$), frequency and intensity of vomiting ($p < 0.001$), and median time to onset of emesis (2.8 hours versus 11.6 hours; $p < 0.001$). No patient receiving placebo vomited fewer than three times, whereas 79% of the patients receiving ondansetron vomited fewer than three times and 14% achieved a complete response. Reported adverse effects of ondansetron and placebo included headache (15% versus 21%) and diarrhea (7% versus 14%). The occurrence of delayed nausea and vomiting (24 to 72 hours after cisplatin administration) was evaluated by patient report in 24 patients. Eleven patients (85%) in the ondansetron group and six patients (55%) in the placebo group (most of whom received rescue antiemetics) experienced at least one episode of delayed vomiting ($p < 0.05$). On the basis of these results, the researchers concluded that ondansetron was effective in preventing acute nausea and vomiting due to cisplatin and that ondansetron did not prevent delayed nausea and vomiting, either because of its short half-life or because delayed nausea and vomiting is caused by a different mechanism.

Ondansetron has been compared with metoclopramide in cisplatin-treated patients.[51,66,67] Marty et al.[66] conducted a double-blind crossover trial in which 97 patients who were naive to antineoplastic drugs and scheduled to receive high-dose cisplatin were randomized to receive ondansetron for 24 hours or metoclopramide for eight hours followed by a placebo infusion for 16 hours. Patients were crossed over to the alternate antiemetic during the second course of cisplatin. Patients were monitored for 24 hours and then used diary cards to report symptoms on days 2 through 6. Seventy-six patients were evaluable for antiemetic efficacy. Ondansetron treatment produced significantly more major responses and more complete responses than metoclopramide treatment. No nausea was suffered by 38% and 20% of the patients in the ondansetron and metoclopramide groups, respectively. The time of peak emesis in patients receiving metoclopramide was between three and four hours after cisplatin administration. There was no obvious peak time of emesis in patients receiving ondansetron; instead, the patients who vomited did so between 6 and 24 hours or later after cisplatin administration. Statistical analysis showed no evidence of treatment-by-period interaction for efficacy, but it did show a trend toward treatment-by-period interaction for patient preference of antiemetic, with patients somewhat more likely to prefer the agent they received first. The incidence and severity of delayed nausea and vomiting according to patient reports were equivalent in both groups. Adverse effects in the ondansetron and metoclopramide groups, respectively, included dystonic reactions (0% versus 3%), headache (17% versus 14%), sedation (6% versus 13%), diarrhea (3% versus 7%), elevated aminotransferases (7% versus 4%), and increased bilirubin (1 patient in each group).

The most recent study to be published[51] was conducted in 121 patients who were naive to antineoplastic drugs. The study design and antiemetic doses were identical to those in the study by Marty et al.[66] This study included an optional delayed phase in which patients could receive either oral metoclopramide 20 mg three times daily or oral ondansetron 8 mg three times daily for five days beginning immediately after the antiemetic infusion was complete. Patients were monitored for 24 hours and then used diary cards to report symptoms on days 2 through 6. Nausea was recorded on a graded scale. Ninety-five patients were evaluable for antiemetic efficacy during the acute phase. Significantly more ondansetron courses than metoclopramide courses resulted in major responses during the first 24 hours (72% versus 41%; $p < 0.001$). Overall complete response rates were not reported. Median time to onset of emesis was 21 hours with ondansetron and 4.5 hours with metoclopramide ($p < 0.001$). Nausea grades were significantly lower in the ondansetron group compared with the metoclopramide group ($p = 0.04$). Statistical analysis showed no evidence of a treatment-by-period interaction. During the delayed phase, there was no statistically significant difference in emetic episodes between the metoclopramide and ondansetron groups (63% success versus 56% success). Nausea scores in the delayed phase were significantly lower for patients receiving metoclopramide ($p = 0.016$). The researchers performed an additional analysis that showed that the success rates for women and men were 65% and 95%, respectively, with the ondansetron courses and 31% and 65%, respectively, with the metoclopramide courses. These rates were not related to the other antineoplastic drugs administered and are in agreement with previous data.[11,45,49] Reported adverse effects of ondansetron and metoclopramide included headache (20% versus 10%), constipation (10% versus 0%), sedation (10% versus 17%), dry mouth (10% versus 8%), and diarrhea (8% versus 16%). Extrapyramidal adverse effects were observed during 6% of the metoclopramide courses but were not reported during the ondansetron courses. Elevated serum aminotransferases occurred in five patients each receiving ondansetron and metoclopramide.

Although ondansetron appeared to be much more effective than metoclopramide in the two studies described above, some points require clarification. First, the potential for a treatment-by-period interaction in the study by Marty et al.[66] compelled the researchers to analyze the results of the first treatment period only, providing a parallel-groups comparison. No significant differences between major response rates for patients in the ondansetron and metoclopramide groups were found in this comparison (73% versus 51%; $p = 0.061$), and the researchers concluded that a larger, parallel-groups study should be conducted. Second, although the literature suggests that continuous-infusion metoclopramide is equivalent in efficacy to intermittent infusions, the optimal dose for continuous-infusion metoclopramide has not been found.[3] Thus, it is possible that the metoclopramide dose was not sufficient for a valid comparison. This possibility is further evidenced by the fact that single-agent studies with intermittent high-dose metoclopramide (2 mg/kg every two hours for five doses or 3 mg/kg every two hours for two doses) have achieved major response rates of 64% to 67% in patients receiving cisplatin 120 mg/sq m over 20 minutes,[8] a much higher success rate than that seen in the studies by Marty et al.[66] and de Mulder et al.[51] Finally, the ondansetron doses used were not the doses that have been approved by the FDA, so the comparisons made in these two studies do not provide useful data.

To determine the relative efficacies of ondansetron and metoclopramide, Hainsworth et al.[67] conducted a trial that employed standard doses of both agents in a well-controlled fashion. Three hundred seven patients who were naive to antineoplastic drugs were randomized to receive either ondansetron or metoclopramide. Groups were comparable with respect to age, gender, and additional emetogenic antineoplastic therapy received. Potential biases in the study include a single-blind design and inconsistent infusion times for cisplatin (cisplatin was infused over three hours or less; comparability of groups with respect to infusion time was not reported). Subjective satisfaction with control of nausea and vomiting was measured by visual analogue scale. Complete response was achieved in more ondansetron than metoclopramide patients, but the difference was not statistically significant; however, a significantly higher rate of major response was achieved in patients who received ondansetron (p = 0.03). Satisfaction with control of nausea and vomiting was rated as 87 mm and 64.5 mm in the ondansetron and metoclopramide groups, respectively ($p < 0.001$). As seen in other studies, there was a significant difference in the time to onset of emesis; the medians for the ondansetron and metclopramide groups were 20.5 hours and 5.25 hours, respectively ($p < 0.001$). There was no attempt to assess delayed nausea and vomiting. Adverse effects were more common overall in the metoclopramide group than the ondansetron group (69% versus 48%; $p < 0.001$), with extrapyramidal adverse effects in 12% versus 0%, diarrhea in 44% versus 25% ($p < 0.001$), headache in 7% versus 16%, and increased serum levels of aspartate aminotransferase (AST) in 2% versus 8%. This study gives the first indication that ondansetron may in fact be more effective than standard high-dose metoclopramide; however, these data must be confirmed.

Reports have appeared that suggest the combination of dexamethasone and ondansetron is better than ondansetron alone.[68-70] The first two published reports were based on unblinded, uncontrolled trials of the combination in patients who had not responded to single-agent ondansetron[68,69] or single-agent dexamethasone.[69] A variety of antineoplastic regimens were administered, including cisplatin-containing regimens. Ondansetron and dexamethasone were given in variable doses by i.v.[68] and oral administration.[68,69] One trial reported that the combined use of ondansetron and dexamethasone increased the complete response rate from 0% to 64%[69]; the other trial reported an increase from 0% to 100%.[68] Because these trials were not conducted under blinded conditons, the true value of adding dexamethasone to ondansetron regimens is still unclear. A study that prospectively evaluated the addition of dexamethasone to ondansetron has been published in abstract form.[70] This was a crossover study in 89 patients who were naive to antineoplastic drugs and scheduled to receive cisplatin 50 to 120 mg/sq m. Patients were randomized to receive ondansetron 0.15 mg/kg i.v. every two hours for three doses with either dexamethasone 20 mg or placebo i.v. 45 minutes before cisplatin administration. Complete response rates in the ondansetron-only group compared with the ondansetron and dexamethasone group were 64% versus 91% (p = 0.0005). Adverse effects were mild and did not differ between the two groups.

Multiple-Day Courses of Cisplatin. Kris et al.[57] studied the safety and efficacy of ondansetron in 12 pretreated patients scheduled to receive cisplatin 20–25 mg/sq m over 15 minutes on four or five consecutive days. Patients were given ondansetron 0.15 mg/kg every two hours for three doses each day beginning 30 minutes before cisplatin administration. Complete response rates per day ranged from 75% on day 1 to 33% on day 3, whereas major response rates ranged from 92% on days 1 and 2 to 50% on day 4. Analysis of total emetic control over the five-day period showed that only one patient had a complete response; 25% had major responses, and 67% failed to respond.

A nonrandomized trial was conducted in 36 patients who received cisplatin 20–40 mg/sq m over 30 minutes each day for four or five days.[9] The three consecutive groups of patients were as follows: group A—12 patients who were naive to antineoplastic drugs and received ondansetron 0.15 mg/kg every six hours for three daily doses; group B—12 pretreated patients who received ondansetron 0.15 mg/kg every six hours for three daily doses; and group C—12 patients who were naive to antineoplastic drugs and received ondansetron 0.15 mg/kg every two hours for three daily doses. Efficacy was evaluated as the number of emetic episodes per 24-hour period. Overall, 29% of the 35 evaluable patients experienced no emetic episodes during the four-to-five day study period, and 51% achieved a major response. No significant differences among the three groups were reported. Of those patients who had been previously treated with antineoplastic drugs, 25% had a complete response and 42% had a major response. Patients who had not previously received antineoplastic drugs responded better than previously treated patients on all study days. In general, the best responses were seen on day 1, with variable or declining responses thereafter. These results were consistent with the results of Kris et al.[57] Adverse effects included headache (14%) and asymptomatic and transient increases in serum bilirubin (71% of patients who initially had normal levels), serum alanine aminotransferase (ALT) (26%), and AST (31%).

Results of another trial of ondansetron in patients receiving multiple-day courses of cisplatin were recently published in abstract form.[71] One hundred four patients who were naive to antineoplastic drugs and scheduled to receive cisplatin 20–40 mg/sq m for four or five days were randomized to receive i.v. ondansetron in a dose of 0.015 mg/kg, 0.15 mg/kg, or 0.30 mg/kg every four hours for three daily doses in a double-blind fashion. Efficacy was evaluated as the number of emetic episodes during each 24-hour period. A statistically significant difference was found between the 0.015-mg/kg group and the 0.15-mg/kg group with respect to the percentage of patients who failed to respond to treatment (more than five emetic episodes) on any study day (47% versus 29%; $p = 0.047$). Complete responses over the entire period were 23%, 21%, and 29% in the low-dose, medium-dose, and high-dose groups, respectively; day 1 responses were 69%, 81%, and 89%. Adverse effects included headache (20%), constipation (15%), and diarrhea (5%). No abnormalities in laboratory values were noted.

Results of a trial comparing ondansetron with metoclopramide in patients receiving multiple-day infusions of cisplatin were recently published in abstract form.[72] This was a randomized, double-blind trial in 45 male patients who were naive to antineoplastic drugs undergoing treatment with cisplatin therapy 20–40 mg/sq m for four to five days. Patients received metoclopramide 1 mg/kg every four hours for three daily doses (22 patients) or ondansetron 0.15 mg/kg every four hours for three daily doses (23 patients). Efficacy was assessed as the number of emetic episodes during each 24-hour period. Comparisons were made between groups for complete response rates and for rate of failure (more than five emetic episodes during any one 24-hour period). Overall, the failure rates for the ondansetron group and metoclopramide group for the entire study period were 9% and 50%, respectively ($p = 0.002$). The difference in complete response rates on day 1 was also statistically significantly in favor of ondansetron (78% versus 14%; $p < 0.001$). Complete response rates on days 2 through 5 were not reported. Adverse effects in the ondansetron and metoclopramide groups, respectively, included headache (39% versus 18%), extrapyramidal adverse effects (13% versus 73%), insomnia (13% versus 9%), diarrhea (9% versus 36%), constipation (9% versus 0%), and transiently increased AST (30% versus 18%) and ALT (39% versus 9%). Confirmation of these results will be necessary because of the surprisingly low response rates with metoclopramide and the very low failure rates with ondansetron compared with those observed in the studies described previously.

Prophylaxis of Delayed Cisplatin-Induced Emesis. The importance of delayed cisplatin-induced nausea and vomiting was brought to light by Kris et al. in 1985.[2] These investigators found that only 26% of patients who received cisplatin 120 mg/sq m remained free from vomiting during the 24–120 hours after treatment, even though 63% of patients did not vomit during the first 24 hours after treatment. A similar trial in which patients received aggressive therapy with antiemetics on the day of cisplatin administration but did not receive antiemetics on the following days showed that only 11% of patients remained free from vomiting 24–96 hours after treatment with cisplatin.[73] These studies show that prophylaxis of acute emesis is not sufficient to prevent delayed nausea and vomiting caused by cisplatin. Additionally, studies have shown that the control of delayed nausea and vomiting not only affects quality of life[6] but also affects the incidence of acute nausea and vomiting with subsequent courses of antineoplastic therapy.[74] Several trials have evaluated the control of delayed nausea and vomiting with ondansetron in a controlled or uncontrolled fashion.

Three groups of investigators evaluated ondansetron (in an uncontrolled fashion) as a prophylactic for delayed nausea and vomiting induced by cisplatin.[51,60,66] In one study,[60] patients who had achieved a complete or major response during the 24 hours after cisplatin administration were given oral ondansetron 8 mg or 12 mg three times daily for the next five days. Two patients received the lower dose and both were classified as treatment failures. Six patients received the higher dose; four were classified as treatment failures. Overall, prophylaxis of delayed nausea and vomiting with oral ondansetron failed in six of eight patients, and the investigators concluded that oral ondansetron was not effective in this capacity. Two trials that compared the efficacies of continuous-infusion ondansetron and metoclopramide for the prophylaxis of acute nausea and vomiting also measured the effects of ondansetron on delayed nausea and vomiting, as described earlier.[51,66] Marty et al.[50] allowed patients no antiemetics after the first 24 hours, while de Mulder et al.[65] allowed either oral ondansetron or oral metoclopramide. Neither of the trials found a difference between metoclopramide and ondansetron with respect to the incidence or severity of delayed nausea and vomiting due to cisplatin. Although the complete response rates during the delayed phase for these trials (35–43%) was much higher than the rate reported by Kris et al.,[57] the difference is probably related to the lower doses of cisplatin used in the trials conducted by Marty et al. and de Mulder et al.

Results of the only study that prospectively evaluated the efficacy of oral ondansetron for the prophylaxis of delayed nausea and vomiting in a controlled fashion were recently published in abstract form.[75] Forty-eight patients who had two or fewer emetic episodes in the 24 hours after administration of cisplatin

120 mg/sq m were randomized to receive ondansetron 16 mg orally three times daily (30 patients) or placebo three times daily (18 patients) on a double-blind basis for four days beginning 24 hours after cisplatin administration. Evaluations were performed by telephone and by diary cards. The number of emetic episodes per 24-hour period, nausea as scored by the visual analogue scale, and adverse effects were documented. Complete response in ondansetron and placebo patients, respectively, was achieved in 67% versus 39% on day 1, 59% versus 44% on day 2, 78% versus 39% on day 3, and 74% versus 50% on day 4. The only statistically significant difference was on day 3 ($p = 0.009$). The overall complete response rate for the four-day period was not reported. No difference was found between ondansetron and placebo in the control of nausea. Adverse effects included headache and constipation (similar incidence in both groups) and diarrhea (five patients in the ondansetron group and one patient in the placebo group). This is the first indication that ondansetron may be effective for the prophylaxis of delayed cisplatin-induced emesis, but its comparative efficacy with other regimens[73] must be studied.

Non-Cisplatin-Containing Antineoplastic Therapy. Many antiemetic trials have been conducted in patients receiving non-cisplatin-containing antineoplastic therapy. Most of these trials are difficult to evaluate and compare because of patient and treatment diversity among groups.[14,76-84] Antiemetic trials frequently study patients receiving cyclophosphamide or anthracycline antibiotics because these agents are relatively emetogenic. Studies have shown that 92% to 100% of patients receiving cyclophosphamide 500–600 mg/sq m without antiemetics[24] or cyclophosphamide 50–75 mg/kg with phenothiazine-type antiemetics[85] typically vomit four to eight times during the first 24 hours. After 24 hours, however, most patients are free from nausea and emesis. Overall, metoclopramide therapy has resulted in complete response rates ranging from 22%[83] to 60%[78] when the drug is given in doses of 20 mg (regardless of patient weight) up to 2 mg/kg in patients receiving combinations of cyclophosphamide, doxorubicin, and other emetogenic antineoplastic drugs. Complete response rates of up to 86% have been shown when corticosteroids are used alone during combination therapy with cyclophosphamide, methotrexate, and fluorouracil.[78,82]

The efficacy of ondansetron for the prophylaxis of nausea and vomiting caused by cyclophosphamide with or without an anthracycline has been studied by a number of investigators (Table 4). Kaasa et al.[86] studied 93 patients who were naive to antineoplastic drugs and scheduled to receive cyclophosphamide with either doxorubicin or epirubicin. This was a randomized, parallel-groups study in which patients received ondansetron or metoclopramide. Nine patients were not evaluable. Complete response during the first 24 hours was achieved by significantly more ondansetron patients than metoclopramide patients ($p = 0.027$); however, there was no significant difference between the groups with respect to the number of major responses. Nausea was assessed on a graded scale and was controlled more often in the ondansetron group (85% had none or mild) than the metoclopramide group (57% had none or mild; $p = 0.008$). On days 2 and 3, emetic control was similar in both groups; major responses were seen in 76% and 68% of the ondansetron and metoclopramide patients, respectively. Adverse effects included headache (10% of the ondansetron group) and restlessness and anxiety (5% of the metoclopramide group). No abnormalities in laboratory values were seen.

A similar trial[87] was conducted in 75 patients with breast cancer who were scheduled to receive cyclophosphamide and either doxorubicin or epirubicin as part of combination therapy. This was a double-blind, crossover study in which patients were randomized to receive either ondansetron or metoclopramide. The alternate antiemetic was given during the next course of therapy. The number of emetic episodes was recorded by the patient, as was nausea on a graded scale. Statistical analysis showed evidence of a treatment-by-period interaction for antiemetic efficacy, so results for the first treatment course in 68 evaluable patients were analyzed. Compared with patients who received metoclopramide, significantly more patients who received ondansetron achieved complete responses or major responses ($p < 0.001$). A crossover analysis performed for nausea scores showed a significant difference in favor of ondansetron (median increase from baseline was 15 mm for ondansetron and 33 mm for metoclopramide; $p < 0.001$). Patient preference was also in favor of ondansetron (63% versus 26%, $p = 0.001$). Adverse effects in the ondansetron and metoclopramide groups, respectively, included headache (8% versus 7%), sedation (4% versus 8%), transient, asymptomatic changes in serum aminotransferases (3% versus 5%), and extrapyramidal symptoms (0% versus 3%).

Cubeddu et al.[24] studied 20 patients who were naive to antineoplastic drugs and scheduled to receive cyclophosphamide. This was a randomized, double-blind, parallel-groups trial comparing ondansetron with placebo. The number of emetic episodes during each 24-hour period was recorded for four days; nausea and overall satisfaction with treatment were measured by the visual analogue scale. Patients with severe nausea and vomiting could receive rescue antiemetic treatment. All patients receiving placebo vomited during the first 24 hours, whereas 70% of the patients receiving ondansetron suffered no emetic episodes during that period ($p = 0.008$). Posttreatment nausea scores were also significantly in favor of ondansetron, with averages of 7.7 mm versus 66.1 mm in the ondansetron and placebo groups, respectively ($p < 0.001$). Satisfaction with antiemetic therapy was higher in the ondansetron group than the metoclopramide group. There was no difference in the number of emetic episodes in the 24 to 96 hours after antineoplastic therapy;

Table 4.
Comparative Trials of Ondansetron in Patients Receiving Non-Cisplatin-Containing Antineoplastic Therapy

Reference	No. Patients	Antineoplastic Regimen[a]	Antiemetic Regimen: Ondansetron	Antiemetic Regimen: Control	% Response[b] Ondansetron MR	% Response[b] Ondansetron CR	% Response[b] Control MR	% Response[b] Control CR
86	93	CTX >500 mg/sq m plus Dox >40 mg/sq m or Epi >40 mg/sq m	8 mg i.v. before antineoplastics, followed by 8 mg p.o. t.i.d. × 3–5 days	Metoclopramide 60 mg i.v. before antineoplastics, followed by 20 mg p.o. t.i.d. × 3–5 days	80	65	62	41
87	75	CTX 500 mg/sq m plus Dox 50 mg/sq m or Epi 50–100 mg/sq m	4 mg i.v. and 4 mg p.o. before antineoplastics, followed by 8 mg p.o. Q8h × 5 days	Metoclopramide 60 mg i.v. and 20 mg p.o. before antineoplastics, followed by 20 mg p.o. Q8h × 5 days	86	66	42	27
24	20	CTX 500–600 mg/sq m	0.15 mg/kg i.v. Q4h × 3 doses[c]	Placebo	70	70	20	0
88	80	CTX 100 mg/sq m p.o. daily × 15 days	8 mg p.o. t.i.d. × 15 days[c]	Placebo	NR	63	NR	29
89	60	CTX ≥ 500 mg/sq m plus Dox ≥ 50 mg/sq m over 48–72 hours	1 mg Q4h × 3 doses on day 1,[c] followed by 8 mg Q8h × 3 doses on day 2		65	55		
			4 mg Q4h × 3 doses on day 1,[c] followed by 4 mg Q8h × 3 doses on day 2		70	65		
			8 mg Q4h × 3 doses on day 1,[c] followed by 1 mg Q8h × 3 doses on day 2		95	85		
91	12	Ifos 4000–6000 mg/sq m over 24 hours	4 mg i.v. Q6h × 7 doses[c] (6 patients who were chemotherapy-naive)		83	33		
			8 mg i.v. Q6h × 7 doses[c] (6 patients with previous exposure to antineoplastic agents who were refractory to metoclopramide)		83	50		
94	33	Mel 140 or 200 mg/sq m[d] plus MPred 1500 mg daily × 5 days	8 mg i.v. immediately followed by 1 mg/hr × 48 hours, then 8 mg p.o. q.i.d. × 5 days		53	24		
			12 mg i.v. immediately followed by 3 mg/hr × 24 hours, then 8 mg p.o. Q8h × 6 days		31	6		

[a] CTX = cyclophosphamide, Dox = doxorubicin, Epi = epirubicin, Ifos = Ifosfamide, Mel = melphalan, MPred = methylprednisolone.
[b] MR = major response, CR = complete response, NR = not reported.
[c] First dose administered before first antineoplastic dose.
[d] Six patients received melphalan 140 mg/sq m; 27 patients received melphalan 200 mg/sq m with autologous bone marrow transplant.

the complete response rates in the placebo and ondansetron groups were 60% and 70%, respectively, during this period. Adverse effects were more common in the placebo group than the ondansetron group and included diarrhea (30% versus 10%), headache (20% versus 10%), and cholestatic jaundice in one placebo patient that abated after two weeks.

A randomized, placebo-controlled trial of oral ondansetron was conducted in 80 women (72 of whom were evaluable).[88] Cyclophosphamide was given orally on days 1 through 14 as part of combination therapy with methotrexate and fluorouracil. Placebo or ondansetron was given as antiemetic therapy. Patients recorded the number of emetic episodes in each 24-hour period and the severity of nausea (on a graded scale). Compared with women in the placebo group, significantly more women who received ondansetron experienced complete responses over the entire 15-day period ($p < 0.01$). Of the patients receiving placebo, 29% withdrew because of treatment failure, compared with 5% of the patients receiving ondansetron. Mild or absent nausea was reported by 47% of the patients receiving ondansetron and 24% of the patients receiving placebo. Adverse effects were not listed.

Another study was conducted in 60 patients scheduled to receive cyclophosphamide 500 mg/sq m or more by i.v. administration and doxorubicin 50 mg/sq m or more over 48–72 hours by i.v. administration.[89] Ondansetron was given for two days. The number of emetic episodes during the 48-hour study period was recorded. Complete response rates ranged from 55% in the low-dose group to 85% in the high-dose group;

major response rates ranged from 65% to 95%. Nausea was negligible in all groups on day 1 and increased slightly in the low-dose and moderate-dose groups on day 2 (medians of 6.0 mm and 8.5 mm, respectively). Adverse effects were mild and not dose related: headache (17%), abdominal cramps (8%), diarrhea (5%), fatigue (3%), and transient increases in serum aminotransferases (3%). Although no statistical analysis was performed and the groups were small, this study indicates that ondansetron may be more effective in higher doses in these patients.

These studies show that ondansetron is effective in controlling nausea and vomiting caused by cyclophosphamide and anthracyclines. Two issues require clarification before the true place of ondansetron therapy in these patients can be understood. First, the appropriateness of such low doses of metoclopramide in the control group must be questioned. The investigators who conducted the studies described above argued that the doses of metoclopramide studied are the doses most commonly used in this group of patients. However, in a seminar given on ondansetron,[90] Gralla stated that although these may be commonly used doses, they are lower than the doses that have been proven to be effective; thus, many of the comparisons may not provide useful information. Second, a number of studies have shown high antiemetic response rates with corticosteroids in patients receiving cyclophosphamide or an anthracycline, or both.[78,82] It is possible that more useful information regarding ondansetron would come from comparisons with corticosteroids.

Ondansetron has been studied for the prophylaxis of ifosfamide-induced nausea and vomiting.[91] Twelve patients who were to receive ifosfamide were studied; six patients were naive to antineoplastic drugs and six patients had been refractory to metoclopramide. Patients were monitored for 42 hours, during which time the patients recorded the number of emetic episodes and the nausea score according to the visual analogue scale. Complete response rates were 33% in the treatment-naive group and 50% in the metoclopramide-refractory group, whereas the major response rate was 83% in both groups. Nausea was slightly more severe at 42 hours than at 24 hours in both groups. Adverse effects included dry mouth and headache (both in one patient). Minor elevations in liver function test results occurred in 58% of patients; these were not considered important by the researchers. The researchers concluded that ondansetron was effective in controlling ifosfamide-induced nausea and vomiting. However, because other studies[92,93] have shown that 50% to 94% of patients who receive ifosfamide have no nausea or vomiting or only mild to moderate nausea or vomiting with standard antiemetics, it is impossible to know how effective ondansetron is without a comparative trial.

Viner et al.[94] studied the safety and efficacy of ondansetron in 33 patients receiving high-dose melphalan; all patients had previously received melphalan. Methylprednisolone was given as part of the antineoplastic regimen. Overall, 42% of the patients suffered two or fewer emetic episodes over the entire seven-day period with no apparent dose–response relationship. The only reported adverse effect was dizziness, which occurred in 3% of patients. Because high-dose melphalan has been reported to cause nausea and vomiting in nearly all patients[95,96] it appears that the combination of ondansetron and high-dose methylprednisolone may be effective in these patients.

Use in Radiation Therapy. Ondansetron has been studied for the prophylaxis of radiation-induced emesis. Pilot studies using daily doses of 8 to 24 mg in three or four divided doses showed that ondansetron was safe, but efficacy was difficult to show because of the lack of a placebo control.[97] No placebo-controlled trials have been conducted, but ondansetron has been compared with low-dose metoclopramide in patients receiving single high doses of radiation to the upper abdomen. Ninety-seven patients were randomized to receive ondansetron 8 mg or metoclopramide 10 mg given three times daily. The rate of complete control of emesis was significantly higher in the ondansetron group than in the metoclopramide group (97% versus 45%; $p < 0.001$).[97] Although ondansetron appears to have some activity against radiation-induced emesis, its true efficacy compared with placebo and with effective doses of metoclopramide is still in question.

Use in Children. The safety and efficacy of ondansetron in children have been evaluated.[98-100] Nine children aged 8 to 18 years who had previously received antineoplastic therapy were given ondansetron 0.15 mg/kg i.v. every four hours for three doses.[98] The type of antineoplastic therapy given was not reported. Five patients had a complete response, and two others had major responses. No adverse effects were reported.

Another trial included 30 patients ages 2 to 16 years who received 31 courses of antineoplastic therapy for solid tumors.[99] This was an open trial to evaluate the efficacy and safety of ondansetron in a variety of antineoplastic-therapy regimens. Ondansetron was given as a 5 mg/sq m i.v. loading dose, followed by 1 to 4 mg orally every eight hours (dose based on body surface area) for five days. Twelve patients were naive to antineoplastic drugs. Patients were monitored in the hospital for 24 hours, and then the patients or their parents used questionnaires to record the number of emetic episodes in each 24-hour period and the severity of the nausea (on a graded scale). Complete response was seen in 71% of the patients during the first 24 hours, and major response was seen in 87% of the patients. On days 2 through 5, however, 64% of the patients who had received cisplatin or ifosfamide (30% overall) stopped responding to ondansetron, despite continued treatment. Results in terms of nausea were not presented. Adverse effects included transient increases in serum aminotransferases in four patients, headache in two patients, diarrhea in three patients, and abdominal pain in two patients.

A study was performed in children scheduled to

receive cyclophosphamide and cytarabine.[100] This was an open, noncomparative trial in 20 patients designed to evaluate the safety and efficacy of ondansetron. Twenty children aged 4 to 18 years were scheduled to receive cyclophosphamide 1000 mg/sq m on day 1 with cytarabine 75 mg/sq m on days 2 through 5 as part of their combination antineoplastic therapy. Nine patients were naive to antineoplastic drugs. An i.v. loading dose of ondansetron was given immediately before antineoplastic therapy: 5 mg/sq m in group A (10 patients) and 3 mg/sq m in group B (10 patients). Ondansetron was then given in a dose of 2 to 4 mg (based on body surface area) orally every eight hours for 13 doses. Monitoring was performed by a nurse for six to eight hours, and then by the patient or the patient's parents; nausea (assessed on a graded scale) and the number of emetic episodes per 24-hour period were recorded. Overall, 90% of patients achieved a complete response on day 1 of therapy, and 75% achieved complete response on days 2 through 5. Nausea was graded as absent in 17 patients and mild in 2 patients on day 1; on days 2 through 5 it was absent in 50% and mild in 50%. Adverse effects included increased serum alkaline phosphatase in one patient, increased serum bilirubin in four patients, and increased ALT in nine patients.

Adverse Effects

The adverse effects of ondansetron appear to be quite mild. Headache is the most common adverse effect reported in clinical trials, with an incidence of up to 43%. Although headache has been reported to be dose related, some studies comparing ondansetron with placebo or metoclopramide have shown a similar or higher incidence of headache in the control group.[21,24,75,87] Liver function abnormalities are typically reported in up to 25% of patients; one trial reported a 71% incidence.[9] These abnormalities are transient and asymptomatic, and they have been reported in similar numbers in the control group in a number of controlled trials.[51,71,86,87] In addition, one recent study[101] found that cisplatin itself may cause liver function abnormalities; the incidence of apparent hepatotoxicity increased as the cisplatin dose increased. Liver function abnormalities have not been shown to be a clinical problem thus far, but it is likely that the importance of this potential toxicity will become clearer after more patients have been treated with ondansetron. Constipation has been reported in the more recent trials, whereas the earlier trials contained no mention of this adverse effect. Only after much study was constipation found to be a relatively common adverse effect of ondansetron, occurring in approximately 10% of patients.[102] This adverse effect appears to be due to the effect of ondansetron on gut motility.[35] Diarrhea reportedly occurs in approximately 22% of patients treated with ondansetron.[102] Sedation appears to be common but is reportedly mild. Postmarketing surveillance will be important in further delineating the adverse-effect profile of ondansetron.

Pharmaceutical Information

Ondansetron hydrochloride dihydrate is an aqueous solution and is available as 2 mg/mL in 20-mL multiple-dose vials. The solution has a pH of 3.3–4.0, is buffered with sodium citrate and citric acid, and is preserved with methylparaben and propylparaben. Its stability is most effectively maintained when it is stored at room temperature (25 °C) and protected from light. Substantial degradation may occur at higher temperatures (100 °C).[103]

Dilute solutions of ondansetron 8 mg/500 mL in polyvinyl chloride (PVC) bags were shown to be physically and chemically stable for 48 hours when stored under refrigeration (4 °C) or at room temperature under normal lighting conditions. Additionally, a concentrated solution of 8 mg/100 mL (in 0.9% sodium chloride injection or 5% dextrose injection) was noted to be stable for seven days under the same conditions as above except protected from light. Infusions for administration are usually placed in 50 mL of 5% dextrose injection or 0.9% sodium chloride injection and infused over 15 minutes.[102,103] The manufacturer does not recommend that infusions be protected from light when administered to patients.

Ondansetron may be given by slow i.v. injection or as an infusion. It is compatible with the following diluents: 0.9% sodium chloride injection, 5% dextrose injection, 5% dextrose and 0.9% sodium chloride injection, 5% dextrose and 0.45% sodium chloride injection, and 3% sodium chloride injection.[102] Infusions are stable in PVC bags or type 1 glass bottles. Dilute solutions may be prepared in plastic syringes and stored either at room temperature or at 4 °C.[103]

Ondansetron may be given as a continuous infusion concurrently with some drugs when it is administered through the Y-site of the infusion set.[104]

The oral preparation of ondansetron is still investigational. The tablets contain 4 mg or 8 mg of active drug.

Indications and Dosage

Ondansetron is indicated for the prevention of nausea and vomiting associated with single-day courses of emetogenic antineoplastic therapy. Ondansetron is indicated for use in adults and in children aged 4 to 18 years. Ondansetron is not currently indicated for use in patients receiving multiple-day courses of antineoplastic therapy or for the prophylaxis of delayed nausea and vomiting.

The standard dose of ondansetron is 0.15 mg/kg i.v. every four hours for three doses, beginning 30 minutes before antineoplastic therapy. No dose modification is necessary for children, elderly patients, or patients with hepatic or renal dysfunction.

The oral formulation of ondansetron has been studied extensively in other countries but is not currently available in the United States.[102]

Cost

The cost of Zofran is $165 per 20-mL vial. Metoclopramide, available in generic form, costs an average of $19.50 per 30-mL vial (150 mg).[105] The standard doses of ondansetron and high-dose metoclopramide (2 mg/kg every two hours for five doses) in a 70-kg patient would cost approximately $136 and $91, respectively. Thus, a standard course of ondansetron is approximately 50% more expensive than a standard course of high-dose metoclopramide.

Formulary Recommendation

Ondansetron appears to be a major breakthrough in the prophylaxis of nausea and vomiting induced by antineoplastic therapy. Studies with strict inclusion and exclusion criteria show excellent rates of complete control in patients receiving single-day antineoplastic therapy, equivalent to or possibly better than those achieved with metoclopramide. Because of the high cost of ondansetron, however, the benefits of this new drug must be weighed against the added cost to the patient and the institution.

Conclusion

At the current time, data are not sufficient to show superiority of ondansetron over high-dose metoclopramide. The greatest advantage of ondansetron over metoclopramide appears to be its lack of important adverse effects. Although the incidence and severity of adverse effects will undoubtedly become clearer after more patients have been treated, these effects are likely to be less problematic with ondansetron than with metoclopramide. Thus, it appears that ondansetron will be the antiemetic of choice in selected patients in whom the risk of adverse effects from high-dose metoclopramide outweighs the added cost of ondansetron, such as children, young adults, and those who have previously experienced adverse effects with metoclopramide. If further studies show that ondansetron is more effective than metoclopramide, then the higher cost of ondansetron will have to be balanced against quality-of-life issues and the cost of extended hospitalizations.

Further studies are needed in the area of antiemetic prophylaxis and treatment in patients receiving antineoplastic therapy. Combinations of synergistic antiemetics must be used in an attempt to provide a higher rate of complete control of acute nausea and vomiting. Delayed and anticipatory nausea and vomiting are symptoms that have not received much attention until recently, but they will be important areas in which to study new antiemetics. Future study must also be directed at achieving complete control of nausea and vomiting even in patients who receive multiple courses of emetogenic antineoplastic therapy.

References

1. Grunberg SM. Making chemotherapy easier. *N Engl J Med.* 1990; 322:846-8.
2. Kris MG, Gralla RJ, Clark RA et al. Incidence, course, and severity of delayed nausea and vomiting following the administration of high-dose cisplatin. *J Clin Oncol.* 1985; 3:1379-84.
3. Merrifield KR, Chaffee BJ. Recent advances in the management of nausea and vomiting caused by antineoplastic agents. *Clin Pharm.* 1989; 8:187-99.
4. Triozzi PL, Laszlo J. Optimum management of nausea and vomiting in cancer chemotherapy. *Drugs.* 1987; 34:136-49.
5. Coates A, Abraham S, Kaye SB et al. On the receiving end—patient perception of the side effects of cancer chemotherapy. *Eur J Cancer Clin Oncol.* 1983; 19:203-8.
6. Lindley CM, Hirsch JD, O'Neill CV et al. Impact of chemotherapy-induced emesis on quality of life. *Pharmacotherapy.* 1990; 10:243. Abstract.
7. Gralla RJ, Itri LM, Pisko SE et al. Antiemetic efficacy of high-dose metoclopramide: randomized trials with placebo and prochlorperazine in patients with chemotherapy-induced nausea and vomiting. *N Engl J Med.* 1981; 305:905-9.
8. Kris MG, Gralla RJ, Tyson LB et al. Improved control of cisplatin-induced emesis with high-dose metoclopramide and with combinations of metoclopramide, dexamethasone, and diphenhydramine. *Cancer.* 1985; 55:527-34.
9. Einhorn LH, Nagy C, Werner K et al. Ondansetron: a new antiemetic for patients receiving cisplatin chemotherapy. *J Clin Oncol.* 1990; 8:731-5.
10. De Haan LD, de Mulder PHM, Beex LVAM et al. The efficacy of GR38032F, an antagonist of 5-hydroxytryptamine-3 (5-HT_3) in the prophylaxis of cisplatin (CDDP)-induced nausea and vomiting. *Eur J Cancer Clin Oncol.* 1988; 24:1383-4. Letter.
11. Olver IN, Simon RM, Aisner J. Antiemetic studies: a methodological discussion. *Cancer Treat Rep.* 1986; 70:555-63.
12. Allen JC, Gralla R, Reilly L et al. Metoclopramide: dose-related toxicity and preliminary antiemetic studies in children receiving cancer chemotherapy. *J Clin Oncol.* 1985; 3:1136-41.
13. Kris MG, Tyson LB, Gralla RJ et al. Extrapyramidal reactions with high-dose metoclopramide. *N Engl J Med.* 1983; 309:433. Letter.
14. Gagen M, Gochnour D, Young D et al. A randomized trial of metoclopramide and a combination of dexamethasone and lorazepam for prevention of chemotherapy-induced vomiting. *J Clin Oncol.* 1984; 2:696-701.
15. Mackinnon JWM, Collin DT. The chemistry of ondansetron. *Eur J Cancer Clin Oncol.* 1989; 25(Suppl 1):S61.
16. Butler A, Hill JM, Ireland SJ et al. Pharmacological properties of GR38032F, a novel antagonist at 5-HT_3 receptors. *Br J Pharmacol.* 1988; 94:397-412.
17. Brittain RT, Butler A, Coates IH et al. GR38032F, a novel selective $5HT_3$ receptor antagonist. *Br J Pharmacol.* 1987; 90:87.
18. Koulu M, Sjoholm B, Lappalainen J et al. Effects of acute GR38032F (odansetron [sic]), a 5-HT_3 receptor antagonist, on dopamine and serotonin metabolism in mesolimbic and nigrostriatal dopaminergic neurons. *Eur J Pharmacol.* 1989; 169:321-4.
19. Higgins GA, Kilpatrick GJ, Bunce KT et al. 5-HT_3 receptor antagonists injected into the area postrema inhibit cisplatin-induced emesis in the ferret. *Br J Pharmacol.* 1989; 97:247-55.
20. Tyers MB, Bunce KT, Humphrey PPA. Pharmacological and anti-emetic properties of ondansetron. *Eur J Cancer Clin Oncol.* 1989; 25(Suppl 1):S15-S19.
21. Cubeddu LX, Hoffmann IS, Fuenmayor NT et al. Efficacy of ondansetron (GR 38032F) and the role of serotonin in cisplatin-induced nausea and vomiting. *N Engl J Med.* 1990; 322:810-6.
22. Fozard JR. Neuronal 5-HT receptors in the periphery. *Neuropharmacology.* 1984; 23:1473-86.
23. Khojasteh A, Sartiano G, Tapazoglou E et al. Ondansetron

for the prevention of emesis induced by high-dose cisplatin. *Cancer*. 1990; 66:1101-5.

24. Cubeddu LX, Hoffmann IS, Fuenmayor NT et al. Antagonism of serotonin S3 receptors with ondansetron prevents nausea and emesis induced by cyclophosphamide-containing chemotherapy regimens. *J Clin Oncol*. 1990; 8:1721-7.
25. Andrews PLR, Bailey HE, Hawthorn J et al. GR38032F, a novel $5HT_3$ receptor antagonist, can abolish emesis induced by cyclophosphamide or radiation in the ferret. *Br J Pharmacol*. 1987; 91:417.
26. Barnes JM, Costall B, Kelly ME et al. GR 38032F improves performance in a mouse habituation test, and inhibits cholinergic-linked deficits. *Br J Pharmacol*. 1989; 98(Suppl):693.
27. Florczyk AP, Schurig JE, Bradner WT. Cisplatin-induced emesis in the ferret: a new animal model. *Cancer Treat Rep*. 1982; 66:187-9.
28. Leonard RCF, Soukop M. Anti-emetics and cancer chemotherapy. *Br J Cancer*. 1990; 61:349-50.
29. Costall B, Domeney AM, Gunning SJ et al. GR38032F: a potent and novel inhibitor of cisplatin-induced emesis in the ferret. *Br J Pharmacol*. 1987; 90:90.
30. Stables R, Andrews PLR, Bailey HE et al. Antiemetic properties of the $5HT_3$-receptor antagonist, GR38032F. *Cancer Treat Rev*. 1987; 14:333-6.
31. Costall B, Coughlan J, Kelly ME et al. Scopolamine-induced deficits in a t-maze reinforced alternation task are attenuated by $5\text{-}HT_3$ receptor antagonists. *Br J Pharmacol*. 1989; 98(Suppl):636P.
32. Costall B, Naylor RJ, Tyers MB. The psychopharmacology of $5\text{-}HT_3$ receptors. *Pharmacol Ther*. 1990; 47:181-202.
33. Blackwell CP, Harding SM. The clinical pharmacology of ondansetron.*Eur J Cancer Clin Oncol*. 1989; 25(Suppl 1):S21-S24.
34. Nielsen OH, Hvid-Jacobsen K, Lund P et al. Gastric emptying and subjective symptoms of nausea: lack of effects of a 5-hydroxytryptamine-3-antagonist ondansetron on gastric emptying in patients with gastric stasis syndrome. *Digestion*. 1990; 46:89-96.
35. Talley NJ, Phillips SF, Haddad A et al. Effect of selective $5HT_3$ antagonist (GR38032F) on small intestinal transit and release of gastrointestinal peptides. *Dig Dis Sci*. 1989; 34:1511-5.
36. Talley NJ, Phillips SF, Haddad A et al. GR38032F (ondansetron), a selective $5\text{-}HT_3$ receptor antagonist, slows colonic transit in healthy man. *Dig Dis Sci*. 1990; 35:477-80.
37. Saynor DA, Dixon CM. The metabolism of ondansetron. *Eur J Cancer Clin Oncol*. 1989; 25(Suppl 1):S75-S77.
38. Priestman TJ, Upadhyaya BK, Palmer JL. The pharmacokinetics of ondansetron (OD) in the elderly. *Proc Am Soc Clin Oncol*. 1990; 9:79. Abstract.
39. Bryson JC, DeBussey SS, Brouwer KR et al. Single and multiple oral dose pharmacokinetics (PK) of GR-C507/75 (GR38032): a novel compound effective in the treatment of chemotherapy-induced nausea (N) and vomiting (V). *Proc Am Soc Clin Oncol*. 1988; 7:69. Abstract.
40. Pritchard JF, Bryson JC, Kernodle AE et al. Influence of age and gender on the pharmacokinetics of ondansetron, a $5HT_3$ antagonist. *Clin Pharmacol Ther*. 1990; 47:161.
41. Colthup PV, Palmer JL. The determination in plasma and pharmacokinetics of ondansetron. *Eur J Cancer Clin Oncol*. 1989; 25(Suppl 1):S71-S74.
42. Lazarus HM, Bryson JC, Lemon E et al. Antiemetic efficacy and pharmacokinetic analyses of the serotonin antagonist ondansetron (GR38032F) during multiple-day chemotherapy with cisplatin prior to autologous bone marrow transplantation. *J Natl Cancer Inst*. 1990; 82:1776-8.
43. Blumer JL, Shurin S, Patrick S et al. Evaluation of pharmacokinetics, safety, and efficacy of ondansetron in children receiving chemotherapy. *Proc Am Soc Clin Oncol*. 1990; 9:332. Abstract.
44. Marty M, Pouillart P, Droz JP et al. The $5\text{-}HT_3$ antagonist GR38032F is superior to high-dose metoclopramide (MCL) in the prophylaxis of acute cisplatin-induced nausea and vomiting. *Proc Am Soc Clin Oncol*. 1989; 8:324. Abstract.
45. Pater JL, Willan AR. Methodologic issues in trials of antiemetics. *J Clin Oncol*. 1984; 2:484-7.
46. Kleinbaum DG, Kupper LL. Summary of methods for testing hypotheses in multiple regression. In: Kleinbaum DG, Kupper LL, eds. Applied regression analysis and other multivariable methods. Belmont, CA: Wadsworth; 1978:176-87.
47. Sullivan JR, Leyden MJ, Bell R. Decreased cisplatin induced nausea and vomiting with alcohol ingestion. *N Engl J Med*. 1983; 309:796.
48. D'Acquisto RW, Tyson LB, Gralla RJ et al. The influence of a chronic high alcohol intake on chemotherapy-induced nausea and vomiting. *Proc Am Soc Clin Oncol*. 1986; 5:256. Abstract.
49. Carey MP, Burish TG, Brenner DE. Delta-9-tetrahydrocannabinol in cancer chemotherapy: research problems and issues. *Ann Intern Med*. 1983; 99:106-14.
50. Jordan NS, Schauer PK, Schauer A et al. The effect of administration rate on cisplatin-induced emesis. *J Clin Oncol*. 1985; 3:559-61.
51. De Mulder PHM, Seynaeve C, Vermorken JB et al. Ondansetron compared with high-dose metoclopramide in prophylaxis of acute and delayed cisplatin-induced nausea and vomiting. *Ann Intern Med*. 1990; 113:834-40.
52. Cunningham D, Hawthorn J, Pople A et al. Prevention of emesis in patients receiving cytotoxic drugs by GR38032F, a selective $5\text{-}HT_3$ receptor antagonist. *Lancet*. 1987; 1:1461-3.
53. Kris MG, Gralla RJ, Clark RA et al. Dose-ranging evaluation of the serotonin antagonist GR-C507/75 (GR38032F) when used as an antiemetic in patients receiving anticancer chemotherapy. *J Clin Oncol*. 1988; 6:659-62.
54. Schmoll HJ. The role of ondansetron in the treatment of emesis induced by non-cisplatin-containing chemotherapy regimens. *Eur J Cancer Clin Oncol*. 1989; 25(Suppl 1):S35-S39.
55. Seynaeve C, van Liessum P, Verweij J et al. Control by GR38032F of acute and delayed nausea (N) and vomiting (V) induced by non-cisplatin chemotherapy. *Invest New Drugs*. 1989; 7:437. Abstract.
56. Grunberg SM, Stevenson LL, Russell CA et al. Dose ranging phase I study of the serotonin antagonist GR38032F for prevention of cisplatin-induced nausea and vomiting. *J Clin Oncol*. 1989; 7:1137-41.
57. Kris MG, Gralla RJ, Clark RA et al. Phase II trials of the serotonin antagonist GR38032F for the control of vomiting caused by cisplatin. *J Natl Cancer Inst*. 1989; 81:42-6.
58. Hesketh PJ, Murphy WK, Lester EP et al. GR 38032F (GR-C507/75): a novel compound effective in the prevention of acute cisplatin-induced emesis. *J Clin Oncol*. 1989; 7:700-5.
59. Marty M, Droz JP, Pouillart P et al. GR38032F, a $5HT_3$ receptor antagonist, in the prophylaxis of acute cisplatin-induced nausea and vomiting. *Cancer Chemother Pharmacol*. 1989; 23:389-91.
60. Smith DB, Newlands ES, Rustin GJS et al. A phase I/II study of the $5\text{-}HT_3$ antagonist GR38032F in the anti-emetic prophylaxis of patients receiving high-dose cisplatin chemotherapy. *Cancer Chemother Pharmacol*. 1990; 25:291-4.
61. Van Liessum PA, Seynaeve C, de Mulder PH et al. Ondansetron in the prophylaxis of nausea and vomiting induced by cisplatin. *Eur J Cancer*. 1990; 26:769-70. Letter.
62. Hait WN. Ondansetron and cisplatin-induced nausea and vomiting. *N Engl J Med*. 1990; 323:1485. Letter.
63. Cubeddu LX, Hoffmann IS, Fuenmayor NT et al. Ondansetron and cisplatin-induced nausea and vomiting—reply. *N Engl J Med*. 1990; 323:1486. Letter.
64. Editors. Ondansetron and cisplatin-induced nausea and vomiting—reply. *N Engl J Med*. 1990; 323:1486. Letter.
65. Marty M. Ondansetron and cisplatin-induced nausea and vomiting—reply. *N Engl J Med*. 1990; 323:1486. Letter.
66. Marty M, Pouillart P, Scholl S et al. Comparison of the 5-hydroxytryptamine$_3$ (serotonin) antagonist ondansetron (GR 38032F) with high-dose metoclopramide in the control

of cisplatin-induced emesis. *N Engl J Med.* 1990; 322:816-21.
67. Hainsworth J, Pendergrass K, Harvey W et al. Ondansetron: more effective than metoclopramide in the prevention of cisplatin-induced nausea and vomiting. *J Clin Oncol.* 1991; 9:(in press).
68. Cunningham D, Turner A, Hawthorn J et al. Ondansetron with and without dexamethasone to treat chemotherapy-induced emesis. *Lancet.* 1989; 1:1323.
69. Smith DB, Newlands ES, Spruyt OW et al. Ondansetron (GR38032F) plus dexamethasone: effective anti-emetic prophylaxis for patients receiving cytotoxic chemotherapy. *Br J Cancer.* 1990; 61:323-4.
70. Roila F, Tonato M, Cognetti F et al. A double-blind multicenter randomized crossover study comparing the antiemetic efficacy and tolerability of ondansetron (OND) vs OND plus dexamethasone (DEX) in cisplatin (CDDP) treated cancer patients (PTS). *Proc Am Soc Clin Oncol.* 1990; 9:339. Abstract.
71. Burton G, Huang A, Lazarus H et al. A double-blind randomized comparison of three doses of IV ondansetron for prevention of emesis induced by multi-day cisplatin therapy. *Proc Am Soc Clin Oncol.* 1990; 9:328. Abstract.
72. Sledge GW, Einhorn LH, Nagy C et al. Randomized trial of ondansetron (OND) and metoclopramide (MCP) as antiemetic therapy for cisplatin-based chemotherapy. *Proc Am Soc Clin Oncol.* 1990; 9:323. Abstract.
73. Kris MG, Gralla RJ, Tyson LB et al. Controlling delayed vomiting: double-blind, randomized trial comparing placebo, dexamethasone alone, and metoclopramide plus dexamethasone in patients receiving cisplatin. *J Clin Oncol.* 1989; 7:108-14.
74. Morrow GR. Prevalence and correlates of anticipatory nausea and vomiting in chemotherapy patients. *J Natl Cancer Inst.* 1982; 68:585-8.
75. Gandara DR, Harvey WH, Monaghan GG et al. Efficacy of ondansetron in the prevention of delayed emesis following high dose cisplatin (DDP). *Proc Am Soc Clin Oncol.* 1990; 9:328. Abstract.
76. Roila F, Basurto C, Minotti V et al. Methylprednisolone versus metoclopramide for prevention of nausea and vomiting in breast cancer patients treated with intravenous cyclophosphamide methotrexate 5-fluorouracil: a double-blind randomized study. *Oncology.* 1988; 45:346-9.
77. Strum SB, McDermed JE, Pileggi J et al. Intravenous metoclopramide: prevention of chemotherapy-induced nausea and vomiting. *Cancer.* 1984; 53:1432-9.
78. Roila F, Tonato M, Basurto C et al. Double-blind controlled trial of the antiemetic efficacy and toxicity of methylprednisolone (MP), metoclopramide (MTC) and domperidone (DMP) in breast cancer patients treated with i.v. CMF. *Eur J Cancer Clin Oncol.* 1987; 23:615-7.
79. David M, Durand M, Chauvergne J et al. Cyclophosphamide, methotrexate, and 5-FU (CMF)-induced nausea and vomiting: a controlled study with high-dose metoclopramide. *Cancer Treat Rep.* 1984; 68:921-2.
80. Gez E, Goodman S, Isacson R et al. High-dose metoclopramide and dexamethasone as an antiemetic in chemotherapy of breast cancer. *Oncology.* 1986; 43:173-5.
81. Gez E, Warner-Efraty E, Ben-Yosef R et al. High-dose metoclopramide and dexamethasone as an antiemetic in outpatients receiving chemotherapy for breast cancer. *Oncology.* 1987; 44:237-9.
82. Ibrahim EM, Al-Idrissi HY, Ibrahim A et al. Antiemetic efficacy of high-dose dexamethasone: randomized, double-blind, crossover study with high-dose metoclopramide in patients receiving cancer chemotherapy. *Eur J Cancer Clin Oncol.* 1986; 22:283-8.
83. Edge SB, Funkhouser WK, Berman A et al. High-dose oral and intravenous metoclopramide in doxorubicin/cyclophosphamide-induced emesis. *Am J Clin Oncol.* 1987; 10:257-63.
84. Cox R, Newman CE, Leyland MJ. Metoclopramide in the reduction of nausea and vomiting associated with combined chemotherapy. *Cancer Chemother Pharmacol.* 1982; 8:133-5.
85. Fetting JH, Grochow LB, Folstein MF et al. The course of nausea and vomiting after high-dose cyclophosphamide. *Cancer Treat Rep.* 1982; 66:1487-93.
86. Kaasa S, Kvaloy S, Dicato MA et al. A comparison of ondansetron with metoclopramide in the prophylaxis of chemotherapy-induced nausea and vomiting: a randomized, double-blind study. *Eur J Cancer.* 1990; 26:311-4.
87. Bonneterre J, Chevallier B, Metz R et al. A randomized double-blind comparison of ondansetron and metoclopramide in the prophylaxis of emesis induced by cyclophosphamide, fluorouracil, and doxorubicin or epirubicin chemotherapy. *J Clin Oncol.* 1990; 8:1063-9.
88. Buser K, Joss R, Piquet D et al. A randomized, double-blind comparison of oral ondansetron and placebo in the prophylaxis of CMF-induced nausea and vomiting. *Proc Am Soc Clin Oncol.* 1990; 9:331. Abstract.
89. Fraschini G, Esparza L, Ciociola A et al. Evaluation of three oral dosages of ondansetron (GR38032F) in the prevention of emesis associated with doxorubicin-cyclophosphamide chemotherapy. *Proc Am Soc Clin Oncol.* 1990; 9:328. Abstract.
90. Anon. Discussion. *Eur J Cancer Clin Oncol.* 1989; 25(Suppl):S51-S54.
91. Green JA, Watkin SW, Hammond P et al. The efficacy and safety of GR38032F in the prophylaxis of ifosfamide-induced nausea and vomiting. *Cancer Chemother Pharmacol.* 1989; 24:137-9.
92. Bramwell VH, Mouridsen HT, Santoro A et al. Cyclophosphamide versus ifosfamide: final report of a randomised phase II trial in adult soft tissue sarcomas. *Eur J Cancer Clin Oncol.* 1987; 23:311-21.
93. Mortan LR, Harrison EF, Hawke JE et al. Toxicity of single vs fractionated-dose ifosfamide in non-small cell lung cancer: a multi-centre study. *Semin Oncol.* 1982; 9(Suppl 4):66-70.
94. Viner CV, Selby PJ, Zulian GB et al. Ondansetron—a new safe and effective antiemetic in patients receiving high-dose melphalan. *Cancer Chemother Pharmacol.* 1990; 25:449-53.
95. Selby PJ, McElwain TJ, Nandi A et al. Multiple myeloma treated with high dose melphalan. *Br J Haematol.* 1987; 66:55-62.
96. Selby PJ, Mbidde EK, Maitland J et al. High dose melphalan and autologous bone marrow transplantation in treatment of refractory Hodgkin's disease. *J Clin Oncol.* 1988; 6:612.
97. Priestman TJ. Clinical studies with ondansetron in the control of radiation-induced emesis. *Eur J Cancer Clin Oncol.* 1989; 25(Suppl 1):S29-S33.
98. Blumer JL, Shurin S, Patrick S et al. Evaluation of pharmacokinetics, safety, and efficacy of ondansetron in children receiving chemotherapy. *Proc Am Soc Clin Oncol.* 1990: 9:332. Abstract.
99. Pinkerton CR, Williams D, Wootton C et al. 5-HT_3 antagonist ondansetron—an effective outpatient antiemetic in cancer treatment. *Arch Dis Child.* 1990; 65:822-5.
100. Carden PA, Mitchell SL, Waters KD et al. Prevention of cyclophosphamide/cytarabine-induced emesis with ondansetron in children with leukemia. *J Clin Oncol.* 1990; 8:1531-5.
101. Hesketh PJ, Twaddell R, Finn A. A possible role for cisplatin (DDP) in the transient hepatic enzyme elevations noted after ondansetron administration. *Proc Am Soc Clin Oncol.* 1990; 9:323. Abstract.
102. Glaxo Pharmaceuticals. Zofran package insert. Research Triangle Park, NC; 1991 Feb.
103. Leak RE, Woodford JD. Pharmaceutical development of ondansetron injection. *Eur J Cancer Clin Oncol.* 1989; 25(Suppl 1):S67-S69.
104. Trissel LA, Tramonte SM, Grilley BJ. Visual compatibility of ondansetron hydrochloride with selected drugs during simulated Y-site injection. *Am J Hosp Pharm.* 1991; 48:988-92.
105. American Druggist blue book. Edelstein E, ed. New York: Hearst; 1990.

Alternatives in the treatment of memory loss in patients with Alzheimer's disease

BURGUNDA W. VOLGER

Abstract: The pathophysiology, symptomatology, and treatment of memory loss in patients with Alzheimer's disease are described.

Alzheimer's disease is characterized by cerebral cortical atrophy, neuronal loss, neurofibrillary tangles, and neuritic plaques. The primary neuropharmacologic defect involves reduced activity of the enzyme choline acetyltransferase, causing reduced synthesis of acetylcholine (ACh). Other neurotransmitters known to be compromised in patients with Alzheimer's disease include norepinephrine, serotonin, dopamine, and somatostatin. Initially, components of short-term memory and immediate recall are lost. Eventually, memory loss is so severe that patients lose the ability to care for themselves. A definite diagnosis of Alzheimer's disease can be made only at autopsy.

Three pharmacologic approaches to enhancing cholinergic function include increasing ACh production by increasing the availability of ACh precursors (lecithin, choline); inhibiting ACh degradation by inhibiting acetylcholinesterase (physostigmine, tacrine hydrochloride); and directly stimulating cholinergic receptors by using cholinomimetic agents (arecoline, RS-86). However, results of studies involving these agents are conflicting: no consistent benefit has been shown in patients with Alzheimer's disease. Although therapy with tacrine hydrochloride has been beneficial in some patients, it has not been effective in all cases and has the potential to cause serious adverse effects.

Despite the research in patients with Alzheimer's disease, no agent has yet been found that produces consistent improvement in the memory loss associated with this disease.

Index terms: Acetylcholinesterase inhibitors; Alzheimer's disease; Amino acids; Arecoline; Choline; Lecithin; Mechanism of action; Memory disorders; Parasympathomimetic agents; Physostigmine; RS-86; Tacrine hydrochloride
Clin Pharm. 1991; 10:447-56

Alzheimer's disease is a devastating disease causing progressive dementia that affects approximately 10% of individuals over the age of 65 years.[1] It was first described in 1907 by Alois Alzheimer and is now the most common cause of dementia[2] and the fourth leading cause of death.[3,4] It is estimated that 1.6 million people currently suffer from severe dementia, and an additional 1 to 5 million people suffer from mild to moderate dementia.[5] These numbers are expected to increase as the average age of the population increases. Because severe dementia often requires long-term care, the costs to society are tremendous. In 1985 alone, the estimated annual costs for the care of patients with dementia was \$24 to \$48 billion.[5] This article will describe the pathophysiology, symptomatology, and treatment of memory loss in patients with Alzheimer's disease. The discussion of treatment will focus on the cholinergic agents, specifically tacrine hydrochloride, the newest agent studied. Therapy with tacrine hydrochloride may potentially benefit some patients, although study results are conflicting. Other alternatives in therapy will be briefly discussed.

Etiology and Pathophysiology

Although there are several proposed causes of Alz-

BURGUNDA W. VOLGER, PHARM.D., is Director, Drug Information and Investigational Drug Services, University of Michigan Hospitals, Ann Arbor, and Clinical Assistant Professor of Pharmacy, College of Pharmacy, University of Michigan.
Address reprint requests to Dr. Volger at the Department of Pharmacy Services, University of Michigan Hospitals, UH B2D301/0008, 1500 East Medical Center Drive, Ann Arbor, MI 48109-0008.
Adapted from an article that appeared in the February 1991 issue of the *Michigan Drug Letter*, a publication of the Department of Pharmacy Services, University of Michigan Medical Center, Ann Arbor.
This is article **680-204-9112** in the **ASHP Continuing Education System**; it qualifies for 1.0 hour of continuing-education credit. See page 475 for learning objectives and test questions.

heimer's disease, including environmental toxins, biochemical deficiencies in the brain, acceleration of normal aging, and infectious agents, the exact cause is still unknown.[6] Aluminum has been implicated as a causative agent for Alzheimer's disease, but this idea remains controversial.[2,6-9] Increased aluminum levels have been found in the nuclei of neurons that bear neurofibrillary tangles (abnormal neurons where cytoplasm is filled with filamentous structures).[9] However, a high intake of aluminum has not been shown to cause deterioration in patients with Alzheimer's disease.[9] In addition, patients with chronic renal failure are known to have excessively high brain levels of aluminum, yet they are not predisposed to developing Alzheimer's disease.[10]

Alzheimer's disease is characterized by various structural changes, including cerebral cortical atrophy, neuronal loss, neurofibrillary tangles, and neuritic plaques (clusters of degenerating nerve terminals).[2] The loss of neurons seen with Alzheimer's disease is more severe than that seen with normal aging.[6] Atrophy typically occurs in the temporal, parietal, and frontal regions of the brain. A high density of plaques and tangles is seen in the cortex and the hippocampus, two regions that are responsible for memory function. Therefore, damage to these areas would result in loss of memory. Reduced cerebral blood flow[11] and decreased cerebral glucose metabolism[12] have been reported in patients with Alzheimer's disease. The reduced blood flow correlates with the severity of Alzheimer's disease, but not with age. The reductions in blood flow and glucose metabolism may be secondary to neuronal loss and decreased neuronal metabolism.[11]

In addition to the structural changes seen in patients with Alzheimer's disease, there are several neuropharmacologic alterations. The most consistent defect involves reduced activity of the enzyme choline acetyltransferase, causing a reduction in the synthesis of acetylcholine (ACh). Francis et al.[13] evaluated the role of cholinergic neurons in Alzheimer's disease. They found a significant correlation between the synthesis of ACh and the degree of cognitive impairment, which supports the idea that the presynaptic cholinergic system is compromised in patients with Alzheimer's disease. Other neurotransmitters known to be compromised in patients with Alzheimer's disease include norepinephrine, serotonin, dopamine, and somatostatin.[2,7,14,15] This fact may affect the therapeutic approach to managing patients with Alzheimer's disease.

Diagnosis

The diagnosis of Alzheimer's disease is one of exclusion. The differential diagnosis should include delirium and memory loss from other causes, multi-infarct dementia, focal neurological disease, depression, normal pressure hydrocephalus, Creutzfeldt-Jakob disease, and poor adaptive social behavior.[2,3] A definite diagnosis of Alzheimer's disease can be made only at autopsy, where neuritic plaques and neurofibrillary tangles can be noted. Unfortunately, there is no laboratory test available for the diagnosis of Alzheimer's disease. Patients should undergo a complete physical, neurological, and neuropsychological examination to determine the cause of dementia and delirium. Because there is a relationship between Down's syndrome and Alzheimer's disease (linked to a defect in chromosome 21),[6,16,17] a complete family history should be obtained. Patients with a family history for Alzheimer's disease have at least a fourfold greater risk of developing the disease,[3,18] suggesting a hereditary component. Patients who have signs and symptoms of depression should undergo a trial of antidepressant therapy.

Clinical Manifestations

The clinical onset of Alzheimer's disease is often subtle, with the first signs and symptoms (e.g., forgetfulness) being noted by family members. Often patients exhibit unusual behavioral reactions such as anxiety or depression. Initially, daily events, names, words, and other components of short-term memory and immediate recall are forgotten.[2] As the disease progresses, patients tend to become irritable and sensitive to psychosocial and environmental stresses. Affect and mood become labile, with the reaction commonly being anger, anxiety, denial, or depression. Eventually, memory loss is so severe that patients lose the ability to care for themselves. Institutionalization is often required to provide adequate care for the patient. It is not unusual for patients with Alzheimer's disease to experience "sundowner's syndrome," a worsening of the symptoms at night[2]; this may occur because sensory input is typically reduced in the evening hours, so patients have more difficulty orienting themselves. The prognosis for patients with Alzheimer's disease is poor; the average duration of the disease is nine years from onset until death.[19] The life expectancy of a patient with Alzheimer's disease is one half to one third that of an unaffected individual because of infectious and nutritional complications associated with a long-term disability.[3,19]

Treatment

The initial treatment modality for patients with Alzheimer's disease is nondrug therapy. The patient should be in a consistent environment; the lifestyle should provide stability and minimize confusion and daily changes in routine.[2,3] Patients should be encouraged to perform at their maximum level, using the skills that remain intact.[3,18] Reminder notes can be placed in strategic locations to assist with daily activities.

Many patients will require pharmacologic therapy for behavior management sometime during their illness. Because the exact cause of Alzheimer's disease is unknown, it is difficult to implement an effective therapeutic regimen. In the past, pharmacotherapy for symptomatic control of Alzheimer's disease was nonspecific and included vasodilators (e.g., ergoloid mesylates such as Hydergine [Sandoz]),[20] antidepressants, antipsychotics, and anxiolytics.[3,18] Now, based on the known cholinergic deficits in patients with Alzheimer's disease, many treatments have focused on enhancing cholinergic function.

Agents That Enhance Cholinergic Function

Three approaches to enhancing cholinergic function have been extensively evaluated: increasing ACh production by increasing the availability of ACh precursors (lecithin, choline); inhibiting ACh degradation by inhibiting the enzyme acetylcholinesterase (physostigmine, tacrine hydrochloride); and directly stimulating cholinergic receptors by using cholinomimetic agents (arecoline, RS-86 [spiro-(1-methyl-4-piperidyl)-*N*-ethyl succinimide hydrobromide]). The limitation of using cholinergic precursors or acetylcholinesterase inhibitors is that intact cholinergic neurons are required to synthesize ACh. Theoretically then, these agents may be more beneficial in the early stages of Alzheimer's disease, before extensive neural degeneration has occurred.[2] Cholinomimetic agents do not depend on intact presynaptic neurons; they act solely on the postsynaptic neurons and may be advantageous in more advanced stages of Alzheimer's disease.

Trials evaluating cholinergic enhancers are summarized in Table 1. Efficacy is difficult to assess because the studies often were unblinded and involved short-term therapy in small numbers of patients at different stages of Alzheimer's disease. In addition, measurements of improvement are often subjective; even when consistent, objective tests are used, a significant improvement in the test score does not necessarily mean clinical improvement.[18] A more complete description of some of the tests used to measure response can be found elsewhere.[44,45] The results of these studies are conflicting; cholinergic precursors and cholinomimetic agents have not consistently proved to be beneficial in patients with Alzheimer's disease.

Additional agents that enhance cholinergic function have been investigated. Acetyl-L-carnitine (Sigma-Tau), a substance structurally related to ACh, is thought to act on neural transmission. The addition of the acetyl group to L-carnitine increases the ability of the substance to bind to neuroreceptors.[46] Data from Phase III clinical trials suggest that acetyl-L-carnitine may slow the progression of Alzheimer's disease or improve cognition in some patients.[47,48] Velnacrine (HP 029, Hoechst-Roussel), a derivative of tacrine hydrochloride, also has central cholinomimetic activity. The safety and pharmacokinetic profiles of velnacrine have been established,[49,50] and the drug will soon

Table 1.
Trials Evaluating Cholinergic Enhancers in Patients with Alzheimer's Disease

Reference	Study Design[a]	No. Patients	Age (yr)	Severity of Disease	Treatment	Length of Therapy	Results
21	PC	7	NR[b]	Mild to moderate	Choline 50, 100, 200 mg/kg/day p.o. in 4 doses or placebo	2 weeks	No improvement
22	DB, PC	52	Mean = 74	NR	Lecithin (95% PTC[c]) 25 g/day p.o. or placebo	6 months	Positive effect
23	DB, PC, X	10	65–82	NR	Lecithin (95% PTC) 4, 12, 20, g/day p.o. or placebo	1 week with each treatment	No improvement
24	DB, PC, X	7	54–73	Mild to moderate	Lecithin (53% PTC) 35 g/day p.o. or placebo	2 weeks	No improvement
25	DB, PC, X	15	47–85	Moderate	Lecithin (55% PTC) 10 g/day p.o. or placebo	3 months	No improvement
26	DB, PC, X	13	54–81	Mild	Lecithin (95% PTC) 10–20 g/day p.o. or placebo	3 weeks	No improvement or deterioration
27	DB, PC, X	11	Mean = 65.5	NR	Lecithin 35 g/day p.o. or placebo	5 months	No improvement
28	DB, PC, X	12	53–89	NR	Physostigmine[d] 0.5–3 mg (maximum 15 mg/day) p.o. q 2 h × 6 or placebo	4 days	No significant improvement; some patients responded favorably, others did not
29	O	5	NR	NR	Physostigmine[d] 1 mg p.o. q 2 h × 6	17 months–3 years	Variable: 2 improved, 2 had no change, 1 deteriorated
30	DB, PC	10	52–76	Moderate to severe	Physostigmine[d] 0.5–2 mg p.o. q 2 h × 6 or placebo	3–5 days	Improvement in 7 of 10 who completed trial
31	DB, PC, X	6	55–63	Mild	Lecithin (35% PTC) 10.8 g/day p.o. plus physostigmine[d] 2–2.5 mg p.o. q 2 h × 6 or placebo	2–3 days	Positive response in all patients

Continued on next page

Table 1 *(continued)*

Reference	Study Design[a]	No. Patients	Age (yr)	Severity of Disease	Treatment	Length of Therapy	Results
32	DB, PC, X	10	50–68	NR	Physostigmine[d] 0.125–0.5 mg i.v. or placebo	1 dose	Positive response in 8 of 10 patients
33	DB, PC, X	8	NR	NR	Lecithin (35% PTC) 10.8 g/day plus physostigmine[d] 1–2.5 mg p.o. q 2 h × 6 or placebo	NR	Positive response in all 8 patients
34	DB, PC	16	56–80	Mild to moderate	Physostigmine[d] 8–16 mg/day p.o. or placebo	6 weeks	Positive response in 7 of 10 patients receiving drug; no response in 6 patients receiving placebo
35	DB, PC	11	NR	Mild to moderate	Physostigmine[d] 0.25–1 mg i.v, arecoline 2–4 mg i.v., or placebo	1 dose	Dose-dependent improvement
36	DB, PC, X	8	55–68	Mild to moderate	RS-86 4–5 mg/day p.o. or placebo	8 days	Slight improvement in some patients; no significant improvements noted
37	DB, PC, X	12	54–78	NR	RS-86 1.5–4.5 mg/day p.o. or placebo	14 days	Improvement in 7 of 12, no improvement in 5 of 12; patients with less severe disease at start of trial had greatest improvement
38	O	12	42–85	Moderate	Tacrine hydrochloride 0.25–1.5 mg/kg i.v.	Single-dose infusions	Variable; 9 patients improved, 3 had no change
39	R	10	57–71	NR	4 treatment groups: lecithin + tacrine hydrochloride; lecithin + placebo tacrine hydrochloride; placebo lecithin + tacrine hydrochloride; placebo lecithin + placebo tacrine hydrochloride. Tacrine hydrochloride dose 10 mg p.o. × 3 doses; lecithin (92% PTC) 20 g p.o. × 3 doses	All patients received each treatment for 1 day	Neither drug alone nor the combination produced any significant improvement
40	DB, PC, X	17	Mean = 70.7	Moderate to severe	Tacrine hydrochloride[d] 25–200 mg/day p.o. or placebo plus lecithin at least 10 g/day p.o.	3 weeks	Improvement in 16 of 17 during tacrine hydrochloride administration; no improvement noted with placebo
41	O	52	51–85	Moderate	Tacrine hydrochloride 25–100 mg/day p.o. plus lecithin (75% PTC) 4.7 g/day p.o.	8 weeks	Significant improvement in cognitive and functional status; no change in behavior
42	DB, PC, X	52	51–88	Moderate	Tacrine hydrochloride[d] 85 mg/day (mean) p.o. or placebo plus lecithin (75% PTC) 4.7 g/day p.o.	8 weeks	No significant improvement
43	DB, PC, X	10	Mean = 70.3	NR	Tacrine hydrochloride[d] 100–250 mg/day p.o. or placebo plus lecithin (55% PTC) 30 g/day p.o.	7 days	No significant improvement

[a] PC = placebo controlled, DB = double blind, X = crossover, O = open label, R = randomized.
[b] NR = not reported.
[c] PTC = phosphatidylcholine.
[d] Optimum dosage determined from dose-finding phase.

enter Phase III clinical trials. Anecdotal evidence in 375 patients participating in Phase II clinical trials indicates a 30% to 50% response rate.[51]

Tacrine Hydrochloride. Tacrine hydrochloride (tetrahydroaminoacridine) is an investigational agent (new drug application submitted by Warner-Lambert) that has been studied over the past decade for the management of Alzheimer's disease. Although its mechanism of action is not entirely known, it reversibly inhibits acetylcholinesterase, thereby increasing the concentration of ACh in the cerebrospinal fluid.[52,53] In addition, tacrine hydrochloride is thought to block potassium channels and inhibit sodium activation in the axon.[52-55] These effects on the ion channel may facilitate the release of ACh at the neuromuscular junction.

The pharmacokinetic limitations seen with physostigmine (i.e., half-life of two hours requiring administration every two hours) are not seen with tacrine hydrochloride. The physiologic effects of tacrine hydrochloride are usually seen within one to two hours and last for at least four hours.[52,56] Tacrine hydrochloride is rapidly absorbed, readily penetrates the blood–brain barrier, and is cleared by the liver.[56]

The adverse-effect profile of tacrine hydrochloride is similar to that of physostigmine, which is not surprising because both agents inhibit the action of acetylcholinesterase. Increasing peripheral concentrations of ACh can result in decreased heart rate, nausea, belching, diarrhea, and diaphoresis. Adverse effects are usually more pronounced with higher doses of tacrine hydrochloride, although this is not always the case. Because the cholinergic system exerts a depressant effect, depression associated with Alzheimer's disease might be expected to be worsened by tacrine hydrochloride; however, this does not occur.[57] By far the most serious adverse effect associated with tacrine hydrochloride is the reversible increase in liver function test results to at least three times the normal values, suggesting hepatotoxicity.[53] Early trials with tacrine hydrochloride were stopped because of this evidence of hepatotoxicity.[58] In subsequent trials, the maximum daily dose of tacrine hydrochloride (up to 200 mg) was lowered to 100 mg to minimize the likelihood of hepatotoxicity occurring.

Summers et al.[38] first studied the effect of tacrine hydrochloride in patients with Alzheimer's disease in 1981. They evaluated 12 patients (age 42 to 85 years, mean = 72 years) who had had two or more of the following symptoms for at least three months: impaired orientation, impaired recent or remote memory, and deterioration of intellectual functioning. Patients were excluded when they had dementia secondary to another cause (e.g., cardiovascular disease, alcoholism, epilepsy). The severity of each subject's dementia was retrospectively evaluated and staged into one of six categories (0 = history of dementia or confusion, VI = bedridden and unable to respond to simple commands). Tacrine hydrochloride was administered intravenously over one hour in doses ranging from 0.25 to 1.5 mg/kg. The initial dose was 0.5 mg/kg, with adjustments made on the basis of response and adverse effects. At doses of 1 to 1.5 mg/kg, glycopyrrolate (a peripherally acting anticholinergic agent) was concomitantly administered to reduce the incidence of nausea and emesis. Response was measured at baseline and at 1, 6, and 24 hours postinfusion. Response was evaluated according to results of the Orientation Test (12-item test of basic orientation, scores of <8 indicate dementia) and the Names Learning Test (12-item test of paired association repeated five times, scores of <44 indicate dementia). Global improvement was defined as a one-stage change in dementia staging. All subjects had at least stage III disease at baseline. The average change in staging was 1.5 levels; nine patients improved and three patients showed no change. Results for the Orientation Test showed that tacrine hydrochloride 0.25 to 0.5 mg/kg significantly improved memory in patients with stage III Alzheimer's disease. This effect was maximal six hours after the infusion. Nausea and diaphoresis were noted in four patients and emesis in an additional two patients, all at doses of at least 1 mg/kg. Although these results were viewed with caution because of limitations of the trial (small sample size, retrospective staging at baseline, unblinded), they spurred interest in the potential use of tacrine hydrochloride in patients with Alzheimer's disease.

In 1982, Kaye et al.[39] evaluated the effect of lecithin and tacrine hydrochloride combination therapy on memory in 10 subjects (age 57 to 71 years, mean = 61.5 years) who met the *Diagnostic and Statistical Manual of Mental Disorders, Third Edition* (DSM-III)[59] criteria for primary degenerative dementia and had a mean score for the Wechsler Memory Quotient of 75.9 ± 4.4 (range = 57 to 99). All patients had had dementia for at least six months and were unable to work, but they could care for themselves. Patients were randomized to four treatment groups: lecithin plus tacrine hydrochloride; lecithin plus placebo tacrine hydrochloride; placebo lecithin plus tacrine hydrochloride; or placebo lecithin plus placebo tacrine hydrochloride. All patients received each regimen with a 56-hour washout period between trials. Lecithin (92% phosphatidylcholine) 20 g and tacrine hydrochloride 10 mg were administered three times daily for one day. Response was assessed according to the Serial Learning Test, Prompt Recall Procedure, and Free Recall of Random and Related Words Test. The Serial Learning Test scores improved with combination therapy, but not significantly. Prompt Recall Procedure and Free Recall Scores did not change in any of the four treatment groups. The authors observed that patients who were initially less impaired had an increase in their Serial Learning Test scores, but the improvement in memory was not significant and normal behavior was not restored. Neither drug alone nor the combination therapy produced any significant changes in the measured responses.

Long-term oral administration of tacrine hydrochloride to 17 patients in the middle to late stages of Alzheimer's disease was evaluated in three phases by Summers et al.[40] Phase 1 evaluated the diagnosis of Alzheimer's disease and assessed the optimum dose of tacrine hydrochloride in an unblinded manner. Tacrine hydrochloride therapy was initiated at 25 mg per day, and the dosage was increased by 25 to 50 mg per day (to a maximum dosage of 200 mg per day) over 7 to 10 days. Clinical improvement was assessed according to the Orientation Test, Names Learning Test, and Global Improvement Score. All patients also received at least 10 g of lecithin daily. Fifteen of the 17 patients entered phase 2, which was a randomized, double-blind, three-week, crossover study of tacrine hydrochloride versus placebo. Tacrine hydrochloride was administered at the optimum dose identified in phase 1. Before tacrine hydrochloride administration, the mean stage was IV (severe deficit due to Alzheimer's disease). During tacrine hydrochloride administration, the mean stage was II (16 of 17 patients improved); no change in staging was noted with placebo administration. Responses to all three tests significantly improved with tacrine hydrochloride compared with baseline and placebo. Placebo administration produced no change in responses compared with baseline. Twelve of the 15 patients who improved in phase 2 participated in phase 3, a long-term assessment of tacrine hydrochloride administered at the optimum dose; placebo was not used. At the time a report of this study was published, the average duration of therapy in phase 3 was 12.6 months (range = 3 to 26 months). Results for phase 3 were not reported. Adverse effects included nausea, vomiting, diarrhea, and diaphoresis, all of which were seen at dosages of 150 to 200 mg/day. Although the results of this trial are promising, they were cautiously evaluated by peers[60] because of methodological shortcomings such as inclusion criteria that did not reflect current practice and incomplete reporting of results.

A multicenter, uncontrolled, unblinded trial was initiated in Canada to evaluate the effects of tacrine hydrochloride in patients with Alzheimer's disease. In the dose-finding evaluation,[41] 52 patients (age 51 to 85 years, mean = 67 years) with probable or definitive Alzheimer's disease (according to criteria established by the National Institute of Neurological and Communicative Disorders and Stroke and the Alzheimer's Disease and Related Disorders Association [NINCDS and ADRDA])[61] were evaluated. All patients were at stage IV or V according to the Reisburg Global Deterioration Scale. Tacrine hydrochloride therapy was initiated at 25 mg daily, and the dosage was increased by 25 mg every two weeks over eight weeks, to a maximum of 100 mg daily. All patients also received lecithin (75% phosphatidylcholine) 4.7 g daily, which was started two weeks before tacrine hydrochloride therapy. Patients were evaluated every two weeks according to the Mini-Mental State Examination (MMSE), the Modified Mini-Mental State Examination (3MSE), and the Rapid Disability Rating Scale-II (RDRS-II). Before the start of therapy and after each dosage change, the Behavioral Scale for Alzheimer's Disease (BEH-AD) and Hierarchic Dementia Scale (HDS) were also used to assess the response to therapy. Blood was collected every two weeks for determinations of serum tacrine hydrochloride and lecithin concentrations and liver function. Six patients dropped out of the study, two because of increases in liver function test results to more than three times the normal upper limit. The maximum daily dosage (100 mg) was reached in 38 patients; 8 patients could not tolerate more than 75 mg daily because of gastrointestinal adverse effects. Significant improvement was noted in the MMSE, 3MSE, and RDRS-II scores at eight weeks compared with baseline. These improvements did not last; measurements returned to baseline four weeks after therapy was discontinued. The authors noted that no change in behavior was seen as measured by the BEH-AD; however, there were significant improvements seen in cognitive (MMSE, 3MSE) and functional (RDRS-II) scores.

The same authors evaluated the efficacy of tacrine hydrochloride in 52 patients (age, 51 to 88 years, mean = 67 years) with a diagnosis of Alzheimer's disease at stage IV or V (according to NINCDS and ADRDA criteria).[42] After a 10-week dose adjustment phase similar to that of the previous study,[41] the patients entered a 24-week, double-blind phase. After a four-week washout period, patients were randomized to receive tacrine hydrochloride at their optimum dosage or placebo for eight weeks. Therapy was crossed over for an additional eight weeks after a second four-week washout period. All patients also received lecithin (75% phosphatidylcholine) 4.7 g daily throughout the study. Patients were evaluated every other week according to the MMSE, 3MSE, and RDRS-II. At the beginning and end of each eight-week phase, the BEH-AD and HDS were also used to measure the response to therapy. Adverse effects and liver function tests were monitored throughout the trial. Six patients did not complete the dose adjustment phase and an additional seven patients did not complete the double-blind phase. Elevations in serum alanine aminotransferase concentrations to more than three times the normal upper limit as early as the sixth week of the dose adjustment phase were seen in nine (17%) patients receiving tacrine hydrochloride dosages of 75–100 mg daily. Liver function test results returned to normal levels within one to six weeks after discontinuation of tacrine hydrochloride therapy in all of these patients. Adverse effects were seen in 35% of patients in the double-blind phase and included abdominal cramping, nausea, diarrhea, and polyuria. Significant improvement was seen on the MMSE after four weeks of tacrine hydrochloride therapy at a mean dose of 85 mg. No significant improvement was noted in any other weeks of evaluation according to the MMSE or any other scale, including the BEH-AD and HDS.

In a recent report by Fitten et al.,[43] the efficacy of short-term and long-term tacrine hydrochloride therapy was evaluated in 10 patients (mean age = 70.3

years) with Alzheimer's disease (according to NINCDS and ADRDA criteria). After a dose-finding phase, patients were randomized to receive their optimal dosage of tacrine hydrochloride (range = 100 to 250 mg daily) or placebo in a double-blind trial for seven days. Therapy was crossed over after a seven-day washout period. Throughout the trial, patients received lecithin (55% phosphatidylcholine) 30 g daily. In this short-term phase, vital signs were measured daily, and the MMSE was administered twice weekly. Several other neuropsychologic tests were administered once weekly, including the Fuld Object Memory Test, Digit Span Test, Trail-Making Test, Immediate and Delayed Paragraph Recall, Name-Learning Test, and Orientation Test. There was no significant improvement in any of the test results with tacrine hydrochloride therapy. Adverse effects were most common at dosages greater than 125 mg daily and included nausea, vomiting, and diaphoresis; four (40%) patients had increases in liver function test results (alanine aminotransferase 45 to 368 U/L, normal 3 to 36 U/L; aspartate aminotransferase 60 to 150 U/L, normal 8 to 40 U/L) that persisted for 3 to 12 weeks after discontinuation of tacrine hydrochloride therapy. Four months after the short-term phase, the remaining six patients entered the double-blind, crossover, long-term phase. After new baseline data were obtained, patients were randomized to receive their previously determined optimal dosage or placebo for five two-week intervals: one interval with placebo and four intervals with tacrine hydrochloride. All patients also received lecithin (75% phosphatidylcholine) 9 g daily. Neuropsychological tests were conducted at the end of each two-week period. Only one patient showed clinically important signs of cognitive improvement as evidenced by the MMSE scores, spouse ratings, and change in clinical stage (from stage VI to V). Two additional patients showed modest improvement in cognitive test scores, but no clinical improvement.

The efficacy of tacrine hydrochloride in patients with Alzheimer's disease has been evaluated over the past decade. Although initial reports spurred much interest and hope, further trials revealed a less optimistic picture and the potential for serious adverse effects. Tacrine hydrochloride therapy has been beneficial in some patients, but it has not proved to be a panacea, as was originally hoped. Because it acts on the enzyme acetylcholinesterase, it depends on intact cholinergic neurons to synthesize ACh. Therefore, it may be more beneficial in the early stages of Alzheimer's disease.

Other Investigational Agents

The efficacy of a variety of additional agents has been evaluated in the management of Alzheimer's disease. To date, most of these agents have not proved to be effective, although many of the trials have been with small numbers of subjects.

Although vasopressin and its synthetic analogue desmopressin appear to improve attention and memory in nondemented subjects,[62,63] their use has been less beneficial in patients with Alzheimer's disease.[64-66] Vasopressin is thought to enhance memory through its ability to stimulate release of endogenous adrenocorticotropic hormone (ACTH).[62] This idea led Soininen et al.[67] to conduct a double-blind, placebo-controlled trial to study the effect of a synthetic analogue of ACTH (Org 2766, Organon International B.V.) on memory in 77 patients with Alzheimer's disease. Treatment continued for six months with no significant difference between drug and placebo according to any of the rating scales. Instead, there was a progression of dementia in both groups.

Opiate antagonists may influence memory and attention,[68] which led to the suggestion that they could relieve the symptoms of dementia. Reisberg et al.[69] evaluated in a double-blind, placebo-controlled study the effect of intravenous naloxone hydrochloride (1, 5, or 10 mg administered in random order) in seven patients with moderate to severe Alzheimer's disease. Significant improvement compared with baseline was seen in responses to the Brief Cognitive Rating Scale and a variety of psychometric assessments. The results of this study suggest that narcotic antagonists may have a beneficial effect on cognition in patients with Alzheimer's disease. Because of the short half-life of naloxone and the need for intravenous administration, subsequent trials were conducted with naltrexone, an oral narcotic antagonist with a longer half-life. Although the results with naltrexone have been conflicting,[70] it appears that the drug does not improve cognitive function in patients with Alzheimer's disease.[71,72]

It is well known that there is increased monoamine oxidase (MAO) type B activity in patients with Alzheimer's disease.[73-75] The biologic importance of this finding is unknown, but it has led to trials evaluating selegiline hydrochloride in patients with Alzheimer's disease. Selegiline hydrochloride is a reversible MAO inhibitor that is relatively selective for MAO type B; however, at higher dosages (>40 mg daily) MAO type A is also inhibited. In a double-blind, crossover trial, Piccinin et al.[76] evaluated the effect of selegiline hydrochloride 10 mg daily versus placebo in 20 patients with Alzheimer's disease as diagnosed by DSM-III criteria. Patients served as their own controls, receiving each treatment for three months with no washout between treatments. A series of neuropsychological evaluations were done at baseline and at the end of each treatment period. Significant improvement was noted with word fluency, digit span, long-term spatial memory, and letter cancellation tests. Adverse effects were minimal and included excitation, dizziness, and orthostatic hypotension. The results of this study support the findings of an earlier trial[77] and suggest that further trials of long-term selegiline hydrochloride administration with larger patient populations may be warranted.

Piracetam (UCB), an agent developed in 1967, was the first of a new class of drugs known as the nootropics. Although the mechanism of action of these agents is unknown, they may facilitate learning and memory and prevent cognitive impairment.[78] Several trials have been conducted to evaluate the efficacy of piracetam in combination with choline; results have not been favorable.[78-80] Aniracetam (Hoffmann-La Roche), a substance related to piracetam, also has not proven to be effective in patients with Alzheimer's disease.[81]

Other agents that have been studied in patients with Alzheimer's disease include 4-aminopyridine,[82] S-adenosyl-L-methionine,[83] phosphatidylserine (Fidia Research Laboratories),[84] clonidine,[85] guanfacine[86] and a somatostatin analogue (L363, 586, Merck Sharp & Dohme).[87] None of these agents have been shown to produce substantial improvement in symptoms in patients with Alzheimer's disease.

The newest agent that has stimulated interest in research for Alzheimer's disease is nerve growth factor. Although most of the studies to date have used a product obtained from purified mouse salivary glands,[88] a product that is a clone of human nerve growth factor is being developed (Syntex Corporation and Genentech).[89] Nerve growth factor acts by stimulating choline acetyltransferase activity, thereby increasing the synthesis of ACh.[88,90,91] It is hoped that nerve growth factor will correct the ACh deficits seen in patients with Alzheimer's disease, improving memory and slowing disease progression.[88] As with most agents that work by enhancing cholinergic function, nerve growth factor would most likely work best in patients with early stages of disease. It would not correct damage that has already occurred but rather would slow disease progression.[89] Because it is a protein, nerve growth factor does not cross the blood–brain barrier. A mechanism for drug delivery to the brain is still being investigated. Potential solutions include implantable drug infusion pumps, polymer drug delivery systems, or neural tissue transplantation.[92]

Conclusion

Despite the research in patients with Alzheimer's disease, no agent has yet been found that produces consistent improvement in symptoms. Research has primarily been targeted at improving central nervous system cholinergic function. The most widely studied agent is tacrine hydrochloride, but results have been disappointing. It is now known that other neurotransmitter systems are also deficient in patients with Alzheimer's disease. However, results of research involving these other neurotransmitters have also been disappointing. Continued research in patients with Alzheimer's disease is needed in an effort to control the symptoms of this severely disabling disease of the elderly.

References

1. Evans DA, Funkenstein HH, Albert MS et al. Prevalence of Alzheimer's disease in a community population of older persons. *JAMA*. 1989; 262:2551-6.
2. Ereshefsky L, Rospond R, Jann M. Organic brain syndromes, Alzheimer type. In: DePiro JT, Talbert RL, Hayes PE et al., eds. Pharmacotherapy—a pathophysiologic approach. New York: Elsevier; 1989:678-96.
3. Kerzner LJ. Diagnosis and treatment of Alzheimer's disease. *Adv Intern Med*. 1984; 29:447-70.
4. Hesp B, Resch JF. The medicinal chemist's approach to CNS drug discovery. In: Meltzer HY, ed. Psychopharmacology—the third generation of progress. New York: Raven Press; 1987:1645-7.
5. Anon. Alzheimer disease—California, 1985–1987. *MMWR*. 1990; 39:105-7.
6. Mozar HN, Bal DG, Howard JT. Perspectives on the etiology of Alzheimer's disease. *JAMA*. 1987; 257:1503-7.
7. Wilcock GK. Recent research into dementia. *Age Ageing*. 1988; 17:73-86.
8. McDermott JR, Smith AI, Iqbal K et al. Brain aluminum in aging and Alzheimer's disease. *Neurology*. 1979; 29:809-14.
9. Shore D, Wyatt RJ. Aluminum and Alzheimer's disease. *J Nerv Ment Dis*. 1983; 171:553-8.
10. Arieff AI, Cooper JD, Armstrong D et al. Dementia, renal failure, and brain aluminum. *Ann Intern Med*. 1979; 90:741-7.
11. Tachibana H, Meyer JS, Kitagawa Y et al. Effects of aging on cerebral blood flow in dementia. *J Am Geriatr Soc*. 1984; 32:114-9.
12. Foster NL, Chase TN, Mansi L et al. Cortical abnormalities in Alzheimer's disease. *Ann Neurol*. 1984; 16:649-54.
13. Francis PT, Palmer AM, Simms NR et al. Neurochemical studies of early-onset Alzheimer's disease. *N Engl J Med*. 1985; 313:7-11.
14. Tamminga CA, Foster NL, Chase TN. Reduced brain somatostatin levels in Alzheimer's disease. *N Engl J Med*. 1985; 313:1294-5. Letter.
15. Beal MF, Mazurek MF, Tran VT et al. Reduced numbers of somatostatin receptors in the cerebral cortex in Alzheimer's disease. *Science*. 1985; 229:289-91.
16. Selkoe DJ. Deciphering Alzheimer's disease: the amyloid precursor protein yields new clues. *Science*. 1990; 248:1058-60.
17. Cutler NR, Heston LL, Davies P et al. Alzheimer's disease and Down's syndrome: new insights. *Ann Intern Med*. 1985; 103:56 -78.
18. Rathmann KL, Conner CS. Alzheimer's disease: clinical features, pathogenesis, and treatment. *Drug Intell Clin Pharm*. 1984; 18:684-91.
19. Walsh JS, Welch HG, Larson EB. Survival of outpatients with Alzheimer-type dementia. *Ann Intern Med*. 1990; 113:429-34.
20. Thompson TL, Filley CM, Mitchell WD et al. Lack of efficacy of Hydergine in patients with Alzheimer's disease. *N Engl J Med*. 1990; 323:445-8.
21. Thal LJ, Rosen W, Sharpless NS et al. Choline chloride in Alzheimer's disease. *Ann Neurol*. 1981; 10:580. Letter.
22. Levy R, Little A, Chuaqui P et al. Early results from double blind, placebo controlled trial of high dose phosphatidylcholine in Alzheimer's disease. *Lancet*. 1983; 1:987-8. Letter.
23. Brinkman SD, Pomara N, Goodnick PJ et al. A dose-ranging study of lecithin in the treatment of primary degenerative dementia (Alzheimer's disease). *J Clin Psychopharmacol*. 1982; 2:281-5.
24. Brinkman SD, Smith RC, Meyer JS et al. Lecithin and memory training in suspected Alzheimer's disease. *J Gerontol*. 1982; 37:4-9.
25. Etienne P, Dastoor D, Gauthier S et al. Alzheimer disease: lack of effect of lecithin treatment for 3 months. *Neurology*. 1981; 31:1552-4.
26. Weintraub S, Mesulam MM, Auty R et al. Lecithin in the treatment of Alzheimer's disease. *Arch Neurol*. 1983; 40:527-8. Letter.
27. Smith RC, Reisberg B. Pharmacologic treatment of Alzheimer's-type dementia: new approaches. *Psychopharmacol Bull*. 1984; 20:542-5.

28. Jenike MA, Albert MS, Heller H et al. Oral physostigmine treatment for patients with presenile and senile dementia of the Alzheimer's type: a double-blind placebo-controlled trial. *J Clin Psychiatry*. 1990; 51:3-7.
29. Beller SA, Overall JE, Rhoades HM et al. Long-term outpatient treatment of senile dementia with oral physostigmine. *J Clin Psychiatry*. 1988; 49:400-4.
30. Mohs RC, Davis BM, Johns CA et al. Oral physostigmine treatment of patients with Alzheimer's disease. *Am J Psychiatry*. 1985; 142:28-33.
31. Thal LJ, Fuld PA, Masur DM et al. Oral physostigmine and lecithin improve memory in Alzheimer's disease. *Ann Neurol*. 1983; 13:491-6.
32. Davis KL, Mohs RC. Enhancement of memory processes in Alzheimer's disease with multiple-dose intravenous physostigmine. *Am J Psychiatry*. 1982; 139:1421-4.
33. Thal LJ, Fuld PA. Memory enhancement with oral physostigmine in Alzheimer's disease. *N Engl J Med*. 1983; 308:720-1. Letter.
34. Thal LJ, Masur DM, Blau AD et al. Chronic oral physostigmine without lecithin improves memory in Alzheimer's disease. *J Am Geriatr Soc*. 1989; 37:42-8.
35. Christie JE, Shering A, Ferguson J et al. Physostigmine and arecholine: effects of intravenous infusions in Alzheimer presenile dementia. *Br J Psychiatr*. 1981; 138:46-50.
36. Bruno G, Mohr E, Gillespie M et al. Muscarinic agonist therapy of Alzheimer's disease. *Arch Neurol*. 1986; 43:659-61.
37. Hollander E, Davidson M, Mohs RC et al. RS 86 in the treatment of Alzheimer's disease: cognitive and biological effects. *Biol Psychiatry*. 1987; 22:1067-78.
38. Summers WK, Viesselman JO, March GM et al. Use of THA in treatment of Alzheimer-like dementia: pilot study in twelve patients. *Biol Psychiatry*. 1981; 16:145-53.
39. Kaye WH, Sitaram N, Weingartner H et al. Modest facilitation of memory in dementia with combined lecithin and anticholinesterase treatment. *Biol Psychiatry*. 1982; 17:275-80.
40. Summers WK, Majovski LV, Marsh GM et al. Oral tetrahydroaminoacridine in long-term treatment of senile dementia, Alzheimer type. *N Engl J Med*. 1986; 315:1241-5.
41. Gauthier S, Bouchard R, Bacher Y et al. Progress report on the Canadian multicentre trial of tetrahydroaminoacridine with lecithin in Alzheimer's disease. *Can J Neurol Sci*. 1989; 16:543-6.
42. Gauthier S, Bouchard R, Lamontagne A et al. Tetrahydroaminoacridine-lecithin combination treatment in patients with intermediate-stage Alzheimer's disease. *N Engl J Med*. 1990; 322:1272-6.
43. Fitten LJ, Perryman KM, Gross PL et al. Treatment of Alzheimer's disease with short- and long-term oral THA and lecithin: a double-blind study. *Am J Psychiatry*. 1990; 147:239-42.
44. *Psychopharmacol Bull*. 1988; 24(Sep):501-828.
45. Crook T, Ferris S, Bartus R, eds. Assessment in geriatric psychopharmacology. New Canaan, CT: Mark Powley; 1983.
46. Anon. Alzheimer's disease. *Wellcome Trends Hosp Pharm*. 1989; 11(Aug):14-6.
47. Rai G, Wright G, Scott L et al. Double-blind, placebo controlled study of acetyl-L-carnitine in patients with Alzheimer's dementia. *Curr Med Res Opin*. 1990; 11:638-47.
48. Anon. Sigma-Tau acetyl-L-carnitine Alzheimer's multicenter trials. *FDC Rep*. 1990; 52(Mar 19):T&G12.
49. Puri SK, Hsu RS, Ho I et al. Single dose safety, tolerance, and pharmacokinetics of HP 029 in healthy young men: a potential Alzheimer agent. *J Clin Pharmacol*. 1989; 29:278-84.
50. Puri SK, Hsu RS, Ho I et al. The effect of food on the bioavailability of velnacrine (HP 029) in healthy elderly men: a potential Alzheimer agent. *J Clin Pharmacol*. 1989; 29:956-60.
51. Anon. Hoechst-Roussel velnacrine maleate phase III trial in Alzheimer's. *FDC Rep*. 1990; 52(Apr 9):T&G5-6.
52. Sattin A, Muhoberac BB, Aprison MH et al. Tetrahydroaminoacridine (THA) as a pharmacological probe in Alzheimer's disease and other neurodegenerative disorders. *Med Hypotheses*. 1989; 29:155-9.
53. Kumar V, Becker RE. Clinical pharmacology of tetrahydroaminoacridine: a possible therapeutic agent for Alzheimer's disease. *Int J Clin Pharmacol Ther Tox*. 1989; 27:478-85.
54. Drukarch B, Kits KS, Van der Meer EG et al. 9-Amino-1,2,3,4-tetrahydroacridine (THA), an alleged drug for the treatment of Alzheimer's disease, inhibits acetylcholinesterase activity and slows outward K+ current. *Eur J Pharmacol*. 1987; 141:153-7.
55. Freeman SE, Lau WM, Szilagyi M. Blockade of a cardiac K+ channel by tacrine: interactions with muscarinic and adenosine receptors. *Eur J Clin Pharmacol*. 1988; 154:59-65.
56. Forsyth DR, Wilcock GK, Morgan RA et al. Pharmacokinetics of tacrine hydrochloride in Alzheimer's disease. *Clin Pharmacol Ther*. 1989; 46:634-41.
57. Vida S, Gauthier L, Gauthier S. Canadian collaborative study of tetrahydroaminoacridine (THA) and lecithin treatment of Alzheimer's disease: effect on mood. *Can J Psychiatry*. 1989; 34:165-70.
58. Marx JL. Alzheimer's drug trial put on hold. *Science*. 1987; 238:1041-2.
59. American Psychiatric Association. Quick reference to the diagnostic criteria from DSM-III. Washington, DC: American Psychiatric Press; 1980:66-8.
60. Pirozzolo FJ, Baskin DS, Swihart AA et al. Oral tetrahydroaminoacridine in the treatment of senile dementia, Alzheimer's type. *N Engl J Med*. 1987; 316:1603-5. Letter.
61. McKhann G, Drachman D, Folstein M et al. Clinical diagnosis of Alzheimer's disease: report of the NINCDS-ADRDA work group under the auspices of Department of Health and Human Services task force on Alzheimer's disease. *Neurology*. 1984; 34:939-44.
62. Legros JJ, Gilot P, Seron X et al. Influence of vasopressin on learning and memory. *Lancet*. 1978; 1:41-2. Letter.
63. Weingartner H, Gold P, Ballenger JC et al. Effects of vasopressin on human memory functions. *Science*. 1981; 211:601-3.
64. Jolles J. Neuropeptides and the treatment of cognitive deficits in aging and dementia. *Progress Brain Res*. 1986; 70:429-41.
65. Tinklenberg JR, Pfefferbaum A, Berger PA. L-Desamino-D-arginine vasopressin (DDAVP) in cognitively impaired patients. *Psychopharmacol Bull*. 1981; 17:206-7.
66. Durso R, Fedio P, Brouwers P et al. Lysine vasopressin in Alzheimer disease. *Neurology*. 1982; 32:674-7.
67. Soininen H, Koskinen T, Helkala EL et al. Treatment of Alzheimer's disease with a synthetic ACTH 4-9 analog. *Neurology*. 1985; 35:1348-51.
68. Gallagher M, King RA, Young NB. Opiate antagonists improve spatial memory. *Science*. 1983; 221:975-6.
69. Reisberg B, Ferris SH, Anand R et al. Effects of naloxone in senile dementia: a double-blind trial. *N Engl J Med*. 1983; 308:721-2. Letter.
70. Tennant FS. Preliminary observations on naltrexone for treatment of Alzheimer's type dementia. *J Am Geriatr Soc*. 1987; 35:369-70. Letter.
71. Pomara N, Roberts R, Rhiew HB et al. Multiple, single-dose naltrexone administrations fail to affect overall cognitive functioning and plasma cortisol in individuals with probable Alzheimer's disease. *Neurobiol Aging*. 1985; 6:233-6.
72. Hyman B, Eslinger PJ, Damasio AR. Effect of naltrexone on senile dementia of the Alzheimer type. *J Neurol Neurosurg Psychiatry*. 1985; 48:1169-71.
73. Adolfsson R, Gottfries CG, Oreland L et al. Increased activity of brain and platelet monoamine oxidase in dementia of Alzheimer type. *Life Sci*. 1980; 27:1029-34.
74. Smith RC, Ho BT, Kralik P et al. Platelet monoamine oxidase in Alzheimer's disease. *J Gerontol*. 1982; 37:572-4.
75. Alexopoulos GS, Lieberman KW, Young RC. Platelet MAO activity in primary degenerative dementia. *Am J Psychiatry*. 1984; 141:97-9.
76. Piccinin GL, Finali G, Piccirilli M. Neuropsychological effects of L-deprenyl in Alzheimer's type dementia. *Clin Neurophar-*

macol. 1990; 13:147-63.
77. Tariot PN, Sunderland T, Weingartner H et al. Cognitive effects of L-deprenyl in Alzheimer's disease. *Psychopharmacology.* 1987; 91:489-95.
78. Growdon JH, Corkin S, Huff FJ. Piracetam combined with lecithin in the treatment of Alzheimer's disease. *Neurobiol Aging.* 1986; 7:269-76.
79. Friedman E, Sherman KA, Ferris SH et al. Clinical response to choline plus piracetam in senile dementia: relation to red-cell choline levels. *N Engl J Med.* 1981; 304:1490-1. Letter.
80. Corona GL, Cucchi ML, Frattini P et al. Clinical and biochemical responses to therapy in Alzheimer's disease and multi-infarct dementia. *Eur Arch Psychiatr Neurol Sci.* 1989; 239:79-86.
81. Sourander LB, Portin R, Molsa P et al. Senile dementia of the Alzheimer type treated with aniracetam: a new nootropic agent. *Psychopharmacology.* 1987; 91:90-5.
82. Davidson M, Zemishlany Z, Mohs RC et al. 4-Aminopyridine in the treatment of Alzheimer's disease. *Biol Psychiatry.* 1988; 23:485-90.
83. Cohen BM, Satlin A, Zubenko GS. *S*-adenosyl-L-methionine in the treatment of Alzheimer's disease. *J Clin Psychopharmacol.* 1988; 8:43-7.
84. Amaducci L, SMID Group. Phosphatidylserine in the treatment of Alzheimer's disease: results of a multicenter study. *Psychopharmacol Bull.* 1988; 24:130-4.
85. Mohr E, Schlegel J, Fabbrini G et al. Clonidine treatment of Alzheimer's disease. *Arch Neurol.* 1989; 46:376-8.
86. Schlegel J, Mohr E, Williams J et al. Guanfacine treatment of Alzheimer's disease. *Clin Neuropharmacol.* 1989; 12:124-8.
87. Cutler NR, Haxby JV, Narang PK et al. Evaluation of an analogue of somatostatin (L363,586) in Alzheimer's disease. *N Engl J Med.* 1985; 312:725. Letter.
88. Harbaugh RE. Nerve growth factor as a potential treatment in Alzheimer's disease. *Biomed Pharmacother.* 1989; 43:483-5.
89. Marx J. NGF and Alzheimer's: hopes and fears. *Science.* 1990; 247:408-10.
90. Hefti F, Weiner WJ. Nerve growth factor and Alzheimer's disease. *Ann Neurol.* 1986; 20:275-81.
91. Hefti F. Is Alzheimer's disease caused by lack of nerve growth factor? *Ann Neurol.* 1983; 13:109-10. Letter.
92. Harbaugh RE. Novel CNS-directed drug delivery systems in Alzheimer's disease and other neurological disorders. *Neurobiol Aging.* 1989; 10:623-9.

Treatment of delirium in the critically ill patient

DOUGLAS N. FISH

Abstract: The clinical use of neuroleptics, benzodiazepines, narcotic analgesics, barbiturates, and neuromuscular blockers to manage delirium and agitation in the intensive-care setting is reviewed.

Delirium is the most commonly encountered mental disturbance in critically ill patients and may be precipitated by factors such as physical illness, medications, pain, and emotional stress. If agitation cannot be controlled through nonpharmacologic means, pharmacologic intervention may be necessary.

Haloperidol is the neuroleptic of choice for rapid control of delirium and agitation in the critically ill patient. It has few adverse effects in most patients, even at high doses, although it can cause extrapyramidal symptoms. Among the benzodiazepines, lorazepam should be considered a first-line agent. It may be used alone or in combination with haloperidol (or another neuroleptic). Midazolam is suitable for administration by continuous i.v. infusion in the intensive-care setting because of its water solubility, short half-life, and short duration of action. The sedative effects of narcotics may be advantageous in patients with both agitation and pain. Barbiturates are not recommended for routine use in the treatment of delirium and agitation. The use of neuromuscular blocking agents such as pancuronium bromide and metocurine iodide may be necessary when other therapies have failed.

Haloperidol and the benzodiazepines, alone or in combination, are the drugs of choice for treatment of acute agitation and delirium in critically ill patients.

Index terms: Barbiturates; Benzodiazepines; Delirium; Haloperidol; Hospitals; Opiates; Psychotherapeutic agents; Skeletal muscle relaxants
Clin Pharm. 1991; 10:456-66

The development of acute mental status changes is common in the severely ill patient. These disturbances may be manifested as delirium and psychosis, fear, anxiety, and depression. Effective control of delirium or agitation is necessary to reduce the risk of physical harm to the patient, as well as to improve the quality of care during the hospital stay. Physical restraints and pharmacologic sedation are commonly used to protect i.v. lines, respiratory equipment, indwelling catheters, chest tubes, nasogastric tubes, and other devices often necessary for managing a patient's medical care. In addition, such measures often are required to control agitation or delirium during certain diagnostic and patient-care procedures. This review will describe the clinical use of neuroleptics, benzodiazepines, narcotic analgesics, barbiturates, and neuromuscular blockers

DOUGLAS N. FISH, PHARM.D., is Fellow in Infectious Disease/Critical Care, Department of Pharmacy Practice (M/C 886), College of Pharmacy, University of Illinois at Chicago, 833 South Wood Street, Chicago, IL 60612. At the time this manuscript was written he was a clinical pharmacy resident, Duke University Medical Center, Durham, NC.

The assistance of Karen Young, Diane E. Klumpe, Pharm.D., and Chris C. Rudd, Pharm.D., in the preparation and review of this manuscript is acknowledged.

for the management of delirium and agitation in the intensive-care setting. Relative advantages and disadvantages of these drugs will be discussed, as well as currently suggested guidelines for proper choice and dosage of specific agents.

Definition and Etiology

Delirium is the most commonly encountered mental disturbance in critically ill patients. A prior history of psychiatric disturbances is not predictive of development of delirium in this patient population. Although the overall incidence of delirium is reported to range from 7%[1] to 57%,[2] the risk increases substantially in seriously ill persons over the age of 50 years.[3] Some studies report that 10–15% of patients aged 65 years or older experience acute delirium after general surgical procedures.[4]

Delirium may develop insidiously over weeks to months but is most often acute in onset. A lucid interval of one to three days, during which no abnormalities are noted in the patient, may precede admission to the intensive-care unit (ICU). This period may be followed by the abrupt onset of agitation and other mental status changes. The clinical presentation of delirium may include (1) disordered or incoherent speech, irritability, and sensory misperceptions (hallucinations, delusions, and misidentifications); (2) fluctuating periods of restlessness, agitation, and lethargy; (3) alterations in the sleep–wake cycle, with a mixture of insomnia and hypersomnia; and (4) variable disturbances in concentration, memory, and orientation. Incoherent mumbling interspersed with shouting, extreme suspicion, hostility, and often combativeness add to the difficult management of the delirious patient. For unexplained reasons, the clinical manifestations of delirium are generally worse at night.[5]

Although the cause of delirium is often never determined, the clinician must systematically exclude diverse underlying factors that may contribute to acute mental status changes. Organic causes such as underlying pathology or drug toxicity must be identified and corrected. Medical illness of any type can be associated with alterations in central nervous system function, with the mental disturbances improving after the illness is resolved.

Among the chief causes of altered mental status in the critically ill patient are adverse drug reactions and important drug–drug interactions.[6] Numerous drugs have been implicated in the development of delirium or agitation (see Table 1). Drugs with anticholinergic properties (e.g., atropine, antihistamines) may be particularly troublesome, especially in older patients.[14,15] Mental status abnormalities have occurred in 5% of patients receiving prednisone 40 mg/day (or the equivalent) and in up to 20% of patients given prednisone 80 mg/day.[28] Normeperidine, a metabolite of meperidine, can incite delirium, tremors, myoclonus, and seizures.[37,38] Cardiovascular drugs, such as lidocaine,[33] procainamide,[46] propranolol,[47,48] and digoxin,[29] are often implicated as the cause of alterations in mental status. Cimetidine and ranitidine may produce central nervous system disturbances including delirium, hallucinations, paranoia, agitation, and confusional states.[24,25,50] Cimetidine also inhibits the cytochrome P-450 enzyme system of the liver and can increase the toxic potential of drugs metabolized by this pathway (e.g., benzodiazepines, barbiturates, lidocaine, narcotic analgesics).[53-57] Antimicrobials such as penicillins[44,45] and imipenem–cilastatin[30] add further to the long list of drugs that may cause delirium. On the other hand, withdrawal from certain drugs such as alcohol, benzodiazepines, and narcotics may also cause severe agitation, delirium, and combativeness.[4-6,58,59] Although it is difficult to differentiate drug-induced mental status changes from those that have other causes, patients should be carefully assessed for potential adverse drug effects, drug–drug interactions, and drug withdrawal reactions.

Table 1.
Drugs Commonly Used in the Intensive-Care Unit That Have Been Reported to Cause Psychosis and Delirium

Acyclovir[7]	Ketoconazole[32]
Aminocaproic acid[8]	Lidocaine[33]
Amphotericin B[9]	Methyldopa[34]
Anticonvulsants[10–13]	Metoclopramide[35]
Anticholinergic agents[14,15]	Metronidazole[36]
Antihistamines[16]	Narcotic analgesics[37,38]
Benzodiazepines[17–19]	Nifedipine[39]
Captopril[20]	Nitroprusside sodium[40]
Cephalosporins[21–23]	Nonsteroidal anti-inflammatory agents[41–43]
Cimetidine[24,25]	Penicillin[44,45]
Ciprofloxacin[26]	Procainamide[46]
Clonidine[27]	Propranolol[47,48]
Corticosteroids[28]	Quinidine sulfate[49]
Digitalis[29]	Ranitidine[50]
Imipenem–cilastatin[30]	Theophylline[51]
Ketamine[31]	Trimethoprim–sulfamethoxazole[52]

In addition to physical illness and medications, other factors may cause mental disturbances in the critically ill patient. These include emotional stress, sleep deprivation, pain, prolonged noise, crowding of the patient, change in environment, and day–night disorientation. The importance of these factors and their management are currently the subject of intense research.[5,60-62]

Patients behaving abnormally in the intensive-care setting are often given the diagnosis "ICU psychosis." Although this term implies that environmental features of the critical-care unit are inherently capable of inducing psychosis, the occurrence of true functional psychosis in the ICU is rare. Many clinicians contend that a diagnosis of ICU psychosis should not be given without a thorough search for the underlying cause of the condition.[4-6]

Pharmacologic Treatment

How to properly manage and treat delirium is controversial. Controlling agitation through nonpharmacologic means (i.e., nonthreatening environment, correction of organic causes, use of physical restraints) is desirable. If these efforts are ineffective, pharmacologic intervention may be necessary. The primary objective of drug therapy is to achieve and maintain safe and rapid behavioral control so that necessary medical care can be provided. The choice of drug, dosage, and route of administration depends on the severity of the agitation, the ability of the patient to cooperate with the ICU staff, the patient's overall physical condition, and the patient's concurrent drug therapy. Fear, anxiety, or depression must be distinguished from delirium because the drugs of choice and dosages used to treat these disorders differ substantially from those used to treat delirium.

Patients with delirium or acute agitation often require immediate sedation with rapidly acting drugs, and onset of action is an important consideration in drug selection. Duration of action is also an important factor in choosing an appropriate agent. Although drugs with long durations of action require less frequent administration and reduced effort on the part of pharmacy and nursing staffs, they may be less advantageous if prolonged or excessive sedation occurs. Although many of the drugs useful in treating agitation may be administered orally, acute delirium with extreme agitation requires i.v. or i.m. therapy. In these situations, i.v. administration is preferable to i.m. administration for the following reasons[5]: (1) Drug absorption after i.m. injection may be erratic and unpredictable, resulting in inconsistent plasma concentrations and pharmacologic effects. (2) Drug absorption from distal muscles may be reduced in cases of hemodynamic compromise. (3) Repeated, painful i.m. injections may further agitate the delirious patient. (4) Intramuscular injections may interfere with interpretation of clinically important muscle enzyme studies. (5) In patients with a bleeding diathesis, i.m. injections are undesirable. (6) Intravenous administration provides more rapid and reliable pharmacologic effects.

Neuroleptics

The use of neuroleptic drugs to treat acute agitation and delirium has received a great deal of attention. These agents have excellent efficacy, an extremely high therapeutic index (ratio of a toxic dose to a dose that produces a therapeutic effect), and little effect on respiration. They are not addictive, and there is limited potential for patients to develop tolerance to their beneficial effects.[63-65]

Pharmacokinetics. These drugs are quickly and reliably absorbed after both oral and i.m. administration, although plasma concentrations after administration demonstrate considerable interpatient variability. Peak blood concentrations are achieved in as little as 10–30 minutes after i.m. injection and two to six hours after an oral dose. Neuroleptics are metabolized in the liver by microsomal-enzyme oxidation and are eliminated in the bile and urine as both active and inactive products. Substantial enterohepatic circulation occurs, with half-lives of individual agents ranging from 20 hours (haloperidol) to 60 hours (chlorpromazine).[63] The pharmacokinetic half-life and the pharmacologic duration of action are not highly correlated for these agents. In spite of their long half-lives, these drugs often require frequent administration to control delirium effectively.

Selection. There is no convincing evidence that any one of the neuroleptic agents is more effective than another for the treatment of delirium or that an agent with more sedative potential is better than one with less sedative potential for the control of agitated patients.[5] The selection of a particular neuroleptic agent depends instead on the relative adverse-effect profiles of individual agents and the familiarity of the practitioner with each drug.

Neuroleptic drugs are characterized as either low potency or high potency. In general, low-potency agents tend to produce more sedative, hypotensive, and anticholinergic effects. Although sedative effects may be useful when delirium is compounded by underlying anxiety, pain, or emotional stress, excessive sedation should be avoided because it interferes with subsequent evaluation of alterations in mental status. Hypotensive effects that result from antagonism of peripheral α-adrenergic receptors may be devastating in ICU patients with hemodynamic instability. Anticholinergic adverse effects could induce additional mental status alterations and exacerbate the delirium. Two low-potency agents, thioridazine and mesoridazine, have quinidine-like adverse effects with substantial potential for causing serious ventricular arrhythmias when used in high dosages.[63,66-68]

As a result of their unsuitable adverse-effect profiles, low-potency agents have generally fallen out of widespread use in favor of high-potency drugs. In contrast to the low-potency agents, high-potency neuroleptics have a greater potential for causing extrapyramidal adverse effects, but they have substantially fewer anticholinergic, sedative, and cardiovascular effects. In most critically ill patients, hypotension and anticholinergic effects can be more serious than extrapyramidal reactions. Although extrapyramidal adverse effects are undesirable, they are rarely life threatening and can be managed with dosage reduction or antiparkinsonian drugs.[63,65]

Tolerance to many of the neuroleptic-induced adverse effects, including those discussed above, develops with continued use in patients receiving long-term therapy. However, treatment of acute delirium may not continue long enough for this tolerance to develop. Patients with substantial hemodynamic instability may not be able to compensate adequately for neuroleptic-associated cardiovascular changes and therefore may continue to be at risk for these adverse effects during prolonged therapy with neuroleptic agents.[63,64]

In addition to the adverse effects already discussed, two additional adverse reactions deserve mention.

First, all currently used neuroleptics have been associated with the development of tardive dyskinesia. This syndrome occurs almost exclusively in patients exposed to these drugs over periods of months to years. There have been no reported occurrences of tardive dyskinesia when these drugs have been used for short-term sedation and control of delirium. A second uncommon adverse reaction is neuroleptic malignant syndrome (NMS). This serious idiosyncratic reaction is characterized by four clinical features: muscular rigidity, hyperpyrexia, autonomic instability, and marked changes in mental status. Although a thorough discussion of NMS is beyond the scope of this review, the clinician should be aware that NMS could occur during neuroleptic therapy. Over 100 cases of NMS have been reported in the literature to date, implicating virtually all of the currently used neuroleptics. The development of NMS does not seem to be related to the use of low-potency versus high-potency agents.[69,70]

Although any of the currently available neuroleptic agents may be used in the treatment of delirium, most of the available literature describes the use of three agents in particular: haloperidol, droperidol, and chlorpromazine.

Haloperidol

This high-potency agent is considered by many clinicians to be the drug of choice for rapid control of agitation and delirium in the critically ill patient. Haloperidol may be given orally, intravenously, or intramuscularly. Although haloperidol has a somewhat slower onset of action than diazepam when given i.v. (10–30 minutes versus 1–5 minutes), it has advantages over other drugs. Unlike benzodiazepines, low-potency neuroleptics, narcotic analgesics, and barbiturates, haloperidol minimally impairs hemodynamic and respiratory function. Its mild clinical effects on heart rate, blood pressure, pulmonary artery pressure, and respiration are especially desirable in severely ill patients with impaired cardiovascular or respiratory status. Unlike low-potency neuroleptics, haloperidol has minimal anticholinergic effects and little potential for exacerbating delirium.[63]

Haloperidol undergoes metabolic reduction to form the metabolite known as reduced haloperidol. Although some data suggest that reduced haloperidol may be pharmacologically active, more recent work has shown that reduced haloperidol may exert its activity through in vivo interconversion to the parent compound. The clinical importance of this metabolite is currently unclear.[71-74]

The mechanism by which haloperidol reduces delirium is not clear. Clinical improvement may be due to its sedative or antipsychotic properties or both. Some studies suggest that actions other than blockade of central dopamine receptors may be responsible for haloperidol's calming effect in patients with delirium.[65,72,75]

Route of Administration. Like other antipsychotics, haloperidol is rapidly absorbed after both oral and i.m. administration. As noted earlier, however, rapid control of acute delirium with extreme agitation is best accomplished with i.v. administration. Although the i.v. route is not included in FDA-approved labeling for haloperidol, there is now extensive literature examining the administration of the drug by this route. Haloperidol may be safely given by rapid, direct i.v. injection.[5] Although administration over longer periods offers no known advantage, doses have also been given in 30–50 mL of fluid as an i.v. infusion. Because heparin sodium forms a precipitate when combined with haloperidol lactate (the injectable salt), heparin infusions should be stopped and i.v. lines or heparin locks should be flushed with 0.9% sodium chloride injection or 5% dextrose injection before and after haloperidol is administered.[76] Haloperidol decanoate, a long-lasting "depot" form of the drug used for deep i.m. injection, is commercially prepared in a sesame oil vehicle and must not be given intravenously.[63]

Dosage. Several authors have proposed dosage guidelines for i.v. haloperidol in the treatment of acute delirium. The initial i.v. dose varies with the degree of delirium present: 0.5–2 mg for mild agitation, 2–5 mg for moderate agitation, and 10–20 mg for severe agitation. Considering haloperidol's delayed onset of action, doses should be given at intervals of no less than 20–30 minutes.[5,6,75,77] If the initial dose does not produce the desired calming effect after 30 minutes, the same dose may be repeated. If the patient still exhibits uncontrolled agitation 30 minutes after the second dose, the initial dose should be doubled. This increased dose should then be given every 30 minutes until calm is achieved.[5] Alternatively, in severely agitated patients, each successive dose may be doubled and administered at 30-minute intervals until agitation is controlled.[75,77] This process is referred to as "neuroleptization."

Although some authors have stated that bolus i.v. doses larger than 10 mg have no benefit over smaller doses,[78] others have reported giving single i.v. doses as large as 150 mg to achieve adequate control of agitation.[79] Although partial control of agitation is not usually a reasonable endpoint, the smallest possible effective dose should always be used to avoid the adverse effects of haloperidol, especially extrapyramidal symptoms. Large doses may occasionally be needed and can be safely given to patients with close monitoring of clinical status. However, when large doses of haloperidol fail to provide sufficient control, addition of a benzodiazepine may improve efficacy and should be considered (see the section on lorazepam).[4,5,78]

After the delirious patient is calmed, recurrence of agitation signals the need for additional doses of haloperidol. Such doses are usually required within 6–12 hours after the completion of initial neuroleptization, although severely agitated patients may require additional drug within 1–2 hours.[5,6] Because neuroleptization is time consuming and may require the constant attention of health-care professionals, it has been suggested that haloperidol be given on a regular maintenance schedule instead of on an as-needed basis. This regular dosing should then be continued around-the-clock until delirium has completely subsided.[4,6] Eisendrath and Link[80] have recommended that one half of the total dose used for neuroleptization be given in divided doses for initial daily maintenance therapy. Subsequent daily doses should be gradually tapered as the delirium clears. Adams and Fernandez[77] have proposed a different regimen in which the dose used for neuroleptization is repeated on the following day in divided doses. Thereafter, this total dose is cut daily by one third and tapered off over 48–72 hours. The disadvantage of these two regimens, however, is that regularly scheduled, potentially high-dose maintenance therapy without continuous assessment of altered mental status may lead to excessive administration of the drug. Weber et al.[6] have asserted that doses should be individualized and adjusted frequently to ensure that the patient receives the lowest effective dose. This strategy is important in critically ill patients who have rapidly changing clinical conditions. Ideally, the total dose of haloperidol on the second day should be only a fraction of the dose required for neuroleptization. A reasonable starting dose is 5 mg i.v. every six hours for moderate to severe agitation with dose titration based on the degree of continuing agitation. Dosage and frequency of administration must be guided by individual patient response and frequent clinical assessments. Because delirium is often worse at night, another 0.5–5 mg dose may be required in addition to the maintenance dose.[5]

Maximum Dosage. The maximum total daily dosage of i.v. haloperidol has not been established. Adams et al.,[4,78] have reported safely using dosages of i.v. haloperidol ranging from 100 to 480 mg over 24 hours in critically ill cancer patients suffering from delirium. The highest prolonged i.v. haloperidol dosage administered during this study was 240 mg/day for 15 consecutive days. Among agitated cardiac patients in a coronary-care unit who were described by Tesar et al.,[81] one patient received 485 mg of i.v. haloperidol over 8 hours and another patient received 530 mg over 24 hours with a total dosage of 1485 mg during a five-day period. Neither of these patients suffered any apparent adverse effects from such high haloperidol dosages. Stern[79] documented the highest reported dosage: an ICU patient safely received 945 mg of i.v. haloperidol in a single day. One case report mentions a cancer patient suffering from agitated delirium secondary to bilateral occipital cerebral infarctions whose delirium was controlled with a continuous i.v. infusion of haloperidol.[82] Haloperidol was administered at sustained rates of up to 25 mg/hour (600 mg/day), and the patient received 3800 mg over a 10-day period with no adverse effects. Although such case reports confirm that large dosages may be safely given, overaggressive use of haloperidol should nevertheless be avoided.

Adverse Reactions. The use of i.v. haloperidol, even in such extraordinary doses, has been associated with surprisingly few adverse effects. Haloperidol is relatively nonirritating to the veins. Hypotensive episodes after i.v. administration are rare and are almost always caused by hypovolemia. These can be prevented by ensuring adequate volume replacement. Intravenous haloperidol is generally safe for use in patients with a seizure disorder or head trauma and also appears to be the safest agent in patients with chronic obstructive pulmonary disease. Haloperidol has been used safely in patients receiving dopamine and does not block dopamine-mediated increases in renal blood flow. The drug has also been safely used in patients receiving epinephrine infusions, but alternate pressors such as norepinephrine should be used to avoid unopposed β-adrenergic activity and hypotension caused by potential α-adrenergic blockade with high doses of haloperidol. Extremely high doses may prolong the QT interval on the electrocardiogram.[5,63,75,83,84]

As a high-potency neuroleptic, haloperidol has increased potential to cause extrapyramidal symptoms. These are not dose related and are sudden in onset. The most common extrapyramidal symptoms with oral haloperidol therapy are dystonic reactions. Although these reactions usually involve muscles of the back, neck, and face, laryngospasm may also rarely occur.[85] In addition, akathisia may also be seen after haloperidol use. Patients with akathisia often have the clinical symptoms of restlessness, agitation, irritability, and thought or speech disorders; in severe cases psychosis-like behavior may develop. Akathisia may easily be mistaken for continued or worsened delirium, and accurate differentiation is necessary for proper treatment. Both dystonia and akathisia normally respond to standard treatment with anticholinergic agents (i.e., diphenhydramine or benztropine).[63,64] However, akathisia may frequently prove unresponsive to therapy with anticholinergic drugs. Agents such as propranolol and amantadine have been shown to be useful in the treatment of akathisia, although use of these agents may be problematic in the critically ill patient with unstable cardiovascular or renal function, or both.[86-90] Alternatively, haloperidol therapy should be discontinued or the dose should be reduced, and treatment with benzodiazepines should be attempted.

Extrapyramidal symptoms are seldom observed with the use of i.v. haloperidol, and Menza et al.[91] have concluded that the incidence of these symptoms after i.v. use is lower than it is after oral or i.m. administration of this drug. The reason for this route-related difference in toxicity is not clear.

Haloperidol therapy is contraindicated in patients with coma, severe toxic central nervous system depression, or a previous history of hypersensitivity to the drug.[63]

Haloperidol has few drug interactions. Additive depressant effects on the central nervous system may be seen when haloperidol is administered concomitantly with analgesics, barbiturates, or anesthetics.

Dementia has been reported with concomitant methyldopa use.[92,93] Patients receiving lithium carbonate have developed acute encephalopathic syndromes when haloperidol was administered concurrently.[94-98] These reactions have been reported to cause irreversible neurological damage in some patients secondary to unknown mechanisms, often when the serum lithium concentrations were within the normal therapeutic range. However, numerous patients have received these drugs concomitantly, and the combination has been shown to be both safe and efficacious. Until further studies provide more definitive information, it appears that the combination may be safely administered with careful monitoring for neurotoxicity.

Place in Therapy. I.V. haloperidol is effective for the treatment of agitation and delirium. Although high doses may occasionally be needed, i.v. haloperidol has few adverse effects in most patients. Many clinicians consider haloperidol, alone or in combination with benzodiazepines, to be the drug of choice for the treatment of delirium.

Other Neuroleptics

Droperidol. Like haloperidol, droperidol is a high-potency butyrophenone neuroleptic agent. It is commonly used during induction and maintenance of anesthesia. Droperidol is also used as an antiemetic during surgical and diagnostic procedures and during administration of antineoplastic drugs. In comparison with haloperidol, droperidol has little antipsychotic action and produces more sedation. In a comparative study of 27 acutely agitated patients,[99] droperidol achieved more rapid and reliable control of agitation than equivalent doses of haloperidol. Unfortunately, droperidol is a more potent α-adrenergic antagonist than haloperidol and is far more likely to cause hypotension, especially when combined with other agents such as benzodiazepines or narcotics. Droperidol may also cause excessive sedation and extrapyramidal symptoms. These adverse effects make droperidol less suitable for use in an intensive-care setting. Until more studies are performed, droperidol cannot be considered first-line therapy for the treatment of delirium. This drug should only be used when delirium is refractory to other more widely used agents.[5,63,64]

Chlorpromazine. Chlorpromazine, a low-potency phenothiazine derivative, was the first neuroleptic that was useful in the treatment of delirium. Because of the availability of haloperidol, chlorpromazine is now used infrequently in the ICU because of its anticholinergic, hypotensive, and proarrhythmic properties. Although chlorpromazine may be given i.v., the incidence of serious adverse effects is lower when it is given i.m. or orally. Typical initial i.m. doses for the control of agitation are 25–50 mg repeated every hour until control is achieved and then every three to six hours as needed. Chlorpromazine, as well as other low-potency agents, should not be considered as first-line treatment but may be useful when agitation is refractory to other drugs.[63,75]

Thiothixene, Trifluoperazine, and Fluphenazine. These high-potency agents have oral and i.m. routes (not i.v.) included in FDA-approved labeling and are effective for control of delirium when used in doses equivalent to those for haloperidol. They appear to offer no advantages over haloperidol, and experience with these agents is extremely limited.[75]

Benzodiazepines

Benzodiazepines have an extraordinary record of safe and efficacious use for several indications. They are popular because of their diverse range of clinical applications, relative lack of serious adverse effects, low addiction potential compared with narcotics and barbiturates, and variety of individual agents and dosage forms from which to choose. Because of their sedative and anxiolytic properties, benzodiazepines may be used to treat delirium in critically ill patients.

Pharmacokinetics. The benzodiazepines are completely absorbed from a functioning gastrointestinal tract after oral administration, although time to peak serum concentration for individual agents can range from 0.5 to 8 hours. With the exception of lorazepam, absorption tends to be erratic after i.m. injection. Rapid uptake of these drugs into the brain and other highly perfused organs occurs, followed by redistribution into less well perfused tissues such as muscle and fat. These distribution characteristics give benzodiazepines administered by the i.v. or i.m. route a rapid onset of action, but peak effects are generally brief. The benzodiazepines are extensively metabolized in the liver, and elimination rates of most of these drugs are prolonged considerably in patients with severe hepatic disease. With the exception of lorazepam and oxazepam, the benzodiazepines are metabolized to pharmacologically active products with long half-lives that significantly extend the total duration of their action.[6,17,63]

Adverse Effects. In general, benzodiazepines have mild clinical toxicity. Most of the commonly observed adverse effects are related to the drugs' pharmacologic mechanisms of action and include sedation, lightheadedness, motor incoordination, ataxia, confusion, and impairment of mental performance. Anterograde amnesia is also common,[100,101] although this adverse effect may actually be beneficial in patients for whom pain, anxiety, or emotional stress are underlying factors in the development of mental disturbances. Other adverse effects may include weakness, headache, blurred vision, chest and joint pains, and nausea and vomiting. In addition to the adverse effects listed above, two other effects are important in severely ill patients: paradoxical central nervous system excitation and depression of the cardiovascular and respiratory systems. Paradoxical central nervous system reactions include increased hostility and irritability, vivid or disturbing dreams, anxiety, euphoria, hallucinations, paranoia, and restlessness. Although the overall incidence of such paradoxical responses is low, they occur more frequently in the elderly, in patients with liver disease or a low serum albumin concentration, in patients receiving high doses of these drugs, and in patients who are hypersensitive to benzodiazepines. The appearance of these adverse effects warrants dosage reduction or selection of an alternative agent; the frequency of cross-sensitivity among benzodiazepines in producing paradoxical effects is not known.[17,63]

Although studies in normal, healthy subjects have shown that benzodiazepines have minimal effects on cardiovascular and respiratory function, their mild depressant effects may become more important when these drugs are used in the intensive-care setting. Administration of benzodiazepines by injection may produce shallow respiration, apnea, hypotension, bradycardia, or cardiac arrest. Premature ventricular contractions and other arrhythmias have also been reported. These effects are seen particularly in elderly or severely ill patients who have compromised pulmonary function or unstable cardiovascular status. The severity of these depressant effects is drug specific and frequently dose related. Because sedation of the delirious ICU patient often requires large and frequent doses of these drugs, careful monitoring of respiratory and cardiovascular functions is mandatory.[6,17,63,75]

As stated earlier, benzodiazepines are relatively unlikely to cause physical dependence when used for the short-term management of delirium. Although the benzodiazepine withdrawal syndrome is typically associated with chronic use, withdrawal symptoms have been reported for virtually all benzodiazepines commonly used in the ICU.[102-107] Symptoms of withdrawal closely resemble symptoms of delirium (e.g., irritability, insomnia, disturbances in concentration, confusion, hostility, and sensory disturbances). Thus, although uncommon, the benzodiazepine withdrawal syndrome should be considered as a possibility in those patients suffering from apparent recurrence of delirium after the discontinuation of benzodiazepine therapy.

Benzodiazepines interact infrequently with other drugs. Additive effects are seen with other drugs that have a depressant effect on the central nervous system (e.g., narcotic analgesics, anticonvulsants), and marked sedation may result. Concurrent use of valproic acid may cause psychotic episodes[11,108]; however, these episodes may be due to valproic acid alone and may not represent a true drug interaction. The abovementioned effects of the benzodiazepines on cardiovascular and respiratory function may also be potentiated by other drugs, including narcotic analgesics, which may produce the same effects.[17,63]

Selection. In the intensive-care setting, benzodiazepines offer two advantages not shared by neuroleptic agents: an extremely rapid onset of sedative effect and an unequaled amount of clinical experience with the drugs. When used judiciously, benzodiazepines are effective in managing acute agitation and delirium. They may be used as single agents or in combination with neuroleptics or narcotic analgesics. Because no single benzodiazepine is clearly more efficacious than any other, choice of a drug is determined primarily by chemical properties, pharmacokinetic considerations, and individual clinicians' prior experiences with drugs in this pharmacologic class. The most frequently used benzodiazepines in the ICU are diazepam, lorazepam, and midazolam.

Diazepam

Diazepam has been used in the intensive-care setting for many years and remains the standard with which all other benzodiazepines are compared. Diazepam controls agitation and delirium effectively in doses of 5–10 mg i.v. every three to four hours with dosage and frequency of administration titrated to patient response. Onset of action is rapid, usually within one to five minutes. Diazepam, however, has several properties that may be disadvantageous in the critically ill patient. These include considerable pain on injection and slow, erratic absorption when given i.m.; a relatively high frequency of thrombophlebitis when administered i.v.; a long half-life (20–60 hours) compared with that of newer benzodiazepines; and the presence of pharmacologically active metabolites, one of which (desmethyldiazepam) has an elimination half-life as long as 200 hours. Substantial accumulation of parent drug and metabolites occurs in the presence of hepatic disease, resulting in a prolonged half-life and duration of action. Diazepam may also cause more cardiorespiratory depression than the other benzodiazepines, especially when given i.v. and administered at rates greater than 5 mg/min. Because of these disadvantages, diazepam is no longer considered the benzodiazepine of choice for control of agitation and delirium in the critically ill patient; however, it is still a useful alternative to lorazepam and midazolam.[6,17,63,75]

Lorazepam

In contrast to diazepam, lorazepam has several advantages in the intensive-care setting. It is the only benzodiazepine that is reliably absorbed after i.m. injection, although the i.v. route is still usually preferable in ICU patients. Secondly, lorazepam has a relatively short half-life of 15–20 hours and has no active metabolites. In addition, lorazepam is primarily eliminated through conjugation with glucuronic acid and does not rely on hepatic cytochrome P-450 enzyme oxidation. Lorazepam is believed by many to have fewer adverse effects on cardiovascular and respiratory function than the other benzodiazepines, but depressant effects on these systems are still common in patients with hemodynamic instability or pulmonary dysfunction. Caution must still be exercised when lorazepam is used in seriously ill patients.[4,17,63,75,78,109]

Like diazepam, lorazepam produces prompt effects when administered by injection. The onset of action is

1–5 minutes after i.v. injection and 15–30 minutes after i.m. injection. Before i.v. administration, lorazepam should be diluted with an equal volume of sterile water for injection, 5% dextrose injection, or 0.9% sodium chloride injection. The maximum rate of administration should be 2 mg/min to minimize the risk of hypotension.[63]

Dosage varies depending on the degree of agitation and is adjusted according to patient response. The manufacturer recommends a maximum single dose of 4 mg i.v. or i.m., but Modell[110] reported administration of 80 mg i.v. as a single dose given over 40 minutes with no adverse effects noted. Clinical judgment and patient response remain the best guidelines for selecting appropriate dosages.

Several authors have advocated the use of lorazepam in combination with haloperidol for two reasons.[4,64,78,111] First, combining these drugs may allow lower total doses of each to be used with increased efficacy and fewer adverse effects. Second, some researchers believe that this combination is synergistic; haloperidol is a dopamine receptor antagonist, whereas lorazepam potentiates the actions of γ-aminobutyric acid (also a dopamine antagonist). Some authors recommend adding lorazepam only after high doses of haloperidol have been ineffective, whereas others recommend using both drugs in combination at the outset of therapy. Adams et al.[4,78] recommends beginning treatment with haloperidol 3 mg i.v. and lorazepam 0.5–1 mg i.v. These doses are then doubled and repeated in 30 minutes if the patient shows little or no response. Successive doses can be doubled every 30 minutes until sufficient control is achieved. Using this method, Adams[4] reported total 24-hour dosages ranging from 100 to 480 mg of haloperidol and up to 480 mg of lorazepam in critically ill cancer patients. Adams et al.[78] reported giving cancer patients total 24-hour dosages of haloperidol 480 mg i.v. and lorazepam 240 mg i.v. These large dosages effectively controlled severe agitation with no apparent adverse effects. These reports illustrate that lorazepam may be safely used in large doses, if necessary. Overaggressive use of lorazepam should be avoided, however, because of the increased risk of important adverse effects on cardiovascular and pulmonary function in critically ill patients. As with haloperidol, large doses of lorazepam should be used with caution.

Lorazepam is a safe and effective drug for the treatment of delirium and agitation and should be considered as a first-line agent. It may be used alone or in combination with haloperidol (or another neuroleptic). This choice depends on physician preference, severity of agitation, and patient response to use of a single agent.

Midazolam

Midazolam is a relatively new benzodiazepine that has gained considerable popularity for induction and maintenance of general anesthesia, preoperative sedation, and conscious sedation before various procedures. Midazolam is distinguished from other currently available benzodiazepines by a much shorter half-life (one to two hours), a shorter duration of action, an extremely short onset of action after i.v. or i.m. injection, a low frequency of pain or thrombophlebitis on injection, and increased water solubility that allows greater stability in aqueous solutions. Midazolam is particularly suitable for administration by constant i.v. infusion in the intensive-care setting because of its water solubility, short half-life, and short duration of action.

Although profound hypotension and apnea have been reported, the cardiovascular and respiratory depressant effects of midazolam are generally mild. Commonly observed fluctuations in respiratory rate and volume, pulse rate, and especially blood pressure are more likely to be clinically important in patients who are critically ill, suffering from chronic obstructive pulmonary disease, receiving concurrent narcotic medications, or receiving high dosages of midazolam. This high-risk group encompasses virtually all ICU patients, and constant patient monitoring is a necessity.[63,112-115] Adverse central nervous system effects in the form of hostility and hallucinations have been reported after a single dose of midazolam.[19]

Although the overall experience with midazolam in controlling acute agitation and delirium is still limited, published reports have shown that the drug is safe and effective. The recommended starting dosage is 1–5 mg/hour by constant i.v. infusion, with adjustment upward according to patient response. Shapiro et al.[116] reported effective control of agitation in ICU patients with various high-dose, continuous-infusion midazolam regimens supplemented by bolus doses of 0.05 mg/kg and infusion rate increases as needed for continued agitation. Westphal et al.[117] and Geller et al.[118] reported that continuous i.v. infusions of midazolam 1–15 mg/hr effectively controlled agitation in patients after cardiac and other major surgeries. While receiving midazolam, these patients also required decreased total narcotic dosages for maintenance of sedation and analgesia. Of note, Lineaweaver et al.[119] reported no ill effects in a patient with delirium tremens who received a total dosage of midazolam 2850 mg over a five-day period.

As more clinical experience is gained, short-term use of midazolam in the ICU will probably continue to increase. Until more evaluable literature is available, however, midazolam cannot be routinely recommended as first-line therapy for controlling agitation and delirium in ICU patients.

Narcotics

Narcotics such as morphine, meperidine, and fentanyl are frequently used in the intensive-care setting. Their sedative effects may be advantageous in patients with both agitation and pain. If pain is the underlying cause of a patient's agitation, effective pain control with narcotic analgesics may obviate the need for other agents such as neuroleptics or benzodiazepines. Conversely, effective management of anxiety may also reduce the need for powerful analgesics. Because narcotic agents also have important depressant effects on cardiopulmonary function and bowel motility, caution must be used when administering these agents concurrently with other drugs that have similar pharmacologic effects. In addition, these drugs also can induce delirium or aggravate the signs and symptoms of preexisting delirium.[37,38,63,75]

Barbiturates

Although barbiturates such as phenobarbital, secobarbital, and pentobarbital have been used to control agitation and delirium through sedation, no literature currently supports their use for this purpose. The barbiturates as a class possess many disadvantages in relation to more commonly used drugs, including long half-lives; development of tolerance; withdrawal symptoms after long-term use; important interactions with many drugs by induction of hepatic metabolic enzymes; a high incidence of adverse effects such as excess sedation, severe hypotension, and severe respiratory depression; and risk of potentially fatal overdose. For these reasons, many authors now state that the barbiturates have no place in the treatment of delirium and agitation. Their routine use is not recommended.[5,63,75]

Neuromuscular Blockers

The use of neuromuscular blocking agents such as pancuronium bromide and metocurine iodide may be necessary when other therapies have failed. In cases of life-threatening agitation and delirium (for example, in a mechanically ventilated patient), pharmacologic paralysis may be indicated for proper medical management. Induction and maintenance of paralysis carry attendant risks, and other measures should be tried before resorting to this procedure.[75] It must be noted that neuromuscular blocking agents have no effect on consciousness, pain threshold, or cerebration. Therefore, they can only be used in patients in whom the necessary anesthesia, analgesia, or sedation is induced and maintained.

Conclusion

Delirium and agitation are common in critically ill patients. These symptoms may have a variety of causes that must be systematically investigated and appropriately treated. Haloperidol and benzodiazepines, alone or in combination, are the drugs of choice for treatment of acute agitation and delirium in ICU patients. The choice of an individual agent is often personalized and depends on each patient's clinical condition.

References

1. Hale M, Koss N, Kertein M et al. Psychiatric complications in surgical ICU. *Crit Care Med.* 1977; 5:199-203.
2. Blachy PH, Starr A. Post-cardiotomy delirium. *Am J Psychiatry.* 1964; 121:371-5.
3. Nadleson T. The psychiatrist in the surgical intensive care unit. *Arch Surg.* 1976; 111:113-7.
4. Adams F. Neuropsychiatric evaluation and treatment of delirium in the critically ill cancer patient. *Cancer Bull.* 1984; 36:156-60.
5. Cassem EH, Lake CR, Boyer WF. Psychopharmacology in the ICU. In: Chernow B, ed. The pharmacologic approach to the critically ill patient. 2nd ed. Baltimore, MD: Williams & Wilkins; 1988:491-510.
6. Weber RJ, Oszko MA, Bolender BJ et al. The intensive care unit syndrome: causes, treatment, and prevention. *Drug Intell Clin Pharm.* 1985; 19:13-20.
7. Tomson CR, Goodiship THJ, Rodger RSC. Psychiatric side effects of acyclovir in patients with chronic renal failure. *Lancet.* 1985; 1:385-6.
8. Wysenbeek AJ, Sella A, Blum I et al. Acute delirious state after epsilon-aminocaproic acid administration. *Clin Toxicol.* 1979; 14:93-5.
9. Winn RE, Bower JH, Richards JF. Acute toxic delirium: neurotoxicity of intrathecal administration of amphotericin B. *Arch Intern Med.* 1979; 139:706-7.
10. Saloman M. Acute carbamazepine encephalopathy. *JAMA.* 1975; 231:915.
11. Alvarez N, Hazlett J, Courcelle R. Behavioral changes produced by valproic acid. *Clin Electroencephalogr.* 1982; 13:50-3.
12. McLellan DL, Swash M. Choreoathetosis and encephalopathy induced by phenytoin. *Br Med J.* 1974; 2:204-5.
13. Miller WI. Phenytoin chronic toxicity and associated psychosis. *Drug Intell Clin Pharm.* 1988; 22:1003-4.
14. Greenblatt DJ, Shader RI. Anticholinergics. *N Engl J Med.* 1973; 288:1215-9.
15. Tune LE, Damlouji NF, Holland A et al. Association of post operative delirium with raised serum levels of anticholinergic drugs. *Lancet.* 1981; 2:651-2.
16. Douglas WW. Histamine and 5-hydroxytryptamine (serotonin) and their antagonists. In: Goodman and Gilman's the pharmacological basis of therapeutics. 7th ed. Gilman AG, Goodman LS, Rall TW et al, eds. New York: Macmillan; 1985:618-24.
17. Harvey SC: Hypnotics and sedatives. In: Goodman and Gilman's the pharmacological basis of therapeutics. 7th ed. Gilman AG, Goodman LS, Rall TW et al, eds. New York: Macmillan; 1985:340-51.
18. Hall RC, Joffe JR. Aberrant response to diazepam: a new syndrome. *Am J Psychiatry.* 1972; 129:738-42.
19. Burnakis TG, Berman DE. Hostility and hallucinations as a consequence of midazolam administration. *DICP.* 1989; 23:671-2.
20. Gillman MA, Sandyk R. Reversal of captopril-induced psychosis with naloxone. *Am J Psychiatry.* 1985; 142:270.
21. Vincken W. Psychotic reaction to cefuroxime. *Lancet.* 1984; 1:965.
22. Saker BM, Musk AW, Haywood EF et al. Reversible toxic psychosis after cephalexin. *Med J Aust.* 1973; 1:497-8.
23. Al-Zahawi MF, Sprott MS, Hendrick DJ. Hallucinations in association with ceftazidime. *Br Med J.* 1988; 297:858.
24. Adler LE, Sudju L, Wilets G. Cimetidine toxicity manifested as paranoia and hallucinations. *Am J Psychiatry.* 1980; 137:1112-3.
25. Schentag JJ, Cerra FB, Calleri G et al. Pharmacokinetic and clinical studies in patients with cimetidine-induced mental confusion. *Lancet.* 1979; 1:177-81.
26. Altes J, Gasco J, de Antonio J et al. Ciprofloxacin and delirium. *Ann Intern Med.* 1989; 110:170-1.
27. Brown MJ, Salmon D, Rendell M. Clonidine hallucinations. *Ann Intern Med.* 1980; 93:456-7.

28. The Boston Collaborative Drug Surveillance Program. Acute adverse reactions to prednisone in relation to dosage. *Clin Pharmacol Ther*. 1972; 13:694-98.
29. Shear MK, Sacks MH. Digitalis delirium: report of two cases. *Am J Psychiatry*. 1978; 135:109-10.
30. Calandra GB, Brown KR, Grad LC et al. Review of adverse experiences and tolerability in the first 2516 patients treated with imipenem/cilastatin. *Am J Med*. 1985; 78(Suppl 6A):73-8.
31. Dundee JW, Knox JWD, Black GW et al. Ketamine as an induction agent in anaesthetics. *Lancet*. 1970; 1:1370-1.
32. Fisch RZ, Lahad A. Adverse psychiatric reaction to ketoconazole. *Am J Psychiatry*. 1989; 146:939-40.
33. Turner WM. Lidocaine and psychotic reactions. *Ann Intern Med*. 1982; 97:149-50.
34. Endo M, Hirai K, Ohara M. Paranoid-hallucinatory state induced in a depressive patient by methyldopa: a case report. *Psychoneuroendocrinology*. 1978; 3:211-5.
35. Fishbain DA, Rogers A. Delirium secondary to metoclopramide. *J Clin Psychopharmacol*. 1987; 7:281-2.
36. Schentag JJ, Ziemniak JA, Greco JM et al. Mental confusion in a patient treated with metronidazole—a concentration-related effect? *Pharmacotherapy*. 1982; 2:384-7.
37. Morisy L, Platle D. Hazards of high-dose meperidine. *JAMA*. 1986; 255:467-8.
38. Kaiko RF, Foley KM, Grabinski PY et al. Central nervous system excitatory effects of meperidine in cancer patients. *Ann Neurol*. 1983; 13:180-5.
39. Ahmad S. Nifedipine-induced acute psychosis. *J Am Geriatr Soc*. 1984; 32:408.
40. Cohn JN, Burke LP. Nitroprusside. *Ann Intern Med*. 1979; 91:752-7.
41. Carney MWP. Paranoid psychosis with indomethacin. *Br Med J*. 1977; 1:994-5.
42. Kruis R, Barger R. Paranoid psychosis with sulindac. *JAMA*. 1980; 243:1420.
43. Griffith JD, Smith CH, Smith RC. Paranoid psychosis in a patient receiving ibuprofen, a prostaglandin synthesis inhibitor: a case report. *J Clin Psychiatry*. 1982; 43:499-500.
44. Nichols PJ. Neurotoxicity of penicillin. *J Antimicrob Chemother*. 1980; 6:161-5.
45. Raichle ME, Kutt H, Louis S et al. Neurotoxicity of intravenously administered penicillin G. *Arch Neurol*. 1971; 25:232-9.
46. McCrum ID, Guidry JR. Procainamide-induced psychosis. *JAMA*. 1978; 240:1265-6.
47. Fleminger R. Visual hallucinations and illusions with propranolol. *Br Med J*. 1978; 1:1182.
48. Gershon ES, Goldstein RE, Moss AJ et al. Psychosis with ordinary doses of propranolol. *Ann Intern Med*. 1979; 90:938-9.
49. Gilbert GJ. Quinidine dementia. *JAMA*. 1977; 237:2093-4.
50. Price W, Coli L, Brandstetter RD et al. Ranitidine-associated hallucinations. *Eur J Clin Pharmacol*. 1985; 29:375-76.
51. Wasser WG, Brondheim HE, Richardson BK. Theophylline madness. *Ann Intern Med*. 1981; 95:191.
52. Mermel LA, Doro JM, Kabadi UM. Acute psychosis in a patient receiving trimethoprim–sulfamethoxazole intravenously. *J Clin Psychiatry*. 1986; 47:269-70.
53. Klotz U, Reimann I. Elevation of steady-state diazepam levels by cimetidine. *Clin Pharmacol Ther*. 1981; 30:513-7.
54. Desmond PV, Patwardhan RV, Schenker S et al. Cimetidine impairs elimination of chlordiazepoxide (Librium) in man. *Ann Intern Med*. 1980; 93:266-8.
55. Klotz U, Arvela P, Rosenkranz B. Effect of single doses of cimetidine and ranitidine on the steady-state plasma levels of midazolam. *Clin Pharmacol Ther*. 1985; 38:652-5.
56. Bauer LA, Edwards WAD, Randolph FP et al. Cimetidine-induced decrease in lidocaine metabolism. *Am Heart J*. 1984; 108:413-5.
57. Fine A, Churchill D. Potentially lethal interaction of cimetidine and morphine. *Can Med Assoc J*. 1981; 124:1434-6.
58. Busto U, Sellers EM, Naranjo CA et al. Withdrawal reaction after long-term therapeutic use of benzodiazepines. *N Engl J Med*. 1986; 315:854-9.
59. Finley PR, Nolan PE. Precipitation of benzodiazepine withdrawal following sudden discontinuation of midazolam. *DICP*. 1989; 23:151-2.
60. Baker CF. Sensory overload and noise in the ICU: sources of environmental stress. *Crit Care Q*. 1984; 6:66-80.
61. Gowan NJ. The perceptual world of the intensive care unit: an overview of some environmental considerations in the helping relationship. *Heart Lung*. 1979; 8:340-4.
62. Helion MC, Gordon SH, Nunnery SL. The correlation between sleep deprivation and the intensive care unit syndrome. *Heart Lung*. 1980; 9:464-8.
63. AHFS drug information 89. McEvoy GK, ed. Central nervous system agents. Bethesda, MD: American Society of Hospital Pharmacists; 1989:981-1305.
64. Dubin WR, Feld JA. Rapid tranquilization of the violent patient. *Am J Emerg Med*. 1989; 7:313-20.
65. Baldessarini RJ. Drugs and the treatment of psychiatric disorders. In: Goodman and Gilman's the pharmacological basis of therapeutics. 7th ed. Gilman AG, Goodman LS, Rall TW et al. eds. New York: Macmillan; 1985:391-412.
66. Eikayan U, Frishman W. Cardiovascular effects of phenothiazines. *Am Heart J*. 1980; 100:397-401.
67. Salama AA. Complete heart block associated with mesoridazine in lithium combination. *J Clin Psychiatry*. 1987; 48:123.
68. Kiriike N, Maeda Y, Nishiwaki S et al. Iatrogenic torsade de pointes induced by thioridazine. *Biol Psychiatry*. 1987; 22:99-103.
69. Shaler A, Munitz H. The neuroleptic malignant syndrome: agent and host interaction. *Acta Psychiatr Scand*. 1986; 73:337-47.
70. Harsch HH. Neuroleptic malignant syndrome: physiological and laboratory findings in a series of nine cases. *J Clin Psychiatry*. 1987; 48:328-33.
71. Korp ER, Wyatt RJ. Reduced haloperidol: effects on striatal dopamine metabolism and conversion to haloperidol in the rat. *Psychopharmacology*. 1984; 83:34-7.
72. Korp ER, Costakos DT, Wyatt RJ. Interconversions of haloperidol and reduced haloperidol in guinea pig and rat liver microsomes. *Biochem Pharmacol*. 1985; 34:2923-7.
73. Midha KK, Hawes EM, Hubbard JW et al. Interconversion between haloperidol and reduced haloperidol in man. *J Clin Psychopharmacol*. 1987; 7:362-4.
74. Ereshefsky L, Davis CM, Harrington CA et al. Haloperidol and reduced haloperidol plasma levels in selected schizophrenic patients. *J Clin Psychopharmacol*. 1984; 4:138-42.
75. Tesar GE, Stern TA. Rapid tranquilization of the agitated intensive care unit patient. *J Intensive Care Med*. 1988; 3:195-201.
76. Schutz VH, Schroder F. Heparin sodium compatibility with simultaneous administration of other drugs. *Krankenhauspharmazie*. 1985; 6:7-11. Translation.
77. Adams S, Fernandez F. Intravenous use of haloperidol. *Hosp Pharm*. 1987; 22:306-7. Letter.
78. Adams F, Fernandez F, Andersson BS. Emergency pharmacotherapy of delirium in the critically ill cancer patient. *Psychosomatics*. 1986; 27(Suppl 1):33-7.
79. Stern TA. The management of anxiety and depression following myocardial infarction. *Mt. Sinai J Med (NY)*. 1985; 52:623-33.
80. Eisendrath SI, Link N. Mental changes in the ICU: detection and management. *Drug Ther Hosp Ed*. 1983; 8(Oct):18-9, 23-6.
81. Tesar GE, Murray GB, Cassem NH. Use of high-dose intravenous haloperidol in the treatment of agitated cardiac patients. *J Clin Psychopharmacol*. 1985; 5:344-7.
82. Fernandez F, Holmes VF, Adams F et al. Treatment of severe, refractory agitation with a haloperidol drip. *J Clin Psychiatry*. 1988; 49:239-41.
83. Cameron OG. Safe use of haloperidol in a patient with cardiac dysrhythmia. *Am J Psychiatry*. 1978; 135:1244.

84. Donlan PT, Hopkin J, Schaffer CB et al. Cardiovascular safety of rapid treatment with intramuscular haloperidol. *Am J Psychiatry*. 1979; 136:233-4.
85. Flaherty JA, Lahmeyer HW. Laryngeal-pharyngeal dystonia as a possible cause of asphyxia with haloperidol treatment. *Am J Psychiatry*. 1978; 135:1414-5.
86. Van Putten T, Marder SR. Behavioral toxicity of antipsychotic drugs. *J Clin Psychiatry*. 1987; 48(Suppl 9):13-9.
87. Marsden CD, Jenner P. The pathophysiology of extrapyramidal side-effects of neuroleptic drugs. *Psychol Med*. 1980; 10:55-72.
88. Fann WE, Lake CR. Amantadine versus trihexyphenidyl in the treatment of neuroleptic-induced parkinsonism. *Am J Psychiatry*. 1976; 133:940-3.
89. Allen RM, Lane JD, Brauchi JT. Amantadine reduces haloperidol-induced dopamine receptor hypersensitivity in the striatum. *Eur J Pharmacol*. 1980; 65:313-5.
90. Adler L, Angrist B, Peselow E et al. A controlled assessment of propranolol in the treatment of neuroleptic induced akathisia. *Br J Psychiatry*. 1986; 149:42-5.
91. Menza MA, Murray GB, Holmes VF et al. Decreased extrapyramidal symptoms with intravenous haloperidol. *J Clin Psychiatry*. 1987; 48:278-80.
92. Thornton WE. Dementia induced by methyldopa with haloperidol. *N Engl J Med*. 1976; 294:1222.
93. Nadel I, Wallach M. Drug interaction between haloperidol and methyldopa. *Br J Psychiatry*. 1979; 135:484.
94. Thomas CJ. Brain damage with lithium/haloperidol. *Br J Psychiatry*. 1979; 134:552.
95. Cohen WJ, Cohen NH. Lithium carbonate, haloperidol, and irreversible brain damage. *JAMA*. 1974; 230:1283-7.
96. Spring G, Frankel M. New data on lithium and haloperidol incompatibility. *Am J Psychiatry*. 1981; 138:818-21.
97. Keitner GI, Shahzad R. Reversible neurotoxicity with combined lithium and haloperidol administration. *J Clin Psychopharmacol*. 1984; 4:104-5.
98. Miller F, Menninger J. Lithium-neuroleptic neurotoxicity is dose dependent. *J Clin Psychopharmacol*. 1987; 7:89-91.
99. Resnick M, Burton BT. Droperidol vs. haloperidol in the initial management of acutely agitated patients. *J Clin Psychiatry*. 1984; 45:298-9.
100. George KA, Dundee JW. Relative amnesic actions of diazepam, flunitrazepam, and lorazepam in man. *Br J Clin Pharmacol*. 1977; 4:45-50.
101. Dundee JW, Wilson JB. Amnesic action of midazolam. *Anaesthesia*. 1980; 35:459-61.
102. Falk JL, Tang M. Development of physical dependence on midazolam following oral self-administration. *Pharmacol Biochem Behav*. 1987; 26:797-800.
103. Howe JG. Lorazepam withdrawal seizures. *Br Med J*. 1981; 280:1163-4.
104. Barton DF. More on lorazepam withdrawal. *Drug Intell Clin Pharm*. 1981; 92:94-6.
105. Owen RT, Tyrer P. Benzodiazepine dependence: a review of the evidence. *Drugs*. 1983; 25:383-98.
106. Levy AB. Delirium and seizures due to abrupt alprazolam withdrawal: case report. *J Clin Psychiatry*. 1984; 45:38-9.
107. DeBard ML. Diazepam withdrawal syndrome: a case with psychosis, seizures, and coma. *Am J Psychiatry*. 1979; 136:104-5.
108. Bellman MH, Ross EM. Side effects of sodium valproate. *Br Med J*. 1977; 1:1662. Letter.
109. Leppik IE, Derivan AT, Homan RW et al. Double-blind study of lorazepam and diazepam in status epilepticus. *JAMA*. 1983; 249:1452-4.
110. Modell JG. Further experience and observations with lorazepam in the management of behavioral agitation. *J Clin Psychopharmacol*. 1986; 6:355-87.
111. Salzman C, Green AI, Rodriguez-Villa F et al. Benzodiazepines combined with neuroleptics for management of severe disruptive behavior. *Psychosomatics*. 1986; 27(Suppl 1):17-21.
112. Dornauer RJ, Aston R. Update: midazolam maleate, a new water-soluble benzodiazepine. *JAMA*. 1983; 249:650-2.
113. Greenblatt DJ, Abernethy DR. Midazolam pharmacology and pharmacokinetics. *Anesthesiol Rev*. 1985; 12(May-Jun):17-20.
114. Khanderia U, Pandit SK. Use of midazolam hydrochloride in anesthesia. *Clin Pharm*. 1987; 6:533-47.
115. Reves JG, Samuelson PN, Gelman S et al. Cardiovascular effects of midazolam. *Anesthesiol Rev*. 1985; 12(May-Jun):24-8.
116. Shapiro JM, Westphal BA, White PF et al. Midazolam infusion for sedation in the intensive care unit: effect on adrenal function. *Anesthesiology*. 1986; 64:394-8.
117. Westphal LM, Cheng EY, White PF et al. Use of midazolam infusion for sedation following cardiac surgery. *Anesthesiology*. 1987; 67:257-62.
118. Geller E. Midazolam infusion and the benzodiazepine antagonist flumazenil for sedation of intensive care patients. *Resuscitation*. 1988; 16(Suppl):S31-S39.
119. Lineaweaver WC, Anderson K, Hing DN. Massive doses of midazolam infusion for delirium tremens without respiratory depression. *Crit Care Med*. 1988; 16:294-5.

Health Care for the Elderly

The explosive growth of the elderly population (65 years of age and older) poses unique problems for the medical community. In the United States in 1900, there were about 3 million people aged 65 years and older, which was 4% of the population. By 1984, there were 28 million elderly, constituting about 12% of the population.

Although those figures are dramatic enough, the prospects for the next several decades are even more staggering. By the year 2020, the number of elderly persons will rise to over 64 million. . . .

Therefore, one of the most important tasks that the medical community faces today is to prepare for the problems in caring for the elderly in the 1990s and the early 21st century.

—Anon. American Medical Association white paper on elderly health. Report of the Council on Scientific Affairs. *Arch Intern Med*. 1990; 150:2459-72.

Therapy Update

Ethnicity and psychotropic drugs

WILLIAM S. BOND

Abstract: The literature concerning the effect of race and ethnicity on the pharmacokinetics of psychotropic drugs is reviewed, and recommendations concerning the use of these agents are presented.

While no differences in the pharmacokinetics or dosage requirements of antipsychotic drugs have been demonstrated among black, Hispanic, and white persons, Asians seem to have a lower threshold for both the therapeutic and adverse effects of antipsychotic drugs than do Caucasians. Use of lower than usual initial dosages of antipsychotic drugs in Asian patients appears to be prudent. Although ethnicity may have an effect on antidepressant drug pharmacology and dosage requirements, the available data are not sufficiently convincing to make any dosage recommendations. Claims that Asians require lower dosages of lithium than do other ethnic groups are not supported by the available evidence. Higher plasma benzodiazepine concentrations and lower drug clearance observed in Asians compared with Caucasians are consistent with clinical observations of lower dosage requirements for Asian patients; smaller than usual dosages of these agents are recommended for Asian patients.

Interracial pharmacokinetic and pharmacodynamic differences for psychotropic drugs can affect clinical outcomes. Further study of this issue is warranted.

Index terms: Asians; Benzodiazepines; Blood levels; Caucasians; Dosage; Ethnic groups; Excretion; Negroes; Pharmacogenetics; Pharmacokinetics; Psychotherapeutic agents; Race
Clin Pharm. 1990; 10:467-70

Ethnic or racial background is usually not considered in decisions regarding psychotropic drug dosage. A growing body of evidence, however, indicates that the pharmacokinetics and pharmacodynamics of these agents may differ substantially among different races, and that these differences can affect clinical outcome. Differences between Asian and Caucasian groups are especially well documented. This paper reviews the literature concerning this subject and presents recommendations regarding the clinical use of psychotropic drugs in different racial or ethnic groups.

Antipsychotic Drugs

Comparisons of antipsychotic pharmacology in Caucasians and other racial groups reveal both similarities and potentially important differences. Single-dose pharmacokinetic studies of trifluoperazine,[1] fluphenazine,[2] and haloperidol[3] report wide interindividual variations but no major differences between healthy black and white subjects. Therapeutic antipsychotic drug dosages prescribed for Hispanic patients have not been observed to be significantly different from those used for white and black patients.[4]

In contrast, clinical reports indicate major differences between Asian and Caucasian psychiatric patients both in therapeutic antipsychotic dosages and in pharmacokinetic and pharmacodynamic factors. With some exceptions,[5] clinical observations and surveys[6-9] have suggested that, as compared with Caucasians, Asian patients generally require lower doses of antipsychotic drugs and tend to have a lower neuroleptic threshold (defined as the highest dose at which the patient did not require anticholinergic medication and manifested minimal extrapyramidal symptoms).[7,10]

The observation that Asian patients require lower dosages than do Caucasians is strengthened by pharmacokinetic studies of haloperidol that report higher plasma or serum drug concentrations in Asian patients, even when differences in weight and body surface area are controlled.[11,12] Increased absorption and reduced hepatic hydroxylation capacity account in part for these higher levels.[13] Pharmacodynamic factors (i.e., dopamine-receptor-mediated responses) also

WILLIAM S. BOND, PHARM.D., is Professor of Clinical Pharmacy, Philadelphia College of Pharmacy and Science, Woodland Avenue at 43rd Street, Philadelphia, PA 19104.

The Therapy Update *section provides concise analytical reviews of narrowly defined, important topics in pharmacotherapy. Priority is given to articles that focus on new or emerging standards in drug therapy. Articles are not intended to be comprehensive reviews of drugs or of disease states and their treatment.*

play a role in dosage differences, as evidenced by more prominent antipsychotic-induced prolactin responses[12] and lower thresholds for therapeutic (e.g., reduction in Brief Psychiatric Rating Scale scores) and adverse antipsychotic effects in Asian individuals than in Caucasians.[14]

Available data indicate that one should start with lower than usual antipsychotic drug dosages in Asian patients and increase dosages gradually. Further longitudinal assessments of therapeutic dosages and of pharmacokinetic and pharmacodynamic variables using antipsychotic drugs other than haloperidol are needed. In addition, certain factors such as receptor density and affinity, brain drug concentrations, and protein binding have been assessed only indirectly, if at all. The recent finding by Zhou et al.[15] of lower levels of α_1-acid glycoprotein in Chinese than in Caucasian subjects makes determination of possible interracial differences in protein binding particularly important, given that binding of basic drugs like antipsychotic and antidepressant agents is generally extensive.[16] Finally, interracial comparative studies must control for differences in body weight and surface area, the influence of other prescribed and nonprescribed drugs, foodstuffs (e.g., caffeine-containing foods), and social habits (e.g., smoking, alcohol ingestion) that may affect hepatic enzyme metabolizing activity.

Antidepressant Drugs

Very little published information exists concerning differences in antidepressant pharmacology among blacks, Caucasians, and Hispanics. A study by Ziegler and Biggs,[17] which reported that plasma nortriptyline concentrations were 50% higher in black patients than in white patients, has been criticized for improper correction of plasma concentrations on the basis of weight.[18] No patient weights were given in that report. Critics of the report point out that if the black patients weighed more than the white patients, this difference might explain the difference in drug concentrations.

Studies suggest a lower tricyclic antidepressant dosage requirement and increased sensitivity to the anticholinergic effects of these agents in Hispanics than in Caucasian patients.[19,20] However, a single-dose study comparing the plasma nortriptyline levels and clearance rates in healthy Hispanic and Caucasian volunteers failed to demonstrate any major differences between the two groups.[21]

Survey data collected from multiple Asian countries indicate that both imipramine and amitriptyline are used in much lower dosage ranges than is customary in the United States.[22] From these data, an imipramine hydrochloride dosage range of 1.4 to 2.7 mg/kg of body weight was calculated; this is approximately half that found therapeutic for many Caucasian patients (i.e., 3.5 mg/kg).[23]

This survey information is consistent with the results of some single-dose pharmacokinetic studies that found that Asians achieve significantly higher plasma concentrations of tricyclic antidepressants[24-26] and have lower clearance rates than do Caucasians.[26] The studies by Allen et al.[25] and Rudorfer et al.,[26] however, did not adjust the dosage for patient weight. This seems to be an important factor, since subsequent comparisons in which dosage was based on body weight found no significant pharmacokinetic differences between the two groups.[27,28] In addition, while 30% of Asians have been found to have a deficiency of debrisoquin hydroxylation, and the ability to hydroxylate debrisoquin is closely linked with the ability to hydroxylate nortriptyline,[29] no such problem has been found in the hepatic metabolism of tricyclic antidepressants by Asians; the drug fraction metabolized to the hydroxylated form and the clearance of drug by hydroxylation are not different for Caucasians and Asians.[26,28]

Firm recommendations regarding the clinical use of tricyclic antidepressant drugs in different ethnic groups cannot be made from the available information. Pharmacokinetic and pharmacodynamic investigations with larger patient samples and control of dosage for body weight, drug interactions, and environmental variables such as diet, smoking, and alcohol use are needed before the existence of ethnic differences in antidepressant metabolism and response can be definitively determined.

Other Psychotropic Drugs

There is little evidence to support claims made by Takahashi[30] and others[8] that Asian patients require lower dosages of lithium and respond to lower plasma lithium levels than do Caucasians for the treatment and prophylaxis of bipolar illness. No direct comparative studies have been published. Lithium dosage varies considerably among individuals. The serum concentrations of lithium required for treatment or prophylaxis of bipolar illness are also quite variable, and the relationship between serum lithium concentration and clinical outcome remains obscure.[31,32] The interval between the last dose and the drawing of the blood sample has an important effect on reported lithium concentrations, and none of the studies have taken this variable into account. The observation by Honda and Suzuki[33] that Caucasians in the United States have higher lithium clearances and larger volumes of distribution than do Japanese is based on a short-term study of a small number of patients. Other published pharmacokinetic data[34] show little difference for these values.

There is no convincing evidence for differences in required lithium dosage or plasma levels in different racial groups. Direct comparative studies are needed that evaluate the relationship between clinical response and pharmacokinetic and pharmacodynamic measures.

Survey data indicate that Asians are prescribed significantly lower benzodiazepine dosages than are Caucasians.[9] Single-dose pharmacokinetic studies of alprazolam and diazepam support this finding. Lin et al.[35] found that Asians manifested significantly higher plasma levels, lower clearances, and longer half-lives for alprazolam than did Caucasians. These interracial differences persisted when adjustments had been made for body surface area and when Caucasians were compared with American-born and foreign-born Asians. Kumana et al.[36] reported smaller volumes of distribution and higher mean serum diazepam and desmethyldiazepam concentrations in Chinese volunteers compared with Caucasians. Drug clearance was similar in the two groups. In this study, the greater amount of body fat in Caucasians was an important factor accounting for ethnic differences in the disposition of diazepam, a highly lipid-soluble drug. Ghoneim et al.[37] also observed a smaller volume of distribution for diazepam and higher serum concentrations of diazepam and desmethyldiazepam in Asians than in Caucasians. Clearance adjusted for body weight was slower in the Asian group as well. Protein binding and drug elimination half-life were similar in both groups.

Cognitive and psychomotor effects after a single dose of diazepam were similar in Asian and Caucasian subjects.[37] If, as these investigators point out, long-term therapy causes greater accumulation of benzodiazepine in Asians, as might be expected from these pharmacokinetic differences, more central nervous system depression would occur in Asians than in Caucasians.

Smaller initial dosages of benzodiazepines should probably be prescribed for Asian patients than for Caucasians until the effects of the drugs are appreciated. Pharmacokinetic variables and cognitive and psychomotor effects of intermediate- and long-term benzodiazepine treatment in Asians, Caucasians, and other racial groups need to be investigated.

Conclusion

Available pharmacokinetic and pharmacodynamic information supports clinical observations and surveys that indicate that Asian patients require lower dosages of antipsychotic drugs and benzodiazepines than do other ethnic groups. The role of ethnicity in the clinical use of antidepressants remains unclear because of the limited data comparing antidepressant pharmacology in blacks, Caucasians, and Hispanics and the conflicting pharmacokinetic data for Asian and Caucasian individuals. Claims that Asians require lower dosages of lithium than do other ethnic groups are not supported by the available evidence.

The ethnic background of patients needs to be considered in the design of clinical investigations of the safety and efficacy of psychotropic drugs. The influence of ethnicity on psychotropic drug disposition and effect will become increasingly important in clinical practice, given the continued immigration to the United States of large numbers of people of different ethnic backgrounds.

References

1. Midha KK, Hawes EM, Hubbard JW et al. A pharmacokinetic study of trifluoperazine in two ethnic populations. *Psychopharmacology*. 1988; 95:333-8.
2. Midha KK, Hawes EM, Hubbard JW et al. Variation in the single-dose pharmacokinetics of fluphenazine in psychiatric patients. *Psychopharmacology*. 1988; 96:206-11.
3. Midha KK, Chakraborty BS, Ganes DA et al. Intersubject variation in the pharmacokinetics of haloperidol and reduced haloperidol. *J Clin Psychopharmacol*. 1989; 9:98-104.
4. Adams GL, Dworkin RJ, Rosenberg SD. Diagnosis and pharmacotherapy issues in the case of Hispanics in the public sector. *Am J Psychiatry*. 1984; 141:970-4.
5. Sramek JJ, Sayles MA, Simpson GM. Neuroleptic dosage for Asians: a failure to replicate. *Am J Psychiatry*. 1986; 143:535-6.
6. Yamamoto J, Fung D, Lo S et al. Psychopharmacology for Asian Americans and Pacific Islanders. *Psychopharmacol Bull*. 1979; 15:29-31.
7. Lin KM, Finder E. Neuroleptic dosage for Asians. *Am J Psychiatry*. 1983; 140:490-1.
8. Okuma T. Differential sensitivity to the effects of psychotropic drugs: psychotics vs. normals; Asian vs. western populations. *Folia Psychiatr Neurol Jpn*. 1981; 35:79-87.
9. Rosenblat R, Tang SW. Do oriental psychiatric patients receive different dosages of psychotropic medication when compared with occidentals? *Can J Psychiatry*. 1987; 32:270-4.
10. Binder RL, Levy R. Extrapyramidal reactions in Asians. *Am J Psychiatry*. 1981; 138:1243-4.
11. Potkin SG, Shen Y, Pardes H et al. Haloperidol concentrations elevated in Chinese patients. *Psychiatry Res*. 1984; 12:167-72.
12. Lin KM, Poland RE, Lau JK et al. Haloperidol and prolactin concentrations in Asians and Caucasians. *J Clin Psychopharmacol*. 1988; 8:195-201.
13. Chang WH, Chen TY, Lee CF et al. Low plasma reduced haloperidol/haloperidol ratios in Chinese patients. *Biol Psychiatry*. 1987; 22:1406-8.
14. Lin KM, Poland RE, Nuccio I et al. A longitudinal assessment of haloperidol doses and serum concentrations in Asian and Caucasian schizophrenic patients. *Am J Psychiatry*. 1989; 146:1307-11.
15. Zhou HH, Adedoyin A, Wilkinson GR. Differences in plasma binding of drugs between Caucasians and Chinese subjects. *Clin Pharmacol Ther*. 1990; 48:10-7.
16. Kremer JMH, Wilting J, Janssen LHH. Drug binding to human alpha-1-acid glycoprotein in health and disease. *Pharmacol Rev*. 1988; 40:1-47.
17. Ziegler VE, Biggs JT. Tricyclic plasma levels. *JAMA*. 1977; 238:2167-9.
18. Rifkin A, Klein DF, Quitkin F. Possible effect of race on tricyclic plasma levels. *JAMA*. 1978; 239:1845-6.
19. Marcos L, Cancro R. Pharmacotherapy of Hispanic depressed patients: clinical observations. *Am J Psychother*. 1982; 26:4.
20. Escobar JI, Tuason VB. Antidepressant agents: a cross-cultural study. *Psychopharmacol Bull*. 1980; 16:49-52.
21. Gaviria M, Gil AA, Javaid JI. Nortriptyline kinetics in Hispanic and Anglo subjects. *J Clin Psychopharmacol*. 1986; 6:227-31.
22. Yamashita I, Asano Y. Tricyclic antidepressants: therapeutic

plasma level. *Psychopharmacol Bull*. 1979; 15:40-1.

23. Glassman AH, Perel JM, Shostak M et al. Clinical implications of imipramine plasma levels for depressive illness. *Arch Gen Psychiatry*. 1977; 34:197-204.
24. Kishimoto A, Hollister LE. Nortriptyline kinetics in Japanese and Americans. *J Clin Psychopharmacol*. 1984; 4:171-2.
25. Allen JJ, Vaddadi KS, Rack PH. Differences in the effects of clomipramine on English and Asian volunteers. Preliminary report on a pilot study. *Postgrad Med J*. 1977; 53(Suppl 4): 79-86.
26. Rudorfer MB, Lane EA, Chang WH et al. Desipramine pharmacokinetics in Chinese and Caucasian volunteers. *Br J Clin Pharmacol*. 1984; 17:433-4.
27. Pi EH, Simpson GH, Cooper TB. Pharmacokinetics of desipramine in Caucasian and Asian volunteers. *Am J Psychiatry*. 1986; 143:1174-6.
28. Pi EH, Tran-Johnson TK, Walker NR et al. Pharmacokinetics of desipramine in Asian and Caucasian volunteers. *Psychopharmacol Bull*. 1989; 23: 483-7.
29. Kalow W. Ethnic differences in drug metabolism. *Clin Pharmacokinet*. 1982; 7:373-400.
30. Takahashi R. Lithium treatment in affective disorders: therapeutic plasma level. *Psychopharmacol Bull*. 1979; 15:32-4.
31. Sashidharan SP. The relationship between serum lithium levels and clinical response. *Ther Drug Monit*. 1982; 4:249-64.
32. Gelenberg AJ, Carroll JA, Baudhuin MG et al. The meaning of serum lithium levels in maintenance therapy of mood disorders: a review of the literature. *J Clin Psychiatry*. 1989; 50(Suppl 12):17-22.
33. Honda Y, Suzuki T. Transcultural pharmacokinetic study on Li concentration in plasma and saliva. *Psychopharmacol Bull*. 1979; 15:37-9.
34. Baldessarini RJ. Chemotherapy in psychiatry. Cambridge, MA: Harvard Univ; 1985.
35. Lin KM, Lau JK, Smith R et al. Comparison of alprazolam plasma levels in normal Asian and Caucasian male volunteers. *Psychopharmacol*. 1988; 96:365-9.
36. Kumana CR, Lauder IJ, Chan M et al. Differences in diazepam pharmacokinetics in Chinese and white Caucasians—relation to body lipid stores. *Eur J Clin Pharmacol*. 1987; 32:211-5.
37. Ghoneim MM, Korttila K, Chiang CK et al. Diazepam effects and kinetics in Caucasians and Orientals. *Clin Pharmacol Ther*. 1981; 29:749-56.

DUE Criteria

The DUE Criteria *section of* Clinical Pharmacy *features model drug-use evaluation criteria that may be employed as a component of a comprehensive quality assurance program. The criteria sets are presented in the format used in the ASHP book* Criteria for Drug Use Evaluation. *Some of the criteria sets will have been originally published in that book; others will be presented here for the first time and published in future volumes of the ASHP book. The practitioners who developed a criteria set are acknowledged.*

In selecting drug products for coverage in DUE Criteria, *priority is given to products that have been recently marketed, those that are frequently prescribed, those that have high potential risk associated with their use, and those that are expensive. When feasible, a criteria set will be linked with a Drug Review that appears in the same issue.*

These criteria sets are a starting point for the development of DUE criteria for a specific practice setting. Readers are encouraged to modify the model criteria to fit their own circumstances.

Criteria for use of ondansetron hydrochloride in adult and pediatric inpatients and adult outpatients[a]

Element	Standard 100%	Standard 0%	Exception[b] or Critical Preventive/ Responsive Measure[c]	Sources of Information
Justification for Use				
1. Prevention of acute-onset nausea and vomiting associated with highly emetogenic cancer chemotherapy regimens[1–10]	X		1A. None	1. History and physical (H&P), physician orders, progress notes
Critical (Process) Indicators				
2. Other drug and nondrug causes of pre-existing nausea and vomiting identified	X		2A. None	2. H&P, physician orders, progress notes, medication administration record (MAR), nursing notes
3. Appropriate adult dosage: 0.15 mg/kg administered intravenously over 15 min beginning 30 min before start of cancer chemotherapy and repeated after 4 and 8 hr[3,5,7–10]	X		3A. Standardized doses used based on patient weight: if <70 kg, 8 mg; if 70–80 kg, 10 mg; and if >80 kg, 12 mg 3B. Second and third doses administered to adult patient 2 and 4 hr after initial ondansetron dose to facilitate outpatient use[7,9,11] 3C. Initial 8-mg dose administered over 15 min beginning 30 min before start of cancer chemotherapy followed by 1 mg/hr as continuous infusion for 24 hr[4,10]	3, 3A–C. Physician orders, progress notes, MAR
4. Appropriate pediatric dosage: 0.15 mg/kg administered intravenously over 15 min beginning 30 min before start of cancer chemotherapy and repeated after 4 and 8 hr[2,5,12]	X		4A. None	4. Physician orders, progress notes, MAR

Prepared by Steven C. Hartwig, M.S., Drug Usage Evaluation Coordinator, The Ohio State University (OSU) Hospitals, and Clinical Instructor, OSU College of Pharmacy, Columbus.

 0278-2677/91/0601-0471$00.75.

Element	Standard 100%	Standard 0%	Exception[b] or Critical Preventive/ Responsive Measure[c]	Sources of Information
5. Ondansetron dose diluted in 50 mL of 5% dextrose injection or 0.9% sodium chloride injection[5]	X		5A. Ondansetron dose diluted in 10% mannitol injection, Ringer's injection, 0.3% potassium chloride and 0.9% sodium chloride injection, 0.3% potassium chloride and 5% dextrose injection, 5% dextrose and 0.9% sodium chloride injection, 5% dextrose and 0.45% sodium chloride injection, or 3% sodium chloride injection[5,13]	5, 5A. Physician notes, MAR
Complications				
6. Headache[1,4,5,7–10]		X	6A. Identify other drug and nondrug causes 6B. Provide supportive care and symptomatic therapy	6. Progress notes, nursing notes 6A, B. Physician orders, progress notes, MAR, nursing notes
7. Diarrhea[4,5,10,14]		X	7A. Identify other drug and nondrug causes 7B. Provide supportive care and symptomatic therapy	7. Progress notes, nursing notes 7A, B. Physician orders, progress notes, MAR, nursing notes
8. Constipation[4,14]		X	8A. Identify other drug and nondrug causes 8B. Provide supportive care and symptomatic therapy	8. Progress notes, nursing notes 8A, B. Physician orders, progress notes, MAR, nursing notes
9. Sedation[1,4,9,10,14]		X	9A. Identify other drug and nondrug causes 9B. Provide supportive care 9C. Caution patient to avoid activities requiring full state of alertness	9. Progress notes, nursing notes 9A, B. Physician orders, progress notes, MAR, nursing notes 9C. Physician orders, progress notes, nursing notes
Outcome Measures				
10. Prevention of cancer chemotherapy-induced nausea and emesis	X		10A. One or two episodes of emesis 10B. Subjective reduction in nausea in patient with history of cancer chemotherapy-induced nausea 10C. Patient lost to follow-up	10, 10A. Progress notes, nursing notes 10B. H&P, progress notes, nursing notes 10C. Progress notes
11. Cancer chemotherapy course completed as scheduled			11A. Medical contraindications to continuation of chemotherapy 11B. Patient died 11C. Patient lost to follow-up	11. Physician orders, progress notes, MAR, nursing notes 11A–C. Progress notes

[a] Criteria address justification for use (indications), critical (process) indicators, complications of therapy, and patient outcome. Each criterion consists of an element, a standard, exceptions to the standard, and sources of information. The element is the minimum level of evidence needed to show that patient care was optimal. The standard defines the deviation from an element that is acceptable. If no deviation is acceptable, the standard is 100%. Exceptions are circumstances in which deviation is allowable. Sources of information listed are the most reliable sources. Sources pertaining to an element or exception are identified by the number assigned to the element or exception (e.g., 5, 5A).

[b] For justification for use and critical (process) indicators.

[c] For complications and outcome measures.

References

1. Bonneterre J, Chevallier B, Metz R et al. A randomized double-blind comparison of ondansetron and metoclopramide in the prophylaxis of emesis induced by cyclophosphamide, fluorouracil, and doxorubicin or epirubicin chemotherapy. *J Clin Oncol*. 1990; 8:1063–9.
2. Carden PA, Mitchell SL, Waters KD et al. Prevention of cyclophosphamide/cytarabine-induced emesis with ondansetron in children with leukemia. *J Clin Oncol*. 1990; 8:1531–5.
3. Cubeddu LX, Hoffman IS, Fuenmayor NT et al. Efficacy of ondansetron (GR 38032F) and the role of serotonin in cisplatin-induced nausea and vomiting. *N Engl J Med*. 1990; 322:810–6.
4. De Mulder PHM, Seynaeve C, Vermorken JB et al. Ondansetron compared with high-dose metoclopramide in prophylaxis of acute and delayed cisplatin-induced nausea and vomiting. A multicenter, randomized, double-blind, crossover study. *Ann Intern Med*. 1990; 113:834–40.

5. Glaxo Pharmaceuticals. Zofran package insert. Research Triangle Park, NC; 1991 January.
6. Schmoll HJ. The role of ondansetron in the treatment of emesis induced by noncisplatin-containing chemotherapy regimens. *Eur J Cancer Clin Oncol*. 1989; 25(Suppl 1):S35–S39.
7. Einhorn LH, Nagy C, Werner K et al. Ondansetron: a new antiemetic for patients receiving cisplatin chemotherapy. *J Clin Oncol*. 1990; 8:731–5.
8. Grunberg SM, Stevenson LL, Russell CA et al. Dose ranging phase I study of the serotonin antagonist GR38032F for prevention of cisplatin-induced nausea and vomiting. *J Clin Oncol*. 1989; 7:1137–41.
9. Kris MG, Gralla RJ, Clark RA et al. Dose-ranging evaluation of the serotonin antagonist GR-C507/75 (GR38032F) when used as an antiemetic in patients receiving anticancer chemotherapy. *J Clin Oncol*. 1988; 6:659–62.
10. Marty M, Pouillart P, Scholl S et al. Comparison of the 5-hydroxytryptamine$_3$ (serotonin) antagonist ondansetron (GR38032F) with high-dose metoclopramide in the control of cisplatin-induced emesis. *N Engl J Med*. 1990; 322:816–21.
11. Kris MG, Gralla RJ, Clark RA et al. Phase II trials of the serotonin antagonist GR38032F for the control of vomiting caused by cisplatin. *J Natl Cancer Inst*. 1989; 81:42–6.
12. Blumer JL, Shurin S, Patrick et al. Evaluation of pharmacokinetics, safety, and efficacy of ondansetron in children receiving chemotherapy. *Proc Am Soc Clin Oncol*. 1990; 9:332. Abstract.
13. Leak RE, Woodford JD. Pharmaceutical development of ondansetron injection. *Eur J Cancer Clin Oncol*. 1989; 25(Suppl 1):S67–S69.
14. Smith RN. Safety of ondansetron. *Eur J Cancer Clin Oncol*. 1989; 25(Suppl 1):S47–S50.

CP Continuing Education

The ASHP Continuing-Education System gives readers a self-assessment mechanism for selected articles in Clinical Pharmacy *and* AJHP. *It allows readers to obtain continuing-education credit for these articles.*

For the purpose of CE-credit enrollment, a blank answer sheet is published at the end of each installment of the column for the CE articles in that issue. An enrollee accumulates these answer sheets until the enrollment is submitted, using the form that is published in the June and December issues of Clinical Pharmacy *and in the June and December issues of* AJHP. *Any combination of tests within an 18-month period, from both* Clinical Pharmacy *and* AJHP, *may be included in an enrollment. More complete details about enrollment in the system appear in the semiannual enrollment form.*

Article 680-204-9113 (see page 430)
Qualifies for 1.0 hour of CE credit

Ondansetron—the first of a new class of antiemetic agents

Learning Objectives

After studying this article, the reader should be able to

1. Describe the mechanism of action and pharmacology of ondansetron and the mechanisms by which antineoplastic drugs cause nausea and vomiting.
2. Compare pharmacokinetic values of ondansetron in different age groups.
3. Describe the administration guidelines of ondansetron.
4. Describe the comparative efficacies of ondansetron and metoclopramide in patients treated with various antineoplastic drugs.
5. Identify the types and incidences of adverse effects incurred with both ondansetron and metoclopramide.

Self-assessment Questions

For each question there is only one best answer.

1. The central binding site of action of ondansetron is postulated to be
   a. In the enterochromaffin cells of the gut.
   b. In the area postrema of the medulla.
   c. In the diaphragm.
   d. In the vagus nerve.
2. Cisplatin is thought to cause nausea and vomiting as a result of
   a. Local irritation of the GI tract.
   b. Stimulation of dopamine receptors in the chemoreceptor trigger zone.
   c. Its neurotoxic metabolites.
   d. Serotonin release from enterochromaffin cells in the gut and subsequent stimulation of receptors in the area postrema.
3. Pharmacokinetic values of ondansetron
   a. Are significantly different in children compared with adults.
   b. May change if the patient is a heavy smoker.
   c. Follow Michaelis-Menton kinetics.
   d. Are somewhat different in the elderly; however, no dosage change is recommended.
4. Serum concentrations of ondansetron
   a. Should be measured routinely, especially in the elderly.
   b. Can be used to compare the efficacy of ondansetron with metoclopramide.
   c. Do not appear to correlate with antiemetic activity.
   d. Are useful for evaluating potential drug interactions.
5. Ondansetron for intravenous administration
   a. Must be diluted in at least 500 mL of 5% dextrose injection.
   b. May be infused in 50 mL of 5% dextrose or 0.9% sodium chloride injection.
   c. Should be prepared in glass containers only.
   d. Should be administered undiluted by rapid i.v. push.
6. Ondansetron is approved in the United States for administration by
   a. Continuous i.v. infusion.
   b. Intermittent i.v. infusion.
   c. I.M. injection.
   d. Oral tablet.
7. Which of the following statements correctly compares ondansetron with metoclopramide?
   a. Ondansetron has been shown to be superior to metoclopramide in antiemetic efficacy in all studies.
   b. Ondansetron has been shown to be inferior to metoclopramide in antiemetic efficacy in all studies.
   c. Ondansetron is less likely than metoclopramide to cause bothersome adverse effects.
   d. Ondansetron therapy costs approximately the same as high-dose metoclopramide therapy.
8. Ondansetron has been studied in patients with nausea and vomiting induced by
   a. Cisplatin.

ASHP journal CE instructions and enrollment form

Instructions

1. The system is flexible. You may select any combination of tests from the *American Journal of Hospital Pharmacy* and *Clinical Pharmacy* to give you the number of credits you need.
2. An Answer Sheet is published at the end of each installment of the CE column. An Enrollment Form is published in the June and December issues of *AJHP* and *CP*.
3. Complete only one Enrollment Form, but note on the form all the tests you are taking. Staple together all answer sheets for one enrollment.
4. Tests included must have been published within the past 18 months. Once a particular test is included in an enrollment, it may not be included in a subsequent enrollment.
5. The passing score on each test is 70%. Within four weeks of receiving your enrollment, ASHP will mail you a CE letter or notify you that certain tests were failed. Failed tests may be retaken only one time, without additional cost. There are no refunds for failed tests.
6. ASHP is approved by the American Council on Pharmaceutical Education as a provider of continuing pharmaceutical education (Provider Number 680-204). (The following states recognize ACPE-approved providers: AK, AL, AR, AZ, CA, DE, FL, GA, IA, ID, IL, IN, KS, KY, LA, MA, MD, ME, MI, MN, MO, MS, MT, NC, NE, NH, NJ, NM, NV, OH, OR, PA, RI, SC, SD, TN, WA, and WY [also Puerto Rico].) Most states that recognize ACPE-approved providers will accept credit earned through journal CE programs; however, since some states have restrictions on the number of credit hours or CE units they will accept toward the total requirement, it is advised that readers check with their respective state board of pharmacy if they are uncertain about the board's regulations.
7. Send your Enrollment Form, Answer Sheet(s), and check (made payable to ASHP) to:

ASHP CE
American Society of Hospital Pharmacists
4630 Montgomery Avenue
Bethesda, MD 20814

Enrollment Form

Name________________________

Address________________________

City____________ State________ Zip________

Fee Schedule
$5.00/hour
$20.00 minimum/enrollment

Tests included in this enrollment must have been published within the past 18 months.

Test Number	Hours of Credit

Total hours ________
Total fee($) enclosed ________

(Write additional numbers and hours on a separate sheet and attach it to this form.)

ACPE® *The American Society of Hospital Pharmacists is approved by the American Council on Pharmaceutical Education as a provider of continuing pharmaceutical education.*

Current Literature

Drug Reaction Alerts

Drug Reaction Alerts focuses primarily on serious, unlabeled reactions to new chemical entities. The citations are compiled monthly from International Pharmaceutical Abstracts, *which covers over 800 pharmacy and health-related journals worldwide. An address for reprints (when available) follows the name of the corresponding author of each citation.*

Pharmacists may use the FDA Adverse Reaction Report form that appears in most issues of Clinical Pharmacy for submitting reports of adverse drug reactions directly to FDA.

Androgens

Tully MP, Cooper RG, Jayson MI (Rheumatic Diseases Center, Hope Hospital, Salford M6 8HD, England). Intracranial hypertension associated with **stanozolol**. *DICP*. 1990; 24:1234. Case. (60-year-old woman with chronic low back pain; received stanozolol 10 mg daily for nine months; experienced a seizure; blood pressure, 170/110 mm Hg; cerebrospinal fluid pressure, 330 mm water; withdrawal of stanozolol led to patient recovery and discharge from hospital 10 days after seizure)

Antifungals

Gradon JD (Division of Infectious Diseases, Maimonides Medical Center, 4802 Tenth Ave., Brooklyn, NY 11219), Sepkowitz DV. Massive hepatic enlargement with fatty change associated with **ketoconazole**. *DICP*. 1990; 24:1175-6. Case. (37-year-old woman with acquired immunodeficiency syndrome; received ketoconazole 800 mg daily for 12 months as suppressive therapy for cryptococcal meningitis; developed massive hepatic enlargement and elevation of liver function test results; concomitant zidovudine, phenytoin, and sulfamethoxazole in combination with trimethoprim; liver tissue biopsy showed evidence of fatty liver; withdrawal of all medications led to subjective patient improvement but no decrease in liver size; liver function test results remain elevated; undetectable cryptococcal antigen)

Antineoplastic Agents

Devalck C, Ismaili K, Ferster A et al. (Sariban E, Hôpital Universitaire des Enfants, 1020 Brussels, Belgium). Acute **ifosfamide**-induced proximal tubular toxic reaction. *J Pediatr*. 1991; 118:325-6. Case. (female child with metastatic mesenchymoma of liver; received ifosfamide 3 g/sq m/day and mesna 3.6 g/sq m/day with hyperhydration for three days; developed decreased serum potassium, phosphorus, and bicarbonate concentrations and transient signs of renal insufficiency two days after completion of ifosfamide therapy; concomitant vincristine and actinomycin D; positive rechallenge with ifosfamide 3 g/sq m/day and mesna three months later; renal tissue biopsy showed areas of focal proximal tubular sclerosis indicative of toxic tubulopathy; therapy with daily oral supplements of potassium, phosphorus, and bicarbonate led to patient recovery and no signs of glomerular or tubular dysfunction six months later)

Antithyroid Drugs

Peter SA (State University of New York's Health Science Center, 1717 Ditmas Ave., Brooklyn, NY 11226). **Propylthiouracil**-associated hepatitis. *J Nat Med Assoc*. 1991; 83:75-7. Case. (43-year-old woman with Graves' disease; received propylthiouracil 600 mg daily then 300 mg daily for three months; developed hepatitis; withdrawal of propylthiouracil did not stop decline in patient's liver function; liver function test results began to show improvement 12 days after withdrawal of propylthiouracil)

Cardiac Drugs

Ahn CS (Nuclear Medicine Service, Veterans Affairs Medical Center, Brockton, MA 02401), Tow DE. Intrahepatic cholestasis due to hypersensitivity reaction to **procainamide**. *Arch Intern Med*. 1990; 150:2589-90. Case. (71-year-old man with premature ventricular contractions; received procainamide in doses ranging from 375 mg every three hours to 750 mg every six hours for six days; developed intrahepatic cholestasis; concomitant pancrelipase and albuterol; procainamide replaced with tocainamide 400 mg twice daily; no evidence of jaundice nine months later)

Hanston P (Department of Intensive Care, University Hospital St. Luc, Hippocrate Ave. 10, B-1200 Brussels, Belgium), Evrard P, Mahieu P et al. **Flecainide**-associated interstitial pneumonitis. *Lancet*. 1991; 337:371-2. Case. (49-year-old man with ventricular arrhythmias; received flecainide 150 mg twice daily for one year; developed pulmonary complications; withdrawal of flecainide led to nondetectable concentrations of drug in serum after nine days and in bronchoalveolar lavage sample after 27 days; patient died from cardiac arrhythmia 66 days after withdrawal of flecainide; results of microscopic examination of lungs at autopsy were indicative of interstitial pneumonitis; detectable concentrations of flecainide found in hepatic and pulmonary tissues but not in renal tissues)

Mattingly PM (Department of Pharmacotherapy and Research, Tampa General Hospital, P.O. Box 1289, Davis Island, Tampa, FL 33601), Burnette PK, Weston MW et al. Pancytopenia secondary to short-term, high-dose intravenous infusion of **amrinone**. *DICP*. 1990; 24:1172-4. Case. (64-year-old man with congestive heart failure; received amrinone 5–10 µg/kg/min as continuous intravenous infusions in short courses over several days; developed pancytopenia; concomitant furosemide, potassium chloride, aspirin, amiodarone, mexiletine, and dopamine; after six days of therapy with amrinone, hemoglobin was 8.2 g/dL, hematocrit was 25%, white blood cell count was 4.3×10^9/L, and red blood cell count was 2.9×10^{12}/L; withdrawal of amrinone and therapy with transfusions of packed red blood cells led to return of hematologic values to baseline after eight days)

Continued on page 481

Continued from page 478

Cathartics and Laxatives

Beuers U, Spengler U (Department of Medicine II, Klinikum Grosshadern, University of Munich, 8000 Munich 70, FRG), Pape GR. Hepatitis after chronic abuse of **senna**. *Lancet*. 1991; 337:372-3. Case. (26-year-old woman; self-medicated with extract of senna fruits equivalent to sennoside B 100 mg daily and a laxative tea equivalent to folia sennae 10 g twice weekly; developed toxic hepatitis; withdrawal of extract and tea led to decrease in serum aminotransferases to 20–40 U/L within one week; positive rechallenge)

Drug Interactions

Davis RL (College of Pharmacy, University of New Mexico, Albuquerque, NM 87131), Berman W, Wernly JA et al. **Warfarin–nafcillin** interaction. *J Pediatr*. 1991; 118:300-3. Case. (10-year-old girl who received nafcillin 750 mg every six hours by i.v. injection for treatment of bacterial endocarditis; 10 days later received warfarin 2.5 mg each evening and heparin by continuous i.v. infusion for anticoagulation after cardiac surgery; warfarin dose gradually increased to 7.5 mg each evening based on lack of increase in prothrombin time at lower doses; withdrawal of nafcillin after 19 days of concomitant warfarin and nafcillin therapy led to gradual increase in prothrombin time; adjustment of warfarin dose to 5 mg daily alternating with 2.5 mg daily led to prothrombin time of 19 seconds)

Pedersen-Bjergaard U, Myhre J (Gentofte Hospital, University of Copenhagen, DK-2900 Hellerup, Denmark). Severe hypocalcemia after treatment with diphosphonate and aminoglycoside. *Br Med J*. 1991; 302:295. Case. (62-year-old woman with multiple myeloma who received **clodronic acid** 2400 mg/day for 13 days for treatment of hypercalcemia; developed marginal hypocalcemia and clodronic acid was withdrawn for several weeks; received **netilmicin** up to 200 mg/day for 15 days for treatment of enterobacter septicemia; developed hypocalcemia that regressed after withdrawal of netilmicin; reinstitution of clodronic acid for seven days led to severe hypocalcemia; withdrawal of clodronic acid and therapy with calcium, diazepam, and phenobarbital led to control of tetany but hypocalcemia persisted; progression of underlying neoplasm led to patient death)

Seaton TL, Celum CL, Black DJ (Department of Pharmacy Practice, School of Pharmacy, SC-69, University of Washington, Seattle, WA 98195). Possible potentiation of **warfarin** by **fluconazole**. *DICP*. 1990; 24:1177-8. Case. (68-year-old woman with severe rheumatoid arthritis and mitral valve replacement who received warfarin for 20 years, most recently at 2–4 mg/day; received fluconazole 100 mg twice daily for eight days for treatment of candidal wound infection; experienced increased prothrombin time and gastrointestinal bleeding; concomitant ranitidine, prednisone, ferrous sulfate, furosemide, digoxin, enalapril, metoprolol, hydroxychloroquine, and aspirin; withdrawal of warfarin and administration of fresh frozen plasma allowed patient to complete 21-day course of therapy with fluconazole; two days after completion of fluconazole therapy, warfarin was reinstituted at 2–4 mg/day with stable coagulation values)

Zornberg GL (McLean Hospital, Belmont, MA 02178), Bodkin JA, Cohen BM. Severe adverse interaction between pethidine and **selegiline**. *Lancet*. 1991; 337:246. Case. (56-year-old man with Parkinson's disease who received selegiline 5 mg twice daily; received **meperidine** 75–150 mg/day with hydroxyzine for pain relief after elective surgical procedure; experienced increasing restlessness and irritability on second postoperative day; progressed to delirium with fluctuations between stupor and severe agitation on fourth postoperative day; concomitant pergolide, carbidopa in combination with levodopa, imipramine, and desipramine; withdrawal of meperidine on fourth postoperative day and of selegiline on fifth postoperative day led to resolution of symptoms by ninth day)

Drugs, Adverse Reactions

Williams I (Academic Department of Genito-Urinary Medicine, University College and Middlesex School of Medicine, London W1N 8AA, England), Weller IV, Malin A et al. **Thalidomide** hypersensitivity in AIDS. *Lancet*. 1991; 337:436-7. Cases. (three men with stage 4 human immunodeficiency viral infections; received thalidomide 100–200 mg/day for treatment of persistent ulcerative stomatitis resistant to topical therapy; developed widespread erythematous macular rash; withdrawal of thalidomide led to resolution of reactions; positive rechallenge in two patients)

Heavy Metal Antagonists

Mehta J (Blood Research Centre, Vivina Building SA, S.V. Road, 400 058 Bombay, India), Singhal S, Revankar R et al. Fatal systemic lupus erythematosus in patient taking oral iron chelator L1. *Lancet*. 1991; 337:298. Cases. (18-year-old man with β-thalassemia and 12-year-old girl with thalassemia major; received **1,2-dimethyl-3-hydroxypyrid-4-one**; man developed hepatomegaly with positive tests for antinuclear antibodies and antibodies to histones but negative test for dsDNA antibody; withdrawal of 1,2-dimethyl-3-hydroxypyrid-4-one led to decrease in hepatomegaly but increase in antinuclear antibody titer; therapy with prednisolone 40 mg/day led to improvement but symptoms of systemic lupus erythematosus remained; symptoms worsened after development of urinary tract infection and man died after cardiac arrest; girl did not develop symptoms of systemic lupus erythematosus but had positive tests for antinuclear antibody and antibodies to histones; 1,2-dimethyl-3-hydroxypyrid-4-one withdrawn immediately)

Hypotensive Agents

Hammarstrom L (Department of Clinical Immunology, Huddinge Hospital, S-14186 Huddinge, Sweden), Smith CI, Berg U. **Captopril**-induced IgA deficiency. *Lancet*. 1991; 337:436. Case. (10-year-old girl with hypertension caused by glomerulonephritis; received captopril 6.25 mg/day for four months then increased to 18.75 mg/day; experienced decrease in serum IgA concentration after one-half year and nondetectable serum IgA concentration within one year; concomitant propranolol, furosemide, and prednisolone; receipt of kidney graft and withdrawal of captopril led to slow return of serum IgA concentration to normal range)

Immunosuppressive Agents

Frayha HH, Nazer H, Kalloghlian A et al. (Sabbah R, Department of Pediatrics, Pathology, and Hematology/Oncology, King Faisal Specialist Hospital and Research Center, 11211 Riyadh, Saudi Arabia). Lymphoproliferative disorder in a liver transplant patient of **FK 506**). *Lancet*. 1991; 337:296-7. Case. (6-month-old child with orthotopic liver transplantation; received FK 506 1 mg twice daily for eight months; developed fever, hepatosplenomegaly, and widespread lymphadenopathy; concomitant nystatin, hydrochlorothiazide, co-trimoxazole, and fludrocortisone; decrease in dose of FK 506 followed by withdrawal led to decrease in sizes of lymph nodes and spleen and improvement in hematologic values)

Rello J, Vallverdu I, Coll P et al. (Net A, Department of Intensive Care, Service de Medicine Intensiva, Hospital de la Santa Creu i Sant Pau, Avenue Sant Antoni M Claret 167, 08025 Barcelona, Spain). Aseptic meningitis associated with **muromonab-CD3**. *DICP*. 1990; 24: 1233. Case. (22-year-old man with acute transplant rejection two years after orthotopic heart transplantation; received muromonab-CD3 for seven days; developed meningitis; withdrawal of muromonab-CD3 led to resolution of symptoms without antimicrobial therapy; negative cerebrospinal fluid cultures for bacterial, mycobacterial, fungal, and viral pathogens)

Books Received

Books are listed as soon as received; selected books may be reviewed in Book Reviews in subsequent issues.

Advances in Pain Research and Therapy, Volume 18: The Design of Analgesic Clinical Trials, edited by Mitchell B. Max, Russell K. Portenoy, and Eugene M. Laska. Published by Raven Press, 1185 Avenue of the Americas, New York, NY 10036, 1991. xxi + 729 p. Price $122.

Drug Interactions & Updates, 1991, by Philip D. Hansten and John R. Horn. Published by Lea & Febiger, 100 Chester Field Parkway, Malvern, PA 19355-9725, 1990. xi + 522 p. (Price $70 (U.S.), $80 (elsewhere).

Handbook of Drug Therapy in Liver and Kidney Disease, edited by Robert W. Schrier and John G. Gambertoglio. Published by Little, Brown and Company, 34 Beacon Street, Boston, MA 02108, 1991. xi + 388 p. Price $34.50.

Manual of Clinical Microbiology, Fifth Edition, edited by Albert Balows, William J. Hausler, Jr., Kenneth L. Herrmann et al. Published by the American Society for Microbiology, 1325 Massachusetts Avenue, N.W., Washington, DC 20005, 1991. xix + 1364 p. Price $64 (ASM members), $84 (nonmembers), hardbound; $56 (ASM members), $73 (nonmembers), softbound.

Patient Compliance in Medical Practice and Clinical Trials, Joyce A. Cramer and Bert Spilker, editors. Published by Raven Press, 1185 Avenue of the Americas, New York, NY 10036, 1991. xvii + 414 p. Price $65.

USP DI, 11th Edition. Volume I (two books): Drug Information for the Health Care Professional. Volume II: Advice for the Patient—Drug Information in Lay Language. Volume III: Approved Drug Products and Legal Requirements. Published by The United States Pharmacopeial Convention, Inc., 12601 Twinbrook Parkway, Rockville, MD 20852, 1991. Volume IA and IB: 3304 p. total. Volume II: 1624 p. Volume III: 1016 p. Price (including monthly updates) $195, complete set; $130, Vol. I and II; $110, Vol. I only; $42, Vol. II only; $75, Vol. III only.

Advertising Index

Adria Laboratories
Idamycin, 482, inside back cover, outside back cover
American Society of Hospital Pharmacists
CiteSearch, 416
Clinical Pharmacy, 428
Concepts in Immunology and Immunotherapeutics, 420
Criteria for Drug Use Evaluation, Volumes 1 & 2, 476
Pocket Guide to Injectable Drugs, 1991 Edition, 470
Baxter Healthcare Corporation, Hyland Division
Gammagard, 412-414
Burroughs Wellcome Company
Zovirax I.V., 408-410
Department of Veterans Affairs (Richmond)
Positions Available, 415
Eisenhower Medical Center
Position Available, 416
Glaxo Inc.
Zofran, 421-426
Eli Lilly and Company
Hospital Division, inside front cover
Roerig, A Division of Pfizer Pharmaceuticals
Diflucan, 407
Unasyn, 418-420

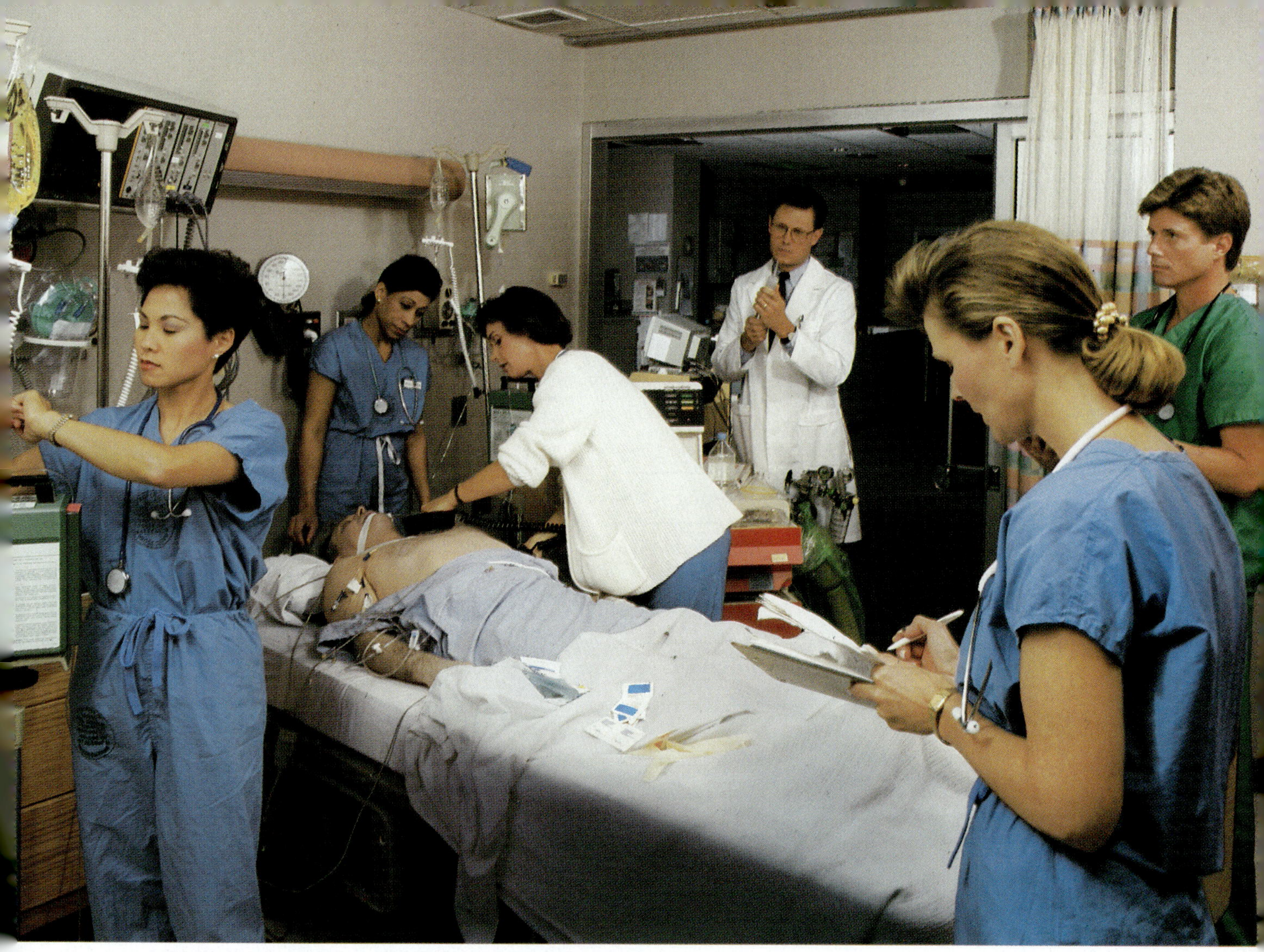

News

Conference attendees told ISIS-3 shows equal efficacy, safety differences among thrombolytics 486
William A. Check

Fludarabine approved for marketing 496

Enzyme replacement therapy approved for Gaucher's disease 496

News Briefs 498

Upcoming Specialty Meetings 498

Conference attendees told ISIS-3 shows equal efficacy, safety differences among thrombolytics

Probably the most important message of the Third International Study of Infarct Survival (ISIS-3), reported at the 40th Annual Scientific Session of the American College of Cardiology in March, is that cardiac mortality in the United States would be substantially reduced if many more patients having a myocardial infarction (MI) were treated within a few hours of the onset of chest pain with a thrombolytic agent plus aspirin. This is true of all three thrombolytics: streptokinase, tissue plasminogen activator (t-PA), and anistreplase. "Small differences in the safety of different thrombolytics are much less important than the large benefits of thrombolytics," trial organizers concluded.

Senior ISIS-3 investigator Peter Sleight, M.D., Professor of Cardiovascular Medicine at Oxford University, estimated that use of a thrombolytic agent plus aspirin can save 5 lives for every 100 patients treated, reducing the mortality rate to about 10%.

Jeffrey L. Anderson, M.D., Professor of Medicine at the University of Utah, agreed that the potential benefit of thrombolytic agents is more important than any differences among them. "If anything, thrombolysis is being underutilized [in the United States]," said Anderson. Thrombolysis is appropriate for 40–50% of MI patients but is used in only 20–25% of patients in the United States. "You can give any of the three agents and come out ahead," he stressed.

Moreover, a meta-analysis by ISIS-3 biostatistician Richard Peto, FRS, Co-Director of the Clinical Trials Service Unit at Oxford, suggested that the benefits of thrombolysis extend to groups of MI patients not now considered candidates for thrombolytic therapy.

But the drugs may not be equivalent in every respect. Results of ISIS-3 suggest that there is a slight but real increase in the incidence of strokes, particularly cerebral hemorrhage, with t-PA and anistreplase. ISIS-3 investigator Rory Collins, MBBS, Codirector of the Clinical Trials Service Unit at Oxford, noted that "the excess risk with t-PA does not appear to be balanced by any mortality gain at all."

Genentech, which markets t-PA (alteplase), found fault with the trial's design. The t-PA used in ISIS-3 was duteplase, a two-stranded form of t-PA made by Burroughs Wellcome, not Genentech's single-stranded t-PA, they objected. And, Genentech claimed, t-PA functions best with immediate intravenous administration of heparin, not administration of heparin subcutaneously at four hours, as it was given in ISIS-3. But ISIS investigators countered these arguments and stuck by their conclusions.

ISIS-3 enrolled 46,000 patients in 20 countries; 42,000 were randomized to receive one of the thrombolytics. All patients received aspirin (one-half tablet at the start of thrombolytic therapy, followed by one-half tablet daily for one month). Half of them received heparin, which was started at four hours and given subcutaneously at a dosage of 12,500 units twice daily for one week.

Five-week mortality figures were 10.3% for t-PA, 10.5% for streptokinase, and 10.6% for anistreplase. These trivial differences can be attributed to "the play of chance," said Peto.

Sleight noted that these mortality rates were higher than in the Thrombolysis in Myocardial Infarction (TIMI) trial, in which t-PA was used. But he noted that TIMI excluded patients over 70 years of age. In ISIS-3 there were 2500 older patients, and they had a mortality rate of

A significant excess of strokes in hospital was seen with t-PA (1.5%) and anistreplase (1.4%) compared with streptokinase (1.1%). This difference translates into 100 more strokes for t-PA for every 20,000 patients treated.

25%, much higher than the average.

Advanced age is not in itself a contraindication to thrombolysis, said Peto, based on the combined results of ISIS-3 and last year's Italian thrombolysis trial, GISSI-2, involving a total of 42,000 patients. Even patients over age 75 had a reduction in mortality proportional to that seen in younger patients. And, because baseline mortality is higher in older patients, the absolute number of lives saved by treating them is actually greater than from treating younger persons. Also, Peto said, patients who had an ECG showing bundle-branch block benefited at least as much from thrombolysis as those who had the traditional treatment indication, ST segment elevation.

It was in the area of cerebrovascular complications that differences among the three thrombolytic agents arose. A significant excess of strokes in hospital was seen with t-PA (1.5%) and anistreplase (1.4%), compared with streptokinase (1.1%). This difference translates into 100 more strokes for t-PA for every 20,000 patients treated.

Specifically, there was a significant excess of cerebral bleeds for t-PA (0.7%) and anistreplase (0.6%) compared with streptokinase (0.3%). Two thirds were confirmed by autopsy findings or by computed-tomography scans. Most of the excess was seen on day 1 or 2 after thrombolysis. Although small, the excess adds up to a significantly increased risk—3 to 4 cerebral bleeds per 1000 patients treated with t-PA or anistreplase.

Putting these data into perspective, Harvey White, FRACP, of Green Lane Hospital in Auckland, New Zealand, echoed Sleight's comments. The increase in bleeding is "dimensionally smaller than the reduction in mortality," he said; "the emphasis should be on giving treatment."

A double-edged effect was seen when patients who received heparin were compared with those who did not. Mortality in patients receiving heparin plus aspirin was slightly less than that in patients receiving aspirin alone (10% versus 10.5%), reported Collins. He called this "a very moderate effect." On the debit side, he noted that heparin added 2 cerebral bleeds for every 1000 patients, which he termed "a real hazard." On balance, Collins concluded, the data favor addition of this specific heparin regimen to aspirin therapy but do not extend to an earlier, more intensive intravenous heparin regimen.

In fact, Sleight suggested, "Most American physicians ought seriously to re-examine" the use of early, high-dose intravenous heparin, because it might be dangerous.

But one prominent American cardiologist was not convinced. "I still believe that if you're not using intravenous heparin with t-PA, you don't maximize the results," said Robert Roberts, M.D., Chief of Cardiology at Baylor College of Medicine. Roberts cited the TIMI results, in which t-PA plus early, high-dose intravenous heparin produced a higher 90-minute coronary artery patency rate than did streptokinase.

"It's not patency you're after, it's being alive and not having a disabling stroke," countered Sleight. In his view, emphasis on 90-minute patency rates is misplaced. He pointed out that by 18 hours all agents open the same fraction of arteries. That, he believes, is why mortality rates are the same with streptokinase and t-PA.

And Collins pointed to a subgroup of 3000 patients in ISIS-3 whose physicians chose to give them immediate intravenous heparin. Among these patients there was no difference in mortality between t-PA and streptokinase. But there was a "disturbing doubling of the stroke risk" relative to patients receiving subcutaneous heparin, said Collins.

Responding to Genentech's objection that results of ISIS-3 do not apply to alteplase, since duteplase was the form of t-PA used, Sleight noted that duteplase produced 90-minute patency rates that are similar to those

On balance, Collins concluded, the data favor addition of this specific heparin regimen to aspirin therapy but do not extend to an earlier, more intensive intravenous heparin regimen.

produced by alteplase in clinical trials in which it was used at the doses employed in ISIS-3.

One point on which virtually everyone agrees is that all MI patients without explicit contraindications should receive aspirin starting immediately upon admission. Most evidence favors a dosage of 160 mg/day. "Aspirin should be given at acute MI, which is not the case in the U.S. today," said Charles H. Hennekens, M.D., Associate Professor of Medicine at Harvard Medical School. In trials in which aspirin was added to streptokinase or t-PA, Dr. Hennekens said, "more lives were saved with aspirin than with thrombolytics."

Some estimates of aspirin use in American MI patients

Continued on page 496

Gammagard®
Immune Globulin Intravenous (Human)

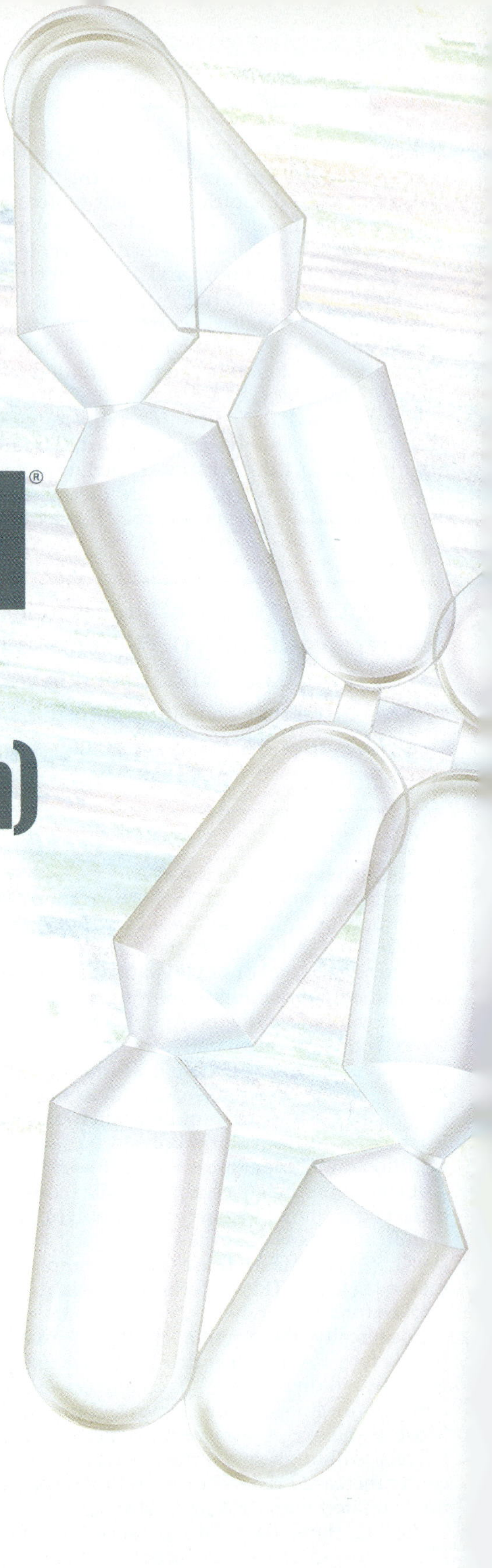

EXOSURF® Neonatal™

(COLFOSCERIL PALMITATE, CETYL ALCOHOL, TYLOXAPOL)

For Intratracheal Suspension / 10 mL vials

PLEASE CONSULT FULL PRODUCT INFORMATION BEFORE PRESCRIBING.

INDICATIONS AND USAGE: Exosurf Neonatal is indicated for:

1. **Prophylactic** treatment of infants with birth weights of less than 1350 grams who are at risk of developing RDS (see PRECAUTIONS),
2. **Prophylactic** treatment of infants with birth weights greater than 1350 grams who have evidence of pulmonary immaturity, and
3. **Rescue** treatment of infants who have developed RDS.

CONTRAINDICATIONS: There are no known contraindications to treatment with Exosurf Neonatal.

WARNINGS: Intratracheal Administration Only: Exosurf Neonatal should be administered only by instillation into the trachea. **General:** The use of Exosurf Neonatal requires expert clinical care by experienced neonatologists and other clinicians who are accomplished at neonatal intubation and ventilatory management. Adequate personnel, facilities, equipment, and medications are required to optimize perinatal outcome in premature infants. Instillation of Exosurf Neonatal should be performed **only** by trained medical personnel experienced in airway and clinical management of unstable premature infants. Vigilant clinical attention should be given to all infants prior to, during, and after administration of Exosurf Neonatal. **Acute Effects:** Exosurf Neonatal can rapidly affect oxygenation and lung compliance. **Lung Compliance:** If chest expansion improves substantially after dosing, peak ventilator inspiratory pressures should be reduced immediately, without waiting for confirmation of respiratory improvement by blood gas assessment. Failure to reduce inspiratory ventilator pressures rapidly in such instances can result in lung overdistention and fatal pulmonary air leak. **Hyperoxia:** If the infant becomes pink and transcutaneous oxygen saturation is in excess of 95%, FiO_2 should be reduced in small but repeated steps (until saturation is 90 to 95%) without waiting for confirmation of elevated arterial pO_2 by blood gas assessment. Failure to reduce FiO_2 in such instances can result in hyperoxia. **Hypocarbia:** If arterial or transcutaneous CO_2 measurements are <30 torr, the ventilator rate should be reduced at once. Failure to reduce ventilator rates in such instances can result in marked hypocarbia, which is known to reduce brain blood flow. **Pulmonary Hemorrhage:** In the single study conducted in infants weighing <700 grams at birth, the incidence of pulmonary hemorrhage (10% vs 2% in the placebo group) was significantly increased in the Exosurf Neonatal group. None of the five studies involving infants with birth weights >700 grams showed a significant increase in pulmonary hemorrhage in the Exosurf Neonatal group. In a cross-study analysis of these five studies, pulmonary hemorrhage was reported for 1% (14/1420) of infants in the placebo group and 2% (27/1411) of infants in the Exosurf Neonatal group. Fatal pulmonary hemorrhage occurred in three infants; two in the Exosurf Neonatal group and one in the placebo group. Mortality from all causes among infants who developed pulmonary hemorrhage was 43% in the placebo group and 37% in the Exosurf Neonatal group. Pulmonary hemorrhage in both Exosurf Neonatal and placebo infants was more frequent in infants who were younger, smaller, male, or who had a patent ductus arteriosus. Pulmonary hemorrhage typically occurred in the first 2 days of life in both treatment groups. In more than 7700 infants in the open, uncontrolled study, pulmonary hemorrhage was reported in 4%, but fatal pulmonary hemorrhage was reported rarely (0.4%). In the controlled clinical studies, Exosurf Neonatal treated infants who received steroids more than 24 hours prior to delivery or indomethacin postnatally had a lower rate of pulmonary hemorrhage than other Exosurf Neonatal treated infants. Attention should be paid to early and aggressive diagnosis and treatment (unless contraindicated) of patent ductus arteriosus during the first 2 days of life (while the ductus arteriosus is often clinically silent). Other potentially protective measures include attempting to decrease FiO_2 preferentially over ventilator pressures during the first 24 to 48 hours after dosing, and attempting to decrease PEEP minimally for at least 48 hours after dosing. **Mucous Plugs:** Infants whose ventilation becomes markedly impaired during or shortly after dosing may have mucous plugging of the endotracheal tube, particularly if pulmonary secretions were prominent prior to drug administration. Suctioning of all infants prior to dosing may lessen the chance of mucous plugs obstructing the endotracheal tube. If endotracheal tube obstruction from such plugs is suspected, and suctioning is unsuccessful in removing the obstruction, the blocked endotracheal tube should be replaced immediately.

PRECAUTIONS:

General: In the controlled clinical studies, infants known prenatally or postnatally to have major congenital anomalies, or who were suspected of having congenital infection, were excluded from entry. However, these disorders cannot be recognized early in life in all cases, and a few infants with these conditions were entered. The benefits of Exosurf Neonatal in the affected infants who received drug appeared to be similar to the benefits observed in infants without anomalies or occult infection. **Prophylactic Treatment-Infants <700 Grams:** In infants weighing 500 to 700 grams, a single prophylactic dose of Exosurf Neonatal significantly: improved FiO_2 and ventilator settings, reduced pneumothorax, and reduced death from RDS, but increased pulmonary hemorrhage (see WARNINGS). Overall mortality did not differ significantly between the placebo and Exosurf Neonatal groups (see Table 1 in full product information). Data on multiple doses in infants in this weight class are not yet available. Accordingly, clinicians should carefully evaluate the potential risks and benefits of Exosurf Neonatal administration in these infants. **Rescue Treatment-Number of Doses:** A small number of infants with RDS have received more than two doses of Exosurf Neonatal as rescue treatment. Definitive data on the safety and efficacy of these additional doses are not available. **Carcinogenesis, Mutagenesis, Impairment of Fertility:** Exosurf Neonatal at concentrations up to 10,000 μg/plate was not mutagenic in the Ames Salmonella assay. Long-term studies have not been performed in animals to evaluate the carcinogenic potential of Exosurf Neonatal. The effects of Exosurf Neonatal on fertility have not been studied.

ADVERSE REACTIONS:

General: Premature birth is associated with a high incidence of morbidity and mortality. Despite significant reductions in overall mortality associated with Exosurf Neonatal, some infants who received Exosurf Neonatal developed severe complications and either survived with permanent handicaps or died.

In controlled clinical studies evaluating the safety and efficacy of Exosurf Neonatal, numerous safety assessments were made. In infants receiving Exosurf Neonatal, pulmonary hemorrhage, apnea and use of methylxanthines were increased. A number of other adverse events were significantly reduced in the Exosurf Neonatal group, particularly various forms of pulmonary air leak and use of pancuronium. Tables 3 and 4 summarize the results of the major safety evaluations from the controlled clinical studies.

Table 3: Safety Assessments[a]—Prophylactic Treatment

Number of Doses:	Single Dose		Single Dose		Single Dose		1 vs 3 Doses	
Birth Weight Range:	500 to 700 grams		700 to 1350 grams		700 to 1100 grams		700 to 1100 grams	
Treatment Group:	Placebo (Air)	EXOSURF	Placebo (Air)	EXOSURF	Placebo (Air)	EXOSURF	EXOSURF 1 Dose	EXOSURF 3 Doses
Number of Infants:	N=108	N=107	N=193	N=192	N=222	N=224	N=356	N=360
	% of Infants		% of Infants		% of Infants		% of Infants	
Intraventricular Hemorrhage (IVH)								
Overall	51	57	31	27	36	36	38	35
Severe IVH	26	25	10	8	13	14	9	9
Pulmonary Air Leak (PAL)								
Overall	52	48	16	11	32	25	29	27
Pneumothorax	23	10*	5	6	19	11*	14	12
Pneumopericardium	1	4	2	0	<1	1	1	1
Pneumomediastinum	2	1	2	3	7	1**	3	2
Pulmonary Interstitial Emphysema	43	44	13	7*	26	20	23	22
Death from PAL	4	6	<1	<1	2	1	2	1
Patent Ductus Arteriosus	49	53	66	70	50	55	59	57
Necrotizing Enterocolitis	2	4	11	13	3	4	6	2*
Pulmonary Hemorrhage	2	10**	2	4	1	4	4	6
Congenital Pneumonia	4	4	2	4	2	2	1	1
Nosocomial Pneumonia	10	10	2	4	4	7	14	15
Non-Pulmonary Infections	33	35	34	39	28	29	35	34
Sepsis	30	34	30	34	23	24	30	27
Death From Sepsis	4	4	3	3	1	2	3	2
Meningitis	4	6	3	1	2	3	1	2
Other Infections	7	4	5	3	6	10	10	11
Major Anomalies	3	1	2	4	7	4	4	4

Table 3: Safety Assessments[a]—Prophylactic Treatment (Cont.)

Number of Doses:	Single Dose		Single Dose		Single Dose		1 vs 3 Doses	
Birth Weight Range:	500 to 700 grams		700 to 1350 grams		700 to 1100 grams		700 to 1100 grams	
Treatment Group:	Placebo (Air)	EXOSURF	Placebo (Air)	EXOSURF	Placebo (Air)	EXOSURF	EXOSURF 1 Dose	EXOSURF 3 Doses
Number of Infants:	N=108	N=107	N=193	N=192	N=222	N=224	N=356	N=360
	% of Infants		% of Infants		% of Infants		% of Infants	
Hypotension	70	77	52	47	59	62	54	50
Hyperbilirubinemia	22	21	63	61	27	31	20	21
Exchange Transfusion	4	3	1	2	2	2	3	1
Thrombocytopenia[b]	21	25	not available		9	8	12	10
Persistent Fetal Circulation	0	1	1	1	0	2*	1	<1
Seizures	11	8	2	2	11	9	6	5
Apnea	34	33	76	73	55	65*	62	68
Drug Therapy								
Antibiotics	96	99	98	96	98	99	>99	99
Diuretics	55	60	39	37	59	63	64	65
Anticonvulsants	14	18	23	24	20	16	9	8
Inotropes	46	40	20	20	26	20	28	27
Sedatives	62	71	65	64	63	57	52	52
Pancuronium	19	11	22	14*	19	13*	15	11
Methylxanthines	38	43	77	77	61	72*	75	82*

[a] All parameters were examined with "as-treated" analyses.
[b] Thrombocytopenia requiring platelet transfusion.
* $p<0.05$
** $p<0.01$

Table 4: Safety Assessments[a]—Rescue Treatment

Number of Doses:	Two Doses		Two Doses	
Birth Weight Range:	700 to 1350 grams		1250 grams and above	
Treatment Group:	Placebo (Air)	EXOSURF	Placebo (Air)	EXOSURF
Number of Infants:	N=213	N=206	N=622	N=615
	% of Infants		% of Infants	
Intraventricular Hemorrhage (IVH)				
Overall	48	52	23	18*
Severe IVH	13	9	5	4
Pulmonary Air Leak (PAL)				
Overall	54	34***	30	18***
Pneumothorax	29	20*	20	10***
Pneumopericardium	4	1	1	2
Pneumomediastinum	8	4	5	2**
Pulmonary Interstitial Emphysema	48	25***	24	13***
Death from PAL	7	3	<1	1
Patent Ductus Arteriosus	66	57	54	45*
Necrotizing Enterocolitis	3	3	1	2
Pulmonary Hemorrhage	3	1	<1	1
Congenital Pneumonia	2	3	2	2
Nosocomial Pneumonia	5	7	2	2
Non-Pulmonary Infections	19	22	13	13
Sepsis	15	17	8	8
Death From Sepsis	<1	<1	1	<1
Meningitis	1	<1	1	<1*
Other Infections	5	8	5	6
Major Anomalies	3	3	4	4
Hypotension	62	57	50	39**
Hyperbilirubinemia	17	19	12	10
Exchange Transfusion	3	4	1	2
Thrombocytopenia[b]	10	11	4	<1**
Persistent Fetal Circulation	1	1	6	2**
Seizures	10	10	6	3*
Apnea	48	65**	37	44*
Drug Therapy				
Antibiotics	100	99	98	98
Diuretics	60	65	45	34***
Anticonvulsants	17	17	10	5**
Inotropes	36	31	27	16***
Sedatives	72	68	76	64***
Pancuronium	34	17**	33	15***
Methylxanthines	62	74**	49	53

[a] All parameters were examined with "as-treated" analyses.
[b] Thrombocytopenia requiring platelet transfusion.
* $p<0.05$
** $p<0.01$
*** $p<0.001$

Pulmonary Hemorrhage: See WARNINGS. **Abnormal Laboratory Values:** Abnormal laboratory values are common in critically ill, mechanically ventilated, premature infants. A higher incidence of abnormal laboratory values in the Exosurf Neonatal group was not reported. **Events During Dosing:** Data on events during dosing are available from more than 8800 infants in the open, uncontrolled clinical study (Table 5).

Table 5: Events During Dosing in the Open, Uncontrolled Study[a]

Treatment Type:	Prophylactic Treatment	Rescue Treatment
Number of Infants:	N=1127	N=7711
	% of Infants	% of Infants
Reflux of Exosurf	20	31
Drop in O_2 saturation ($\geq 20\%$)	6	22
Rise in O_2 saturation ($\geq 10\%$)	5	6
Drop in transcutaneous pO_2 (≥ 20 mm Hg)	1	8
Rise in transcutaneous pO_2 (≥ 20 mm Hg)	2	5
Drop in transcutaneous pCO_2 (≥ 20 mm Hg)	<1	1
Rise in transcutaneous pCO_2 (≥ 20 mm Hg)	1	3
Bradycardia (<60 beats/min)	1	3
Tachycardia (>200 beats/min)	<1	<1
Gagging	1	5
Mucous Plugs	<1	<1

[a] Infants may have experienced more than one event.
Investigators were prohibited from adjusting FiO_2 and/or ventilator settings during dosing unless significant clinical deterioration occurred.

Reflux: Reflux of Exosurf Neonatal into the endotracheal tube during dosing has been observed and may be associated with rapid drug administration. If reflux occurs, drug administration should be halted and, if necessary, peak inspiratory pressure on the ventilator should be increased by 4 to 5 cm H_2O until the endotracheal tube clears. ***>20% Drop in Transcutaneous Oxygen Saturation:*** If transcutaneous oxygen saturation declines during dosing, drug administration should be halted and, if necessary, peak inspiratory pressure on the ventilator should be increased by 4 to 5 cm H_2O for 1 to 2 minutes. In addition, increases of FiO_2 may be required for 1 to 2 minutes. ***Mucous Plugs:*** See WARNINGS.

DOSAGE AND ADMINISTRATION: See full product information.

Wellcome
BURROUGHS WELLCOME CO., Research Triangle Park, NC 27709

Printed in U.S.A. EX-Y01228

Continued from page 487

are as low as 20%. Why don't all physicians give aspirin at the time of an MI? "Aspirin is too cheap," Peto suggested, only half-facetiously.

At a symposium on thrombolysis during the ACC meeting, panelists were asked which thrombolytic agent they now favor, based on results of clinical trials to date. "All of them are probably equal," said Anderson. He cited three criteria for distinguishing the drugs: cost, where there are already "clear differences"; safety, which is "beginning to become more interesting"; and convenience, which he called "the major advantage for anistreplase." (Anistreplase is given as a rapid 5- to 10-minute injection, rather than a one- to three-hour infusion, as are streptokinase and t-PA. For this reason it appears promising for use in outpatient settings, such as in ambulances.)

White responded, "I use streptokinase as the cheapest drug. [Anistreplase] has the advantage of convenience and getting the drug in as quickly as possible. t-PA is very expensive and there is a question of cerebral bleeds that comes up again and again." (Approximate U.S. costs per dose are $220 for streptokinase, $1700 for anistreplase, and $2200 for alteplase.)

One point on which virtually everyone agrees is that all MI patients without explicit contraindications should receive aspirin starting immediately upon admission.

Elliot Rapaport, M.D., Chief of the Cardiology Division at San Francisco General Hospital, also emphasized the cost differential. "Clearly there is a distinct cost advantage to using streptokinase, and we take advantage of that," he said.

Summarizing the current state of knowledge, Sleight pointed out that ISIS-3 and GISSI-2 yielded very similar results. In both large international trials there was no mortality difference between streptokinase and t-PA and there was a slight but significant excess of cerebral bleeds with t-PA. "I hope that the combination of these two massive studies is going to change practice," Sleight concluded. But, in Roberts's opinion, "I suspect it won't change anything. American doctors will wait for the results of American studies first."

An American study is now getting under way. Called GUSTO (Global Utilization of Streptokinase and t-PA in Occluded Coronary Arteries) and sponsored by Genentech, it will enroll 33,000 patients. Subjects will receive either alteplase 100 mg given over 90 minutes or streptokinase 1.5 million units infused over 60 minutes. All patients will receive an immediate 5000-unit intravenous bolus dose of heparin followed by 1000 units/hour for 24 hours. All will also receive aspirin. A unique feature of this trial is that a third group of patients will receive a combined regimen of alteplase and streptokinase. The primary endpoints of GUSTO will be 30-day and one-year mortality.

GUSTO will certainly not settle all questions. For instance, it will not show whether immediate administration of heparin provides a better outcome with t-PA than administration of heparin at four hours. Nor can it prove which is the most effective thrombolytic agent, since anistreplase is not included. All that is certain, White predicts, is that, "Whatever is the best regimen in GUSTO, we will still need another trial."

William A. Check
Clinical Pharmacy Correspondent

Fludarabine approved for marketing

Fludarabine phosphate (Fludara, Berlex Laboratories, Inc.) was granted marketing approval in April for use in patients with B-cell chronic lymphocytic leukemia (CLL) who have not responded to or have had disease progression during standard therapy. Fludarabine has been available to patients with refractory or relapsed CLL since 1989 under the National Cancer Institute's Group C compassionate-use program. The drug was granted orphan status in 1988.

Fludarabine is a fluorinated nucleotide analogue of vidarabine. Within minutes after intravenous administration, fludarabine is converted to the active metabolite 2-fluoro-vidarabine.

Complete response rates of 13% were reported for two open-label studies of fludarabine in patients with CLL refractory to at least one standard drug regimen; partial response rates for these two studies were 35% (M. D. Anderson Cancer Center study) and 19% (Southwest Oncology Group study). The median duration of disease control was 91 weeks and 65 weeks, respectively. The median survival of all patients treated with fludarabine was 43 weeks and 52 weeks, respectively.

The most common adverse events associated with fludarabine therapy are myelosuppression (neutropenia, thrombocytopenia, and anemia), fever and chills, infection, and nausea and vomiting. Severe neurologic toxicity has been reported rarely in patients receiving fludarabine at recommended dosages.

The recommended dosage of fludarabine phosphate is 25 mg/sq m, given as a 30-minute intravenous infusion daily for five days. Courses should be repeated every 28 days. The optimal duration of therapy has not been established. Administration of three additional cycles of therapy after maximal response has been achieved is recommended.

Fludara is supplied as a lyophilized solid cake containing 50 mg of fludarabine phosphate; the product is packaged in single-vial cartons in packages of five.

Enzyme replacement therapy approved for Gaucher's disease

FDA has approved marketing of alglucerase (Ceredase, Genzyme Corporation) for the treatment of Gaucher's disease, a genetic condition characterized by a deficiency of β-glucocerebrosidase, an enzyme required for degradation of the glycolipid glucocerebroside. Alglucerase is indicated for long-term enzyme replace-

Continued on page 498

Continued from page 496

ment therapy in patients with type I Gaucher's disease who have symptoms resulting from moderate to severe anemia, thrombocytopenia, bone disease, or enlargement of the spleen or liver.

Alglucerase is a modified form of the human enzyme. The product is prepared from pooled human tissue. The product was designated an orphan product and has been available to patients through a treatment IND program.

News Briefs

- Labeled indications for **intravenous immune globulin** (Gammar IV, Armour Pharmaceutical Company) have been expanded to include use in patients with defective antibody synthesis, usually associated with primary immune deficiency.

- Free single copies of the report of the **NIH Consensus Development Conference on Diagnosis and Management of Asymptomatic Primary Hyperparathyroidism** can be obtained from William H. Hall, Director of Communications, Office of Medical Applications of Research, National Institutes of Health, Building 1, Room 259, Bethesda, MD 20892 (301-496-1143).

- Copies of the 1991 report of **"New Medicines in Development for Arthritis"** can be obtained by writing to Editor, New Medicines in Development for Arthritis, Pharmaceutical Manufacturers Association, 1100 15th Street, N.W., Washington, DC 20005. The report lists drugs that are being developed for treatment of gout, juvenile rheumatoid arthritis, lupus, osteoarthritis, osteoporosis, Paget's disease, rheumatoid arthritis, scleroderma, and spondylitis. For each drug, the manufacturer, indication, and stage of development are listed. The information is based on PMA-sponsored surveys of government and industry sources.

- A report analyzing the morbidity and mortality among patients receiving encainide, flecainide, or placebo in the **Cardiac Arrhythmia Suppression Trial** (CAST) was published in the March 21, 1991, issue of the *New England Journal of Medicine.*

- *Immunology and Allergy Practice* has announced a contest, sponsored by Janssen Pharmaceutica, for **case reports related to allergy, clinical immunology, obstructive pulmonary disorders, or related ear, nose, and throat problems.** A $400 prize will be awarded for the best paper in each of the following categories: a physician in private practice; a physician in academia; a physician in training; and nurses, paramedical personnel, and persons with Ph.D. or Pharm.D. degrees. An original and two copies of the paper, along with a note indicating the category of the submission, should be submitted to Gerald L. Klein, M.D., Associate Editor, *Immunology and Allergy Practice*, 2067 West Vista Way, Suite 140, Vista, CA 92083. The deadline for submissions is December 31, 1991.

Upcoming Specialty Meetings

American Society for Pharmacology and Experimental Therapeutics. San Diego, CA, August 16–20. Contact ASPET, 9650 Rockville Pike, Bethesda, MD 20814; 301-530-7060.

American Academy of Pain Management. Baltimore, MD, August 29–September 1. Contact AAPM, 3600 Sisk Road, Suite 2-D, Modesto, CA 95356; 209-545-0754.

American Academy of Family Physicians. Washington, DC, September 26–29. Contact R. Graham, M.D., 8880 Ward Parkway, Kansas City, MO 64114; 816-333-9700.

American Society for Microbiology. Chicago, IL, September 29–October 2. Contact ASM, 1325 Massachusetts Avenue, N.W., Washington, DC 20005; 202-737-3600.

Cancer Symposium (15th). Sponsored by the Scripps Memorial Hospital Cancer Center. San Diego, CA, October 3–5. Contact Meeting Management, Cancer Symposium, 5665 Oberlin Drive, Suite 110, San Diego, CA 92121.

Child Neurology Society. Portland, OR, October 3–5. Contact M. E. Currey, 475 Cleveland Avenue North, Suite 275, St. Paul, MN 55104; 612-641-1584.

American College of Emergency Physicians. Boston, MA, October 7–10. Contact J. C. Johnson, M.D., ACEP, P.O. Box 619911, Dallas, TX 75261.

American Society of Internal Medicine. Washington, DC, October 9–13. Contact ASIM, 1101 Vermont Avenue, N.W., Suite 500, Washington, DC 20005; 202-289-1700.

American College of Nutrition. Clearwater Beach, FL, October 11–14. Contact M. S. Seelig, M.D., M.P.H., 722 Robert E. Lee Drive, Wilmington, NC 28412; 919-452-1222.

American College of Clinical Pharmacology. Atlanta, GA, October 14–16. Contact J. M. Bertolet, 175 Strafford Avenue, Suite 1, Wayne, PA 18087; 215-687-7711.

American Academy of Child and Adolescent Psychiatry. San Francisco, CA, October 16–20. Contact AACAP, 3615 Wisconsin Avenue, N.W., Washington, DC 20016; 202-966-7300.

Letters

Labetalol for treatment of hypertension in a child 500
Denis Y. Ishisaka, Charles D. Yonan, Ben F. Housel

Antimicrobial dosages in guidelines for prevention of bacterial endocarditis 501
Julie McMorrow, Paul R. Jones, Milap C. Nahata

Correction 501

The Letters *column is a forum for rapid exchange of ideas among readers of* Clinical Pharmacy. *Liberal criteria are applied in the review of submissions to encourage contributions to this column.*

The Letters *column includes the following types of contributions: (1) comments, addenda, and minor updates on previously published work, (2) alerts on potential problems related to drug therapy or clinical research, (3) observations or comments on trends in drug therapy or clinical research, and (4) brief expressions of opinion about controversies in drug therapy or clinical research.*

Letters need not be submitted with the journal's manuscript checklist. The following conditions, however, must be adhered to: (1) the body of the letter must be no longer than two typewritten pages, (2) the use of references, tables, and illustrations should be minimized, (3) the authors' names, affiliations, and mailing addresses must be typed at the end of the letter in the format used by Clinical Pharmacy, *and (4) the entire letter (including references, tables, and authors' names) must be typed double-spaced on plain white paper (not letterhead). Following acceptance of a letter, the authors are required to sign an exclusive publication statement and a copyright transferal form.*

Labetalol for treatment of hypertension in a child

There is little documentation of the use of labetalol for the treatment of hypertension in children. We report the successful use of this drug in a child with renal-artery stenosis.

A five-year-old, 28-kg boy was found to have a blood pressure (BP) of 150/120 mm Hg during a school physical examination; his hypertension was subsequently determined to be caused by renal-artery stenosis. Balloon angioplasty of the stenosis was performed four months after diagnosis, but there was no change in BP. While the patient was taking propranolol hydrochloride 10 mg and hydralazine hydrochloride 25 mg t.i.d. p.o., his systolic and diastolic BPs were 116–130 and 70–80 mm Hg, respectively, and his pulse dropped below 60 beats/min at times. The propranolol dosage was not increased because of the bradycardic episodes and adverse effects—predominantly fatigue and gastrointestinal upset—attributed to the drug. The child was hospitalized to have captopril therapy started. On admission, his BP was 130/77 mm Hg, and his pulse was 86 beats/min.

The starting dosage of oral captopril was 7 mg q.i.d., given as a solution. The dosage was gradually increased as long as the systolic BP was >110 mm Hg; the maximum dosage given was 50 mg t.i.d. (as tablets). Hydralazine and propranolol were withheld while the child's response to the first captopril dose was observed. Administration of hydralazine hydrochloride was resumed, and the dosage reached 40 mg t.i.d. p.o. Oral propranolol hydrochloride therapy was also resumed at the previous dosage of 10 mg t.i.d. and was gradually withdrawn over two days. The goal of therapy (systolic BP <110 mm Hg, diastolic BP 70–80 mm Hg, pulse 80–100 beats/min) was not achieved with captopril and hydralazine (systolic BP >100 mm Hg, diastolic BP 80 mm Hg, pulse >100 beats/min).

Oral labetalol hydrochloride therapy was started with 500 mg given on the first day (200 mg, then 150 mg 8 and 16 hours later); the BP fell to an average of 92/42 mm Hg, and the pulse was 90–100 beats/min. On day 2 of labetalol therapy, hydralazine was withdrawn. On the same day, the patient started having episodes of emesis, which prompted reduction of labetalol dosage to 150 mg p.o. every eight hours. Although the emesis, which lasted until day 5 of labetalol therapy, was initially thought to be induced by labetalol, it was later attributed to viral gastroenteritis. The child was discharged from the hospital taking oral captopril 50 mg and labetalol hydrochloride 150 mg t.i.d. One week after discharge, the BP was 108/80 mm Hg, and the pulse was 84 beats/min. No adverse drug effects were noted.

We based this patient's initial labetalol dosage on an

abstract by Jureidini,[1] who used labetalol in six 4- to 14-year-old children with pheochromocytoma or renal hypertension who had not been successfully treated with other β–adrenergic blockers and hydralazine (with or without diuretics). The initial labetalol hydrochloride dosage was 20 mg/kg/day in three or four daily doses and was increased as needed to 40 mg/kg/day. Labetalol was effective in three children; two required only labetalol and diuretic therapy to achieve a normal BP. The only reported adverse effect was mild scalp tingling in one child. In another report, an eight-year-old child received labetalol, but the response of this patient was not specifically reported.[2] Mueller and Solhaug[3] described the use of labetalol in pediatric hypertensive emergencies. Constant i.v. infusions of labetalol hydrochloride (0.4–1.5 mg/kg/hr) were used for 8–38 hours and reduced BP in two patients without producing adverse effects. In two other patients, intermittent i.v. bolus doses of 0.3–0.6 mg/kg controlled BP without causing adverse effects.

We used labetalol hoping that it would not produce adverse effects similar to those attributed in this patient to propranolol. Labetalol was more tolerable and at least as effective as propranolol. Further studies are needed to define the optimal use of labetalol in children.

1. Jureidini K. Oral labetalol in a child with phaeochromocytoma and five children with renal hypertension. *Aust N Z J Med.* 1980; 10:479. Abstract.
2. New Zealand Hypertension Study Group. A multi-centre study of labetalol in hypertension. *N Z Med J.* 1981; 93:215-8.
3. Mueller JB, Solhaug MJ. Labetalol in pediatric hypertensive emergencies. *Pediatr Res.* 1988; 23:543A. Abstract.

Denis Y. Ishisaka, Pharm.D., Clinical Pharmacist in Pediatrics
University of California, Davis Medical Center
2315 Stockton Boulevard
Sacramento, CA 95817

Charles D. Yonan, Pharm.D. Degree Candidate
University of California, San Francisco School of Pharmacy

Ben F. Housel, M.D.
Department of Emergency Medicine
University of California, Davis Medical Center

Antimicrobial dosages in guidelines for prevention of bacterial endocarditis

The updated American Heart Association (AHA) guidelines for the prevention of bacterial endocarditis,[1] summarized in the March issue of *Clinical Pharmacy,*[2] reflect an increased recognition of factors that affect antimicrobial pharmacokinetics and patient compliance. We offer the following thoughts, some of which we have expressed elsewhere,[3,4] on the recommended dosage and administration of the erythromycins and of vancomycin.

The doses of erythromycin ethylsuccinate and erythromycin stearate recommended for penicillin-allergic patients appear not to be therapeutically equivalent.[3] AHA recommends an initial adult erythromycin dose of 800 mg when the ethylsuccinate ester is used or 1 g when the stearate salt is used. However, when the ethylsuccinate ester is used, erythromycin 1.6 g is more likely than 800 mg to produce serum erythromycin concentrations similar to those achieved with 1 g of erythromycin as stearate.[5] Similarly, an initial pediatric erythromycin dose of 30 mg/kg (as ethylsuccinate) is more likely than the AHA-recommended 20 mg/kg (as ethylsuccinate) to produce concentrations similar to those achieved with the recommended 20-mg/kg dose of erythromycin as stearate. If the erythromycin ethylsuccinate doses recommended by AHA are considered adequate for prophylaxis, perhaps the erythromycin stearate doses should be reduced accordingly. Erythromycin estolate and enteric-coated-pellet formulations of erythromycin base—in dosages similar to those specified for the stearate salt—may also be suitable for prevention of endocarditis.[3]

AHA recommends giving i.v. vancomycin over one hour to adults and suggests an initial pediatric dose of 20 mg/kg (as hydrochloride). These statements could be interpreted as recommending that vancomycin be infused at 20 mg/kg/hr in children. It may be more appropriate to extend the infusion duration to 1.5–2 hours (a rate of 10–13 mg/kg/hr) for the initial pediatric dose.[4,6] The one-hour infusion duration, however, is suitable for the subsequent recommended pediatric dose of 10 mg/kg.

1. Dajani AS, Bisno AL, Chung KJ et al. Prevention of bacterial endocarditis: recommendations by the American Heart Association. *JAMA.* 1990; 264:2919-22.
2. Anon. New recommendations for prevention of bacterial endocarditis include amoxicillin use. *Clin Pharm.* 1991; 10:168,175. News.
3. McMorrow J, Nahata MC. Prevention of bacterial endocarditis. *JAMA.* 1991; 265:1687-8. Letter.
4. McMorrow J, Nahata MC. Prevention and management of bacterial endocarditis. *J Pharm Pract.* 1991; 4:(in press).
5. AHFS drug information 90. McEvoy GK, ed. Erythromycins. Bethesda, MD: American Society of Hospital Pharmacists; 1990:178-83.
6. Nelson JD. 1991–1992 Pocketbook of pediatric antimicrobial therapy. 9th ed. Baltimore, MD: Williams & Wilkins; 1991.

Julie McMorrow, Pharm.D., ASHP Fellow in Critical Care Drug Therapy

Paul R. Jones, Clinical Pharmacist

Milap C. Nahata, Pharm.D., Professor of Pharmacy and Pediatrics
Colleges of Pharmacy and Medicine

The Ohio State University
500 West 12th Avenue
Columbus, OH 43210

Correction

Current issues in the treatment of epilepsy (May 1991, Therapy Review). On page 339, the recommended concentration of phenytoin in 0.9% sodium chloride injection is 6.6 mg/mL or less.

Therapy Reviews

Therapy of acute thromboembolism with heparin and warfarin

BARRY L. CARTER

Abstract: The indications, efficacy, dosage, administration, and monitoring of heparin and warfarin therapy for acute thromboembolic events are reviewed, with emphasis on recent changes in treatment recommendations.

High-dose heparin therapy is indicated for acute deep-vein thrombosis and pulmonary embolism. Heparin therapy as an adjunct to thrombolytic agents for acute myocardial infarction is becoming increasingly accepted. Heparin therapy for acute thromboembolic events consists of a dosage that elevates the activated partial thromboplastin time to 1.5 to 2.0 times the control value; formerly, 1.5 to 2.5 times control was considered therapeutic. The recommended heparin dosage is a bolus dose of 70–100 units/kg followed by an infusion of 15–25 units/kg/hr. To prevent recurrent thromboembolism, most patients require long-term therapy following acute treatment; this typically consists of warfarin, which should be initiated on day 1 or 2 of heparin therapy whenever possible. For most indications, the intensity of warfarin has been reduced to a dosage that elevates the prothrombin time to 1.3 to 1.5 times control. Alternative therapies (low-molecular-weight heparins) and routes (subcutaneous heparin) should be further investigated.

Current recommendations for heparin and warfarin therapy of acute thromboembolism include reduced intensity of both drugs and shortened duration of therapy. Since the therapeutic ranges for both heparin and warfarin therapy have been compressed, closer monitoring may be necessary to achieve and maintain adequate anticoagulation.

Index terms: Anticoagulants; Dosage; Heparin; Protocols; Thromboembolism; Warfarin
Clin Pharm. 1991; 10:503-18

Guidelines for the use of anticoagulants have evolved rapidly in recent years. Carter, Jones, and Waickman[1] reviewed anticoagulation for pulmonary embolism (PE) and deep-vein thrombosis (DVT) in *Clinical Pharmacy* in 1985. Since then, consensus conferences on anticoagulation and prevention of venous thrombosis and pulmonary embolism have been convened by the American College of Chest Physicians and the National Heart, Lung, and Blood Institute.[2-4] The purpose of this paper is to provide an update on the therapeutic use of heparin and warfarin for acute thromboembolism. This review will not consider controversial therapy, such as the use of heparin for unstable angina, transient ischemic attacks, or strokes; for these indications, aspirin is generally preferred over anticoagulants. Pathophysiology and diagnostic issues that have been covered in other publications[1,5-10] will not be discussed here.

Heparin Pharmacology

Heparin is composed of sulfated mucopolysaccharide polymers with various molecular weights, charges, and primary sugar sequences.[11] This heterogeneity can result in differences in physical properties among different manufacturers' products or lots.

Heparin catalyzes the reaction between antithrombin III (AT III) and serine proteases in the clotting cascade (activated factors IXa, Xa, XIa, and XIIa and thrombin). This reaction proceeds almost instantane-

BARRY L. CARTER, PHARM.D., is Associate Professor, College of Pharmacy, University of Houston, Houston, TX, and Adjunct Associate Professor, Department of Family Medicine, Baylor College of Medicine, Houston.

Address reprint requests to Dr. Carter at the College of Pharmacy, University of Houston, 1441 Moursund Street, Houston, TX 77030.

The assistance of Jean M. Nappi, Pharm.D., and Margaret A. Noyes, Pharm.D., in manuscript review, of Kathryn Hale in literature review, and of Phi Hoang for artwork is acknowledged.

This is article **680-204-9115** in the **ASHP Continuing Education System**; it qualifies for 1.0 hour of continuing-education credit. See page 552 for learning objectives and test questions.

ously and prevents the activated clotting factors from activating their respective substrates, thereby halting further coagulation.[1] The binding of heparin to AT III requires a specific decasaccharide sequence. Sequences of 16 to 20 monosaccharides demonstrate maximum antithrombin activity.[11] The activity of heparin cofactor II is also accelerated by heparin and may contribute to the inactivation of serine proteases.

The traditional view of heparin's mechanism of action has been that the drug does not cause clot lysis but rather prevents extension of the clot by serving as a cofactor for AT III, which inhibits clotting[1]; thus, heparin promotes thrombus resolution by allowing naturally occurring thrombolytics to slowly lyse the clot. Data from recent studies have suggested, however, that the antithrombotic activity may be due to the ability of heparin to change the electronegativity of the endothelial surface, which then inhibits platelet adhesion and clotting factors.[11] There is also limited experimental evidence that heparin may cause a release of endogenous tissue plasminogen activator from the endothelium, which could promote thrombolysis.[11,12] These mechanisms require additional investigation.

Low-molecular-weight (LMW) heparins are currently being studied for the treatment of acute venous thrombosis.[11,13-16] The molecular weight of heparin is large and variable (3,000 to 30,000). LMW heparins are extracted from heparin and have molecular weights between 1,200 and 15,000, with less variability than is seen with heparin. These drugs have been developed in an attempt to reduce bleeding (decrease the anticoagulant effect) while retaining, or even enhancing, the antithrombotic effect. The half-life of activity of one LMW heparin was found to be 4 hours.[16] Dosages of LMW heparins that prevent thrombosis do not significantly prolong the activated partial thromboplastin time (APTT).[11,16] In animals, LMW heparins have been associated with less bleeding than has heparin, but they require additional study in humans.

Use of Heparin after Acute Myocardial Infarction

Heparin alone is not as effective as thrombolytics for treatment of acute coronary occlusion. However, heparin is commonly administered as adjuvant therapy with thrombolytics after acute myocardial infarction.[17-33] The need for early heparin therapy in combination with thrombolytics is becoming increasingly apparent,[23,24,27-29] for several reasons. First, even with thrombolysis, the ruptured endothelium continues to be a potent stimulant for coagulation.[27] Thus, the mechanism of reocclusion may be the same as that which initiated the coronary thrombus. The usefulness of early heparin treatment probably relates to the antithrombin effects of heparin, which inhibit new coagulation on re-exposed endothelium after thrombolysis. Second, thrombolytics may promote coagulation by increasing platelet aggregation.[30]

Heparin therapy to prevent early reocclusion may be more important with alteplase than with streptokinase. Alteplase is not only more clot specific than streptokinase but also produces fewer fibrin degradation products for shorter periods of time.[27] Fibrin degradation products have potent anticoagulant activity.

The importance of adequate early heparin therapy as an adjunct to alteplase has recently been demonstrated in two trials. Bleich et al.[27] compared coronary patency three days after alteplase administration in patients who were randomized to receive alteplase plus immediate intravenous heparin therapy (bolus dose followed by continuous intravenous infusion) or alteplase alone. Significantly more coronary arteries were patent in the heparin group (30 of 42 patients, or 71%) than in the control group (18 of 42 patients, or 43%). The recently completed Heparin–Aspirin Reperfusion Trial (HART)[29] compared heparin with aspirin in 205 patients who had received alteplase. Patients were randomly assigned to low-dose aspirin (80 mg daily) or intravenous heparin (5000-unit bolus followed by infusion adjusted to maintain an APTT of 1.5–2.0 times control). Patency was measured at a mean of 18 hours after initiation of therapy in the heparin group and 17.8 hours after initiation in the aspirin group. Significantly more affected arteries were patent in the heparin-treated group (82 of 100 patients) than in the aspirin-treated group (48 of 93 patients). In those who initially had patent arteries, patency was assessed again at 7 days; in this subgroup there was no difference in patency between patients receiving aspirin and those receiving heparin. These findings suggest that early and rapid anticoagulation with heparin may be critical in order to reduce the risk of reocclusion with alteplase. There is reason to suspect that heparin may also benefit patients who receive streptokinase, but this remains to be established. Although these studies have helped to clarify this controversial role for heparin, additional data are needed to determine the most appropriate regimen.

The Gruppo Italiano per lo Studio della Sopravvivenza nell' Infarto Miocardico trial (GISSI-2)[24] used heparin 12,500 units s.c. twice daily beginning 12 hours after administration of either alteplase or streptokinase. This study has been criticized because the heparin regimen was delayed.[30] The above data[27-30] suggest that an intravenous bolus dose of heparin should be administered at the initiation of thrombolytic therapy or early in the course of treatment. The heparin infusion may be started during the thrombolytic infusion or immediately after completion of the thrombolytic infusion. Most studies adjusted the APTT to 1.5–2.0 times control (or 1.5–2.0 times the patient's baseline APTT). It has been suggested that heparin be administered for 7–10 days. However, some investigators have used heparin for 72 hours. The optimal duration and intensity are yet to be established. If an invasive procedure such as angiography is performed, the infusion rate can be reduced 50% for two or three hours before the procedure and then reestablished immediately after removal of the catheter.[29] While the therapeutic range for heparin after acute myocardial infarction is still being established, the techniques for determining dosage and monitoring therapy will generally be the same as those for heparin use in DVT and PE.

High-dose heparin has also been used empirically as adjunctive therapy during percutaneous transluminal coronary angioplasty[34]; APTT was maintained at 1.5 to 2.5 times control. The placement of intracoronary stents to prevent reocclusion is being investigated[34]; in patients receiving stents, high-dose heparin has been given for four days, followed by warfarin for six months.

Heparin Therapy of Deep-Vein Thrombosis and Pulmonary Embolism

Heparin has clearly been shown to reduce morbidity and mortality in patients with venous thromboembolic events including DVT and PE.[1] Because of the potential for clot extension, all patients with calf-vein thrombosis should also receive anticoagulants.[35,36]

The major goal of heparin therapy for DVT is to rapidly establish anticoagulation to prevent proximal extension of the thrombus and embolization.[1] The importance of rapid anticoagulation was demonstrated by Hull and associates,[37] who compared continuous intravenous heparin with intermittent subcutaneous heparin in proximal-vein thrombosis of the leg. In that study, subcutaneous administration of heparin was much less effective than intravenous administration, which the investigators attributed to inadequate anticoagulation with the subcutaneous regimen. Recurrence was documented by venography and ventilation–perfusion scans. The risk of recurrent thromboembolism was 15 times higher (24.5% versus 1.6%) when anticoagulation was inadequate (APTT < 1.5 times control) in the first 24 hours of therapy. While information on intensity of early heparin therapy and subsequent recurrences of thromboembolism is limited, the study by Hull et al., plus an uncontrolled trial,[38] provide support for early aggressive use of heparin in doses that rapidly achieve an APTT of at least 1.5 times control.

If it is accepted that early and sustained therapeutic APTTs are important for efficacy, is this the standard in clinical practice? It has frequently been observed that APTTs are subtherapeutic in many patients. This is supported by a recent study by Wheeler et al.,[39] which outlines all the common mistakes and misconceptions with heparin therapy. These investigators identified 65 patients who received heparin in three affiliated hospitals. Problems identified included the following:

- There was a long delay from early symptoms of thrombosis or embolism until a diagnostic test was performed (mean, 98 hours).
- Only 29% of patients were treated with heparin at the initial suspicion of thrombosis.
- Initiation of heparin after a positive diagnostic test was delayed by a mean of 13 hours (range, 0.5–144 hours).
- The bolus dose was often inadequate, and 8% of patients received no bolus dose.
- Only 45% of APTTs were greater than 1.5 times control in the first 24 hours. It was not until day 6 that 80% were therapeutic.
- The first APTT was not obtained for a mean of 12 hours after the start of heparin.
- Many subtherapeutic APTTs (mean, 1.2 times control) were followed by no change in heparin therapy, an increase in the infusion rate only, or administration of a bolus dose only.
- When the APTT was excessive, the infusion was often stopped for too long or the dosage reduced too much, resulting in subtherapeutic APTTs (56% of patients).

These findings can be attributed to a healthy respect for—or even fear of—heparin and a lack of understanding of the pharmacokinetics of the drug. As stated by Wheeler et al., it is unlikely that these findings are unique to their institutions. The timid use of heparin may predispose patients to a higher risk of recurrent thromboembolism. Comprehensive, sustained clinical pharmacy services could help to prevent many of these problems. This was suggested by a study of pharmacist-directed heparin therapy in a California hospital[40]; the authors found that the time to therapeutic effect and the time patients' APTTs or activated coagulation times were outside the therapeutic range were shorter in the pharmacist-directed group than in the control group. A survey of pharmacist-managed therapy in all California hospitals[41] showed that 20% of hospitals had a pharmacist who regulated heparin therapy. In these centers, 41% of heparin-treated patients were managed by a pharmacist.

Heparin Dosing

After intravenous administration, the half-life of heparin is about 90 minutes (range, 0.5–2.5 hours).[1,42] The drug undergoes dose-dependent elimination, and the half-life is prolonged at higher dosages.[42] Heparin clearance is related to body weight.[42] Studies have shown that heparin requirements are increased in smokers, persons with AT III deficiency, and males.[42,43] Heparin requirements have been observed to be higher in patients with PE, but this has not been a consistent finding, nor is a diagnosis of PE a reliable predictor of heparin dosage.[1,44] While these patient characteristics may assist with empirical dosage selection, wide intersubject variability persists. Body weight has been the best predictor of dosage.

An algorithm for treating acute thromboembolic events with heparin and warfarin is displayed in Figure 1. Several changes have been made in the algorithm since it was published in 1985.[1] The first is that the therapeutic range for APTT has been revised to 1.5 to 2.0 times control.[35] Another change is a recommendation that all patients should receive an initial hepa-

Figure 1. Algorithm for the acute management of deep-vein thrombosis (DVT) or pulmonary embolism (PE) (adapted from reference 1). APTT = activated partial thromboplastin time; PT = prothrombin time. This algorithm could also be used for other acute thromboembolic events when heparin and long-term warfarin are the agents of choice.

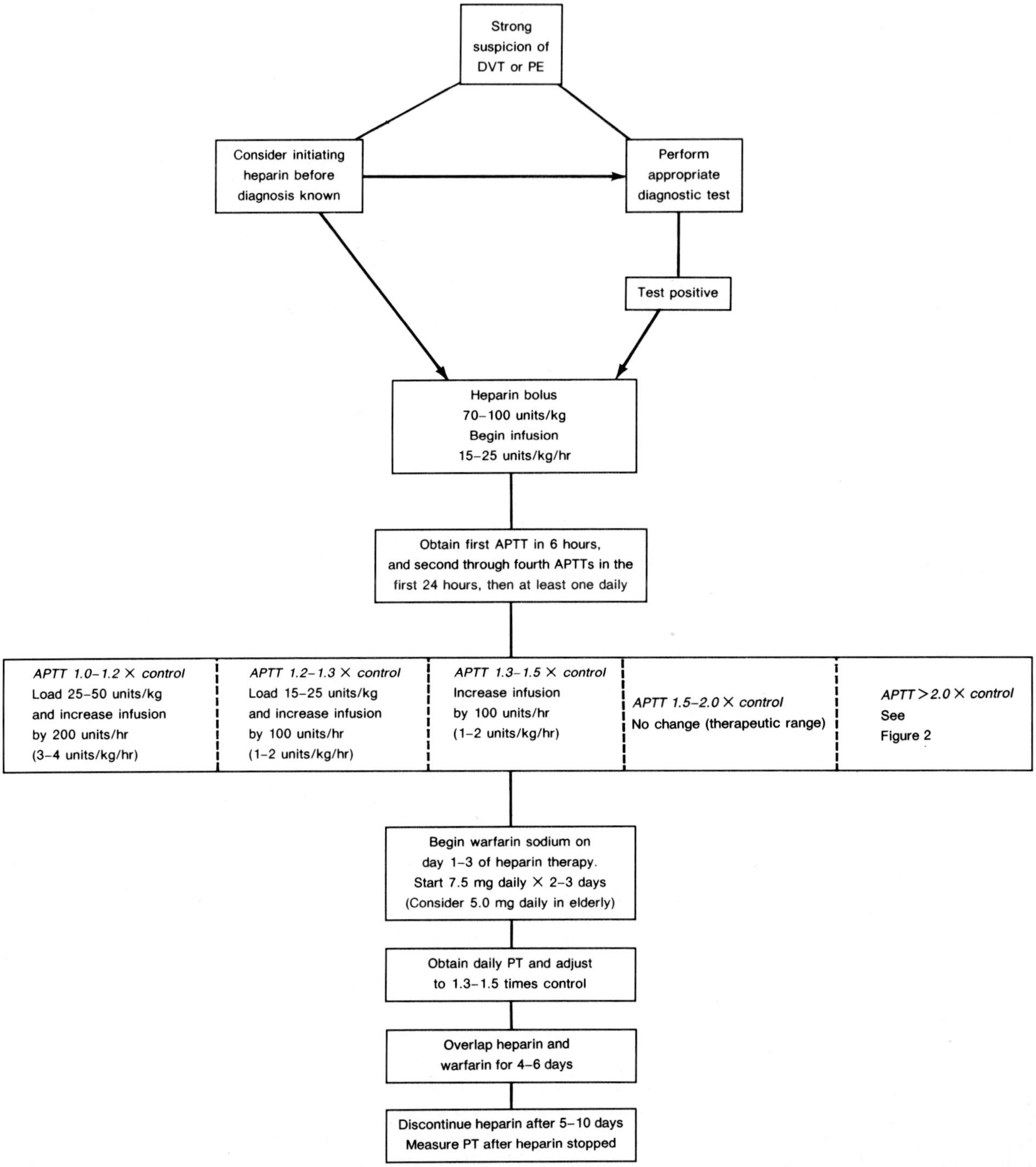

rin infusion of 15–25 units/kg/hr, regardless of the severity of the thromboembolic event. While the heparin requirements in some studies have been 10–20 units/kg/hr, dosages below 20 units/kg/hr may result in subtherapeutic APTTs in up to 25% of patients.[1,39] In several studies, 40,000 units in the first 24 hours (30,000 units in patients at risk of bleeding) was used in order to achieve rapid anticoagulation.[36,37,45,46] This corresponds to an infusion rate of 1500 units per hour. Depending on the patient's weight, the algorithm dosage corresponds to 900 to 2000 units per hour. An initial infusion of 1000 units per hour, a dosage commonly used, is too low for the majority of patients and will delay the time to therapeutic APTT. Low dosages (900–1000 units per hour) should be reserved for patients at high risk of bleeding and the elderly. Saya et al.[40] described heparin infusion calculations based on estimated blood volume (Table 1). In morbid obesity,

Table 1.
Heparin Infusion Dosages Based on Patient's Estimated Blood Volume[a]

Weight (lb)	Heparin Dosage (units/hr) for Indicated Height (inches) 60	62	64	66	68	70	72	74
Men								
100	841	875	911	949	989	1032	1078	1126
110	878	912	947	985	1026	1069	1114	1162
120	915	948	984	1022	1063	1106	1151	1199
130	951	985	1021	1059	1099	1142	1188	1236
140	988	1021	1057	1095	1136	1179	1228	1272
150	1024	1058	1093	1132	1172	1215	1260	1309
160	1061	1094	1130	1168	1209	1252	1297	1345
170	1097	1131	1167	1205	1245	1288	1334	1382
180	1134	1168	1203	1242	1282	1325	1370	1418
190	1171	1204	1240	1278	1319	1362	1407	1455
200	1207	1241	1277	1314	1355	1389	1444	1492
210	1244	1277	1313	1351	1392	1435	1480	1528
220	1280	1314	1350	1388	1428	1471	1517	1574
230	1316	1350	1386	1424	1465	1508	1553	1601
240	1354	1387	1423	1461	1501	1544	1590	1638
250	1390	1424	1459	1498	1538	1581	1626	1675
260	1427	1460	1496	1534	1575	1618	1663	1711
270	1463	1497	1533	1571	1611	1654	1700	1748
280	1500	1533	1569	1607	1648	1691	1736	1784
290	1536	1570	1606	1644	1684	1727	1773	1821
300	1573	1607	1642	1680	1721	1764	1809	1857
310	1610	1643	1679	1717	1758	1800	1846	1894
Women								
80	662	694	729	766	805	847	891	938
90	699	732	767	804	843	884	929	975
100	737	769	804	841	880	922	966	1013
110	774	807	842	879	918	960	1004	1050
120	812	845	879	916	956	997	1041	1088
130	850	882	917	954	993	1035	1079	1125
140	887	920	954	991	1031	1072	1116	1163
150	925	957	992	1029	1068	1110	1154	1201
160	962	995	1030	1067	1106	1148	1192	1238
170	1000	1032	1067	1104	1144	1185	1229	1276
180	1038	1070	1105	1142	1181	1223	1267	1314
190	1075	1108	1142	1179	1219	1260	1304	1351
200	1113	1145	1180	1217	1256	1298	1342	1389
210	1150	1183	1218	1255	1294	1336	1380	1426
220	1189	1220	1255	1292	1331	1373	1417	1464
230	1225	1258	1293	1330	1369	1411	1455	1501
240	1263	1296	1330	1367	1407	1448	1492	1539
250	1300	1333	1368	1405	1444	1486	1530	1577
260	1338	1371	1406	1443	1482	1523	1568	1614
270	1376	1408	1443	1480	1519	1561	1605	1652
280	1413	1446	1480	1518	1557	1599	1643	1689
290	1451	1484	1518	1555	1595	1636	1680	1727

[a] Adapted from reference 40, with permission.

the heparin requirement has been reported to be as high as 4000 units per hour.[47]

Methods have been studied that predict heparin dosage from pharmacokinetic data or from heparin concentrations after an initial dose.[1,42,48-51] Groce et al.[49] studied empirical dosage adjustments using the APTT versus a two-point predictive method. These investigators found that 65% of APTTs were subtherapeutic in the group that received dosage adjustments based on the APTT, whereas no APTT was subtherapeutic at any time with the predictive method. In addition, resolution of symptoms was significantly faster and duration of hospitalization significantly shorter in the two-point predictive group. Predictive methods may offer major advantages for heparin dosage adjustments; further study is needed to compare recurrence rates, duration of hospitalization, and bleeding risks in larger populations.

The initial APTT should be obtained six hours after the initiation of the infusion.[1,35] Most patients will be near their steady-state heparin concentration at this time, since the mean heparin half-life is 90 minutes. However, there is a great deal of intersubject variability in clearance. The drug also undergoes dose-dependent elimination, and the half-life is prolonged at higher dosages.[42,50] Several APTTs should be obtained within the first 24 hours to make further adjustments and ensure a rapid therapeutic response. The APTT should be determined twice daily until stabilized and then once daily. If a change in the heparin dosage is made, an APTT should be obtained within six to eight hours. Frequent monitoring may be necessary until stabilization occurs.

It is common to withhold heparin for too long or to reduce the infusion rate too much when the APTT is excessive.[39] Figure 2 displays an algorithm for reducing the heparin dosage when the APTT is excessive. Obviously, clinical judgment should also guide any dosage adjustment. This algorithm can be used when there is no bleeding or only minor bleeding. For more severe bleeding episodes, the clinician should consider reversing the effect of heparin with protamine sulfate or fresh frozen plasma, especially if the APTT is greater than 3 times control.

Duration of Heparin Therapy

The duration of i.v. heparin therapy has conventionally been 10 to 14 days. However, in many settings the trend has been to use shorter courses in an attempt to decrease the hospital stay and reduce the risk of thrombocytopenia. More recent recommendations suggest a duration of 5 to 10 days, even though limiting heparin therapy to five days may have contributed to a high recurrence rate in at least one study.[52] The timing of warfarin initiation during the course of heparin therapy can influence the duration of i.v. heparin therapy. Gallus et al.[45] compared early initiation of warfarin (mean, day 1 of heparin therapy) and late initiation of warfarin (mean, day 7 of heparin therapy) in patients with acute venous thrombosis or pulmonary embolism. Heparin was discontinued as soon as the prothrombin time (PT) was therapeutic. The mean duration of heparin treatment was 4.1 days in the early group ($n = 139$) and 9.5 days in the late group ($n = 127$). Recurrences were 3.6% and 4.7%, respectively, as measured by ventilation–perfusion lung scans and ^{125}I fibrinogen leg scans. These differences were not significant.

Hull and colleagues[46] recently published the results of a double-blind, randomized trial to determine if 5 days of i.v. heparin therapy is as effective as 10 days. Patients with proximal venous thrombosis received a

Figure 2. Algorithm for managing excessive anticoagulation with heparin. Recommendations are for patients who are not bleeding or for those with minor bleeding. APTT = activated partial thromboplastin time. Depending upon the laboratory control, these APTT ranges correspond to the following times: 2.0–2.5 = 70–100 seconds; 2.5–3.5 = 88–140 seconds; >3.5 = >122–140 seconds.

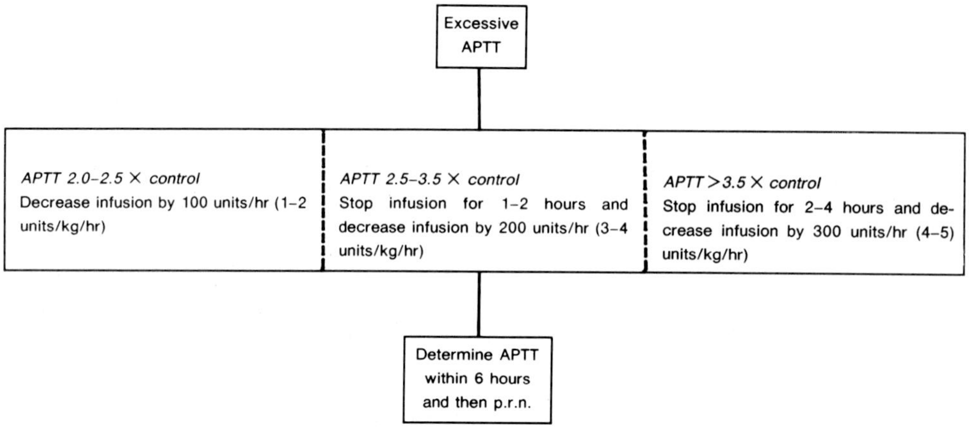

bolus dose of 5000 units of heparin followed by a continuous infusion. The APTT was adjusted to 1.8 to 2.8 times control. Patients who were at low risk of bleeding received 40,000 units whereas those at high risk received 30,000 units in the first 24 hours. Patients were randomized to receive a long course of heparin (10 days, $n = 100$) or a short course (5 days, $n = 99$). Warfarin was started either on day 1 (short-course group) or day 5 (long-course group). Investigator blinding was maintained by a clinical pharmacist who made adjustments in the heparin infusions and the warfarin doses. The frequency of recurrence was 7.0% in the long-course group and 7.1% in the short-course group. Bleeding occurred more frequently in the long-course group.

These two studies suggest that five days of heparin therapy (with warfarin started on day 1) may be sufficient for patients with venous thrombosis. This is reflected in the algorithm (Figure 1). Longer treatment might be reserved for patients with recurrent events or those with genetic coagulation abnormalities. Heparin and warfarin should be overlapped for at least four days; therefore, most patients will require at least five days of heparin. This is the rationale for using 5–10 days in the algorithm.

In the United States, most centers use a continuous infusion of heparin. Intermittent injections of heparin are favored in other countries. The continuous infusion has several advantages over the intermittent injection technique.[1]

Subcutaneous Heparin for Acute Thromboembolic Events

Heparin has also been administered subcutaneously for acute thromboembolic events. This route has typically been used when venous access cannot be achieved. It is less desirable because the response to s.c. heparin has been unpredictable and resulted in more recurrent thromboembolic events.[1,37,53] In the study by Hull et al.,[37] the higher recurrence rate (19% with s.c. heparin sodium versus 5% with i.v. heparin sodium) was attributed to inadequate anticoagulation early in the course of s.c. administration. Following an i.v. bolus dose of 5,000 units, 15,000 units given s.c. every 12 hours (adjusted to maintain a therapeutic APTT) was found to be inadequate.

Some investigators have reported that higher initial heparin dosages are necessary with s.c. administration.[37,53] However, factors other than the route of administration may have influenced their findings. The results of studies with heparin sodium showed inferior early anticoagulation compared with results for heparin calcium.[37,53-55] Bentley et al.[55] compared s.c. heparin calcium with i.v. heparin sodium in patients with calf-vein thrombosis. The initial dosage in all patients was 40,000 units in the first 24 hours (except for women over 55 years of age, who received 30,000 units). Subcutaneous heparin calcium was superior to i.v. heparin sodium with regard to limiting the extension of calf-vein thrombi ($p < 0.01$). In a second study, s.c. heparin calcium (initial dose of 15,000 units, then adjusted to maintain the APTT at 50–70 seconds) was found to be equivalent to i.v. heparin calcium (initial 5000-unit bolus dose, then 1250 units per hour).[54]

Walker and colleagues[56] administered s.c. heparin calcium or i.v. heparin sodium randomly to 100 patients with deep-vein thrombosis of the legs. In both groups, 250 units/kg was administered in the first 12 hours. Phlebography was performed to examine the change in thrombus size. More thrombi were reduced in size in the s.c. heparin calcium group, and more increased in size in the i.v. heparin sodium group. However, interpretation is difficult because clotting time was 10–20% longer in the s.c. group after day three than in the i.v. group, and the daily heparin dose was 20% higher.

These studies suggest that heparin calcium may be more efficacious than heparin sodium, especially when both are given subcutaneously. Further studies are needed to resolve this issue. If heparin calcium is superior to heparin sodium, the mechanism is unclear;

the difference may be due to different pharmacodynamic properties. These theories have yet to be proved. When compared with s.c. heparin sodium, s.c. heparin calcium showed superior efficacy in spite of lower bioavailability.[57,58] Peak heparin concentrations and overall serum levels were lower with heparin calcium, and the effects on clotting time were less than those seen with heparin sodium.

Higher doses should be used if the subcutaneous route is chosen. The initial dose should be an i.v. bolus of 5,000 units, followed by at least 16,500 to 20,000 units s.c. every 12 hours. The dosage should be adjusted rapidly to achieve an APTT of 1.5 to 2.0 times control. The APTT should be obtained six hours after a dose (midpoint of the dosing interval). The method of administration has previously been described.[1]

Adverse Reactions to Heparin

Thrombocytopenia. Heparin has been reported to cause thrombocytopenia in up to 30% of patients who receive the drug.[1] More reliable estimates range from 1% to 5%.[6,43,59-62] Two types of thrombocytopenia have been described, and there may also be a third distinct type.[62] The first type occurs rapidly after single i.v. doses of heparin in animals. This mild thrombocytopenia is reversible and is probably caused by a reversible clumping of platelets.

An early mild thrombocytopenia occurs within the first four days of heparin therapy.[61,62] Platelet counts typically drop to 100,000–150,000/cu mm. The patients remain asymptomatic, and the thrombocytopenia is often transient, even when heparin is continued. The mechanism for this reaction is not clear.

The severe, delayed type of thrombocytopenia usually occurs 6 to 12 days after the start of heparin therapy and rapidly recurs with rechallenge. Thrombocytopenia has occurred with intravenous heparin administration and low-dose prophylaxis.[63] The platelet counts drop below 100,000/cu mm, and patients may develop gangrene, stroke, myocardial infarction, and disseminated intravascular coagulation. The mechanism of thrombosis is presumed to be secondary to marked platelet aggregation.[64] While clinically overt thrombosis is uncommon, subclinical thrombi may develop in most patients.[65] The fact that this severe form of thrombocytopenia develops later in therapy is one rationale for shorter courses of heparin. This type of thrombocytopenia is consistent with an immunologic phenomenon causing injury to platelets and vascular endothelial cells.[62,65] Several reports have suggested that bovine lung heparin causes thrombocytopenia much more frequently than porcine heparin. However, recent investigations suggest that there is no difference between products.[59-62]

Platelet counts should be monitored at least every two or three days for all patients receiving heparin. Daily platelet counts for the first three weeks of heparin therapy have been recommended.[43] If the platelet count falls below 100,000/cu mm, heparin should be discontinued immediately. Some patients with heparin-induced thrombocytopenia have been treated with LMW heparins, with varying success.[11,62,66] Other therapies have included thrombolytic agents, aspirin, and dextran.[62] Frame and colleagues[67] recently reported the effects of intravenous immune globulin followed by platelet transfusion in a patient with severe thrombocytopenia. The patient's platelet count recovered within two days after this therapy. Additional investigation will be necessary to confirm these results.

Osteoporosis. High doses of heparin administered for longer than five months have been associated with osteoporosis and bone fractures.[68-70] Osteoporosis has been observed with daily doses in excess of 15,000 units. The mechanism for the bone loss is not known, but a recent case report of a bone biopsy suggested that the osteoporosis was reversible after discontinuation of heparin.[70]

Liver Function Test Abnormalities. Heparin has been reported to increase liver enzyme levels. While several studies have reported elevations in liver function test results, the mechanism and significance are still not apparent. Dukes et al.[71] reported that serum aminotransferase concentrations increased in 95% of 86 patients treated with heparin. Alanine aminotransferase and aspartate aminotransferase increased to excessive levels in 59% and 27% of patients, respectively. There was no relationship to heparin source, patient age, daily dosage, or total heparin received. Other investigators have noted a relationship between dosage and liver enzyme levels. Lactate dehydrogenase concentration was increased above normal in 35% of patients. However, there were no clinical signs of hepatic dysfunction. In 20% of the patients, the abnormal values returned to normal despite continued heparin treatment. These laboratory values should be monitored at baseline, on day 5, and at the end of acute heparin therapy.

Bleeding. Bleeding is the most common adverse reaction to heparin and may occur in up to 20% of patients treated with acute, high-dose heparin therapy. The relationship between bleeding risk and APTT is not predictable, partly because bleeding is related to other factors such as the effect of heparin on platelets and coexisting conditions.[35] However, there is sufficient evidence to suggest that bleeding risk increases up to threefold with an APTT between 2.0 and 2.9 times control and eightfold with APTT greater than 3.0 times control.[1,72] Data also suggest that the risk of bleeding is lower with a constant infusion than with intermittent injections.[1] The risk of bleeding is higher when heparin is given with thrombolytics.[27,29]

As shown in Figure 2, heparin dosage should be modified when anticoagulation is excessive and bleeding is minor. For severe bleeding, protamine sulfate is the drug of choice. One milligram of i.v. protamine sulfate will neutralize approximately 90 units of beef lung heparin and 115 units of pork intestinal mucosa heparin. If protamine sulfate is given 30 minutes or more after the last heparin dose, the protamine sulfate dose should be estimated based on the approximate amount of heparin remaining (mean half-life, 90 minutes). Protamine sulfate must be given slowly to avoid hypotension and shock. Excessive doses of protamine sulfate have anticoagulant effects, and doses greater than 100 mg should be avoided.

Other Adverse Reactions. Other common adverse reactions to heparin include fever, chills, rash, and urticaria.

Monitoring Heparin Therapy

Key factors that should be monitored in patients receiving heparin therapy are listed in Table 2. The primary test for monitoring heparin therapy is the APTT, which measures the intrinsic clotting system (factors VIII, IX, XI, and XII) and clotting factors in the final common pathway (II, X, and V). The test is performed by adding calcium chloride, an activator such as diatomaceous earth, and partial thromboplastin to the patient's plasma. Partial thromboplastin is a rabbit-brain phospholipid that mimics platelet phospholipid.[73] The sensitivity and precision of the APTT depend upon the reagents and instrumentation and vary among laboratories.[74]

When warfarin is added to a heparin regimen the APTT can be elevated further. One study found a strong relationship between the increase in the PT and the corresponding increase in the APTT.[75] With warfarin therapy, the average PT ratio of 1.87 corresponded to an APTT of 1.79. Therefore, adjustment in the heparin dosage may be necessary after warfarin is started. In addition, heparin requirements may decline after two to three days, which may also necessitate dosage reductions.

In some settings, the activated clotting time (ACT) is used to monitor heparin therapy. This test has the advantage that it can be performed at the bedside.[1,50]

Although the APTT is the established and recommended test for monitoring heparin therapy, it may not accurately predict bleeding or recurrent thromboembolism.[11,76] Tests that more accurately predict these outcomes would be desirable. A modified version of the APTT has recently been studied (Heptest).[77] While this test measures several clotting factors, it is more specific for anti-Xa activity than for activity of other clotting factors. Until the role of this or other alternatives to the APTT has been clearly defined, the APTT (or the activated clotting time) should be used to monitor heparin therapy.

Conversion to Long-term Therapy

Short-term anticoagulation with heparin (<14 days) results in an unacceptably high rate of thromboembolic recurrence in many instances.[1,36] Therefore, therapy is often continued for several months with warfarin (for DVT or PE) or aspirin (for acute myocardial infarction).

Table 2.
Factors To Be Monitored in Patients Receiving Intravenous Heparin Therapy

Signs and symptoms of thromboembolism
Signs and symptoms of bleeding (include urinalysis and stool for occult blood)
Activated partial thromboplastin time (monitor at baseline, two to four times on day 1 of therapy, twice daily until controlled, then daily)
Platelet count (baseline, then every two to three days)
Hemoglobin and hematocrit (baseline, then every two to three days)
Total heparin dosage ordered and actual dosage given per hour, per shift, and per day
Alanine aminotransferase, aspartate aminotransferase, lactate dehydrogenase (baseline, day 5, and day 7 or 10)

For DVT or PE, intravenous heparin may be converted to twice-daily subcutaneous injections. The dosage is adjusted to maintain the APTT ratio at 1.5, after which APTT monitoring can be discontinued.[1,3] However, a cost–benefit assessment in patients with proximal venous thrombosis suggested that oral warfarin was preferable to s.c. heparin.[78] Therefore, s.c. heparin should be reserved for patients who cannot have PT determinations or for patients who are pregnant. Thus, warfarin is generally the drug of choice for long-term therapy to prevent recurrent thromboembolism.

Overlapping Heparin and Warfarin. Heparin and warfarin therapy should be overlapped for four to six days (Figure 1).[1,35,37,43,79] There are several important reasons for this overlap:

1. Heparin reduces AT III levels.
2. Warfarin reduces protein C levels.
3. The antithrombotic effect of warfarin is delayed for four days (until factors II, IX, and X decline).
4. An early "therapeutic" PT may be due to an early drop in factor VII and this may not indicate true anticoagulation.

While these findings have all been documented, it has not been demonstrated that a shorter overlap increases the thrombotic risk.

Heparin-induced decreases in AT III levels[43,80] are probably of little significance while the patient is receiving heparin. However, when heparin is discontinued the anticoagulant effects of the drug terminate rapidly. It may take three days for the AT III level to return to baseline. Thus, the patient may be hypercoagulable for several days after heparin is discontinued. The reduction in AT III is even more dramatic in patients with AT III deficiency.[80]

Warfarin inhibits the synthesis of the vitamin K-dependent clotting factors II, VII, IX, and X.[1] However, the anticoagulant proteins C and S are also vitamin K dependent and are depressed by warfarin.[81,82] When warfarin therapy is started, factor VII and protein C levels decline rapidly within the first 12 to 24 hours.[81-83] Therapeutic reductions in factors IX and X, however, do not occur for four to six days. The antithrombotic effects of warfarin relate to suppression of factors IX and X.[43,82] Thus, patients may be hypercoagulable for the first three to four days of warfarin therapy, since the protein C level is low and factors IX and X remain elevated. This relationship is exaggerated when a loading dose of warfarin sodium is given. Hypercoagulability has been associated with the warfarin-induced skin necrosis that occurs in patients with pre-existing protein C deficiencies.[84,85]

It is common practice for some clinicians to discontinue heparin on day 2 or 3 of warfarin therapy when the first "therapeutic" PT is achieved. However, the PT test is substantially influenced by factor VII. If this "therapeutic" PT is achieved before the fourth day of warfarin therapy, the patient may not be anticoagulated because factors IX and X have not yet reached their nadir. For all of these reasons, the minimum overlap of heparin and warfarin should be four days, regardless of whether the PT is "therapeutic." It may be necessary to extend the overlap to five to six days if PTs are not in the therapeutic range on day 4.

When To Initiate Warfarin. Warfarin can be started at any time, as long as the minimum overlap with heparin is achieved. However, since shorter hospitalization is generally preferred, warfarin must be started early. This is especially important if heparin therapy is shortened to five days. Several studies have demonstrated that initiating heparin and warfarin together on day 1 is both safe and effective.[36,45,46,86,87]

Two studies have found that beginning warfarin on days 1 to 3 of heparin therapy reduces the length of hospitalization.[86,87] Rosiello and coworkers[87] performed a retrospective study in 38 patients with angiographically documented pulmonary embolism. Patients were categorized into early warfarin (day 0.1 to 3.0 of heparin therapy; mean, 1.7 days) or late warfarin (day 3.1 to 8.6 of heparin therapy; mean, 5.2 days). The duration of heparin therapy was significantly shorter in the early warfarin group (7.4 versus 10.5 days). There was a significant reduction in the duration of hospitalization in the early warfarin group (2.2 days), which reduced costs an average of $1076 per patient. These authors estimated that the cost avoidance would be $86 million per year if warfarin were started early in the course of heparin therapy for all patients with pulmonary embolism in the United States.

These data indicate that warfarin should be started on day 1 of therapy or as soon as a diagnosis is confirmed. The latest that warfarin should be started would be day 3 of heparin therapy.

Warfarin Products

Several studies have suggested that various warfarin products have less than 10–20% variation in bioavailability from the reference standard.[88-91] However, the impact of switching brands was documented at one hospital, where the pharmacy switched from dispensing Coumadin (Du Pont) to Panwarfin (Abbott) without informing the medical staff and nursing staff.[92] The hospital's anticoagulation clinic personnel noticed more difficulty with patient control before they discovered that a different product was being dispensed. A retrospective analysis showed an increase in clinic visits due to poorer control after the product switch, accompanied by greater dosage variability.

Although the differences in bioavailability among warfarin products are small, they may be clinically important for patients controlled on the drug.[88] The fact that one study found less than 20% variation between products[91] is not reassuring. Therefore, product substitution should not occur once a patient has been stabilized on one brand of warfarin. All departments should be informed and involved in the decision when an institution decides to change brands.

Warfarin Dosing

The pharmacokinetics and pharmacodynamics of warfarin are extremely complex, with a great deal of intersubject variability.[88,93] Loading doses of warfarin are no longer considered acceptable.[1,83] Conventionally, therapy is initiated by administering warfarin sodium 10 mg daily for two to three days and adjusted according to response.[1] However, this 10-mg dose could be considered a loading dose since the average warfarin sodium dosage with lower intensity therapy is about 5.5 to 6 mg daily. Therefore, the algorithm in Figure 1 suggests warfarin sodium 7.5 mg daily for two to three days. Because mean doses in the elderly are lower,[94] the dosage should be decreased in patients over age 65.

Warfarin dosing remains largely empirical. Often the key to making adjustments is not the PT after three doses of warfarin, but rather the rate of increase in the PT.[88] An experienced clinician can examine the rate of increase of the initial daily PTs and make efficient dosage modifications. The most common mistake made by clinicians is to make an excessive dosage change that results in subtherapeutic or elevated PTs several days later. This has become even more problematic since the established therapeutic range has been compressed from that recommended before 1985. The key is to make very small dosage adjustments, such as 2.5 to 5.0 mg per week (10–15%), unless the warfarin requirements are anticipated to be far outside the norm.

Some authors have advocated the use of dosage prediction techniques for achieving better dosage estimations and more rapid stabilization. It has even been suggested that one of these techniques should be used for every patient receiving warfarin,[88] but I do not think these techniques can be justified at this time.

Numerous equations based on simple linear regression have been developed for predicting warfarin dosage.[1,95-102] These have yielded statistically significant correlations between predicted and actual dosages. However, when the difference in predicted versus actual dosage is examined, the rate of inaccurate predictions exceeds 35%.[101,103,104] Hence, these techniques are unsatisfactory for predicting warfarin dosage requirements.

Several computer techniques that model warfarin response have been described.[104-112] Carter and coworkers[104,105] described the use of an analog computer to model warfarin response and predict daily dosages and compared the computer-predicted dosages to those prescribed by physicians. The number of therapeutic PTs was greater in the patients whose dosages were predicted by the analog computer.[104] However, a substantial number of predictions were not accurate.[105]

Computer programs that use Bayesian forecasting have also been described.[106-112] Only one study has compared use of such a program with physician dosing.[109] White et al.[109] found that the computer-dosed group required significantly shorter times to achieve a therapeutic PT and to achieve a stable PT and had a significantly reduced length of stay. However, in other reports, the examination of predicted versus actual dosage (or PT ratio) shows a great deal of variability and error.[106,107]

Proponents of dosage prediction techniques often fail to acknowledge a critical fact: These techniques were typically developed for a therapeutic PT ratio of 1.5 to 2.5. The current recommendation for most thromboembolic events is 1.3 to 1.5. The error associated with predictive techniques for this narrow range is unacceptable. White et al.[109] stated in their study methodology that, "Acknowledging the difficulty of dosing warfarin and the inherent imprecision in the measurement of a prothrombin time, it was arbitrarily decided that an error of approximately 4–5 seconds was acceptable." Therefore, the therapeutic range that they considered acceptable was actually 1.4–2.2.

No computer method has been compared with predictions made by a clinician experienced with warfarin therapy (e.g., a consultant). There is insufficient evidence that any predictive method provides a substantial improvement in dosage predictions. There is also concern that a computer might be relied on in spite of inaccurate predictions. For example, a recent study found serious prediction errors (predictions up to 50 mg per day) with the Data-Med program.[112] Because of these concerns, dosage prediction techniques should still be considered investigational until well-controlled trials demonstrate their utility with the lower therapeutic range for warfarin therapy.

Intensity of Warfarin Therapy

Previously, the therapeutic PT range for warfarin (using rabbit-brain thromboplastin) was considered to be 1.5 to 2.5 times control. In a 1985 review of DVT and PE, the recommended PT range was 1.3 to 2.0 times control.[1] The two subsequent American College of Chest Physicians consensus conferences suggested a lower intensity of anticoagulation with warfarin to maintain the PT at 1.3 to 1.5 times control. This was based on results of well-controlled trials.[1,2,37,46,113,114]

Table 3.
Recommended Therapeutic Ranges for Prothrombin Time Ratio (PTr) and International Normalized Ratio (INR) in Patients Receiving Warfarin Therapy[113]

PTr[a]	INR[b]	Indications
1.3–1.5	2.0–3.0	Treatment of deep-vein thrombosis
		Treatment of pulmonary embolism
		Prophylaxis for
		Acute myocardial infarction
		High-risk surgery
		Systemic embolism
		Bioprosthetic heart valves
		Valvular heart disease
		Atrial fibrillation
1.5–2.0	3.0–4.5	Recurrent systemic embolism
		Mechanical prosthetic valves

[a] PTr = ratio of patient's prothrombin time to control prothrombin time.
[b] The exact conversion of an INR of 2.0–3.0 depends on the sensitivity of the thromboplastin, but it approximates a PT of 1.3–1.6; the exact conversion of an INR of 3.0–4.5 is a PT ratio of 1.6–1.9.

The only indications for a range of 1.5 to 2.0 times control were prevention of recurrent systemic embolism and therapy for patients with mechanical heart valves (Table 3).

Serious confusion exists about therapeutic PT ranges because methods for determining PT may use thromboplastins of different origins.[1,113-117] Throughout the world, thromboplastins are used that are derived from sources differing in their responsiveness to warfarin. Therefore, therapeutic ranges for thromboplastins from different sources varied markedly. In the 1960s, changes in the source of thromboplastin in the United States resulted in an increased intensity of warfarin therapy that was not generally recognized. To standardize thromboplastins, the World Health Organization established a standardized reporting system for the PT in 1982 called the International Normalized Ratio (INR). In order to convert a PT ratio to an INR, the sensitivity of the thromboplastin must be known. Commercial manufacturers of thromboplastins and laboratories are beginning to supply these values.[118,119] A nomogram for conversion of a PT to an INR is available.[113] An international committee has recommended that editors and reviewers of scientific papers should no longer accept PT values unless an INR is presented as well.[118]

One major concern with maintaining a PT ratio of 1.3 is the variability associated with the PT test using North American thromboplastins. Clinicians must appreciate this variability, especially between laboratories, when low-intensity warfarin therapy is used.

Monitoring Warfarin Therapy

Recently, a rapid method for determining the PT with capillary whole blood (Coumatrak Protime Test System, Biotrak, Inc., Mountain View, CA) has been described.[120-122] Blood is obtained by a finger-stick and applied to a cartridge with a capillary channel. Blood flows through the capillary and mixes with the thromboplastin. A portable laser photometer then measures the time for the blood to clot. Investigators found good correlations between PTs measured by this system and by reference laboratories.[120,121] This method dramatically reduced the time required to determine the PT. A major advantage is that the test can be performed at the bedside or in an anticoagulation clinic. One study allowed patients to make their own modifications in warfarin dosage at home.[122] This type of home-based monitoring will require reliable patients and should be investigated more extensively.

Other methods for monitoring warfarin therapy include specific clotting factor assays.[88,123] These may offer better predictability of anticoagulant or antithrombotic effects. These assays have not yet been adopted in clinical practice.

Adverse Reactions to Warfarin

Bleeding. The major risk with long-term warfarin therapy is bleeding.[1] The risk of all bleeding (major and minor) ranges between 6% and 29%.[124-127] The incidence of major bleeding (fatal or life-threatening) has been 2% to 8% in various studies.[124-126] Fatal hemorrhage is usually due to cerebral bleeding, and this is much more common in patients who receive the drug for stroke.[125,126] In a review of clinical trials, Levine et al.[126] reported that the risk of fatal bleeding was less than 1.0% for patients with atrial fibrillation, ischemic heart disease, or venous thromboembolism. However, 1.7% of patients with prosthetic valves and 4.8% with ischemic cerebrovascular disease had fatal bleeding. Hypertension has also been found to be a risk factor for cerebrovascular hemorrhage.[125,126]

In a retrospective, cohort study, risk factors for major bleeding included age over 65 years, history of stroke, history of gastrointestinal bleeding, a serious comorbid condition, and atrial fibrillation.[125] Females and those over 60 years of age have been found to have significantly increased risk in several, but not all, studies.[1,124,127] Landefeld and Goldman[125] found that the cumulative risk of major bleeding was 11% after 12 months of therapy and 22% after 48 months. Minor bleeding occurred in 9% at 12 months and 41% at 48 months. In this study, which included various indications for warfarin, the risk of major bleeding was greatest during the first month of therapy. The risk of major bleeding was 3% per month for the first month, 0.8% per month for months 2–12, and 0.3% per month after 12 months of therapy. However, this is in contrast to the findings of Bussey et al.,[128] who evaluated patients in an anticoagulation clinic who had started warfarin therapy within the past two months. The risk of major hemorrhage was 0.02 episode per patient year; for minor hemorrhage, it was 0.15 episode per patient year. However, this study may have missed patients who were at high risk of bleeding during the first month of therapy and had not yet been referred to the anticoagulation clinic. Bleeding risk may also have been reduced because of close control and follow-up in this anticoagulation clinic.

The most common site of bleeding is the gastrointestinal tract.[125,126] However, hematuria is also common. In many of these cases of gastrointestinal bleeding or hematuria, correctable lesions can be identified, many of which are malignant or premalignant.[129,130] Most cases of upper gastrointestinal bleeding are due to peptic ulcer disease.[130]

The intensity of warfarin therapy clearly influences the risk of bleeding.[1,124,126,129,131-133] This has been the major rationale for less-intense warfarin therapy in the past seven years in the United States. The risk of bleeding escalates with PT ratios greater than 1.5. However, bleeding can occur at any level of anticoagulation and often occurs within the therapeutic PT range.

Concomitant aspirin therapy (500 mg daily) substantially increases the risk of bleeding.[124,126,134] This combination should be avoided whenever possible. Dipyridamole does not appear to increase bleeding risk and is preferable to aspirin when antiplatelet effects are desired (e.g., in patients with prosthetic cardiac valves).

Skin Necrosis. Warfarin has been reported to cause skin necrosis that typically involves the breast, buttocks, thighs, and penis.[84,85,135] This adverse reaction generally occurs early in the course of warfarin therapy and often involves patients with hereditary protein C deficiencies.[94,95] The skin necrosis is thought to be due to hypercoagulability, capillary thrombosis, and necrosis that result from the rapid drop in protein C that occurs when warfarin is started.

Purple Toes Syndrome. The purple toes syndrome has been reported rarely in patients receiving warfarin.[136-138] The toes become purple and painful. The purple areas frequently blanch with pressure and fade with elevation, and the color often fluctuates from hour to hour.[138] The syndrome may involve other areas of the feet. This adverse effect typically occurs three to eight weeks after the start of warfarin therapy. Biopsy data suggest that the mechanism is related to cholesterol microembolization that occurs from the rupture of atherosclerotic plaques. Several patients have reportedly developed renal failure and died as a possible consequence of the microemboli.[138] Therefore, warfarin should be discontinued, whenever possible, if the purple toes syndrome occurs.

Teratogenicity. Finally, warfarin is teratogenic.[1] Generally, heparin is preferred to warfarin for long-term treatment in pregnant patients.

Discharge and Follow-up

Heparin can influence the PT. One study found that the PT often declined significantly when heparin was discontinued.[139,140] Therefore, the PT should be measured approximately six to eight hours after the discontinuation of heparin and then daily until discharge.

In an attempt to shorten hospitalization, warfarin therapy often is not stabilized before discharge. In such cases, depending on the level of stability, the PT

Figure 3. Algorithm for management of long-term warfarin therapy after hospital discharge (adapted from reference 1). PTr = prothrombin time ratio (patient's PT to control PT); PE = pulmonary embolism; DVT = deep-vein thrombosis. The therapeutic range for most indications is a PT ratio of 1.3 to 1.5; however, for recurrent thromboembolism and mechanical heart valves the suggested range is 1.5 to 2.0. Maximum time between PT determinations should be four to eight weeks.

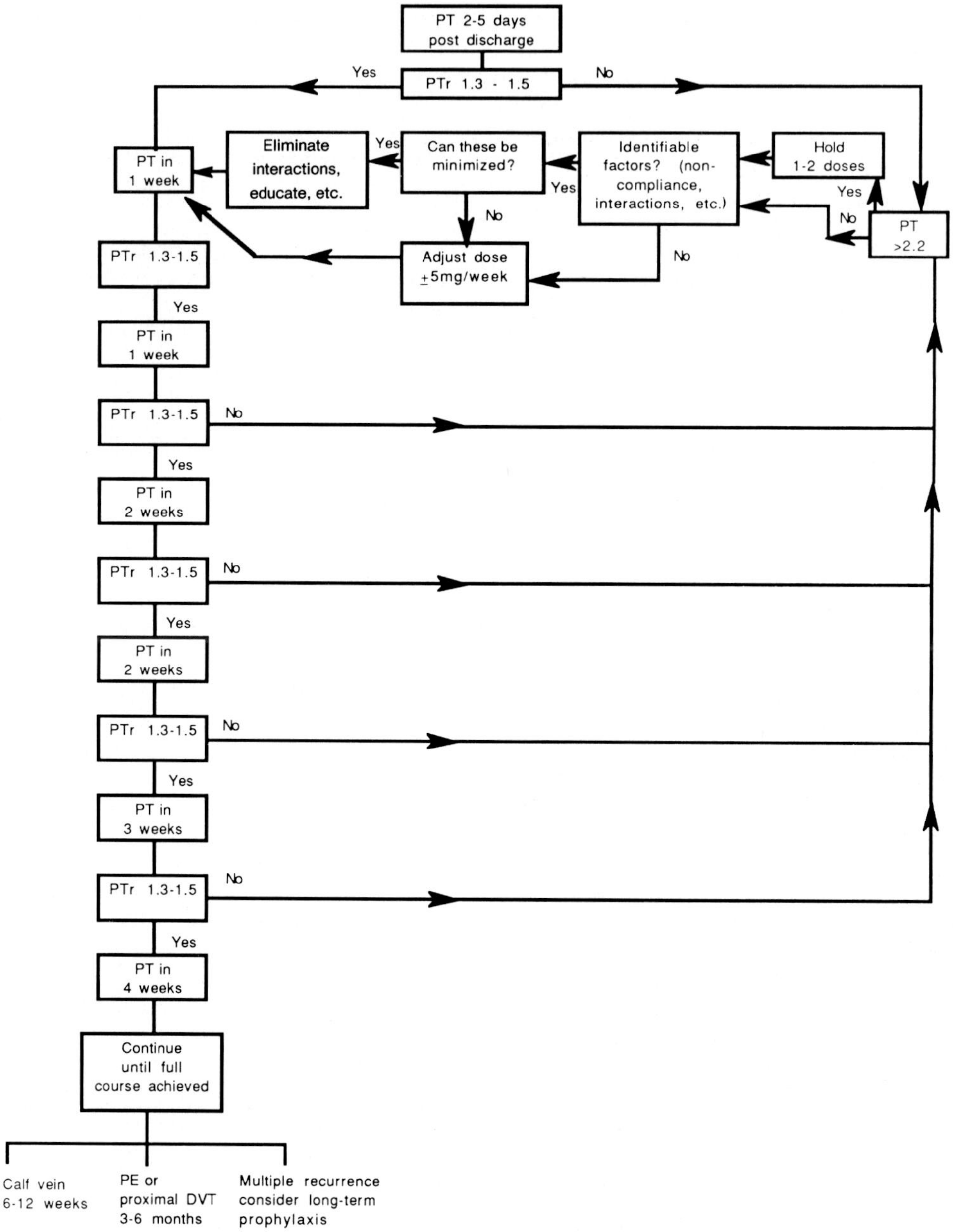

should be measured two to five days after discharge (Figure 3). Warfarin requirements frequently change after discharge and during long-term therapy. Therefore, close follow-up is essential. After several weekly PT determinations, the interval between PT measurements can gradually be increased. If at any time the PT is outside the desired range, the warfarin dosage should be re-evaluated and weekly PT determinations reinstituted. It is my opinion that well-stabilized patients should be seen at least once a month. This has been standard practice in many anticoagulation clinics. However, Rospond and colleagues[128,141] recently have questioned the need for monthly monitoring in stabilized patients. In their study in an anticoagulation clinic, the results indicated that less frequent monitoring might be acceptable for well-controlled patients.

The duration of warfarin therapy following acute PE or DVT should be three to six months.[1,6,35] However, clinical practice and small studies have often used courses as short as three to six weeks.[142] Often, high recurrence rates (>10%) have been found when short courses were given, and recurrence has been assessed based on clinical symptoms, which are not reliable. The only indication for courses shorter than three months is the presence of a risk factor that can be eliminated. In patients who have continuing risk factors (e.g., AT III deficiency, cancer) or multiple recurrences, anticoagulation may be required indefinitely.

The duration of therapy for calf-vein thrombosis is still not well defined. It may be possible to treat this condition for as little as six weeks.[1,6] In symptomatic patients, however, a minimum of three months is recommended.[35,36,143]

Conclusion

In the past five years, important new information about heparin and warfarin has been generated that has led to changes in the use of these drugs for acute thromboembolic events. Recommendations include reduced intensity of both heparin and warfarin therapy, shortened duration of therapy, and increased attention to alternative therapies (low-molecular-weight heparins) and routes (subcutaneous heparin). Since the therapeutic ranges for both heparin and warfarin therapy have been compressed, closer monitoring may be necessary to achieve and maintain adequate anticoagulation.

References

1. Carter BL, Jones ME, Waickman LA. Pathophysiology and treatment of deep-vein thrombosis and pulmonary embolism. *Clin Pharm.* 1985; 4:279-96.
2. American College of Chest Physicians and National Heart, Lung, and Blood Institute National Conference on Antithrombotic Therapy. *Arch Intern Med.* 1986; 146:462-72.
3. 2nd American College of Chest Physicians Conference on Antithrombotic Therapy. *Chest.* 1989; 95(Suppl 2):1S-169S.
4. Consensus Conference. Prevention of venous thrombosis and pulmonary embolism. *JAMA.* 1986; 256:744-9.
5. Rodvold DK, Quandt CM, Friedenberg WR. Thromboembolic disorders. In: DiPiro JT, Talbert RL, Hayes PE et al., eds. Pharmacotherapy: a pathophysiologic approach. New York: Elsevier; 1989; 324-45.
6. Mohr DN, Ryu JH, Litin SC et al. Recent advances in the management of venous thromboembolism. *Mayo Clin Proc.* 1988; 63:281-90.
7. Philbrick JT, Becker DM. Calf deep venous thrombosis: a wolf in sheep's clothing? *Arch Intern Med.* 1988; 148:2131-8.
8. Huisman MV, Buller HR, ten Cate JW et al. Management of clinically suspected acute venous thrombosis in outpatients with serial impedance plethysmography in a community hospital setting. *Arch Intern Med.* 1989; 149:511-3.
9. Bergqvist D. Postoperative thromboembolism: frequency, etiology, prophylaxis. Berlin: Springer-Verlag; 1983; 1-230.
10. Melamed AJ, Suarez J. Detection and prevention of deep venous thrombosis. *Drug Intell Clin Pharm.* 1988; 22:107-14.
11. Cines DB. Heparin: do we understand its antithrombotic actions? *Chest.* 1986; 89:420-6.
12. Huber K, Resch I, Rosc D et al. Heparin induced increase of t-PA antigen plasma levels in patients with unstable angina: no evidence for clinical benefit of heparinization during the initial phase of treatment. *Thromb Res.* 1989; 55:779-84.
13. Siegbahn A, Y-Hassan S, Boberg J et al. Subcutaneous treatment of deep venous thrombosis with low molecular weight heparin. A dose finding study with LMWH-Novo. *Thromb Res.* 1989; 55:767-78.
14. Harenberg J, Heene DL. Pharmacology and special clinical applications of low-molecular-weight heparins. *Am J Hematol.* 1988; 29:233-40.
15. Doutremepuich C, Guyot M, Lalanne MC et al. Comparative pharmacology of low molecular weight heparins: implications of manufacturing processes on biological effects. *Thromb Res.* 1989; 55:419-26.
16. Harenberg J, Giese C, Dempfle CE et al. Biological activity and safety of the subcutaneous administration of high doses of low molecular weight heparin for 8 days in human volunteers. *Thromb Haemost.* 1989; 61:357-62.
17. White HD, Rivers JT, Maslowski AH et al. Effect of intravenous streptokinase as compared with that of tissue plasminogen activator on left ventricular function after first myocardial infarction. *N Engl J Med.* 1989; 320:817-21.
18. Chesebro JH, Knatterud G, Roberts R et al. Thrombolysis in myocardial infarction (TIMI) trial, phase I: a comparison between intravenous tissue plasminogen activator and intravenous streptokinase. *Circulation.* 1987; 76:142-54.
19. The TIMI Study Group. Comparison of invasive and conservative strategies after treatment with intravenous tissue plasminogen activator in acute myocardial infarction: results of the thrombolysis in myocardial infarction (TIMI) phase II trial. *N Engl J Med.* 1989; 320:618-27.
20. Col JJ, Col-De Beys CM, Renkin JP et al. Pharmacokinetics, thrombolytic efficacy and hemorrhagic risk of different streptokinase regimens in heparin-treated acute myocardial infarction. *Am J Cardiol.* 1989; 63:1185-92.
21. Cercek B, Lew AS, Hod H et al. Enhancement of thrombolysis with tissue-type plasminogen activator by pretreatment with heparin. *Circulation.* 1986; 74:583-7.
22. ISIS (International Studies of Infarct Survival) Pilot Study Investigators. Randomized factorial trial of high-dose intravenous streptokinase, of oral aspirin and of intravenous heparin in acute myocardial infarction. *Eur Heart J.* 1987; 8:634-42.
23. The SCATI Group. Randomised controlled trial of subcutaneous calcium-heparin in acute myocardial infarction. *Lancet.* 1989; 2:182-6.
24. Gruppo Italiano per lo Studio della Sopravvivenza nell' Infarto Miocardico. GISSI-2: a factorial randomised trial of alteplase versus streptokinase and heparin versus no heparin among 12,490 patients with acute myocardial infarction. *Lancet.* 1990; 336:65-71.
25. Meinertz T, Kasper W, Schumacher M et al. The German multicenter trial of anisoylated plasminogen streptokinase activator complex versus heparin for acute myocardial infarction. *Am J Cardiol.* 1988; 62:347-51.
26. Fuster V, Stein B, Badimon L et al. Antithrombotic therapy after myocardial reperfusion in acute myocardial infarction. *J Am Coll Cardiol.* 1988; 12:78A-84A.
27. Bleich SD, Nichols TC, Schumacher RR et al. Effect of heparin on coronary arterial patency after thrombolysis with tissue plasminogen activator in acute myocardial infarction. *Am J Cardiol.* 1990; 66:1412-7.
28. Eisenberg PR, Sherman LA, Jaffe AS. Paradoxic elevation of fibrinopeptide A after streptokinase: evidence for continued thrombosis despite intense fibrinolysis. *J Am Coll Cardiol.* 1987; 10:527-9.
29. Hsia J, Hamilton WP, Kleiman N et al. A comparison between heparin and low-dose aspirin as adjunctive therapy with tissue plasminogen activator for acute myocardial infarction. *N Engl J Med.* 1990; 323:1433-7.
30. White HD. GISSI-2 and the heparin controversy. *Lancet.* 1990; 336:297-8.
31. Kaplan K, Davison R, Parker M et al. Role of heparin after intravenous thrombolytic therapy for acute myocardial infarction. *Am J Cardiol.* 1987; 59:241-4.
32. Topol EJ, George BS, Kereiakes DJ et al. A randomized controlled trial of intravenous tissue plasminogen activator and early intravenous heparin in acute myocardial infarction. *Circulation.* 1989; 79:281-6.
33. ISIS-2 (Second International Study of Infarct Survival) Collaborative Group. Randomised trial of intravenous streptokinase, oral aspirin, both or neither among 17,187 cases of

suspected acute myocardial infarction: ISIS-2. *Lancet*. 1988; 2:349-60.
34. Holmes DR Jr, Vlietstra RE, Reiter SJ et al. Advances in interventional cardiology. *Mayo Clin Proc*. 1990; 65:565-83.
35. Hyers TM, Hull RD, Weg JG. Antithrombotic therapy for venous thromboembolic disease. *Chest*. 1989; 95(Suppl 2):37S-51S.
36. Lagerstedt CI, Olsson CG, Fagher BO et al. Need for long-term anticoagulant treatment in symptomatic calf-vein thrombosis. *Lancet*. 1985; 2:515-8.
37. Hull RD, Raskob GE, Hirsh J et al. Continuous intravenous heparin compared with intermittent subcutaneous heparin in the initial treatment of proximal-vein thrombosis. *N Engl J Med*. 1986; 315:1109-14.
38. Basu D, Gallus A, Hirsh J et al. A prospective study of the value of monitoring heparin treatment with the activated partial thromboplastin time. *N Engl J Med*. 1972; 287:324-7.
39. Wheeler AP, Jaquiss RDB, Newman JH. Physician practices in the treatment of pulmonary embolism and deep venous thrombosis. *Arch Intern Med*. 1988; 148:1321-5.
40. Saya FG, Coleman LT, Martinoff JT. Pharmacist-directed heparin therapy using a standard dosing and monitoring protocol. *Am J Hosp Pharm*. 1985; 42:1965-9.
41. Guglielmo BJ, Schweigert BF, Kishi DT. Pharmacist-managed drug therapy in California hospitals. *Am J Hosp Pharm*. 1989; 46:1366-9.
42. Cipolle RJ, Seifert RD, Neilan BA et al. Heparin kinetics: variables related to disposition and dosage. *Clin Pharmacol Ther*. 1981; 29:387-93.
43. Wessler S, Gitel SN. Pharmacology of heparin and warfarin. *J Am Coll Cardiol*. 1986; 8:10B-20B.
44. Tenero DM, Bell HE, Deitz PA et al. Comparative dosage and toxicity of heparin sodium in the treatment of patients with pulmonary embolism versus deep-vein thrombosis. *Clin Pharm*. 1989; 8:40-3.
45. Gallus A, Jackaman J, Tillett J et al. Safety and efficacy of warfarin started early after submassive venous thrombosis or pulmonary embolism. *Lancet*. 1986; 2:1293-6.
46. Hull RD, Raskob GE, Rosenbloom D et al. Heparin for 5 days as compared with 10 days in the initial treatment of proximal venous thrombosis. *N Engl J Med*. 1990; 322:1260-4.
47. Ellison MJ, Sawyer WT, Mills TC. Calculation of heparin dosage in a morbidly obese woman. *Clin Pharm*. 1989; 8:65-8.
48. Chenella FC, Gill MA, Kern JW et al. Improved method for estimating initial heparin infusion rates. *Am J Hosp Pharm*. 1979; 36:782-4.
49. Groce JB, Gal P, Douglas JB et al. Heparin dosage adjustment in patients with deep-vein thrombosis using heparin concentrations rather than activated partial thromboplastin time. *Clin Pharm*. 1987; 6:216-22.
50. Cipolle RJ, Rodvold KA. Heparin. In: Evans WE, Schentag JJ, Jusko WJ eds. Applied pharmacokinetics: principles of therapeutic drug monitoring. Spokane, WA: Applied Therapeutics; 1986:908-43.
51. Mungall D, Floyd R. Bayesian forecasting of APTT response to continuously infused heparin with and without warfarin administration. *J Clin Pharmacol*. 1989; 29:1043-7.
52. Holmgren K, Andersson G, Fagrell B et al. One month versus six month therapy with oral anticoagulants after symptomatic deep vein thrombosis. *Acta Med Scand*. 1985; 218:279-84.
53. Andersson G, Fagrell B, Holmgren K et al. Subcutaneous administration of heparin: a randomised comparison with intravenous administration of heparin to patients with deep-vein thrombosis. *Thromb Res*. 1982; 27:631-9.
54. Doyle DJ, Turpie GG, Hirsh J et al. Adjusted subcutaneous heparin or continuous intravenous heparin in patients with acute deep vein thrombosis. *Ann Intern Med*. 1987; 107:441-5.
55. Bentley PG, Kakkar VV, Scully MF et al. An objective study of alternative methods of heparin administration. *Thromb Res*. 1980; 18:177-87.
56. Walker MG, Shaw JW, Thomson GJL et al. Subcutaneous calcium heparin versus intravenous sodium heparin in treatment of established acute deep vein thrombosis of the legs: a multicentre prospective randomised trial. *Br Med J*. 1987; 294:1189-92.
57. Thomas DP, Sagar S, Stamatakis JD et al. Plasma heparin levels after administration of calcium and sodium salts of heparin. *Thromb Res*. 1976; 9:241-8.
58. Low J, Briggs JC. Comparative plasma heparin levels after subcutaneous sodium and calcium heparin. *Thromb Haemost*. 1978; 40:397-406.
59. Rao AK, White GC, Sherman L et al. Low incidence of thrombocytopenia with porcine mucosal heparin: a prospective multicenter study. *Arch Intern Med*. 1989; 149:1285-8.
60. Bailey RT, Ursick JA, Heim KL et al. Heparin-associated thrombocytopenia: a prospective comparison of bovine lung heparin, manufactured by a new process, and porcine intestinal heparin. *Drug Intell Clin Pharm*. 1986; 20:374-8.
61. Green D. Heparin-induced thrombocytopenia. *Med J Aust*. 1986; 144:37-9.
62. Cola C, Ansell J. Heparin-induced thrombocytopenia and arterial thrombosis: alternative therapies. *Am Heart J*. 1990; 119:368-74.
63. Cottingham JK, Wheelock JB. Heparin-associated thrombocytopenia: a complication of low-dose heparin prophylaxis. *Military Med*. 1989; 154:242-4.
64. White PW, Sadd JR, Nensel RE. Thrombotic complications of heparin therapy: including six cases of heparin-induced skin necrosis. *Ann Surg*. 1979; 190:595-608.
65. Cines DB, Tomaski A, Tannenbaum S. Immune endothelial-cell injury in heparin-associated thrombocytopenia. *N Engl J Med*. 1987; 316:581-9.
66. Gouault-Heilmann M, Huet Y, Adnot S et al. Low molecular weight heparin fractions as an alternative therapy in heparin-induced thrombocytopenia. *Haemostasis*. 1987; 17:134-40.
67. Frame JN, Mulvey KP, Phares JC et al. Correction of severe heparin-associated thrombocytopenia with intravenous immunoglobulin. *Ann Intern Med*. 1989; 111:946-7.
68. Howell R, Fidler J, Letsky E et al. The risks of antenatal subcutaneous heparin prophylaxis: a controlled trial. *Br J Obstet Gynecol*. 1983; 90:1124-8.
69. Griffith GC, Nichols G, Asher JD et al. Heparin osteoporosis. *JAMA*. 1965; 193:91-4.
70. Zimran A, Shilo S, Fisher D et al. Histomorphometric evaluation of reversible heparin-induced osteoporosis in pregnancy. *Arch Intern Med*. 1986; 146:386-8.
71. Dukes GE Jr, Sanders SW, Russo J Jr et al. Transaminase elevations in patients receiving bovine or porcine heparin. *Ann Intern Med*. 1984; 100:646-50.
72. Landefeld CS, Cook EF, Flatley M et al. Identification and preliminary validation of predictors of major bleeding in hospitalized patients starting anticoagulant therapy. *Am J Med*. 1987; 82:703-13.
73. Fritsma, GA. Clot-based assays of coagulation. In: Corriveau DM, Fritsma GA, eds. Hemostasis and thrombosis in the clinical laboratory. Philadelphia: Lippincott; 1988:92-127.
74. Carter BL. Hematology: coagulation. In: Traub SL, ed. Basic skills in interpreting clinical laboratory data. Bethesda, MD: American Society of Hospital Pharmacists; 1991 (in press).
75. Hauser VM, Rozek SL. Effect of warfarin on the activated partial thromboplastin time. *Drug Intell Clin Pharm*. 1986; 20:964-7.
76. Meisenberg B. Heparin for proximal-vein thrombosis. *N Engl J Med*. 1986; 316:1162.
77. Bara L, Combe-Tamzali S, Conard J et al. Laboratory monitoring of a low molecular weight heparin (Enoxaparin) with a new clotting test (Heptest). *Haemostasis*. 1987; 17:127-33.
78. Hull RD, Raskob GE, Hirsh J et al. A cost-effectiveness analysis of alternative approaches for long-term treatment of proximal venous thrombosis. *JAMA*. 1984; 252:235-9.
79. Hull R, Delmore T, Carter C et al. Adjusted subcutaneous heparin versus warfarin sodium in the long-term treatment of venous thromboembolism. *N Engl J Med*. 1982; 306:189-94.

80. Marciniak E, Gockerman JP. Heparin-induced decrease in circulating antithrombin-III. *Lancet*. 1977; 2:581-4.
81. Weiss P, Soff GA, Halkin H et al. Decline of proteins C and S and factors II, VII, IX and X during the initiation of warfarin therapy. *Thromb Res*. 1987; 45:783-90.
82. Epstein DJ, Bergum PW, Bajaj SP et al. Radioimmunoassays for protein C and factor X: plasma antigen levels in abnormal hemostatic states. *Am J Clin Pathol*. 1984; 82:573-81.
83. O'Reilly RA, Aggeler PM. Studies on coumarin anticoagulant drugs: initiation of warfarin therapy without a loading dose. *Circulation*. 1968; 38:169-77.
84. Horn JR, Danziger LH, David RJ. Warfarin-induced skin necrosis: report of four cases. *Am J Hosp Pharm*. 1981; 38:1763-8.
85. McGehee WG, Klotz TA, Epstein DJ et al. Coumarin necrosis associated with hereditary protein C deficiency. *Ann Intern Med*. 1984; 101:59-60.
86. Self TH, Bauman JH, Brown JR et al. Concurrent initiation of heparin and warfarin therapy. *Am Heart J*. 1981; 102:470-1.
87. Rosiello RA, Chan CK, Tencza F et al. Timing of oral anticoagulation therapy in the treatment of angiographically proven acute pulmonary embolism. *Arch Intern Med*. 1987; 147:1469-73.
88. Porter RS, Sawyer WT, Lowenthal DT. Warfarin. In: Evans WE, Schentag JJ, Jusko WJ, eds. Applied pharmacokinetics: principles of therapeutic drug monitoring. Spokane, WA: Applied Therapeutics; 1986:1057-1104.
89. Wagner JG, Welling PG, Lee KP et al. In vivo and in vitro availability of commercial warfarin tablets. *J Pharm Sci*. 1971; 60:666-77.
90. Ruedy J, Davies RO, Gagnon MA. Drug bioavailability. *Can Med Assoc J*. 1976; 115:105.
91. Muller FO, Steyn JM, Hundt HKL et al. Warfarin bio-availability: a comparison of 4 products. *S Afr Med J*. 1988; 74:566-7.
92. Richton-Hewett S, Foster E, Apstein CS. Medical and economic consequences of a blinded oral anticoagulant brand change at a municipal hospital. *Arch Intern Med*. 1988; 148:806-8.
93. Shetty HGM, Fennerty AG, Routledge PA. Clinical pharmacokinetic considerations in the control of oral anticoagulant therapy. *Clin Pharmacokinet*. 1989; 16:238-53.
94 Routledge PA, Chapman DH, Davies DM et al. Pharmacokinetics and pharmacodynamics of warfarin at steady state. *Br J Clin Pharmacol*. 1979; 8:243-7.
95. Williams DB, Karl RC. A simple technique for predicting daily maintenance dose of warfarin. *Am J Surg*. 1979; 137:572-6.
96. Miller DR, Brown MA. Predicting warfarin maintenance dosage based on initial response. *Am J Hosp Pharm*. 1979; 36:1351-5.
97. Sawyer WT. Predictability of warfarin dose requirements: theoretical considerations. *J Pharm Sci*. 1979; 68:432-4.
98. Routledge PA, Davies DM, Bell SM et al. Predicting patients' warfarin requirements. *Lancet*. 1977; 2:854-5.
99. Gordon BM, Wiser TH, Davis RJ. Warfarin maintenance-dose prediction based upon initial anticoagulant response. *Clin Pharm*. 1984; 3:297-9.
100. Holford NHG. Clinical pharmacokinetics and pharmacodynamics of warfarin: understanding the dose–effect relationship. *Clin Pharmacokinet*. 1986; 11:483-504.
101. Jupe DML, Peterson GM, Coleman RL et al. Warfarin dosage requirements: prospective clinical trial of a method for prediction from the response to a single dose. *Br J Clin Pharmacol*. 1988; 25:607-10.
102. Sawyer WT, Poe TE, Canaday BR et al. Multicenter evaluation of six methods for predicting warfarin maintenance-dose requirements from initial response. *Clin Pharm*. 1985; 4:440-6.
103. Carter BL, Reinders TP, Hamilton RA. Prediction of maintenance warfarin dosage from initial patient response. *Drug Intell Clin Pharm*. 1983; 17:23-6.
104. Carter BL, Taylor JW, Becker A. Evaluation of three dosage-prediction methods for initial in-hospital stabilization of warfarin therapy. *Clin Pharm*. 1987; 6:37-45.
105. Carter BL, Barr W, Rock W et al. Warfarin dosage predictions assisted by the analog computer. *Ther Drug Monit*. 1988; 10:69-73.
106. Doyle DA, Ludden TM, Carter BL et al. Evaluation of a Bayesian regression program for predicting warfarin response. *Ther Drug Monit*. 1989; 11:276-84.
107. Svec JM, Coleman RW, Mungall DR et al. Bayesian pharmacokinetic/pharmacodynamic forecasting of prothrombin response to warfarin therapy: preliminary evaluation. *Ther Drug Monit*. 1985; 7:174-80.
108. Sheiner LB. Computer-aided long-term anticoagulation therapy. *Comput Biomed Res*. 1969; 2:507-18.
109. White RH, Hong R, Venook AP et al. Initiation of warfarin therapy: comparison of physician dosing with computer-assisted dosing. *J Gen Intern Med*. 1987; 2:141-8.
110. Murray B, Coleman R, McWaters D et al. Pharmacodynamics of warfarin at steady state. *Ther Drug Monit*. 1987; 9:1-5.
111. Lee C, Coleman RW, Mungall DR. Effect of using warfarin plasma concentrations in Bayesian forecasting of prothrombin-time response. *Clin Pharm*. 1987; 6:406-12.
112. Noer BL, Tortorice KL, Angaran DM. Evaluation of a computer warfarin dosing program. *Pharmacotherapy*. 1989; 9:175. Abstract.
113. Hirsh J, Poller L, Deykin D et al. Optimal therapeutic range for oral anticoagulants. *Chest*. 1989; 95(Suppl 2):5S-11S.
114. Hirsh J, Deykin D, Poller L. "Therapeutic range" for oral anticoagulant therapy. *Chest*. 1986; 89(Suppl 2):11S-15S.
115. Loeliger EA, Lewis SM. Progress in laboratory control of oral anticoagulants. *Lancet*. 1982; 2:318-20.
116. Loeliger EA. The optimal therapeutic range in oral anticoagulation: history and proposal. *Thromb Haemost*. 1979; 42:1141-52.
117. Poller L. Oral anticoagulants reassessed. *Br Med J*. 1982; 284:1425-6.
118. Loeliger EA. ICSH/ICTH recommendations for reporting prothrombin time in oral anticoagulant control. *Thromb Haemost*. 1985; 53:155-6.
119. Palareti G, Coccheri S, Poggi M et al. Oral anticoagulant therapy control: evidence that INR expression improves the inter-laboratory comparability of results—the Bologna oral anticoagulant control exercise. *Thromb Haemost*. 1987; 58:905-10.
120. Weibert RT, Adler DS. Evaluation of a capillary whole-blood prothrombin time measurement system. *Clin Pharm*. 1989; 8:864-7.
121. Lucas, FV, Duncan A, Jay R et al. A novel whole blood capillary technic for measuring the prothrombin time. *Am J Clin Pathol*. 1987; 88:442-6.
122. Ansell J, Holden A, Knapic N. Patient self-management of oral anticoagulation guided by capillary (fingerstick) whole blood prothrombin times. *Arch Intern Med*. 1989; 149:2509-11.
123. Furie B, Liebman HA, Blanchard RA et al. Comparison of the native prothrombin antigen and the prothrombin time for monitoring oral anticoagulant therapy. *Blood*. 1984; 64:445-51.
124. Petitti DB, Strom BL, Melmon KL. Prothrombin time ratio and other factors associated with bleeding in patients treated with warfarin. *J Clin Epidemiol*. 1989; 42:759-64.
125. Landefeld CS, Goldman L. Major bleeding in outpatients treated with warfarin: incidence and prediction by factors known at the start of outpatient therapy. *Am J Med*. 1989; 87:144-52.
126. Levine MN, Raskob G, Hirsh J. Hemorrhagic complications of long-term anticoagulant therapy. *Chest*. 1989; 95(Suppl 2):26S-36S.
127. Gurwitz JH, Goldberg RJ, Holden A et al. Age-related risks of long-term oral anticoagulant therapy. *Arch Intern Med*. 1988; 148:1733-6.
128. Bussey HI, Rospond RM, Quandt CM et al. The safety and effectiveness of long-term warfarin therapy in an anticoagu-

lation clinic. *Pharmacotherapy*. 1989; 9:214-9.
129. Landefeld CS, Rosenblatt MW, Goldman L. Bleeding in outpatients treated with warfarin: relation to the prothrombin time and important remediable lesions. *Am J Med*. 1989; 87:153-9.
130. Wilcox CM, Truss CD. Gastrointestinal bleeding in patients receiving long-term anticoagulant therapy. *Am J Med*. 1988; 84:683-90.
131. Francis CW, Marder VJ, McCollister EC et al. Two step warfarin therapy: prevention of postoperative venous thrombosis without excessive bleeding. *JAMA*. 1983; 249:374-8.
132. Saour JN, Sieck JO, Mamo LAR et al. Trial of different intensities of anticoagulation in patients with prosthetic heart valves. *N Engl J Med*. 1990; 322:428-32.
133. Turpie AGG, Gunstensen J, Hirsh J et al. Randomised comparison of two intensities of oral anticoagulant therapy after tissue heart valve replacement. *Lancet*. 1988; 1:1242-5.
134. Chesebro JH, Fuster V, Elveback LR et al. Trial of combined warfarin plus dipyridamole or aspirin therapy in prosthetic heart valve replacement: danger of aspirin compared with dipyridamole. *Am J Cardiol*. 1983; 51:1537-41.
135. Kandrotas RJ, Deterding J. Genital necrosis secondary to warfarin therapy. *Pharmacotherapy*. 1988; 8:351-4.
136. Feder W, Auerback R. "Purple toes": an uncommon sequela of oral coumarin drug therapy. *Ann Intern Med*. 1961; 55:911-7.
137. Lebsack CS, Wiebert RT. "Purple toes" syndrome. *Postgrad Med*. 1982; 71:81-4.
138. Hyman BT, Landas SK, Ashman RF et al. Warfarin-related purple toes syndrome and cholesterol microembolization. *Am J Med*. 1987; 82:1233-7.
139. Sawyer WT, Raasch RH. Effect of heparin on prothrombin time. *Clin Pharm*. 1984; 3:192-4.
140. Lutomski DM, Djuric PE, Draeger RW. Warfarin therapy: the effect of heparin on prothrombin times. *Arch Intern Med*. 1987; 147:432-3.
141. Rospond RM, Quandt CM, Clark GM et al. Evaluation of factors associated with stability of anticoagulation therapy. *Pharmacotherapy*. 1989; 9:207-13.
142. Fennerty AG, Dolben J, Thomas P et al. A comparison of 3 and 6 weeks' anticoagulation in the treatment of venous thromboembolism. *Clin Lab Haematol*. 1987; 9:17-21.
143. Hull RD, Hirsh J, Carter CJ et al. Diagnostic efficacy of impedance plethysmography for clinically suspected deep vein thrombosis: a randomized trial. *Ann Intern Med*. 1985; 102:21-8.

Pharmacologic management of endometriosis

EMMANUEL SALTIEL AND SUSAN M. GARABEDIAN-RUFFALO

Abstract: The incidence, pathogenesis, staging, and treatment of endometriosis are reviewed, with an emphasis on pharmacologic management of this condition.

Endometriosis—the presence of ectopic endometrial tissue—can be found in 15–25% of infertile women and may be found in 1–5% of all women between menarche and menopause. Although the pathogenesis of endometriosis is uncertain, the most tenable etiologic theory is a combination of celomic metaplasia and retrograde menstruation. Staging is based on the American Fertility Society classification scheme, with stage I being the mildest and stage IV the most severe form of the disease.

The management of endometriosis depends on the extent of the disease, the severity of the symptoms, the age of the patient, and the patient's desire for future fertility. Treatment modalities include expectant management, surgery, induction of a pseudopregnancy state with hormonal therapy (e.g., oral contraceptives), or induction of a pseudomenopausal state. The induction of a pseudomenopausal state with the use of oral danazol gained widespread favor in the 1970s as the treatment of choice in patients with endometriosis, but therapy is often associated with unpleasant adverse effects. Gonadotropin-releasing hormone (GnRH) agonists may provide a safe and clinically effective alternative to danazol therapy in patients with endometriosis. Results of a multicenter study comparing nafarelin with danazol for treatment of endometriosis indicated no significant differences between treatment groups with respect to improvements in disease state and symptomatology. The most common adverse effect associated with nafarelin therapy is hot flashes.

The GnRH agonist nafarelin is as effective as danazol or oral contraceptives for the treatment of endometriosis and causes fewer adverse reactions. GnRH agonists may replace danazol as the treatment of choice in patients with endometriosis.

Index terms: Androgens; Contraceptives, oral; Danazol; Endometriosis; Goserelin agonists; Nafarelin
Clin Pharm. 1991; 10:518-31

EMMANUEL SALTIEL, PHARM.D., is Clinical Coordinator, Pharmacy Services, Cedars-Sinai Medical Center, and Assistant Clinical Professor, School of Pharmacy, University of Southern California, Los Angeles. SUSAN M. GARABEDIAN-RUFFALO, PHARM.D., is Assistant Professor of Clinical Pharmacy Practice, School of Pharmacy, University of Southern California.

Address reprint requests to Dr. Saltiel at the Cedars-Sinai Medical Center, Department of Pharmacy, 8700 Beverly Boulevard, Los Angeles, CA 90048.

This is **article 680-204-9118** in the **ASHP Continuing Education System**; it qualifies for 1.0 hour of continuing-education credit. See page 553 for learning objectives and test questions.

Since its original histologic description by von Rokitansky in 1860[1] and its naming by Sampson in 1921,[2] endometriosis—the finding of ectopic endometrial tissue—has been extensively studied. Despite advances made in the knowledge of the disease, it remains poorly understood. Its natural course is uncertain, its precise etiology is not known, its clinical presentation is variable, and treatment strategies are by no means agreed upon.

The incidence of endometriosis depends on the population and method of study (Table 1).[3-6] According to Dawood,[3] the incidence of endometriosis seems to be increasing, and this increase is both real (because of a current trend of postponing conception) and apparent (because of an increase in the number of laparoscopy procedures and an increased awareness of the disease). Perhaps 1% to 5% of all women between menarche and menopause have endometriosis, and at least 20% of those who undergo laparoscopy are so diagnosed.[4,7] Nulliparity (60–70% of all women with endometriosis) and family history are risk factors.[3,8]

Dysmenorrhea (26–63%), deep dyspareunia (12–27%), menstrual irregularities (12–14%), and infertility (20–50%) are the most common complaints in women with endometriosis.[9] Less frequently, urinary symptoms (dysuria, urgency, and hematuria) may be reported.

Although the likelihood and severity of dysmenorrhea and dyspareunia do not correlate with the severity of endometriosis, the probability of successful conception does appear to be inversely related to the severity of disease.[3,10] There appears to be an association between endometriosis and infertility: Endometriosis can be found in 15–25% of infertile women, and in women with otherwise unexplained infertility, the incidence may be as high as 80%.[9,10] Of all women with diagnosed endometriosis, 30–40% complain of infertility; this incidence is 20 times greater than that in women without endometriosis.[4,10] The rate of infertility in women with severe endometriosis is over 50%. The exact mechanism of infertility in women with endometriosis is not known; probably more than one mechanism is involved. It is generally accepted that mechanical factors play a role in infertility in women with severe endometriosis. Periovarian and peritubal adhesions or ovarian endometriomas, or both, may interfere mechanically with ovulation, ovum pickup, fertilization, or ovum transport and as a result may prevent conception. The cause or causes of infertility in women with minimal or mild endometriosis are less clear. A variety of factors associated with alterations in sexual function, ovulation, ovum transport, fertilization and implantation may be involved.[11]

Endometriosis can have a substantial economic impact on the individual patient (e.g., lost work time) and on the overall health care system. Endometriosis as a single diagnosis accounted for an estimated 582,000 hospital days in 1980.[11]

The purpose of this article is to review the incidence, pathogenesis, staging, and treatment of endometriosis, with an emphasis on pharmacologic management of this condition.

Table 1.
Incidence of Endometriosis in Various Populations[a]

Year	Population	Incidence (%)
1949	Women undergoing pelvic operations	5–15
1949	Women undergoing routine examination of the ovaries	16.8
1976–82	Symptomatic teenagers undergoing laparoscopy	47–65
1977	All women undergoing "major gynecologic procedures"	33–50
1978	All women undergoing gynecologic laparoscopies	18
1980	Women who had a first-degree relative with endometriosis	7
1980	Women who did not have a first-degree relative with endometriosis	1
1980	All menstruating women	4–17
1981	Women whose fallopian tubes were previously ligated within 4 cm of the proximal end	74
1981	Women whose fallopian tubes were previously ligated more than 4 cm from the proximal end	20
1982	All women between menarche and menopause	5
1982	Women who had elective sterilization	21
1983	All women undergoing laparoscopy	20

[a] Adapted from references 3–6.

Pathogenesis

Theories of Pathogenesis. The pathogenesis of endometriosis remains uncertain. Theories include celomic metaplasia and retrograde menstruation, heredity, direct implantation, luteinized unruptured follicle syndrome, and elevated prostaglandin levels. The major etiologic theories are celomic metaplasia and retrograde menstruation, as well as genetic factors.

According to the celomic metaplasia theory, undifferentiated celomic epithelial cells remain dormant on the peritoneal surface until the ovaries begin to function. They respond to cyclic stimulation by ovarian estrogen and progesterone in a manner similar to that of normal endometrial cells (Figure 1)[12] and eventually can be identified as definite lesions on the peritoneal surface. The longer cyclic stimulation and withdrawal persist without a break (e.g., pregnancy), the larger the lesions can become.[13] The celomic metaplasia theory can account for all sites of endometriosis.

The most widely accepted explanation of the cause of endometriosis is the retrograde flow of menstrual fluid with subsequent implantation of viable fragments within the pelvic cavity.[3] Retrograde menstruation can account for the frequent sites of endometriosis in the posterior aspects of the pelvis. Retrograde menstruation does not explain the extrapelvic sites of

Figure 1. The menstrual cycle. FSH = follicle-stimulating hormone; LH = luteinizing hormone; HCG = human chorionic gonadotropin. (Reprinted with permission from reference 12.)

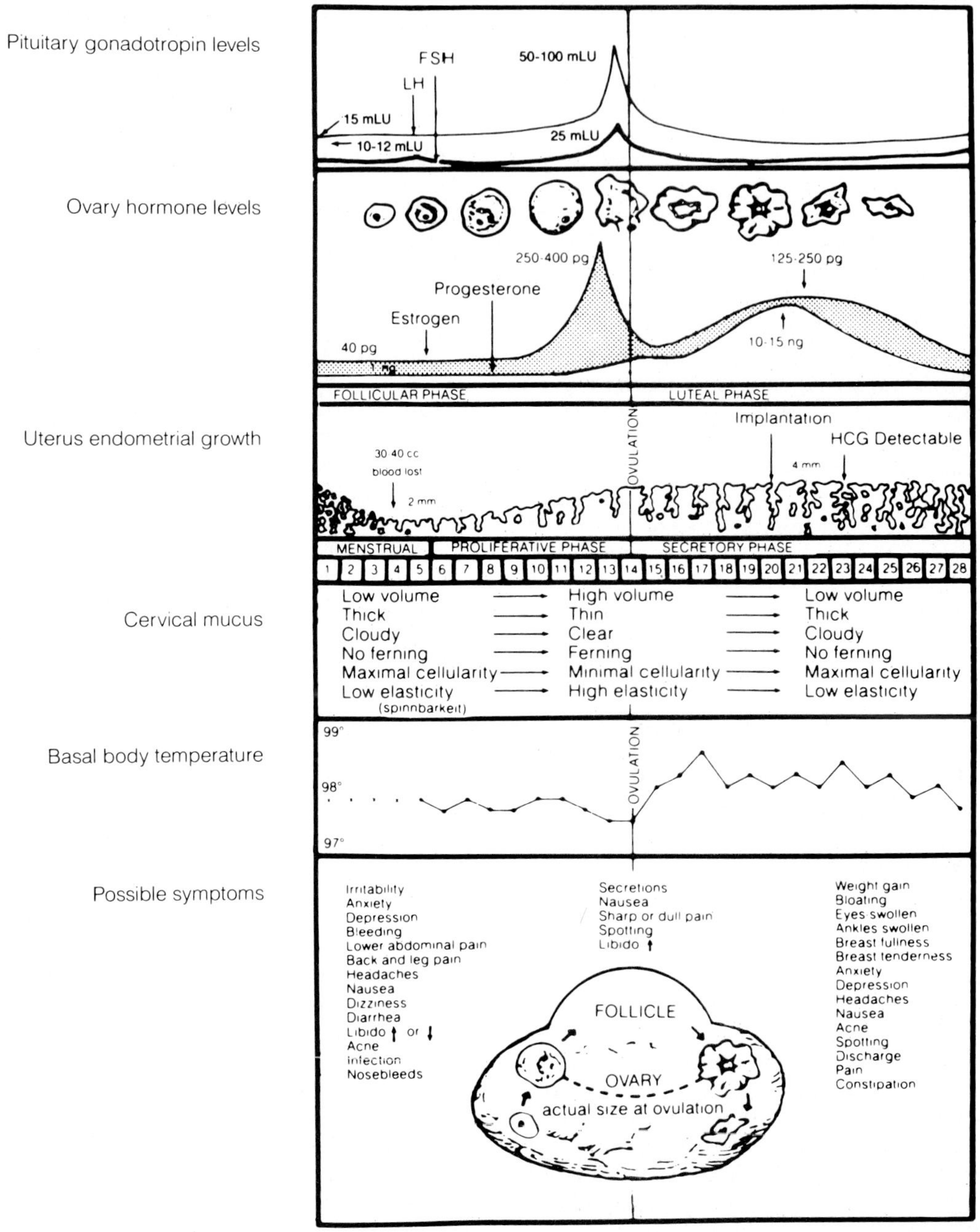

endometriosis; therefore, the most tenable etiologic theory is a combination of celomic metaplasia and retrograde menstruation. Table 2 lists the sites and frequency of extrapelvic endometriosis.

Heredity may be a factor in the development of endometriosis. Interviews of 123 women who had been treated for endometriosis showed a 5.8% incidence of endometriosis among female siblings over 18 years of age.[15] There was an 8.1% risk when the mother had endometriosis and a 7% risk when the female sibling or mother had endometriosis. In contrast, the risk of endometriosis was 1% in these women's sisters-in-law and 0.9% in their mothers-in-law.[16] Although the precise genetic mechanism is unknown, it may account for the small number of patients who have both endometriosis and a family history of the disease but not for the majority of patients who have endometriosis and a negative family history.

Pathologic Findings and Classification of Endometriosis. The gross appearance of endometriosis is variable, depending on the stage of the disease and the length of time it has existed. Minimal lesions appear as bluish-red spots, each surrounded by a ring of puckered scar tissue, scattered over the pelvic peritoneal surfaces. As a result of repeated cyclic stimulation, these small foci may grow to larger lesions

Table 2.
Sites and Frequency of Extrapelvic Endometriosis[a]

Site	Estimated Frequency (% Women with Endometriosis)
Intestine	≤12
Appendix	<1.0 to 1.4
Sigmoid	0.8
Omentum	0.6
Small intestine	0.1 to 0.2
Cervix	2.5
Rectovaginal septum	1.6
Urinary tract	0.5 to 1.0
Inguinal area	0.8
Incisional	0.2 to 0.8
Lung and pleura	51[b]

[a] Adapted from reference 14.
[b] Percentage of women with extrapelvic endometriosis.

known as endometriomas. These endometriomas may continue to grow, coalesce, and lead to the development of scar tissue and adhesions between adjacent peritoneal tissues. Ovarian involvement can vary from microscopic cysts to a large loculated structure measuring up to 10 cm in diameter.[13] Hemorrhage into an ovarian cyst or a corpus luteum cyst is termed "chocolate cyst."

The diagnosis and classification of endometriosis are based on laparoscopy. The clinical classification of endometriosis is essential for determining prognosis, selecting therapy, and assessing the result of treatment.

The American Fertility Society (AFS) classification scheme is based on a 20-point scale that grossly evaluates 15 potential areas of disease involvement to place the patient's disease into one of four stages.[3,10,13] In the staging process, the peritoneum, the ovaries, and the fallopian tubes are quantitatively assessed for endometrial tissue as well as for adhesions. The more extensive the disease, the higher the score. Stage I is referred to as minimal disease, stage II as mild disease, stage III as moderate disease, and stage IV as severe disease. It should be noted that the AFS classification was revised in 1985. The newer classification system attempts to differentiate between deep and superficial lesions and between unilateral and bilateral involvement. Thus, earlier trial results may be at variance with more recent studies because of a different patient population.

Management of Endometriosis

The management of women with endometriosis depends on the extent of the disease (i.e., the AFS classification), the severity of the symptoms, the age of the patient, and the patient's desire for future fertility. Treatment modalities include expectant management, surgery, induction of a pseudopregnancy state with hormonal therapy, or induction of a pseudomenopausal state.

Expectant Management

Expectant management, or watchful waiting, may be the most appropriate form of therapy (or nontherapy) in selected patients. For example, in women with mild to moderate endometriosis and complaints of infertility, expectant management combined with identification and correction of other infertility factors has been shown to produce pregnancy rates as high as those achieved with medical therapy or conservative surgery.[15,17-19] Indeed, 52% of women with mild disease and 25% of those with moderate disease may conceive without surgical or pharmacologic therapy.[20]

Surgery

Surgical management of endometriosis is indicated in the following situations: (1) for confirmation of the diagnosis; (2) for tubal occlusion or peritubal, pelvic, or ovarian adhesions when fertility is desired; (3) for chocolate cysts of the ovary; (4) for intractable pelvic pain unrelieved by medical therapy; and (5) in cases of failed medical therapy.[3]

The major benefit of laparoscopic cautery or laser surgery, the simplest form of surgical therapy, is that it provides treatment at the time of diagnosis, reducing the need for subsequent, more invasive surgical procedures. However, this type of surgical therapy has no effect on very small lesions (microfoci), very large lesions, and dense adhesions. In addition, treatment is frequently incomplete, and keen surgical skills are required to prevent complications.[10]

Conservative surgery is indicated in women who wish to maintain their reproductive function. Any or all of the following procedures can be performed: (1) ovarian cystectomy for chocolate cysts; (2) lysis of adhesions and salpingoplasty for tubal involvement; (3) cauterization of pelvic peritoneal lesions at noncritical sites; and (4) microsurgical techniques. Many of these procedures can be done with the laparoscope.[3] The advantage of conservative surgery is that it is effective in advanced cases of endometriosis, even when the disease is associated with adhesions. The disadvantages include a requirement of microsurgical skill, a lack of effect on microfoci, and a risk of postoperative adhesions.[10]

Definitive or complete surgery is indicated in women who do not want to maintain their reproductive function or in whom all previous medical and surgical efforts have failed. The surgery includes total hysterectomy and bilateral salpingo-oophorectomy.[3]

Definitive surgery is the only form of treatment that is curative and is not associated with recurrence. However, it does terminate reproductive function and therefore is only performed in carefully selected patients.[10] Estrogen replacement therapy can be initiated for menopausal symptoms within a few days of surgery if all endometriosis has been removed. Approximately 2% of patients may have postmenopausal endometriosis, usually in association with either endogenous estrogen sources or exogenously administered estrogens.[3]

Induction of Pseudopregnancy

Because endometrial implants (like normal endometrial tissue) are supported by ovarian hormones,[21] manipulation of these hormones is the basis for the medical treatment of endometriosis. Karnaky's use of stilbestrol in 1948[22] established the concept of ovarian suppression as a treatment for endometriosis. This concept led to the pseudopregnancy regimens first established by Kistner in 1958.[23] Hormonal therapy eliminates the repeated cyclic variations in ovarian estrogen and progesterone that stimulate periodic growth and disintegration of the ectopic endometrium. Although high-dose combination oral contraceptives were effective at relieving dysmenorrhea and pelvic pain, frequent adverse effects often precluded continued therapy. Such adverse effects included abdominal swelling and mastalgia in up to 100% of users.[24]

It was soon discovered that low-dose combination oral contraceptives were equally efficacious and were associated with a far lower frequency of adverse effects. Any combination containing 30 to 35 μg of ethinyl estradiol can be used. Treatment is started as one tablet daily and increased to two tablets daily if breakthrough bleeding occurs. The short-term goal of therapy is amenorrhea, and therapy is continued for six to nine months. Pathologically, therapy is associated with decidualization, necrobiosis, and resorption of the endometriotic tissue.[25]

Continuous progestational therapy can also be used and may be associated with fewer adverse effects than the estrogen–progestogen combinations.[24] Medroxyprogesterone acetate given orally (30–100 mg/day) or i.m. as a depot (100 mg every two weeks or 200 mg monthly) is frequently used.[24-26] More recently, gestrinone, a synthetic trienic 10-norsteroid progestin, has been investigated for the treatment of endometriosis with favorable results. Dosages ranging from 1.25 mg twice weekly to 2.5 mg three times weekly have been demonstrated to be as effective as alternative hormonal treatments.[27-30]

The adverse effects of all pseudopregnancy regimens are often problematic and include water retention, weight gain, oily skin, acne, and infrequent, mild hirsutism.[3,10] Nausea may occur in up to 40% of patients but usually subsides over a few days.[23] Breakthrough bleeding may occur in 25% of women receiving progestin therapy and may respond to the addition of ethinyl estradiol 20–30 μg daily.[3,10]

The goal of pseudopregnancy therapy is to induce an adynamic endometrium with no cyclical changes and no bleeding. While suppressing endogenous hormonal release, however, these agents may directly stimulate endometrial growth, and increased pain may be noted in the first two or three weeks.[31] Symptomatic improvement is seen in 60–94% of patients, and posttreatment pregnancy rates of 43–55% can be expected.[3,10,31] Treatment is continued for six to nine months. Most investigators have reported a recurrence rate of 5–10% annually, with a first-year recurrence rate of up to 17–18%.[3]

Thus, pseudopregnancy may be helpful as short-term therapy with possible long-term benefit in some women. This form of hormonal therapy is less costly than other forms of medical management, but the many potential complications of continuous use of combination oral contraceptives (e.g., risk of thromboembolism) must be considered before selection of pseudopregnancy therapy for endometriosis.

The use of progestational agents alone reduces the risks associated with estrogen therapy (e.g., thromboembolic disease). However, their effects on hypothalamic function and ovarian suppression are less predictable than the effects of combination therapy. Breakthrough bleeding is a major concern. The use of the depot form of medroxyprogesterone acetate, 200 mg given monthly, may be advantageous in older women not interested in becoming pregnant and in whom surgery is contraindicated. However, because prolonged posttreatment amenorrhea may occur, progestational therapy is not recommended in women who want to become pregnant.[10] Additionally, the use of high doses of medroxyprogesterone acetate has been associated with deleterious alterations in lipoprotein concentrations, including a 26% decrease in high-density-lipoprotein (HDL) cholesterol and a 12% decrease in apolipoprotein A-1.[32]

Induction of Pseudomenopause

The induction of a pseudomenopausal state with the use of oral danazol gained widespread favor in the 1970s as the medical treatment of choice in patients with endometriosis. More recently, GnRH agonists have been studied for the relief of pain and reduction of endometriotic lesions in patients with endometriosis (Tables 3 and 4). In 1982, Meldrum and his colleagues[43] demonstrated the efficacy of daily s.c. 100-μg injections of a GnRH agonist in five women with endometriosis who were treated for 28 days. The efficacy of GnRH agonists given intranasally[44-46] or s.c.[47] for the treatment of endometriosis has been further demonstrated in small series of patients treated for up to 31 weeks, with subjective and objective improvement documented in uncontrolled trials. Although several GnRH agonists have been studied for the treatment of endometriosis, this discussion will be limited to nafarelin, which is the first drug in this class to carry FDA-approved labeling for this indication. Additionally, the largest study to date compared nafarelin with danazol. None of the other GnRH agonists has been compared with nafarelin, none of the studies used as many patients as were enrolled in the nafarelin–danazol trial, and none of these drugs is labeled for use in the treatment of endometriosis.

Efficacy of Danazol. Therapy with danazol, an

Table 3.
Gonadotropin-Releasing Hormone (GnRH) Agonists Evaluated for Treatment of Endometriosis[a]

GnRH Agonist	Half-life in Humans (min)	Relative Potency[b]	Routes of Administration in Humans
Typtorelin depot (Decapeptyl, Ferring)	50	100	s.c., i.m.
Buserelin (Suprefact, Hoechst-Roussel)	75[c]	Not determined	s.c. induction, followed by intranasal dosing t.i.d.
Histrelin (Ortho)	<60	100	s.c.
Leuprolide (Lupron, Abbott, TAP)	180[d]	15	s.c., intranasal
Nafarelin (Synarel, Syntex)	240	200	Intranasal b.i.d.
Goserelin (Zoladex, ICI)	N.A.[e,f]	N.A.	s.c., i.m.

[a] Reprinted with permission from reference 33.
[b] Potency is determined by the estrus suppression test in rats and is expressed relative to that of native GnRH, which has a potency of 1 (leuprolide potency is determined by a test that measures increases in circulating luteinizing hormone in rats).
[c] Dose = 1000 μg s.c. or 500 μg i.v.
[d] Dose = 1000 μg s.c.
[e] N.A. = not available.
[f] Dose = 3.6 mg/month given as depot i.m. injection.

Table 4.
Gonadotropin-Releasing Hormone (GnRH) Agonist Regimens Studied in the Treatment of Endometriosis

Regimen	Reference
Leuprolide Acetate	
3.75 mg i.m. (depot) every 4 weeks for 20 weeks	34
0.5 mg s.c. daily for three months, followed by 3.75 mg i.m. (depot) every month for six months	37
0.5 mg s.c. daily for six months	37
3.75 mg i.m. (depot) every month for 20 weeks	41
0.5 mg s.c. daily for seven days, followed by 0.4 mg intranasally four times daily for 25 weeks	42
Buserelin (As the Acetate Salt)	
0.3 mg intranasally three times daily for 24 weeks	38
0.2 mg s.c. daily for six months	39
0.4 mg intranasally three times daily for six months	39
Goserelin	
3.6 mg s.c. (depot) every month for six months	40
[D-Trp^{6},des-Gly-NH$_{2}$^{10}] LH-RH ethylamide	
500 mg s.c. daily for one month, followed by 250 mg s.c. daily for eight months	34
[(Imbzl)-D-His^{6},Pro^{9}-NEt] GnRH	
0.1 mg s.c. daily for 24 weeks	36

isoxazol derivative of 17-α-ethinyl testosterone, suppresses the midcycle spikes in luteinizing hormone (LH) and follicle-stimulating hormone (FSH), lowers basal LH and FSH levels, reduces serum estradiol and progesterone concentrations, and results in an atrophic endometrium, like that seen during menopause.[3,10] One specific action deserves mention because it clearly is not shared by GnRH agonists. Danazol (200 mg four times daily) suppresses autoantibodies observed in the sera of 40–60% of women with endometriosis.[48,49] This is not entirely surprising because danazol is known to suppress antiplatelet antibodies when used to treat idiopathic thrombocytopenic purpura[50] and autoantibodies when used to treat systemic lupus erythematosus.[51] In one small trial, an apparent association was seen between a reduction in autoantibody concentration and fertility.[49] Five of ten patients treated with danazol conceived. Three of the five patients initially had marked elevations of more than five autoantibodies, and in all three of these patients, the autoantibody levels decreased during therapy. No such association was seen with the GnRH agonist, suggesting that danazol may be more effective than GnRH agonists to treat endometriosis and infertility associated with a high autoantibody concentration. However, these data require confirmation by other trials before formal recommendations can be made about product selection in patients with endometriosis and elevated autoantibodies.

Danazol, in dosages ranging from 100 to 800 mg daily, is associated with symptomatic improvement in 70–95% of patients[3,10,52] and with laparoscopic evidence of disease regression in 85–95% of patients. Daily dosages of less than 800 mg, however, are associated with variable results, lower pregnancy rates, and higher relapse rates.[3] In one recent retrospective trial, however, danazol therapy was clearly less effective than conservative surgery (operative laparoscopy) in producing complete disease resolution in women with minimal or mild endometriosis.[53]

Fertility rates with danazol have been quite variable and seem to depend on disease stage: Pregnancy rates have been reported to be 70–83% for women with mild disease (although in one trial, a rather dismal 26% was reported),[53] 37–73% for women with moderate disease, and 27–33% for women with severe disease.[54-57] In one trial, the use of danazol preoperatively and postoperatively was associated with a greater pregnancy rate (53%) than preoperative or postoperative therapy alone (22%).[56] Although no comparative trials have been performed, the pregnancy rates associated with danazol therapy appear to be higher than those achieved with pseudopregnancy therapy. Disease recurs in 5–23% of patients receiving danazol during the first year after treatment and in 5–9% per year thereafter.[3,54,57] However, recurrence rates as high as 30–40% have been reported.[54,55]

Efficacy of GnRH Agonists. *Physiologic Effects of GnRH.* GnRH controls pituitary secretion of LH and FSH. During the follicular phase of the menstrual cycle, GnRH is normally released in pulses every 60 to 90 minutes, with the amplitude of release increasing until ovulation. The frequency then slows markedly during the luteal phase. This pulsatile release of GnRH from the median eminence in the arcuate and periventricular nuclei of the medial basal hypothalamus stimulates anterior pituitary release of LH and FSH.[33,58] In response to GnRH stimulation during the follicular phase, FSH is released and stimulates the development of ovarian follicles, whereas the small amount of secreted LH stimulates estrogen secretion from these developing follicles (Figures 1 and 2). As serum estrogen levels increase during the follicular phase, GnRH is further stimulated, which further increases LH secretion. Subsequently, most of the developing follicles atrophy while the dominant follicle matures, producing even more estrogen. Estrogen causes endometrial growth as well as growth and maturity of the uterine glands and uterine mucosa. When estrogen levels exceed 200 pg/mL for at least 50 hours, the pituitary gland is stimulated to produce a surge of LH. This dramatic increase in LH concentrations causes the final maturation of the ovarian follicle, ovulation itself, and the formation of the corpus luteum.

After ovulation, the ovaries enter the luteal phase of the menstrual cycle. During this phase, the corpus luteum produces estrogen and progesterone. Progesterone causes thickening of the endometrium, further maturation of the uterine glands, and stimulation of the uterine glands to secrete a thick fluid to prepare for implantation. If implantation does not occur, the corpus luteum regresses with an attendant reduction in serum estrogen and progesterone levels. When hormonal levels drop, the endometrium cannot be maintained and menstruation occurs.[22,23]

Nafarelin. Nafarelin acts as a GnRH agonist by binding to the GnRH receptors on the gonadotrophs of the anterior pituitary, stimulating gonadotropin release. This initial rise in gonadotropin levels is then followed by a profound suppression of pituitary release of gonadotropins. Ovarian estrogen secretion is completely eliminated, and serum estradiol is reduced to castration levels, similar to the levels in patients who have undergone bilateral oophorectomy[43] and far lower than levels achieved with alternative forms of medical therapy for endometriosis.[59] For this reason, nafarelin therapy is sometimes referred to as medical oophorectomy. The hypogonadal state is achieved within two to six weeks of therapy (Figure 3).[9,60] The hormonal changes lead to glandular involution and stromal atrophy of endometriotic implants.[9]

Initiation of short-term nafarelin therapy results in a profound increase in FSH that persists for three weeks and an increase in LH, which remains elevated even longer. Serum estradiol levels rise rapidly, as much as ninefold, and can remain elevated for up to three weeks (Figure 4). Continued administration results in receptor desensitization or down-regulation, with reduced levels of LH, FSH, and steroid production (Figures 5 and 6).

In an uncontrolled pilot trial, Schriock and coworkers[60] assessed the benefit of six months of treatment with nafarelin (as the acetate salt) 500 µg b.i.d. intranasally in eight women with endometriosis.[60] Three of the patients had had no previous treatment for endometriosis, and five had previously received danazol (terminated at least three months before this trial). All eight women reported a complete loss of or marked decrease in pain during treatment, with substantial symptomatic relief usually occurring by week 4 and maximal relief achieved by week 12. Seven of the women who underwent repeat laparoscopy ($n = 5$) or laparotomy ($n = 2$) had decreases in their clinical staging and active disease scores after therapy. No endometrial implants were found in five of the seven patients after therapy. One patient had a single, small endometriotic implant in the cul-de-sac after treat-

Figure 2. The hypothalamic–pituitary–gonadal axis.

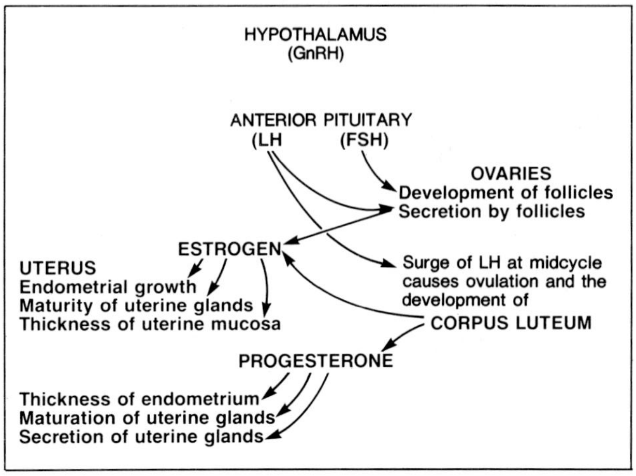

Figure 3. Mean ± S.D. basal concentrations of estradiol (E_2) in eight women with endometriosis during treatment with nafarelin (therapy begun in follicular phase of menstrual cycle). Mean estradiol concentration in postmenopausal women was 12.2 ± 4.1 µg/mL. (Reprinted with permission from reference 60.)

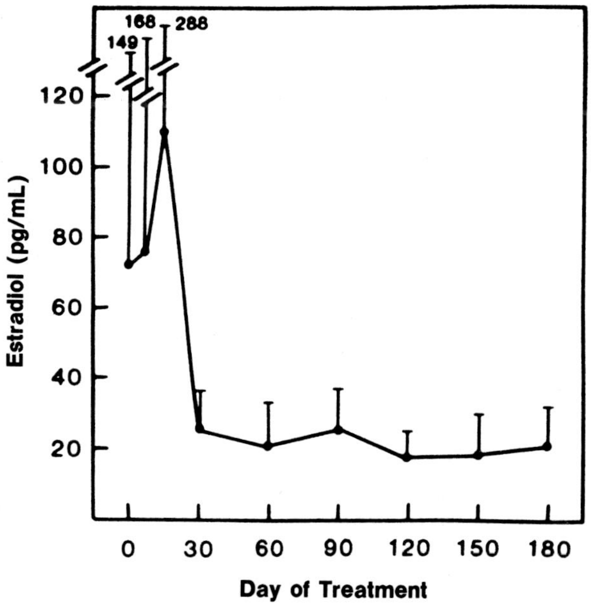

Figure 4. Mean ± S.E. serum estradiol (E_2) concentrations before and during the administration of nafarelin (as the acetate salt) 125 µg/day (n = 12), 250 µg/day (n = 8), or 1000 µg/day (n = 7). (Reprinted with permission from reference 61.)

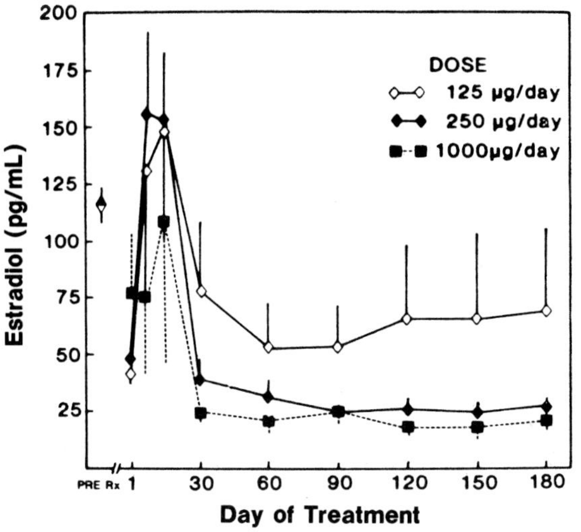

ment. The remaining patient had persistent, active disease involving one fallopian tube and was the only patient with an ovarian endometrioma. All patients experienced hot flashes during therapy. Three patients required dosage reduction (one half of the original dose) because of the severity of the hot flashes. In all three cases, the hot flashes subsided in intensity. Other adverse effects included vaginal dryness (four patients), mild transient headaches (five patients), and mild transient depression (two patients). Within three to six months after completion of the treatment course, partial and complete recurrence of dysmenorrhea occurred in four and two of the women, respectively. The mean time from discontinuation of treatment until the first ovulatory menses was 47 ± 8 days, with a range of 36 to 57 days.

In an uncontrolled trial, Brzynski and Comite[63] treated 11 women with infertility of two to eight years' duration and laparoscopic evidence of endometriosis with intranasal nafarelin (as the acetate salt) 400 µg/day (five patients) or 800 µg/day (six patients) for six months. Severity of illness, as assessed by pelvic examination, improved significantly: The AFS stage improved in 6 of the 11 patients with a complete response in 3 patients. Excluding the women who had stage IV disease, four of six patients (67%) had clinical improvement as assessed by a reduction in the AFS score, and five of six patients (83%) conceived. The major adverse effect of treatment, hot flashes, was reported in 10 women. Bone mass was not significantly reduced.

Comparison of Nafarelin with Danazol. A multicenter, randomized, double-blind study was performed comparing two doses of intranasal nafarelin with oral danazol 800 mg/day.[64] A total of 236 women with endometriosis were randomized to receive nafarelin (as the acetate salt) 200 µg (77 patients) or 400

Figure 5. Schematic of GnRH agonist-induced down-regulation of the pituitary gonadotropins luteinizing hormone (LH) and follicle-stimulating hormone (FSH) over the first 14 days of therapy. (Reprinted with permission from reference 62.)

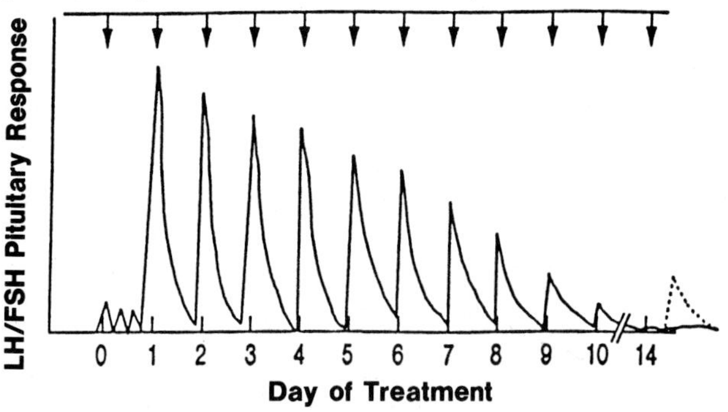

Figure 6. Schematic of GnRH agonist-induced down-regulation of the pituitary gonadotropins luteinizing hormone (LH) and follicle-stimulating hormone (FSH) over two months of therapy. (Reprinted with permission from reference 62.)

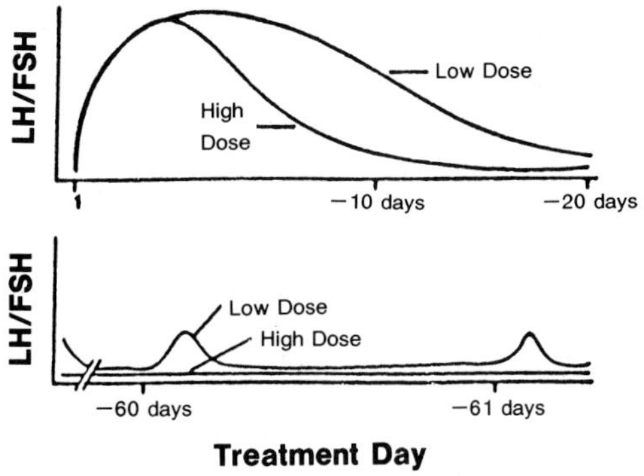

µg (79 patients) twice daily or danazol 200 mg four times daily (80 patients). Eleven patients (seven receiving nafarelin, four receiving danazol) withdrew because of hot flashes, two withdrew because of a rapid rise in aminotransferases (danazol), and one withdrew because of inefficacy of therapy (danazol). Nine patients were excluded from the analysis of efficacy for reasons not related to the study of drugs. Thus, 213 patients were evaluated. At baseline, 45% of the patients had stage III or stage IV disease according to the revised AFS classification scheme, and 42% reported severe or very severe symptoms. The groups were well matched for disease characteristics, including stage of disease, age, and nulliparous status. Fifteen percent of the women treated with the higher dose of nafarelin had a history of pelvic inflammatory disease, whereas only 4% of those receiving the lower dose of nafarelin and 6% of those receiving danazol had such a history. This was the only demographic difference among the groups.

Each treatment modality was associated with improvement in laparoscopic score, with the mean improvement being approximately 43%. The improvements were significant (p = 0.0001), but there were no significant differences among groups. In the subset of women with stage III or stage IV disease, 30–56% re-

Figure 7. Mean laparoscopic scores in 213 patients before and after treatment with nafarelin (as the acetate salt) 800 μg/day or 400 μg/day or danazol 800 mg/day. (Adapted with permission from reference 64.)

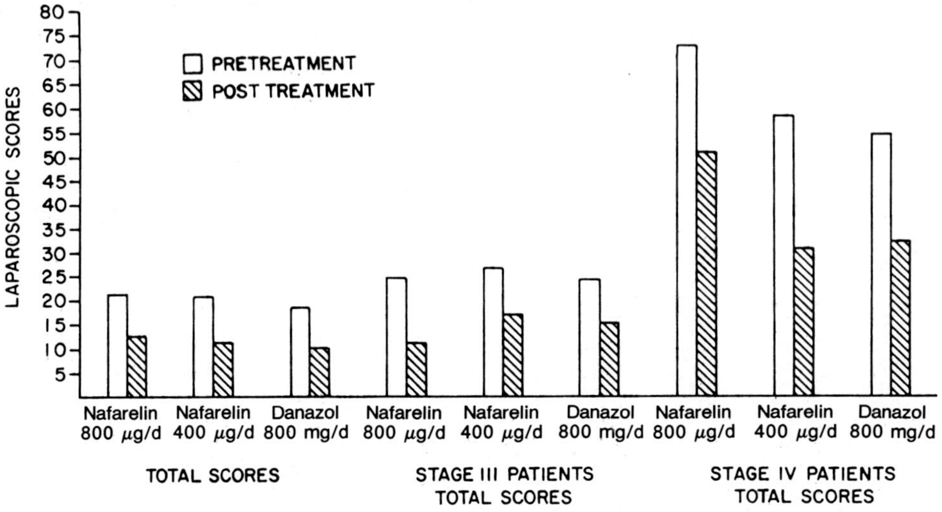

ductions in mean laparoscopic scores were found (Figure 7). Complete resolution occurred in 20% of the patients receiving nafarelin 800 μg/day, compared with 8% of patients receiving nafarelin 400 μg/day and 16% of patients receiving danazol 800 mg/day. Complete remission in patients receiving nafarelin 800 μg/day depended on the initial severity of the disease: The remission rate was 50% in those with stage I disease, 20% in those with stage II disease, 5% in those with stage III disease, and 0% in those with stage IV disease. Complete remission in patients receiving nafarelin 400 μg/day occurred in 13% of those with stage I disease, 13% of those with stage II disease, 0% of those with stage III disease, and 10% of those with stage IV disease. Complete remission figures for women receiving danazol were 26% (stage I), 25% (stage II), 5% (stage III), and 0% (stage IV). The only intergroup difference with respect to change in disease state that approached statistical significance (p = 0.06) was between nafarelin 800 μg/day and nafarelin 400 μg/day in the women with stage I disease; the higher dose was associated with an increased frequency of complete remission.

At the conclusion of the treatment course, the number of patients with stage 0 or stage I disease had increased significantly ($p < 0.001$), and the number with stage III or IV had decreased significantly ($p < 0.001$). There were no significant differences among groups. When stratum-adjusted analysis of variance was applied, differences in response to treatment between the group receiving nafarelin 800 μg/day and the group receiving nafarelin 400 μg/day ($p = 0.02$) approached the required significance level of 0.016 for multiple testing.

Symptomatology improved rapidly in all three treatment groups within the first month, with more than 80% reporting no symptoms or mild ones. The changes were significant ($p = 0.001$), with no significant differences among groups. Six months after the conclusion of the treatment course, 202 of the patients were evaluated for symptoms. Of these, 73% and 77% of those who took 400 μg and 800 μg of nafarelin, respectively, and 78% of those who took danazol still reported no or only mild symptoms of endometriosis. No patient reported very severe symptoms, and only 2–3% of patients reported severe symptoms. There were no significant differences in the rate of clinical relapse among any of the groups.

Of the 149 patients who attempted to become pregnant, 58% succeeded. Of those followed for 12 months after therapy, 52% and 30% of the patients receiving the higher and lower dose of nafarelin, respectively, and 36% of those receiving danazol were successful. The differences among the treatment groups were not significant. The incidence of weight gain and edema was greater in patients receiving danazol ($p \leq 0.001$).

Adverse Effects of Therapy. *Danazol.* A broad range of adverse effects, often more annoying than hazardous, are associated with danazol use in more than 85% of women receiving the drug.[43,65] These can be divided into androgenic effects, antiestrogenic effects, and idiopathic effects (Table 5). The most frequent adverse effect of danazol is weight gain. Ten-pound weight gains are common; however, it is not uncommon for women to gain 20 to 30 pounds while receiving danazol therapy.[66-68] Weight gain is most rapid in the first two months of therapy and may plateau by the fourth month. The weight gain is reversible after discontinuation of danazol therapy.[31] Despite the frequency of these adverse effects, only 3–7% of women require discontinuation of therapy.[57,66]

Danazol in dosages of 600 to 800 mg/day has demonstrated negative effects on the plasma lipoprotein profile, including a 14–41% increase in low-density-lipoprotein (LDL) cholesterol and a 45–53% decrease in HDL cholesterol. These effects are manifested after two to four weeks of treatment and are reversible within four to eight weeks after discontinuation of therapy.[32,68-70] Other adverse effects noted with danazol therapy include reductions in apolipoproteins A-1 (29%) and A-2 (12%) and a 17% increase in apolipoprotein B over a six-month course.[32] Patients who receive long-term or repeated courses of danazol and develop adverse effects in their serum lipid profiles may be at increased risk of cardiovascular complications.

The usual dosage of danazol is 800 mg/day, administered four times daily, generally for a six-month to nine-month period. Lower dosages, such as 400–600 mg/day, can sometimes be effective in relieving symptoms and are often attempted to reduce the incidence or severity of adverse effects. However, these lower dosages are also associated with lower fertility rates and higher rates of disease recurrence.[3,31]

Nafarelin. The safety and tolerability of nafarelin have been determined from review of approximately 267 patients in clinical trials.[60,61,63,64,68,71] In general, nafarelin is well tolerated, with relatively few patients requiring discontinuation of therapy or dosage reduction because of adverse effects. Hot flashes, which are related to estradiol suppression, are the most commonly reported adverse effect attributable to nafarelin therapy in patients being treated for endometriosis. This effect appears to be dose dependent.

In the multicenter trial comparing nafarelin (as the acetate salt) 800 µg/day and 400 µg/day with danazol 800 mg/day, hot flashes were the predominant adverse effect associated with both forms of therapy.[64] Hot flashes were reported in 90% of those receiving nafarelin; the hot flashes were deemed to be acceptable in 80% to 90% of the women. Hot flashes were also reported in 91% to 100% of women in other studies,[60,63] necessitating dosage reduction from 1000 µg/day to 500 µg/day in 37.5% of the patients in one trial.[60] The dose relationship of this phenomenon was made even more clear by results of a dose-finding study by Monroe.[61] A total of 32 patients were given one of three dosages of nafarelin intranasally for six months. Hot flashes were reported in 35%, 65%, and 100% of women receiving 125 µg/day, 250 µg/day, and 1000 µg/day, respectively. It appears that the incidence and severity of hot flashes can be greatly diminished by the concurrent use of an oral progestin such as norethindrone in dosages of up to 3.5 mg/day.[72] However, this benefit must be weighed against the negative effects of progestins on serum lipid profiles.

Other symptoms of hypoestrogenism, including vaginal dryness, superficial dyspareunia, and decreased libido, have been reported in patients receiving nafarelin therapy.[58,64] Vaginal dryness was reported in four of eight women receiving 1000 µg/day in one study[60] and in two of eight women receiving 1000 µg/day in another trial.[61] Headache, emotional lability, and insomnia have also been reported.[58,60,64] In the multicenter trial, these three adverse effects were reported in approximately 19%, 15%, and 8%, respectively, of the patients receiving nafarelin.[64] Weight

Table 5.
Adverse Reactions to Danazol 800 mg/day[a]

Adverse Effects	% Patients Reporting Adverse Effect
Androgenic	
Acne	17–20
Edema	6
Weight gain (5–10 kg)	5–55
Hirsutism	6–20
Voice changes	3
Oily skin	3
Antiestrogenic	
Flushes and sweats	15
Uterine spotting	10
Decreased breast size	5–30
Change in libido	5
Atrophic vaginitis	3
Idiopathic	
Gastrointestinal disturbance	8
Weakness, dizziness	8
Muscle aches or cramps	4
Skin rashes	3
Headaches	2

[a] Adapted with permission from reference 3.

gain, edema, and myalgias have been reported infrequently[64] or not at all[60,63] in trials of nafarelin.

An unexpected finding in three clinical trials of nafarelin in patients with endometriosis was a fall in the total polymorphonuclear leukocyte count.[60,61,73] In one trial, three transient episodes of reduced polymorphonuclear leukocyte count were recorded.[73] In each of two trials, the leukocyte cell count remained low in one patient after discontinuation of therapy, despite a negative workup.[60,61] In one of these studies, two of three groups receiving nafarelin had statistically significant decreases in mean neutrophil count.[61] In neither study, however, was there an increased susceptibility to infection. Thus, reports of leukopenia may represent a laboratory aberration.

The effects of nafarelin on bone metabolism are controversial. Several studies of the effects of GnRH agonists on bone metabolism have produced conflicting results. Because prolonged periods of hypoestrogenism, including the postmenopausal period, are associated with bone calcium resorption, loss of bone mineral content, and the development of osteoporosis, several authors have addressed this concern in studies with GnRH analogues. GnRH therapy is associated with increases in urinary calcium excretion to postmenopausal levels.[43,44] Tummon and coworkers[74] reported that six months of therapy with danazol or GnRH therapy did not change vertebral (L1-L4) bone mineral content as measured by photon absorptiometry,[74] whereas Cann et al.[75] reported that nafarelin in daily doses of 400 µg to 800 µg was associated with a 6.9–7.4% decrease in vertebral mineral density as quantitated by computed axial tomography, with no change in cortical bone mass. Most recently, Johansen and her coinvestigators,[71] using single and dual photon absorptiometry to measure bone mass in the fore-

Table 6.
Costs of Endometriosis Treatment Regimens

Treatment Regimen	Average Wholesale Price (AWP) per Month of Treatment ($)[a]
Ethinyl estradiol 35 μg plus norethindrone 1 mg (Norinyl 1/35, Syntex) orally once daily	18.48 (28 days)
Medroxyprogesterone acetate (generic) 30 mg orally once daily	21.20
Medroxyprogesterone acetate (Depo-Provera, Upjohn[b]) 200 mg i.m. monthly	13.37
Nafarelin (as the acetate salt) (Synarel, Syntex) 200 μg intranasally twice daily	235.00
Danazol (generic, Rugby) 200 mg orally four times daily	211.26
Danazol (Danocrine, Winthrop) 200 mg orally four times daily	245.02
Leuprolide acetate[c] (Lupron, TAP) 3.75 mg i.m. monthly	315.00
Goserelin (Zoladex, ICI) 3.6 mg s.c. every 28 days	318.75

[a] All costs are AWP per updated *American Druggist Blue Book* (January 29, 1991).
[b] 100 mg/mL; 5-mL vial costs $433.43.
[c] If one half of a 7.5-mg vial is used, the cost would be $196.88.

arm and spine, respectively, demonstrated that six months of therapy with nafarelin 400 μg/day resulted in a 2–6% reduction in all bone mass measurements.[71] These alterations are comparable to those found in breast-feeding women up to six months postpartum.[76] In both trials the alterations in bone mass were fully reversible within six months after discontinuation of therapy.[71,75] Therefore, bone mass alterations may be clinically important only in women being treated continuously or repeatedly with nafarelin.

Surrey and colleagues[72] studied the concurrent use of a progestin with a GnRH agonist to determine whether the progestin diminished the adverse effect of GnRH on bone loss. In their noncontrolled trial, the use of norethindrone in daily doses of up to 3.5 mg with a GnRH agonist for six months was associated with no cortical bone loss in the distal one third of the radius as assessed by single photon absorptiometry, but was associated with some bone loss (5.6%) in the lumbar spine as assessed by quantitative computed tomography. The authors speculated that higher dosages of norethindrone may abolish bone loss associated with GnRH agonist therapy and should be seriously considered in the treatment of women with endometriosis.[72] Improvements in pain and AFS classification scores were similar in patients receiving combination therapy and historical controls who received GnRH agonist therapy alone. In another trial, Riis and colleagues[77] demonstrated that patients who concurrently received nafarelin with norethindrone 1.2 mg/day had no bone loss (except at the distal forearm) compared with untreated controls, whereas therapy with nafarelin alone was associated with 2–6% bone loss.

According to the package insert for nafarelin, "Mean total vertebral mass, re-examined by dual photon absorptiometry six months after completion of treatment, was 1.4% below pretreatment levels. Since studies have not been completed for more than six months of therapy, the manufacturer further recommends that retreatment cannot be recommended since safety data beyond six months are not available."[78]

The serum alkaline phosphatase level may increase with nafarelin therapy but generally not above the upper limit of normal.[33,71] Unlike danazol, nafarelin is not associated with adverse alterations in serum lipoproteins,[33,68] although one study demonstrated a 16% increase in total cholesterol and a 23% increase in LDL cholesterol with no change in HDL cholesterol.[71]

Cost of Medical Therapy

Table 6 shows the most current *American Druggist Blue Book* average wholesale prices of one month of treatment with nafarelin, danazol, leuprolide, goserelin, medroxyprogesterone acetate, or ethinyl estradiol–norethindrone.

Patient Information

Nafarelin is commercially available as an intranasal spray with each spray containing 200 μg. Patient instruction is key to optimal use. A nafarelin demonstration kit is available from Syntex Laboratories. In addition to specific instructions regarding the use of the nasal inhalation unit, the potential adverse effects of nafarelin therapy should be described to the patient (Table 7). The patient should be warned about nasal stinging, hot flashes, and vaginal dryness that may occur during therapy. It should be made clear that these reactions are not dangerous, although they may be annoying. Patients should be reassured that these effects are reversible once the course of therapy is completed. Compliance with the nafarelin regimen should be reinforced. Additionally, the patient will need to be told that her menstrual cycle should restart within five to eight weeks after she completes the course of nafarelin therapy. The safe use of nafarelin during pregnancy has not been established; therefore, patients should use a nonhormonal method of contraception concurrently.[78] If a patient becomes pregnant during treatment with nafarelin, she should discontinue treatment and consult her physician.[78] In addition, patients with intercurrent rhinitis that requires the use of a topical nasal decongestant should be advised to use the decongestant at least 30 minutes after nafarelin administration to decrease the possibility of

Table 7.
Patient Instructions for Intranasal Administration of Nafarelin

1. Gently clear your nasal passages by blowing your nose before using nafarelin.
2. After removing the dust cap, insert the tip of the container into one nostril.
3. Tilt your head forward slightly, keeping the bottle upright.
4. Close the other nostril and squeeze container gently while you inhale through your nose. Inhale through your nose while you squeeze and for several seconds thereafter.
5. Relax and breathe out through your mouth.
6. You may experience some stinging in your nose. This effect should not be severe and may diminish over the course of therapy.
7. Hot flashes are common with this medication. These occurrences are not dangerous but may be uncomfortable. If they are bothersome to you, contact your pharmacist or physician.
8. Vaginal dryness may occur during therapy. If this occurs and disrupts intercourse, you may try a water-based lubricant, such as K-Y Jelly. If intercourse is still uncomfortable, contact your pharmacist or physician.
9. After the course of therapy prescribed by your physician (usually six months), your usual menstrual cycle should begin within five to eight weeks.
10. The manufacturer recommends that a nonhormonal method of contraception be used concurrently with nafarelin therapy.

reducing nafarelin absorption.[78] Similarly, patients started on danazol or oral contraceptives should be advised of the potential adverse effects of these agents (see discussions above).

Guidelines for Drug Selection

Based on the preceding discussion, it is apparent that GnRH agonists are the medical treatment of choice for women with endometriosis. They are as effective as danazol or oral contraceptive agents and cause fewer adverse reactions. In selecting a GnRH agonist, it should be kept in mind that nafarelin is easy to use and gives patients independence from monthly office visits and i.m. injections, but it does require patient education because of its intranasal formulation. For patients in whom poor compliance is anticipated, the use of i.m. depot leuprolide should be considered. If financial considerations are overriding, the use of oral contraceptives may be a reasonable first step.

Conclusion

Endometriosis affects a substantial percentage of women, producing pain as well as infertility. Medical management of endometriosis can relieve the patient's symptoms, reduce the size and number of endometriotic lesions, and improve fertility.

Management of the patient with endometriosis depends on the extent of disease, the severity of symptoms, the patient's age, and her desire for future fertility. Pharmacologic treatment includes induction of a pseudopregnancy state with hormonal therapy or induction of a pseudomenopausal state with either danazol or a GnRH agonist.

The GnRH agonists may replace danazol as the treatment of choice in patients with endometriosis because of their favorable dosage schedule and decreased incidence of adverse effects.

References

1. Von Rokitansky C. Ueber uterusdrusen-neubildung in uterus and ovarialsarcomen. *Zkk Gesellsch d Aerzte zu Wien*. 1860; 37:577. Cited in: Ridley JH. The histogenesis of endometriosis: a review of facts and fancies. *Obstet Gynecol Surv*. 1968; 23:1-35.
2. Sampson JA. Perforating hemorrhagic (chocolate) cysts of the ovary, their importance and especially their relation to pelvic adenomas of the endometrial type. *Arch Surg*. 1921; 3:245-323.
3. Dawood MY. Endometriosis. In: Gold JJ, Josimovich JB, eds. Gynecologic endocrinology. New York: Plenum; 1987:387-404.
4. Booker MW. Endometriosis. *Br J Hosp Med*. 1988; 39 (May):440-5.
5. Ranney B. Etiology, prevention, and inhibition of endometriosis. *Clin Obstet Gynecol*. 1980; 23:875-80.
6. Simpson JL, Elias S, Malinak LR et al. Heritable aspects of endometriosis. *Am J Obstet Gynecol*. 1980; 137:327-31.
7. Schneider GT. Endometriosis: an update. In: Studd J, ed. Progress in obstetrics and gynecology. Edinburgh: Churchill Livingstone; 1983:246-56.
8. Luciano AA, Pitkin RM. Endometriosis: approaches to diagnosis and treatment. *Surg Annu*. 1984; 16:297-312.
9. Hurst BS, Rock JA. Endometriosis: pathophysiology, diagnosis, and treatment. *Obstet Gynecol Surv*. 1989; 44:297-304.
10. Dmowski WP. Endometriosis. In: Glass RH, ed. Office gynecology. Baltimore: Williams & Wilkins; 1987:317-36.
11. National Center for Health Statistics, McCarthy E. Inpatient utilization of short-stay hospitals by diagnosis: United States, 1980. Hyattsville, MD: National Center for Health Statistics, 1982; DHHS publication no. (PHS) 83-1735. (Vital and health statistics; series 13: Data from the National Health Survey, no. 74).
12. Hatcher RA, Stewart GK, Stewart F et al. Contraceptive technology 1986–87. 13th ed. New York: Irvington Publishers; 1986.
13. Mattox JH. Endometriosis. In: Wilson JR, Carrington ER, eds. Obstetrics and gynecology. 8th ed. St. Louis: Mosby; 1987:122-32.
14. Markham SM, Carpenter SE, Rock JA. Extrapelvic endometriosis. *Obstet Gynecol Clin North Am*. 1989; 16:193-219.
15. Schenken RS, Malinak LR. Conservative surgery versus expectant management for the infertile patient with mild endometriosis. *Fertil Steril*. 1982; 37:183-6.
16. Simpson JL, Elias S, Malinak LR et al. Heritable aspects of endometriosis. I. Genetic studies. *Am J Obstet Gynecol*. 1980; 137:327-9.
17. Portuondo JA, Echanojauregui AD, Herran C et al. Early conception in patients with untreated mild endometriosis. *Fertil Steril*. 1983; 39:22-5.
18. Schmidt CL. Endometriosis: a reappraisal of pathogenesis and treatment. *Fertil Steril*. 1985; 44:157-73.
19. Hull ME, Moghissi KS, Magyar DM et al. Comparison of different treatment modalities of endometriosis in infertile women. *Fertil Steril*. 1987; 47:40-4.
20. Olive DL, Stohs GF, Metzger DA et al. Expectant management and hydrotubations in the treatment of endometriosis-associated infertility. *Fertil Steril*. 1985; 44:35-41.
21. DiZerega GS, Barber DL, Hodgen GD. Endometriosis: role of ovarian steroids in initiation, maintenance, and suppression. *Fertil Steril*. 1980; 33:649-53.
22. Karnaky KJ. The use of stilbestrol for endometriosis. *South*

Med J. 1948; 41:1109-11.
23. Kistner RW. The use of progestins in the treatment of endometriosis. *Am J Obstet Gynecol.* 1958; 75:264-78.
24. Metzger DA, Luciano AA. Hormonal therapy of endometriosis. *Obstet Gynecol Clin North Am.* 1989; 16:105-22.
25. Moghissi KS. Pseudopregnancy induced by estrogen-progestogen or progestogens alone in the treatment of endometriosis. *Prog Clin Biol Res.* 1990; 323:221-32.
26. Kauppila AJI, Telimaa S, Ronnberg L. Steroidal drugs in endometriosis. *Acta Obstet Gynecol Scand Suppl.* 1989; 150:7-13.
27. Cooke ID, Thomas EJ. The medical treatment of mild endometriosis. *Acta Obstet Gynecol Scand Suppl.* 1989; 150:27-30.
28. Venturini PL, Bertolini S, Brunenghi MCM et al. Endocrine, metabolic, and clinical effects of gestrinone in women with endometriosis. *Fertil Steril.* 1989; 52:589-95.
29. Hornstein MD, Gleason RE, Barbieri RL. A randomized double-blind prospective trial of two doses of gestrinone in the treatment of endometriosis. *Fertil Steril.* 1990; 53:237-41.
30. Fedele L, Bianchi S, Viezzoli T et al. Gestrinone versus danazol in the treatment of endometriosis. *Fertil Steril.* 1989; 51:781-5.
31. Raible MD. Pathophysiology and treatment of endometriosis. *Am J Hosp Pharm.* 1981; 38:1696-701.
32. Telimaa S, Penttila I, Puolakka J et al. Circulating lipid and lipoprotein concentrations during danazol and high-dose medroxyprogesterone acetate therapy of endometriosis. *Fertil Steril.* 1989; 52:31-5.
33. Henzl MR. Gonadotropin-releasing hormone (GnRH) agonists in the management of endometriosis: a review. *Clin Obstet Gynecol.* 1988; 31:840-56.
34. Dlugi AM, Miller JD, Knittle J et al. Lupron depot (leuprolide acetate for depot suspension) in the treatment of endometriosis: a randomized, placebo-controlled, double-blind study. *Fertil Steril.* 1990; 54:419-27.
35. Dupont A, Dupont P, Belanger A et al. Hormonal and biochemical changes during treatment of endometriosis with the luteinizing hormone-releasing hormone (LH-RH) agonist [D-Trp^6, des-Gly-NH_2^{10}] LH-RH ethylamide. *Fertil Steril.* 1990; 54:227-32.
36. Cedars MI, Lu JK, Medrum DR et al. Treatment of endometriosis with a long-acting gonadotropin-releasing hormone agonist plus medroxyprogesterone acetate. *Obstet Gynecol.* 1990; 75:641-5.
37. Rivlin ME, Miller JD, Kreuger RP et al. Leuprolide acetate in the management of ureteral obstruction caused by endometriosis. *Obstet Gynecol.* 1990; 75:532-8.
38. Franssen AMH, Kauer FM, Chada DR et al. Endometriosis: treatment with gonadotropin-releasing hormone agonist buserelin. *Fertil Steril.* 1989; 51:401-8.
39. Dmowski WP, Radwanska E, Binor Z et al. Ovarian suppression induced with buserelin or danazol in the management of endometriosis: a randomized comparative trial. *Fertil Steril.* 1989; 51:395-400.
40. Tummon IS, Pepping ME, Bing Z et al. A randomized, prospective comparison of endocrine changes induced with intranasal leuprolide or danazol for the treatment of endometriosis. *Fertil Steril.* 1989; 51:390-4.
41. Dlugi AM, Miller JD, Knittle J et al. Lupron depot (leuprolide acetate for depot suspension) in the treatment of endometriosis: a randomized placebo-controlled, double-blind study. *Fertil Steril.* 1990; 54:419-27.
42. Venturini PL, Fasce V, Constantini S et al. Treatment of endometriosis with goserelin depot, a long-acting gonadotropin-releasing hormone agonist analog: endocrine and clinical results. *Fertil Steril.* 1990; 54:1021-7.
43. Meldrum VR, Chang RJ, Lu J et al. "Medical ovariectomy" using a long-acting GnRH agonist: a possible new approach in the treatment of endometriosis. *J Clin Endocrinol Metab.* 1982; 54:1081-3.
44. Lemay A, Sandow J, Bureau M et al. Prevention of follicular maturation in endometriosis by subcutaneous administration of luteinizing hormone-releasing hormone agonist started in the luteal phase. *Fertil Steril.* 1988; 49:410-7.
45. Lemay A, Quesnel G. Potential new treatment of endometriosis: reversible inhibition of pituitary-ovarian function by chronic intranasal administration of a luteinizing hormone-releasing hormone (LHRH) agonist. *Fertil Steril.* 1982; 38:376-9.
46. Pring DW, Maresh M, Fraser AC. Luteinizing hormone-releasing hormone agonist in women with endometriosis. *Br Med J.* 1983; 287:1718-9.
47. Lemay A, Maheux R, Foure N et al. Reversible hypogonadism induced by luteinizing hormone-releasing hormone (LHRH) agonist (buserelin) as a new therapeutic approach for endometriosis. *Fertil Steril.* 1984; 41:863-9.
48. Gleicher N, El-Roeiy A, Confino E et al. Autoantibodies in reproductive failure: I. Is endometriosis an autoimmune disease? *Obstet Gynecol.* 1987; 70:115-9.
49. El-Roeiy A, Dmowski WP, Gleicher N et al. Danazol but not gonadotropin-releasing hormone agonists suppresses autoantibodies in endometriosis. *Fertil Steril.* 1988; 50:864-71.
50. Ahn YS, Harrington WJ, Simon SR et al. Danazol for the treatment of idiopathic thrombocytopenic purpura. *N Engl J Med.* 1983; 308:1396-7.
51. Agnello V, Pariser K, Gell J. Preliminary observations on danazol therapy of systemic lupus erythematosus: effects on DNA antibodies, thrombocytopenia and complement. *J Rheumatol.* 1983; 10:682-5.
52. Mandanes AE, Farber M. Danazol. *Ann Intern Med.* 1982; 96:625-30.
53. Fayez JA, Collazo LM, Vernon C. Comparison of different modalities of treatment for minimal and mild endometriosis. *Am J Obstet Gynecol.* 1988; 159:927-32.
54. Dmowski WP, Cohen MR. Antigonadotropin (danazol) in the treatment of endometriosis: evaluation of posttreatment fertility and three-year follow-up data. *Am J Obstet Gynecol.* 1978; 130:41-8.
55. Puelo JG, Hammond CB. Conservative therapy of endometriosis externa: the effects of danazol therapy. *Fertil Steril.* 1983; 40:164-9.
56. Madelenat P, Dubuisson JB, Foulot H et al. Severe endometriosis. *Contrib Gynecol Obstet.* 1987; 16:356-64.
57. Daniell JF, Christianson C. Combined laparoscopic surgery and danazol therapy for pelvic endometriosis. *Fertil Steril.* 1981; 35:521-5.
58. Erickson LD, Ory SJ. GnRH analogues in the treatment of endometriosis. *Obstet Gynecol Clin North Am.* 1989; 16:123-45.
59. Meldrum DR, Partridge WM, Karow WG et al. Hormonal effects of danazol and medical oophorectomy in endometriosis. *Obstet Gynecol.* 1983; 62:480-5.
60. Schriock E, Monroe SE, Henzl M et al. Treatment of endometriosis with a potent agonist of gonadotropin-releasing hormone (nafarelin). *Fertil Steril.* 1985; 44:583-8.
61. Monroe SE, Blumenfeld Z, Andreyko JL et al. Dose-dependent inhibition of pituitary-ovarian function during administration of a gonadotropin-releasing hormone agonistic analog (nafarelin). *J Clin Endocrinol Metab.* 1986; 63:1334-41.
62. Hodgen GD. General applications of GnRH agonists in gynecology: past, present, and future. *Obstet Gynecol Surv.* 1989; 44:293-6.
63. Brzynski RG, Comite F. Nafarelin, an intranasal GnRH analog, for infertility associated with endometriosis. Paper presented at the 43rd Annual Meeting of the American Fertility Society. Reno, NV: 1987 Sep 30.
64. Henzl MR, Corson SL, Moghissi K et al. Administration of nasal nafarelin as compared with oral danazol for endometriosis. A multicenter double-blind comparative clinical trial. *N Engl J Med.* 1988; 318:485-9.
65. Barbieri RL, Evans S, Kistner RW. Danazol in the treatment of endometriosis: analysis of 100 cases with a 4-year follow-up. *Fertil Steril.* 1982; 37:737-46.
66. Buttram VC, Reiter RC, Ward S. Treatment of endometriosis with danazol: report of a 6-year prospective study. *Fertil Steril.* 1985; 43:353-60.

67. Biberoglu KO, Behrman SJ. Dosage aspects of danazol therapy in endometriosis: short-term and long-term effectiveness. *Am J Obstet Gynecol.* 1981; 139:645-54.
68 Burry KA, Patton PE, Illingsworth DR. Metabolic changes during medical treatment of endometriosis: nafarelin acetate versus danazol. *Am J Obstet Gynecol.* 1989; 160:1454-61.
69. Fahraeus L, Larsson U, Ljunberg S et al. Profound alterations of the lipoprotein metabolism during danazol treatment in premenopausal women. *Fertil Steril.* 1984; 42:52-7.
70. Dlugi AM, Rufo S, D'Amico JF et al. A comparison of the effects of buserelin versus danazol on plasma lipoproteins during treatment of pelvic endometriosis. *Fertil Steril.* 1988; 49:913-6.
71. Johansen JS, Riis BJ, Hassager C et al. The effect of gonadotropin-releasing hormone agonist analog (nafarelin) on bone metabolism. *J Clin Endocrinol.* 1988; 67:701-6.
72. Surrey ES, Gambone JC, Lu JKH et al. The effects of combining norethindrone with a gonadotropin-releasing hormone agonist in the treatment of symptomatic endometriosis. *Fertil Steril.* 1990; 53:620-6.
73. Jacobs LA, Thie JL, Fields CS et al. Treatment of endometriosis with the GnRH agonist nafarelin acetate (NA). Paper presented at the annual meeting of the American Fertility Society. Reno, NV: 1987 Sep 29.
74. Tummon IS, Ali A, Pepping ME et al. Bone mineral density in women with endometriosis before and during ovarian suppression with gonadotropin-releasing hormone agonists or danazol. *Fertil Steril.* 1988; 49:792-6.
75. Cann CE, Henzl M, Burry K et al. Reversible bone loss is produced by the GnRH agonist nafarelin. In: Cohn DV, Martin TJ, Meunier PJ, eds. Calcium regulation and bone metabolism: basic and clinical aspects. New York: Elsevier; 1987:123-7.
76. Hayslip CC, Klein TA, Wray L et al. The effects of lactation on bone mineral content in healthy postpartum women. *Obstet Gynecol.* 1989; 73:588-92.
77. Riis BJ, Christiansen C, Johansen JS et al. Is it possible to prevent bone loss in young women treated with luteinizing hormone-releasing hormone agonists? *J Clin Endocrinol Metab.* 1990; 70:920-2.
78. Syntex Laboratories, Inc. Synarel product information. Palo Alto, CA; 1990 Mar.

Research

Pharmacokinetics and pharmacodynamics of glyburide in young and elderly nondiabetic adults

TERRY L. SCHWINGHAMMER, EDWARD J. ANTAL, RENEÉ T. KUBACKA, MARY E. HACKIMER, AND JANN M. JOHNSTON

Abstract: The pharmacokinetics and pharmacodynamics of glyburide were studied in elderly and young nondiabetic adults.

Healthy nondiabetic men and women 18–40 years of age (young subjects) and 60–85 years of age (elderly subjects) were recruited. After an overnight fast, the subjects were given a baseline glucose tolerance test (GTT). The next day, again after a fast, each subject was given a 5-mg oral tablet of glyburide, and the GTT was performed one hour later. Serum glucose, serum insulin, and plasma glyburide concentrations were determined.

Twenty elderly (mean ± S.D. age, 65.7 ± 5.3 years) male (n = 10) and female (n = 10) volunteers and 15 young (22.3 ± 4.5 years) male volunteers were enrolled. Compared with the young subjects, the elderly subjects had slower glyburide absorption, as determined from a lower peak plasma concentration and smaller area under the plasma concentration–time curve from zero to four hours (AUC_{0-4}). The elderly subjects also had a lower glyburide elimination rate constant and higher volume of distribution and a 52% higher free fraction. There was no difference in the glyburide AUC_{0-24} or $AUC_{0-\infty}$ or in oral clearance between the groups. The elderly group had greater increases in serum glucose and insulin concentrations after the baseline GTT. After glyburide administration, the elderly group had a smaller fractional decrease in the glucose AUC_{0-3} from the baseline GTT result than the young subjects. Linear regression analysis of the relationship between the fractional change in glucose concentration and the glyburide AUC_{0-4} showed significantly different slopes between the two groups.

The aging process appears to affect the pharmacokinetics and pharmacodynamics of glyburide.

Index terms: Absorption; Age; Antidiabetic agents; Blood levels; Drugs, body distribution; Excretion; Glyburide; Pharmacodynamics; Pharmacokinetics
Clin Pharm. 1991; 10:532-8

The prevalence of type II diabetes mellitus has been reported to range from 2% in persons 20 to 44 years of age to as high as 17.7% in those between 65 and 74.[1] Although proper weight control and exercise are the preferred forms of therapy initially, oral hypoglycemic agents may be added for patients whose plasma glucose levels do not adequately respond to those measures.[2] However, the physiological changes that accompany aging may affect the disposition of and response to oral hypoglycemics. Decreased hepatic metabolism and renal function in the elderly may impede drug elimination and prolong the hypoglycemic effect.[3] The reduced serum albumin concentrations consistently reported in the elderly may result in an increased free fraction of highly protein-bound drugs like the sulfonylureas.[4,5] An increase in adipose tissue mass relative to total body weight in the aging person may result in an increased volume of distribution of lipid-soluble drugs.[4] In addition to their vulnerability to pharmacokinetic changes, elderly patients have been reported to be particularly susceptible to sulfonylurea-induced hypoglycemia, even in the absence of identifiable contributing factors such as impaired function of excretory organs.[6,7] A change in sensitivity

TERRY L. SCHWINGHAMMER, PHARM.D., is Associate Professor of Pharmacy and Therapeutics, School of Pharmacy, University of Pittsburgh (UP), Pittsburgh, PA. EDWARD J. ANTAL, PH.D., is Director, Clinical Pharmacokinetics, The Upjohn Company, Kalamazoo, MI. RENEÉ T. KUBACKA, PHARM.D., is Associate Professor of Pharmacy and Therapeutics, School of Pharmacy, UP. MARY E. HACKIMER is Education and Research Coordinator, The Pittsburgh Diabetes Center. JANN M. JOHNSTON, M.D., is Chairman, Department of Endocrinology, Mercy Hospital of Pittsburgh.

Address reprint requests to Dr. Schwinghammer at the Department of Pharmacy and Therapeutics, School of Pharmacy, University of Pittsburgh, 907 Salk Hall, Pittsburgh, PA 15261.

The assistance of the staff of the Clinical Research Center at the University of Pittsburgh and of Helen Jarosz and Anna Giancola is acknowledged.

Supported in part by a grant from The Upjohn Company and by NIH/DRR/GCRC grant 5M01RR00056.

Presented in part at the National Meeting of the American Association of Pharmaceutical Scientists, Boston, MA, June 11, 1987.

or pharmacodynamic response may further complicate the use of these drugs in the elderly.[4]

Glyburide is a second-generation oral sulfonylurea hypoglycemic with clinical efficacy comparable to that of first-generation compounds, such as chlorpropamide.[8] It has a shorter duration of action than chlorpropamide and thus lowers the risk of prolonged hypoglycemia in elderly patients.[3] The drug is extensively metabolized by the liver through oxidative pathways involving the cytochrome P-450 system.[9] Two major less active metabolites are produced and excreted by biliary (50%) and renal (50%) routes. As a result, mild to moderate renal failure is unlikely to result in accumulation of the drug.[10] Definitive studies of the influence of hepatic disease on glyburide pharmacokinetics have yet to be conducted, although there is evidence that hepatic oxidative metabolism may decline with age.[4] The drug is more than 99% bound to serum albumin[11]; an increased free fraction could occur as a consequence of decreased serum albumin in the elderly.

Most of the research on glyburide pharmacokinetics has been conducted in relatively young diabetics or young nondiabetic subjects. In this study, we compared the pharmacokinetics and pharmacodynamics of glyburide in healthy elderly nondiabetic subjects with those in healthy young nondiabetic volunteers to determine whether changes in these variables occur with age.

Methods

Subjects. Healthy nondiabetic men and women between 18 and 40 years of age (young subjects) and between 60 and 85 years of age (elderly subjects) were eligible for participation in the study. Each subject underwent a comprehensive physical examination and provided a complete medical history and blood and urine samples for laboratory screening before being enrolled. The research protocol was approved by the institutional review board, and written informed consent was obtained from each subject.

Criteria for exclusion from the study were (1) a history of diabetes mellitus; (2) the presence of active hepatic disease evidenced by a total serum bilirubin concentration of ≥1.8 mg/dL or an abnormal serum concentration of aspartate aminotransferase, alanine aminotransferase, albumin, or total protein; (3) the presence of acute renal disease indicated by a calculated creatinine clearance of 20 mL/min or less; (4) the presence of diseases or the long-term use of drugs known to affect blood glucose control or the action of sulfonylureas; (5) a malabsorption syndrome or active peptic ulcer disease; (6) a history of allergy to or intolerance of sulfa drugs; and (7) the presence of any other chronic diseases that in the judgment of the investigators would preclude a subject's participation in the study.

Treatment. The subjects were maintained on a standard 2800-calorie diet beginning on the day before study day 1. On day 1, after a 10-hour overnight fast, the subjects received an oral, carbonated, caffeine-free drink containing glucose 75 g in 300 mL of water (Koladex, Custom Laboratories, Inc., Baltimore, MD), and a baseline three-hour glucose tolerance test (GTT) was performed. On day 2, again after a 10-hour overnight fast, each subject was given a single 5-mg oral tablet of glyburide (Micronase, The Upjohn Company, Kalamazoo, MI, lot 906RD), followed by 180 mL of water. One hour later, the same GTT was repeated.

Blood Sampling. A heparin lock was inserted into a forearm vein of each subject for withdrawing blood samples. For the GTTs, 3-mL blood samples were collected to determine serum glucose and insulin concentrations at time zero (just before the glucose was given) and 15, 30, 45, 60, 75, 90, 120, 150, and 180 minutes after the glucose was given. Serum was separated from cellular elements by centrifugation and kept frozen at –20 °C until analysis.

To determine glyburide concentrations, 10-mL blood samples were collected just before the glyburide dose was administered and 1, 2, 3, 4, 5, 6, 8, 12, 16, 20, and 24 hours afterward. Plasma was separated and kept frozen at –20 °C until analysis. A 10-mL blood sample was also collected before glyburide administration for protein-binding determinations.

Sample Analysis. Glucose concentrations were measured by the hexokinase method (Centrifichem, Baker Instruments Corporation, Allentown, PA); insulin concentrations were determined by radioimmunoassay (Immuphase Insulin RIA Test Kit, Corning Medical and Scientific, Medfield, MA). Glyburide concentrations were determined by a high-performance liquid chromatographic method.[12] The protein binding of glyburide was determined by equilibrium dialysis with ^{14}C-labeled glyburide and a sac dialysis membrane (SpectraPor4 Dialysis Tubing, Spectrum Medical Industries, Los Angeles, CA). Binding was found to be concentration independent between glyburide concentrations of 1 and 1000 ng/mL.

Data Analysis. Pharmacokinetic values for glyburide were calculated by model-independent methods.[13] The terminal log-linear phase of each plasma glyburide concentration–time curve was identified visually, and each subject's terminal-phase rate constant (k) was estimated by least-squares linear regression analysis. The corresponding biological mean elimination half-life ($t_{1/2}$) was calculated as 0.693 divided by the mean k. The areas under the plasma concentration–time curves from zero to four hours (AUC_{0-4}) and from time zero to the last sampling time (AUC_{0-24}) were calculated by using the linear trapezoidal rule, and the corresponding values for time zero to infinity ($AUC_{0-\infty}$) were calculated as the sum of AUC_{0-24} plus the concentration at the last sampling time divided by the respective k. Individual AUC_{0-4} values for free glyburide ($AUC_{0-4,free}$) were calculated as AUC_{0-4} multiplied by the free fraction. Assuming complete absorption, apparent oral clearance (CL_{oral}) was calculated as the administered dose divided by

$AUC_{0-\infty}$.[14] The apparent volume of distribution by area (V) was calculated as CL_{oral}/k. The maximum and minimum glyburide, glucose, and insulin concentrations (C_{max} and C_{min}, respectively) were determined, as were the times at which C_{max} and C_{min} occurred (t_{max} and t_{min}, respectively).

AUCs of glucose and insulin were determined by using the trapezoidal rule for all samples from zero to three hours (AUC_{0-3}). To correct for differences between age groups in baseline GTT results, the fractional change in AUC_{0-3} between baseline and glyburide days for glucose ($\delta AUC_{glucose}$) and insulin ($\delta AUC_{insulin}$) were equated with (AUC_{0-3} on glyburide day − AUC_{0-3} on baseline day)/AUC_{0-3} on baseline day. The resulting values were then normalized to account for differences in absorption between age groups by dividing individual $\delta AUC_{glucose}$ and $\delta AUC_{insulin}$ values by the respective glyburide AUC_{0-4} and $AUC_{0-4,free}$ values. $\delta AUC_{glucose}$ and $\delta AUC_{insulin}$ were evaluated as a function of the corresponding glyburide AUC_{0-4} and $AUC_{0-4,free}$ values by linear least-squares regression analysis.

Differences between groups were analyzed by Student's t test. An a priori level of significance of < 0.05 was set for all statistical analyses.

Results

Subject Characteristics. Twenty elderly (mean ± S.D. age, 65.7 ± 5.3 years) male ($n = 10$) and female ($n = 10$) volunteers and 15 young (mean ± S.D. age, 22.3 ± 4.5 years) male volunteers met the inclusion criteria and were enrolled; no subjects withdrew from the study before its completion. The young subjects had a significantly higher mean ± S.D. serum albumin concentration than the elderly subjects (4.5 ± 0.2 and 4.2 ± 0.4 g/dL, respectively; $p = 0.0087$). There was no significant difference between the young group and the elderly group in mean ± S.D. body weight (79.0 ± 11.3 and 78.7 ± 16.9 kg, respectively) or mean ± S.D. serum creatinine concentration (1.1 ± 0.1 and 1.0 ± 0.2 mg/dL, respectively).

Pharmacokinetics. Table 1 shows the glyburide pharmacokinetic data for each age group. Plasma glyburide concentration–time curves for the two groups are shown in Figure 1. Glyburide C_{max} in the young subjects ranged from 71 to 253 ng/mL (mean ± S.D., 138 ± 56 ng/mL). C_{max} in the elderly subjects ranged from 29 to 159 ng/mL (mean ± S.D., 95 ± 37 ng/mL; $p = 0.0105$). The mean t_{max} occurred slightly later in the elderly group (3.7 hours) than in the young group (2.9 hours), but the difference was not significant. The mean AUC_{0-4} was significantly smaller in the elderly subjects ($p = 0.038$), but there was no significant difference in AUC_{0-24}, $AUC_{0-\infty}$, or $AUC_{0-4,free}$ between groups. There was no difference in the mean CL_{oral}, but the mean k was significantly lower and the mean V significantly higher in the elderly group. The mean ± S.D. $t_{1/2}$ was significantly longer in the elderly group (9.9 ± 6.7 hours) than in the young group (4.9 ± 3.2 hours). The mean free fraction of glyburide in the elderly subjects was significantly higher than that in the young subjects (0.00299 and 0.00197, respectively; $p = 0.0001$). Serum albumin concentrations were significantly lower in the elderly subjects, and a significant correlation was observed between glyburide free fraction and serum albumin concentration ($r^2 = 0.151$, $p = 0.031$).

Pharmacodynamics. Table 2 shows the pharmacodynamic data calculated for the glucose and insulin responses to the GTT before and after glyburide treatment in each age group. Serum glucose and insulin

Table 1.
Glyburide Pharmacokinetic Data

Variable[a]	Mean ± S.D. Value: Young Subjects ($n = 15$)	Elderly Subjects ($n = 20$)
C_{max} (ng/mL)	138 ± 56	95 ± 37[b]
t_{max} (hr)	2.9 ± 1.5	3.7 ± 1.3
AUC_{0-4} (ng·hr/mL)	273 ± 139	186 ± 99[c]
AUC_{0-24} (ng·hr/mL)	698 ± 284	573 ± 172
$AUC_{0-\infty}$ (ng·hr/mL)	710 ± 296	652 ± 170
$AUC_{0-4,free}$ (ng·hr/mL)	0.538 ± 0.289	0.560 ± 0.306
CL_{oral} (mL/hr/kg)	107 ± 51	111 ± 45
k (hr^{-1})	0.196 ± 0.104	0.091 ± 0.045[d]
V (L/kg)	0.735 ± 0.579	1.477 ± 0.909[e]
Free fraction	0.00197 ± 0.00007	0.00299 ± 0.00017[f]

[a] C_{max} = peak plasma glyburide concentration; t_{max} = time to C_{max}; AUC_{0-4}, AUC_{0-24}, and $AUC_{0-\infty}$ = area under the plasma concentration–time curve from 0 to 4 hours, 0 to 24 hours, and 0 hours to infinity, respectively; $AUC_{0-4,free}$ = AUC_{0-4} for free glyburide; CL_{oral} = apparent oral clearance; k = elimination rate constant; V = volume of distribution by area.

[b] Significantly different from corresponding value for young subjects ($p = 0.0105$).

[c] $p = 0.0381$.

[d] $p = 0.0003$.

[e] $p = 0.0093$.

[f] $p = 0.0001$.

Figure 1. Mean ± S.D. plasma glyburide concentrations after a single 5-mg oral dose in young (dashed line) and elderly (solid line) nondiabetic volunteers.

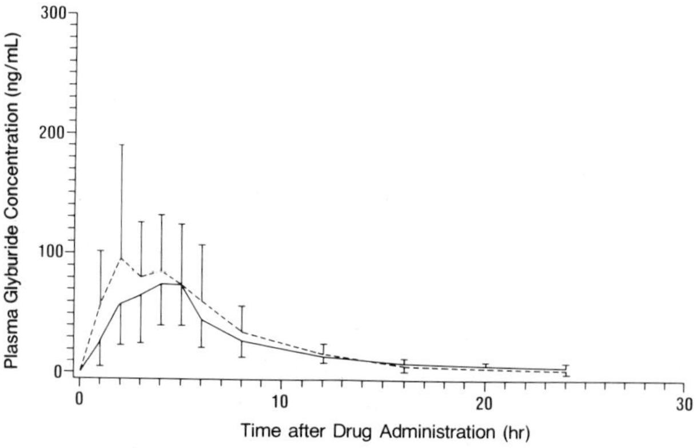

less activity (<50% of isolates were susceptible) against *Ps. aeruginosa* than ciprofloxacin (100% of isolates were susceptible). Imipenem, ciprofloxacin, ofloxacin, and ceftazidime had excellent activity against 10 amikacin-resistant (determined by disk diffusion only) isolates of *S. marcescens*, with median MICs of 1, 0.125, 0.5, and 2 μg/mL, respectively (Table 1).

Discussion

Among 63 amikacin-resistant isolates, the predominant organisms were *Ps. aeruginosa* and *X. maltophilia*, which were most frequently collected from sputum and urine. Overall, the quinolones showed the greatest activity against organisms determined to be amikacin resistant by the agar dilution method.

Findings of amikacin resistance by disk diffusion were not always in agreement with the results of MIC testing. In fact, one third of the isolates identified as amikacin resistant by disk diffusion, especially *X. maltophilia* and *S. marcescens* isolates, were found to be susceptible by MIC testing. This extent of disagreement was unexpected, since disk diffusion results are believed to be reliable predictors of the results of MIC testing, including that involving agar dilution methods.[10] The reason for this discrepancy is unclear. One explanation could be that these isolates were stored at –70 °C and subcultured twice before MIC testing, allowing for a change in the expression of resistance.[11] However, repeat disk diffusion testing recently produced the same results showing amikacin resistance. Other factors that may account for the differences in susceptibility test results include the use of Mueller-Hinton medium from different manufacturers or different lots, storage of the isolates at –70 °C, poor subculturing technique, loss of disk potency, or poor definition of inhibition zone size. Our microbiologists are highly qualified in performing susceptibility studies, antimicrobial-impregnated disks were used only if adequate time remained before the expiration date, and quality control test results were well within acceptable limits.

Metchock et al.[12] recently reported discrepancies between the results of disk diffusion methods and those of the broth microdilution method when used to test the susceptibility of *X. maltophilia*. They reported that up to 24% of the results of the disk diffusion method showing susceptibility of this organism to aminoglycosides and ciprofloxacin were false. This contrasts with our findings, in which MIC testing showed *X. maltophilia* to be susceptible and disk diffusion showed it to be resistant.

In 1977 Craven et al.[11] reported dichotomous results when using disk diffusion (cutoff for resistance, 13 mm) and MIC testing. For four strains of *S. marcescens*, inhibition zone diameters consistently indicated resistance and MIC values often indicated susceptibility. All of our *S. marcescens* isolates identified as amikacin-resistant by disk diffusion were shown to be susceptible by MIC testing. Like Craven et al., we found that MIC testing often indicated susceptibility even though inhibition zone sizes evidenced resistance. Which method is most predictive of clinical outcome is unclear. However, peak serum amikacin concentrations should usually be maintained between 20 and 30 μg/mL. Consequently, even when susceptibility is suggested by MIC testing, an acceptable inhibition quotient (i.e., drug concentration/MIC = 2–4) may not be achievable.

The rate of nosocomial isolation of *X. maltophilia* appears to be increasing, especially among immunocompromised hosts.[6,13] Morrison et al.[14] reviewed the clinical characteristics of nosocomial *X. maltophilia* infection and associated mortality in severely ill patients. They found that 60% of isolates were resistant to all aminoglycosides, 75% were resistant to all semisynthetic penicillins, and 96% were resistant to all cephalosporin antimicrobials. For clinically serious infections, intravenous trimethoprim–sulfamethoxazole is currently the recommended treatment for *X. maltophilia* infection.[15] However, trimethoprim–sulfamethoxazole is not appropriate for all patients, mainly because of hypersensitivity reactions. Our results showed that ciprofloxacin and ofloxacin were the most active antimicrobials against *X. maltophilia* in vitro. The median MIC was 1.0 μg/mL for both quinolones. Disk diffusion testing appeared to detect more amikacin-resistant organisms, whereas MIC testing showed amikacin susceptibility in 27% of isolates identified as resistant by disk diffusion. The clinical usefulness of these quinolones is questionable, however, since only 58%–75% of isolates were susceptible. The mean MIC_{90} (MIC for 90% of isolates) of ciprofloxacin and ofloxacin for *X. maltophilia* is 4 and >2 μg/mL, respectively.[16] Clinical studies are needed to verify the role of these antimicrobials in the treatment of clinically important *X. maltophilia* infection.

Pseudomonas aeruginosa, our second most frequently isolated amikacin-resistant organism, is often implicated in life-threatening nosocomial infections, and double antimicrobial coverage is used to limit the emergence of resistant strains. The susceptibility profiles of the amikacin-resistant *Ps. aeruginosa* isolates differed from those of *X. maltophilia* isolates. Ciprofloxacin was uniformly active against all amikacin-resistant *Ps. aeruginosa* isolates. Ofloxacin, however, was much less active against *Ps. aeruginosa*. This is not surprising, since ofloxacin has been shown to be eight times less active (mean MIC_{90}, 4 μg/mL) than ciprofloxacin (0.5 μg/mL) against the organism.[17] The remaining antimicrobials studied, including ceftazidime, cefoperazone, and imipenem–cilastatin, had only moderate activity. Further study of the synergistic effects of combination therapy is warranted.

Conclusion

Of the antimicrobials tested, ciprofloxacin had the greatest activity against amikacin-resistant organisms in vitro. Clinical studies are needed to elucidate ciprofloxacin's role in the treatment of infections caused by amikacin-resistant isolates.

References

1. Ruiz-Palacios GM, DeLeon SP, Sifuentes J et al. Control of emergence of multi-resistant gram-negative bacilli by exclusive use of amikacin. *Am J Med*. 1986; 80(Suppl 6B):71-5.
2. Gerding DN, Larson TA. Aminoglycoside resistance in gram-negative bacilli during increased amikacin use. *Am J Med*. 1985; 79(Suppl 1A):1-7.
3. Cook LN, Davis RS, Stover BH. Outbreak of amikacin-resistant Enterobacteriaceae in an intensive care nursery. *Pediatrics*. 1980; 65:264-8.
4. Cross AS, Opal S, Kopecko DJ. Progressive increase in antibiotic resistance of gram-negative bacterial isolates. Walter Reed Hospital, 1976 to 1980: specific analysis of gentamicin, tobramycin, and amikacin resistance. *Arch Intern Med*. 1983; 143:2075-80.
5. Gaynes RE, Groisman E, Nelson E et al. Isolation, characterization, and cloning of a plasmid–bovine gene encoding a phosphotransferase that confers high-level amikacin resistance in enteric bacteria. *Antimicrob Agents Chemother*. 1988; 32:1379-84.
6. Zuravleff JJ, Yu VL. Infection caused by *Pseudomonas maltophilia* with emphasis on bacteremia: case reports and a review of the literature. *Rev Infect Dis*. 1982; 4:1236-46.
7. Khardori N, Elting L, Wong E et al. Nosocomial infections due to *Xanthomonas maltophilia* (*Pseudomonas maltophilia*) in patients with cancer. *Rev Infect Dis*. 1990; 12:997-1003.
8. National Committee for Clinical Laboratory Standards. Approved standard M7-A. Performance standards for antimicrobial disc susceptibility tests. 4th ed. Villanova, PA: National Committee for Clinical Laboratory Standards; 1988:75-92.
9. National Committee for Clinical Laboratory Standards. Approved standard M7-A. Methods for dilutional antimicrobial susceptibility tests for bacteria that grow aerobically. 2nd ed. Villanova, PA: National Committee for Clinical Laboratory Standards; 1988:95-116.
10. Bauer AW, Kirby WM, Sherris JC et al. Antibiotic susceptibility testing by a standardized single disc method. *Am J Clin Pathol*. 1966; 45:493-6.
11. Craven PC, Jorgensen JH, Kaspar RL et al. Amikacin therapy of patients with multiply antibiotic-resistant *Serratia marcescens* infections. *Am J Med*. 1977; 62:902-10.
12. Metchock B, Hill B, Maher K et al. Susceptibility of *Xanthomonas* (*Pseudomonas*) *maltophilia* to antimicrobial agents. Paper presented at 28th Interscience Conference on Antimicrobial Agents and Chemotherapy. Los Angeles, CA: 1988 Oct 26.
13. Nagai T. Association of *Pseudomonas maltophilia* with malignant lesions. *J Clin Microbiol*. 1984; 20:1003-5.
14. Morrison AJ, Hoffman KK, Wenzel RP. Associated mortality and clinical characteristics of nosocomial *Pseudomonas maltophilia* in a university hospital. *J Clin Microbiol*. 1986; 24:52-5.
15. Sanford JP. *Pseudomonas* species (including melioidosis and glanders). In: Mandell GL, Douglas RG, Bennett JE, eds. Principles and practice of infectious diseases. New York: Wiley; 1990:1692-6.
16. Auckenthaler K, Michea-Hamzehpour M, Pechiere JC. In-vitro activity of newer quinolones against aerobic bacteria. *J Antimicrob Chemother*. 1986; 17:29-39.
17. Gruneberg RN, Felmughan D, O'Hare MD et al. The comparative in-vitro activity of ofloxacin. *J Antimicrob Chemother*. 1988; 22(C):9-19.

DUE Criteria

The DUE Criteria *section of* Clinical Pharmacy *features model drug-use evaluation criteria that may be employed as a component of a comprehensive quality assurance program. The criteria sets are presented in the format used in the ASHP book* **Criteria for Drug Use Evaluation.** *Some of the criteria sets will have been originally published in that book; others will be presented here for the first time and published in future volumes of the ASHP book. The practitioners who developed a criteria set are acknowledged.*

In selecting drug products for coverage in DUE Criteria, *priority is given to products that have been recently marketed, those that are frequently prescribed, those that have high potential risk associated with their use, and those that are expensive. When feasible, a criteria set will be linked with a Drug Review that appears in the same issue.*

These criteria sets are a starting point for the development of DUE criteria for a specific practice setting. Readers are encouraged to modify the model criteria to fit their own circumstances.

Criteria for use of hetastarch[a]

Element	Standard 100%	Standard 0%	Exception[b] or Critical Preventive/ Responsive Measure[c]	Sources of Information
Justification for Use				
1. Shock due to blood loss, with systolic blood pressure of <90 mm Hg, cardiac index of <2.2 L/min/sq m, or pulmonary artery wedge pressure (PAWP) of <1.5 mm Hg; administered <2 hr after blood loss[1]	X		1A. Circumstances prohibit administration <2 hr after blood loss	1. History and physical (H&P), laboratory reports, nursing notes, progress notes, nursing flow sheets 1A. Progress notes, H&P
or				
2. Shock due to thermal injury involving >10% of body surface area; administered >24 hr after burn[2,3]	X		2A. None	2. H&P, progress notes, nursing notes
or				
3. Hypovolemia due to hemorrhage, burns, sepsis, or surgery[4,5]	X		3A. None	3. Operating room (OR) records, H&P, progress notes, nursing notes
or				
4. Adjunct in leukapheresis to enhance granulocyte yield[6]	X		4A. None	4. Special procedure report, progress notes
or				
5. Pump prime for cardiopulmonary bypass[7–9]	X		5A. None	5. OR records
or				
6. Plasma volume expander after cardiopulmonary bypass[10–13]	X		6A. None	6. OR records, progress notes
Critical (Process) Indicators				
7. Evidence of allergic reaction monitored for continuously[14]	X		7A. None	7. Progress notes, nursing notes
8. Prothrombin time (PT), activated partial thromboplastin time (APTT), hematocrit (Hct), and hemoglobin concentration (Hb) measured within 24 hr of initial hetastarch dose and at least daily during therapy[14]	X		8A. None	8. Progress notes, laboratory reports, physician orders

Prepared by Sharon A. Basile, Pharm.D., Clinical Pharmacist, Internal Medicine, Department of Pharmacy, University Medical Center, and Clinical Assistant Professor, College of Pharmacy, University of Florida Health Science Center/Jacksonville.

 0278-2677/91/0701-0549$00.75.

Element	Standard 100%	Standard 0%	Exception[b] or Critical Preventive/ Responsive Measure[c]	Sources of Information
9. Evidence of vascular overload or hypervolemia, including pulmonary edema, congestive heart failure (CHF), and elevated blood pressure, monitored continuously[14]	X		9A. None	9. Progress notes, nursing notes, nursing flow sheets
10. Serum sodium level measured daily in sodium-restricted patient[14]	X		10A. None	10. Laboratory reports, progress notes
11. If patient received leukapheresis, then complete blood count, total leukocyte and platelet counts, Hct, Hb concentration, PT, and APTT measured immediately before and weekly during treatment[14]	X		11A. None	11. Laboratory reports, progress notes, special procedure report
12. Dosage and rate of administration adjusted for clinical response and blood pressure[14]: a. Usual adult dose: hetastarch 6% in 0.9% sodium chloride injection 30–60 g (500–1000 mL), with total daily dose not to exceed 1.2 g/kg (20 mL/kg) or 90 g (1500 mL) b. Acute hemorrhagic shock: 1.2 g/kg/hr c. Burns or septic shock: <1.2 g/kg/hr d. Severe renal disease (creatinine clearance, <10 mL/min): usual adult dose, but subsequent doses only 25–50% of usual dose e. Leukapheresis: 250–700 mL of hetastarch 6% at constant fixed ratio (usually 1:8) to venous whole blood	X		12A. Hetastarch not used in severe bleeding disorder, severe CHF, or renal failure with oliguria or anuria[14]	12, 12A. Physician orders, progress notes, laboratory reports, medication administration records (MAR), nursing notes, H&P, special procedure report
Complications				
13. Allergic reaction or sensitivity (vomiting, increase in temperature, chills, itching, enlargement of glands, headache, myalgia, peripheral edema, or wheezing)[14]		X	13A. Identify other drug and nondrug causes 13B. Discontinue hetastarch; treat symptomatically	13. Progress notes, nursing notes 13A, B. Progress notes, physician orders, MAR, nursing notes
14. Interference with platelet function (increased PT, APTT, and clotting times)[14]		X	14A. Identify other drug and nondrug causes 14B. Use with caution in patient with thrombocytopenia 14C. Avoid in patient with severe bleeding disorder	14. Laboratory reports, progress notes 14A. Laboratory reports, progress notes, nursing notes, MAR 14B. Laboratory reports, H&P, progress notes 14C. H&P, progress notes, nursing notes
15. Circulatory overload[14]		X	15A. Identify other drug and nondrug causes 15B. Avoid giving >1500 mL of hetastarch per day 15C. Avoid using hetastarch in patient with severe CHF	15. Progress notes, laboratory reports, nursing flow sheets 15A. Progress notes, laboratory reports, nursing flow sheets, MAR, nursing notes 15B. Progress notes, physician orders, MAR 15C. H&P, progress notes, nursing notes
16. Greatly elevated serum sodium level[14]		X	16A. Identify other drug and nondrug causes 16B. Discontinue hetastarch	16. Laboratory reports, progress notes 16A. Laboratory reports, progress notes, nursing notes, MAR 16B. Physician orders, progress notes, MAR

Element	Standard 100%	Standard 0%	Exception[b] or Critical Preventive/ Responsive Measure[c]	Sources of Information
Outcome Measures				
17. Hetastarch discontinued after normalization of blood pressure, cardiac index, and PAWP or evidence of therapeutic response is seen[1]	X		17A. Patient died 17B. Another agent used (albumin or plasma protein fraction)	17. Physician orders, progress notes, nursing flow sheets, nursing notes 17A. Progress notes 17B. Physician orders, progress notes, MAR
18. Administration slowed or stopped in patient exhibiting vascular overload or hypervolemia, excessive blood pressure response, potentially dangerous elevation of serum sodium, or allergic reaction[14]	X		18A. None	18. Physician orders, progress notes, nursing notes, laboratory reports

[a] Criteria address justification for use (indications), critical (process) indicators, complications of therapy, and patient outcome. Each criterion consists of an element, a standard, exceptions to the standard, and sources of information. The element is the minimum level of evidence needed to show that patient care was optimal. The standard defines the deviation from an element that is acceptable. If no deviation is acceptable, the standard is 100%. Exceptions are circumstances in which deviation is allowable. Sources of information listed are the most reliable sources. Sources pertaining to an element or exception are identified by the number assigned to the element or exception (e.g., 1, 1A).

[b] For justification for use and critical (process) indicators.

[c] For complications and outcome measures.

References

1. Haupt MT, Rackow EC. Colloid osmotic pressure and fluid resuscitation with hetastarch, albumin and saline solutions. *Crit Care Med.* 1982; 10:159–62.
2. Waters LM, Christensen MA, Sato RM. Hetastarch: an alternative colloid in burn shock management. *J Burn Care Rehabil.* 1989; 10:11–6.
3. Pruitt BA Jr. Fluid resuscitation for extensively burned patients. *J Trauma.* 1981; 21:690–2.
4. Puri VK, Paidipaty B, White L. Hydroxyethyl starch for resuscitation of patients with hypovolemia and shock. *Crit Care Med.* 1981; 9:833–7.
5. Rackow EC, Kalk JL, Fein A et al. Fluid resuscitation in circulatory shock: a comparison of the cardiorespiratory effects of albumin, hetastarch and saline solutions in patients with hypovolemic and septic shock. *Crit Care Med.* 1983; 11:839–50.
6. Strauss RG, Maguire LC, Koepke JA et al. Properties of neutrophils collected by discontinuous-flow centrifugation leukapheresis employing hydroxyethyl starch. *Transfusion.* 1979; 19:192–6.
7. Saunders CR, Carlisle L, Bick RL. Hydroxyethyl starch versus albumin in cardiopulmonary bypass prime solutions. *Ann Thorac Surg.* 1983; 36:532–9.
8. Palarrzo DA, Parr GVS, Bull AP et al. Hetastarch as a prime for cardiopulmonary bypass. *Soc Thorac Surg.* 1982; 34:680–3.
9. Hicks GL, Jensen LA, Norsen LH et al. Platelet inhibitors and hydroxyethyl starch: safe and cost-effective artery surgery. *Ann Thorac Surg.* 1985; 39:422–5.
10. Kirklin JK, Lell WA, Kouchoukos NT. Hydroxyethyl starch vs. albumin for colloid infusion following cardiopulmonary bypass in patients undergoing myocardial revascularization. *Ann Thorac Surg.* 1984; 37:40–6.
11. Moggio RA, Rha CC, Somberg ED et al. Hemodynamic comparison of albumin and hydroxyethyl starch in postoperative cardiac surgery patients. *Crit Care Med.* 1983; 11:943–5.
12. Munsch CM, MacIntyre E, Machin SJ et al. Hydroxyethyl starch: an alternative to plasma for postoperative volume expansion after cardiac surgery. *Br J Surg.* 1988; 75:675–8.
13. Diehl JT, Lester JL, Cosgrove DM. Clinical comparison of hetastarch and albumin in postoperative cardiac patients. *Soc Thorac Surg.* 1982; 34:674–9.
14. AHFS drug information 89. McEvoy GK, ed. Bethesda, MD: American Society of Hospital Pharmacists; 1989:1370–1.

CP Continuing Education

The ASHP Continuing-Education System gives readers a self-assessment mechanism for selected articles in Clinical Pharmacy *and* AJHP. *It allows readers to obtain continuing-education credit for these articles.*

For the purpose of CE-credit enrollment, a blank answer sheet is published at the end of each installment of the column for the CE articles in that issue. An enrollee accumulates these answer sheets until the enrollment is submitted, using the form that is published in the June and December issues of Clinical Pharmacy *and in the June and December issues of* AJHP. *Any combination of tests within an 18-month period, from both* Clinical Pharmacy *and* AJHP, *may be included in an enrollment. More complete details about enrollment in the system appear in the semiannual enrollment form.*

Article 680-204-9115 (see page 503)
Qualifies for 1.0 hour of CE credit

Therapy of acute thromboembolism with heparin and warfarin

Learning Objectives

After studying this article, the reader should be able to

1. State the indications for warfarin and heparin in the treatment of acute thromboembolic events.
2. Provide recommendations for dosing and monitoring heparin in a patient with an acute thromboembolic event.
3. State four reasons why administration of heparin and warfarin should be overlapped, and explain the regimens for each.
4. Identify the appropriate warfarin dosage intensity for each indication.
5. Provide recommendations for outpatient follow-up and laboratory monitoring of patients starting warfarin therapy.
6. Identify common adverse reactions to heparin and warfarin.

Self-assessment Questions

For each question, there is only one best answer.

1. The minimum duration of intravenous heparin for acute deep-vein thrombosis of the legs should be

   a. 3 days.
   b. 5 days.
   c. 10 days.
   d. 14 days.

2. When alteplase is administered for treatment of acute myocardial infarction, heparin therapy

   a. Is unnecessary.
   b. Should be avoided because of the risk of bleeding if an invasive procedure is required.
   c. Is used to prevent early reocclusion.
   d. Should be given, beginning no earlier than six hours after alteplase is administered.

3. In order to reduce the risk of recurrence of deep-vein thrombosis, which of the following is most important?

   a. Maintain the activated partial thromboplastin time (APTT) at 1.3 times control.
   b. Maintain the APTT at 3.0 times control.
   c. Start warfarin on day 1 of therapy.
   d. Rapidly achieve a therapeutic APTT.

4. A patient has been given an i.v. bolus dose of heparin and an infusion has been started. However, the APTT is still very low (almost control). What should be done to rapidly achieve a therapeutic APTT?

   a. Give another bolus dose.
   b. Increase the infusion rate.
   c. Give a bolus dose and increase the infusion rate.
   d. Give three bolus doses separated by 5–10 minutes.

5. The recommended initial infusion rate of heparin for the treatment of deep-vein thrombosis or pulmonary embolism is

   a. 1000 units/hr.
   b. 10–20 units/kg/hr.
   c. 15–25 units/kg/hr.
   d. 2500 units/hr.

6. One of the best predictors of heparin dosage requirements is

   a. Age.
   b. Body weight.
   c. Smoking status.
   d. Antithrombin III deficiency.

7. The delayed form of thrombocytopenia is

   a. Transient.
   b. Associated with platelet counts between 100,000 and 150,000/cu mm.
   c. Rarely seen in humans.
   d. Probably immunologically mediated.

8. During conversion from heparin to warfarin therapy after an acute thromboembolic event, it is recommended that the two drugs be overlapped for four to six days for all of the following reasons except

   a. Warfarin decreases antithrombin III.

Current Literature

Drug Reaction Alerts

Drug Reaction Alerts focuses primarily on serious, unlabeled reactions to new chemical entities. The citations are compiled monthly from International Pharmaceutical Abstracts, *which covers over 800 pharmacy and health-related journals worldwide. An address for reprints (when available) follows the name of the corresponding author of each citation.*

Pharmacists may use the FDA Adverse Reaction Report form that appears in most issues of Clinical Pharmacy *for submitting reports of adverse drug reactions directly to FDA.*

Antilipemic Agents

Deslypere JP, Vermeulen A (University Hospital, B-9000 Ghent, Belgium). Rhabdomyolysis and **simvastatin**. *Ann Intern Med.* 1991; 114:342. Case. (53-year-old man with hypercholesterolemia; received simvastatin 10 mg/day for two months and increased to 40 mg/day for 21 months; developed rhabdomyolysis; withdrawal of simvastatin led to gradual and complete resolution of clinical and laboratory signs of muscle damage)

Cardiac Drugs

Echt DS, Liebson PR, Mitchell LB et al. (Richardson DW, CAST Coordinating Center, 1107 N.E. 45th, Room 505, Seattle, WA 98105). Mortality and morbidity in patients receiving **encainide, flecainide**, or placebo: Cardiac Arrhythmia Suppression Trial. *N Engl J Med.* 1991; 324:781-8. Study. (randomized placebo-controlled study; 1498 patients from Cardiac Arrhythmia Suppression Trial; 857 patients received encainide or its placebo; 641 patients received flecainide or its placebo; mean follow-up time, 10 months; 89 patients died; 43 patients receiving encainide or flecainide and 16 patients receiving placebo died from cardiac arrhythmias; 17 patients receiving encainide or flecainide and five patients receiving placebo died from nonarrhythmic cardiac causes; three patients receiving encainide or flecainide and five patients receiving placebo died from noncardiac causes)

Moller HU (Department of Ophthalmology, Aarhus Kommunehospital, DK-8000 Aarhus C, Denmark), Thygesen K, Kruit PJ. Corneal deposits associated with **flecainide**. *Br Med J.* 1991; 302:506-7. Cases. (two men, aged 46 and 72 years, with atrial fibrillation; 46-year-old man received flecainide 200–300 mg/day for more than one year; 72-year-old man received flecainide 100–200 mg/day for four months; developed corneal deposits with visual disturbances; withdrawal of flecainide led to improvement in vision; 46-year-old man underwent surgery to abrade opacities; abraded epithelium had same chromatographic appearance as flecainide, as determined by high-performance liquid chromatography)

Drug Interactions

Bartle WR, Blakely JA (University of Toronto, Sunnybrook Health Science Center, North York, Ontario, Canada). Potentiation of **warfarin** anticoagulation by **acetaminophen**. *JAMA.* 1991; 265:1260. Case. (66-year-old woman; received warfarin at an average dose of 3 mg/day and acetaminophen approximately 1.6 g/day for eight days; developed hematuria, gingival hemorrhage, and prolongation of prothrombin time; withdrawal of warfarin and acetaminophen and therapy with 3 units of fresh frozen plasma led to return of prothrombin time to normal range; warfarin reinstituted without incident)

Gastrointestinal Drugs

Santucci L, Farroni F, Fiorucci S et al. (Morelli A, University degli Studi di Perugia, 06100 Perugia, Italy). Gynecomastia during **omeprazole** therapy. *N Engl J Med.* 1991; 324:635. Case. (53-year-old man with duodenal ulcer resistant to standard treatment; received omeprazole 20 mg daily for eight weeks; developed painful bilateral gynecomastia during therapy; serum hormone concentrations and liver function test results within normal ranges; withdrawal of omeprazole led to regression of gynecomastia after approximately four weeks; positive rechallenge)

Oxytocics

Fliers E, Duren DR, van Zwieten PA (Academic Medical Center, 1105 AZ Amsterdam, the Netherlands). A prostaglandin analogue as a probable cause of myocardial infarction in a young woman. *Br Med J.* 1991; 302:416. Case. (32-year-old pregnant woman; received **sulprostone** up to 500 μg/hr as an i.v. injection for labor induction; experienced a myocardial infarction and recovered completely; experienced a second myocardial infarction during coronary angiography and developed severe cardiac failure; therapy with digoxin, furosemide, captopril, and acenocoumarol led to patient's survival; evaluated for heart transplantation)

Advertising Index

American Society of Hospital Pharmacists
AHFS Drug Information 91, 554
Criteria for Drug Use Evaluation, Volumes 1 & 2, 499
European Drug Index, 559
Guidelines for Administration of Intravenous Medications to Pediatric Patients, 548
MedTeach, 531
ASHP Research and Education Foundation
Anticoagulation Clinic Traineeship Program, 557
Baxter Healthcare Corporation, Hyland Division
Gammagard, 488-490
Burroughs Wellcome Company
Exosurf Neonatal, 491-495
Zovirax I.V., 560-562
Department of Veterans Affairs (Richmond)
Positions Available, 563
Eli Lilly and Company
Hospital Division, 485
Methodist Medical Center of Illinois
Position Available, 497
The Pharmacy Council on Cholesterol
10 Cholesterol Battle Strategies, 502
Roerig, A Division of Pfizer Pharmaceuticals
Diflucan, inside front cover
Schering-Plough Corporation
Position Available, 497
SmithKline Beecham
Tagamet, inside back cover, outside back cover
Wyeth-Ayerst Laboratories, Inc.
Ativan Injection, 564-566

News

Guidelines for *Pneumocystis carinii* pneumonia prophylaxis in children issued 569

Gallium marketed for treatment of cancer-related hypercalcemia 573

Two cardiovascular agents, ramipril and isradipine, approved for U.S. market 573

News Briefs 573

Upcoming Specialty Meetings 574

Guidelines for *Pneumocystis carinii* pneumonia prophylaxis in children issued

Guidelines for prophylaxis against *Pneumocystis carinii* pneumonia (PCP) in children infected with human immunodeficiency virus (HIV) have been formulated by a working group convened by the Pediatric HIV Resource Center, Newark, New Jersey, and supported in part by the U.S. Department of Health and Human Services.[1] The document reviews information on the impact of PCP on HIV-infected children, problems in defining appropriate populations for prophylaxis, the relationship between CD4+ cell count and PCP in children with HIV infection, and potential regimens for prophylaxis. Recommendations for prophylaxis are summarized in the following paragraphs. Readers are referred to the full document for a complete discussion of all recommendations.

Indications for Prophylaxis. Prophylaxis should be initiated in HIV-infected children with the following age-adjusted CD4+ cell counts: <1500/cu mm for children 1–11 months, <750/cu mm for children 12–23 months, <500/cu mm for children 24 months to 5 years, and <200/cu mm for children 6 years and older. Any HIV-infected child with a CD4+ percentage of <20%, regardless of the absolute CD4+ cell count, is a candidate for prophylaxis.

Prophylaxis is not recommended during the first month of life because of the risk of adverse effects in neonates and because PCP is rare at this age. However, if the infant is at risk of HIV infection, the CD4+ cell count should be determined. If it is <1500/cu mm, prophylaxis should be begun at one month. If the count is higher, the test should be repeated one month later, and the need for prophylaxis should be re-evaluated.

Whenever a child is found to be HIV seropositive, the CD4+ count should be determined and the need for prophylaxis evaluated. During the first two years of life, the count should be monitored at least every three or four months (monthly if the count is approaching the cutoff levels for prophylaxis). In older children, counts should be monitored at least every six months; the frequency depends on the child's age and CD4+ cell count.

For some children started on prophylaxis, therapy may subsequently be discontinued (e.g., infants who were seropositive initially but are later shown not to be infected; HIV-infected or seropositive children who have

Continued on page 573

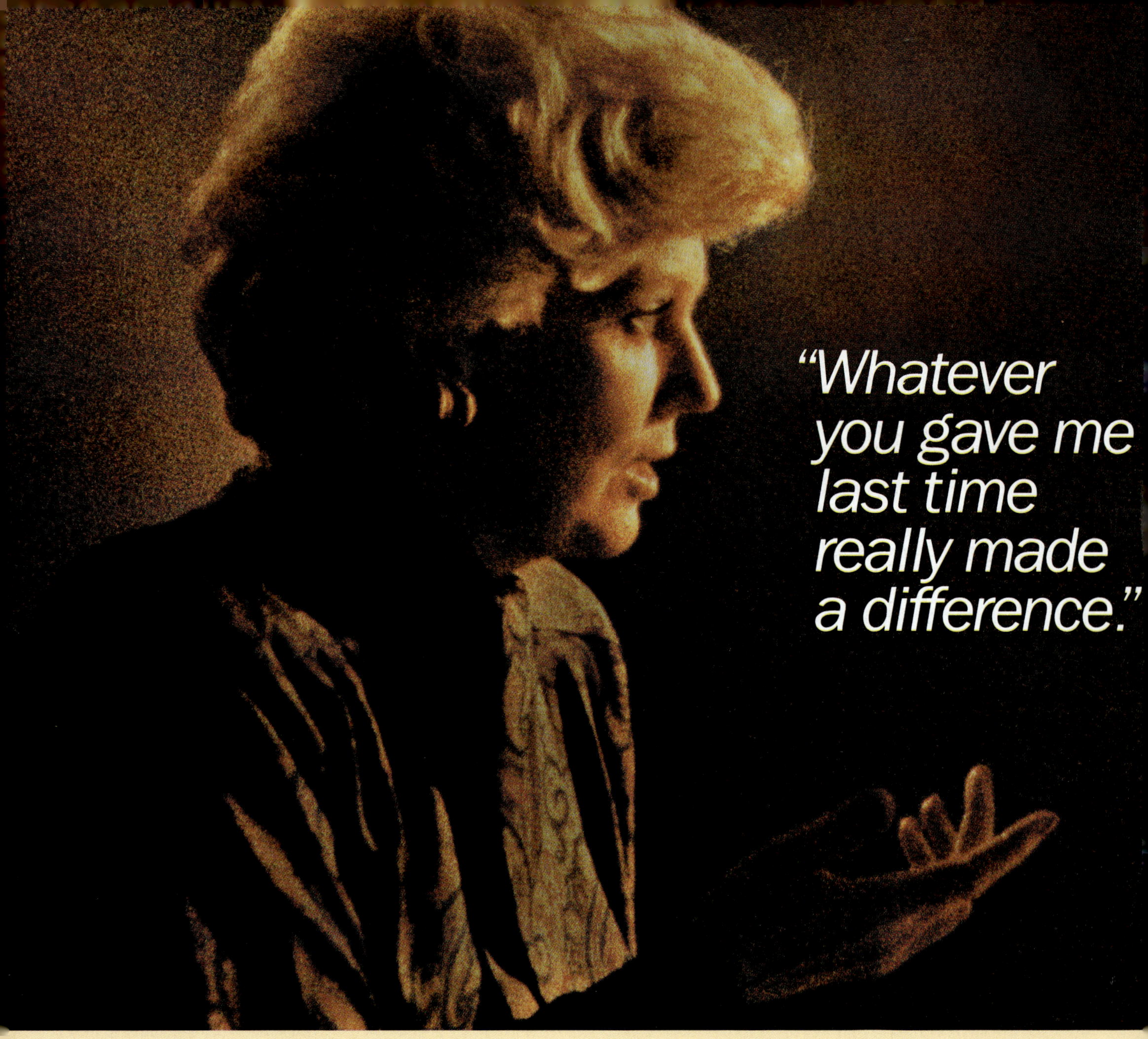
"Whatever you gave me last time really made a difference."

Continued from page 569

CD4+ cell counts above the treatment threshold for two sequential measurements made one month apart, unless special circumstances could have altered the count). A child who has had an episode of PCP should receive lifelong PCP prophylaxis regardless of his or her age or CD4+ cell count.

Recommended Regimens. The recommended regimen is trimethoprim 150 mg/sq m/day with sulfamethoxazole 750 mg/sq m/day (maximum daily dosage, 320 mg and 1600 mg, respectively) given in two divided daily doses on three consecutive days each week. The intermittent regimen is intended to minimize toxicity. Administration of trimethoprim–sulfamethoxazole should be permanently discontinued if life-threatening toxicity occurs. If reactions are less severe, treatment can be interrupted and then restarted within two weeks. Complete blood counts with differential and platelet count should be monitored monthly. Three acceptable alternative regimens are trimethoprim 150 mg/sq m/day with sulfamethoxazole 750 mg/sq m/day given (1) as a single daily dose on three consecutive days each week, (2) in two divided doses every day, and (3) in two divided daily doses three time a week on alternate days.

If trimethoprim–sulfamethoxazole is not tolerated, alternatives include aerosolized pentamidine isethionate 300 mg given via a Respirgard II inhaler monthly (if child is at least five years of age) or dapsone 1 mg/kg (maximum, 100 mg) orally once daily (if child is at least one month of age). Some clinicians use pentamidine isethionate 4 mg/kg i.v. every two to four weeks if neither aerosolized pentamidine nor dapsone is tolerated.

1. Working Group on PCP Prophylaxis in Children. Guidelines for prophylaxis against *Pneumocystis carinii* pneumonia for children infected with human immunodeficiency virus. *MMWR*. 1991; 40(RR-2):1-13.

Gallium marketed for treatment of cancer-related hypercalcemia

Gallium nitrate injection (Ganite, Fujisawa) has been approved for the treatment of symptomatic cancer-related hypercalcemia that has not responded to hydration. The recommended dosage is 200 mg/sq m daily for five days. A lower dosage may be used in patients with mild hypercalcemia. Treatment may be discontinued early if calcium levels return to normal before five days of therapy. Gallium is given as a continuous intravenous infusion. Use of gallium is contraindicated in patients with severe renal impairment.

Increased blood urea nitrogen and serum creatinine concentrations have been reported in 12.5% of patients treated with gallium. Treatment should be discontinued if the creatinine concentration exceeds 2.5 mg/dL. Concurrent use of nephrotoxic agents may increase the risk of toxicity. Up to 79% of patients may develop transient hypophosphatemia. Low serum bicarbonate levels have been reported in 40–50% of patients.

Postmarketing studies will include two studies comparing gallium with pamidronate and etidronate and two pharmacokinetics studies, one in hypercalcemic patients with various degrees of renal dysfunction and one evaluating additional dosages and schedules.

Two cardiovascular agents, ramipril and isradipine, approved for U.S. market

The angiotensin-converting-enzyme inhibitor ramipril (Altace, Hoechst-Roussel Pharmaceuticals Inc. and The Upjohn Company) and the calcium-channel blocker isradipine (DynaCirc, Sandoz and Allen & Hanburys) have been marketed for the treatment of hypertension.

Ramipril. Ramipril is a prodrug that is rapidly de-esterified in the liver to form the active drug ramiprilat. About 60% of an oral dose of ramipril is absorbed. Peak serum ramiprilat concentrations are achieved about three hours after oral administration of ramipril. The extent of protein binding is about 73% for ramipril and 56% for ramiprilat. Ramiprilat is metabolized to inactive compounds. Renal excretion accounts for about 60% of an administered dose; fecal elimination (about 40% of an administered dose) may reflect elimination of unabsorbed drug and biliary excretion of metabolites. Serum concentrations of ramiprilat decline in a triphasic manner. The half-life during the major distribution phase is two to four hours. The half-life corresponding to clearance of ramiprilat is 9–18 hours. Excretion of ramipril and its metabolites may be decreased in patients with renal insufficiency.

In clinical trials, the effective antihypertensive dosage usually fell within the range of 2.5–10 mg once daily. The recommended dosage range is 2.5–20 mg daily. A dosage reduction is suggested in patients with renal insufficiency.

The adverse-effect profile of ramipril is similar to those of other angiotensin-converting-enzyme inhibitors. The most common adverse reactions are headache, dizziness, fatigue, and nausea and vomiting.

Ramipril is available as 1.25-, 2.5-, 5-, and 10-mg hard-gelatin capsules.

Isradipine. Isradipine, a dihydropyridine derivative, is rapidly and nearly completely absorbed after oral administration. Because of extensive first-pass metabolism, the bioavailability of oral 5- to 20-mg doses is about 17%. Peak plasma concentrations are reached in about 2.5 hours. The drug is about 97% bound to plasma proteins. Isradipine is metabolized in the liver to inactive compounds that are excreted in the urine; fecal elimination of unchanged drug accounts for about 10% of a dose. Isradipine undergoes biphasic elimination; the effective elimination half-life is about nine hours. Bioavailability may be increased in elderly persons and patients with hepatic dysfunction.

A dosage of 2.5–7.5 mg twice daily was generally effective in clinical trials involving patients with hypertension. The recommended dosage is 2.5–5 mg twice daily. Most of the adverse effects of isradipine are related to its vasodilatory effects and are more common at higher dosages.

News Briefs

- New **guidelines for rabies prevention** have been issued by the Immunization Practices Advisory Committee of the Centers for Disease Control (*MMWR*. 1991; 40(RR-3):1-19.). Topics include descriptions of available biologic products, rationale and guidelines for postexposure treatment (local wound care and use of rabies vaccine and rabies immune globulin), postexposure treatments commonly used outside the United States, pre-exposure vaccination, postexposure therapy of previously vaccinated persons, unintentional inoculation with modified live rabies virus animal vaccine, and adverse reactions and cautions involving biologic products.

• Labeled indications for **cimetidine** (Tagamet, SmithKline Beecham) have been expanded to include use in healing lesions and relieving symptoms of erosive gastroesophageal reflux disease. The recommended adult oral dosage is 1600 mg daily in divided doses (800 mg twice daily or 400 mg four times daily) for 12 weeks.

• Bristol-Myers Laboratories has filed a new drug application (NDA) for **dideoxyinosine** (ddI). Hoffmann-La Roche has also announced that it is in the process of submitting an NDA for **dideoxycytidine** (ddC).

• Connaught Laboratories, Inc., has begun marketing **cytomegalovirus immune globulin intravenous [human]** (CytoMune-IV), which is manufactured by the Massachusetts Public Health Biologic Laboratories.

• FDA has granted orphan drug status to **intravenous etidronate disodium** (Didronel, MGI Pharma, Inc.) for both the treatment and prevention of osteoporosis in patients receiving total parenteral nutrition.

• A report on **current theories and beneficial clinical practices concerning nutritional support in the care of patients with AIDS** is available. The report was prepared by the Life Sciences Research Office of the Federation of American Societies for Experimental Biology (FASEB). Send requests, along with $15, to Special Publication Office, FASEB, 9650 Rockville Pike, Bethesda, MD 20814.

• Free, single copies of the report of the **NIH Consensus Development Conference on Clinical Use of Botulinum Toxin** can be obtained from William H. Hall, Director of Communications, Office of Medical Applications of Research, National Institutes of Health, Building 1, Room 259, Bethesda, MD 20892; 301-496-1143.

Upcoming Specialty Meetings

13th Annual Meeting of the Society for Medical Decision Making. Rochester, NY, October 20–23; contact SMDM, Office of Continuing Medical Education, George Washington University, 2300 K Street, N.W., Washington, DC 20037; 202-994-8929.

NIH Consensus Development Conference on the Recognition and Treatment of Depression in Late Life. Bethesda, MD, November 4–6; contact Conference Registrar, Prospect Associates, 1801 Rockville Pike, Suite 500, Rockville, MD 20852; 301-468-6338.

Association of Clinical Scientists. Jacksonville, FL, November 13–17; contact F. W. Sunderman, Jr., M.D., Department of Laboratory Medicine, University of Connecticut Medical School, 263 Farmington Avenue, Farmington, CT 06030; 203-679-2328.

Third Triennial Symposium on New Directions in Antiviral Chemotherapy. San Francisco, CA, November 14–16; contact Extension Programs in Medical Education, Registration Office, LS105, UCSF Box 0742, San Francisco, CA 94143-0742; 415-476-5808.

American College of Allergy and Immunology. New York, NY, November 15–20; contact ACAI, 800 East Northwest Highway, Suite 1080, Palatine, IL 60067; 708-359-2800.

American Cancer Society. Atlanta, GA, November 16; contact ACS, 1599 Clifton Road, N.E., Atlanta, GA 30329; 404-320-3333.

The Evolution of Protecting Human Subjects: From Nuremberg to the Nineties. Boston, MA, November 21–22; contact Public Responsibility in Medicine and Research, 132 Boylston Street, Boston, MA 02116; 617-423-4112 (fax, 617-423-1185).

Drug Review

Clinical uses of fentanyl, sufentanil, and alfentanil

MICHAEL A. CLOTZ AND MILAP C. NAHATA

Abstract: The pharmacokinetics, pharmacodynamics, and clinical uses of fentanyl, sufentanil, and alfentanil are reviewed.

The fentanyl derivatives have reduced or eliminated many of the disadvantages of opioid anesthetics, such as incomplete amnesia and undesirable hemodynamic responses to surgery. Fentanyl is 50–100 times as potent as morphine and was the first of the three to be marketed. Sufentanil is even more potent than fentanyl. Alfentanil has the fastest onset of action, followed by sufentanil and then fentanyl. Alfentanil also has the shortest duration of action of the group. Most studies of these agents have been done to assess their role as anesthetics in cardiac surgery. All three provide cardiovascular stability when administered before noxious surgical stimuli, except when given as a single bolus during the induction of anesthesia. All seem to produce adequate anesthesia, particularly when used in combination with nitrous oxide. Because of its short duration of action, alfentanil is preferred for brief procedures or when rapid changes in the level of consciousness are desired. All three agents have also been used for analgesia; epidural administration provides adequate relief of pain. Fentanyl has been formulated as a transdermal patch that seems to provide the same degree of analgesia as a continuous i.v. infusion. Fentanyl has also been formulated as an investigational lozenge that has shown advantages as a preoperative sedative in children.

As more is learned about these agents, their perioperative uses for anesthesia, analgesia, and sedation will continue to be refined.

Index terms: Alfentanil; Analgesics and antipyretics; Fentanyl; Pharmacokinetics; Sufentanil
Clin Pharm. 1991; 10:581-93

Late in the nineteenth century, morphine sulfate in large doses (1–2 mg/kg), in addition to scopolamine in some cases, was administered to surgical patients as a sole anesthetic. This practice, while popular initially, was associated with substantial morbidity and mortality. As a result, opioids in anesthesia practice were relegated to being a component of "balanced anesthesia" consisting of small to moderate doses of opioids supplemented by hypnotics, muscle relaxants, and inhalational anesthetics. In 1969 Lowenstein et al.[1] reintroduced high-dose opioid anesthesia when they used high-dose morphine as the sole anesthetic for patients undergoing cardiovascular surgery. Several drawbacks, including incomplete amnesia, a hypertensive response to surgical stimuli, hypotension and vasodilation secondary to histamine release, and bradycardia have limited morphine's popularity as a "complete" anesthetic, however.

These disadvantages illustrated the need for more potent yet less toxic agents if opioids were to be used as primary anesthetic agents. This led to the development of the synthetic opioid fentanyl in 1960. Fentanyl, which is chemically related to meperidine, has approximately 600 times the analgesic potency of meperidine and is 50–100 times as potent as morphine.[2] Sufentanil, first synthesized in 1974, is even more potent than fentanyl yet has a shorter duration of action. Animal studies suggest that very potent doses of sufentanil can be administered without severe adverse effects.[3] Alfentanil, first synthesized in 1978, is faster in onset than fentanyl and has approximately one third the duration of action but is only approximately one fourth as potent. Two other synthetic opioids, lofentanil and carfentanil, are each 20–30 times as potent as fentanyl.

Fentanyl (available as the citrate salt; Sublimaze, Janssen; other manufacturers), sufentanil (as the citrate salt; Sufenta, Janssen), and alfentanil (as the hydrochloride salt; Alfenta, Janssen) are also now being used more frequently as postoperative analgesics and

MICHAEL A. CLOTZ, PHARM.D., is Clinical Pharmacist, Children's Hospital, Columbus, OH; when this review was written he was a fellow in pediatric pharmacotherapy, Children's Hospital and College of Pharmacy, The Ohio State University (OSU), Columbus. MILAP C. NAHATA, PHARM.D., is Professor of Pharmacy and Pediatrics, Colleges of Pharmacy and Medicine, OSU, and Wexner Institute for Pediatric Research, Children's Hospital.

The contributions of J. David Martino, M.D., are acknowledged.

Address reprint requests to Dr. Nahata at the College of Pharmacy, The Ohio State University, 500 W. 12th Avenue, Columbus, OH 43210.

This is **article 680-204-9114** in the **ASHP Continuing Education System**; it qualifies for 1.0 hour of continuing-education credit. See page 638 for learning objectives and test questions.

as sedatives for patients requiring mechanical ventilation. They are also being explored as premedications for surgery and other painful procedures. This article reviews the properties and uses of fentanyl, sufentanil, and alfentanil for anesthesia, analgesia, and sedation.

Pharmacokinetics

An extensive review of the pharmacokinetic properties of fentanyl, sufentanil, and alfentanil has been presented by Mather.[2] In addition, Larijani and Goldberg[4] briefly discussed the pharmacokinetics of all these drugs in their review of alfentanil. The purpose of this article is to emphasize only the important aspects and summarize new information.

Physicochemical Properties. The physicochemical properties of the fentanyl derivatives (Table 1) have a major influence on their different pharmacokinetic and pharmacodynamic characteristics. Sufentanil is the most lipid-soluble member of the group.[3,4] Fentanyl is less lipid soluble than sufentanil but more lipid soluble than alfentanil.[6] Alfentanil is still far more lipid soluble than morphine.[6] Conversely, alfentanil has the lowest ionization constant and thus has the greatest percentage un-ionized at physiological pH.[6] Sufentanil is less un-ionized at a pH of 7.4, while fentanyl is the least un-ionized at physiological pH.[3,4,6]

Table 1.
Physicochemical Properties of Fentanyl, Alfentanil, and Sufentanil[4,5]

Property	Fentanyl	Sufentanil	Alfentanil
pK_a	8.4	8.4	6.5
% Un-ionized at pH 7.4	9	8.5	89
Free fraction (%)	16	10	8
Lipid solubility[a]	8913	9550	145

[a] Octanol:water partition coefficient (relative to morphine, where morphine = 1).

Absorption. The fentanyl derivatives are most commonly administered by the intravenous route. While little has been done to investigate absorption via the gastrointestinal tract, absorption via other routes including epidural, transdermal, and oral transmucosal has been studied.

Epidural Absorption. The opioids are frequently used epidurally to produce anesthesia and relief of acute or chronic pain.[7] Several investigators have attempted to measure the systemic absorption of the fentanyl derivatives after epidural administration. After doses of up to 150 μg of fentanyl were administered epidurally, concentrations in plasma remained less than 1.1 ng/mL and were not detectable in some patients.[8-10] Similarly, plasma sufentanil concentrations were very low or undetectable in patients receiving the drug epidurally.[11-14] The degree of absorption appears to be dose dependent.[13] The addition of epinephrine to sufentanil therapy decreases concentrations of the opioid in plasma, although not significantly.[11,13]

Transdermal Absorption. The physicochemical properties of fentanyl make it suitable for transdermal delivery. Fentanyl has been formulated as a transdermal patch for use as a constant-release analgesic. Concentrations do not reach a peak and plateau until 12–15 hours or longer after application.[15-17] At an equal dose rate (100 μg/hr), fentanyl concentrations produced by the transdermal formulation are significantly lower for up to eight hours after application than those produced by intravenous infusions.[18,19]

Oral Transmucosal Absorption. Oral transmucosal fentanyl citrate is being investigated as a preoperative sedative. Stanley et al.[20] evaluated the plasma concentrations achieved and found interpatient variability, but concluded that peak concentrations are dose dependent. Also, the time to achieve peak concentrations was significantly shorter in a group that sucked on the delivery system fast than in a slow-sucking group.

Distribution. The differences in distribution among the drugs of this class can be attributed to their physicochemical differences. After intravenous administration, fentanyl is rapidly and extensively distributed to highly perfused organs.[2] The steady-state volume of distribution of fentanyl is 2–3 L/kg.[21] Alfentanil is not as widely distributed as fentanyl; the volume of distribution is 0.4–1 L/kg.[21,22] Animal studies suggest that ion trapping in tissues (as the agent is less ionized at pH 7.4) and alfentanil's stronger affinity for plasma proteins than tissue proteins are responsible for the drug's small volume of distribution.[6] The volume of distribution of sufentanil, 1.7–2.5 L/kg, is intermediate between those of alfentanil and fentanyl.[23,24]

The fentanyl derivatives are highly bound to plasma proteins. Fentanyl binds primarily to α_1-acid glycoprotein and is 80–85% bound to α_1-acid glycoprotein or albumin.[6,21,25] The binding of fentanyl in vitro seems to be pH dependent; the percentage bound increases with increasing pH (range, 7.2–7.6).[25] Sufentanil also is highly bound to α_1-acid glycoprotein. Overall, sufentanil is approximately 93% plasma protein bound, and binding decreases with increasing pH.[6] Alfentanil also has a very strong affinity for α_1-acid glycoprotein. The free fraction of alfentanil is directly related to the concentration of α_1-acid glycoprotein.[4] At clinically encountered concentrations (0.4–100 ng/mL), approximately 88% of alfentanil is bound to plasma protein. At higher alfentanil concentrations (10–100 μg/mL), <60% is bound to plasma protein, presumably because of saturation of binding sites.[21]

Metabolism and Elimination. The major route of elimination of these agents is hepatic metabolism.[2,25,26] Less than 6% of the total body clearance of fentanyl is due to renal mechanisms.[25,27] Even smaller percentages of alfentanil and sufentanil are excreted unchanged in the urine.[2,28] The clearance of fentanyl approximates hepatic blood flow in healthy males.[21] The rate-limiting step for the elimination of fentanyl is redistribution from the peripheral compartment. This explains the relatively long elimination half-life of fentanyl after repeated or prolonged administration.[25] The hepatic clearance of alfentanil is slower than that of fentanyl. However, because of its smaller volume of distribution, alfentanil's overall rate of elimination is higher than that of fentanyl.[21,29] The clearance of sufentanil is slower than fentanyl's but faster than alfentanil's.[3,27] Conversely, the elimination half-life of sufentanil is shorter than fentanyl's but longer than alfentanil's.

Factors Affecting Pharmacokinetics. *Type of Surgery.* Hudson et al.[30] determined the pharmacokinetics of sufentanil in 10 patients undergoing abdominal aorta surgery.[30] The authors found a longer elimination half-life in these patients than in other surgical patients (12.1 and 2.7 hours, respectively). The subjects also had a larger volume of distribution (8.7 L/kg) relative to values previously reported (1.7 L/kg). Decreased hepatic blood flow, greater age, the infusion of large volumes of fluids, and a greater proportion of adipose tissue in the subjects may have contributed to these differences.

Cardiopulmonary bypass (CPB) can cause profound alterations in the disposition of the fentanyl derivatives. These changes can be ascribed to hemodilution, hypothermic slowing of metabolism, and sequestration in the bypass circuit.[31] Because of hemodilution, the concentrations of fentanyl and sufentanil decrease markedly after the initiation of CPB.[32-34] Concentrations then remain relatively constant and increase slightly upon the termination of CPB and rewarming of the patient. The elimination of the drugs after CPB is slower than would be expected in other surgical patients.[31] The volume of distribution, elimination half-life, and free fraction of alfentanil increase by a factor of 2–4 during CPB.[5] These alterations are associated with changes in the concentration of α_1-acid glycoprotein.

Age. A great deal of variation in the pharmacokinetics of these drugs exists among age groups. Compared with adults, infants and children have a shorter distribution half-life, larger central volume of distribution, larger steady-state volume of distribution, and faster clearance of fentanyl.[35-38] As with fentanyl, children have a smaller apparent steady-state volume of distribution, smaller initial volume of distribution, and shorter distribution and elimination half-lives of alfentanil than adults.[39-41] Meistelman et al.[40] found no differences in total body clearance of alfentanil between children and adults, while others have reported a greater clearance in children.[39,42] Premature neonates have a significantly longer elimination half-life and a lower total body clearance of alfentanil than children older than nine months.[43]

Evaluations of sufentanil pharmacokinetics in children have yielded variable results, and no direct comparisons have been made between children and adults. It appears that children older than one month and adults have similar sufentanil volumes of distribution and total body clearances.[44,45] In one study, the elimination half-life for children was shorter than published values for adults.[44] Infants less than one month of age have a significantly larger steady-state volume of distribution, longer distribution and elimination half-lives, and slower total body clearance of sufentanil than older children and adults.[45]

Elderly adults are reported to have a smaller volume of distribution of fentanyl than young adults.[46] Some researchers have found no change in clearance and elimination half-life with increasing age[46,47]; others have reported a significant decrease in total body clearance and increase in elimination half-life of alfentanil with increasing age.[48,49]

Hepatic or Renal Disease. Since the opioids are extensively metabolized by the liver, hepatic dysfunction should dramatically affect the disposition of these agents. However, Chauvin et al.[50] found no alteration in pharmacokinetic variables after a single dose of sufentanil was given to patients with uncomplicated cirrhosis. In another study, however, the elimination half-life of alfentanil was more than doubled in cirrhotic patients compared with subjects with normal renal and hepatic function.[51] The effects of multiple doses were not evaluated. Davis et al.[52] were unable to detect differences in alfentanil pharmacokinetic variables between healthy children and those with cholestatic liver disease. This lack of change was probably due to the fact that hepatocellular function remains intact in patients with cholestatic liver disease. A significant decrease in total alfentanil clearance was seen in three patients who underwent liver transplantation. Whether this decrease in clearance was due to allograft injury during organ procurement, decreased hepatic clearance, massive blood transfusion, altered protein binding, or increased volume of distribution is not known.

Theoretically, the derangements in plasma protein concentrations seen in renal dysfunction can alter the disposition of the highly protein-bound fentanyl derivatives.[2] However, no alterations in the clearance or elimination half-life of alfentanil were seen in patients with chronic renal failure.[52,53] One investigator found a larger volume of distribution of alfentanil in patients with chronic renal failure than in controls.[53] The pharmacokinetics of sufentanil also seem to be unaffected by chronic renal failure.[54] However, while no significant differences were found between patients with renal failure and controls, total clearance and elimination half-life varied more in renal failure patients.[54]

Pharmacodynamics

Potency. Fentanyl has 50–100 times the analgesic potency of morphine.[2] Alfentanil is only one fourth to one tenth as potent as fentanyl after a bolus dose.[4] Sufentanil is 5–10 times as potent as fentanyl[2,3] and 20–40 times as potent as alfentanil.[4] Carfentanil and lofentanil are extremely potent, having 20–30 times the potency of fentanyl.[2] Whether extreme potency represents an advantage remains to be seen. While potency is an important consideration, there is wide variability in opioid requirements among patients.

Onset of Action. The time to unresponsiveness or

unconsciousness has been used as a marker of the time to onset of action of these agents.[55] Many factors affect the time to onset of action, including dose and rate of administration. All the drugs in this class can produce unconsciousness within five minutes.[4,56,57] Alfentanil has a faster onset of action than fentanyl.[4,56,58] Sufentanil, because of its greater lipid solubility, also seems to act more quickly than fentanyl.[57,59]

Specific Effects. *Central Nervous System Effects.* The fentanyl derivatives are typical opioids in that they are pure μ-receptor agonists. The actions of the drugs in this class are qualitatively similar.[60] The opioids produce analgesia and sedation. Whether opioids alone can prevent awareness and produce complete amnesia is under debate.[61-63] The electroencephalogram (EEG) provides a reliable measurement of the CNS effects of opioids. Alfentanil, sufentanil, and fentanyl cause a predictable, progressive slowing of the EEG.[56,64] Using spectral edge analysis, Scott et al.[56] developed a continuous, noninvasive method of measuring CNS effects. Investigators have used this method in an attempt to correlate plasma concentrations of the opioids with CNS effects (EEG).

Cardiovascular Effects. Some investigators have reported an increase in heart rate when these agents are given in combination with pancuronium[65-68] but not when they are administered with vecuronium or metocurine; this is not unexpected because of pancuronium's vagolytic properties.[67,68] No depression in myocardial contractility (ejection fraction) has been noted with the use of these agents.[69-71] Surgical stimulation, including tracheal intubation, skin incision, intraoperative manipulation, and skin closure, produces a sympathetic stress response producing hypertension and tachycardia. The fentanyl derivatives effectively block the sympathetic stress response to surgical stimulation, providing hemodynamic stability.[66,72,73] These effects seem to be related to the dose and the plasma concentration.

Hormonal Effects. The stress response described above is the result of the release of endogenous catecholamines, cortisol, glucose, and other hormones in response to surgical manipulation.[55] Davis et al.[44] showed that sufentanil was successful in preventing significant increases in catecholamine concentrations in response to surgical stimuli. Likewise, fentanyl prevents increases in circulating concentrations of adrenocorticotropic hormone, growth hormone, cortisol, and glucose in response to surgical manipulation.[74]

Concentration–Effect Relationship. There have been attempts to correlate plasma concentrations of these opioids with their effects. Scott et al.[56] correlated serum concentrations of fentanyl and alfentanil with the spectral edge of the EEG. They found a lag time between changes in the EEG and changes in serum opioid concentrations. This lag time was greater for fentanyl than for alfentanil; theoretically, this could be due to fentanyl's greater lipid solubility.

Shafer and colleagues[75] found that alfentanil 200 ng/mL (supplemented by nitrous oxide) was an effective concentration for 50% of patients (CP_{50}) undergoing intra-abdominal surgery; the CP_{95} was 400 ng/mL. Ausems and coworkers[76] further measured effective concentrations of alfentanil for anesthesia in patients undergoing general surgery. A concentration of 475 ng/mL, in combination with 60% nitrous oxide, was necessary to block the response to tracheal intubation in half of their 37 patients. The alfentanil CP_{50}'s for skin incision and skin closure were 275 and 150 ng/mL, respectively. The CP_{50} for intraoperative stimuli was dependent on the surgical procedure and ranged from 270 to 412 ng/mL. The CP_{50} for acceptable spontaneous respiration was 223 ng/mL.

According to Hug,[5] fentanyl concentrations greater than 1 ng/mL produce slight analgesia and ventilatory depression, concentrations greater than 3 ng/mL produce further analgesia and a 50% decrease in the ventilatory response to carbon dioxide, and concentrations greater than 20 ng/mL produce unconsciousness.

A sufentanil CP_{50} of 1.08 ng/mL was suggested by Marty et al.[77] to be necessary for suppressing the response to tracheal intubation. To suppress responses to intraoperative manipulation, sufentanil concentrations ranging from 0.2 to 2.3 ng/mL were necessary, and the CP_{50} for satisfactory respiration was 0.25 ng/mL.

Adverse Effects

After rapid intravenous administration, the fentanyl derivatives cause bradycardia and hypotension, although to a lesser extent than morphine.[60,67,78-80] The mechanism seems to be vagal stimulation, and these effects can be prevented by premedication with vagolytic agents, such as atropine. The mechanism by which morphine produces hypotension is histamine release, a phenomenon not observed with the fentanyl derivatives.[55,79,81] After bolus administration, the potent opioids produce chest wall rigidity that can make ventilation difficult or impossible. Pretreatment with a muscle relaxant can usually prevent this adverse effect.[79]

When the fentanyl derivatives were introduced, claims were made of short durations of action allowing for rapid recovery after administration was stopped. Soon after high-dose fentanyl became a popular anesthetic, reports appeared of delayed respiratory depression and muscular rigidity (two to six hours postoperatively).[82-85] These effects are probably due to secondary peaks in plasma fentanyl concentrations many hours after injection.[84-86] Stoekel and coworkers[85] hypothesized that enterohepatic recirculation is responsible for this event, but this is unlikely because of fentanyl's high hepatic extraction ratio.[21] Other more probable explanations include redistribution from adipose tissue and muscle and absorption from the gastrointestinal tract.[84] This phenomenon is more likely to occur when hypothermia (and rewarming) or acidosis occur in the postoperative period.[87,88] Similarly, postoperative respiratory depression and rigidity have been reported with sufentanil therapy.[89-91] This is not surprising, since sufentanil, while having a smaller volume of distribution than fentanyl, is still widely distributed.

Alfentanil, because of its very small volume of distribution, should produce these effects infrequently. However, Mahla et al.[92] reported two cases of delayed respiratory depression occurring approximately 45 minutes after discontinuation of an alfentanil infusion for anesthesia in spinal fusion surgery. The infusions were lengthy (five to more than eight hours). The contribution of this long infusion time to the respiratory depression is not known. Jaffe and Coalson[93] reported another case of recurrent respiratory depression after a 93-minute infusion of alfentanil for anesthesia. This effect was reversed by naloxone in all three patients. A mechanism that produces a secondary peak in the alfentanil concentration sufficient to produce delayed respiratory depression has yet to be elucidated.

There have been several reports of seizures or seizure-like activity after the use of sufentanil.[71,94-97] Since no concomitant EEG recording was documented in four of these reports,[71,95-97] it is unclear whether these episodes consisted of generalized tonic–clonic seizures, myoclonus, or atypical muscle rigidity. Bowdle[94] reported one case of generalized myoclonus in the absence of cortical seizure activity in an EEG recording. Katz and colleagues[98] described a patient who developed seizure-like activity once after receiving sufentanil and again three days later after being given fentanyl. EEG recording during the fentanyl-associated incident did not show unusual CNS activity. Strong and Matson[99] reported a case of seizure activity after alfentanil treatment. The patient had received a fairly small dose, which makes it less likely that the activity represented muscle rigidity. However, pre-existing cerebral infarction and Todd's paralysis could not be ruled out as contributing factors. A detailed review of the possible proconvulsant effects of the opioid anesthetics has been published.[100]

Other common adverse effects of these agents include facial itching, nausea, vomiting, and decreased gastrointestinal tract motility.

Use of Fentanyl, Sufentanil, and Alfentanil for Anesthesia

Cardiovascular Procedures. Since Lowenstein et al.[1] first described the use of high-dose morphine for anesthesia in cardiac surgery, there has been much interest in investigating the newer opioids for this use. The newer opioids have replaced morphine in cardiovascular surgery primarily because of their greater potency and specificity in blocking the hormonal stress response to surgery. All the stress responses would have an adverse effect on an individual with coronary artery disease. Studies of the use of fentanyl and sufentanil in cardiovascular procedures are summarized in Table 2.

In early evaluations, low-dose fentanyl (30–75 μg/kg) failed to block hemodynamic responses to surgical stimuli.[70,101,102] However, Sprigge et al.[66] found that 100 μg/kg administered as a bolus followed by a short infusion was effective in producing cardiovascular stability during cardiovascular surgery. Zurick et al.[65] found that fentanyl 150 μg/kg was effective in controlling responses to stimuli and provided greater coronary artery perfusion than halothane.

Sufentanil has also been evaluated for use in cardiovascular procedures. As with fentanyl, the results have been mixed. When given as a single bolus for the induction of anesthesia, sufentanil does not seem to be effective in these procedures,[71,104] probably owing to the interval between administration and stimuli such as sternotomy.

Comparative trials of fentanyl, sufentanil, and alfentanil have been performed (Table 3). Sufentanil seems to be as effective or more effective than fentanyl or alfentanil in providing cardiovascular stability.[60,105-108] Fentanyl and alfentanil are equivalent in their ability to provide cardiovascular stability.[107,108] There is evidence that all three of these opioids provide adequate anesthesia in coronary artery surgery, particularly when supplemental doses are administered before noxious stimulation begins.

Other Procedures. While the bulk of investigations have centered on the use of the newer opioids in cardiovascular surgery, these agents have shown usefulness in many other surgical procedures. Pathak and colleagues[109] found that the total opioid requirement was less in spinal fusion patients receiving morphine or fentanyl by continuous infusion than by intermittent bolus injections. In addition, wake-up tests, used to assess spinal cord function, were performed more smoothly and repeatedly in the infusion groups. All the patients who received fentanyl infusions were able to be extubated in the operating room.

Rucquoi and Camu[78] found that cardiovascular stability was provided by large doses of alfentanil and fentanyl in patients undergoing lower abdominal surgery. Doses of 30 and 120 μg of fentanyl and alfentanil per kilogram, respectively, were used after the induction of anesthesia and again immediately before the surgical incision. Both fentanyl and alfentanil lowered the heart rate, mean arterial blood pressure, and cardiac index during the period between the first dose and the skin incision. After the second dose the same responses were evident, but only for 20 minutes in the alfentanil-treated group, compared with the entire one-hour observation period for the patients given fentanyl. Stuart-Taylor and Sleigh[110] found that an alfentanil infusion of 7.5 μg/kg/min for 10 minutes followed by 0.75 μg/kg/min for the duration of surgery necessitated less use of volatile agents than did 50–100-μg bolus doses of fentanyl. The authors, however, did not report the number and size of doses in the fentanyl group.

Clark et al.[111] reported that fentanyl or sufentanil, in combination with nitrous oxide, produced hemody-

Table 2.
Summary of Trials of Fentanyl and Sufentanil in Cardiovascular Procedures

Reference	No. Patients	Dosage	Observations[a]
Fentanyl (as the Citrate Salt)			
69	10	50 μg/kg at 100–200 μg/min	Doses escalated by >30 μg/kg produced decreased CI and LVSWI
101	12	50 μg/kg at 200 μg/min (observations made after 10-μg/kg and 50-μg/kg doses); supplemental dose of 250–500 μg/kg given before noxious stimuli	Total doses of 50–89 μg/kg failed to block hemodynamic responses to intubation, skin incision, and sternotomy
102	9	100 μg/kg at 200 μg/min up to 10 μg/kg, then 300 μg/min up to 100 μg/kg	Significant increases in MAP and HR and significant decrease in SV at sternotomy
66	10	60 μg/kg (30-μg/kg bolus, then 0.3 μg/kg/min)	Fewer patients in the 100-μg/kg group responded to intubation and surgical stimulation, but the difference was not statistically significant
	10	90 μg/kg (40-μg/kg bolus, then 0.4 μg/kg/min)	
	10	100 μg/kg (50-μg/kg bolus, then 0.5 μg/kg/min)	
65	10	150 μg/kg at 1500–2000 μg/min	Increase in HR after intubation; no change in SBP, DBP, or MAP; better coronary artery perfusion compared with patients given halothane and nitrous oxide
Sufentanil (as the Citrate Salt)			
103	40	15 μg/kg over 2 minutes	Significant decrease in SBP after induction of anesthesia and after skin incision; significant increase in DBP after sternotomy
104	8	1.8 μg/kg (1-μg/kg bolus, then 0.015 μg/kg/min)	Neither dosage prevented hypertensive response to sternotomy
	8	17.5 μg/kg (10-μg/kg bolus, then 0.15 μg/kg/min)	
71[b]	5	5-μg/kg induction dose, with 1-μg/kg supplements before noxious stimuli	Significant increase in SBP after intubation, incision, and sternotomy
	5	10-μg/kg induction dose, with 2-μg/kg supplements before noxious stimuli	Significant increase in HR after sternotomy in 5- and 10-μg/kg groups
	10	20-μg/kg induction dose, with 5-μg/kg supplements before noxious stimuli	
44[b]	20	15 μg/kg over 1 minute	No significant increase in HR or BP after skin incision and sternotomy

[a] CI = cardiac index, LVSWI = left ventricular stroke work index, SBP = systolic blood pressure, HR = heart rate, SV = stroke volume, DBP = diastolic blood pressure, MAP = mean arterial blood pressure, BP = blood pressure.
[b] Pediatric investigation.

namic and hormonal stability during general surgery. The patients were first given sufentanil 1 μg/kg or fentanyl 7 μg/kg. Thereafter, either opioid was given in increments of 25 and 100 μg when heart rate or systolic blood pressure increased more than 15% from baseline. No differences during surgery were noted between the two groups, but respiratory drive was significantly depressed in the fentanyl group postoperatively. Also, the fentanyl group experienced significantly more pain at 30 but not 60 minutes postoperatively, and the time to extubation was shorter in the sufentanil group.

Ausems and colleagues[73] compared intermittent bolus injections of alfentanil 1–2 mg with a continuous infusion of alfentanil, both in combination with nitrous oxide, in patients having lower abdominal surgery. The computer-assisted infusion device was designed to produce a target plasma drug concentration chosen by the anesthesiologist by giving bolus doses and increasing the infusion rate when anesthesia was determined to be inadequate and to interrupt the infusion or decrease the rate if less anesthesia was indicated. The infusion produced greater hemodynamic stability than did the intermittent boluses. No patients in the infusion group required naloxone for inadequate ventilation postoperatively, compared with 5 of 10 patients in the bolus dose group.

Because of its duration of action, alfentanil should be an acceptable anesthetic for short surgical procedures. However, Hull and Jacobson[112] failed to detect differences in recovery characteristics between 45 women who received 700 μg of alfentanil and 45 women who received 100 μg of fentanyl for short (6.21–9.78-min) gynecological procedures. More patients in the alfentanil group became apneic after the induction of anesthesia. The authors suggested that the apnea may have been averted and the recovery characteristics more favorable if multiple, smaller doses had been given.

Cartwright[113] compared recovery after anesthesia with nitrous oxide plus halothane (mean concentration, 1.8%) with recovery after 500 μg of alfentanil initially followed by supplements of 200 μg if necessary. The duration of anesthesia was similar for both groups. The mean ± S.D. time to recovery, defined as the interval between discontinuation of the nitrous oxide and the point at which patients could open their eyes and state their names, was significantly shorter for the alfentanil group (5.6 ± 1.1 min) than the halothane group (10.1 ± 1.1 min). Apnea was a major

Table 3.
Summary of Comparative Trials of Alfentanil, Sufentanil, and Fentanyl for Cardiovascular Procedures

Reference	No. Patients	Opioid[a]	Dosage	Observations[b]
60	18	S	12.9 μg/kg	Significant increases in MAP and SBP during sternotomy and sternal spreading in F group; increases not seen in S group
	19	F	122 μg/kg	
105	20	S	5 μg/kg over 1 minute, with 2.5-μg/kg supplements before noxious stimuli	Significantly lower MAP and LVSWI after induction of anesthesia in S group than in F group; no marked hemodynamic response to surgical stimuli in either group
	20	F	25 μg/kg over 1 minute, with 25-μg/kg supplements before noxious stimuli	
106[c]	11	S	5 μg/kg over 5–10 minutes	Significant increase in DBP and MBP in all groups after sternotomy; significant increase in MAP in F group; significant decrease in HR in S group
	10	S	10 μg/kg over 5–10 minutes	
	10	F	50 μg/kg over 5–10 minutes	
	10	F	75 μg/kg over 5–10 minutes	
107	10	A	40-μg/kg bolus, then 6 μg/kg/min (total, 1379 μg/kg)	No significant differences in hemodynamic responses to surgical stimuli
	9	F	48-μg/kg bolus, then 0.3 μg/kg/min (total, 110 μg/kg)	
108	8	S	15-μg/kg induction dose and 5 μg/kg before skin incision	All three agents provided adequate hemodynamic stability
	7	F	75-μg/kg induction dose and 25 μg/kg before skin incision	
	8	A	125-μg/kg induction dose followed by 0.5-μg/kg/hr continuous infusion	

[a] S = sufentanil, F = fentanyl, A = alfentanil.
[b] MAP = mean arterial blood pressure, SBP = systolic blood pressure, LVSWI = left ventricular stroke work index, DBP = diastolic blood pressure, MBP = mean blood pressure, HR = heart rate.
[c] Pediatric investigation.

problem in the alfentanil group, occurring in 22 of 39 patients, compared with only 1 of 34 subjects who received halothane.

Welling and Donegan[114] reported on the use of alfentanil and droperidol for craniotomy to remove epileptogenic foci in four patients. Because there is risk of damaging vital areas of the brain, especially speech, memory, and motor areas, patient responses to electrical stimulation are evaluated by electrocorticography. Patient cooperativeness is essential during these portions of the procedure, so an anesthetic technique that is easily adjustable to maintain a comfortable yet cooperative patient is essential. Using alfentanil boluses of 5–7.5 μg/kg followed by infusions of 1.0–2.0 μg/kg/min, the authors were able to provide adequate anesthesia during periods of maximum stimulation. When cortical mapping was to be performed, the infusion rate was decreased to 0.25–0.5 μg/kg/min. This produced a responsive yet comfortable patient within two minutes.

From the available information for general surgery, all three of the newer opioids, usually in combination with nitrous oxide, are acceptable anesthetics. When alfentanil is used, continuous infusion may produce a more stable anesthetic course than intermittent bolus doses. For short procedures or when rapidly changing levels of anesthesia are needed, alfentanil appears to be an acceptable agent.

Use of Fentanyl, Sufentanil, and Alfentanil for Analgesia

Labor and Delivery. Use of the newer opioids for analgesia during labor and delivery has been investigated. These studies have almost exclusively involved epidural administration of these agents either alone or in combination with local anesthetics. Carrie et al.[8] administered 150–200 μg of fentanyl (infusion rate not reported) epidurally to 38 women who requested analgesia in the first stage of labor. The initial dose of fentanyl provided adequate analgesia (assessed with a 10-point visual analogue scale) for up to 90 minutes. Nine patients required two doses, and six subjects requested a third dose of fentanyl 90 minutes after the previous dose. The subsequent dose(s), while not providing as dramatic a relief of pain as the first, still produced considerable analgesia. Except for mild pruritus, no adverse effects were noted. All the infants except one had Apgar scores of 7–10 at one minute.

Justins and coworkers[115] compared epidural fentanyl 80 μg plus bupivacaine hydrochloride 12 mg with epidural bupivacaine alone in the first stage of labor. The addition of fentanyl provided significantly faster onset of analgesia and more satisfactory analgesia than did bupivacaine alone. The only difference in adverse effects was that the fentanyl group experienced more itching than the control group. Subsequently, Justins and colleagues[9] compared epidural fentanyl 80 μg plus bupivacaine hydrochloride 12 mg with intramuscular fentanyl 100 μg plus epidural bupivacaine hydrochloride 12 mg for analgesia in the first stage of labor in a randomized, double-blind study. At 10 minutes, the patients in the epidural fentanyl group had significantly less pain than the intramuscular fentanyl group. Furthermore, significantly more patients in the intramuscular fentanyl group

(62%) required supplemental epidural bupivacaine than in the other group (16%). There were no differences in adverse effects, and neonatal status was not adversely affected in either group.

Vella et al.[116] administered bupivacaine epidurally in addition to fentanyl 80 μg either intravenously or epidurally in women who required analgesia in the first stage of labor. Significantly more patients in the intravenous fentanyl group (75%) required supplemental bupivacaine than did patients in the epidural fentanyl group (30%). The pain score (rated with a visual analogue scale) declined more rapidly in the epidural fentanyl group but was significantly lower than that in the intravenous fentanyl group at 20 minutes. Of the 20 patients in the intravenous fentanyl group, 11 had received supplemental bupivacaine by 20 minutes, compared with only 4 in the epidural fentanyl group. There were no differences in adverse effects between the groups; the most common reactions were hypotension, nausea, vomiting, and itching.

Gaffud and colleagues[117] administered 0.5% bupivacaine hydrochloride (mean dose, 118 mg) alone or in combination with 100 μg of fentanyl (mean dose of bupivacaine hydrochloride, 110 mg) epidurally to 20 patients undergoing repeat cesarean section in a double-blind, randomized study. More patients in the bupivacaine-alone group experienced pain during the procedure and required supplemental analgesia. Significantly fewer patients in the bupivacaine plus fentanyl group required analgesics after skin incision. Similarly, Preston et al.[10] found that fewer mothers who received epidural fentanyl 1 μg/kg plus lidocaine experienced pain during nonemergent cesarean section than mothers who received epidural lidocaine in 0.9% sodium chloride injection. Five of the 15 subjects in the lidocaine plus sodium chloride injection group required intravenous opioids to control intraoperative pain, compared with none in the fentanyl plus lidocaine group. Adverse effects were not different between the groups, and no adverse effects were noted in the neonates.

Phillips[14] compared a continuous epidural infusion of sufentanil 10 μg/hr plus bupivacaine hydrochloride 12.5 mg/hr with bupivacaine hydrochloride 12.5 mg/hr alone for labor and delivery. The time to onset of analgesia was similar between the two groups, but the patients in the sufentanil plus bupivacaine group had a significantly lower pain score and greater reduction in the pain score than the bupivacaine-alone group. The bupivacaine-alone group required higher infusion rates and more supplemental doses of bupivacaine. Pruritus occurred significantly more often in the sufentanil plus bupivacaine group but was detected only upon questioning and was not severe enough to require treatment. No adverse neonatal effects were noted in either group.

Other Severe Pain. Duthie and colleagues[118] administered fentanyl 100 μg/hr intravenously to 45 patients undergoing orthopedic, cardiac, or abdominal procedures or procedures expected to last longer than four hours. The infusions were begun at the beginning of the operation and continued for 24 hours. Assessment of pain on a 4-point scale at 8, 12, and 24 hours revealed an incidence of severe pain of 7% in the orthopedic group, 15% in the abdominal group, and none in the prolonged-procedure group. The incidence of pain in the cardiac group was not reported. Since this was primarily a pharmacokinetic study, no control group was used.

Chudnofsky et al.[119] reported on the use of fentanyl in 841 patients in their emergency department over a 3.5-year period. Orthopedic procedures and incision and drainage of abscesses accounted for nearly 70% of fentanyl use. The doses ranged from 25 to 1400 μg. Adverse effects were rare and included nausea, vomiting, urticaria, and itching. More serious adverse effects occurred in nine patients. Six of these developed respiratory depression, and three experienced hypotension. However, two of the patients who developed hypotension and four of those who developed respiratory depression were intoxicated on entering the emergency department. The third patient who became hypotensive had received 100 mg of labetalol hydrochloride intravenously 40 minutes before being given fentanyl. All the adverse effects were transient and did not require hospital admission. This low incidence of adverse effects does not obviate the need for very close patient monitoring when fentanyl is used.

Epidural administration of opioids has become a popular method of producing analgesia while attempting to reduce the systemic adverse effects. Chrubasik et al.[120] compared epidural fentanyl, alfentanil, and morphine for the treatment of postoperative pain. When the patients complained of pain, morphine sulfate, fentanyl, and alfentanil boluses and infusions of 2 mg and 0.2 mg/hr, 100 μg and 20 μg/hr, and 1 mg and 200 μg/hr, respectively, were provided. The infusion rates were decreased or extra bolus doses were administered depending on the level of pain, which was assessed with a visual analogue scale. Alfentanil and fentanyl produced a significantly faster onset of analgesia than morphine. Adverse effects were mild and included pruritus, nausea, vomiting, and urinary retention. There were no significant differences in adverse effects between the groups.

Cohen and colleagues[13] found that intravenous and epidural sufentanil both produced rapid onset of analgesia and that epidural sufentanil had a significantly longer duration of action after cesarean section. In a randomized, double-blind study, patients received 50 μg of sufentanil epidurally or 10 μg intravenously. Epidural administration caused significantly more pruritus than did intravenous administration.

Rosen and coworkers[121] administered either morphine sulfate 5 mg or sufentanil 30, 45, or 60 μg epidurally for the relief of pain after cesarean section. The subjects receiving sufentanil had a significantly faster onset of analgesia than those receiving morphine. Morphine, however, produced a significantly longer duration of pain relief than any of the doses of sufentanil. Also, the groups given 30 or 45 μg of sufentanil required significantly more supplemental analgesics than the morphine group. There were no significant differences in any variable among the sufentanil groups.

Sufentanil has also been evaluated for pain relief after epidural administration in children. Beniabed and coworkers[12] administered sufentanil 0.75 μg/kg epidurally to 15 children for the relief of pain after urologic procedures. Although the onset of action after a single injection was rapid (mean ± S.D., 3 ± 0.3 min), the duration of action was short (198 ± 19 min). Pruritus occurred in three children and nausea and vomiting in five.

The effectiveness of transdermally administered fentanyl for managing postoperative pain has been evaluated. Holley and Van Steennis[122] placed a transdermal patch designed to deliver fentanyl 100 μg/hr on eight subjects two hours before the induction of anesthesia. Anesthesia was induced with 300 μg of intravenous fentanyl and maintained with enflurane and nitrous oxide. The transdermal patch was left in place for 24 hours. Postoperative morphine requirements were similar to those of a group of patients receiving fentanyl 100 μg/hr intravenously, with 60% of the morphine given in the first six hours postoperatively before fentanyl concentrations reached a plateau. Respiratory depression was the only adverse effect that was discussed, and it did not occur in the transdermal patch group.

In a double-blind study, Caplan et al.[17] compared transdermal fentanyl with placebo for the treatment of postoperative pain. The transdermal patch was designed to deliver fentanyl at 75 μg/hr. During the 24-hour period when the patches were in place, patients receiving fentanyl required significantly less morphine and had significantly lower pain scores on a visual analogue scale than patients given placebo. These differences persisted in the 12-hour observation period after the patches were removed. The only adverse effect that was significantly more prominent in the fentanyl group was vomiting (30% versus 73%).

Use of Fentanyl, Sufentanil, and Alfentanil as Sedatives

Sedation of the Mechanically Ventilated Patient. The goal of sedation in the intensive-care unit is to make the patient as comfortable as possible while maintaining compliance with imposed ventilation. The ideal agent would provide cardiovascular stability, have a rapid onset and cessation of action, and be convenient to administer, preferably by continuous infusion. Fentanyl and alfentanil theoretically meet these requirements.

No controlled trial of fentanyl for prolonged sedation in the intensive-care unit has been reported. However, because of its relatively rapid onset of action, ease of administration, and relatively short duration of action, fentanyl is the sedative of choice in some institutions, particularly for neonates.[123] Fears of prolonged duration of action after repeated or prolonged administration[84-86] have not been validated nor refuted by means of clinical trials. Shafer et al.[124] reported a case in which a patient required an increasing rate of fentanyl infusion to remain sedated. The infusion rate and plasma fentanyl concentrations eventually reached those associated with general anesthesia, yet the subject remained easy to arouse.

Because of its small volume of distribution and short elimination half-life, alfentanil may be more reliable (in terms of cessation of action) than fentanyl as a continuous-infusion sedative in the intensive-care unit. Cohen[125] reviewed his experience with alfentanil infusions in 34 intensive-care patients. Mean infusion rates ranged from 0.11 to 2.09 μg/kg/min. Four patients required an atracurium infusion, and all the patients received supplemental doses of diazepam 0.1 mg/kg. The quality of sedation was rated good or perfect 98% of the time and acceptable in all cases; however, brief periods of inadequate sedation were reported in eight patients. The contribution of diazepam to sedation cannot be ignored. No adverse effects were reported. Yate et al.[126] reported on the use of alfentanil infusions for sedation and analgesia in 10 postoperative patients who required mechanical ventilation. After receiving a bolus of 1 mg, the patients were administered a continuous infusion of 0.25 μg/kg/min for an average of 796 minutes. Spontaneous respiration returned after a mean of 35 minutes, and the patients were extubated about two hours after the infusion was stopped. Only one patient required supplemental midazolam because he persisted in fighting the ventilator. Vomiting was the only adverse effect, which occurred in three patients after the infusion ended.

Cohen and Kelly[127] administered alfentanil at rates of 0.08–2.5 μg/kg/min to 16 patients who required sedation while receiving assisted ventilation. Bolus doses of 3 μg/kg were administered before procedures such as tracheal suctioning and if sedation was subjectively judged to be inadequate. Supplemental diazepam was administered when necessary. Patients over 50 years of age required a mean infusion rate of 0.4 μg/kg/min, while those younger than 50 needed a mean infusion rate of 1 μg/kg/min. The investigators judged the quality of sedation to be good, and no untoward effects were reported. All the patients were awake before the infusion was discontinued, but no details on tapering of the infusion were provided. Sinclair and coworkers[128] administered a loading dose of alfentanil 50 μg/kg followed by an initial continuous infusion of 24 μg/kg/hr to 14 intensive-care patients who required mechanical ventilation for more than 12 hours. The infusion rate was decreased if the nurse believed that the patient was too sedated; the rate was increased or a dose of midazolam 2.5–5.0 mg (as the hydrochloride salt) was given if the patient was inadequately sedated. This regimen was effective for 11 of the 14 patients. No adverse effects were reported.

From the published reports, it appears that alfentanil may be a suitable agent for the sedation of mechanically ventilated patients. For now, though, lack of controlled trials and the cost of the drug may limit its widespread use for this purpose. Fentanyl is being used in these patients, but the lack of published trials prohibits specific recommendations of fentanyl for this purpose. It theoretically should be effective, but one must be cautious of the probability of fentanyl accumulation with prolonged administration.

Preoperative Sedation. In children, preoperative sedation poses a difficult problem. Intramuscular or intravenous administration of agents may compound the apprehension and fear that are already present. The absorption of oral preanesthetic agents is variable, and a large volume of liquid usually must be given. A noninjectable dosage form that would provide reliable absorption would obviate these problems. Fentanyl citrate has been formulated as a lozenge for oral transmucosal administration. Clinical evaluations of oral transmucosal fentanyl citrate (OTFC), an investigational product, have been performed in adult volunteers and pediatric patients. Stanley et al.[20] studied 28 adult volunteers receiving OTFC in doses of 5 mg (n = 7), 4 mg (n = 3), 2 mg (n = 8), 1 mg (n = 2), or 0.5 mg (n = 8). The subjects were assessed for changes in heart rate, systolic blood pressure, diastolic blood pressure, and pain threshold (evaluated with a graded electrical stimulus). Sedation occurred within 10 minutes after drug administration. This effect was dose related and reached its peak at approximately 90 minutes. No clinically important changes in heart rate or blood pressure were associated with any dose throughout the study. Respiratory changes evidenced by significant reductions in respiratory rate and oxygen saturation and increases in end-tidal carbon dioxide content were minimal at the lower doses. End-tidal carbon dioxide was significantly elevated and respiratory rate significantly decreased in the patients receiving the 4- and 5-mg doses. The level of electrical current perceived as painful increased (reflecting increasing analgesia) in all groups in a dose-related fashion. While the 4- and 5-mg doses were not suitable for clinical use because of undesired respiratory depression, the lower doses (0.5–2.0 mg [5–30 µg/kg]) could provide sedation and analgesia without causing clinically important adverse effects.

To determine which dose of OTFC might be suitable for premedication in children, Streisand and coworkers[129] compared four dose ranges in 47 children. The patients received 5–10, 10–15, 15–20, or 20–25 µg of OTFC per kilogram about 60 minutes before the planned induction of anesthesia. Evaluations were made preoperatively, during induction, and in the recovery room. Respiratory rate, oxygen saturation, blood pressure, and heart rate were monitored. The investigators and the parents evaluated the patients for anxiety and activity. The group given 15–20 µg/kg was judged to have had the best response, because most of these children became sedated and cooperative, and adverse effects were limited to mild facial itching. Conversely, the group given 20–25 µg/kg had clinically important respiratory depression; in 25% of these patients, oxygen saturation declined to <89%.

Feld et al.[130] compared OTFC 15–20 µg/kg with placebo in 40 children undergoing surgery. OTFC produced significantly less anxiety and more sedation than placebo. Respiratory rate was reduced in the fentanyl group, but no significant difference in oxygen saturation was noted. There was a higher incidence of nausea and facial pruritus in the OTFC group.

Nelson and colleagues[131] administered OTFC 15–20 µg/kg, a commonly given oral premedication (meperidine hydrochloride 1.5 mg/kg, diazepam 0.2 mg/kg, and atropine sulfate 0.02 mg/kg), or no premedication to 60 children. Effectiveness in reducing anxiety and activity before surgery and the ease of induction of anesthesia were evaluated. Activity and anxiety scores improved significantly with OTFC but not with the common oral premedication compared with the controls (no premedication). Minimum activity and anxiety occurred at 28.6 and 18.1 minutes, respectively, after OTFC administration. Children given no premedication had increasing activity and anxiety scores in the holding area as they waited to go into the operating room. The patients' status before induction and status on emergence from anesthesia were not significantly different among the three groups.

Henderson and colleagues[132] administered sufentanil 1.5, 3.0, and 4.5 µg/kg intranasally to 80 children as a preanesthetic in a placebo-controlled double-blind trial. Patients who received sufentanil were more easily separated from their parents and were more calm than patients given placebo. Patients who received 4.5 µg/kg had a significantly larger decrease in ventilatory compliance perioperatively and a greater incidence of vomiting postoperatively than any of the other groups. Administration of a shorter acting agent, such as midazolam or alfentanil, may be preferable in this situation.[133]

Formulary Recommendations

Alfentanil has a place on the formulary of institutions that perform short surgical procedures; its relatively short duration of action makes it a superior agent for these procedures. Sufentanil seems to be preferable to alfentanil and fentanyl for cardiovascular procedures and thus has a place on the formulary of institutions that perform cardiovascular surgery. Because of the greater experience with fentanyl for analgesia and sedation and the relatively low cost of this agent (it is generically available), fentanyl can be a part of any hospital's formulary.

Conclusion

The introduction of the newer, more potent opioids has added considerably to the clinician's armamentarium against pain. Most experience with these agents has been in the areas of induction and maintenance of anesthesia. Their use for anesthesia in cardiovascular surgery has been extensively studied. Sufentanil seems to be the most useful of the group in providing cardiovascular stability throughout the operative period. When doses of these agents are given just before noxious stimuli, however, there does not seem to be a difference among the agents. For general surgery, all the agents appear to provide an adequate depth of anesthesia. For short procedures, alfentanil seems to be the drug of choice.

The use of these agents for sedation and analgesia has also been investigated. All three drugs provide adequate analgesia when given intramuscularly or intravenously. Much study of epidural administration has been done. Although the agents provide sufficient analgesia when given by this route, if prolonged analgesia is required, as for postoperative pain relief, continuous epidural infusions are preferred to epidural bolus injections because of the short duration of action of the latter. Transdermally administered fentanyl is promising, but more experience with this route is required before concrete recommendations can be made.

Sedation of the mechanically ventilated patient requires an agent that provides analgesia and cardiovascular stability and is easy to administer. Fentanyl and alfentanil have met these objectives. Because of its short duration of action, alfentanil has been more thoroughly evaluated than fentanyl. In the available studies, alfentanil provided adequate sedation and a very rapid cessation of action. Preoperative sedation, especially of children, is difficult to achieve; oral transmucosal fentanyl citrate may ultimately offer a solution.

References

1. Lowenstein E, Hallowell P, Levine FH et al. Cardiovascular responses to large doses of intravenous morphine in man. *N Engl J Med*. 1969; 281:1389-93.
2. Mather LE. Clinical pharmacokinetics of fentanyl and its newer derivatives. *Clin Pharmacokinet*. 1983; 8:422-46.
3. Rosow CE. Sufentanil citrate: a new opioid analgesic for use in anesthesia. *Pharmacotherapy*. 1984; 4:11-9.
4. Larijani GE, Goldberg ME. Alfentanil hydrochloride: a new short-acting narcotic analgesic for surgical procedures. *Clin Pharm*. 1987; 6:275-82.
5. Hug CC. Pharmacokinetics and dynamics of narcotic analgesics. In: Prys-Roberts C, Hug CC, eds. Pharmacokinetics of anaesthesia. Oxford, England: Blackwell Scientific; 1984:187-234.
6. Meuldermans WE, Hurkmans RM, Heykants JJ. Plasma protein binding and distribution of fentanyl, sufentanil, alfentanil, and lofentanil in blood. *Arch Int Pharmacodyn Ther*. 1982; 257:4-19.
7. Yaksh TL. Spinal opiate analgesia: characteristics and principles of action. *Pain*. 1981; 11:293-346.
8. Carrie LE, O'Sullivan GM. Epidural fentanyl in labour. *Anaesthesia*. 1981; 36:965-9.
9. Justins DM, Knott C, Luthman J et al. Epidural vs intramuscular fentanyl: analgesia and pharmacokinetics in labour. *Anaesthesia*. 1983; 38:937-42.
10. Preston PG, Rosen MA, Hughes SC et al. Epidural anesthesia with fentanyl and lidocaine for cesarean section: maternal effects and neonatal outcome. *Anesthesiology*. 1988; 68:938-43.
11. Klepper ID, Sherrill DL, Boetger CL et al. Analgesic and respiratory effects of extradural sufentanil in volunteers and the influence of adrenaline as an adjuvant. *Br J Anaesth*. 1987; 59:1147-56.
12. Beniabed M, Ecoffey C, Levron JC et al. Analgesia and ventilatory response to CO_2 following epidural sufentanil in children. *Anesthesiology*. 1987; 67:948-51.
13. Cohen SE, Tan S, White PF. Sufentanil analgesia following cesarean section: epidural versus intravenous administration. *Anesthesiology*. 1988; 68:129-34.
14. Phillips G. Continuous infusion epidural analgesia in labor: the effect of adding sufentanil to 0.125% bupivacaine. *Anesth Analg*. 1988; 67:462-5.
15. Larijani GE, Bell SD, Goldberg ME et al. Pharmacokinetics of fentanyl following transdermal application. *Anesthesiology*. 1988; 69:A363. Abstract.
16. Varvel JR, Shafer SL, Hwang SS et al. Absorption characteristics of transdermally administered fentanyl. *Anesthesiology*. 1989; 70:928-34.
17. Caplan RA, Ready B, Oden RV et al. Transdermal fentanyl for postoperative pain management: a double-blind placebo study. *JAMA*. 1989; 261:1036-9.
18. Duthie DJ, Rowbotham DJ, Wyld R et al. Plasma fentanyl concentrations during transdermal delivery of fentanyl to surgical patients. *Br J Anaesth*. 1988; 60:614-8.
19. Nimmo WS, Duthie DJ. Plasma fentanyl concentrations after transdermal or IV infusion of fentanyl. *Anesthesiology*. 1986; 65:A559. Abstract.
20. Stanley TH, Hague B, Mock DL et al. Oral transmucosal fentanyl citrate (lollipop) premedication in human volunteers. *Anesth Analg*. 1989; 69:21-7.
21. Bower S, Hull CJ. Comparative pharmacokinetics of fentanyl and alfentanil. *Br J Anaesth*. 1982; 54:871-7.
22. Meuldermans W, Van Peer A, Hendrickx J et al. Alfentanil pharmacokinetics and metabolism in humans. *Anesthesiology*. 1988; 69:527-34.
23. Bovill JG, Sebel PS, Blackburn CL et al. Kinetics of alfentanil and sufentanil: a comparison. *Anesthesiology*. 1981; 55:A174. Abstract.
24. Bovill JG, Sebel PS, Blackburn CL et al. The pharmacokinetics of sufentanil in surgical patients. *Anesthesiology*. 1984; 61:502-6.
25. McClain DA, Hug CC. Intravenous fentanyl kinetics. *Clin Pharmacol Ther*. 1980; 28:106-14.
26. Bovill JG, Odoom J, Heykants J. Biotransformation of alfentanil in man. *Anesthesiology*. 1988; 69:A467. Abstract.
27. Bovill JG, Sebel PS. Pharmacokinetics of high-dose fentanyl: a study in patients undergoing cardiac surgery. *Br J Anaesth*. 1980; 52:795-801.
28. Davis PJ, Cook DR. Clinical pharmacokinetics of the newer intravenous anaesthetic agents. *Clin Pharmacokinet*. 1986; 11:18-35.
29. Bovill JG, Sebel PS, Blackburn CL et al. The pharmacokinetics of alfentanil (R39209): a new opioid analgesic. *Anesthesiology*. 1982; 57:439-43.
30. Hudson RJ, Bergstrom RG, Thomson IR et al. Pharmacokinetics of sufentanil in patients undergoing abdominal aortic surgery. *Anesthesiology*. 1989; 70:426-31.
31. Holley FO, Ponganis KV, Stanski DR. Effect of cardiopulmonary bypass on the pharmacokinetics of drugs. *Clin Pharmacokinet*. 1982; 7:234-51.
32. Koska AJ, Romagnoli A, Kramer WG. Effect of cardiopulmonary bypass on fentanyl distribution and elimination. *Clin Pharmacol Ther*. 1981: 29:100-5.
33. Flezzani P, Alvis MJ, Jacobs JR et al. Sufentanil disposition during cardiopulmonary bypass. *Can J Anaesth*. 1987; 34:566-9.
34. Okutani R, Philbin DM, Rosow CE et al. Effect of hypothermic hemodilutional cardiopulmonary bypass on plasma sufentanil and catecholamine concentrations in humans. *Anesth Analg*. 1988; 67:667-70.
35. Johnson KL, Erickson JP, Holley FO et al. Fentanyl pharmacokinetics in the pediatric population. *Anesthesiology*. 1984; 61:A441. Abstract.
36. Koehntop DE, Rodman JH, Brundage DM et al. Pharmacokinetics of fentanyl in neonates. *Anesth Analg*. 1986;

65:227-32.
37. Singleton MA, Rosen JI, Fisher DM. Plasma concentrations of fentanyl in infants, children and adults. *Can J Anaesth.* 1987; 34:152-5.
38. Gauntlett IS, Fisher DM, Hertzka RE et al. Pharmacokinetics of fentanyl in neonatal humans and lambs: effects of age. *Anesthesiology.* 1988; 69:683-7.
39. Sale JP, Goresky GV, Koren G et al. Pharmacokinetics of alfentanil in children. *Anesth Analg.* 1986; 65:S129. Abstract.
40. Meistelman C, Saint-Maurice C, Lepaul M et al. A comparison of alfentanil pharmacokinetics in children and adults. *Anesthesiology.* 1987;66:13-6.
41. Goresky GV, Koren G, Sabourin MA et al. The pharmacokinetics of alfentanil in children. *Anesthesiology.* 1987; 67:654-9.
42. Roure P, Jean N, Leclerc AC et al. Pharmacokinetics of alfentanil in children undergoing surgery. *Br J Anaesth.* 1987; 59:1437-40.
43. Davis PJ, Killian A, Stiller RL et al. Pharmacokinetics of alfentanil in newborn premature infants and older children. *Dev Pharmacol Ther.* 1989; 13:21-7.
44. Davis PJ, Cook DR, Stiller RL et al. Pharmacokinetics and pharmacodynamics of high-dose sufentanil in infants and children undergoing cardiac surgery. *Anesth Analg.* 1987; 66:203-8.
45. Greeley WJ, de Bruijn NP, Davis DP. Sufentanil pharmacokinetics in pediatric cardiovascular patients. *Anesth Analg.* 1987; 66:1067-72.
46. Singleton MA, Rosen JI, Fisher DM. Pharmacokinetics of fentanyl in the elderly. *Br J Anaesth.* 1988; 60:619-22.
47. Scott JC, Stanski DR. Decreased fentanyl and alfentanil dose requirements with age. A simultaneous pharmacokinetic and pharmacodynamic evaluation. *J Pharmacol Exp Ther.* 1987; 240:159-66.
48. Helmers H, Van Peer A, Woestenborghs R et al. Alfentanil kinetics in the elderly. *Clin Pharmacol Ther.* 1984; 36:239-43.
49. Lemmens HJ, Bovill JG, Hennis PJ et al. Influence of age on the pharmacokinetics of alfentanil. *Anesthesiology.* 1988; 69:A629. Abstract.
50. Chauvin M, Haberer JP, Spielvogel C et al. Sufentanil pharmacokinetics in patients with cirrhosis. *Anesth Analg.* 1989; 68:1-4.
51. Ferrier C, Marty J, Bouffard Y et al. Alfentanil pharmacokinetics in patients with cirrhosis. *Anesthesiology.* 1985; 62:480-4.
52. Davis PJ, Stiller RL, Cook DR et al. Effects of cholestatic hepatic disease and chronic renal failure on alfentanil pharmacokinetics in children. *Anesth Analg.* 1989; 68:579-83.
53. Chauvin M, Lebrault C, Levron JC et al. Pharmacokinetics of alfentanil in chronic renal failure. *Anesth Analg.* 1987; 66:53-6.
54. Davis PJ, Stiller RL, Cook DR et al. Pharmacokinetics of sufentanil in adolescent patients with chronic renal failure. *Anesth Analg.* 1988; 67:268-71.
55. Stanley TH. Opiate anaesthesia. *Anaesth Intensive Care.* 1987; 15:38-59.
56. Scott JC, Ponganis KV, Stanski DR. EEG quantitation of narcotic effect: the comparative pharmacodynamics of fentanyl and alfentanil. *Anesthesiology.* 1985; 62:234-41.
57. Sanford TJ, Smith NT, Dec-Silver H et al. A comparison of morphine, fentanyl, and sufentanil anesthesia for cardiac surgery: induction, emergence, and extubation. *Anesth Analg.* 1986; 65:259-66.
58. Smith NT, Quinn ML, Westover CJ et al. The EEG's of alfentanil, sufentanil, and fentanyl: a quantitative comparison. *Anesth Analg.* 1986; 66:S145. Abstract.
59. De Lange S, Boscoe MJ, Stanley TH. Comparison of sufentanil–O_2 and fentanyl–O_2 for coronary artery surgery. *Anesthesiology.* 1982; 56:112-8.
60. Rosow C. Alfentanil. *Semin Anesth.* 1988; 7:107-12.
61. Lowenstein E, Philbin DM. Narcotic "anesthesia" in the eighties. *Anesthesiology.* 1981; 55:195-7. Editorial.
62. Wong KC. Narcotics are not expected to produce unconsciousness and amnesia. *Anesth Analg.* 1983; 62:625-6. Editorial.
63. Hilgenberg JC. Intraoperative awareness during high-dose fentanyl–oxygen anesthesia. *Anesthesiology.* 1981; 54:341-3.
64. Bovill JG, Sebel PS, Wauquier et al. Electroencephalographic effects of sufentanil anaesthesia in man. *Br J Anaesth.* 1982; 54:45-52.
65. Zurick AM, Urzua J, Yared JP et al. Comparison of hemodynamic and hormonal effects of large single-dose fentanyl anesthesia and halothane/nitrous oxide anesthesia for coronary artery surgery. *Anesth Analg.* 1982; 61:521-6.
66. Sprigge JS, Wyands JE, Whalley DG et al. Fentanyl infusion anesthesia for aortocoronary bypass surgery: plasma levels and hemodynamic response. *Anesth Analg.* 1982; 61:972-8.
67. Gravlee GP, Ramsey FM, Roy RC et al. Rapid administration of a narcotic and neuromuscular blocker: a hemodynamic comparison of fentanyl, sufentanil, pancuronium, and vecuronium. *Anesth Analg.* 1988; 67:39-47.
68. Estafanous FG, Zurick AM. Hemodynamic effects of sufentanil/metocurine versus sufentanil/pancuronium in patients undergoing coronary artery surgery. *Cleve Clin Q.* 1985; 52:391-7.
69. Hicks HC, Mowbray AG, Yhap EO. Cardiovascular effects of and catecholamine responses to high dose fentanyl–O_2 anesthesia in patients with ischemic coronary artery disease. *Anesth Analg.* 1981; 60:563-8.
70. Wyands JE, Wong P, Whalley DG et al. Oxygen–fentanyl anesthesia in patients with poor left ventricular function: hemodynamics and plasma fentanyl concentrations. *Anesth Analg.* 1983; 62:476-82.
71. Moore RA, Yang SS, McNicholas KW et al. Hemodynamic and anesthetic effects of sufentanil as the sole anesthetic for pediatric cardiovascular surgery. *Anesthesiology.* 1985; 62:725-31.
72. Kay B, Nolan D, Mayall R et al. The effect of sufentanil on the cardiovascular responses to tracheal intubation. *Anaesthesia.* 1987; 42:382-6.
73. Ausems ME, Vuyk J, Hug CC et al. Comparison of a computer-assisted infusion versus intermittent bolus administration of alfentanil as a supplement to nitrous oxide for lower abdominal surgery. *Anesthesiology.* 1988; 68:851-61.
74. Lacoumenta S, Yeo TH, Burrin JM et al. Fentanyl and the β-endorphin, ACTH and glucoregulatory hormonal response to surgery. *Br J Anaesth.* 1987; 59:713-20.
75. Shafer A, Sung ML, White PF. Pharmacokinetics and pharmacodynamics of alfentanil infusions during general anesthesia. *Anesth Analg.* 1986; 65:1021-8.
76. Ausems ME, Hug CC, Stanski DR et al. Plasma concentrations of alfentanil required to supplement nitrous oxide anesthesia for general surgery. *Anesthesiology.* 1986; 65:362-73.
77. Marty J, Couderc E, Servin F et al. Plasma concentrations of sufentanil required to suppress hemodynamic responses to noxious stimuli during nitrous oxide anesthesia. *Anesthesiology.* 1988; 69:A631. Abstract.
78. Rucquoi M, Camu F. Cardiovascular responses to large doses of alfentanil and fentanyl. *Br J Anaesth.* 1983; 55:223S-230S.
79. Rosow CE, Philbin DM, Keegan CR et al. Hemodynamics and histamine release during induction with sufentanil or fentanyl. *Anesthesiology.* 1984; 60:489-91.
80. Spiess BD, Sathoff RH, El-Ganzouri AR et al. High dose sufentanil: four cases of sudden hypotension on induction. *Anesth Analg.* 1986; 65:703-5.
81. Flacke JW, Flacke WE, Bloor BC et al. Histamine release by four narcotics: a double-blind study in humans. *Anesth Analg.* 1987; 66:723-30.
82. Adams AP, Pybus DA. Delayed respiratory depression after use of fentanyl during anaesthesia. *Br Med J.* 1978; 1:278-9.
83. Christian CM, Waller JL, Moldenhauer CC. Postoperative rigidity following fentanyl anesthesia. *Anesthesiology.* 1983; 58:275-7.
84. Becker LD, Paulson BA, Miller RD et al. Biphasic respiratory

depression after fentanyl–droperidol or fentanyl alone used to supplement nitrous oxide anesthesia. *Anesthesiology*. 1976; 44:291-6.
85. Stoekel H, Hengstmann JH, Schuttler J. Pharmacokinetics of fentanyl as a possible explanation for the recurrence of respiratory depression. *Br J Anaesth*. 1979; 51:741-4.
86. McQuay HJ, Moore RA, Patterson GM et al. Plasma fentanyl concentrations and clinical observations during and after operation. *Br J Anaesth*. 1979; 51:543-50.
87. Klausner JM, Caspi J, Lelcuk S et al. Delayed muscular rigidity and respiratory depression following fentanyl anesthesia. *Arch Surg*. 1988; 123:66-7.
88. Caspi J, Klausner JM, Safadi T et al. Delayed respiratory depression following fentanyl anesthesia for cardiac surgery. *Crit Care Med*. 1988; 16:238-40.
89. Robinson D. Respiratory arrest after recovery from anaesthesia supplemented with sufentanil. *Can J Anaesth*. 1988; 35:101-2. Letter.
90. Chang J, Fish KJ. Acute respiratory arrest and rigidity after anesthesia with sufentanil: a case report. *Anesthesiology*. 1985; 63:710-1.
91. Goldberg M, Ishuak S, Garcia C et al. Postoperative rigidity following sufentanil administration. *Anesthesiology*. 1985; 63:199-201.
92. Mahla ME, White SE, Moneta MD. Delayed respiratory depression after alfentanil. *Anesthesiology*. 1988; 69:593-5.
93. Jaffe RS, Coalson D. Recurrent respiratory depression after alfentanil administration. *Anesthesiology*. 1989; 70:151-3.
94. Bowdle TA. Myoclonus following sufentanil without EEG seizure activity. *Anesthesiology*. 1987; 67:593-5.
95. Rosman EJ, Capan LM, Turndorf H. Another case of probable seizure after sufentanil. *Anesth Analg*. 1987; 66:922. Letter.
96. Brian JE, Seifen AB. Tonic–clonic activity after sufentanil. *Anesth Analg*. 1987; 66:481. Letter.
97. Molbegott LP, Flashburg MH, Karasic HL et al. Probable seizures after sufentanil. *Anesth Analg*. 1987; 66:91-3.
98. Katz RI, Eide TR, Hartman A et al. Two instances of seizure-like activity in the same patient with two different narcotics. *Anesth Analg*. 1988; 67:289-90.
99. Strong WE, Matson M. Probable seizure after alfentanil. *Anesth Analg*. 1989; 68:692-3.
100. Modica PA, Tempelhoff R, White PF. Pro- and anticonvulsant effects of anesthetics (part I). *Anesth Analg*. 1990; 70:303-15.
101. Waller JL, Hug CC, Nagle DM et al. Hemodynamic changes during fentanyl–oxygen anesthesia for aortocoronary bypass operation. *Anesthesiology*. 1981; 55:212-7.
102. Sonntag H, Larsen R, Hilfiker O et al. Myocardial blood flow and oxygen consumption during high-dose fentanyl anesthesia in patients with coronary artery disease. *Anesthesiology*. 1982; 56:417-21.
103. Sebel PS, Bovil JG. Cardiovascular effects of sufentanil anesthesia. *Anesth Analg*. 1982; 61:115-9.
104. Sonntag H, Stephan H, Lange H et al. Sufentanil does not block sympathetic responses to surgical stimuli in patients having coronary artery revascularization surgery. *Anesth Analg*. 1989; 68:584-92.
105. Matthews HM, Furness G, Carson IW et al. Comparison of sufentanil–oxygen and fentanyl–oxygen anaesthesia for coronary artery bypass grafting. *Br J Anaesth*. 1988; 60:530-5.
106. Hickey PR, Hansen DD. Fentanyl– and sufentanil–oxygen–pancuronium anesthesia for cardiac surgery in infants. *Anesth Analg*. 1984; 63:117-24.
107. Hynynen M, Takkunen O, Salmenpera M et al. Continuous infusion of fentanyl or alfentanil for coronary artery surgery. *Br J Anaesth*. 1986; 58:1252-9.
108. Bovill JG, Warren PJ, Schuller JL et al. Comparison of fentanyl, sufentanil, and alfentanil anesthesia in patients undergoing valvular heart surgery. *Anesth Analg*. 1984; 63:1081-6.
109. Pathak KS, Brown RH, Nash CL et al. Continuous opioid infusion for scoliosis fusion surgery. *Anesth Analg*. 1983; 62:841-5.
110. Stuart-Taylor ME, Sleigh JW. Alfentanil infusions. Comparison of bolus administration of fentanyl with three alfentanil infusion regimens. *Anaesthesia*. 1987; 42:1218-22.
111. Clark NJ, Meuleman T, Liu WS et al. Comparison of sufentanil–N_2O and fentanyl–N_2O in patients without cardiac disease undergoing general surgery. *Anesthesiology*. 1987; 66:130-5.
112. Hull CJ, Jacobson L. A clinical trial of alfentanil as an adjuvant for short anaesthetic procedures. *Br J Anaesth*. 1983; 55:173S-178S.
113. Cartwright DP. Recovery after anaesthesia with alfentanil or halothane. *Can Anaesth Soc J*. 1985; 32:479-83.
114. Welling EC, Donegan J. Neuroleptanalgesia using alfentanil for awake craniotomy. *Anesth Analg*. 1989; 68:57-60.
115. Justins DM, Francis D, Houlton PG et al. A controlled trial of extradural fentanyl in labour. *Br J Anaesth*. 1982; 54:409-14.
116. Vella LM, Willatts DG, Knott C et al. Epidural fentanyl in labour: an evaluation of the systemic contribution to analgesia. *Anaesthesia*. 1985; 40:741-7.
117. Gaffud MP, Bansal P, Lawton C et al. Surgical analgesia for cesarean delivery with epidural bupivacaine and fentanyl. *Anesthesiology*. 1986; 65:331-4.
118. Duthie DJ, McLaren AD, Nimmo WS. Pharmacokinetics of fentanyl during constant rate i.v. infusion for the relief of pain after surgery. *Br J Anaesth*. 1986; 58:950-6.
119. Chudnofsky CR, Wright SW, Dronen SC et al. The safety of fentanyl use in the emergency department. *Ann Emerg Med*. 1989; 18:635-9.
120. Chrubasik J, Wust H, Schulte-Monting J et al. Relative analgesic potency of epidural fentanyl, alfentanil, and morphine in treatment of postoperative pain. *Anesthesiology*. 1988; 68:929-33.
121. Rosen MA, Dailey PA, Hughes SC et al. Epidural sufentanil for postoperative analgesia after cesarean section. *Anesthesiology*. 1988; 68:448-53.
122. Holley FO, van Steennis CA. Postoperative analgesia with fentanyl: pharmacokinetics and pharmacodynamics of constant-rate i.v. and transdermal delivery. *Br J Anaesth*. 1988; 60:608-13.
123. Bell SG, Ellis LJ. Use of fentanyl for sedation of mechanically ventilated neonates. *Neonatal Netw*. 1987; 16:27-31.
124. Shafer A, White PF, Schuttler J et al. Use of a fentanyl infusion in the intensive care unit: tolerance to its anesthetic effects? *Anesthesiology*. 1983; 59:245-8.
125. Cohen AT. Experience with alfentanil infusion as an intensive care sedative analgesic. *Eur J Anaesth*. 1987; Suppl 1:63-6.
126. Yate PM, Thomas D, Sebel PS. Alfentanil infusion for sedation and analgesia in intensive care. *Lancet*. 1984; 2:396-7.
127. Cohen AT, Kelly DR. Assessment of alfentanil by intravenous infusion as long-term sedation in intensive care. *Anaesthesia*. 1987; 42:545-8.
128. Sinclair ME, Sear JW, Summerfield RJ et al. Alfentanil infusions on the intensive therapy unit. *Intensive Care Med*. 1988; 14:55-9.
129. Streisand JB, Stanley TH, Hague B et al. Oral transmucosal fentanyl citrate premedication in children. *Anesth Analg*. 1989; 69:28-34.
130. Feld LH, Champeau MW, van Steennis CA et al. Preanesthetic medication in children: a comparison of oral transmucosal fentanyl citrate versus placebo. *Anesthesiology*. 1989; 71:374-7.
131. Nelson PS, Streisand JB, Mulder SM et al. Comparison of oral transmucosal fentanyl citrate and an oral solution of meperidine, diazepam, and atropine for premedication in children. *Anesthesiology*. 1989; 70:616-21.
132. Henderson JM, Brodsky DA, Fisher DM et al. Pre-induction of anesthesia in pediatric patients with nasally administered sufentanil. *Anesthesiology*. 1988; 68:671-5.
133. Stanley TH. New routes of administration and new delivery systems of anesthetics. *Anesthesiology*. 1988; 68:665-8. Editorial.

Therapy Review

Drug use during breast-feeding

Philip O. Anderson

Abstract: The physicochemical and pharmacokinetic factors involved in transfer of drugs into breast milk are reviewed.

Passage of drugs into milk can best be viewed as a two-compartment system. Various ratios of the drug concentration values in the two compartments and ratios of maternal-to-infant intake have been described. Knowledge of the limitations of these methods is necessary to properly interpret and apply the literature on drug excretion into breast milk. Factors involved in choosing a drug for a nursing mother are listed, a stepwise approach to minimizing transfer of drug to the infant is presented, and the literature on the excretion of specific drugs into milk is reviewed. Generally, drugs given to nursing mothers reach infants in much smaller amounts than drugs given to pregnant women. Decisions about nursing during drug therapy and the choice of drug therapy in a nursing mother should be based on the dosage and duration of therapy, age of the infant, quantity of milk consumed, experience with the drug in infants, degree of oral absorption of the drug by the infant, potential long-term effects, possible interference with lactation, and non-dose-related toxicities (e.g., potential allergic reactions).

Too often, the mother's need for a medication is perceived as a reason to discontinue nursing. By understanding the principles of drug passage into breast milk and systematically evaluating the mother's needs, infant factors, and the data on specific drugs, clinicians can usually devise treatment plans that allow nursing while minimizing the risks to the infant.

Index terms: Contraindications; Excretion; Lactation; Pediatrics; Pharmacokinetics; Reference books; Toxicity
Clin Pharm. 1991; 10:594-624

In recent years, there has been a growing appreciation of the benefits of breast-feeding for the infant and mother.[1,2] As a consequence, the number of women who nurse their infants has steadily increased in the United States from 22% in 1971 to over 60% today.[1,3] The duration of nursing, however, is often suboptimal.[1] Recent surveys in Western countries indicate that 90–99% of women who are breast-feeding receive a medication during the first week postpartum.[4] Surveys in Norway found that 17–25% of women nursing at four months postpartum had taken a medication during the previous two weeks and 5% of nursing mothers were receiving long-term drug therapy.[4,5] Health-care providers frequently are faced with questions concerning the use of medications during breast-feeding. Although maternal medication use is often viewed as a reason for early discontinuation of nursing, it usually need not be.

Passage of Drugs into Milk

A drug given to a nursing mother follows a complex path on its way to the infant. It may be partially inactivated in the mother's liver, excreted in her urine, or distributed and protein bound to such an extent that her free serum drug concentation is low. Drugs that must be administered to the mother by injection because of poor oral bioavailability may not be orally bioavailable in the infant either. If any of the drug is absorbed by the infant, it is subject to hepatic metabolism, renal excretion, protein binding, and tissue distribution. Therefore, as a general rule, drugs given to nursing mothers reach infants in much smaller amounts than drugs given to pregnant women, whose bloodstream is separated from that of the fetus only by the placenta (which is quite permeable to many drugs). This fact is often overlooked by lay persons

Philip O. Anderson, Pharm.D., FASHP, is Director, Drug Information Service, Department of Pharmacy, University of California San Diego Medical Center, San Diego, CA.

Reprints may be ordered from the American Society of Hospital Pharmacists, 4630 Montgomery Avenue, Bethesda, MD 20814 for $10 each. Direct the requests to Customer Service and specify code R611. Reprints are not available from Dr. Anderson.

The following colleagues are acknowledged for their review of the manuscript and many helpful suggestions: James E. Knoben, Pharm.D., M.P.H., James R. Lane, Jr., Pharm.D., Robert E. Pachorek, Pharm.D., William G. Troutman, Pharm.D., and Verónica Valdés, M.D. Additional thanks go to Audrey J. Naylor, M.D., D.P.H., Ruth Wester, and the other Wellstart staff members for their continuing support and encouragement.

This is **article 680-204-9116** in the **ASHP Continuing Education System**; it qualifies for 1.0 hour of continuing-education credit. See page 639 for learning objectives and test questions.

Permission to reprint the list of drugs from the *Handbook of Clinical Drug Data* was granted by Drug Intelligence Publications, Inc.

and health-care professionals alike in their thinking about drug use during the perinatal period.[5]

Drugs pass across the mammary epithelium by passive diffusion down a concentration gradient formed by the nonionized, free drug on each side of the membrane.[6,7] The membrane acts as a semipermeable lipid barrier, similar to other membranes in the body. It contains small pores that allow drugs with molecular weights of less than approximately 200 to pass unimpeded in an aqueous phase.[7] Larger drug molecules must dissolve in the outer lipid membrane of the epithelial cells, diffuse across the aqueous interior of the cell, dissolve in and pass through the opposite cell membrane, and then pass into the milk.[7] Although active or facilitated transport processes have been described for the passage of some endogenous substances across some membranes in the body, no drugs are known to enter human milk by these mechanisms. However, the complexity of the fluids on both sides of the mammary epithelium results in several simultaneous equilibration processes.

Ion Trapping. The most important equilibration process occurs across the mammary epithelium between the unbound, nonionized drug in the bloodstream and the aqueous phase of the milk. Because the pH of milk is typically slightly acid relative to that of plasma, the pH partition theory predicts that the ionized form of a weak base concentrates in milk in a process commonly called "ion trapping."[7] Conversely, a weak acid is "trapped" in plasma because of the relatively greater concentration of the ionized form there. Ion trapping affects weak acids with a pK_a of approximately 8 or less and weak bases with a pK_a of 6 or greater.[8] Weaker acids and bases act as nonelectrolytes and do not undergo ion trapping.

Protein Binding. Both plasma and milk contain proteins that can bind drugs. The total plasma protein concentration is approximately 75 g/L, whereas milk contains approximately 8–9 grams of protein per liter.[9] Of the plasma proteins, 45 g/L is albumin, a major drug-binding protein. The albumin concentration in milk is only about 0.4 g/L. The major proteins in milk are casein, α-lactalbumin, lactoferrin, and immunoglobulin A; casein is apparently the major drug-binding protein.[10,11] None of these proteins binds drugs well; quantitatively important binding of drugs to milk proteins does not occur except in the case of drugs that are also extensively bound to plasma proteins.[10-12] The net effect of protein binding is that highly protein-bound drugs tend to remain in the plasma and to pass into the milk in low concentrations.

Lipid Partitioning. Unlike plasma, milk contains emulsified fat, ranging from 3% to 5%.[13] Milk fat can concentrate lipid-soluble drugs, causing the total amount of drug in milk to increase. For highly lipid-soluble drugs such as diazepam and chlorpromazine, well over half of the total amount of drug in milk is found in milk fat.[14,15] Nevertheless, because the amount of fat in milk is low compared with the total volume of milk, the net effect of lipid partitioning on the total amount of drug reaching the infant is usually relatively small. It is important to keep lipid partitioning in mind, however, when designing or evaluating studies on drug excretion into breast milk. Drug concentrations in skim milk are sometimes measured and reported. Failure to account for the drug in milk fat can markedly distort the results of a study.

Non-Steady-State Conditions. All of the previous discussion relates to constant, steady-state conditions in which plasma and milk drug concentrations have come to equilibrium. Because constant plasma concentations are the exception during drug therapy (e.g., continuous infusions, good extended-release products, transdermal patches), other factors must be taken into account during intermittent drug administration to the mother. The shorter the half-life of a drug, the greater the fluctuations in plasma concentrations during intermittent administration. A drug that enters the milk rapidly will achieve a greater initial concentration in milk relative to the plasma concentration than a drug that enters slowly. Because milk is produced and periodically emptied from the breast during nursing, slowly equilibrating drugs may never achieve high concentrations in milk. The physicochemical factors that determine the rate of passage into milk are the drug's lipid solubility and its molecular weight. Lipid solubility is important because the drug must dissolve in the lipid mammary epithelial cell membrane (on both entering and exiting the cell), whereas low molecular weight favors rapid diffusion across the aqueous interior of the cell.[7,8] The rate of blood flow to the breasts may also affect the rate of passage into milk for some drugs.

Another factor that comes into play during intermittent drug administration is the retrograde diffusion of drugs from the milk back into plasma. Studies in animals indicate that drugs instilled into the udder pass out of the milk and are detectable in the plasma.[16,17] The rate and extent of passage appear to be determined by the same physicochemical factors governing passage from the plasma into milk.

An important clinical correlate that is often misunderstood is the utility of pumping the breasts and discarding the milk to hasten the disappearance of some unwanted substance from the milk. Many mothers and some prescribers have the impression that once a drug has passed into the milk, it will remain there until the breast is emptied. However, because of retrograde diffusion, this is not the case. Furthermore, diffusion into milk is a minor route of drug elimination (usually less than 1% of a maternal dose).[18] For both of these reasons, "pumping and dumping" is not a useful maneuver for expediting drug elimination from milk.

Pharmacokinetic Models

Several authors have proposed pharmacokinetic models to describe the passage of drugs into breast milk.[19-21] The two-compartment open pharmacokinetic model, in which the central compartment represents

Figure 1. Two-compartment model of drug excretion into breast milk.

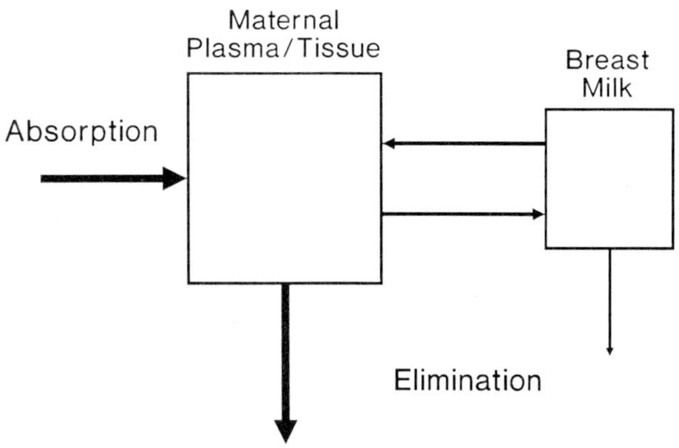

maternal fluids and tissues and the peripheral compartment represents breast milk, aids the understanding of drug passage into milk (Figure 1). This model differs from a standard two-compartment open model in which the second compartment would eventually come to equilibrium with the central compartment. The peripheral compartment (breast milk) is periodically emptied and replenished as nursing and milk production occur. Three-compartment and four-compartment models have also been presented.[20,22,23] Results of work available only in abstract form indicate that three-compartment models may be adequate to describe the behavior of most drugs.[24] However, these more complex models do not seem any more useful than the two-compartment model for conceptualizing most drugs' passage into milk.[19] Noncompartmental analysis has also been used and is probably the best method of deriving all clinically important data.[25] In addition to the models proposed for drugs, a model has been proposed for gases, such as those that may be inhaled in the work place.[26]

Infant Factors

Infant factors can be important in determining the safety of using a particular drug in a nursing mother because infants do not absorb and eliminate drugs in the same ways as adults. Neonates may absorb some rather large and complex molecules, such as proteins.[27,28] Although this ability allows passage of antibodies to the infant from the mother (a primary advantage of nursing), absorption of some otherwise unabsorbable drug molecules theoretically may also occur. However, this latter point has not been studied. Other factors that can influence drug absorption are the infant's higher gastric pH, GI flora and GI transit time, and reduced amounts of bile salts and pancreatic enzymes.[29]

The affinity of neonatal plasma proteins for drugs is also less than that of older infants and children, leading to increased free drug concentrations.[29,30] Newborns also have a greater percentage of body water and extracellular fluid volume than older children and adults.[29,30] Both hepatic metabolism and renal excretion of drugs are low in newborns. Hepatic metabolic capacity matures within weeks to equal or surpass adult levels.[30] Glomerular filtration rate matures over two to five months to adult levels.[30]

All of the above factors can lead to prolonged drug half-lives in neonates that may allow drugs to accumulate to unexpectedly high concentrations with repeated dosing. This effect may be magnified in preterm infants, whose metabolic and renal excretory capacities are less than those of full-term neonates.[30]

Additionally, infant responses to medications are sometimes different from those of older children and adults. These differences may result from immature enzyme systems, differences in the number or affinity of drug receptors, immaturity of the nervous system, increased permeability of some membranes such as the blood–brain barrier, or other factors.[29]

Methods of Estimating Infant Drug Exposure

Milk/Plasma Ratio. The milk-to-plasma (M/P) ratio has often been used as an index of the extent of drug passage into breast milk. This term is derived from early animal studies that were designed to elucidate the principles of drug passage into milk. These studies measured drug concentrations in plasma and milk ultrafiltrate (i.e., unbound drug in the aqueous portion) during equilibrium (i.e., continuous infusion) conditions. Rasmussen,[31] who is credited with much of this work, pointed out in 1973 that calculations of the M/P ratio at non-steady-state conditions "give no absolutely reliable expression of the relationship between the concentation of drugs in milk and plasma." To make matters worse, there is no standard definition for the M/P ratio, and various authors have applied the term differently. Unfortunately, the M/P ratio has become widely used in the clinical literature and must be understood to avoid erroneous conclusions.

In the past, the term has most often been taken to mean the number obtained by dividing the drug concentration in milk by a simultaneously obtained plasma drug concentration (M/P_{point} ratio). Because the rates of drug passage into and out of milk vary with lipid solubility and molecular weight, the milk concentration–time curve may lag behind the plasma concentration–time curve. Drugs that are more water soluble or have a higher molecular weight, or both, are more sluggish in their passage into and out of milk than drugs that are more lipid soluble or have a lower molecular weight, or both.[32,33] This lag time leads to an M/P_{point} ratio that can vary considerably during the dosing interval.

Clinical studies[32,33] and computer simulations[23] have clearly demonstrated this phenomenon. Use of an M/P ratio calculated in this fashion can be quite misleading, because the value of an M/P_{point} ratio can be extremely dependent on the time of sampling with respect to the dose. Time dependency is most pronounced for drugs that achieve higher concentrations in milk than in plasma. Other potential problems with the M/P_{point} ratio occur because the ratio calculated after a single dose can differ from that calculated after multiple doses.[23] Work in animals has also demonstrated that the M/P_{point} ratio varies markedly according to the route of administration.[34] The M/P_{point} ratio, although frequently used, is of doubtful value as a clinical tool.

More recently, the ratio of areas under the milk and plasma concentration–time curves (AUCs) has been used to define the M/P ratio (M/P_{AUC}) for a drug.[4,8] This method provides a time-integrated average estimate of the M/P ratio that may more reliably predict the average excretion of drugs into milk under steady-state conditions.

The most important point is that the M/P ratio, regardless of the method of calculation, is merely a means to an end, not an end in itself. Even the most carefully measured M/P ratio has no inherent clinical meaning. In the absence of a measured drug concentration in milk, the M/P ratio can be used to calculate average or worst-case milk drug concentrations, as shown in equation 1:

$$\text{Drug concentration in milk} = \text{maternal plasma drug concentration} \times \text{M/P ratio} \quad (1)$$

Use of the average (or mid-dosing-interval) maternal plasma drug concentration and the M/P_{AUC} ratio in the above equation would provide an estimate of the average drug concentration in milk. Use of the peak maternal plasma drug concentration and the M/P_{point} ratio at the peak time would provide a worst-case estimate of the drug concentration in milk; a report of drug concentration in milk at the peak time is preferable to this estimate, though.

Percentage of Maternal Dose. Like the M/P ratio, the percentage of the maternal dose that an infant receives has been used to summarize clinical data and assess the safety of a drug during breast-feeding. It is not as directly applicable as the percentage of the usual therapeutic infant dose for indicating infant drug exposure, but a number of authors have used the percentage of maternal dose to estimate the risk to the infant.[4,18] Unfortunately, the definition of percentage of maternal dose, like the M/P ratio, has not been standardized.

The value is usually calculated by dividing the estimated amount of drug excreted into milk during a stated time period (which varies by author) by the maternal dose and multiplying by 100 to derive a percentage. In general, the dose in milk is calculated either from milk drug concentrations measured in a clinical trial or by use of some form of the M/P ratio together with an estimate of milk intake. The method of estimating milk intake has varied among authors, with some using a constant value (e.g., 0.8 or 1 L of milk per day, independent of infant age or weight), in their calculations and others using weight-adjusted values (e.g., 150 mL/kg/day). The method of expressing dosage has also varied among authors, with some using the absolute doses in their calculations and some using milligram-per-kilogram doses. The latter method is preferable and has been used to provide the best current compilations of these values.[18,35]

Although it is perhaps somewhat more useful than the M/P ratio, the percentage of maternal dose is best viewed as a means of estimating the dose to the infant via milk rather than being predictive of the desirability of nursing during maternal drug use. A major reason that the percentage of maternal dose is not optimal when used alone is that this method is based on the presumption that maternal and infant drug pharmacokinetics and pharmacodynamics are the same. Not only is this usually untrue, but the difference between the two varies with the infant's age, as described previously.

Infant Dosage. More relevant than either of the above ratios is the dosage of drug received by an infant in breast milk that is given by equation 2:

$$\text{Infant dosage} = \text{drug concentration in milk} \times \text{volume of milk ingested} \quad (2)$$

If instantaneous milk drug concentrations and milk volumes could be determined and instantaneous infant doses could be calculated and added up for the entire nursing period, the exact infant dosage would be known. Computer simulations that use this method have been performed.[19]

Because such precise knowledge is a clinical impossibility, estimates of drug concentration and milk volume must be made. When clinical studies are available, dosage and milk concentration data should be used to estimate the drug concentration in milk in a specific patient by adjusting the maternal plasma and milk concentration estimates for the actual dose given. The assumption that the drug concentration in milk is linearly related to the maternal dose appears usually to be correct.

An estimate of ingested milk volume can also be made. A completely breast-fed infant daily ingests a mean ± S.D. milk volume of 661 ± 175 mL (coefficient of variation, 26%) in the second week postpartum and 787 ± 88 mL (coefficient of variation, 11%) between the second and fifth months.[36] An average value of 150 mL/kg/day is often used to estimate daily infant milk intake.[4,18] Because the coefficients of variation of estimated infant milk intake are large, a larger value of 190–230 mL/kg/day could be used to ensure capturing intakes of the majority of infants.

When the average estimate of ingested milk volume (150 mL/kg/day) and the average dose-adjusted milk concentration for a drug (approximately the concentration at the midpoint of the dosing interval) are used, an average drug dosage received by the infant can be calculated. This calculation would be most useful for long-term therapy with drugs that may accumulate. For more toxic drugs, of which a single dose might bring about an adverse effect in an infant, a larger estimate of ingested milk volume (e.g., 230 mL/kg/day) can be used with the dose-adjusted peak milk concentration for a drug to estimate the maximum expected dose that a nursing infant might ingest. Once the infant's dose is estimated, this dose can be compared with the infant dose (or adult dose if the infant dose is unknown) in milligrams per kilogram to determine whether the infant is likely to receive a pharmacologically important amount of drug via breast milk. Because the dose in milk refers to the drug alone, an adjustment must be made if the dose is usually expressed in terms of a salt form.

Estimation of Infant Serum Concentration. The infant serum concentration is possibly the most direct measure of infant risk from a drug in breast milk. The average infant serum concentration ($C_{ss_{ave}}$) can be estimated from equation 3:

$$C_{ss_{ave}} = F \times \text{infant dosage}/\text{CL} \quad (3)$$

where F is the bioavailability fraction and CL is the drug clearance of the infant. Equations 1, 2, and 3 can be combined to create equations 4 and 5, which provide an estimate of the average infant plasma concentration.

$$C_{ss_{ave}} = F \times \text{drug concentration in milk} \times \text{volume of milk ingested}/\text{CL} \quad (4)$$

$$C_{ss_{ave}} = F \times \text{maternal plasma drug concentration} \times \text{M/P ratio} \times \text{volume of milk ingested}/\text{CL} \quad (5)$$

The estimates provided by these equations may be useful measures of infant drug exposure when the plasma concentration–effect relationship and the other data in the equation are available. If drug concentration in milk is known, then equation 4 is preferred over the other equations.

Prediction of Drug Passage into Milk Based on Physicochemical Factors

As the relationship of the physical and chemical properties of drugs to their passage into milk has been elucidated, attempts have been made to predict passage of drugs into milk based solely on their physicochemical properties. The first such attempt was made by Meskin and Lien in 1985.[37] They used least-squares regression to correlate various functions of the molecular weight, octanol/water (o/w) partition coefficient, and the degree of dissociation (for acids and bases) with the M/P_{point} ratio of several acidic and basic drugs. Their equations of best fit were able to account for only 65% of the variance for acidic drugs and 64% for basic drugs. Protein binding was not explicitly included as a variable; however, it was implicitly included because lipid solubility is a determinant of a drug's affinity for proteins. The use of the M/P_{point} ratio from various studies as an endpoint was a major fault of this study. No prospective validation of the equations has been reported.

Fleishaker et al.[12] proposed a diffusional model to predict the average steady-state M/P ratio (defined by the authors as M/P_{point} ratio during continuous infusion or M/P_{AUC} ratio with multiple intermittent administration). The model predicts the M/P ratio from the pK_a, the measured milk protein-binding value, and the measured skim-milk/whole-milk concentration ratio. This latter value provides a measure of drug partitioning into milk fat.[14] The model demonstrated good prospective prediction ability in constant-infusion and single i.v. dose studies in rabbits,[38] even after artificial manipulation of serum protein binding.[39] This model was used to determine the effects of postpartum changes in serum and milk proteins on the M/P ratio in a small group of postpartum women.[40] Effects on the M/P ratio were small and were subject to great interindividual variability.

A different approach has been taken by Atkinson and Begg,[15] who developed methods of predicting milk lipid-partitioning values from o/w partition coefficients and milk protein-binding values from plasma protein binding.[9,10] Partitioning into milk lipids is directly related to the o/w partition coefficient,[15] and drug binding to milk proteins has a curvilinear relationship to the plasma protein binding of the drug.[10]

Using these methods, Atkinson and Begg developed a physiologically based method of predicting the M/P_{AUC} ratio from the pK_a, the o/w partition coefficient, and the extent of plasma protein binding.[8] Equations were developed based on multiple linear regression analysis that accounted for 93.6% of the variance for weak acids and 82.9% of the variance for weak bases. They found that the ion-trapping effect on acids and bases was the major determinant of the M/P_{AUC} ratio, with protein binding and lipid partitioning having lesser roles.

This model is appealing because of its potential to make clinically useful predictions from readily available physicochemical data. However, its predictions are associated with wide 95% confidence intervals in retrospective predictions of literature M/P_{AUC} ratio values. The 95% confidence intervals encompass a range of prediction errors of 230–340% for basic drugs and 510–570% for acidic drugs. Several factors may have caused this variability, including (1) lack of pharmacokinetically rigorous human studies to provide accurate and reproducible endpoints (e.g., consistent M/P_{AUC} ratios), (2) use in some cases of non-steady-state M/P_{AUC} ratios, and (3) large variations in reported values for pK_a, o/w partition coefficients, and plasma protein binding. This model has not been prospectively tested in animals or humans or directly compared with the Fleishaker model.

Limitations of Prediction Methods

Individual Variability. Individual variation will always remain a major limiting factor in the ability of any method to accurately predict passage of drugs into milk in a specific individual in the clinical setting. Interindividual and intraindividual variabilities with respect to factors affecting drug excretion into milk are relatively large and include variations in milk protein, pH, and fat content. Table 1 shows the values measured in one study.[12] During the first few days postpartum, protein-rich colostrum is secreted and may bind drugs in a way different from that of mature milk (compare patients 1–4 with patients 5–8). Note also that several subjects had milk pH values that were slightly alkaline with respect to plasma pH, which would reverse the typical pattern of ion trapping.

A recent paper reported that milk pH varies with the time postpartum.[42] Colostrum pH approximates that of plasma, but milk pH rapidly drops to between 7.0 and 7.1 in the first two weeks postpartum; it then gradually increases to about 7.4 by one year postpartum. However, the preliminary work for this study showed that the measured pH of milk depended on the method of collection. The pattern described above was for aerobically collected milk samples. The pH of milk collected anaerobically was about 0.27 pH units less (more acidic) than that of aerobically collected samples.[42] Other studies in rabbits[38] and humans[43,44] have produced similar results. This difference appears to be caused by carbon dioxide dissolved in milk, which is rapidly released in air.[42] Because pH partitioning and ion trapping occur within the breast, the pH of milk relevant to drug partitioning may be lower than previously thought.

The milk fat content also varies considerably between the first flow of milk during a feeding (foremilk) and the last portion of the flow (hindmilk). Hindmilk contains about two to three times as much fat as foremilk.[36,45] Fat content may also vary in the same woman at different times of day, although supporting data are conflicting.[45,46] The fat content of milk also undergoes a slight, gradual increase with the duration of nursing.[13,47,48] As discussed previously, the volume of milk ingested also varies considerably.

Presence of Metabolites. None of the previously described prediction methods takes into account the presence of metabolites. Active metabolites in milk can add to the overall pharmacologic effect in the infant. In addition, some inactive metabolites are pharmacologically important to the infant. For example, glucuronide esters can be excreted into milk and deconjugated in the infant's GI tract to the active moiety, which is then absorbed.[49] The presence of active or potentially active metabolites in the milk not only adds to the total dose that the infant receives, but also tends to lengthen the duration of the peak drug concentration in milk, making it difficult to coordinate nursing times with low drug concentrations.

Prediction versus Measurement

Two lessons can be learned from the knowledge of our poor prediction ability. First, applying estimates based on population values (regardless of how they are derived) to a specific mother–child pair will occasionally be misleading because of the variability in the factors listed above. Weak acids and bases are particularly subject to occasional large prediction errors because of variability in milk pH. Second, with so few good clinical studies available and such a large amount of interindividual variability in drug excretion for many drugs, the clinical literature probably does not provide a much better estimate of drug passage into milk than estimates based on good physicochemical models.

Regardless of the inability to make precise predictions, average population values may be useful, particularly when two drugs are being compared with each other to determine which is the safer. Because drug doses in milk are usually quite small, a prediction error of 200–300%. (i.e., three to four times as much drug in milk as predicted) may also be only a small dose.

Breast-feeding mothers occasionally request that their milk be analyzed to determine whether it is safe to nurse their infant during drug therapy. Because of the time-related variability in drug excretion as well as the special analytic difficulties (and cost) involved in measuring drug concentrations in milk, such analysis is not recommended as useful. Possible exceptions are to rule out excessive concentrations of persistent environmental contaminants in the milk of mothers who may have had an unusually high exposure in the past[50] and after single doses of a radiopharmaceutical, in which case radioactivity can be directly measured to help determine when resumption of nursing is safe.[51]

Table 1.
Interindividual Variability of Breast Milk[a]

Patient	Time[b]	Milk pH	Creamatocrit[c] (v/v%)	Total Protein (g/dL)
1	3 days	7.54	8.86	2.55
2	7 days	6.97	12.45	2.38
3	10 days	7.14	8.13	1.58
4	11 days	7.21	7.99	2.03
5	1 month	7.49	3.49	0.93
6	3 months	7.46	8.65	0.99
7	4 months	7.13	6.53	1.01
8	4 months	7.62	8.34	0.92

[a] Adapted from reference 12.
[b] Reported as postpartum days or months.
[c] Creamatocrit is a measure of milk fat performed by centrifuging milk in a capillary tube and reading the result like a hematocrit.[41]

Effects of Drugs on Lactation

In addition to the effects of drugs on the infant, the potential effects of drugs on lactation should be considered. Drugs can affect lactation by either central or peripheral mechanisms.[4,52,53] Many drugs affect prolactin secretion centrally. Those that decrease prolactin secretion may interfere with nursing by decreasing the milk yield, which in turn may result in inadequate infant weight gain, necessitate supplementation, or cause early cessation of breast-feeding.[54] Many of these drugs affect prolactin by altering CNS dopamine metabolism and uptake. High central dopamine concentrations are associated with decreased serum prolactin concentrations and lactation inhibition.[54] Dopaminergic agents such as bromocriptine have been used to suppress lactation in mothers who do not want to nurse. Dopamine antagonists, such as the neuroleptics, can cause galactorrhea. The dopamine antagonists metoclopramide and sulpiride have been used therapeutically to increase the milk supply in the mothers of premature infants and in adoptive mothers.[54]

The cerebral paraventricular and supraoptic nuclei control oxytocin synthesis and release.[55] They receive excitatory cholinergic and inhibitory noradrenergic neurons from other parts of the brain. Therefore, sufficiently large doses of centrally acting anticholinergic agents might be expected to inhibit milk ejection. However, study of this phenomenon has not been reported in humans. Sympathomimetics can decrease milk production, probably by centrally decreasing suckling-induced oxytocin and prolactin release and peripherally reducing mammary blood flow.[54-57]

Peripherally, sex hormones (except progesterone) directly affect the breast to decrease lactation. Estrogens and estrogen with androgen combinations were used clinically to suppress lactation before the advent of bromocriptine.

Factors To Consider When Choosing a Drug for a Nursing Mother

Lists of drugs that are acceptable and unacceptable during breast-feeding abound. However, a number of drug and nondrug factors may affect decisions about nursing during drug therapy in a specific mother–infant pair. All of these factors should be considered before prescribing.

Dosage and Duration of Therapy. The dosing regimen of the drug to be given to the mother can often be the deciding factor in whether to discontinue nursing. Dosages of some drugs vary over a wide range for different indications. Even drugs that are potentially harmful to the infant may not contraindicate nursing or may require only a short abstinence period after a low dose or a short duration of therapy. Conversely, a drug that is usually safe during nursing may potentially be problematic when it is given in a high dose or for a long duration.

Age of the Infant. Newborn, and especially premature, infants may be more susceptible than older infants to the pharmacologic effects of drugs in breast milk. Also, newborn infants are more likely to be exclusively breast-fed than older infants.

Quantity of Milk Consumed. As infants grow older, breast milk may become a quantitatively less important part of their diet. Supplemental fluids and food are introduced and eventually become the major source of the baby's nutrition. A one-year-old baby may only nurse once or twice daily for psychological reasons rather than nutrition. The dosage of drug ingested by such an infant will be much less than the dosage ingested by a completely breast-fed one-month-old infant.

Experience with the Drug in Infants. A long history of use of a drug in infants allows a more confident prediction of the risks to the infant from the drug in milk. There is usually little or no information on the dosage, safety, or pharmacokinetics in infants of newly marketed drugs.

Oral Absorption by the Infant. Many drugs are poorly absorbed by the oral route and must be administered to the mother by injection to achieve therapeutic effects. The infant receives these drugs orally and would not be expected to absorb them. This fact alone may allow determination of the safety of some drugs during breast-feeding. Common examples of this type of drug are insulin, aminoglycoside antibiotics, and magnesium sulfate.

Potential Long-Term Effects. When potent agents are given to the mother for a prolonged period of time during nursing, concern arises as to the long-term consequences of even small amounts of the drugs in milk. Potent hormonal or CNS agents may not cause immediate effects in the nursing infant but may subtly affect growth and development. Unfortunately, few studies have been performed that evaluate the long-term effects of long-term maternal drug therapy on the nursing infant. It is prudent to attempt to minimize the exposure of the infant to agents that may potentially affect his or her development in the absence of information indicating their safety.

Possible Interference with Lactation. Certain drugs may decrease the supply of breast milk, causing early cessation of nursing or a need for greater supplementation with formula. This effect may occasionally be sufficiently subtle to go unrecognized and result in undernourishment and suboptimal growth of the infant.

Non-Dose-Related Toxicities. The most frequent concern about drug use during breast-feeding is that the infant will receive a pharmacologically important dose of the drug. However, unwanted effects that are not related to the dose of drug ingested by the infant may also occur. Allergic sensitization of the infant to drugs ingested by the mother is one such phenomenon. Although only a few cases have been reported in the literature, allergic sensitization is expected to happen occasionally. When potentially sensitizing drugs such as penicillins are prescribed for the mother, it is worthwhile to consider warning her to watch for rashes and other signs of allergy in her infant.

Antimicrobials may affect the infant's GI flora. Particular concern has been expressed about the third-generation cephalosporins, which have potent activity against enteric organisms. Although these drugs are not orally absorbed, they are acid stable and thus can pass along the infant's GI tract in an active form.[58] Nursing mothers should be warned to watch for signs of thrush, diarrhea, or diaper rash in their infants while taking antimicrobial agents.

Infants with glucose-6-phosphate dehydrogenase (G6PD) deficiency are susceptible to hemolytic anemia caused by small amounts of offending agents in breast milk. There have been reports of hemolysis due to maternal ingestion of fava beans, dipyrone, dapsone, or long-acting sulfonamides. Hemolysis due to these same agents (which cause hemolysis because of their oxidizing potential) may occur in premature or newborn infants because of the susceptibility of their red blood cells to oxidative stress. Other apparently non-dose-related (possibly allergic) adverse reactions include aplastic anemia due to chloramphenicol and agranulocytosis due to phenothiazines. Although these rare reactions do not necessarily contraindicate nursing, extra monitoring of the infant may be required.

Stepwise Approach to Minimizing Infant Exposure

Prescribers all too frequently admonish a mother to stop nursing immediately when they prescribe a drug or drugs for her. This admonishment is usually the result of unwarranted anxiety about the specific drug and a lack of knowledge about breast-feeding. Abrupt weaning can be psychologically and physically traumatic for both infant and mother. Such harsh, abrupt action is usually not necessary. Often, alternative maternal drug therapies that present a lower risk to the nursing infant are available.

The Drug Information Service of the University of California San Diego Medical Center answers approximately 1000 questions annually on drugs and breast-feeding from health-care professionals and lay persons. What follows is a systematic approach to answering these questions. This approach was developed over the past 10 years, often in consultation with the lactation professionals at Wellstart/The San Diego Lactation Program. The goal is to minimize infant exposure to drugs in breast milk with minimal disruption of nursing. This list should be used in a stepwise fashion from top to bottom, in conjunction with the available information on the specific drugs being considered for the mother and the factors discussed above.

Withhold the Drug. Some drug therapy is not essential and could be foregone with the mother's cooperation. Examples are the use of phenazopyridine (a known cause of methemoglobinemia and hemolysis) with antimicrobial therapy for urinary-tract infections and the use of multi-ingredient cold products to treat one or two symptoms.

Delay Therapy. For a mother who is about to wean her infant, elective drug use (e.g., a radiopharmaceutical diagnostic procedure) or elective surgery might be delayed.

Choose Drugs That Pass Poorly into Milk. In some relatively homogeneous classes of drugs (e.g., β-adrenergic blocking agents), there are large differences among class members in the amount of drug distribution into milk. Choosing a drug that is distributed poorly into milk and has no active or potentially active metabolites can greatly minimize the infant's drug dosage.

Choose an Alternative Route of Administration. Minimization of maternal drug concentrations in blood will also minimize drug concentrations in milk and the infant's dose. Local application of drugs to the affected maternal site often helps attain this goal. Inhaled or topically applied corticosteroids and inhaled bronchodilators and nasal decongestants rather than oral products are examples of such changes in route of administration.

Avoid Nursing at Times of Peak Drug Concentrations in Milk. Coordination of drug dosing times with nursing times to avoid nursing during the periods of peak drug concentration in breast milk can minimize infant exposure. A general rule is that peak concentrations usually occur in milk approximately one to three hours after an oral dose. Two compilations contain a list of times to the peak drug concentration in milk for specific agents.[4,18] Nursing just before a dose is taken may help avoid this peak time in older infants. With newborn infants, nursing may be so frequent and irregular that this avoidance strategy may not be successful. This strategy works best for drugs with short half-lives in non-extended-release dosage forms. Long-acting drugs and extended-release products may not have a distinct peak in plasma or milk. Besides adding to the overall dosage to the infant, the passage of active or potentially active metabolites into milk usually occurs after a long and unpredictable time lag, making it difficult to time feedings to avoid peak drug concentrations in milk. If there is concern that an infant may be receiving clinically important doses of a drug in milk, the infant's plasma drug concentration can be measured.

Administer the Drug before the Infant's Longest Sleep Period. In the case of long-acting drugs that can be given once daily, maternal administration just before the infant's longest sleep period may help minimize the infant dose. An example is the tricyclic antidepressants, which can be given once daily after the last feeding of the day. A middle-of-the-night bottle feeding can be substituted, if necessary.

Temporarily Withhold Breast-feeding. Sometimes, drug therapy is temporary (e.g., use of sedatives or anesthetics for dental or surgical procedures or use of diagnostic agents). Because these procedures are often elective, the mother might choose to pump extra milk before the procedure and refrigerate the milk for use during the period of abstinence from nursing. Formula could also be substituted temporarily. Some mothers may be able to use a lactating friend or relative as a milk donor or temporary "wet nurse." As previously explained, pumping and discarding the milk during the time of nursing abstinence does not substantially hasten the disappearance of drug from the milk in most cases. Pumping the breasts may be necessary to relieve engorgement and its attendant pain and to maintain milk flow, however. Abstinence may also lead to difficulties in resuming nursing once the infant becomes accustomed to an alternative method of feeding.

The length of time that breast-feeding should be withheld depends on the drug. When the primary concern is that potentially toxic serum drug concentrations will accumulate in the infant during multiple days of maternal drug therapy, breast-feeding might be reinstituted as early as one to two maternal drug half-lives (50–75% elimination) after the last dose. With highly toxic drugs, when even a small dose might be harmful, a delay of four to five maternal drug half-lives (94–97% elimination) or longer may be advisable.

Discontinue Nursing. A small minority of drugs that are necessary for the mother's health are too toxic to allow nursing. In these cases (e.g., antineoplastic therapy), it is usually in the best interest of both the mother and the infant to discontinue breast-feeding altogether.

Sources of Information

Numerous reviews on drug use during breast-feeding have been published. However, a few are of particular importance. The American Academy of Pediatrics (AAP) Committee on Drugs recently published an updated version of its list.[59] This list is useful because the AAP is considered an authority. The fact that a drug is listed as safe by the AAP is often persuasive to a prescriber who is otherwise unwilling to allow a mother to nurse during drug therapy. Shortcomings of the list are the lack of differentiation with respect to the age of the infant, lack of consideration of the effects of drugs on lactation, incompleteness of the list, and failure to compare alternatives within a drug class.

A widely used source is the book *Drugs in Pregnancy and Lactation*.[60] It provides data from the primary literature and lists the AAP recommendation for the drug.

By far, the most detailed source is the book *Drugs and Human Lactation*, compiled by the World Health Organization working group.[4] Each drug listing occupies about two pages and explains all quantitative and qualitative aspects of the drug based on all reliable published studies. The cost of the book (approximately $230) may be an impediment to its purchase.

A recent review article by Atkinson and Begg contains a comprehensive list of drug data presented in a brief, standardized format.[18] It provides quantitative data including M/P_{AUC} ratios, times to peak concentration in milk, and percentages of maternal dose. The data are updated annually and published in tabular format in the *Clinical Pharmacokinetics Handbook of Drug Data*.[35]

Specific Drug Information

All of the previously mentioned references consider individual drugs but do not compare drugs within classes or make recommendations for the choice of drugs. The following list does not attempt to duplicate the excellent quantitative presentation of data in *Drugs and Human Lactation* and the *Clinical Pharmacokinetics Handbook of Drug Data*. Quantitative data, when necessary, can be obtained from the original study or one of the above sources.

The list presents guidelines as to the choice of drugs within drug classes (whenever possible) and any special patient-management considerations. In compiling the list, an attempt was made to include literature reports on as many drugs as possible, without using any exclusion criteria for the quality of the report. However, editorial comments indicate this author's opinion of study flaws and limitations. Judgments about the appropriateness of the drugs for use during nursing were made with the assumption that the infant is full-term and is exclusively breast-fed. As mentioned previously, greater caution should be used in pre-term infants, while older, partially breast-fed infants tolerate drugs in milk better. The assumption was also made that usual drug doses are given to the mother; very high dosage regimens may carry more risk to the infant than that indicated.

Many drugs have not been studied during lactation or have only been studied by the manufacturer and not reported in the literature. Without good published data, the product's package insert should be consulted for an appraisal of at least the drug's medicolegal status with respect to use in nursing mothers.

Analgesics and Antipyretics

Acetaminophen. The amount of acetaminophen excreted into milk is small.[61-64] One case of rash, apparently due to acetaminophen in milk, was reported in a breast-fed infant.[65] Acetaminophen is usually safe and is a good analgesic choice during nursing.

Narcotics. Single analgesic doses of most narcotics are excreted in breast milk in amounts that seem small. The following drugs, doses, and routes of administration have been studied: butorphanol tartrate 1–2 mg i.m. and 8 mg p.o.,[66] codeine phosphate or sulfate 60 mg p.o.,[62,67] fentanyl citrate 50–100 µg i.v. or 100 µg epidurally,[68,69] nalbuphine hydrochloride 20 mg i.m.,[70] oxycodone hydrochloride 5–10 mg p.o.,[71] propoxyphene hydrochloride 65 mg p.o.,[72] and sufentanil 50 µg epidurally.[69]

Meperidine given during delivery interferes with the early establishment of breast-feeding because of infant sedation.[73] Single postpartum doses of 50–100 mg of meperidine hydrochloride appear to be safe,[74,75] but repeated doses result in rather high concentrations of meperidine and normeperidine in milk.[76,77] Meperidine causes more neurobehavioral depression in breast-fed neonates than equivalent doses of morphine given by the same route.[77] Morphine sulfate 10–15 mg in single parenteral doses (most patients received i.v. plus i.m. doses) produced only low concentrations in milk,[78] but repeated doses may result in drug accumulation in infant plasma to near therapeutic concentrations.[79] Morphine glucuronides in milk may contribute to the infant's serum concentrations via deconjugation to the active drug. One small series of cases and a retrospective study suggest that postpartum maternal opiates (oral codeine or propoxyphene with or without prior i.m. meperidine) delivered to the infant via breast milk may be a causative factor in episodes of apnea, bradycardia, and cyanosis during the first week of life.[80,81] It appears to be prudent to avoid administering narcotics to mothers when their breast-fed infants have had such an episode and to minimize narcotic use in the perinatal period. Epidural administration or the use of patient-controlled analgesia may help minimize infant dosage.

Heroin abuse can result in high enough drug concentrations in milk to cause addiction or alleviate withdrawal symptoms in infants; however, breast-feeding is not reliable enough to be used as a method of preventing withdrawal.[82,83]

Although most authorities do not consider methadone maintenance a contraindication to breast-feeding,[84-86] it is best to avoid breast-feeding for two to six hours after the dose, when peak milk concentrations occur.[87] One death has been reported in a malnourished five-week-old infant whose mother received methadone maintenance. Methadone was detected in the infant at autopsy, but it is unclear whether the drug contributed to the infant's death.[88]

Nonsteroidal Anti-inflammatory Drugs (NSAIDs). Amounts of most NSAIDs in milk are low because they are weak acids that are extensively protein bound in plasma. However, short-acting agents are preferred for nursing mothers, particularly during the neonatal period. Some agents have active metabolites (e.g., sulindac) or glucuronide metabolites (e.g., salicylate, fenoprofen, ketoprofen) that can add to infant intake.[89] Prolonged bleeding time, hemorrhage, and acute anemia occurred in a seven-day-old infant whose mother was taking naproxen,[90] but naproxen is probably safe after the neonatal period.[89,91] Indomethacin may have caused convulsions in one neonate.[92] Dipyrone, a dangerous analgesic found in many foreign products, and its metabolites are found in milk,[93] and it caused cyanosis in one breast-fed infant.[94] Long-acting agents such as diflunisal, piroxicam, and sulindac should be avoided, at least in mothers of neonates, although amounts of piroxicam in milk are low.[89,95,96] The more toxic NSAIDs such as indomethacin, phenylbutazone, and mefenamic acid should also be avoided.[89,97-100]

The amount of tolmetin in one woman's milk was low.[101] Ketorolac milk concentrations were low after ingestion of ketorolac tromethamine 10 mg orally four times daily for two days,[102] but concentrations in milk after i.m. or i.v. administration have not been studied. Limited data indicate that levels of fenoprofen are low in milk.[103]

Ibuprofen and flurbiprofen have the best documentation of safety during breast-feeding. Amounts of ibuprofen in milk are unmeasurable after doses of up to 1.6 g/day,[104,105] and amounts of flurbiprofen are low to undetectable after doses of up to 50 mg three times daily.[106,107] Diclofenac was not detected in milk after a single dose of diclofenac sodium 50 mg i.m. or 100 mg/day orally for one week; it also appears to be a good choice.[108,109]

Salicylate. Salicylate enters milk in low concentrations relative to those in plasma, although its glucuronide metabolite increases the concentrations.[62,110,111] Doses greater than 1 g of a salicylate result in markedly higher salicylate concentrations in milk.[112] A nine-week-old infant who was only about 50% breast-fed attained a serum salicylate concentration of 65 mg/L during maternal use of aspirin 2.4 g/day.[113] There is a report of metabolic acidosis caused by salicylate in a 16-day-old breast-fed infant whose mother was taking aspirin 650 mg every four hours for arthritis[114]; however, it is unclear whether salicylate in milk was the sole cause. The risk of Reye's syndrome due to salicylate in milk is unknown. NSAIDs such as ibuprofen are preferable to aspirin for long-term therapy. However, if a salicylate is used for long-term maternal therapy, infant plasma concentrations of salicylate should be monitored, particularly in neonates. Although acetaminophen or ibuprofen is preferred, occasional analgesic doses of aspirin should pose no hazards to the infant except for the potential antiplatelet effect. Avoidance of breast-feeding for one to two hours after a dose should obviate this effect.

Anticholinergic Agents

Excretion of anticholinergic agents into milk has not been well studied, but they are weak bases that could concentrate in milk. Theoretical hazards include anticholinergic effects such as drying of secretions, temperature elevations, and CNS disturbances in the infant. Infants should be carefully observed when anticholinergics are given to the mother. Centrally acting anticholinergics may also inhibit milk ejection.

Anticoagulants

Maternal therapy with indandiones (e.g., phenindione) is contraindicated because infant hemorrhage has occurred,[115] although only minute amounts of drug were found in milk after a single, small dose.[116] Although no documentation exists, it is unlikely that heparin passes into milk or is absorbed orally by the infant because of its high molecular weight and negative charge. Amounts of warfarin in milk are of no clinical consequence with maternal doses of warfarin sodium 12 mg/day or less, probably because of extensive protein binding.[117-119] Higher doses have not been studied. Other coumarin derivatives (e.g., dicumarol, acenocoumarol) also appear to be safe.[120-123]

Anticonvulsants

In breast-fed infants, anticonvulsants occasionally achieve plasma concentrations that produce effects; mild drowsiness is common in the infants of mothers taking anticonvulsants, especially in the early neonatal period.[124] Breast-feeding can mitigate withdrawal symptoms in infants whose mothers took anticonvulsants during pregnancy[125]; withdrawal symptoms have been observed after abrupt weaning.[126] The long-term effects of exposure are not well studied. Plasma concentration monitoring in breast-fed infants may be indicated, particularly in infants who are excessively drowsy, feed poorly, or do not gain an adequate amount of weight. Withholding breast-feeding in the early neonatal period has been suggested to minimize sedation.[124] Alternating breast-feeding and bottle feeding has also been suggested to minimize sedation if it occurs.[127] However, administering all or most of the day's dose at bedtime and providing bottle feeding(s) at night may cause less disruption of nursing.

Carbamazepine. Carbamazepine and its major metabolite are excreted in milk and can be detected in nursing infants' plasma. Concentrations are usually low but near the therapeutic range in some infants, although no dose-related effects have been reported.[124,128-131] A case of cholestatic hepatitis, probably an idiosyncratic reaction to carbamazepine, occurred in a three-week-old infant who was exposed to the drug transplacentally as well as via nursing.[132] This apparent non-dose-related toxicity resolved after cessation of nursing. Carbamazepine can be used during lactation, but occasional measurements of infant plasma drug concentrations may be indicated, as well as close observation of the infant for jaundice and other signs of possible adverse idiosyncratic effects.

Clonazepam. Milk and infant plasma concentrations of clonazepam have been measured in only two infants.[133,134] Plasma concentrations were low and no effects were noted, but monitoring of infant plasma drug concentrations may be indicated.

Ethosuximide. Breast-fed infants may attain plasma ethosuximide concentrations near the therapeutic range, and some infants may show signs of drowsiness or fussiness.[131,135-138] Breast-feeding should be undertaken with caution, and the mother's plasma drug concentrations should be kept as low as possible while remaining in the therapeutic range. Measurements of the infant's plasma drug concentrations are indicated.

Phenobarbital. Phenobarbital has a pK_a near the pH of plasma; therefore, variations in milk pH cause marked changes in the amount of drug transferred to milk. Although phenobarbital is generally safe, drowsiness that potentially could lead to feeding difficulties can occur.[124,136,139,140] Phenobarbital and primidone in milk may have contributed to a suffocation death in one infant.[141] Breast-feeding can prevent withdrawal symptoms in infants whose mothers took phenobarbital during pregnancy,[125] and withdrawal symptoms have been observed after abrupt weaning.[126] Phenobarbital can be used in low to moderate doses, but infant behavior, weight gain, and probably plasma drug concentrations should be monitored.[125] Giving all or most of the day's dose at bedtime and providing bottle feeding(s) at night may cause less disruption of nursing.

Phenytoin. Phenytoin is a highly protein-bound weak acid and is excreted into milk in small amounts.[124,131,136,142] Rarely, infants may experience idiosyncratic reactions such as cyanosis and methemoglobinemia,[143] but infants generally tolerate phenytoin in milk.[144]

Primidone. Primidone and its metabolites (phenylethylmalonamide, phenobarbital, and parahydroxyphenobarbital) appear in milk in relatively large amounts.[124,125,136,145] Breast-feeding can prevent withdrawal symptoms in infants whose mothers took anticonvulsants during pregnancy,[125] and withdrawal symptoms have been observed after abrupt weaning.[126,146] Primidone and phenobarbital in milk may have contributed to suffocation death in one infant,[141] and feeding difficulties have been reported in breast-fed infants whose mothers were taking primidone.[147] Primidone can be used in low to moderate doses, but infant behavior and plasma drug concentrations should be closely monitored.[125]

Valproic Acid. Valproic acid passes into milk in low concentrations, and no effects have been noted in infants.[148-151] Infants should be observed for rare idiosyncratic effects such as hepatotoxicity.

Antihistamine Drugs

There are few studies of antihistamine use during lactation. Triprolidine[152] and loratidine[153] are excreted in unimportant amounts. Clemastine may have caused drowsiness in one breast-fed infant,[154] and a long-acting dexbrompheniramine and pseudoephedrine combination caused irritability, crying, and disturbed sleep in another.[155] Cyproheptadine lowers maternal serum prolactin[156] and should be avoided.

Single bedtime doses of antihistamines (preferably short-acting drugs that are used safely in infants) after the last feeding of the day may be adequate for many women and minimize the amount the infant receives. Frequent use of high doses, extended-release products, or combinations with sympathomimetic agents should be avoided. Nasal cromolyn, beclomethasone, or flunisolide is a good alternative.

Anti-infective Agents

Aminoglycosides. Aminoglycosides are polar and pass poorly and irregularly into milk; milk concentrations do not fluctuate as widely or as rapidly as plasma concentrations after i.v. or i.m. administration.[157-162] Systemic effects in infants are unlikely because of the small amounts in milk and poor oral absorption; however, infants should be observed for disruptions of the GI flora, such as thrush and diarrhea.

Antimalarials. Breast-feeding should be undertaken cautiously during daily therapy with chloroquine or hydroxychloroquine, because the importance of the small amounts of drug and metabolites in milk is unclear and accumulation may occur.[163-170] Weekly prophylactic doses are probably safe because the amount of drug in milk is less than the infant prophylactic dose. Small amounts of quinine in milk are unlikely to harm the infant, although allergic reactions may occasionally occur.[171,172] Pyrimethamine appears to be safe and may be excreted in milk in sufficient quantities to treat or protect infants younger than six months of age against malaria; however, breast-feeding is not a reliable method of drug administration.[165,173-175] Mefloquine appears in milk in small amounts after a single dose but has not been studied after weekly dosing for prophylaxis of malaria.[176]

Antituberculars. Antituberculars appear to pass into milk in small quantities. Caution is advised when these agents are used in nursing mothers because many of these drugs can cause hepatic damage. However, inadequate maternal therapy probably poses a much greater risk to the infant than that posed by the drugs in milk. The mother may take single daily doses of many of these drugs at bedtime and substitute a bottle for a nighttime feeding to minimize infant exposure.

Cycloserine is excreted in milk in small amounts, and no adverse reactions have been reported in infants.[177,178] Ethambutol has not been adequately studied.[178] Isoniazid is excreted in milk in amounts that are less than those given to treat an infant.[178,179] Pyrazinamide concentrations in the milk of one woman were low and would have given the baby less than a therapeutic dose.[180] Rifampin has not been well studied, but amounts in milk appear to be small.[178]

Cephalosporins. Cephalosporins appear in milk in trace amounts that could lead to disruption of the GI flora or allergic sensitization.[181-189] Breast-feeding is safe with first-generation and second-generation agents. The risk may be greater with third-generation cephalosporins and similar agents (e.g., moxalactam, aztreonam), which are much more active against normal GI flora.[58,185,190-196] Infants exposed to cephalosporins in milk should be observed for thrush, diarrhea, or rashes.

Penicillins. Penicillins appear in milk in trace amounts that could lead to allergic sensitization, allergic reactions in previously sensitized infants, or disruption of the GI flora.[161,185,197-203] Unless the infant is allergic to penicillin, breast-feeding is generally safe during maternal therapy with the penicillins. Infants exposed to penicillins in milk should be observed for rashes, thrush, or diarrhea.

Quinolones. Ciprofloxacin, ofloxacin, and pefloxacin are slightly concentrated in milk, but absolute concentrations are low.[204,205] Whether these amounts are dangerous for infants is not known.

Norfloxacin was undetectable in milk in one study.[206] Until more safety data are obtained, the fluoroquinolones are probably best avoided during nursing. Nalidixic acid is excreted in minute amounts in milk but has been associated with one case of hemolytic anemia in a breast-fed infant and should be avoided, at least in neonates and G6PD-deficient infants.[207,208]

Sulfonamides. The long-acting sulfonamide sulfamethoxypyridazine has caused hemolysis in a G6PD-deficient infant.[209] Sulfonamides also may cause kernicterus in neonates. Sulfamethoxazole, with or without trimethoprim, and sulfisoxazole can be used safely by nursing mothers of older, healthy, full-term infants.[210,211]

Sulfones. Dapsone in milk apparently caused hemolytic anemia in one infant.[212] Newborns and G6PD-deficient infants are particularly susceptible to dapsone hemolysis. Older infants may be able to tolerate the amounts present in milk.[165,212]

Tetracyclines. Calcium in milk apparently inhibits absorption of the small amounts of tetracycline in milk.[162,213] Infant absorption and plasma concentrations have not been reported with other tetracyclines, but infants would only receive a few milligrams per day of demeclocycline, doxycycline, or minocycline with usual maternal doses.[214-218] Doxycycline concentrations in milk progressively increased with duration of therapy in one study.[216] Although other drugs are preferred for most infections, tetracyclines can be used for a short period of time (7–10 days); prolonged or repeat courses should be avoided during nursing.

Urinary Germicides. Methenamine hippurate and methenamine mandelate pass into milk in small quantities and seem safe to use.[219,220] Nitrofurantoin is excreted in milk in pharmacologically unimportant amounts, but its use should be avoided in mothers of premature infants and infants with G6PD deficiency.[221]

Miscellaneous Anti-infective Agents

Acyclovir. Acyclovir is concentrated in milk; an infant would receive 1–2 mg/day with typical oral maternal dosages.[222,223] Topical acyclovir applied to small areas of the mother's body should pose no risk to the infant. However, it is uncertain whether oral or i.v. acyclovir therapy in the mother is safe for the infant.

Amantadine. Amantadine is a dopamine agonist that decreases maternal serum prolactin and may decrease lactation.[224] The drug is probably best avoided during nursing.

Antimony. Milk concentrations of antimony after maternal therapy with sodium stibogluconate are low. Although it is prudent to avoid nursing during therapy, the risk to the infant is probably not great if breast-feeding is continued.[225]

Chloramphenicol. Chloramphenicol concentrations are not sufficient to induce "gray baby" syndrome but may be enough to cause rare idiosyncratic aplastic anemia.[226,227] Additionally, a number of adverse reactions in infants, including refusal of the breast, falling asleep during feeding, and vomiting after feeding, have occurred.[228] Breast-feeding is contraindicated during maternal chloramphenicol treatment.

Clindamycin. Clindamycin is excreted variably in small amounts in milk.[229,230] It is not certain what effects these amounts may have on infants' GI flora (e.g., induction of pseudomembranous colitis), but a single case of bloody stools in an infant with normal stool flora was reported during maternal clindamycin use.[231] Clindamycin is best avoided if possible, but a few days of therapy with close monitoring of the infant is probably acceptable.

Clofazimine. A breast-fed infant developed the typical skin discoloration and became hypermelanotic during maternal clofazimine use. The skin returned to normal five months after the end of therapy.[232]

Erythromycin. Erythromycin is excreted in milk in amounts smaller than a typical infant dose.[162] One case of pyloric stenosis was reported in a breast-fed infant, but the drug is usually safe.[233]

Mebendazole. Two days after a mother passed a roundworm in her stool and began mebendazole therapy, lactation ceased.[234] Whether the drug played any role in the lactation cessation is questionable. Although not studied during lactation, the drug is poorly absorbed orally and is unlikely to cause adverse effects in a breast-fed infant.

Metronidazole. Metronidazole and its hydroxy metabolite are found in the plasma of nursing infants in concentrations that are 10–20% of maternal plasma concentrations.[235,236] Anecdotal cases of diarrhea and isolation of *Candida* species from breast-fed infants have been reported,[236,237] but most infants do not have immediate reactions.[235,238] Because of the theoretical risk of carcinogenicity and the relatively high infant plasma concentrations achieved, it seems prudent to avoid the drug in nursing mothers. If it is essential to treat trichomoniasis, metronidazole may be given as a single 2-g dose, and an alternative feeding method should be used for the next 24 hours.[239] Furazolidone, which is poorly absorbed orally, is FDA-approved for use in infants and can be used as an alternative treatment for maternal giardiasis if the infant is over one month of age.

Praziquantel. Only a small amount of praziquantel reaches the infant, and use of the drug during nursing appears to be safe.[240]

Trimethoprim. Trimethoprim is excreted in milk, and infants receive about 0.75–1 mg daily with usual maternal doses; this amount is probably not harmful.[210,241]

Vancomycin. A small amount of vancomycin was detected in the milk of one mother.[242] Because the drug is not orally absorbed, its use during nursing seems safe.

Antineoplastics and Immunosuppressants

Breast-feeding is generally considered to be contraindicated in women receiving antineoplastic drugs. Breast-feeding during azathioprine and corticosteroid immunosuppressive therapy has been performed safely in a limited number of cases.

Azathioprine. Three infants were safely breast-fed during maternal azathioprine use (75–100 mg/day) after renal transplantation.[243,244] Low concentrations of the azathioprine metabolite mercaptopurine were found in milk. Breast-feeding can be undertaken with close infant monitoring during immunosuppressive therapy.

Busulfan. Busulfan in a dose of 4 mg daily for five weeks was taken by one woman while breast-feeding with no apparent adverse effects on her infant's leukocytes or hemoglobin.[245] This case is by no means conclusive, however, and breast-feeding is not recommended.

Cisplatin. In one patient, platinum was not detected in milk at any time after an i.v. infusion of 100 mg/sq m.[246] In another patient, milk platinum concentration was 0.9 mg/L 19.5 hours after her third daily dose of 20 mg/sq m.[247] Because the platinum may be in a reactive form, nursing is not recommended.[247]

Cyclophosphamide. Cyclophosphamide is detectable in milk,[248] and two cases of bone marrow depression have been reported in infants of women who nursed while receiving the drug.[249,250] Breast-feeding is not recommended.

Cyclosporine. Milk concentrations of cyclosporine are lower than those in maternal plasma, but there is no information on the safety of maternal cyclosporine therapy during breast-feeding.[251-253] Breast-feeding should be avoided until further data become available.

Doxorubicin. Doxorubicin and its primary active metabolite, doxorubicinol, appear in rather large amounts in milk.[246] Breast-feeding is not recommended.

Hydroxyurea. Hydroxyurea is excreted in small amounts in milk, but breast-feeding is not advised.[254]

Methotrexate. Methotrexate was measured in milk in one patient.[255] The authors concluded that breast-feeding presents little hazard if bottle feeding is not possible; however, this case is not conclusive. Low weekly doses for arthritis probably pose a relatively small risk to the breast-fed infant.

Vincristine. Intramammary vincristine in goats decreases milk volume and alters milk composition, probably by inhibiting lactose synthesis.[256] The only report of vincristine use by a lactating human does not mention an effect on lactation.[249] Breast-feeding is not advisable.

Cardiovascular Drugs

β-Adrenergic Blocking Agents. The excretion of β blockers in breast milk has been extensively studied.[49,257-277] The infant's dose varies greatly among the different compounds, allowing a range of choices among the agents. Somewhat counterintuitively, the most water-soluble drugs reach the infant in the greatest amounts. This situation occurs because plasma protein binding, which is directly related to lipid solubility, is the primary determinant of the extent of passage.[8,257] Moreover, the water-soluble agents have the longest half-lives and are more likely to accumulate in infants. Maternal therapy with atenolol resulted in cyanosis and bradycardia in one breast-fed neonate[276]; hypotension, bradycardia, and transient tachypnea were reported in another infant whose mother was taking acebutolol.[273] These two drugs, as well as betaxolol, nadolol, sotalol, and timolol, should be avoided in nursing mothers of younger infants and when high doses are required. Oxprenolol and mepindolol excretion in milk is intermediate, and these drugs should probably be avoided during the neonatal period. Propranolol, metoprolol, and labetalol (and its isomer, dilevalol) are excreted in milk in low enough quantities to allow nursing even in the neonatal period.

Calcium-Channel-Blocking Agents. One case report indicates that only small amounts of diltiazem are excreted into milk.[278] More data are needed to judge the safety of diltiazem therapy in nursing mothers. Two case reports indicate that only small amounts of nifedipine enter milk.[279,280] A study of three mothers likewise found only small amounts of nitrendipine in milk.[281] Although these drugs appear safe for use in nursing mothers, caution should be exercised until more data are available. Several case reports indicate that the amounts of verapamil and norverapamil in milk and infant plasma are low.[282-285] Use of verapamil while breast-feeding appears to be safe. Tiapamil concentrations in milk are also low.[286]

Antiarrhythmics. Some antiarrhythmics reach near-therapeutic concentrations in breast-fed infants. Although two infants safely breast-fed during maternal amiodarone therapy, infant plasma concentrations were relatively high and breast-feeding should probably be discontinued when amiodarone therapy is required.[287-289] Data on disopyramide indicate that infants may receive relatively large doses of the drug and its metabolite, with infant plasma concentrations below but near the therapeutic range.[290-293] Disopyramide may be used cautiously during lactation if other alternatives are unacceptable. The infant should be observed for anticholinergic symptoms, and perhaps the infant's plasma disopyramide concentrations should be measured. Sparse data from one patient indicate that tocainide may be concentrated in milk and should be used with caution during nursing.[294]

There are several alternative antiarrhythmics that may have less potential to harm the infant. Bretylium tosylate 400 mg orally every eight hours was taken by one mother while nursing with no apparent effects on her infant; more data are needed before it can be concluded that infant exposure to bretylium is safe, though.[295] Lidocaine concentrations in milk during continuous i.v. therapy are low and should pose no hazard to the infant by this route or during use as a local anesthetic.[296] Amounts of flecainide in milk are small and are unlikely to affect the infant.[297,298] Concentrations of mexiletine in milk are low and cannot be detected in the plasma of breast-fed infants,[299,300] but poor feeding may have occurred in one infant.[301] Procainamide and its active metabolite, *N*-acetylprocainamide, are more concentrated in milk than in plasma, but absolute amounts are small.[302] Procainamide should be used with caution until it has been better studied. The amounts of quinidine excreted in milk appear to be unimportant; data are not conclusive, however.[303]

Digoxin. Infants receive trivial doses of digoxin via breast milk; breast-feeding is safe during digoxin therapy.[304-307]

Hypotensive Agents. Certain antihypertensives are less desirable than others during nursing. Milk concentrations of clonidine are much higher than maternal plasma concentrations, and breast-fed infants have plasma concentrations approaching those of the mother.[308] Although no adverse effects have been reported in breast-fed infants, clonidine should be used only with great caution during breast-feeding. Clonidine and guanfacine may also decrease maternal prolactin secretion.[53] Reserpine may cause infant nasal stuffiness and increased tracheobronchial secretions. Because safer alternatives are available, reserpine should be avoided.[309]

The angiotensin-converting enzyme (ACE) inhibitors captopril and enalapril are found in small amounts in milk, and no adverse effects have occurred in infants.[310-312] Milk ACE activity was in the normal range after a dose of enalapril.[311] Limited data indicate that low-dose, short-term use of hydralazine (e.g., for a few days postpartum) is probably safe.[313] Several studies indicate that methyldopa is excreted in unimportant amounts.[314-316] There is limited information on minoxidil in milk, but the amounts appear to be low.[317] However, minoxidil should be used with caution, particularly when therapy involves large doses and long-term use.

Diuretics

Low doses of short-acting thiazide-type diuretics should pose no problems to the infant or suppress lactation,[318,319] although thrombocytopenia or allergic reactions to sulfonamide diuretics might theoretically occur. Large doses of short-acting thiazide-type diuretics or usual doses of loop diuretics or long-acting thiazide-type diuretics (e.g., chlorthalidone, bendroflumethiazide) can suppress lactation and should be avoided.[320-322] Long-acting agents may also accumulate in infants' plasma.[323] Acetazolamide appears in milk in small amounts that are unlikely to harm the infant.[324] The amounts of spironolactone and its metabolites in milk appear to be unimportant.[325]

Ergot Alkaloids

Bromocriptine. Most ergot alkaloids have dopaminergic activity that can suppress maternal prolactin release and lactation.[326] Bromocriptine is used therapeutically for this purpose, a practice that has been criticized because of its potentially serious toxicity.[327,328] The related agents cabergoline, lisuride, terguride, metergoline, and dihydroergocristine have also been used to inhibit lactation.[329-333] Rebound galactorrhea has been reported after withdrawal of high-dose bromocriptine.[334] Mothers who decide to nurse after receiving bromocriptine should probably wait up to a week before breast-feeding because of the drug's long half-life.

Ergonovine and Methylergonovine. Although ergonovine can lower postpartum serum prolactin concentrations,[335-338] methylergonovine apparently does not,[339,340] nor is methylergonovine found in milk in important quantities.[341] Short-term, low-dose regimens of these agents immediately postpartum pose no hazard to the infant, but methylergonovine is preferred because it does not inhibit lactation.[339,340,342] Courses of these drugs given several days postpartum to treat late postpartum uterine bleeding may expose the infant to greater risk because of the larger amount of milk consumed at this age; ergot alkaloids are known to have caused adverse effects in infants.[343]

Ergotamine. Ergotamine therapy daily for six days postpartum did not affect lactation or infant weight in one study.[342] However, the excretion of ergotamine into milk has not been studied. Its use probably should be avoided during lactation, because older ergot preparations produced toxic effects in infants.[343]

Gastrointestinal Drugs

Antidiarrheals. Nonabsorbable products such as kaolin–pectin, psyllium, and other fibers and gums, which may also be useful in firming watery stools, are the preferred agents in nursing mothers. Diphenoxylate excretion into milk has not been studied. Based on the excretion into milk of other narcotic agents, a few small doses of diphenoxylate should be acceptable. Bismuth subsalicylate should be avoided because of systemic salicylate absorption. Loperamide excretion into milk has not been studied.

Mesalamine Derivatives. Small amounts of sulfasalazine and sulfapyridine have been found in milk and infant's plasma after oral sulfasalazine use.[344-347] The sulfapyridine released should cause no bilirubin displacement. Bloody diarrhea occurred in one infant whose mother was taking sulfasalazine,[347] and diarrhea occurred in the infant of a mother using mesalamine suppositories.[348] Small amounts of mesalamine and large amounts of its metabolite were found in milk after oral doses of mesalamine.[349] Mesalamine and its derivatives (e.g., sulfasalazine) may be used cautiously during nursing with close observation of the infant, especially in the case of higher doses.

Cathartics and Laxatives. Old studies indicate that some anthraquinone derivatives, such as aloe and cascara, should be avoided during nursing because of a laxative effect in breast-fed infants.[350] Laxatives that are nonabsorbable or poorly absorbed, such as bulk forming (e.g., psyllium), osmotic (e.g., magnesium or phosphate salts), or stool-softening (e.g., docusate) types, are preferred during lactation. Use of senna in moderate doses appears to be acceptable in nursing mothers if other measures fail.[351,352] Bisacodyl is virtually unabsorbed from the GI tract and should be safe.

Histamine H_2-Receptor Antagonists. Cimetidine is concentrated in milk because of ion trapping[32]; ranitidine is also concentrated, but to a lesser extent.[33,353] Cimetidine should probably be avoided during nursing; ranitidine might best be taken as a single dose at bedtime with avoidance of night feedings. Famotidine, nizatidine, and roxatidine are less concentrated in milk and may be preferable during nursing.[354-356] However, sucralfate, which is virtually nonabsorbable, may be preferable to all H_2-receptor antagonists.

Gastrokinetic Agents. Metoclopramide elevates maternal serum prolactin via central dopaminergic antagonism and results in increased milk production and a more rapid transition from colostrum to mature milk.[357-359] Metoclopramide may be used therapeutically in mothers who are producing insufficient quantities of milk, such as the mothers of premature or sick infants or adoptive mothers.[357,360,361] Elevation of prolactin may be less effective in maintaining milk production later in the puerperium.[362]

Metoclopramide is concentrated in milk because of ion trapping.[363,364] Although infant doses are low, some nursing infants' serum prolactin concentrations are elevated.[364] Concern has been raised because of possible defects in neural development in newborn animals exposed to dopamine receptor antagonists.[4,365] Avoiding breast-feeding for three to four hours after the dose and limiting the duration of therapy to 10–14 days should minimize infant exposure when metoclopramide use is essential.

Domperidone also increases maternal serum prolactin concentrations. Concentrations of domperidone in milk are lower than those of metoclopramide,[365] but domperidone has not been used clinically to enhance lactation. Cisapride concentrations in milk are low, but cisapride's effects on maternal serum prolactin and on infants are not known.[366]

Hormones and Synthetic Substitutes

Buserelin. Buserelin is a luteinizing-hormone-releasing hormone that has been investigated as a postpartum contraceptive.[367,368] The minute amounts in milk appear to have no biologic activity in the nursing infant.

Contraceptives. Frequently, the older, high-estrogen contraceptives suppressed lactation sufficiently to necessitate either supplementary feeding or discontinuation of breast-feeding, especially when the contraceptives were administered immediately postpartum.[369,370] When the currently available low-estrogen plus progestin combination contraceptives are administered beginning at six weeks postpartum, a dramatic effect is usually not seen, but long-term negative effects on milk yield and infant growth occur.[371-374] These effects can lead to early feeding supplementation and discontinuation of breast-feeding. Low-dose, progestin-only contraceptives may actually enhance milk supply and extend the duration of lactation.[372-376] Levonorgestrel implants likewise appear to have no adverse effect on milk yield.[377-379]

Rarely, breast enlargement in infants and proliferation of the vaginal epithelium in female infants have been attributed to use of combination oral contraceptives; however, a causal relationship has not been firmly established.[380-383] One case of megaloblastic anemia in an infant, possibly due to contraceptive steroids in milk, was reported.[384] Assays of estrogens and progestins in milk show that both are found in low concentrations.[385-389] Although these substances are present in milk in small amounts and are readily metabolized by infants,[390] there is some concern over the long-term effects of steroids on the development of breast-fed infants.[391] A long-term (eight-year) follow-up of breast-fed infants of mothers taking contraceptives containing 50 μg of ethinyl estradiol found no adverse effects on the infants' development or behavior.[371] Mean infant serum levonorgestrel concentrations are approximately 10% of maternal serum concentrations during maternal use of levonorgestrel implants[392]; infant growth may undergo a slight, transient depression (but within the normal range) after insertion of the implants, but longer-term development is not affected.[377-379] If hormonal contraception is used, an oral, low-dose, progestin-only type or levonorgestrel implants are preferred because of their lack of detrimental effects on lactation. In mothers who exclusively breast-feed their infants, the efficacy of oral progestin-only contraceptives is equal to that of the combination products.

Corticosteroids. Prednisone and prednisolone excretion into milk appears to be minimal with doses of 20 mg/day or less and is small with even large single oral doses.[393,394] When prednisone doses are larger than 20 mg/day or when therapy will be long term, it seems prudent to use prednisolone (which avoids the double peak in milk caused by the prodrug) rather than prednisone and to avoid nursing for three to four hours after a dose.[393,395] Three infants have been breast-fed during long-term maternal use of methylprednisolone 6–8 mg/day with apparent safety.[243,244] Large i.v. doses of corticosteroids and administration of long-acting agents such as dexamethasone have not been studied, and caution is warranted regarding these uses in nursing mothers. Depot injections, inhaled beclomethasone, or topical corticosteroids should present little or no risk to the infant because of the low maternal serum concentrations achieved. Topical application of a corticosteroid directly to the mother's nipples resulted in symptoms of corticosteroid excess in one nursing infant, however.[396]

Desmopressin. Desmopressin is excreted in small amounts in milk and is unlikely to be well absorbed orally by the infant.[397]

Insulin. Diabetic mothers using insulin may nurse their infants.[398] However, it has been empirically found that these women may need to reduce their insulin dose to approximately 75% of their prepregnancy dose.[398-400]

Oxytocin. Oxytocin administered as a nasal spray brings about milk ejection, thus facilitating lactation and increasing milk volume in mothers of premature infants and adoptive mothers.[401] Use should be limited to a few days, because psychological dependence on the spray can develop in the mother. Water intoxication and seizures occurred in one woman who overused it.[402]

Progesterone. Progesterone used as a contraceptive via implants or intrauterine devices transfers little drug to the breast-fed infant.[403] Milk progesterone concentrations have not been measured after higher doses given to treat premenstrual syndrome.

Prostaglandins. Prostaglandins E_2, $F_{2\alpha}$, 6-keto-prostaglandin $F_{1\alpha}$, and thromboxane B_2 have been found in fresh human milk.[404-406] They appear to be stable in milk and gastric fluid, where they may provide a natural cytoprotective effect to the infant.[407] Therapeutically, prostaglandin E_2 has been investigated as a method of inhibiting lactation and engorgement with mixed results.[408,409] Like oxytocin, prostaglandin $F_{2\alpha}$ administered nasally increases milk ejection.[410]

Thyroid and Antithyroid Agents. *Thyroid.* Thyroid hormones are necessary for normal lactation.[4] It appears that levothyroxine passes into milk poorly, whereas liothyronine may pass in more physiologically important amounts.[411-413] Milk concentrations of thyroid hormones have not been measured after exogenous administration, but physiologic replacement doses of levothyroxine to a breast-feeding mother are not expected to result in excessive thyroid administration to the infant. Replacement therapy with liothyronine or supraphysiologic maternal levothyroxine doses may transfer larger amounts of liothyronine to the infant.[413]

Antithyroid. Propylthiouracil passes poorly into milk and does not affect nursing infants.[414] Methimazole passes into milk more freely and has a longer half-life than propylthiouracil; thus, it is a less desirable alternative.[414] Methimazole in low doses of ≤10 mg/day or carbimazole (a methimazole prodrug) ≤15 mg/day may be used.[414-416] A potential for idiosyncratic reactions and hypothyroidism exists, however, and measurement of the infant's serum thyroxine and thyroid-stimulating hormone concentrations every two to four weeks is prudent when these drugs are used in nursing mothers.[414] Propylthiouracil is the drug of choice during lactation because of its minimal excretion into milk, at least in doses up to 300 mg/day.[414,417]

Psychotherapeutic Agents

Antidepressants. Heterocyclic antidepressants have not been thoroughly studied during lactation. Respiratory depression has been reported in one breast-fed infant whose mother was taking doxepin 25 mg three times a day,[418] but an infant whose mother was taking 150 mg at night had no problems.[419] Maternal doses of amitriptyline up to 150 mg/day, desipramine 300 mg/day, imipramine 200 mg/day, or nortriptyline 125 mg/day have not caused observable effects in the few infants studied.[420-425] The tertiary amines resulted in late peaks of the corresponding secondary amine metabolite in milk.

A single 50-mg dose of trazodone,[426] amoxapine 250 mg/day,[427] or maprotiline hydrochloride 100–150 mg/day[428] produced low drug concentrations in milk, but the effects of these drugs on infants have not been studied. Fluoxetine has been inadequately studied,[429] but the long half-lives of the drug and its metabolite warn against its use.

No agreement exists on the advisability of therapy with tricyclic antidepressants and related antidepressants during lactation. Some authors have recommended against the use of these agents because of potential (but undemonstrated) long-term effects on the infant's neurological development.[430-432] Others, including the AAP, consider these drugs to be acceptable.[59,433] Infant exposure to the tricyclic antidepressants can be minimized by using a secondary amine (i.e., nortriptyline or desipramine) and by giving the drug as a single dose at bedtime, skipping nighttime feeding(s) if possible. Monitoring of the infant is warranted when these drugs are used during breast-feeding.

There are no data on the amounts of monoamine oxidase inhibitors (MAOIs) excreted into milk. These drugs reportedly inhibit lactation.[434] Because of their potential toxicity, MAOIs should be avoided during nursing.

Tranquilizers. Haloperidol has been studied in only two patients; researchers found small quantities of drug that did not affect the infants, but long-term effects are unknown.[435,436] Phenothiazines and thioxanthines pass into milk somewhat unpredictably but usually in small amounts.[434,437-440] Drowsiness has occurred with the more sedating agents, such as chlorpromazine.[438] Other effects, such as extrapyramidal symptoms, may be possible but have not been reported. Follow-up ranging from 15 months to 6 years indicates no long-term effects on infant development.[441-443]

Lithium. Lithium in milk can adversely affect the infant when lithium elimination is impaired, as in cases of dehydration or in neonates and premature infants.[444-446] Neonates may also have lithium in their plasma that was acquired transplacentally. The long-term effects of lithium on infants are not known; some authors consider lithium therapy a contraindication to breast-feeding,[432-434] whereas others do not.[447-449] Lithium can probably be used cautiously in lactating patients who are carefully selected for their ability to monitor their infants. Breast-feeding should be discontinued immediately if the infant appears restless or ill. Measurement of plasma lithium concentrations in the infant can help rule out lithium toxicity.

Sedatives and Hypnotics

Most sedatives and hypnotics pass into breast milk in measurable and potentially important amounts. Sedative and hypnotic intake should be minimized during lactation; agents with unique toxicities in the infant (e.g., bromides, diazepam) should be avoided.

Barbiturates. Barbiturates may stimulate metabolism of endogenous compounds in the infant when small amounts pass into milk. Short-acting agents appear to be preferable to long-acting agents, because smaller amounts are excreted into milk. High single doses may have more potential for causing infant drowsiness than multiple small doses.[139] Typical i.v. doses of thiopental for induction of anesthesia produce low concentrations in milk that do not appear to affect the infant.[450]

Benzodiazepines. Benzodiazepines with long-acting metabolites (e.g., diazepam) can accumulate in infants, especially neonates, because of their immature excretory mechanisms and have caused adverse effects in infants.[451,452] Infant withdrawal symptoms have been reported after abrupt weaning or rapid cessation of long-term alprazolam use during nursing.[453] Long-term benzodiazepine therapy should be avoided if possible during breast-feeding, particularly in the neonatal period. When therapy is essential, the short-acting agents oxazepam and lorazepam appear to be preferable.[44,454-457] Midazolam and its active metabolite attain low levels in milk only transiently after a 15-mg oral dose,[44] but i.v. administration has not been studied. Breast milk should be withheld for six to eight hours after a single dose of diazepam for short procedures, such as dental work or endoscopy. Interesting recent work has found that diazepam and several other benzodiazepine-like substances occur naturally in breast milk in very small but not necessarily meaningless amounts.[458] The source of these compounds and their physiologic effects are not clear.

Miscellaneous Sedatives and Hypnotics. Bromides have caused infant drowsiness and rash during breast-feeding and should be avoided.[459] Chloral hydrate and its active metabolite, trichloroethanol, appear in milk in doses that approximate an infant sedative dose and are detectable for up to 24 hours after a single dose.[460,461] Glutethimide has been detected in minute amounts 8–12 hours after a dose.[462] Milk halothane concentrations equal or surpass concentrations in maternally inhaled air.[463] Meprobamate concentrations peak in milk at four hours, which is two hours after peak maternal plasma concentrations.[464] Amounts of propofol in milk are small and may not have good oral bioavailability in the infant.[465]

Miscellaneous Agents

Baclofen. Baclofen appears in milk in small amounts, and it may be used in nursing mothers with caution.[466]

Bupivacaine. Bupivacaine is undetectable in milk when administered to the mother by the intrapleural or epidural route.[467,468]

Colchicine. Excretion of colchicine in human milk has not been studied, but the drug decreases milk production and alters milk composition in animals when infused into the udder.[469,470] It should probably be avoided while breast-feeding.

Fluorescein. Fluorescein is detectable in milk after i.v. or topical administration.[471,472] After i.v. administration, it had a half-life of 62 hours in milk in one mother. The drug may present a risk to neonates who are undergoing phototherapy. Temporarily withholding nursing may be appropriate.

Fluoride. Fluoride concentrations in milk are low and virtually unrelated to maternal intake.[473] Although there are no definitive studies, most authors recommend fluoride supplementation in breast-fed infants as defined in the AAP guidelines.[474-476]

Gold. Gold is excreted in milk and has been detected in the blood and urine of some nursing infants.[477-482] The weight-adjusted infant dose may be greater than the maternal dose, but the exact amount of gold that infants absorb is not clear.[482] Sufficient amounts are absorbed, however, to potentially cause adverse effects. Opinions vary, but gold therapy is at least a reason to carefully monitor the breast-fed infant and may be a reason for withholding breast-feeding.[480-482]

Herbals. Use of herbal products seems to be increasing among persons who view them as safer or more natural alternatives to pharmaceutical products. For the most part, these products have not been scientifically studied during lactation, but the potential exists for herbal products to have all of the properties of pharmaceuticals, ranging from clinical usefulness to toxicity. One herbal product that is fairly widely used as a galactagogue is fenugreek.[483] It appears to be quite safe (it is also used as the flavoring agent in artificial maple syrup) and has been shown to have oxytocic activity in animals.[484] Recently, androgenization (black pubic hair, hair over the entire forehead, and swollen, red nipples) occurred in the newborn son of a mother who was taking a large daily dosage of a Siberian ginseng product that also produced testosterone-like effects in her.[485,486] Symptoms did not subside until after nursing was discontinued. In addition to their pharmacologic effects, other possible effects of herbals are alteration of the taste or composition of milk[483] and allergenicity.[487]

Iodides, Inorganic and Organic. Inorganic iodides are contraindicated during breast-feeding because of possible thyroid suppression and rashes.[67,343] Topical and vaginal povidone iodine in nursing mothers results in elevated milk iodine concentrations and thyroid suppression in nursing infants.[488-491] Povidone iodine preparations should not be used while nursing. Large amounts of iodine are excreted in milk for weeks after bipedal lymphangiography with ethiodized oil, and nursing should be discontinued after this procedure.[492] Iopanoic acid contains free iodide that can be detected in milk.[493] Diatrizoate,[494,495] gadopentetate,[496] iodamide,[495] iohexol,[497] metrizoate,[497] and metrizamide[498] are detectable in milk after i.v. administration. Although no adverse effects have been reported in infants, breast-feeding should probably be withheld for 24–36 hours after administration of a contrast medium.

Levodopa. Levodopa decreases serum prolactin in nonnursing women with hyperprolactinemia and galactorrhea.[499] It decreases serum prolactin in a dose-dependent fashion and inhibits lactation in high doses in animals.[500] It is likely that levodopa would interfere with lactation in nursing mothers. Effects in breast-fed infants have not been studied.

Lindane. Lindane was excreted in milk at up to 30 times the background concentration after maternal topical application of a 0.3% emulsion daily for three days.[501] Concentrations remained elevated over usual background concentrations for at least seven days. Alternative drugs (e.g., permethrin, pyrethrins) are preferred for use by breast-feeding women.

Magnesium. It has been observed that some mothers have difficulty in establishing a milk supply and some infants have difficulty in nursing after the mothers have received magnesium sulfate infusions for the treatment of pre-eclampsia or eclampsia. These phenomena have not been studied, but infant drowsiness due to placentally transferred magnesium may be involved. Therapy with i.v. magnesium increases milk magnesium concentrations only slightly. Oral absorption of magnesium is poor, and maternal magnesium therapy is not a contraindication to breast-feeding.[502]

Neostigmine. Six infants of mothers treated with neostigmine for myasthenia gravis were reportedly breast-fed successfully. Neostigmine could not be found in milk.[503]

Noscapine. Noscapine concentrations in milk are low and are unlikely to affect nursing infants.[504]

Pentoxifylline. The amounts of pentoxifylline in milk appear to be small, but caution should be used until further experience is gained.[505]

Pravastatin. Limited data indicate that negligible amounts of pravastatin and its major active metabolite are excreted into milk.[506]

Pyridostigmine. Pyridostigmine has been used safely during breast-feeding in three patients with myasthenia gravis.[507,508]

Pyridoxine. High-dose pyridoxine hydrochloride (600 mg/day in three doses) has been used therapeutically to suppress lactation,[509,510] although it is often not effective.[511-513] With usual doses found in foods and low-dose vitamin supplements, pyridoxine has no effect on prolactin or lactation.[514]

Retinoids. The primary active metabolite of etretinate, acitretin, passes into breast milk in a quantity sufficient to recommend avoidance of nursing while taking either etretinate or acitretin.[515] Although there is no information on use during lactation, the manufacturers of topical tretinoin and oral isotretinoin state that these agents are not compatible with nursing. Based on the systemic bioavailability of tretinoin applied topically to a small area such as the face,[516] it seems unlikely that harmful amounts reach the infant via breast milk. Caution should be used to avoid contact of the infant's skin with treated areas of the mother's skin, regardless of whether she is nursing.

Sympathomimetic Agents. Infant irritability, crying, and disturbed sleep occurred during maternal intake of a long-acting preparation containing pseudoephedrine and dexbrompheniramine.[155] However, pseudoephedrine excretion into milk is minimal.[152] In animals, sympathomimetic vasoconstrictors decrease milk flow by central inhibition of secretion and release of oxytocin and by peripheral vasoconstriction, which limits the access of oxytocin to myoepithelial cells in the breast.[55,56] Norepinephrine may also decrease prolactin release.[57] Although these effects are not well documented in humans, lactation inhibition seems to occur occasionally with oral decongestants; therefore, sympathomimetic nasal sprays are recommended over oral decongestant products. Use of oral terbutaline results in low milk terbutaline concentrations,[517] causes no symptoms in breast-fed infants,[518,519] and is not expected to decrease milk supply. β_2-Adrenergic-receptor agonists are probably safe to use orally, but inhaler products should transfer less drug to the infant and are preferred.

Theophylline. Maternal theophylline use may occasionally cause irritability and fretful sleep in infants.[520] Newborn infants are most likely to be affected because of their slow elimination and low plasma protein binding of theophylline.[19,22] Extended-release products or continuous infusion may tend to maximize the infant dose, but infant plasma concentrations remain below the therapeutic range in most cases.[22] There is no need to avoid theophylline products; however, maternal plasma concentrations should be kept in the lower part of the therapeutic range, and infant plasma concentrations may be measured if apparent adverse effects occur. The related drug dyphylline is excreted into milk in greater amounts and is best avoided.[521]

Tolbutamide. Tolbutamide is excreted in small amounts that should cause no harm.[522] No information is available on the other more potent or long-acting oral sulfonylurea agents.

Vaccines. Much contradictory literature on poliovirus has been published regarding the possibility that antibodies in milk could prevent active immunization in infants. It has been recommended that breast-feeding of newborns be withheld for six hours before and after immunization[523]; however, when infants are immunized after six weeks of age, breast-feeding has a negligible effect on antibody titers.[524,525] Breast-fed infants have a better antibody response to bacillus Calmette-Gúerin, *Haemophilus influenzae* type b, and poliovirus vaccines and to diphtheria and tetanus toxoids than those who are not breast-fed.[526-528] Rubella vaccine is transferred into milk and results in an immune response in about one-half of infants; however, this response appears to be of little consequence.[529,530] Breast-feeding is not a contraindication to the use of any vaccine in the mother.[531]

Drugs for Nonmedical Use

Alcohol. Alcohol equilibrates rapidly between blood and milk; milk concentrations are about equal to simultaneously determined blood concentrations.[532,533] Potential effects on infants vary depending on the pattern of use. One case of drunkenness (deep, unarousable sleep with snoring, deep respiration, no reaction to pain, inability to suck, excessive perspiration, and a feeble pulse) was reported in an eight-day-old infant whose mother drank 750 mL of port wine in a 24-hour period.[343,534] A case of pseudo-Cushing's syndrome has been reported in an infant whose mother drank "at least 50 12-ounce cans of beer weekly plus generous amounts of more concentrated alcoholic beverages."[535] One prospective study suggests that as little as one drink daily can cause slight impairment of the infant's motor development that increases in a dose-dependent fashion.[536]

Alcohol also affects lactation; it inhibits the milk ejection reflex in a dose-dependent fashion, with single doses over 2 g/kg completely blocking suckling-induced oxytocin release.[537,538] Animal studies demonstrated that alcohol consumption resulted in reduced suckling-induced prolactin release and reduced milk yield.[539,540] An unknown substance in beer increases maternal serum prolactin, but this effect also occurs with nonalcoholic beer.[541,542]

Alcohol should be used in moderation during lactation. Nursing should probably be withheld temporarily after alcohol consumption, with the duration dependent on the amount consumed. One to two hours per drink is suggested.

Amphetamines. In one case report of a mother taking amphetamine sulfate 20 mg/day therapeutically, amphetamine concentrations in milk were less than those in plasma, and no adverse effects on the infant were noted.[543] However, there is likely to be substantial intersubject variation in excretion, and concentrations in milk during high-dose amphetamine abuse have not been studied. It is likely that some infants would experience drug-induced behavioral abnormalities, possibly either stimulation or drowsiness and poor feeding.[544] Amphetamine also inhibits prolactin release and, if taken in high doses, could interfere with lactation.[545] A related drug, norpseudoephedrine, is found in the milk of mothers who chew khat, as well as in their infants' urine.[546]

Caffeine. Anecdotal reports of infant jitteriness and difficulty sleeping have been reported with high maternal intake of caffeine (four or five cups of coffee and two or three 480-mL bottles of cola daily in one case, and four mugs of tea, five mugs of coffee, and one cola per day in another), but infant serum caffeine concentrations were not measured.[547,548] Systematic studies have indicated that caffeine is excreted into milk in relatively small amounts and infants are usually not affected, even with rather high maternal intake.[549-552] Effects are more likely in premature and newborn infants because of their greatly diminished ability to metabolize caffeine.[553]

Cocaine. The chemical nature of cocaine and results from animal studies indicate that it would be expected to appear in milk in amounts that might affect the infant.[554] In addition, infants do not possess the plasma cholinesterase needed to metabolize the drug, leading to accumulation. There has been only one report in the literature on the measurement of cocaine in milk and the effects of the drug (vomiting, diarrhea, irritability and dilated pupils) on a breast-fed infant.[555] Cocaine was detectable in milk for 24–36 hours after use. Convulsions occurred in an infant whose mother used topical cocaine to treat sore nipples.[556] Breast-feeding is not recommended when the mother is a chronic cocaine abuser, and even occasional use of cocaine is discouraged during breast-feeding. Breast-feeding should be withheld for at least 24 hours after cocaine use.

Marijuana. Marijuana excretion in milk has not been well studied, but dronabinol may reach rather high concentrations in milk and may be detected in the infant, particularly with heavy maternal use.[557] Short-term effects in infants have not been reported, but a decrement in motor development at one year in the infants of marijuana-smoking mothers was reported in one study.[558] Marijuana also lowers serum prolactin slightly in nonlactating women[559] and oxytocin release in rodents.[560] However, the effect of marijuana on nursing is not known. Breast-feeding should probably be avoided when the mother is a heavy marijuana user and during therapeutic dronabinol use. Breast-feeding should probably be withheld for several hours after occasional marijuana use, and caution should be used to avoid exposing the infant to marijuana smoke.

Phencyclidine. Phencyclidine is concentrated in milk and remains detectable for weeks after heavy use.[561,562] Breast-feeding should be avoided after phencyclidine use, but a sufficient duration of abstinence is undefined.

Tobacco. Nicotine and its metabolite, cotinine, are excreted into breast milk in amounts proportional to the number of cigarettes smoked by the mother.[563-567] The milk of smokers contains higher concentrations of cadmium than the milk of nonsmokers,[568] but other toxins in smoke have not been measured in milk. Maternal smoking appears to increase the frequency of infantile colic.[534,569,570] Smokers also use formula supplements more and wean their infants from breast-feeding earlier than nonsmokers,[565,570-574] in part because nicotine lowers maternal basal prolactin concentrations.[574]

Nursing mothers should be advised to (1) stop or decrease smoking to the greatest degree possible, (2) not smoke just before nursing, and (3) not smoke in the same room with the infant. The AAP statement that smoking is a contraindication to breast-feeding seems overly restrictive because of the benefits of breast-feeding over formula, even in smoking mothers.[568,575,576]

Radiopharmaceuticals

Exposure of the infant to excessive amounts of radioactivity is usually the primary concern raised by maternal use of radiopharmaceuticals, rather than any inherent pharmacologic toxicity of the agent. Breast-feeding should be discontinued, at least temporarily, after administration of a radiopharmaceutical to a nursing mother. The length of time needed for radioactivity to decline (by means of both radioactive decay and maternal excretion) to a safe exposure level in milk depends on several factors: dose, biological half-life, radionuclide half-life, "contamination" with other isotopes, age of the infant, potential for oral absorption of the radionuclide from the infant's GI tract, and the threshold level that is considered safe. Two recent reviews deal comprehensively with the topic of radiopharmaceutical use in nursing mothers.[577,578] Interested readers are referred to these sources for detailed information.

Conclusion

Breast-feeding has numerous, well-established benefits for both the mother and infant, and it is being promoted by many clinicians and organizations. Consequently, the number of mothers choosing to breast-feed is increasing from a low in the early 1970s. Too often, the mother's need for a medication is perceived as a reason to discontinue nursing. This perception is often the result of a lack of knowledge rather than of any known danger. High-quality information on drug use during lactation is being published at an increasing rate, including both theoretical data and information on specific drugs. By understanding the principles of drug passage into breast milk and systematically evaluating the mother's needs, infant factors, and the data on specific drugs, clinicians can usually devise treatment plans that allow nursing while minimizing the risks to the infant. Health-care practitioners involved with the drug treatment of nursing mothers should take the time to perform these simple evaluations to avoid unnecessarily depriving infants of the benefits of breast-feeding.

References

1. American Academy of Pediatrics. Policy statement based on task force report: the promotion of breast-feeding. *Pediatrics*. 1982; 69:654-61.
2. Cunningham AS, Jelliffe DB, Jelliffe EFP. Breast-feeding and health in the 1990s: a global epidemiological review. *J Pediatr*. 1991; 118:659-65.
3. Ford K, Labbok M. Who is breast feeding? Implications of associated social and biomedical variables for research on the consequences of method of infant feeding. *Am J Clin Nutr*. 1990; 52:451-6.
4. Bennett PN, Matheson I, Dukes NMG et al., eds. Drugs and human lactation. Amsterdam: Elsevier; 1988.
5. Matheson I, Kristensen K, Lunde PKM. Drug utilization in breast-feeding women. A survey in Oslo. *Eur J Clin Pharmacol*. 1990; 38:453-9.
6. Miller GE, Banerjee NC, Stowe CM Jr. Diffusion of certain weak organic acids and bases across the bovine mammary gland membrane after systemic administration. *J Pharmacol Exp Ther*. 1967; 157:245-53.
7. Rasmussen F. Excretion of drugs by milk. In: Brodie BB, Gillette JR, eds. Concepts in biochemical pharmacology, part 1. New York: Springer-Verlag; 1971:390-402.
8. Atkinson HC, Begg EJ. Prediction of drug distribution into

human milk from physicochemical characteristics. *Clin Pharmacokinet.* 1990; 18:151-67.
9. Atkinson HC, Begg EJ. The binding of drugs to major human milk whey proteins. *Br J Clin Pharmacol.* 1988; 26:107-9.
10. Atkinson HC, Begg EJ. Prediction of drug concentrations in human skim milk from plasma protein binding and acid-base characteristics. *Br J Clin Pharmacol.* 1988; 25:495-503.
11. Stebler T, Guentert TW. Binding of drugs in milk: the role of casein in milk protein binding. *Pharm Res.* 1990; 7:633-7.
12. Fleishaker JC, Desai N, McNamara PJ. Factors affecting the milk-to-plasma drug concentration ratio in lactating women: physical interactions with protein and fat. *J Pharm Sci.* 1987; 76:189-93.
13. Ferris AM, Jensen RG. Lipids in human milk: a review. 1. Sampling, determination, and content. *J Pediatr Gastroenterol Nutr.* 1984; 3:108-22.
14. Syversen GB, Ratjke SK. Drug distribution within human milk phases. *J Pharm Sci.* 1985; 74:1071-4.
15. Atkinson HC, Begg EJ. Relationship between human milk lipid-ultrafiltrate and octanol-water partition coefficients. *J Pharm Sci.* 1988; 77:796-8.
16. Rasmussen F. Mammary excretion of sulphonamides. *Acta Pharmacol Toxicol.* 1958; 15:138-48.
17. Nouws JFM, Ziv G. Pharmacological aspects of chloramphenicol administration by the intramammary route to lactating dairy cows. *Vet Q.* 1982; 4:23-31.
18. Atkinson HC, Begg EJ, Darlow BA. Drugs in human milk: clinical pharmacokinetic considerations. *Clin Pharmacokinet.* 1988; 14:217-40.
19. Richter O, Reinhardt D. The transference of drugs from breast-feeding mothers to their infants: a pharmacokinetic model. *Biol Res Pregnancy.* 1980; 1:112-7.
20. Wilson JT, ed. Drugs in breast milk. New York: ADIS; 1981:15-36.
21. Tillement JP, Albengres E, Lemaire M. Le lait, compartiment de diffusion d'un médicament. *Thérapie.* 1982; 37:357-62.
22. Stec GP, Greenberger P, Ruo TI et al. Kinetics of theophylline transfer to breast milk. *Clin Pharmacol Ther.* 1980; 28:404-8.
23. Wilson JT, Brown RD, Hinson JL et al. Pharmacokinetic pitfalls in the estimation of the breast milk/plasma ratio for drugs. *Annu Rev Pharmacol Toxicol.* 1985; 25:667-89.
24. Hinson JL, Brown RD, Wilson JT. Drug transfer into milk: model discrimination based upon parity of compartment coefficients. *J Clin Pharmacol.* 1986; 26:545. Abstract.
25. Chaikin P, Chasin M, Kennedy B et al. Suprofen concentrations in human breast milk. *J Clin Pharmacol.* 1983; 23:385-90.
26. Shelly ML, Andersen ME, Fisher JW. An inhalation distribution model for the lactating mother and nursing child. *Toxicol Lett.* 1988; 43:23-9.
27. Walker WA, Hong R. Immunology of the gastrointestinal tract: part I. *J Pediatr.* 1973; 83:517-30.
28. Eastham EJ, Lichauco T, Grady MI et al. Antigenicity of infant formulas: role of immature intestine on protein permeability. *J Pediatr.* 1978; 93:561-4.
29. Milsap RL, Szefler SJ. Special pharmacokinetic considerations in children. In: Evans WE, Schentag JJ, Jusko WJ, eds. Applied pharmacokinetics: principles of therapeutic drug monitoring. 2nd ed. Spokane, WA: Applied Therapeutics; 1986:294-330.
30. Besunder JB, Reed MD, Blumer JL. Principles of drug disposition in the neonate: a critical evaluation of the pharmacokinetic-pharmacodynamic interface (part I). *Clin Pharmacokinet.* 1988; 14:189-216.
31. Rasmussen F. The mechanisms of drug secretion into milk. In: Galli C, Jacini G, Pecile A, eds. Dietary lipids and postnatal development. New York: Raven; 1973:231-45.
32. Somogyi A, Gugler R. Cimetidine excretion into breast milk. *Br J Clin Pharmacol.* 1979; 7:627-9. Letter.
33. Kearns GL, McConnell RF Jr, Trang JM et al. Appearance of ranitidine in breast milk following multiple dosing. *Clin Pharm.* 1985; 4:322-4.
34. Wilson JT, Smith IJ, Hinson JL et al. Fundamental kinetics of drug excretion in breast milk. In: Hamosh M, Goldman AS, eds. Human lactation 2. Maternal and environmental factors. New York: Plenum; 1986:425-35.
35. Atkinson HC, Begg EJ, Darlow BA. Guide to safety of drugs in human milk. In: Mammen GJ, ed. Clinical pharmacokinetics drug data handbook 1990. Auckland: ADIS; 1990:125-64.
36. Neville MC, Keller R, Seacat J et al. Studies in human lactation: milk volumes in lactating women during the onset of lactation and full lactation. *Am J Clin Nutr.* 1988; 48:1375-86.
37. Meskin MS, Lien EJ. QSAR analysis of drug excretion into human breast milk. *J Clin Hosp Pharm.* 1985; 10:269-78.
38. Fleishaker JC, McNamara PJ. *In vivo* evaluation in the lactating rabbit of a model for xenobiotic distribution into breast milk. *J Pharmacol Exp Ther.* 1988; 244:919-24.
39. Fleishaker JC, McNamara PJ. Effect of altered serum protein binding on propranolol distribution into milk in the lactating rabbit. *J Pharmacol Exp Ther.* 1988; 244:925-8.
40. Fleishaker JC, Desai N, McNamara PJ. Possible effect of lactational period on the milk-to-plasma drug concentration ratio in lactating women: results of an in vitro evaluation. *J Pharm Sci.* 1989; 78:137-41.
41. Lucas A, Gibbs JAH, Lyster RLJ et al. Creamatocrit: simple clinical technique for estimating fat concentration and energy value of human milk. *Br Med J.* 1978; 1:1018-20.
42. Morriss FH Jr, Brewer ED, Spedale SB et al. Relationship of human milk pH during course of lactation to concentrations of citrate and fatty acids. *Pediatrics.* 1986; 78:458-64.
43. Allen JC, Neville MC. Ionized calcium in human milk determined with a calcium-selective electrode. *Clin Chem.* 1983; 29:858-61.
44. Matheson I, Lunde PKM, Bredesen JE. Midazolam and nitrazepam in the maternity ward: milk concentrations and clinical effects. *Br J Clin Pharmacol.* 1990; 30:787-93.
45. Hartmann PE, Rattigan S, Saint L et al. Variation in the yield and composition of human milk. *Oxf Rev Reprod Biol.* 1985; 7:118-67.
46. Lammi-Keefe CJ, Ferris AM, Jensen RG. Changes in human milk at 0600, 1000, 1400, 1800, and 2200 h. *J Pediatr Gastroenterol Nutr.* 1990; 11:83-8.
47. Blanc B. Biochemical aspects of human milk—comparison with bovine milk. *World Rev Nutr Diet.* 1981; 36:1-89.
48. Nommsen LA, Lovelady CA, Heinig MJ et al. Determination of energy, protein, lipid, and lactose concentrations in human milk during the first 12 mo of lactation: the DARLING study. *Am J Clin Nutr.* 1991; 53:457-65.
49. Smith MT, Livingstone I, Hooper WD et al. Propranolol, propranolol glucuronide, and naphthoxylacetic acid in breast milk and plasma. *Ther Drug Monit.* 1983; 5:87-93.
50. Wickizer TM, Brilliant LB. Testing for polychlorinated biphenyls in human milk. *Pediatrics.* 1981; 68:411-5.
51. Coakley AJ, Mountford PJ. Nuclear medicine and the nursing mother. *Br Med J.* 1985; 291:159-60. Editorial.
52. Dickey RP. Drugs affecting lactation. *Semin Perinatol.* 1979; 3:279-86.
53. Hell K, Wernze H. Drug-induced changes in prolactin secretion. *Med Toxicol.* 1988; 3:463-98.
54. Ostrom KM. A review of the hormone prolactin during lactation. *Prog Food Nutr Sci.* 1990; 14:1-44.
55. Kaplan CR, Schenken RS. Endocrinology of the breast. In: Mitchell GW Jr, Bassett LW, eds. The female breast and its disorders. Baltimore: Williams & Wilkins; 1990:30-1.
56. Bernabé J, Ricordel M-J. Effets de l'adrénaline et de la phényléphrine sur l'extraction du lait au cours de la traite méchanique de la vache. *Reprod Nutr Dev.* 1985; 25:379-88.
57. Thomas GB, Cummins JT, Doughton BW et al. Direct pituitary inhibition of prolactin secretion by dopamine and noradrenaline in sheep. *J Endocrinol.* 1989; 123:393-402.
58. Miller RD, Keegan KA, Thrupp LD et al. Human breast milk concentration of moxalactam. *Am J Obstet Gynecol.* 1984; 148:348-9.

59. American Academy of Pediatrics. Committee on Drugs. Transfer of drugs and other chemicals into human milk. *Pediatrics*. 1989; 84:924-36.
60. Briggs GG, Freeman RK, Yaffe SJ, comps. Drugs in pregnancy and lactation. 3rd ed. Baltimore: Williams & Wilkins; 1990.
61. Berlin CM Jr, Yaffe SJ, Ragni M. Disposition of acetaminophen in milk, saliva and plasma of lactating women. *Pediatr Pharmacol*. 1980; 1:135-41.
62. Findlay JWA, DeAngelis RL, Kearney MF et al. Analgesic drugs in breast milk and plasma. *Clin Pharmacol Ther*. 1981; 29:625-33.
63. Bitzén P-O, Gustafsson B, Jostell KG et al. Excretion of paracetamol in human breast milk. *Eur J Clin Pharmacol*. 1981; 20:123-5.
64. Notarianni LJ, Oldham HG, Bennett PN. Passage of paracetamol into the breast milk and its subsequent metabolism by the neonate. *Br J Clin Pharmacol* 1987; 24:63-7.
65. Matheson I, Lunde PKM, Notarianni L. Infant rash caused by paracetamol in breast milk? *Pediatrics*. 1985; 76:651-2. Letter.
66. Pittman KA, Smyth RD, Losada M et al. Human perinatal distribution of butorphanol. *Am J Obstet Gynecol*. 1980; 138:797-800.
67. Kwit NT, Hatcher RA. Excretion of drugs in milk. *Am J Dis Child*. 1935; 49:900-4.
68. Leuschen MP, Wolf LJ, Rayburn WF. Fentanyl excretion in breast milk. *Clin Pharm*. 1990; 9:336-7. Letter.
69. Madej TH, Strunin L. Comparison of epidural fentanyl with sufentanil. *Anaesthesia*. 1987; 42:1156-61.
70. Wischnik A, Wetzelsberger N, Lücker PW. Elimination von nalbuphin in die muttermilch. *Arzneimittelforschung*. 1988; 38:1496-8.
71. Marx CM, Pucino F, Carlson JD et al. Oxycodone excretion in human milk in the puerperium. *Drug Intell Clin Pharm*. 1986; 20:474. Abstract.
72. Kunka RL, Venkataramanan R, Stern RM et al. Excretion of propoxyphene and norpropoxyphene in breast milk. *Clin Pharmacol Ther*. 1984; 35:675-80.
73. Righard L, Alade MO. Effect of delivery room routines on success of first breast-feed. *Lancet*. 1990; 336:1105-7.
74. Peiker G, Müller B, Inh W et al. Ausscheidung von pethidin durch die muttermilch. *Zentralbl Gynakol*. 1980; 102:537-41.
75. Freeborn SF, Calvert RT, Black P et al. Saliva and blood pethidine concentrations in the mother and the newborn baby. *Br J Obstet Gynaecol*. 1980; 87:966-9.
76. Quinn PG, Kuhnert BR, Kaine CJ et al. Measurement of meperidine and normeperidine in human breast milk by selected ion monitoring. *Biomed Environ Mass Spectrom*. 1986; 13:133-5.
77. Wittels B, Scott DT, Sinatra RS. Exogenous opioids in human breast milk and acute neonatal neurobehavior: a preliminary study. *Anesthesiology*. 1990; 73:864-9.
78. Feilberg VL, Rosenborg D, Broen Christensen C et al. Excretion of morphine in human breast milk. *Acta Anaesthiol Scand*. 1989; 33:426-8.
79. Robieux I, Koren G, Vandenbergh H et al. Morphine excretion in breast milk and resultant exposure of a nursing infant. *Clin Toxicol*. 1990; 28:365-70.
80. Davis JM, Bhutani VK. Neonatal apnea and maternal codeine use. *Pediatr Res*. 1985; 19:170A. Abstract.
81. Naumburg EG, Meny RG. Breast milk opioids and neonatal apnea. *Am J Dis Child*. 1988; 142:11-2. Letter.
82. Lichtenstein PM. Infant drug addicts. *N Y Med J*. 1915; 102:905.
83. Cobrinik RW, Hood RT Jr, Chusid E. The effect of maternal narcotic addiction on the newborn infant. *Pediatrics*. 1959; 24:288-304.
84. Blinick G, Inturrisi CE, Jerez E et al. Methadone assays in pregnant women and progeny. *Am J Obstet Gynecol*. 1975; 121:617-21.
85. Anon. Methadone in breast milk. *Med Lett Drugs Ther*. 1979; 21:52.
86. Pond SM, Kreek MJ, Tong TG et al. Altered methadone pharmacokinetics in methadone-maintained pregnant women. *J Pharmacol Exp Ther*. 1985; 233:1-6.
87. Kreek MJ, Schecter A, Gutjahr CL et al. Analyses of methadone and other drugs in maternal and neonatal body fluids: use in evaluation of symptoms in a neonate of mother maintained on methadone. *Am J Drug Alcohol Abuse*. 1974; 1:409-19.
88. Smialek JE, Monforte JR, Aronow R et al. Methadone deaths in children: a continuing problem. *JAMA*. 1977; 238:2516-7.
89. Brooks PM, Needs CJ. Antirheumatic drugs in pregnancy and lactation. *Baillieres Clin Rheumatol*. 1990; 4:157-71.
90. Fidalgo I, Correa R, Gomez Carrasco JA et al. Anemia aguda, rectorragia y hematuria asociadas a la ingestión de naproxén. *An Esp Pediatr*. 1989; 30:317-9.
91. Jamali F, Stevens DRS. Naproxen excretion in milk and its uptake by the infant. *Drug Intell Clin Pharm*. 1983; 17:910-1. Letter.
92. Eeg-Olofsson O, Elwin C-E, Steen B. Convulsions in a breast-fed infant after maternal indomethacin. *Lancet*. 1978; 2:215.
93. Zylber-Katz E, Linder N, Granit L et al. Excretion of dipyrone metabolites in human breast milk. *Eur J Clin Pharmacol*. 1986; 30:359-61.
94. Rizzoni G, Furlanut M. Cyanotic crises in a breast-fed infant from mother taking dipyrone. *Human Toxicol*. 1984; 3:505-7.
95. Østensen M. Piroxicam in human milk. *Eur J Clin Pharmacol*. 1983; 25:829-30.
96. Østensen M, Matheson I, Laufen H. Piroxicam in breast milk after long-term treatment. *Eur J Clin Pharmacol*. 1988; 35:567-9.
97. Strobel E, Herrmann B. Zur frage des überganges von oxyphenbutazon in den fetalen kreislauf und die muttermilch. *Arzneimittelforschung*. 1962; 12:302-5.
98. Strobel E, Leuxner E. Über die zulässigkeit der verabreichung von Butazolidin bei schwangeren und wöchnerinnen. *Med Klin*. 1957; 52:1708-10.
99. Buchanan RA, Eaton CJ, Koeff ST et al. The breast milk excretion of mefenamic acid. *Curr Ther Res*. 1968; 10:592-6.
100. Steelman SL, Breault GO, Tocco D et al. Pharmacokinetics of MK-647, a novel salicylate. *Clin Pharmacol Ther*. 1975; 17:245. Abstract.
101. Sagraves R, Waller ES, Goehrs HR. Tolmetin in breast milk. *Drug Intell Clin Pharm*. 1985; 19:55-6. Letter.
102. Wischnik A, Manth SM, Lloyd J et al. The excretion of ketorolac tromethamine into breast milk after multiple oral dosing. *Eur J Clin Pharmacol*. 1989; 36:521-4.
103. Rubin A, Chernish SM, Crabtree R et al. A profile of the physiologic disposition and gastro-intestinal effects of fenoprofen in man. *Curr Med Res Opin*. 1974; 2:529-44.
104. Weibert RT, Townsend RJ, Kaiser DG et al. Lack of ibuprofen secretion into human milk. *Clin Pharm*. 1982; 1:457-8.
105. Townsend RJ, Benedetti TJ, Erickson SH et al. Excretion of ibuprofen into breast milk. *Am J Obstet Gynecol*. 1984; 149:184-6.
106. Cox SR, Forbes KK. Excretion of flurbiprofen into breast milk. *Pharmacotherapy*. 1987; 7:211-5.
107. Smith IJ, Hinson JL, Johnson VA et al. Flurbiprofen in postpartum women: plasma and breast milk disposition. *J Clin Pharmacol*. 1989; 29:174-84.
108. Fowler PD. Voltarol: diclofenac sodium. *Clin Rheum Dis*. 1979; 5:427-64.
109. Sioufi A, Stierlin H, Schweizer A et al. Recent findings concerning clinically relevant pharmacokinetics of diclofenac sodium. In: Kåss E, ed. Voltaren—new findings. Bern: Hans Huber; 1982:19-30.
110. Erickson SH, Oppenheim GL. Aspirin in breast milk. *J Fam Pract*. 1979; 8:189-90.
111. Levy G. Salicylate pharmacokinetics in the human neonate. In: Morselli PL, Garattini S, Sereni F, eds. Basic and therapeutic aspects of perinatal pharmacology. New York: Raven; 1975:319-30.
112. Jamali F, Keshavarz E. Salicylate excretion in breast milk.

Int J Pharm. 1981; 8:285-90.
113. Unsworth J, d'Assis-Fonseca A, Beswick DT et al. Serum salicylate levels in a breast fed infant. *Ann Rheum Dis*. 1987; 46:638-9.
114. Clark JH, Wilson WG. A 16-day-old breast-fed infant with metabolic acidosis caused by salicylate. *Clin Pediatr*. 1981; 20:53-4.
115. Eckstein HB, Jack B. Breast-feeding and anticoagulant therapy. *Lancet*. 1970; 1:672-3.
116. Goguel M, Noël G, Gillet J-Y et al. Thérapeutique anticoagulante et allaitement: étude du passage de la phényl-2-dioxo, 1,3 indane dans le lait maternel. *Rev Fr Gynecol Obstet*. 1970; 65:409-12.
117. Baty JD, Breckenridge A, Lewis PJ et al. May mothers taking warfarin breast feed their infants? *Br J Clin Pharmacol*. 1976; 3:969p.
118. McKenna R, Cole ER, Vasan U. Is warfarin sodium contraindicated in the lactating mother? *J Pediatr*. 1983; 103:325-7.
119. Orme ML'E, Lewis PJ, de Swiet M et al. May mothers given warfarin breast-feed their infants? *Br Med J*. 1977; 1:1564-5.
120. Brambel CE, Hunter RE. Effect of dicumarol on the nursing infant. *Am J Obstet Gynecol*. 1950; 59:1153-9.
121. Illingworth RS, Finch E. Ethyl biscoumacetate (Tromexan) in human milk. *J Obstet Gynaecol Br Commonw*. 1959; 66:487-8.
122. Houwert-de Jong M, Gerards LJ, Tetteroo-Tempelman CAM et al. May mothers taking acenocoumarol breast feed their infants? *Eur J Clin Pharmacol*. 1981; 21:61-4.
123. Fondevila CG, Meschengieser S, Blanco A et al. Effect of acenocoumarine on the breast-fed infant. *Thromb Res*. 1989; 56:29-36.
124. Kaneko S, Suzuki K, Sato T et al. The problems of antiepileptic medication in the neonatal period: is breast-feeding advisable? In: Janz D, Bossi L, Dam M et al, eds. Epilepsy, pregnancy, and the child. New York: Raven; 1982:343-8.
125. Kuhnz W, Koch S, Helge H et al. Primidone and phenobarbital during lactation period in epileptic women: total and free drug serum levels in the nursed infants and their effects on neonatal behavior. *Dev Pharmacol Ther*. 1988; 11:147-54.
126. Knott C, Reynolds F, Clayden G. Infantile spasms on weaning from breast milk containing anticonvulsants. *Lancet*. 1987; 2:272-3. Letter.
127. Brodie MJ. Management of epilepsy during pregnancy and lactation. *Lancet*. 1990; 336:426-7.
128. Niebyl JR, Blake DA, Freeman JM et al. Carbamazepine levels in pregnancy and lactation. *Obstet Gynecol*. 1979; 53:139-40.
129. Kuhnz W, Jäger-Roman E, Rating D et al. Carbamazepine and carbamazepine-10,11-epoxide during pregnancy and postnatal period in epileptic mothers and their nursed infants: pharmacokinetics and clinical effects. *Pediatr Pharmacol*. 1983; 3:199-208.
130. Froescher W, Eichelbaum M, Niesen M et al. Carbamazepine levels in breast milk. *Ther Drug Monit*. 1984; 6:266-71.
131. Meyer FP, Quednow B, Potrafki A et al. Zur pharmakokinetik von antiepileptika in der perinatalperiode. *Zentralbl Gynakol*. 1988; 110:1195-205.
132. Frey B, Schubiger G, Musy JP. Transient cholestatic hepatitis in a neonate associated with carbamazepine exposure during pregnancy and breast-feeding. *Eur J Pediatr*. 1990; 150:136-8.
133. Fisher JB, Edgren BE, Mammel MC et al. Neonatal apnea associated with maternal clonazepam therapy: a case report. *Obstet Gynecol*. 1985; 66(Suppl):34S-35S.
134. Söderman P, Matheson I. Clonazepam in breast milk. *Eur J Pediatr*. 1987; 147:212-3. Letter.
135. Koup JR, Rose JQ, Cohen ME. Ethosuximide pharmacokinetics in a pregnant patient and her newborn. *Epilepsia*. 1978; 19:535-9.
136. Kaneko S, Sato T, Suzuki K. The levels of anticonvulsants in breast milk. *Br J Clin Pharmacol*. 1979; 7:624-7. Letter.
137. Rane A, Tunell R. Ethosuximide in human milk and in plasma of a mother and her nursed infant. *Br J Clin Pharmacol*. 1981; 12:855-8.
138. Kuhnz W, Koch S, Jakob S et al. Ethosuximide in epileptic women during pregnancy and lactation period. Placental transfer, serum concentrations in nursed infants and clinical status. *Br J Clin Pharmacol*. 1984; 18:671-7.
139. Tyson RM, Shrader EA, Perlman HH. Drugs transmitted through breast milk: II. Barbiturates. *J Pediatr*. 1938; 14:86-90.
140. Westernik D, Glerum JH. Scheiding en microbepaling van fenobarbital en fenytoine en modermelk. *Pharm Weekbl*. 1965; 100:577-83.
141. Juul S. Fenemalforgiftning via modermælken? *Ugeskr Laeger*. 1969; 131:2257-8.
142. Steen B, Rane A, Lönnerholm G et al. Phenytoin excretion in human breast milk and plasma levels in nursed infants. *Ther Drug Monit*. 1982; 4:331-4.
143. Finch E, Lorber J. Methaemoglobinaemia in the newborn. *J Obstet Gynaecol Br Emp*. 1954; 61:833-4.
144. Livingston S. Treatment of epilepsy with diphenylhydantoin sodium. *Postgrad Med*. 1956; 20:584-90.
145. Nau H, Rating D, Häuser I et al. Placental transfer and pharmacokinetics of primidone and its metabolites phenobarbital, PEMA and hydroxyphenobarbital in neonates and infants of epileptic mothers. *Eur J Clin Pharmacol*. 1980; 18:31-41.
146. Göpfert-Geyer I, Koch S, Rating D et al. Delivery, gestation, data at birth, and neonatal period in children of epileptic mothers. In: Janz D, Bossi L, Dam M et al., eds. Epilepsy, pregnancy, and the child. New York: Raven; 1982:179-87.
147. Granström M-L, Bardy AH, Hiilesmaa VK. Prolonged feeding difficulties of infants of primidone mothers during neonatal period: preliminary results from the prospective Helsinki study. In: Janz D, Bossi L, Dam M et al., eds. Epilepsy, pregnancy, and the child. New York: Raven; 1982:357-8.
148. Nau H, Rating D, Koch S et al. Valproic acid and its metabolites: placental transfer, neonatal pharmacokinetics, transfer via mother's milk and clinical status in neonates of epileptic mothers. *J Pharmacol Exp Ther*. 1981; 219:768-77.
149. Nau H, Helge H, Luck W. Valproic acid in the perinatal period: decreased maternal serum protein binding results in fetal accumulation and neonatal displacement of the drug and some metabolites. *J Pediatr*. 1984; 104:627-34.
150. Von Unruh GE, Froescher W, Hoffmann F et al. Valproic acid in breast milk: how much is really there? *Ther Drug Monit*. 1984; 6:272-6.
151. Philbert A, Pedersen B, Dam M. Concentration of valproate during pregnancy, in the newborn and in breast milk. *Acta Neurol Scand*. 1985; 72:460-3.
152. Findlay JWA, Butz RF, Sailstad JM et al. Pseudoephedrine and triprolidine in plasma and breast milk of nursing mothers. *Br J Clin Pharmacol*. 1984; 18:901-6.
153. Hilbert J, Radwanski E, Affrime MB et al. Excretion of loratadine in human breast milk. *J Clin Pharmacol*. 1988; 28:234-9.
154. Kok THHG, Taitz LS, Bennett MJ et al. Drowsiness due to clemastine transmitted in breast milk. *Lancet*. 1982; 1:914-5.
155. Mortimer EA Jr. Drug toxicity from breast milk? *Pediatrics*. 1977; 60:780-1. Letter.
156. Wortsman J, Soler NG, Hirschowitz J. Cyproheptadine in the management of the galactorrhea-amenorrhea syndrome. *Ann Intern Med*. 1979; 90:923-5.
157. Fujimori H, Imai S. Studies on dihydrostreptomycin administered to the pregnant and transferred to their fetuses. *J Jpn Obstet Gynecol Soc*. 1957; 4:133-49.
158. Chyo N, Sunada H, Nohara S. Clinical studies of kanamycin applied in the field of obstetrics and gynecology. *Asian Med J*. 1962; 5:265-75.
159. Takase Z, Shirafuji H, Uchida M et al. Laboratory and clinical studies on tobramycin in the field of obstetrics and gynecology. *Chemotherapy (Tokyo)*. 1975; 23:1402. Abstract.

160. Uwaydah M, Bibi S, Salman S. Therapeutic efficacy of tobramycin—a clinical and laboratory evaluation. *J Antimicrob Chemother.* 1975; 1:429-37.
161. Von Kobyletzki D, Sas M, Schmitz G et al. Pharmacokinetic studies with sisomicin in obstetrics. *Infection.* 1979; 7(Suppl 3):S276.
162. Matsuda S. Transfer of antibiotics into maternal milk. *Biol Res Pregnancy.* 1984; 5:57-60.
163. Nation RL, Hackett LP, Dusci LJ et al. Excretion of hydroxychloroquine in human milk. *Br J Clin Pharmacol.* 1984; 17:368-9. Letter.
164. Deturmeny E, Viala A, Durand A et al. Le passage de la chloroquine dans le lait, sur 1 cas. *Therapie.* 1984; 39:438-40. Letter.
165. Edstein MD, Veenendaal JR, Newman K et al. Excretion of chloroquine, dapsone and pyrimethamine in human milk. *Br J Clin Pharmacol.* 1986; 22:733-5.
166. Ogunbona FA, Onyeji CO, Bolaji OO et al. Excretion of chloroquine and desethylchloroquine in human milk. *Br J Clin Pharmacol.* 1987; 23:473-6.
167. Ette EI, Essien EE, Ogonor JI et al. Chloroquine in human milk. *J Clin Pharmacol.* 1987; 27:499-502.
168. Akintonwa A, Gbajumo SA, Biola Mabadeje AF. Placental and milk transfer of chloroquine in humans. *Ther Drug Monit.* 1988; 10:147-9.
169. Østensen M, Brown ND, Chiang PK et al. Hydroxychloroquine in human breast milk. *Eur J Clin Pharmacol.* 1985; 28:357.
170. Witte AMC, Klever HJH, Brabin BJ et al. Field evaluation of the use of an ELISA to detect chloroquine and its metabolites in blood, urine and breast-milk. *Trans R Soc Trop Med Hyg.* 1990; 84:521-5.
171. Terwilliger WG, Hatcher RA. The elimination of morphine and quinine in human milk. *Surg Gynecol Obstet.* 1934; 58:823-6.
172. Phillips RE, Looareesuwan S, White NJ et al. Quinine pharmacokinetics and toxicity in pregnant and lactating women with falciparum malaria. *Br J Clin Pharmacol.* 1986; 21:677-83.
173. Clyde DF, Shute GT, Press J. Transfer of pyrimethamine in human milk. *J Trop Med Hyg.* 1956; 59:277-84.
174. Clyde DF. An examination of factors involved in the transfer of pyrimethamine in human milk. *East Afr Med J.* 1957; 34:81-5.
175. Clyde DF. Prolonged malaria prophylaxis through pyrimethamine in mothers' milk. *East Afr Med J.* 1960; 37:659-60.
176. Edstein MD, Veenendaal JR, Hyslop R. Excretion of mefloquine in human breast milk. *Chemotherapy (Basel).* 1988; 34:165-9.
177. Morton RF, McKenna MH, Charles E. Studies on the absorption, diffusion, and excretion of cycloserine. *Antibiot Annu.* 1955–1956; 3:169-72.
178. Snider DE Jr, Powell KE. Should women taking antituberculosis drugs breast-feed? *Arch Intern Med.* 1984; 144:589-90.
179. Berlin CM Jr, Lee C. Isoniazid and acetylisoniazid disposition in human milk, saliva and plasma (part 1). *Fed Proc.* 1979; 38(Mar 1):426. Abstract.
180. Holdiness MR. Antituberculosis drugs and breast-feeding. *Arch Intern Med.* 1984; 144:1888. Letter.
181. Mischler TW, Corson SL, Larranaga A et al. Cephradine and epicillin in body fluids of lactating and pregnant women. *J Reprod Med.* 1978; 21:130-6.
182. Yoshioka H, Cho K, Takimoto M et al. Transfer of cefazolin into human milk. *J Pediatr.* 1979; 94:151-2.
183. Takase Z, Shirafuji H, Uchida M. Fundamental and clinical studies of cefuroxime in the field of obstetrics and gynecology. *Chemotherapy (Tokyo).* 1979; 27(Suppl 6):600-2.
184. Takase Z, Shirafuji H, Uchida M. Experimental and clinical studies of cefadroxil in the treatment of infections in the field of obstetrics and gynecology. *Chemotherapy (Tokyo).* 1980; 28(Suppl 2):424-31.
185. Kafetzis DA, Siafas CA, Georgakopoulos PA et al. Passage of cephalosporins and amoxicillin into the breast milk. *Acta Paediatr Scand.* 1981; 70:285-8.
186. Dubois M, Delapierre D, Chanteux L et al. A study of the transplacental transfer and the mammary excretion of cefoxitin in humans. *J Clin Pharmacol.* 1981; 21:477-83.
187. Dresse A, Lambotte R, Dubois M et al. Transmammary passage of cefoxitin: additional results. *J Clin Pharmacol.* 1983; 23:438-40.
188. Cho N, Fukunaga K, Kunii K. A study of clinical application of cefmetazole in perinatal period. *Jpn J Antibiot.* 1981; 34:915-24.
189. Lou MA, Wu YH, Jacob LS et al. Penetration of cefonicid into human breast milk and various body fluids and tissues. *Rev Infect Dis.* 1984; 6(Suppl 4):S816-S820.
190. Kafetzis DA, Lazarides CV, Siafas CA et al. Transfer of cefotaxime in human milk and from mother to foetus. *J Antimicrob Chemother.* 1980; 6(Suppl A):135-41.
191. Takase Z, Shirafuji H, Uchida M. Fundamental and clinical studies of cefoperazone (T-1551) in the field of obstetrics and gynecology. *Chemotherapy (Tokyo).* 1980; 28(Suppl 6):825-36.
192. Shimada J, Ueda Y. Moxalactam—absorption, excretion, distribution, and metabolism. *Rev Infect Dis.* 1982; 4(Suppl):S569-S580.
193. Kafetzis DA, Brater DC, Fanourgakis JE et al. Ceftriaxone distribution between maternal blood and fetal blood and tissues at parturition and between blood and milk postpartum. *Antimicrob Agents Chemother.* 1983; 23:870-3.
194. Blanco JD, Jorgensen JH, Castaneda YS et al. Ceftazidime levels in human breast milk. *Antimicrob Agents Chemother.* 1983; 23:479-80.
195. Fleiss PM, Richwald GA, Gordon J et al. Aztreonam in human serum and breast milk. *Br J Clin Pharmacol.* 1985; 19:509-11.
196. Ito K, Hirose R, Tamaya T et al. Pharmacokinetic and clinical studies on aztreonam in the perinatal period. *Jpn J Antibiot.* 1990; 43:719-26.
197. Takase Z, Shirafuji H, Uchida M. Fundamental and clinical studies of mezlocillin in the field of obstetrics and gynecology. *Chemotherapy (Tokyo).* 1979; 27(Suppl 1):375-81.
198. Von Kobyletzki D, Dalhoff A, Lindemeyer H et al. Ticarcillin serum and tissue concentrations in gynecology and obstetrics. *Infection.* 1983; 11:144-9.
199. Baier R, Wolnik L, Puppel H et al. Piperacillin concentrations in milk and serum from lactating women. In: Program and abstracts of the 22nd Interscience Conference on Antimicrobial Agents and Chemotherapy. Washington, DC: American Society for Microbiology; 1982:203. Abstract.
200. Branebjerg PE, Heisterberg L. Blood and milk concentrations of ampicillin in mothers treated with pivampicillin and in their infants. *J Perinat Med.* 1987; 15:555-8.
201. Matheson I, Samseth M, Sande HA. Ampicillin in breast milk during puerperal infections. *Eur J Clin Pharmacol.* 1988; 34:657-9.
202. Matheson I, Samseth M, Løberg R et al. Milk transfer of phenoxymethylpenicillin during puerperal mastitis. *Br J Clin Pharmacol.* 1988; 25:33-40.
203. Campbell AC, McElnay JC, Passmore CM. The excretion of ampicillin in breast milk and its effect on the suckling infant. *Br J Clin Pharmacol.* 1991; 31:230p.
204. Giamerellou H, Kolokythas E, Petrikkos G et al. Pharmacokinetics of three newer quinolones in pregnant and lactating women. *Am J Med.* 1989; 87(Suppl 5A):49S-51S.
205. Cover DL, Mueller BA. Ciprofloxacin penetration into human breast milk: a case report. *DICP.* 1990; 24:703-4.
206. Takase Z, Shirafuji H, Uchida M. Basic and clinical studies of AM-715 in the field of obstetrics and gynecology. *Chemotherapy (Tokyo).* 1981; 29(Suppl 4):697-704.
207. Belton EM, Jones RV. Haemolytic anaemia due to nalidixic acid. *Lancet.* 1965; 2:691. Letter.
208. Traeger A, Peiker G. Excretion of nalidixic acid via mother's milk. *Arch Toxicol Suppl.* 1980; 4:388-90.
209. Harley JD, Robin H. "Late" neonatal jaundice following

maternal treatment with sulfamethoxypyridazine. *Pediatrics*. 1966; 37:855-6. Letter.
210. Miller RD, Salter AJ. The passage of trimethoprim/sulfamethoxazole into breast milk and its significance. In: Daikos CK, ed. Progress in chemotherapy. Vol. 1. Antibacterial chemotherapy. Athens: Hellenic Society for Chemotherapy; 1974:687-91.
211. Kauffman RE, O'Brien C, Gilford P. Sulfisoxazole secretion into human milk. *J Pediatr*. 1980; 97:839-41.
212. Sanders SW, Zone JJ, Foltz RL et al. Hemolytic anemia induced by dapsone transmitted through breast milk. *Ann Intern Med*. 1982; 96:465-6.
213. Posner AC, Prigot A, Konicoff NG. Further observations on the use of tetracycline hydrochloride in prophylaxis and treatment of obstetric infections. In: Antibiotics annual 1954–1955. New York: Medical Encyclopedia; 1954-55:594-8.
214. Von Kobyletzki D, Strauch D. Zur frage der diaplazentaren passage und ausscheidung mit der muttermilch von demethylchlortetracyclin. *Z Geburtshilfe Gynakol*. 1964; 161:292-305.
215. Mizuno S, Takata M, Sano S et al. Studies on minocycline. *Jpn J Antibiot*. 1969; 22:473-9.
216. Tokuda G, Yuasa M, Mihara S et al. Clinical studies of doxycycline in obstetrical and gynecological fields. *Chemotherapy (Tokyo)*. 1969; 17:339-44.
217. Lutziger H. Konzentrationbestimmungen und klinisch wirksamkeit von doxycycline (Vibramycin) in uterus, adnexen und muttermilch. *Ther Umsch*. 1969; 26:476-80.
218. Brogden RN, Speight TM, Avery GS. Minocycline: a review of its antibacterial and pharmacokinetic properties and therapeutic use. *Drugs*. 1975; 9:251-91.
219. Allgén L-G, Holmberg G, Persson B et al. Biological fate of methenamine in man. *Acta Obstet Gynecol Scand*. 1979; 58:287-93.
220. Berger H. Excretion of mandelic acid in breast milk. *Am J Dis Child*. 1941; 61:256-61.
221. Pons G, Rey E, Richard M-O et al. Nitrofurantoin excretion in human milk. *Dev Pharmacol Ther*. 1990; 14:148-52.
222. Lau RJ, Emery MG, Galinsky RE. Unexpected accumulation of acyclovir in breast milk with estimation of infant exposure. *Obstet Gynecol*. 1987; 69:468-71.
223. Meyer LJ, de Miranda P, Sheth N et al. Acyclovir in human breast milk. *Am J Obstet Gynecol*. 1988; 158:586-8.
224. Siever LJ. The effect of amantadine on prolactin levels and galactorrhea on neuroleptic-treated patients. *J Clin Psychopharmacol*. 1981; 1:2-7.
225. Berman JD, Melby PC, Neva FA. Concentration of Pentostam in human breast milk. *Trans R Soc Trop Med Hyg*. 1989; 83:784-5.
226. Havelka J, Hejzlar M, Popov V et al. Excretion of chloramphenicol in human milk. *Chemotherapy (Basel)*. 1968; 13:204-11.
227. Plomp TA, Thiery M, Maes RAA. The passage of thiamphenicol and chloramphenicol into human milk after single and repeated oral administration. *Vet Hum Toxicol*. 1983; 25:167-72.
228. Havelka J, Franková A. Príspevek k vedlejsím úcinkum chloramfenikolu u novorozencu. *Cesk Pediatr*. 1972; 27:31-3.
229. Matsuda S, Mori S, Azuma S. Clinical evaluation of clindamycin in gyneco-obstetrics. *Chemotherapy (Tokyo)*. 1969; 17:899-900.
230. Stéen B, Rane A. Clindamycin passage into human milk. *Br J Clin Pharmacol*. 1982; 13:661-4.
231. Mann CF. Clindamycin and breast-feeding. *Pediatrics*. 1980; 66:1030-1. Letter.
232. Browne SG, Hogerzeil LM. "B 663" in the treatment of leprosy. Preliminary report of a pilot trial. *Lepr Rev*. 1962; 33:6-10.
233. Stang H. Pyloric stenosis associated with erythromycin ingested through breastmilk. *Minn Med*. 1986; 69:669-70,82.
234. Rao TS. Does mebendazole inhibit lactation? *N Z Med J*. 1983; 96:589-90. Letter.
235. Heisterberg L, Branebjerg PE. Blood and milk concentrations of metronidazole in mothers and infants. *J Perinat Med*. 1983; 11:114-20.
236. Passmore CM, McElnay JC, Rainey EA et al. Metronidazole excretion in human milk and its effect on the suckling neonate. *Br J Clin Pharmacol*. 1988; 26:45-51.
237. Clements CJ. Metronidazole and breast feeding. *N Z Med J*. 1980; 92:329. Letter.
238. Gray MS, Kane PO, Squires S. Further observations on metronidazole (Flagyl). *Br J Vener Dis*. 1961; 37:278-9.
239. Erickson SH, Oppenheim GL, Smith GH. Metronidazole in breast milk. *Obstet Gynecol*. 1981; 57:48-50.
240. Pütter J, Held F. Quantitative studies on the occurrence of praziquantel in milk and plasma of lactating women. *Eur J Drug Metab Pharmacokinet*. 1979; 4:193-8.
241. Arnauld R, Soutoul JH, Gallier J et al. Étude du passage de la triméthoprime dans le lait maternel. *Ouest Med*. 1972; 25:959-64.
242. Reyes MP, Ostrea EM Jr, Cabinian AE et al. Vancomycin during pregnancy: does it cause hearing loss or nephrotoxicity in the infant? *Am J Obstet Gynecol*. 1989; 161:977-81.
243. Coulam CB, Moyer TP, Jiang N-S et al. Breast-feeding after renal transplantation. *Transplant Proc*. 1982; 13:605-9.
244. Grekas DM, Vasiliou SS, Lazarides AN. Immunosuppressive therapy and breast-feeding after renal transplantation. *Nephron*. 1984; 37:68. Letter.
245. Bounameaux Y, Durenne JM. Un cas de luecémie chez une femme allaitante: effects du traitement par le Busulfan sur le nourrisson. *Ann Soc Belg Med Trop*. 1964; 44:381-3.
246. Egan PC, Costanza ME, Dodion P et al. Doxorubicin and cisplatin excretion into human milk. *Cancer Treat Rep*. 1985; 69:1387-9.
247. De Vries EGE, van der Zee AGJ, Uges DRA et al. Excretion of platinum into breast milk. *Lancet*. 1989; 1:497. Letter. (Corrected in *Lancet*. 1989; 1:798.)
248. Wiernik PH, Duncan JH. Cyclophosphamide in human milk. *Lancet*. 1971; 1:912. Letter.
249. Amato D, Niblett JS. Neutropenia from cyclophosphamide in breast milk. *Med J Aust*. 1977; 1:383-4.
250. Durodola JI. Administration of cyclophosphamide during late pregnancy and early lactation: a case report. *J Natl Med Assoc*. 1979; 71:165-6.
251. Flechner SM, Katz AR, Rogers AJ et al. The presence of cyclosporine in body tissues and fluids during pregnancy. *Am J Kidney Dis*. 1985; 5:60-3.
252. Lewis GJ, Lamont CAR, Lee HA et al. Successful pregnancy in a renal transplant recipient taking cyclosporin A. *Br Med J*. 1983; 286:603. Letter.
253. Ziegenhagen DJ, Crombach G, Dieckmann M et al. Schwangerschaft unter ciclosporin-medikation nach nierentransplantation. *Dtsch Med Wochenschr*. 1988; 113:260-3.
254. Sylvester RK, Lobell M, Teresi ME et al. Excretion of hydroxyurea into milk. *Cancer*. 1987; 60:2177-8.
255. Johns DG, Rutherford LD, Leighton PC et al. Secretion of methotrexate into human milk. *Am J Obstet Gynecol*. 1972; 112:978-80.
256. Henderson AJ, Faulkner A. The effects of vincristine on milk secretion and milk composition in the goat. *Q J Exp Physiol*. 1985; 70:15-22.
257. Riant P, Urien S, Albengres E et al. High plasma protein binding as a parameter in the selection of betablockers for lactating women. *Biochem Pharmacol*. 1986; 35:4579-81.
258. Michael CA. Use of labetalol in the treatment of severe hypertension during pregnancy. *Br J Clin Pharmacol*. 1979; 8(Suppl):211S-215S.
259. Bauer JH, Pape B, Zajicek J et al. Propranolol in human plasma and breast milk. *Am J Cardiol*. 1979; 43:860-2.
260. Sandström B, Regårdh C-G. Metoprolol excretion into breast milk. *Br J Clin Pharmacol*. 1980; 9:518-9. Letter.
261. Devlin RG, Duchin KL, Fleiss PM. Nadolol in human serum and breast milk. *Br J Clin Pharmacol*. 1981; 12:393-6.
262. Liedholm H, Melander A, Bitzén P-O et al. Accumulation of

atenolol and metoprolol in human breast milk. *Eur J Clin Pharmacol*. 1981; 20:229-31.
263. Taylor EA, Turner P. Anti-hypertensive therapy with propranolol during pregnancy and lactation. *Postgrad Med J*. 1981; 57:427-30.
264. Krause W, Stoppelli I, Milia S et al. Transfer of mepindolol to newborns by breast-feeding mothers after single and repeated daily doses. *Eur J Clin Pharmacol*. 1982; 22:53-5.
265. Fidler J, Smith V, de Swiet M. Excretion of oxprenolol and timolol in breast milk. *Br J Obstet Gynaecol*. 1983; 90:961-5.
266. Thorley KJ, McAinsh J. Levels of the beta-blockers atenolol and propranolol in the breast milk of women treated for hypertension in pregnancy. *Biopharm Drug Dispos*. 1983; 4:299-301.
267. Lustgarten JS, Podos SM. Topical timolol and the nursing mother. *Arch Ophthalmol*. 1983; 101:1381-2.
268. White WB, Andreoli JW, Wong SH et al. Atenolol in human plasma and breast milk. *Obstet Gynecol*. 1984; 63(Suppl):42S-44S.
269. Sioufi A, Hillion D, Lumbroso P et al. Oxprenolol placental transfer, plasma concentrations in newborns and passage into breast milk. *Br J Clin Pharmacol*. 1984; 18:453-6.
270. Lindeberg S, Sandström B, Lundborg P et al. Disposition of the adrenergic blocker metoprolol in the late-pregnant woman, the amniotic fluid, the cord blood and the neonate. *Acta Obstet Gynecol Scand Suppl*. 1984; 118:61-4.
271. Kulas J, Lunell N-O, Rosing U et al. Atenolol and metoprolol. A comparison of their excretion into human breast milk. *Acta Obstet Gynecol Scand Suppl*. 1984; 118:65-9.
272. Lunell NO, Kulas J, Rane A. Transfer of labetalol into amniotic fluid and breast milk in lactating women. *Eur J Clin Pharmacol*. 1985; 28:597-9.
273. Boutroy MJ, Bianchetti G, Dubruc C et al. To nurse when receiving acebutolol: is it dangerous for the neonate? *Eur J Clin Pharmacol*. 1986; 30:737-9.
274. Radwanski E, Nagabhushan N, Affrime MB et al. Secretion of dilevalol in breast milk. *J Clin Pharmacol*. 1988; 28:448-53.
275. Hackett LP, Wojnar-Horton RE, Dusci LJ et al. Excretion of sotalol in breast milk. *Br J Clin Pharmacol*. 1990; 29:277-8. Letter.
276. Schmimmel MS, Eidelman AJ, Wilschanski MA et al. Toxic effects of atenolol consumed during breast feeding. *J Pediatr*. 1989; 114:476-8.
277. Morselli PL, Boutroy MJ, Bianchetti G et al. Placental transfer and perinatal pharmacokinetics of betaxolol. *Eur J Clin Pharmacol*. 1990; 38:477-83.
278. Okada M, Inoue H, Nakamura Y et al. Excretion of diltiazem in human milk. *N Engl J Med*. 1985; 312:992-3. Letter.
279. Ehrenkranz RA, Ackerman BA, Hulse JD. Nifedipine transfer into human milk. *J Pediatr*. 1989; 114:478-80.
280. Penny WJ, Lewis MJ. Nifedipine is excreted in human milk. *Eur J Clin Pharmacol*. 1989; 36:427-8.
281. White WB, Yeh SC, Krol GJ. Nitrendipine in human plasma and breast milk. *Eur J Clin Pharmacol*. 1989; 36:531-4.
282. Andersen HJ. Excretion of verapamil in human milk. *Eur J Clin Pharmacol*. 1983; 25:279-80.
283. Inoue H, Unno N, Ou M-C et al. Level of verapamil in human milk. *Eur J Clin Pharmacol*. 1984; 26:657-8.
284. Miller MR, Withers R, Bhamra R et al. Verapamil and breast-feeding. *Eur J Clin Pharmacol*. 1986; 30:125-6.
285. Anderson P, Bondesson U, Mattiasson I et al. Verapamil and norverapamil in plasma and breast milk during breast feeding. *Eur J Clin Pharmacol*. 1987; 31:625-7.
286. Hartmann D, Lunell N-O, Friedrich G et al. Excretion of tiapamil in breast milk. *Br J Clin Pharmacol*. 1988; 26:183-6.
287. McKenna WJ, Harris L, Rowland E et al. Amiodarone therapy during pregnancy. *Am J Cardiol*. 1983; 51:1231-3.
288. Pitcher D, Leather HM, Storey GCA et al. Amiodarone in pregnancy. *Lancet*. 1983; 1:597-8. Letter.
289. Strunge P, Frandsen J, Andreasen F. Amiodarone during pregnancy. *Eur Heart J*. 1988; 9:106-9.
290. Barnett DB, Hudson SA, McBurney A. Disopyramide and its *N*-monodesalkyl metabolite in breast milk. *Br J Clin Pharmacol*. 1982; 14:310-2.
291. MacKintosh D, Buchanan N. Excretion of disopyramide in human breast milk. *Br J Clin Pharmacol*. 1985; 19:856-7. Letter.
292. Hoppu K, Neuvonen P, Korte T. Disopyramide and breast feeding. *Br J Clin Pharmacol*. 1986; 21:553-4. Letter.
293. Ellsworth AJ, Horn JR, Raisys VA et al. Disopyramide and *N*-monodesalkyl disopyramide in serum and breast milk. *DICP*. 1989; 23:56-7.
294. Wilson JH. Breast milk tocainide levels. *J Cardiovasc Pharmacol*. 1988; 12:497. Letter.
295. Gutgesell M, Overholt E, Boyle R. Oral bretylium tosylate use during pregnancy and subsequent breastfeeding: a case report. *Am J Perinatol*. 1990; 7:144-5.
296. Zeisler JA, Gaarder TD, de Mesquita SA. Lidocaine excretion in breast milk. *Drug Intell Clin Pharm*. 1986; 20:691-3.
297. McQuinn RL, Pisani A, Wafa S et al. Flecainide excretion in human breast milk. *Clin Pharmacol Ther*. 1990; 48:262-7.
298. Wagner X, Jouglard J, Moulin M et al. Coadministration of flecainide acetate and sotalol during pregnancy: lack of teratogenic effects, passage across the placenta, and excretion in human breast milk. *Am Heart J*. 1990; 119:700-2.
299. Timmis AD, Jackson G, Holt DW. Mexiletine for control of ventricular dysrhythmias in pregnancy. *Lancet*. 1980; 2:647-8. Letter.
300. Lewis AM, Patel L, Johnston A et al. Mexiletine in human blood and breast milk. *Postgrad Med J*. 1981; 57:546-7.
301. Lownes HE, Ives TJ. Mexiletine use in pregnancy and lactation. *Am J Obstet Gynecol*. 1987; 157:446-7.
302. Pittard WB III, Glazier H. Procainamide excretion in human milk. *J Pediatr*. 1983; 102:631-3.
303. Hill LM, Malkasian GD Jr. The use of quinidine sulfate throughout pregnancy. *Obstet Gynecol*. 1979; 54:366-8.
304. Loughnan PM. Digoxin excretion in human breast milk. *J Pediatr*. 1978; 92:1019-20.
305. Chan V, Tse TF, Wong V. Transfer of digoxin across the placenta and into breast milk. *Br J Obstet Gynaecol*. 1978; 85:605-9.
306. Finley JP, Waxman MB, Wong PY et al. Digoxin excretion in human milk. *J Pediatr*. 1979; 94:339-40. Letter.
307. Reinhart D, Richter O, Genz T et al. Kinetics of the translactal passage of digoxin from breast feeding mothers to their infants. *Eur J Pediatr*. 1982; 138:49-52.
308. Hartikainen-Sorri A-L, Heikkinen JE, Koivisto M. Pharmacokinetics of clonidine during pregnancy and nursing. *Obstet Gynecol*. 1987; 69:598-600.
309. Knowles JA. Drugs in milk. *Pediatr Curr*. 1972; 21:28-32.
310. Devlin RG, Fleiss PM. Captopril in human blood and breast milk. *J Clin Pharmacol*. 1981; 21:110-3.
311. Huttunen K, Grönhagen-Riska C, Fyhrquist F. Enalapril treatment of a nursing mother with slightly impaired renal function. *Clin Nephrol*. 1989; 31:278. Letter.
312. Redman CWG, Kelly JG, Cooper WD. The excretion of enalapril and enalaprilat in human breast milk. *Eur J Clin Pharmacol*. 1990; 38:99.
313. Liedholm H, Wåhlin-Boll E, Hanson A et al. Transplacental passage and breast milk concentration of hydralazine. *Eur J Clin Pharmacol*. 1982; 21:417-9.
314. Jones HMR, Cummings AJ. A study of the transfer of α-methyldopa to the human foetus and newborn infant. *Br J Clin Pharmacol*. 1978; 6:432-4. Letter.
315. Hauser GJ, Almog S, Tirosh M et al. Effect of α-methyldopa excreted in human milk on the breast-fed infant. *Helv Paediatr Acta*. 1985; 40:83-6.
316. White WB, Andreoli JW, Cohn RD. Alpha-methyldopa disposition in mothers with hypertension and in their breast-fed infants. *Clin Pharmacol Ther*. 1985; 37:387-90.
317. Valdivieso A, Valdés G, Spiro TE et al. Minoxidil in breast milk. *Ann Intern Med*. 1985; 102:135. Letter.
318. Werthmann MW Jr, Krees SV. Excretion of chlorothiazide in human milk. *J Pediatr*. 1972; 81:781-3.
319. Miller ME, Cohn RD, Burghart PH. Hydrochlorothiazide

disposition in a mother and her breast-fed infant. *J Pediatr.* 1982; 101:789-91.
320. Healy M. Suppressing lactation with oral diuretics. *Lancet.* 1961; 1:1353-4. Letter.
321. Stout G. Suppression of lactation. *Br Med J.* 1962; 1:1150. Letter.
322. Cominos DC, Van Der Walt A, Van Rooyen AJL. Suppression of postpartum lactation with furosemide. *S Afr Med J.* 1976; 50:251-2.
323. Mulley BA, Parr GD, Pau WK et al. Placental transfer of chlorthalidone and its elimination in maternal milk. *Eur J Clin Pharmacol.* 1978; 13:129-31.
324. Söderman P, Hartvig P, Fagerlund C. Acetazolamide excretion into human breast milk. *Br J Clin Pharmacol.* 1984; 17:599-600. Letter.
325. Phelps DL, Karim A. Spironolactone: relationship between concentration of dethioacetylated metabolite in human serum and milk. *J Pharm Sci.* 1977; 66:1203.
326. Floss HG, Cassady JM, Robbers JE. Influence of ergot alkaloids on pituitary prolactin and prolactin-dependent processes. *J Pharm Sci.* 1973; 62:699-715.
327. Katz M, Kroll D, Pak I et al. Puerperal hypertension, stroke, and seizures after suppression of lactation with bromocriptine. *Obstet Gynecol.* 1985; 66:822-4.
328. Iffy L, TenHove W, Frisoli G. Acute myocardial infarction in the puerperium in patients receiving bromocriptine. *Am J Obstet Gynecol.* 1986; 155:371-2.
329. Van Dam LJ, Rolland R. Lactation-inhibiting and prolactin-lowering effect of lisuride and bromocriptine: a comparative study. *Eur J Obstet Gynecol Reprod Biol.* 1981; 12:323-30.
330. Giorda G, de Vincentiis S, Motta T et al. Cabergoline versus bromocriptine in suppression of lactation after cesarean delivery. *Gynecol Obstet Invest.* 1991; 31:93-6.
331. Vetr M, Krejcí I. Suppression of lactation with terguride. *Acta Univ Palacki Olomuc Fac Med.* 1988; 119:347-52.
332. Scapin F, Buonaccorsi S, Tronconi G et al. Metergoline versus bromocriptine in the prevention of puerperal lactation: a double-blind clinical trial. *Eur J Clin Pharmacol.* 1982; 22:181-3.
333. De Aloysio D, Pamparana F, Zanotti A et al. Dihydroergocristine in stopping lactation: double-blind study vs bromocriptine. *Gynecol Endocrinol.* 1988; 2:67-71.
334. Pentland B, Sawers JSA. Galactorrhoea after withdrawal of bromocriptine. *Br Med J.* 1980; 281:716. Letter.
335. Canales ES, Garrido JT, Zárate A et al. Effect of ergonovine on prolactin secretion and milk let-down. *Obstet Gynecol.* 1976; 48:228-9.
336. Shane JM, Naftolin F. Effect of ergonovine maleate on puerperal lactation. *Am J Obstet Gynecol.* 1974; 120:129-31.
337. Symes JB. A study on the effect of ergometrine on serum prolactin levels following delivery. *J Obstet Gynaecol.* 1984; 5:36-8.
338. Begley CM. The effect of ergometrine on breast feeding. *Midwifery.* 1990; 6:60-72.
339. Del Pozo E, Brun del Rey R, Hinselmann M. Lack of effect of methyl-ergonovine on postpartum lactation. *Am J Obstet Gynecol.* 1975; 123:845-6.
340. González SP, Gayan BP, Pineda VG et al. Prolactina plasmática en el puerperio y su relación con el usó de maleato de metilergonovina. *Rev Chil Obstet Ginecol.* 1984; 49:149-55.
341. Erkkola R, Kanto J, Allonen H et al. Excretion of methylergometrine (methyergonovine) into the human breast milk. *Int J Clin Pharmacol.* 1978; 16:579-80.
342. Jolivet A, Robyn C, Huraux-Rendu C et al. Effet de dérivés des alcaloïdes de l'ergot siegle sur la sécrétion lactée dans le postpartum imméiat. *J Gynecol Obstet Biol Reprod (Paris).* 1987; 7:129-34.
343. Illingworth RS. Abnormal substances secreted in human milk. *Practitioner.* 1953; 171:533-8.
344. Järnerot G, Into-Malmberg M-B. Sulphasalazine treatment during breast feeding. *Scand J Gastroenterol.* 1979; 147:869-71.
345. Berlin CM Jr, Yaffe SJ. Disposition of salicylazosulfapyridine (Azulfidine) and metabolites in human breast milk. *Dev Pharmacol Ther.* 1980; 1:31-9.
346. Esbjörner E, Järnerot G, Wranne L. Sulphasalazine and sulphapyridine serum levels in children to [sic] mothers treated with sulphasalazine during pregnancy and lactation. *Acta Paediatr Scand.* 1987; 76:137-42.
347. Branski D, Kerem E, Gross-Kieselstein E et al. Bloody diarrhea—a possible complication of sulfasalazine transferred through human breast milk. *J Pediatr Gastroenterol Nutr.* 1986; 5:316-7.
348. Nelis GF. Diarrhoea due to 5-aminosalicylic acid in breast milk. *Lancet.* 1989; 1:383. Letter.
349. Jenss H, Weber P, Hartmann F. 5-Aminosalicylic acid and its metabolite in breast milk during lactation. *Am J Gastroenterol.* 1990; 85:331. Letter.
350. Tyson RM, Shrader EA, Perlman HH. Drugs transmitted through breast milk: part I. Laxatives. *J Pediatr.* 1937; 11:824-32.
351. Werthmann MW Jr, Krees SV. Quantitative excretion of Senokot in human breast milk. *Med Ann Dist Columbia.* 1973; 42:4-5.
352. Faber P, Strenge-Hesse A. Relevance of rhein excretion into breast milk. *Pharmacology.* 1988; 36(Suppl 1):212-20.
353. Riley AJ, Crowley P, Harrison C. Transfer of ranitidine to biological fluids: milk and semen. In: Misiewicz JJ, Wormsley KG, eds. The clinical use of ranitidine. Oxford, England: Medicine Publishing Foundation; 1981:78-81.
354. Courtney TP, Shaw RW, Cedar E et al. Excretion of famotidine in breast milk. *Br J Clin Pharmacol.* 1988; 26:639p.
355. Obermeyer BD, Bergstrom RF, Callaghan JT et al. Secretion of nizatidine into human breast milk after single and multiple doses. *Clin Pharmacol Ther.* 1990; 47:724-30.
356. Bender W, Brockmeier D. Pharmacokinetic characteristics of roxatidine. *J Clin Gastroenterol.* 1989; 11(Suppl 1):S6-S9.
357. Guzmán V, Toscano G, Canales ES et al. Improvement of defective lactation by using oral metoclopramide. *Acta Obstet Gynecol Scand.* 1979; 58:53-5.
358. Kauppila A, Kivinen S, Ylikorkala O. Metoclopramide increases prolactin release and milk secretion in puerperium without stimulating the secretion of thyrotropin and thyroid hormones. *J Clin Endocrinol Metab.* 1981; 52:436-9.
359. De Gezelle H, Ooghe W, Thiery M et al. Metoclopramide and breast milk. *Eur J Obstet Gynecol Reprod Biol.* 1983; 15:31-6.
360. Gupta AP, Gupta PK. Metoclopramide as a lactagogue. *Clin Pediatr.* 1985; 24:269-72.
361. Ehrenkranz RA, Ackerman BA. Metoclopramide effect on faltering milk production by mothers of premature infants. *Pediatrics.* 1986; 78:614-20.
362. Barguño JM, del Pozo E, Cruz M et al. Failure of maintained hyperprolactinemia to improve lactational performance in late puerperium. *J Clin Endocrinol Metab.* 1988; 66:876-9.
363. Lewis PJ, Devenish C, Kahn C. Controlled trial of metoclopramide in the initiation of breast feeding. *Br J Clin Pharmacol.* 1980; 9:217-9. Letter.
364. Kauppila A, Arvela P, Koivisto M et al. Metoclopramide and breast feeding: transfer into milk and the newborn. *Eur J Clin Pharmacol.* 1983; 25:819-23.
365. Hofmeyr GJ, Van Iddekinge B, Blott JA. Domperidone: secretion in breast milk and effect on puerperal prolactin levels. *Br J Obstet Gynecol.* 1985; 92:141-4.
366. Hofmeyr GJ, Sonnendecker EWW. Secretion of the gastrokinetic agent cisapride in human milk. *Eur J Clin Pharmacol.* 1986; 30:735-6.
367. Dewart PJ, McNeilly AS, Smith SK et al. LRH agonist buserelin as a post-partum contraceptive: lack of biological activity of buserelin in breast milk. *Acta Endocrinol (Copenh).* 1987; 114:185-92.
368. Fraser HM, Dewart PJ, Smith SK et al. Luteinizing hormone releasing hormone agonist for contraception in breast feeding women. *J Clin Endocrinol Metab.* 1989; 69:996-1002.
369. Gambrell RD Jr. Immediate postpartum oral contraception.

Obstet Gynecol. 1970; 36:101-6.
370. Kærn T. Effect of an oral contraceptive immediately post partum on initiation of lactation. *Br Med J*. 1967; 3:644-5.
371. Nilsson S, Mellbin T, Hofvander Y et al. Long-term follow-up of children breast-fed by mothers using oral contraceptives. *Contraception*. 1986; 34:443-57.
372. Koetsawang S. The effects of contraceptive methods on the quality and quantity of breast milk. *Int J Gynaecol Obstet*. 1987; 25(Suppl):115-27.
373. Laukaran VH. The effects of contraceptive use on the initiation and duration of lactation. *Int J Gynaecol Obstet*. 1987; 25(Suppl):129-42.
374. World Health Organization (WHO) Task Force on Oral Contraceptives, Special Programme of Research, Development, and Research Training in Human Reproduction. Effects of hormonal contraceptives on breast milk composition and infant growth. *Stud Fam Plann*. 1988; 19:361-9.
375. Zacharias S, Aguilera E, Jiminez J et al. The effects of hormonal and non-hormonal contraceptives on human lactation and on the re-establishment of fertility. *Int J Gynaecol Obstet*. 1987; 25(Suppl):249-55.
376. McCann MF, Moggia AV, Higgins JE et al. The effects of a progestin-only oral contraceptive (levonorgestrel 0.03 mg) on breast-feeding. *Contraception*. 1989; 40:635-48.
377. Díaz S, Herreros C, Juez G et al. Fertility regulation in nursing women: VII. Influence of Norplant levonorgestrel implants upon lactation and infant growth. *Contraception*. 1985; 32:53-74.
378. Shaaban MM, Salem HT, Abdullah KA. Influence of levonorgestrel contraceptive implants, Norplant, initiated early postpartum upon lactation and infant growth. *Contraception*. 1985; 32:623-35.
379. Affandi B, Karmadibrata S, Prihartono J et al. Effect of Norplant on mothers and infants in the postpartum period. *Adv Contracept*. 1986; 2:371-80.
380. Curtis EM. Oral-contraceptive feminization of a normal male infant. *Obstet Gynecol*. 1964; 23:295-6.
381. Lauritzen C. On endocrine effects of oral contraceptives. *Acta Endocrinol (Copenh)*. 1967; 124(Suppl):87-100.
382. Marriq P, Oddo G. La gynécomastie induite chez le nouveau-né par le lait maternel? Un accident rare des contraceptifs oraux. *Nouv Presse Med*. 1974; 3:2579.
383. Madhavapeddi R, Ramachandran P. Side effects of oral contraceptive use in lactating women—enlargement of breast in a breast-fed child. *Contraception*. 1985; 32:437-43.
384. Mandel H, Berant M. Oral contraceptives and breastfeeding: haematological effects on the infant. *Arch Dis Child*. 1985; 60:971-80.
385. Thomas MJ, Danutra V, Read GF et al. The detection and measurement of *d*-norgestrel in human milk using sephadex LH 20 chromatography and radioimmunoassay. *Steroids*. 1977; 30:349-61.
386. Nilsson S, Nygren K-G, Johansson EDB. Transfer of estradiol to human milk. *Am J Obstet Gynecol*. 1978; 132:653-7.
387. Nilsson S, Nygren K-G. Transfer of contraceptive steroids to human milk. *Res Reprod*. 1979; 1:1-2.
388. Toddywalla VS, Mehta S, Virkar KD et al. Release of 19-nortestosterone type of contraceptive steroids through different drug delivery systems into the serum and breast milk of lactating women. *Contraception*. 1980; 21:217-23.
389. Nilsson S, Nygren K-G, Johansson EDB. Megestrol acetate concentrations in plasma and milk during administration of an oral contraceptive containing 4 mg megestrol acetate to nursing women. *Contraception*. 1985; 32:437-43.
390. Nilsson S, Nygren K-G, Johansson EDB. *d*-Norgestrel concentrations in maternal plasma, milk and child plasma during administration of oral contraceptives to nursing women. *Am J Obstet Gynecol*. 1977; 129:178-84.
391. Harlap S. Exposure to contraceptive hormones through breast milk—are there long-term health and behavioral consequences? *Int J Gynaecol Obstet*. 1987; 25(Suppl):47-55.
392. Shaaban MM, Odlind V, Salem HT et al. Levonorgestrel concentrations in maternal and infant serum during use of subdermal levonorgestrel contraceptive implants, Norplant, by nursing mothers. *Contraception*. 1986; 33:357-63.
393. Öst L, Wettrell G, Björkhem I et al. Prednisolone excretion in human milk. *J Pediatr*. 1985; 106:1008-11.
394. Berlin CM Jr, Kaiser DG, Demers L. Excretion of prednisone and prednisolone in human milk. *Pharmacologist*. 1979; 21:264. Abstract.
395. Anderson PO. Corticosteroid use by breast-feeding mothers. *Clin Pharm*. 1987; 6:445.
396. De Stefano P, Bongo C, Borgna-Pignatti C et al. Factitious hypertension with mineralocorticoid excess in an infant. *Helv Paediatr Acta*. 1983; 38:185-9.
397. Burrow GN, Wassenaar W, Robertson GL et al. DDAVP treatment of diabetes insipidus during pregnancy and the post-partum period. *Acta Endocrinol (Copenh)*. 1981; 97:23-5.
398. Neubauer SH. Lactation in insulin-dependent diabetes. *Progr Food Nutr Sci*. 1990; 14:333-70.
399. Alban Davies H, Clark JDA, Dalton KJ et al. Insulin requirements of diabetic women who breast feed. *Br Med J*. 1989; 298:1357-8.
400. Illingworth P, Howie PW, Jung RT. Insulin requirements during breast feeding. *Br Med J*. 1989; 298:1643-4. Letter.
401. Ruis H, Rolland R, Doesburg W et al. Oxytocin enhances onset of lactation among mothers delivering prematurely. *Br Med J*. 1981; 283:340-2.
402. Seifer DB, Sandberg EC, Ueland K et al. Water intoxication and hyponatremic encephalopathy from the use of an oxytocin nasal spray: a case report. *J Reprod Med*. 1985; 30:225-8.
403. Croxatto HB, Díaz S. The place of progesterone in human contraception. *J Steroid Biochem*. 1987; 27:991-4.
404. Reid B, Smith H, Friedman Z. Prostaglandins in human milk. *Pediatrics*. 1980; 66:870-2.
405. Chappell JE, Clandinin MT, Barbe GJ et al. Prostanoid content of human milk: relationships to milk fatty acid content. *Endocrinol Exp*. 1983; 17:351-8.
406. Alzina V, Puig M, de Echániz L et al. Prostaglandins in human milk. *Biol Neonate*. 1986; 50:200-4.
407. Bedrick AD, Britton JR, Johnson S et al. Prostaglandin stability in human milk and infant gastric fluid. *Biol Neonate*. 1989; 56:192-7.
408. Nasi A, de Murtas M, Parodo G et al. Inhibition of lactation by prostaglandin E_2. *Obstet Gynecol Surv*. 1980; 35:619-20.
409. Tulandi T, Gelfand MM, Maiolo LM. Effect of prostaglandin E_2 on puerperal breast discomfort and prolactin secretion. *J Reprod Med*. 1985; 30:176-8.
410. Toppozada MK, El-Rahman HA, Soliman AY. Prostaglandins as milk ejectors: the nose as a new route of administration. *Adv Prostaglandin Thromboxane Leukotriene Res*. 1983; 12:449-54.
411. Sato T, Suzuki Y. Presence of triiodothyronine, no detectable thyroxine and reverse triiodothyronine in human milk. *Endocrinol Jpn*. 1979; 26:507-13.
412. Oberkotter LV, Hahn HB Jr. Thyroid function and human breast milk. *Am J Dis Child*. 1983; 137:1131. Letters.
413. Oberkotter LV. Analysis of term human milk concentrations of 3,5,3'-triiodo-L-thyronine by high-performance liquid chromatography and radioimmunoassay: correlation with circulating serum levels in lactating women. *J Chromatogr*. 1989; 487:445-9.
414. Cooper DS. Antithyroid drugs: to breast-feed or not to breast-feed. *Am J Obstet Gynecol*. 1987; 157:234-5.
415. Lamberg B-A, Ikonen E, Österlund K et al. Antithyroid treatment of maternal hyperthyroidism during lactation. *Clin Endocrinol*. 1984; 21:81-7.
416. Rylance GW, Woods CG, Donnelly MC et al. Carbimazole and breastfeeding. *Lancet*. 1987; 1:928. Letter.
417. Momotani N, Yamashita R, Yoshimoto M et al. Recovery from foetal hypothyroidism: evidence for the safety of breast-feeding while taking propylthiouracil. *Clin Endocrinol*. 1989; 31:591-5.
418. Matheson I, Pande H, Alertsen AR. Respiratory depression

caused by *N*-desmethyldoxepin in breast milk. *Lancet*. 1985; 2:1124. Letter.
419. Kemp J, Ilett KF, Booth J et al. Excretion of doxepin and *N*-desmethyldoxepin in human milk. *Br J Clin Pharmacol*. 1985; 20:497-9.
420. Sovner R, Orsulak PJ. Excretion of imipramine and desipramine in human breast milk. *Am J Psychiatry*. 1979; 136:451-2.
421. Bader TF, Newman K. Amitriptyline in human breast milk and the nursing infant's serum. *Am J Psychiatry*. 1980; 137:855-6.
422. Brixen-Rasmussen L, Halgrener J, Jørgensen A. Amitriptyline and nortriptyline excretion in human breast milk. *Psychopharmacology*. 1982; 76:94-5.
423. Stancer HC, Reed KL. Desipramine and 2-hydroxydesipramine in human breast milk and the nursing infant's serum. *Am J Psychiatry*. 1986; 143:1597-600.
424. Matheson I, Skjæraasen J. Milk concentrations of flupenthixol, nortriptyline and zuclopenthixol and between-breast differences in two patients. *Eur J Clin Pharmacol*. 1988; 35:217-20.
425. Ware MR, DeVane CL. Imipramine treatment of panic disorder during pregnancy. *J Clin Psychiatry*. 1990; 51:482-4.
426. Verbeeck RK, Ross SG, McKenna EA. Excretion of trazodone in breast milk. *Br J Clin Pharmacol*. 1986; 22:367-70.
427. Gelenberg AJ. Amoxapine, a new antidepressant, appears in human milk. *J Nerv Ment Dis*. 1979; 167:635-6.
428. Lloyd AH. Practical considerations in the use of maprotiline (Ludiomil) in general practice. *J Int Med Res*. 1977; 5(Suppl 4):122-38.
429. Isenberg KE. Excretion of fluoxetine in human breast milk. *J Clin Psychiatry*. 1990; 51:169. Letter.
430. Orsulak PJ, Sovner R. Drs. Orsulak and Sovner reply. *Am J Psychiatry*. 1979; 136:1483-4. Letter.
431. Nurenburg HG. An overview of somatic treatment of psychosis during pregnancy and postpartum. *Gen Hosp Psychiatry*. 1989; 11:328-38.
432. Mortola JF. The use of psychotropic agents in pregnancy and lactation. *Psychiatr Clin North Am*. 1989; 12:69-87.
433. Robinson GE, Stewart DE, Flak E. The rational use of psychotropic drugs in pregnancy and postpartum. *Can J Psychiatry*. 1986; 31:183-90.
434. Buist A, Norman TR, Dennerstein L. Breastfeeding and the use of psychotropic medication: a review. *J Affective Disord*. 1990; 19:197-206.
435. Stewart RB, Karas B, Springer PK. Haloperidol excretion in human milk. *Am J Psychiatry*. 1980; 137:849-50.
436. Whalley LJ, Blain PG, Prime JK. Haloperidol secreted in breast milk. *Br Med J*. 1981; 282:1746-7.
437. Citterio C. Riconoscimento e dosaggio di derivati fenotiazinici nella secrezione lattae. *Neuropsichiatria*. 1964; 20:141-6.
438. Wiles DH, Orr MW, Kolakowska T. Chlorpromazine levels in plasma and milk of nursing mothers. *Br J Clin Pharmacol*. 1978; 5:272-3. Letter.
439. Matheson I, Evang A, Overø KF et al. Presence of chlorprothixene and its metabolites in breast milk. *Eur J Clin Pharmacol*. 1984; 27:611-3.
440. Vendelin Olesen O, Bartels U, Hejelm Poulsen J. Perphenazine in breast milk and serum. *Am J Psychiatry*. 1990; 147:1378-9. Letter.
441. Kris EB, Carmichael DM. Chlorpromazine maintenance therapy during pregnancy and confinement. *Psychiatr Q*. 1957; 31:690-5.
442. Kris EB. Children born to mothers maintained on pharmacotherapy during pregnancy and postpartum. *Recent Adv Biol Psychiatry*. 1962; 4:180-7.
443. Ayd FJ Jr. Children born of mothers treated with chlorpromazine during pregnancy. *Clin Med*. 1964; 71:1758-63.
444. Skausig OB, Schou M. Diegivning under lithiumbehandling. *Ugeskr Laeger*. 1977; 139:400-1.
445. Schou M, Weinstein MR. Problems of lithium maintenance treatment during pregnancy, delivery and lactation. *Agressologie*. 1980; 21(special issue A):7-9.
446. Tunnessen WW Jr, Hertz CG. Toxic effects of lithium in newborn infants: a commentary. *J Pediatr*. 1972; 81:804-7.
447. Linden S, Rich CL. The use of lithium during pregnancy and lactation. *J Clin Psychiatry*. 1983; 44:358-61.
448. Villenueve A, Lajeunesse C, Pires A. Lithium, grossesse et allaitement. *Encephale*. 1989; 15:283-6.
449. Schou M. Lithium treatment during pregnancy, delivery, and lactation: an update. *J Clin Psychiatry*. 1990; 51:410-3.
450. Andersen LW, Qvist T, Hertz J et al. Concentrations of thiopentone in mature breast milk and colostrum following an induction dose. *Acta Anaesthesiol Scand*. 1987; 31:30-2.
451. Kanto JH. Use of benzodiazepines during pregnancy, labour and lactation, with particular reference to pharmacokinetic considerations. *Drugs*. 1982; 23:354-80.
452. Wesson DR, Camber S, Harkey M et al. Diazepam and desmethyldiazepam in breast milk. *J Psychoactive Drugs*. 1985; 17:55-6.
453. Anderson PO, McGuire GG. Neonatal alprazolam withdrawal—possible effects of breast feeding. *DICP*. 1990; 23:614. Letter.
454. Wretlind M. Excretion of oxazepam in breast milk. *Eur J Clin Pharmacol*. 1987; 33:209-10.
455. Whitelaw AGL, Cummings AJ, McFadyen IR. Effect of maternal lorazepam on the neonate. *Br Med J*. 1981; 282:1106-8.
456. Summerfield RJ, Nielsen MS. Excretion of lorazepam into breast milk. *Br J Anaesth*. 1985; 57:1042-3. Letter.
457. Dusci LJ, Good SM, Hall RW et al. Excretion of diazepam and its metabolites in human milk during withdrawal from combination high dose diazepam and oxazepam. *Br J Clin Pharmacol*. 1990; 29:123-6.
458. Peña C, Medina JH, Piva M et al. Naturally occurring benzodiazepines in human milk. *Biochem Biophys Res Commun*. 1991; 175:1042-50.
459. Tyson RM, Shrader EA, Perlman HH. Drugs transmitted through breast milk: III. Bromides. *J Pediatr*. 1938; 14:91-3.
460. Bernstine JB, Meyer AE, Bernstine RL. Maternal blood and breast milk estimation following the administration of chloral hydrate during the puerperium. *J Obstet Gynaecol Br Emp*. 1956; 63:228-31.
461. Lacey JH. Dichloralphenazone and breast milk. *Br Med J*. 1971; 4:684. Letter.
462. Curry SH, Riddall D, Gordon JS et al. Disposition of glutethimide in man. *Clin Pharmacol Ther*. 1971; 12:849-57.
463. Coté CJ, Kenepp NB, Reed SB et al. Trace concentrations of halothane in human breast milk. *Br J Anaesth*. 1976; 48:541-3.
464. Ayd FJ. Excretion of psychotropic drugs in human breast milk. *Int Drug Ther Newsl*. 1973; 8:33-40.
465. Dailland P, Cockshott ID, Didier Lirzin J et al. Intravenous propofol during cesarean section: placental transfer, concentrations in breast milk, and neonatal effects. A preliminary study. *Anesthesiology*. 1989; 71:827-34.
466. Eriksson G, Swahn C-G. Concentrations of baclofen in serum and breast milk from a lactating woman. *Scand J Clin Lab Invest*. 1981; 41:185-7.
467. Naulty JS, Ostheimer G, Datta S et al. Bupivacaine in breast milk following epidural anesthesia for vaginal delivery. *Reg Anesth*. 1983; 8:44-5. Abstract.
468. Baker PA, Schroeder D. Interpleural bupivacaine for postoperative pain during lactation. *Anesth Analg*. 1989; 69:400-2.
469. Sokka TK, Patton S. In vivo effects of colchicine on milk fat globule membrane. *Biochim Biophys Acta*. 1983; 731:1-8.
470. Sordillo LM, Oliver SP, Duby RT et al. Effects of colchicine on milk yield, composition, and cellular differentiation during caprine lactogenesis. *Int J Biochem*. 1984; 16:1135-41.
471. Maguire AM, Bennett J. Fluorescein elimination in human breast milk. *Arch Ophthalmol*. 1988; 106:718-9. Letter.
472. Mattern J, Mayer PR. Excretion of fluorescein into breast milk. *Am J Ophthalmol*. 1990; 109:598-9.
473. Spak CJ, Hardell LI, de Chateau P. Fluoride in human milk. *Acta Paediatr Scand*. 1983; 72:699-701.

474. Greene JC. Fluoride supplementation of the breast-fed infant. *JAMA*. 1990; 263:2179. Letter.
475. Berlin CM Jr. Fluoride supplementation for breast-fed infants. *JAMA*. 1990; 263:2371.
476. American Academy of Pediatrics, Committee on Nutrition. Fluoride supplementation. *Pediatrics*. 1986; 77:758-61.
477. Blau SP. Metabolism of gold during lactation. *Arthritis Rheum*. 1973; 16:777-8. Letter.
478. Gottlieb NL. Suggested errata. *Arthritis Rheum*. 1974; 17:1057. Letter.
479. Bell RAF, Dale IM. Gold secretion in maternal milk. *Arthritis Rheum*. 1976; 19:1374. Letter.
480. Østenson M, Skavdal K, Mykelbust G et al. Excretion of gold into human breast milk. *Eur J Clin Pharmacol*. 1986; 31:251-2.
481. Rooney TW, Lorber A, Veng-Pedersen P et al. Gold pharmacokinetics in breast milk and serum of a lactating woman. *J Rheumatol*. 1987; 14:1120-2.
482. Bennett PN, Humphries SJ, Osborne JP et al. Use of sodium aurothiomalate during lactation. *Br J Clin Pharmacol*. 1990; 29:777-9.
483. Fleiss P. Herbal remedies for the breastfeeding mother. *Mothering*. 1988; (Summer):68-71.
484. Anon. Fenugreek. *Lawrence Rev Nat Prod*. 1987; Jul:1-2.
485. Koren G, Randor S, Martin S et al. Maternal ginseng use associated with neonatal androgenization. *JAMA*. 1990; 264:2866. Letter.
486. Koren G. Maternal use of ginseng and neonatal androgenization. *JAMA*. 1991; 265:1828. Letter.
487. Anon. Toxic reactions to plant products sold in health food stores. *Med Lett Drugs Ther*. 1979; 21:29-31.
488. Postellon DC, Aronow R. Iodine in mother's milk. *JAMA*. 1983; 247:463. Letter.
489. Danziger Y, Pertzelan A, Mimouni M. Transient congenital hypothyroidism after topical iodine in pregnancy and lactation. *Arch Dis Child*. 1987; 62:295-6.
490. Delange F, Chanoine JP, Abrassart C et al. Topical iodine, breastfeeding, and neonatal hypothyroidism. *Arch Dis Child*. 1988; 63:106-7. Letter.
491. Arena Ansotegui J, Emparanza Knörr JI, San Millan Vege MJ et al. Sobrecarga iodada al recién nacido por utilizar PVP-iodada para la preparación perineal materna en el parto vaginal. *An Esp Pediatr*. 1989; 30:23-6.
492. Leming PD, Decker SE, Hee SQ et al. Breast milk iodine excretion following a bipedal lymphangiogram (LAG) in a patient with Hodgkin's disease. *Proc Am Soc Clin Oncol*. 1989; 8:339. Abstract.
493. Holmdahl KH. Cholecystography during lactation. *Acta Radiol*. 1956; 45:305-7.
494. Texier F, Roque D'Obrcastel O, Etling N. Teneur en iode du lait humain après une angiographie pulmonaire. *Presse Med*. 1983; 12:769. Letter.
495. FitzJohn TP, Williams DG, Laker MF et al. Intravenous urography during lactation. *Br J Radiol*. 1982; 55:603-5.
496. Schmiedl U, Maravilla KR, Gerlach R et al. Excretion of gadopentetate dimeglumine in human breast milk. *AJR*. 1990; 154:1305-6.
497. Nielsen ST, Matheson I, Rasmussen JN et al. Excretion of iohexol and metrizoate in human breast milk. *Acta Radiol*. 1987; 28:523-6.
498. Ilett KF, Hackett LP, Patterson JW. Excretion of metrizamide in milk. *Br J Radiol*. 1981; 54:537-8. Letter.
499. Board JA, Fierro RJ, Wasserman AJ et al. Effects of α- and β-adrenergic blocking agents on serum prolactin levels in women with hyperprolactinemia and galactorrhea. *Am J Obstet Gynecol*. 1977; 127:285-7.
500. Deis RP, Kann G, Martinet J. Prolactin release and milk removal induced by suckling and milking in lactating ewes is prevented by L-DOPA treatment. *Reprod Nutr Dev*. 1990; 30:605-10.
501. Senger E, Menzel I, Holzmann H. Therapiebedingte lindankonzentration in der muttermilch. *Dermatosen*. 1989; 37:167-70.
502. Cruikshank DP, Varner MW, Pitkin RM. Breast milk magnesium and calcium concentrations following magnesium sulfate treatment. *Am J Obstet Gynecol*. 1982; 143:685-8.
503. Fraser D. Myasthenia gravis and pregnancy. *Proc R Soc Med*. 1963; 56:379-81.
504. Olsson B, Bolme P, Dahlström B et al. Excretion of noscapine in human breast milk. *Eur J Clin Pharmacol*. 1986; 30:213-5.
505. Witter FR, Smith RV. The excretion of pentoxifylline and its metabolites into human breast milk. *Am J Obstet Gynecol*. 1985; 151:1094-7.
506. Pan H, Fleiss P, Moore L et al. Excretion of pravastatin, an HMG CoA reductase inhibitor, in breast milk of lactating women. *J Clin Pharmacol*. 1988; 28:942. Abstract.
507. Skoglund RR, Roberts CC, Huddlestone J. The role of antiacetylcholine receptor antibody in neonatal myasthenia gravis. *Bull Los Angeles Neurol Soc*. 1978; 43:66-9.
508. Hardell L-I, Lindström B, Lönnerholm G et al. Pyridostigmine in human breast milk. *Br J Clin Pharmacol*. 1982; 14:565-7. Letter.
509. Foukas MD. An antilactogenic effect of pyridoxine. *J Obstet Gynaecol Br Commonw*. 1973; 80:718-20.
510. Marcus RG. Suppression of lactation with high doses of pyridoxine. *S Afr Med J*. 1975; 49:2155-6.
511. Canales ES, Soria J, Zárate A et al. The influence of pyridoxine on prolactin secretion and milk production. *Br J Obstet Gynaecol*. 1976; 83:387-8.
512. Macdonald HN, Collins YD, Tobin MJW et al. The failure of pyridoxine in suppression of puerperal lactation. *Br J Obstet Gynaecol*. 1976; 83:54-5.
513. Boes EGM. Inhibition of puerperal lactation: a comparative study of bromocriptine. *S Afr Med J*. 1980; 57:900-3.
514. Andon MB, Howard MP, Moser PB et al. Nutritionally relevant supplementation of vitamin B_6 in lactating women: effect on plasma prolactin. *Pediatrics*. 1985; 76:769-73.
515. Rollman O, Pihl-Lundin I. Acitretin excretion into human breast milk. *Acta Derm Venereol (Stockh)*. 1990; 70:487-90.
516. Zbinden G. Investigations on the toxicity of tretinoin administered systemically to animals. *Acta Derm Venereol Suppl (Stockh)*. 1975; 74:36-40.
517. Boréus LO, de Château P, Lindberg C et al. Terbutaline in breast milk. *Br J Clin Pharmacol*. 1982; 13:731-2. Letter.
518. Lönnerholm G, Lindström B. Terbutaline excretion into breast milk. *Br J Clin Pharmacol*. 1982; 13:729-30. Letter.
519. Lindberg C, Boréus LO, de Château P et al. Transfer of terbutaline into breast milk. *Eur J Respir Dis*. 1984; 85(Suppl 134):87-91.
520. Yurchak AM, Jusko WJ. Theophylline secretion into breast milk. *Pediatrics*. 1976; 57:518-20.
521. Jarboe CH, Cook LN, Malesic I et al. Dyphylline elimination kinetics in lactating women: blood to milk transfer. *J Clin Pharmacol*. 1981; 21:405-10.
522. Moiel RH, Ryan JR. Tolbutamide Orinase in human breast milk. *Clin Pediatr*. 1967; 8:480.
523. Katz M, Plotkin SA. Oral polio immunization of the newborn infant: a possible method for overcoming interference by ingested antibodies. *J Pediatr*. 1968; 73:267-70.
524. Deforest A, Parker PB, DiLiberti JH et al. The effect of breast-feeding on the antibody response of infants to trivalent oral poliovirus vaccine. *J Pediatr*. 1973; 83:93-5.
525. John TJ, Devarajan LV, Luther L et al. Effect of breast-feeding on seroresponse of infants to oral poliovirus vaccination. *Pediatrics*. 1976; 57:47-53.
526. Pabst HF, Godel J, Grace M et al. Effect of breast-feeding on immune response to BCG vaccine. *Lancet*. 1989; 1:295-7.
527. Pabst HF, Spady DW. Effect of breast-feeding on antibody response to conjugate vaccine. *Lancet*. 1990; 336:269-70.
528. Hahn-Zoric M, Fulconis F, Minoli I et al. Antibody responses to parenteral and oral vaccines are impaired by conventional and low protein formulas as compared to breast-feeding. *Acta Pediatr Scand*. 1990; 79:1137-42.
529. Buimovici-Klein E, Hite RL, Byrne T et al. Isolation of rubella virus in milk after postpartum immunization. *J Pedi-*

atr. 1977; 91:939-41.
530. Losonsky GA, Fishaut JM, Strussenberg J et al. Effect of immunization against rubella on lactation products (2 parts). *J Infect Dis.* 1982; 145:654-66.
531. Immunization Practices Advisory Committee. General recommendations on immunization. *MMWR.* 1989; 38:205-27.
532. Kesäniemi YA. Ethanol and acetaldehyde in the milk and peripheral blood of lactating women after ethanol administration. *J Obstet Gynaecol Br Commonw.* 1974; 81:84-6.
533. Lawton ME. Alcohol in breast milk. *Aust N Z J Obstet Gynaecol.* 1985; 25:71-3.
534. Bisdom W. Alcohol and nicotine poisoning in nurslings. *JAMA.* 1937; 109:178. Abstract.
535. Binkiewicz A, Robinson MJ, Senior B. Pseudo-Cushing syndrome caused by alcohol in breast milk. *J Pediatr.* 1978; 93:965-7.
536. Little RE, Anderson KW, Ervin CH et al. Maternal alcohol use during breast-feeding and infant mental and motor development at one year. *N Engl J Med.* 1989; 321:425-30.
537. Wagner G, Fuchs A-R. Effect of ethanol on uterine activity during suckling in post-partum women. *Acta Endocrinol.* 1968; 58:133-41.
538. Cobo E. Effect of different doses of ethanol on the milk-ejecting reflex in lactating women. *Am J Obstet Gynecol.* 1973; 115:817-21.
539. Vilaró S, Viñas O, Remesar X et al. Effects of chronic ethanol consumption on lactational performance in rat: mammary gland and milk composition and pups' growth and metabolism. *Pharmacol Biochem Behav.* 1987; 27:333-9.
540. Subramanian MG, Abel EL. Alcohol inhibits suckling-induced prolactin release and milk yield. *Alcohol.* 1988; 5:95-8.
541. De Rosa G, Corsello SM, Ruffilli MP et al. Prolactin secretion after beer. *Lancet.* 1981; 2:934. Letter.
542. Carlson HE, Wasser HL, Reidelberger RD. Beer-induced prolactin secretion: a clinical and laboratory study of the role of salsolinol. *J Clin Endocrinol Metab.* 1985; 60:673-7.
543. Steiner E, Villén T, Hallberg M et al. Amphetamine secretion in breast milk. *Eur J Clin Pharmacol.* 1984; 27:123-4.
544. Oro AS, Dixon SD. Perinatal cocaine and methamphetamine exposure: maternal and neonatal correlates. *J Pediatr.* 1987; 111:571-8.
545. DeLeo V, Cella SG, Camanni F et al. Prolactin lowering effect of amphetamine in normoprolactinemic subjects and in physiological and pathological hyperprolactinemia. *Horm Metab Res.* 1983; 15:439-43.
546. Kristiansson B, Abdul Ghani N, Eriksson M et al. Use of khat in lactating women: a pilot study on breast-milk secretion. *J Ethnopharmacol.* 1987; 21:85-90.
547. Rivera-Calimlim L. Drugs in breast milk. *Drug Ther.* 1977; 7:59-63.
548. Clement MI. Caffeine and babies. *Br Med J.* 1989; 298:1461.
549. Hildebrandt R, Gundert-Remy U. Lack of pharmacological active saliva levels of caffeine in breast-fed infants. *Pediatr Pharmacol.* 1983; 3:237-44.
550. Ryu JE. Caffeine in human milk and in serum of breast-fed infants. *Dev Pharmacol Ther.* 1985; 8:329-37.
551. Ryu JE. Effect of maternal caffeine consumption on heart rate and sleep time of breast-fed infants. *Dev Pharmacol Ther.* 1985; 8:355-63.
552. Stavchansky S, Combs A, Sagraves R et al. Pharmacokinetics of caffeine in breast milk and plasma after single oral administration of caffeine to lactating mothers. *Biopharm Drug Dispos.* 1988; 9:285-99.
553. Le Guennec J-C, Billon B. Delay in caffeine elimination in breast-fed infants. *Pediatrics.* 1987; 79:264-8.
554. Wiggins RC, Rolsten C, Ruiz B et al. Pharmacokinetics of cocaine: basic studies of route, dosage, pregnancy and lactation. *Neurotoxicology.* 1989; 10:367-82.
555. Chasnoff IJ, Lewis DE, Squires L. Cocaine intoxication in a breast-fed infant. *Pediatrics.* 1987; 80:836-8.
556. Chaney NE, Francke J, Wadlington WB. Cocaine convulsions in a breast-feeding baby. *J Pediatr.* 1988; 112:134-5.
557. Perez-Reyes M, Wall ME. Presence of Δ^9-tetrahydrocannabinol in human milk. *N Engl J Med.* 1982; 307:819-20. Letter.
558. Astley SJ, Little RE. Maternal marijuana use during lactation and infant development at one year. *Neurotoxicol Teratol.* 1990; 12:161-8.
559. Mendelson JH, Mello NK, Ellingboe J. Acute effects of marijuana smoking on prolactin levels in human females. *J Pharmacol Exp Ther.* 1985; 232:220-2.
560. Tyrey L, Murphy LL. Inhibition of suckling-induced milk ejections in the lactating rat by Δ^9-tetrahydrocannabinol. *Endocrinology.* 1988; 123:469-72.
561. Nicholas JM, Lipshitz J, Schreiber EC et al. Phencyclidine: its transfer across the placenta as well as into breast milk. *Am J Obstet Gynecol.* 1982; 143:143-6.
562. Kaufman KR, Petrucha RA, Pitts FN Jr et al. PCP in amniotic fluid and breast milk: case report. *J Clin Psychiatry.* 1983; 44:269-70.
563. Woodward A, Grgurinovich N, Ryan P. Breast feeding and smoking hygiene: major influences on cotinine in urine of smokers' infants. *J Epidemiol Community Health.* 1986; 40:309-15.
564. Luck W, Nau H. Nicotine and cotinine concentrations in the milk of smoking mothers: influence of cigarette consumption and diurnal variation. *Eur J Pediatr.* 1987; 146:21-6.
565. Schwartz-Bickenbach D, Schulte-Hobein B, Abt S et al. Smoking and passive smoking during pregnancy and early infancy: effects on birth weight, lactation period, and cotinine concentrations in mother's milk and infant's urine. *Toxicol Lett.* 1987; 35:73-81.
566. Labrecque M, Marcoux S, Weber J-P et al. Feeding and urine cotinine values in babies whose mothers smoke. *Pediatrics.* 1989; 83:93-7.
567. Dahlström A, Lundell B, Curvall M et al. Nicotine and cotinine concentrations in the nursing mother and her infant. *Acta Paediatr Scand.* 1990; 79:142-7.
568. Radisch B, Luck W, Nau H. Cadmium concentrations in milk and blood of smoking mothers. *Toxicol Lett.* 1987; 36:147-52.
569. Said G, Patois E, Lellouch J. Infantile colic and parental smoking. *Br Med J.* 1984; 289:660.
570. Matheson I, Rivrud GN. The effect of smoking on lactation and infantile colic. *JAMA.* 1989; 261:42-3. Letter.
571. Whichelow MJ, King BE. Breast feeding and smoking. *Arch Dis Child.* 1979; 54:240-1. Letter.
572. Vió del Rio F, Albala C, Salinas J et al. Influencia del habito de fumar en la lactancia materna. *Rev Med Chil.* 1987; 115:611-5.
573. Counsilman JJ, Mackay EV. Cigarette smoking by pregnant women with particular reference to their past and subsequent breast feeding behaviour. *Aust N Z J Obstet Gynaecol.* 1985; 25:101-7.
574. Nyboe Andersen A, Lund-Andersen C, Falck Larsen J et al. Suppressed prolactin but normal neurophysin levels in cigarette smoking breast-feeding women. *Clin Endocrinol.* 1982; 17:363-8.
575. Newman J. Drugs and breast milk. *Pediatrics.* 1990; 86:148. Letter.
576. Chen Y. Synergistic effect of passive smoking and artificial feeding on hospitalization for respiratory illness in early childhood. *Chest.* 1989; 95:1004-7.
577. Romney BM, Nickoloff EL, Esser PD et al. Radionuclide administration to nursing mothers: mathematically derived guidelines. *Radiology.* 1986; 160:549-54.
578. Mountford PJ, Coakley AJ. A review of the secretion of radioactivity in human breast milk: data, quantitative analysis and recommendations. *Nucl Med Commun.* 1989; 10:15-27.

Research

Determination of sedative and amnestic doses of lorazepam in children

DAVID W. HENRY, JOSEPH W. BURWINKLE, AND NEIL E. KLUTMAN

Abstract: An open-label, dose-escalation study was conducted to determine doses of lorazepam required to induce anterograde amnesia and sedation in children without producing excessive toxicity.

Oncology patients 4 to 17 years of age undergoing lumbar puncture or bone marrow aspiration were eligible; a patient could be entered in the study for a second procedure at a different lorazepam dose. A single oral dose of lorazepam was administered 45–60 minutes before the procedure. Starting with 0.02 mg/kg, the same dose was given to three patients; if no dose-limiting effects occurred, dose was increased by 0.01 mg/kg. Before the procedure the patient was shown a toy that he or she was later asked to identify. Immediately after the procedure (usually 60–75 minutes after the lorazepam dose), sedation was assessed on a scale of 0 (alert) to 4 (coma), and the clinician performing the procedure was asked to subjectively evaluate sedation. Patients were rated for amnesia 24 hours after the procedure; a scale of 0 (recalls procedure and toy without prompting) to 4 (recalls nothing since procedure) was used.

Twenty patients received 28 doses of lorazepam. The study was terminated when two patients who received 0.10 mg/kg had excessive ataxia. Sedation was subjectively considered adequate for 24 of the procedures. Sedation and amnesia scores were not well correlated with increased dose. Amnesia occurred in some patients with doses as low as 0.03 mg/kg.

In children undergoing lumbar puncture or bone marrow aspiration, premedication with oral lorazepam 0.02–0.09 mg/kg generally produced adequate sedation for the procedure. Doses higher than 0.09 mg/kg caused an unacceptable degree of ataxia and had no clinical advantage over lower doses.

Index terms: Anxiolytics, sedatives and hypnotics; Dosage; Lorazepam; Pediatrics; Toxicity
Clin Pharm. 1991; 10:625-9

As a premedicant, lorazepam has been used for its anxiolytic, sedative, and amnestic properties. A limited number of studies have been published evaluating the use of lorazepam before painful procedures and the appropriate dose for use in pediatric patients.

Mundeleer[1] studied preoperative use of oral lorazepam in four- to six-year-old children. He determined 0.05 mg/kg of oral lorazepam to be the optimal dose, because of increasing sleepiness and only slightly greater amnesia at 0.06 mg/kg; sedation was minimal with doses below 0.06 mg/kg. Burtles and Astley[2] compared preoperative use of oral lorazepam 0.05 mg/kg versus diazepam and trimeprazine in children 5 to 13 years of age. Using a picture shown before surgery to measure amnesia, they found a 28% frequency of amnesia with lorazepam. Milligan et al.[3] compared 4 mg of oral lorazepam with placebo in patients ranging from 15 to 75 years of age who were undergoing bone marrow biopsies. Patients were asked immediately after the procedure to rate their pain from the procedure. Twenty-four hours later, they were asked again to rate how much pain they remembered experiencing during the procedure. At 24 hours, lorazepam-treated patients rated their pain 60% lower than they did immediately after the procedure, while controls showed no difference. Thirty-six percent of the lorazepam-treated patients had complete lack of recall of the procedure. Relling et al.[4] admin-

DAVID W. HENRY, M.S., is Assistant Professor of Pharmacy Practice, University of Kansas Medical Center (UKMC), Kansas City, KS. JOSEPH W. BURWINKLE, M.S., is Pharmacy Supervisor, Research Medical Center, Kansas City, MO; at the time of this study, he was a Master of Science in Hospital Pharmacy candidate at UKMC. NEIL E. KLUTMAN, PHARM.D., is Assistant Professor of Pharmacy Practice, UKMC.
Address reprint requests to Mr. Henry at the Department of Pharmacy, University of Kansas Medical Center, 39th and Rainbow Boulevard, Kansas City, KS 66103.
Supported in part by the University of Kansas Department of Pediatrics Children's Miracle Network Telethon Fund.
Presented at the American College of Clinical Pharmacy 10th Annual Meeting, Kansas City, MO, August 8, 1989.

istered lorazepam 0.03 mg/kg intravenously to patients undergoing hepatic clearance studies and assessed amnesia by using a picture recognition test. Twenty-four hours after lorazepam was administered, they found a 31% frequency of amnesia for a picture shown 1.5 hours after the dose.

These studies demonstrate the potential utility of lorazepam before painful procedures in children. There are no data, however, concerning the relative importance of sedation and amnesia before painful procedures, and the dosages of lorazepam required to produce sedation and amnesia in children need further study. The purpose of this study was to determine the doses of lorazepam required to induce anterograde amnesia or sedation, without excessive toxicity, in children.

Methods

Experimental Design. An open-label, dose-escalation experimental design was used in this study. A minimum of three patients were studied at each dose level. If no dose-limiting adverse reactions were seen in three consecutive patients at a particular dose, the dose was increased by 0.01 mg/kg, and the new dose was evaluated in the next three subjects. The starting dose of lorazepam was 0.02 mg/kg orally, an amount we thought was safe, based on published pediatric literature.[1-4] If a patient had a dose-limiting adverse reaction, subsequent patients received the same dose until three consecutive patients tolerated the dose without a dose-limiting adverse reaction or until the study was terminated because of dose-limiting adverse reactions.

Dose-limiting adverse reactions were defined prospectively as confusion lasting more than 10 minutes, obtundation, paradoxical excitement to the point of decreased cooperation, ataxia such that the patient required help to ambulate, hallucinations, and incontinence. All untoward reactions were recorded and could be considered dose-limiting if deemed appropriate by the investigator.

Data were collected by three investigators, although all data for a given patient entry were collected by the same investigator.

Patient Selection. Eligible patients were 4- to 17-year-old oncology patients undergoing a painful procedure (lumbar puncture or bone marrow biopsy or aspiration). In order to participate, informed consent of parents and informed assent of children seven years of age or older must have been obtained in accordance with medical center human subjects committee approval.

Patients were allowed to be enrolled in the study twice, but they were required to receive a different dose each time. A minimum of one week must have elapsed between the first and second study doses. Patients were excluded if they had received any central nervous system depressant within 12 hours before or 24 hours after the dose of lorazepam.

Drug Administration and Data Collection. The calculated dose of lorazepam for each patient was prepared by mixing the appropriate volume of lorazepam injection 2 mg/mL (Ativan, Wyeth-Ayerst) with 15 mL of flavored diluent (Roxane). The dose was administered orally 45 to 60 minutes before the scheduled procedure.

Immediately before the medical procedure, the patient was shown one of three objects (a ball, a car, or a stuffed dog) by the data collector and asked to remember the object. Objects to be used were randomly assigned. If a patient was enrolled in the study twice, a different object was used the second time. The patient was informed that the data collector would ask him or her to recall the object after the procedure. The patient was allowed to handle and play with the toy for approximately five minutes.

After completion of the medical procedure (generally 60–75 minutes after lorazepam administration) the data collector assessed baseline recall by asking the patient to recall the object. The data collector also assigned a sedation score based on the following scale[5,6]: 0 = alert, 1 = transient lethargy, 2 = sleeping <50% of time since lorazepam given, 3 = sleeping >50% of time since lorazepam given, or 4 = coma. Additionally, the clinician performing the medical procedure subjectively determined whether the patient was sufficiently sedated, based largely on apparent anxiety and on physical resistance to the procedure. Before the patient left the clinic, the importance of testing the child's memory was explained to the parents, and they were specifically asked to avoid reminding the patient about the procedure and toy.

Twenty-four hours after lorazepam administration, the patient was questioned again by telephone regarding any adverse effects that may have occurred. The patient was asked if he or she remembered undergoing the procedure and to recall the object. If the child did not remember the object, a list of five objects (apple, ball, boat, car, or stuffed dog) was offered orally from which to choose. The investigator assigned an amnesia score based on the following scale: 0 = recalls procedure and object without prompting, 1 = recalls either procedure or object without prompting, 2 = recalls either procedure or object with prompting, 3 = recalls neither procedure nor object, or 4 = recalls nothing since procedure. If the patient was unable to communicate, a parent was interviewed to determine if there was any evidence of recall of the procedures or object. The parent was asked to comment on adverse reactions noted after the administration of lorazepam.

Data Analysis. The maximum tolerated dose was defined as the highest dose tolerated by three consecutive patients without dose-limiting adverse reactions. Additionally, descriptive statistics were used. The mean amnesia score at 24 hours, the mean sedation score, and the mean number of adverse reactions were calculated for each dose level. These values were graphed to determine if a linear dose–response relationship could be identified, and Spearman's rank cor-

Table 1.
Demographic Data, Lorazepam Doses, and Sedation and Amnesia Scores for Study Patients[a]

Dose (mg/kg)	Patient	Weight (kg)	Age (yr)	Scores	
				Sedation[b]	Amnesia[c]
0.02	A	34.1	9	0	0
0.02	B	33.4	8	1	0
0.02	C	18.5	4	0	0
0.03	B	33.4	8	1	0
0.03	D	14.5	4	2	0
0.03	E	19.2	4	1	1
0.04	F	25.0	4	1	0
0.04	C	18.0	4	1	2
0.04	G	19.0	5	1	0
0.05	H	22.6	5	1	1
0.05	I	18.4	4	0	0
0.05	J[d]	29.2	8	1	0
0.06	D	14.4	4	1	0
0.06	K	50.0	17	0	0
0.06	L	43.5	8	0	N.D.[e]
0.06	M	25.7	9	0	0
0.07	N	30.0	7	0	0
0.07	O	24.0	5	1	0
0.07	P[d]	34.0	11	1	0
0.08	I[d]	19.0	4	0	3
0.08	O[d]	23.0	5	0	0
0.08	Q[d]	26.7	9	0	0
0.08	R[d]	23.2	8	1	1
0.09	H	22.8	5	0	3
0.09	S	35.7	6	1	0
0.09	N	29.4	7	1	1
0.10	S	35.7	6	0	0
0.10	T	18.3	5	0	0

[a] Except as noted, patients received lorazepam before lumbar puncture.
[b] Sedation was determined immediately after the procedure, according to the following scale: 0 = alert, 1 = transient lethargy, 2 = sleeping <50% of time since lorazepam given, 3 = sleeping >50% of time since lorazepam given, 4 = coma.
[c] Amnesia was determined 24 hours after the procedure, according to the following scale: 0 = recalls procedure and object without prompting, 1 = recalls either procedure or object without prompting, 2 = recalls either procedure or object with prompting, 3 = recalls neither procedure nor object, 4 = recalls nothing since procedure.
[d] Patient received lorazepam before bone marrow aspiration.
[e] N.D. = no data. Patient unavailable for amnesia assessment.

relation coefficients (r_s) were calculated. The a priori level of significance was <0.01.

Results

Table 1 contains demographic data, doses, and sedation and amnesia scores. Lorazepam was administered to 20 different patients with 28 entries into the study. Of the 28 entries, 27 involved outpatient clinic patients and 1 an inpatient. Ages of patients enrolled ranged from 4 to 17 years, with a mean of 6.5 years ($n = 28$) and a mode of 4 years ($n = 28$). Six of the 28 entries were for bone marrow aspiration and 22 were for lumbar puncture. One patient, patient L, could not be contacted for the 24-hour follow-up questions, so another patient was enrolled at the same dose. Doses for patients Q and R were assigned simultaneously; therefore, there were four patients at the 0.08-mg/kg level. All patients

Table 2.
Mean Scores for Sedation and Amnesia and Mean Number of Adverse Reactions at Each Lorazepam Dose[a]

Dose (mg/kg)	Mean Score		Mean No. Adverse Reactions
	Sedation[b]	Amnesia[c]	
0.02	0.33	0.00	0.00
0.03	1.33	0.33	0.33
0.04	1.00	0.67	1.33
0.05	0.67	0.33	0.67
0.06	0.25[d]	0.00	2.33
0.07	0.67	0.00	2.00
0.08	0.25[d]	1.00[d]	1.50[d]
0.09	0.67	1.33	2.67
0.10	0.00[e]	0.00[e]	2.50[e]

[a] $n = 3$ except as otherwise noted.
[b] Sedation was determined immediately after the procedure; scale is listed in Table 1 footnote b.
[c] Amnesia was determined 24 hours after the procedure; scale is listed in Table 1 footnote c.
[d] $n = 4$.
[e] $n = 2$.

undergoing bone marrow procedures received lidocaine as a local anesthetic. Among patients undergoing lumbar puncture, use of lidocaine for patient O was not recorded, patient K received lidocaine, and no local anesthetic was given for all other patient entries.

All patients remembered the toy immediately after the procedure. Table 2 shows the mean sedation scores, mean amnesia scores (determined a day after drug administration), and the mean number of adverse reactions noted at each dose level of lorazepam.

Values of r_s for dose versus mean amnesia score, dose versus mean sedation score, and the dose versus mean number of adverse reactions were 0.28 ($p > 0.05$), –0.20 ($p > 0.05$), and 0.66 ($p < 0.01$), respectively. The clinicians who performed the procedures rated patients to be sufficiently sedated for 24 (86%) of 28 procedures, with no apparent relationship to dose.

Adverse reactions among the 28 study entries occurred with the following frequencies: vomiting, 50%; ataxia or dizziness, 36%; nausea, 32%; blurred vision, 11%; increased (paradoxical) restlessness, 7%; muscle weakness, 4%; incontinence, 4%; and confusion, 4%. The frequency and degree of ataxia increased as doses were escalated. Ataxia was first judged to be excessive (dose-limiting) in patients S and T, who received 0.10 mg/kg. The study was terminated at that dose.

Discussion

Adverse Reactions. The mean number of adverse reactions appeared to rise steadily with dose ($r_s = 0.66$, $p < 0.01$). We did not, however, include the severity of adverse reactions in the statistical analysis. Our reported frequencies of adverse reactions represent the full range of lorazepam doses that we used. Because typical lorazepam doses can vary widely, we believe that the frequencies and types of reactions that we observed may be consistent with those generally seen in similar patient populations.

The frequencies of nausea and vomiting were high but may not have been related to lorazepam; patients and parents reported that nausea and vomiting were common after procedures when no premedicants were used.

Dizziness or ataxia also occurred frequently. These two adverse reactions were grouped together because of difficulty distinguishing them in many cases. It appeared that dizziness was more common at low doses and ataxia at higher doses; several patients who received low doses were dizzy for only a short time after lorazepam administration. The severity of ataxia was acceptable up to doses of 0.09 mg/kg, since parents and patients were willing to tolerate the ataxia with the perceived benefit. The dose of 0.10 mg/kg produced ataxia judged to be dose limiting and demonstrated no apparent increase in beneficial effects. We considered 0.09 mg/kg to be the maximum tolerated oral dose.

Sedation. Sedation did not increase at lorazepam doses higher than 0.03 mg/kg, and a dose–sedation relationship could not be confirmed. A dose of 0.03 to 0.05 mg/kg is consistent with those that induced sedation in studies by Relling et al.[4] and Burtles and Astley[2] in pediatric patients. Kothary et al.[7] reported 2 mg orally to be an optimal sedative dose in adults (approximately 0.03 mg/kg in a 70-kg adult), but found no dose–response relationship when sedation was rated by observers. In contrast, Shader et al.[8] found a dose–response relationship with self-rated sedation, although they agreed that adequate sedation could be obtained without impairment of consciousness or excessive drowsiness.

Our findings suggest that an oral lorazepam dose of 0.03 mg/kg provides adequate sedation, based on the sedation scale used, and leads to minimal adverse reactions in this population. However, the clinicians who performed the procedures in our study considered sedation to be sufficient 86% of the time, and sedation, in their judgment, showed little correlation with the sedation scale or with the dose. Patients were not asleep, but they generally lay more quietly and struggled less, even while expressing resistance verbally. This implies that a more meaningful scale is required, minimal sedation is adequate, or sedation alone is not an important effect in these patients.

Amnesia. We exposed children to a toy before the medical procedure with the anticipation that the toy would imprint well in the child's memory and would serve as an indicator that the current procedure was the one recalled 24 hours later. (All patients had had previous experience with the procedures.) All patients remembered the toy immediately after the procedure, verifying initial memory of the toy.

Some degree of amnesia occurred in 7 (25%) of the 28 procedures. In all seven cases, the patient could not recall having a procedure the day before. In five of these cases, the patient forgot the procedure but remembered the toy. In two episodes of amnesia, the patient remembered the toy from his or her first entry into the study at a lower dose (patients C and I). Patient C subsequently recalled the correct toy when prompted by the list of toys. Since patients remembered the toy better than the procedure, a shorter initial exposure to the toy may have resulted in better correlation with memory of the procedure. Since all patients had experienced the same procedure previously, it is possible that some patients may have remembered previous procedures along with the toy from the day before. This would cause lower mean amnesia scores (false negatives). An attempt to avoid this was made by asking for details of the previous day's procedure, but this information was used only if it confirmed memory of the procedure.

The highest mean amnesia score (1.33) occurred at 0.09 mg/kg, but overall the mean amnesia score did not correlate well with dose ($r_s = 0.28$). A dose–response relationship in a group of patients can therefore not be confirmed by this study. However, there was some evidence for a dose–response relationship in individual patients who had amnesia. Three patients (C, I, and N) had amnesia only on their second entries into the study at higher doses. One additional patient (H) had an amnesia score of 1 on his first entry and 3 on his second entry at a higher dose.

By using more sensitive tests of memory, Shader et al.[8] and Kothary et al.[7] have demonstrated a dose–response relationship with amnesia in adults receiving lorazepam. A higher frequency of amnesia has been documented in studies using standard clinical memory tests.[1-4] In our study it was evident that the frequency of anterograde amnesia of painful procedures is relatively low and difficult to predict. Therefore, it is important to individualize the dose, based on the first experience, if a second procedure is done. One might start with 0.03 to 0.05 mg/kg and adjust the dose up to the maximum tolerated dose of 0.09 mg/kg orally if necessary to achieve the desired level of amnesia.

Kothary et al.[7] suggested that the amnestic effect caused by benzodiazepines may be independent of the sedative effects. This is consistent with the differences in sedation and amnesia measured in this study. It is unknown whether sedation alone is adequate, or if amnesia is also desirable in premedicating children for painful procedures. Amnesia may be desirable, especially if the child will require a second painful procedure.

Conclusion

In children undergoing lumbar puncture or bone marrow aspiration, premedication with oral lorazepam 0.02–0.10 mg/kg generally produced adequate sedation for the procedure. The degree of sedation was not well correlated with dose. Amnesia, assessed 24 hours after lorazepam administration, was infrequent and not closely associated with dose. Doses higher than 0.09 mg/kg caused an unacceptable degree of ataxia and had no clinical advantage over lower doses.

References

1. Mundeleer P. Child premedication per os with lorazepam. *Acta Anaesthesiol Belg*. 1980; 31(Suppl):187-93.
2. Burtles R, Astley B. Lorazepam in children. *Br J Anaesth*. 1983; 55:275-9.
3. Milligan DW, Howard MR, Judd A. Premedication with lorazepam before bone marrow biopsy. *J Clin Pathol*. 1987; 40:696-8.
4. Relling MV, Mulhern RK, Dodge RK et al. Lorazepam pharmacodynamics and pharmacokinetics in children. *J Pediatr*. 1989; 114:641-6.
5. Oken MM, Creech RH, Tormey DC et al. Toxicity and response criteria of the Eastern Cooperative Oncology Group. *Am J Clin Oncol*. 1982; 5:649-55.
6. Miller AB, Hoogstraten B, Staquet M et al. Reporting results of cancer treatment. *Cancer*. 1981; 47:207-14.
7. Kothary SP, Brown ACD, Pandit UA et al. Time course of antirecall effect of diazepam and lorazepam following oral administration. *Anaesthesia*. 1981; 55:641-4.
8. Shader RI, Dreyfuss D, Gerrein JR et al. Sedative effects and impaired learning and recall after single oral doses of lorazepam. *Clin Pharmacol Ther*. 1986; 39:526-9.

Research Note

Infusion failure caused by phlebitis and extravasation

ALEX WRIGHT AND JOHN HECKER

Clin Pharm. 1991; 10:630-4

Peripheral intravenous infusions often fail prematurely because the i.v. fluid extravasates (infiltrates or "tissues") or the vein becomes phlebitic.[1] Such infusion failure causes discomfort to the patient and increases the workload for hospital staff. Repeated venipuncture reduces the number of venous access sites available for therapy.

Although extravasation has received comparatively little attention in the literature, many papers have described the incidence of phlebitis.[1] Several methods have been used to analyze data from these studies. The most common have been chi-square analysis and *t* tests. Because elective discontinuation of many infusions causes the number that remain (and therefore could fail) to decrease with time, statistical tests have often been performed on data collected at successive time intervals (usually every 12 or 24 hours) to compare incidences of failure.[2,3] Other studies have largely ignored the effects of time,[4-7] or else time to the diagnosis of phlebitis has been analyzed but differences in proportions of infusions developing phlebitis have been ignored.[8] Besides missing the point that elective discontinuation of infusions that are no longer needed reduces the number that potentially could fail, papers on phlebitis have tended to report numerous factors as being "significant" but have rarely attempted to identify interactions between factors.

A statistical technique known as survival analysis has been used to obtain information on diseases such as cancer. There is an analogy between infusions and cancer in that both failure of infusions and death from cancer occur over variable time periods during which there is continuous loss of subjects—through other causes of death for cancer patients and through elective removals for infusions. Survival analysis has been used only rarely for investigating failure of infusions,[9-11] and then mainly for assessing methods of reducing failure. It has rarely been used to evaluate prognostic factors.

There is evidence suggesting that the rate at which infusion fluids are given influences failure of intravenous sites.[12,13] If this is correct, then sites with low flow rates or sites that are used intermittently should have lower failure rates (should last longer). Published information on failure of intravenous sites deals largely with continuous infusions,[1] and less is known about failure of sites used for intermittent drug delivery. In this study we used survival analysis to identify factors in a typical hospital that are important in failure of infusion sites and to confirm the superior survival of intermittent infusions.

Methods. The study was approved by the ethics committee of Lidcombe Hospital, and patients gave oral informed consent. Information including patients' sex and age, time and site of cannulation, and type of intravenous device used was recorded on a standard form by nursing staff members for patients who had cannulas inserted into peripheral hand or arm veins. All patients who gave consent over a six-week period were studied. All cannulations were done by physicians. Sites were inspected each morning by the same nurse investigator, and relevant data including fluids and drugs infused, phlebitic signs, and times and reasons for cannula removal were recorded. Details of the history of sites during the previous 24 hours were obtained from the nursing staff and the patients' records. The duration of use of each site was calculated to the nearest hour from medical and nursing notes. Resited infusions were treated as new sites.

Infusion failure was defined as the occurrence of extravasation or the presence of two or more of the following signs of phlebitis: pain, tenderness on palpation, erythema, swelling, greater warmth than surrounding skin, and presence of a palpable venous cord (cording). Extravasation was diagnosed by marked swelling that subsided within a few hours after the infusion was stopped. Failure was initially analyzed by the life-table (product limit) method, with the level of significance of differences identified by the log-rank

ALEX WRIGHT is Lecturer in Nursing Studies, School of Nursing, Cumberland College and Lidcombe Hospital, Lidcombe, New South Wales, Australia. JOHN HECKER, PH.D., is Senior Lecturer in Physiology, Department of Physiology, The University of New England, Armidale, New South Wales.

Address reprint requests to Mr. Wright at the School of Nursing, Cumberland College, Lidcombe, N.S.W. 2141, Australia.

The assistance of Peter Bell, John Krummins, and other members of the senior nursing staff on the participating wards at Lidcombe Hospital is acknowledged.

test.[14] Cannulas that had been removed electively but had signs of phlebitis or extravasation were considered to have failed. Data about cannulas removed electively that did not have signs of failure were included in the survival analysis.

Life-table analysis calculates for each group of data a survival curve that represents the proportion of infusions surviving at any time. This curve necessarily decreases with time, and it represents the situation in which cannulas are not removed electively but are used until they fail. The half-life for a survival curve, then, is the time for 50% of infusions to fail. Another statistic, the relative risk of failure (RRF), is the ratio of the observed number of failures to the expected number of failures (calculated by life-table analysis). RRF values of less than 1 indicate lower than average failure. The failure ratio (ratio of two RRFs) is presented for paired comparisons, as this statistic is a measure of the magnitude of difference between pairs of failure curves (e.g., a value of 0.5 indicates that one type of infusion is half as likely to fail).

Because it is difficult to separate effects of different factors with univariate analysis alone, we used multivariate survival analysis to confirm the univariate results (BMDP Statistical Software, Los Angeles, CA 90025). The analysis used Cox's proportional hazards model with stepwise, maximum, partial-likelihood ratio selection of variables and default values. This analysis takes into account interactions between factors and selects factors in a stepwise manner until all of the factors selected have a probability of at least $p <$ 0.1. Otherwise, the a priori level of significance was <0.05.

Results. The study included 395 infusion sites in 313 patients. Nearly half (185) of the sites failed, with a half-life of 70 hours. The survival curve indicated few failures during the first day and then an approximately linear loss with time after two days (Figure 1). There was no significant difference when failed sites were divided into three subgroups representing those that failed because of phlebitis, those that extravasated, and those that extravasated with obvious phlebitic signs (Table 1).

Many cannulas were used to give drugs at 6-, 8-, or 12-hour intervals and were flushed with approximately 5 mL of heparin solution (100 units/mL in 0.9% sodium chloride injection) and capped until the next use (intermittent sites). Other cannulas were used to deliver fluid continuously (continuous infusions). A few continuous infusion sites were later used intermittently for short periods; use of these sites was considered to have been stopped when continuous flow was stopped.

Failure of intermittent infusions was significantly less than for continuous infusions (Table 1, Figure 2), with half-lives of 105 and 57 hours, respectively. No significant difference was found when the continuous infusions were divided into one group with one or more types of crystalloid fluids (0.9% sodium chloride, 5% dextrose, 4% dextrose plus 0.18% sodium chloride,

Figure 1. Overall survival of i.v. infusion sites (n = 395).

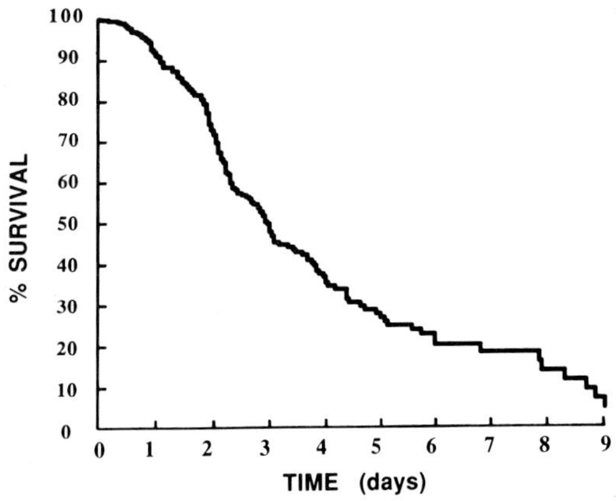

Table 1.
Effect of Selected Variables on Infusion Failure

Variable	No. Infusions	% Failure[a]	Relative Risk of Failure[b]
Infusion type			
Continuous	267	49	1.29
Intermittent	128	41	0.64[c]
Fluid type[d]			
Crystalloid	197	43	1.05
Crystalloid + potassium	50	68	0.93
Crystalloid + blood	20	65	0.89
Cannula type			
Angiocath	344	46	1.01
Dwellcath	51	51	0.94
Hospital service			
Surgical	179	47	1.43
Medical	216	47	0.80[c]
Side of cannula insertion			
Right	170	39	0.87
Left	225	52	1.09
Cannula site			
Hand	163	41	0.92
Wrist	164	50	1.04
Forearm	68	53	1.07
Patient age (yr)			
<56	132	44	1.25
56–71	130	48	0.98
>71	133	48	0.86
Patient sex			
Male	195	41	0.85
Female	200	53	1.16[e]
Cause of infusion failure			
Phlebitis	86	100	0.89
Extravasation	73	100	1.09
Both	26	100	1.22

[a] Failure was defined as the occurrence of extravasation, the presence of at least two signs of phlebitis, or both.

[b] Determined by univariate survival analysis. Relative risk of failure is the observed number of failures divided by the expected number of failures (as calculated by life-table analysis). A value of <1 indicates lower than average failure.

[c] Significantly different ($p < 0.001$, chi-square) from the other value for this type of variable.

[d] Only continuous infusions were analyzed.

[e] Significantly different ($p < 0.01$) from the other value for this type of variable.

Figure 2. Survival of continuous (n = 267) and intermittent (n = 128) i.v. infusion sites.

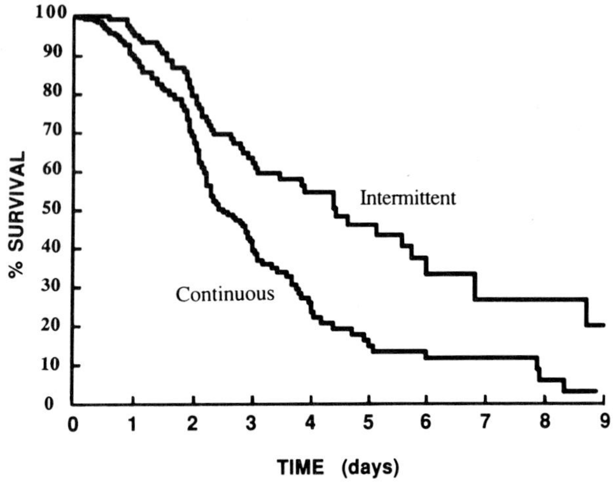

Table 2.
Effect of Drug Therapy on Infusion Failure

Drug(s)[a]	No. Associated Infusions	% Failure	Failure Ratio[b]
Any i.v. antimicrobial	110	61	1.14
Cephalosporins	53	68	1.32
Floxacillin	11	55	0.92
Gentamicin	22	77	1.50
Metronidazole	24	67	1.46
Penicillin or amoxicillin	35	49	0.86
Heparin, bolus	15	47	0.53
Heparin, continuous	18	39	0.46[c]
Heparin (subcutaneous)	63	59	1.07
Selected non-i.v. drugs[d]	95	38	0.57[e]
Anti-inflammatories (oral)	38	39	0.64
Nitrates (oral or percutaneous)	58	41	0.61[c]
Calcium-channel blockers (oral)	58	36	0.50[e]

[a] Unless otherwise noted, drugs were given through an i.v. cannula.
[b] Failure ratio (FR) is the relative risk of failure (RRF) for i.v. sites associated with a listed drug divided by the RRF for sites not associated with the same drug. A FR of <1 indicates better than average survival. RRF is the observed number of failures divided by the expected number of failures.
[c] Significant difference ($p < 0.05$, chi-square) between sites associated and not associated with the listed drug.
[d] Includes oral anti-inflammatory agents, oral and percutaneous nitrates, and oral nifedipine and verapamil.
[e] Significant difference ($p < 0.01$) between sites associated and not associated with the listed drug.

and Hartmann's [lactated Ringer's] solution), a second group with dextrose fluids with potassium (20–30 meq/L), and a third group of infusions with blood or packed cells (usually preceded or followed by crystalloid fluids).

Failure of sites was significantly greater in surgical patients than in medical patients and significantly greater in female than male patients. When sites were divided into three approximately equal groups on the basis of patient age, there was a slight but nonsignificant trend toward lower failure in older patients. The dorsum of the hand was the most common site, followed by the wrist and forearm (including a small number of antecubital cannulas), but there was no significant difference between these sites or between the right and left sides.

Two types of cannulas, Angiocaths (Tuta Labs, Lane Cove, Australia) and Dwellcaths (Terumo Ltd., North Ryde, Sydney, Australia), were used. The most common sizes were 20 gauge for the Angiocaths and 17 gauge for the Dwellcaths. Failure was not significantly different between these types.

The most common intravenous medications were antimicrobials, but there was no significant difference in failure when infusions with and without penicillin or amoxicillin, floxacillin, cephalosporins, aminoglycosides, or metronidazole were analyzed individually or as a group (Table 2). Failure was significantly less in patients who received a group of nonintravenous medications (concomitant medications) consisting of oral and percutaneous nitrates, calcium antagonists (oral nifedipine or verapamil) and oral anti-inflammatory agents such as aspirin and indomethacin. When the three types of medications in this group were analyzed individually, differences were significant when patients received calcium antagonists, nitrates, or both, but not when patients received oral anti-inflammatory agents.

Continuous intravenous heparin given at 18 sites for the treatment of deep-vein thrombosis was associated with significantly decreased failure. A trend to decreased failure when bolus doses of heparin were given for the same purpose was not significant; in 11 instances, heparin boluses were given via intermittent infusion sites, and the difference in failure rate was not significant when these were compared with intermittent sites not receiving heparin boluses. Subcutaneous heparin had no effect.

It was evident from inspection of the data that there were interactions between several of the factors (e.g., more males and more medical patients received intermittent infusions). Factors selected by multivariate analysis as having significant effects ($p < 0.10$) are type of infusion, diagnosis (medical or surgical), calcium antagonists, bolus and continuous i.v. heparin, and sex, although the significance levels for heparin and sex were marginal. Infusion survival was better for intermittent infusions, medical patients, males, and use of calcium antagonists or i.v. heparin.

Discussion. Although extravasation is commonly believed to be caused by the cannula dislodging from the vein or its tip piercing the vein wall, it is more likely to result from phlebitic processes caused by the infusate irritating the vein wall and inducing venoconstriction proximal to the cannula. Such venoconstriction markedly increases the pressure in the vein lumen in the vicinity of the cannula tip, and this tends to cause dilation of and then leakage through the hole made by the cannula.[13] One study showed that local percutaneous administration of nitroglycerin substantially reduced the frequency of infusion extravasation as well as cannula-associated phlebitis.[11] This result would be possible only if extravasation were usually associated with prior constriction of the vein. In the study with nitroglycerin, the magnitude of the decrease in failure was similar for both phlebitis and extravasation. In another study, there was also no difference in the life-table curves for infusions that failed from phlebitis and from extravasation.[12]

Extravasation is easily recognized by the local swelling when sites fail, but diagnosis of phlebitis can be more difficult because it depends on subjective assessment of inflammatory signs that can vary in severity. Several studies have used a scoring system that incorporates the number and severity of such signs,[15] but variation in severity may not be meaningful because its evaluation is influenced by the astuteness of nursing staff. Phlebitis usually results from chemical irritation of the vein wall by the infusate,[1,13] and so, if the infusion is allowed to continue and irritate the vein wall further, phlebitis will increase in severity after it first becomes apparent. Also, there can be marked differences in the assessment of the severity of phlebitic signs between assessors, although assessors usually agree on the presence or absence of phlebitis.[16,17]

Even though many infusions were ended electively, they were classed as failed if they fulfilled our criteria of having either extravasation or two or more phlebitic signs when the cannula was removed. It usually was not possible to determine if unfavorable signs had caused premature cessation of the infusion in elective removal, but the implication is that further use of any sites with two or more phlebitic signs would have been limited. The presence of a single phlebitic sign is a less reliable predictor of failure, since some patients complain of a "tender spot" that may be transitory, is often located at about the position of the cannula tip, and may occasionally be present from the start of an infusion.

The most significant variable found by both methods of analysis was whether the patient was treated by a medical or surgical service. Many medical patients (63%) but few surgical patients (13%) were receiving intermittent infusions. Also, more males (55%) than females (45%) received intermittent infusions. With such interactions, multivariate analysis is the more reliable method.

Animal experiments have shown that local drug-induced venodilation reduces the constrictive response of veins to irritation of the endothelium by infusates.[18] Therefore, it is possible that general vasodilation might also have an effect. Also, systemic anti-inflammatory agents could reduce the degree of irritation, because infusion failure is decreased when steroids are added to infusates.[2,19,20] Our univariate analyses suggested that peripheral vasodilation produced by systemic nitrates and calcium antagonists might decrease infusion failure, although only calcium antagonists were identified by the multivariate analysis.

It is commonly believed that antimicrobials cause infusions to fail, and some surveys have presented supporting data.[4] Our data suggest otherwise. They do, however, support the findings of other investigators that intravenous heparin decreases infusion failure.[2,6,19,21]

We found that whether an infusion was continuous or intermittent had a marked effect on infusion survival. There is little comparable information, but Ferguson et al.[22] found no clinical phlebitis before day 4 with heparin-lock (intermittent) cannulas, while van den Broek et al.[7] found comparatively little phlebitis with heparin-lock cannulas in comparison with continuous infusions. Vein walls are exposed to large volumes of infusate with continuous infusions and thus receive greater irritation.[13] In contrast, intermittent boluses of drugs flushed by a saline solution (with or without heparin) would be less irritant, and there are long periods after drugs are given for the endothelium to recover. Clinical considerations require that many patients receive continuous infusions, but for sites intended only for intermittent drug administration, flushing and capping cannulas after each use would be preferable to the common practice in many wards of using a slow continuous infusion to keep the cannula open.

These results are consistent with our contention[13] that fluids rather than drugs are the main cause of infusion failure, at least with continuous infusions. Crystalloid fluids are mildly acid, typically with pH values of 4.5, although the amounts of titratable acid are relatively small.[23,24] Their irritancy is illustrated by experiments showing that neutralization of fluids markedly prolongs survival of infusions.[19,25,26]

In clinical trials, effects of important confounding factors can be negated either by allocating patients to equal groups according to numbers with these factors or by analytical methods that use stratification to remove their effects. This study shows that relatively few factors need to be considered in experiments testing methods for reducing infusion failure.

Conclusion. I.V. infusion sites were more likely to remain usable when fluid administration was intermittent rather than continuous, when patients were male or were assigned to a medical service, and when patients received continuous i.v. heparin, oral calcium-channel blockers, or non-i.v. nitrates.

References

1. Lewis GBH, Hecker JF. Infusion thrombophlebitis. *Br J Anaesth*. 1985; 57:220-33.
2. Bassan MM, Sheikh-Hamad D. Prevention of lidocaine-infusion phlebitis by heparin and hydrocortisone. *Chest*. 1984; 84:439-41.
3. Holland RB, Leitt MWD, Steffen CM et al. Intravenous cannulas. *Med J Aust*. 1982; 2:86-8.
4. Carey MF, Hollywood D, Duignan JP. Peripheral intravenous cannulation and infusion therapy on a general surgical service—a prospective study. *Ir Med J*. 1986; 79:2-5.
5. Eremin O, Marshall V. Complications of intravenous therapy: reduction by buffering of intravenous fluid preparation. *Med J Aust*. 1977; 2:528-31.

6. Tanner WA, Delaney PV, Hennessy TP. The influence of heparin on intravenous infusions: a prospective study. *Br J Surg*. 1980; 67:311-2.
7. Van den Broek PJ, de Herder-Swinkels JMN, Moffie BG et al. The use of intravenous cannulae and the occurrence of thrombophlebitis. *J Hosp Infect*. 1989; 13:43-53.
8. Hershey CO, Tomford JW, McLaren CE et al. The natural history of intravenous catheter-associated phlebitis. *Arch Intern Med*. 1984; 144:1373-5.
9. Allcutt DA, Lort D, McCollum CN. Final inline filtration for intravenous infusions: a prospective hospital study. *Br J Surg*. 1983; 70:111-3.
10. Tully JL, Friedland GH, Baldini LM et al. Complications of intravenous therapy with steel needles and Teflon catheters. *Am J Med*. 1981; 70:702-6.
11. Wright A, Hecker JF, Lewis GBH. Use of transdermal glyceryl trinitrate to reduce failure of intravenous infusions due to phlebitis and extravasation. *Lancet*. 1985; 2:1148-50.
12. Hecker JF. Failure of infusions from extravasation and phlebitis. *Anaesth Intensive Care*. 1989; 17:433-9.
13. Hecker JF, Fisk GC, Lewis GBH. Phlebitis and extravasation ("tissuing") with intravenous infusions. *Med J Aust*. 1984; 140:659-60.
14. Peto R, Pike MC, Armitage P et al. Design and analysis of randomized clinical trials requiring prolonged observation of each patient. (ii) Analysis and examples. *Br J Cancer*. 1977; 35:1-29.
15. Medical Research Council Report: thrombophlebitis following intravenous infusions. *Lancet*. 1957; 1:595-7.
16. Collin J, Collin C, Constable FL et al. Infusion thrombophlebitis and infection with various cannulas. *Lancet*. 1975; 2:150-2.
17. Lewis GBH, Hecker JF. Infusion thrombophlebitis. *Br J Anaesth*. 1986; 58:466-7.
18. Lewis GBH, Hecker JF. Changes in local venous tone in response to infusions of saline and dextrose solutions. *Anaesth Intensive Care*. 1984; 12:27-32.
19. DeCock C, Vermeij P, Stijnen T. On the efficacy of low dose prednisolone and heparin sodium in the prevention of infusion thrombophlebitis: a double blind trial. *Pharm Weekbl [Sci]*. 1984; 6:88-90.
20. Polak A. Hydrocortisone in the prevention of transfusion thrombophlebitis. *Lancet*. 1956; 1:484.
21. Alpan G, Eyal F, Springer C et al. Heparinization of alimentation solutions administered through peripheral veins in premature infants: a controlled study. *Pediatrics*. 1984; 74:375-8.
22. Ferguson RL, Rosett W, Hodges GR et al. Complications with heparin-lock needles. *Ann Intern Med*. 1976; 85:583-6.
23. Mostert JW. The pH and osmolarity of intravenously used drugs. *JAMA*. 1971; 216:1483.
24. Tse RL. pH of infusion fluids: a predisposing factor in thrombophlebitis. *JAMA*. 1971; 215:642.
25. Bass J, Freeman JB, Makarewicz P et al. Preventing superficial phlebitis during infusion of crystalloid solutions in surgical patients. *Can J Surg*. 1985; 28:124-5.
26. Eremin O, Marshall V. Complications of intravenous therapy: reduction by buffering of intravenous fluid preparation. *Med J Aust*. 1977; 2:528-31.

DUE Criteria

The DUE Criteria *section of* Clinical Pharmacy *features model drug-use evaluation criteria that may be employed as a component of a comprehensive quality assurance program. The criteria sets are presented in the format used in the ASHP book* Criteria for Drug Use Evaluation. *Some of the criteria sets will have been originally published in that book; others will be presented here for the first time and published in future volumes of the ASHP book. The practitioners who developed a criteria set are acknowledged.*

In selecting drug products for coverage in DUE Criteria, *priority is given to products that have been recently marketed, those that are frequently prescribed, those that have high potential risk associated with their use, and those that are expensive. When feasible, a criteria set will be linked with a Drug Review that appears in the same issue.*

These criteria sets are a starting point for the development of DUE criteria for a specific practice setting. Readers are encouraged to modify the model criteria to fit their own circumstances.

Criteria for use of fentanyl citrate, sufentanil citrate, and alfentanil hydrochloride[a]

Element	Standard 100%	Standard 0%	Exception[b] or Critical Preventive/ Responsive Measure[c]	Sources of Information
Justification for Use				
Fentanyl, Sufentanil, and Alfentanil				
1. As analgesic during preoperative, induction, maintenance, and postoperative surgical periods[1–8] or	X		1A. None	1. Anesthesia records, preoperative notes, physician orders, nursing notes, progress notes
2. As opioid component of balanced anesthetic technique[3,4,6–8] or	X		2A. None	2. Anesthesia records, preoperative notes, physician orders, nursing notes, progress notes
3. As opioid supplement to general or regional anesthetic technique[1,3–9] or	X		3A. None	3. Anesthesia records, preoperative notes, physician orders, nursing notes, progress notes
4. To attenuate surgical stress response (e.g., increased heart rate or blood pressure, patient movement); administered with oxygen and neuromuscular blocking agent[4,6–11]	X		4A. None	4. Anesthesia records
Fentanyl and Sufentanil				
5. As complete anesthetic with oxygen in cardiothoracic, neurologic, or orthopedic surgery[1–4] or	X		5A. None	5. Anesthesia records, preoperative notes, physician orders, nursing notes, progress notes
6. As epidural analgesic for postoperative or labor pain[4,9–11]	X		6A. None	6. Anesthesia records, preoperative notes, physician orders, nursing notes, progress notes, labor and delivery records, recovery room records, medication administration record (MAR)

Prepared by Grant B. Satterlee, Pharm.D., Clinical Pharmacist, Surgery/Anesthesiology, Department of Pharmacy, University Medical Center, and Clinical Assistant Professor, College of Pharmacy, University of Florida Health Science Center/Jacksonville, and Irena A. Skora, M.D., Associate Professor of Anesthesiology and Associate Chairperson, Department of Anesthesiology, University of Florida Health Science Center/Jacksonville at University Medical Center.

Element	Standard 100%	Standard 0%	Exception[b] or Critical Preventive/ Responsive Measure[c]	Sources of Information
Fentanyl				
7. As epidural analgesic for cancer pain or other chronic pain[2,4] or	X		7A. None	7. Physician orders, nursing notes, progress notes, MAR
8. As opioid component of neurolept-analgesia[1,2,4] or	X		8A. None	8. Anesthesia records, preoperative notes, physician orders, nursing notes, progress notes
9. To prevent or relieve tachypnea or postoperative emergence delirium[3,9]	X		9A. None	9. Anesthesia records, preoperative notes, physician orders, nursing notes, progress notes
Alfentanil				
10. As alternative to fentanyl and sufentanil when used with inhalational oxygen via incremental i.v. bolus or continuous i.v. infusion in general surgery lasting $\leq$2 hr[7,8] or	X		10A. None	10. Anesthesia records, preoperative notes, physician orders, nursing notes, progress notes
11. To supplement fentanyl or sufentanil anesthesia as incremental i.v. bolus in general surgery during last 20 min of anticipated procedure time[7,8]	X		11A. None	11. Anesthesia records, preoperative notes, physician orders, nursing notes, progress notes
Critical (Process) Indicators				
12. Administered by personnel trained in opioid analgesic use, with resuscitation equipment and opioid antagonists available	X		12A. None	12. Anesthesia records, physician orders, progress notes, institutional policies and procedures
13. No history of hypersensitivity to opioid used	X		13A. None	13. History and physical (H&P), allergies, progress notes, anesthesia records
14. Outpatient warned not to perform tasks that require mental alertness or physical coordination for up to 48 hr after administration	X		14A. None	14. Progress notes, nursing notes
15. Blood pressure, pulse, and respiration monitored continuously during surgical procedure	X		15A. None	15. Anesthesia records, operating room (OR) records, nursing flow sheets, progress notes
16. Not administered for chronic pain control	X		16A. Fentanyl used for cancer pain or other chronic pain[2,4]	16, 16A. H&P, progress notes, physician orders
17. Appropriate dosage[1–11]: a. Fentanyl (as the citrate salt): 2–100 μg/kg i.v. or i.m. b. Sufentanil (as the citrate salt): 1–30 μg/kg i.v. or i.m. with 25–50-μg supplemental bolus doses c. Alfentanil (as the hydrochloride salt): 8–245 μg/kg i.v.	X		17A. Dosage individualized on basis of (1) anesthetic technique, (2) route of administration, (3) surgical procedure, (4) patient age, (5) patient weight, (6) patient clinical status, (7) renal and hepatic function, and (8) concomitant use of central nervous system depressants	17. Anesthesia records, preoperative notes, physician orders, MAR 17A. H&P, progress notes, anesthesia records, preoperative notes, MAR, physician orders, nursing notes, laboratory reports
Complications				
18. Withdrawal symptoms caused by abrupt discontinuation in opioid-dependent patient		X	18A. Provide supportive care	18. Progress notes, H&P, anesthesia records, nursing notes 18A. Progress notes, nursing notes, physician orders, MAR
19. Muscle rigidity (especially truncal)[2,4,7,9,10]		X	19A. Administer i.v. doses slowly (do not push)[4,9] 19B. Administer succinylcholine to terminate effect[9] 19C. Administer nondepolarizing muscle relaxant[9]	19. Anesthesia records, progress notes, nursing notes 19A–C. Anesthesia records, physician orders, progress notes
20. Hypertension during surgical procedure[9]		X	20A. If due to stress, increase dose if possible[9] 20B. Administer vasodilator (e.g., sodium nitroprusside)[4,9] 20C. Consider sedative or hypnotic[9]	20. Anesthesia records, OR records, progress notes 20A–C. Anesthesia records

Element	Standard 100%	Standard 0%	Exception[b] or Critical Preventive/ Responsive Measure[c]	Sources of Information
21. Nausea and vomiting		X	21A. Provide supportive and symptomatic care	21. Anesthesia records, progress notes, nursing notes 21A. Anesthesia records, physician orders, nursing notes
22. Hypotension[9]		X	22A. Administer i.v. doses slowly[9] 22B. Provide supportive care, such as giving i.v. fluid bolus or putting patient in Trendelenburg's position[9]	22, 22A, B. Anesthesia records, OR records, physician orders, nursing notes, progress notes
23. Bradycardia[9]		X	23A. Administer i.v. doses slowly[9] 23B. Administer atropine or glycopyrrolate[9] 23C. Administer pancuronium bromide (0.5–2 mg i.v.)[9]	23, 23A–C. Anesthesia records, OR records, physician orders, nursing notes, progress notes
24. Apnea or respiratory depression[4,9]		X	24A. Administer oxygen[9] 24B. As needed, stimulate patient to breathe, maintain patent airway, and assist or control respiration mechanically[9] 24C. Administer opioid antagonist[9] 24D. Monitor patient postoperatively[9]	24, 24A–D. Nursing notes, progress notes, anesthesia records, OR records
Outcome Measures				
25. Analgesia, as measured by subjective reports of pain relief or objective measures of decreased stress response[9]	X		25A. None	25. Nursing notes, progress notes, anesthesia records
26. Adequate anesthesia, as measured by smooth, steady induction course and emergence, including sedation, amnesia, and analgesia[9]	X		26A. None	26. Nursing notes, progress notes, anesthesia records

[a] Criteria address justifications for use (indications), critical (process) indicators, complications of therapy, and patient outcome. Each criterion consists of an element, a standard, exceptions to the standard, and sources of information. The element is the minimum level of evidence needed to show that patient care was optimal. The standard defines the deviation from an element that is acceptable. If no deviation is acceptable, the standard is 100%. Exceptions are circumstances in which deviation is allowable. Sources of information listed are the most reliable sources. Sources pertaining to an element or exception are identified by the number assigned to the element or exception (e.g., 18, 18A).

[b] For justification for use and critical (process) indicators.

[c] For complications and outcome measures.

References

1. Elkins-Sinn. Fentanyl package insert. Cherry Hill, NJ; 1984 Aug.
2. Gelman CR, Rumack BH, eds. Fentanyl drug evaluation monograph. (Drugdex System, vol. 62.) Denver: Micromedex; 1989.
3. Janssen Pharmaceutica. Sufenta package insert. Piscataway, NJ; 1984 Jun.
4. AHFS drug information 89. McEvoy GK, ed. Bethesda, MD: American Society of Hospital Pharmacists; 1989:1031–2,1048–9.
5. Janssen Pharmaceutica. Alfenta package insert. Piscataway, NJ; 1987 Mar.
6. Gelman CR, Rumack BH, eds. Alfentanil drug evaluation monograph. (Drugdex System, vol. 62.) Denver: Micromedex; 1989.
7. Reitz JA. Alfentanil in anesthesia and analgesics. *Drug Intell Clin Pharm*. 1986; 20:335–41.
8. Larijani GE, Goldberg ME. Alfentanil hydrochloride: a new short-acting narcotic analgesic for surgical procedures. *Clin Pharm*. 1987; 6:275–82.
9. Bailey PL, Stanley TH. Pharmacology of intravenous narcotic anesthetics. In: Miller RD, ed. Anesthesia. 2nd ed. New York: Churchill Livingstone; 1986: 745–97.
10. Monk JP, Beresford R, Ward A. Sufentanil: a review of its pharmacological properties and therapeutic use. *Drugs*. 1988; 36:286–313.
11. Rosow CE. Sufentanil citrate: a new opioid analgesic for use in anesthesia. *Pharmacotherapy*. 1984; 4:11–9.

CP Continuing Education

The ASHP Continuing Education System gives readers a self-assessment mechanism for selected articles in Clinical Pharmacy *and* AJHP. *It allows readers to obtain continuing-education credit for these articles.*

For the purpose of CE-credit enrollment, a blank answer sheet is published at the end of each installment of the column for the CE articles in that issue. An enrollee accumulates these answer sheets until the enrollment is submitted, using the form that is published in the June and December issues of Clinical Pharmacy *and in the June and December issues of* AJHP. *Any combination of tests within an 18-month period, from both* Clinical Pharmacy *and* AJHP, *may be included in an enrollment. More complete details about enrollment in the system appear in the semiannual enrollment form.*

Article 680-204-9114 (see page 581)
Qualifies for 1.0 hour of CE credit

Clinical uses of fentanyl, sufentanil, and alfentanil

Learning Objectives

After studying this article, the reader should be able to

1. Compare and contrast the pharmacokinetic profiles of fentanyl, alfentanil, and sufentanil.
2. Describe the effects that different types of surgery and hepatic and renal dysfunction have on the pharmacokinetics of these agents.
3. Describe the adverse effects of fentanyl, alfentanil, and sufentanil and suggest strategies to avoid them.
4. Recommend an appropriate opioid agent for anesthesia, analgesia, or sedation in a given patient.
5. List three possible indications for oral transmucosal or transdermal dosage forms of fentanyl.

Self-assessment Questions

For each question there is only one best answer.

1. Which of the following statements is (are) true regarding the pharmacokinetics of alfentanil, sufentanil, and fentanyl?
   a. All the fentanyl derivatives are highly bound to plasma proteins.
   b. Alfentanil has the smallest volume of distribution of the agents and fentanyl the largest.
   c. Differences in the distribution of these agents can be attributed to their physicochemical properties.
   d. All of the above alternatives are correct.
   e. None of the above alternatives is correct.

2. Which of the following statements about alteration of the pharmacokinetics of alfentanil, sufentanil, and fentanyl is correct?
   a. Changes in hepatic blood flow secondary to abdominal surgery should have no effect on fentanyl clearance.
   b. Concentrations of fentanyl and sufentanil markedly decrease after cardiopulmonary bypass surgery begins.
   c. Premature neonates have a significantly higher total body clearance of these drugs.
   d. Compared with adults, infants and children have the same total body clearance.
   e. None of the above alternatives is correct.

3. Alfentanil, sufentanil, and fentanyl differ in
   a. Onset of action.
   b. Analgesic efficacy.
   c. Ability to block the hormonal stress response to surgical stimulation.
   d. Ability to produce complete amnesia.
   e. Alternatives a and c are both correct.

4. The adverse-effect profiles of alfentanil, sufentanil, and fentanyl do not include
   a. Facial itching.
   b. Nausea and vomiting.
   c. Bone marrow suppression.
   d. Bradycardia.
   e. Chest wall rigidity.

5. The order of analgesic potency (least to most potent) is
   a. Fentanyl, alfentanil, sufentanil.
   b. Alfentanil, fentanyl, sufentanil.
   c. Fentanyl, sufentanil, alfentanil.
   d. Sufentanil, alfentanil, fentanyl.
   e. The three agents are equally potent.

6. Which of the following statements describe(s) the use of opioid anesthesia for cardiovascular procedures?
   a. High-dose morphine has been replaced by sufentanil and fentanyl as the opioid of choice.
   b. Sufentanil seems slightly better than fentanyl in preventing hypertensive responses to sternotomy.
   c. Alfentanil and fentanyl seem equivalent in their ability to provide hemodynamic stability during cardiovascular procedures.
   d. All of the above alternatives are correct.
   e. None of the above alternatives is correct.

Support the international community of pharmacy through membership in the

International Pharmaceutical Federation (F.I.P.)

What is F.I.P.?

F.I.P. is the international organization of pharmacists and pharmaceutical scientists. Founded in Holland in 1912, F.I.P. is an independent organization that has grown to represent pharmacists of all disciplines.

What are the goals of F.I.P.?

To further the development of pharmacy as a profession and as an applied science, and to extend the role of the pharmacist in health care.

Who are the members of F.I.P.?

Professional and scientific societies and associations; individual pharmacists and pharmaceutical scientists; pharmaceutical groups (libraries, regional societies, pharmacy faculty, pharmaceutical companies); and commercial and industrial companies.

Why become a member of F.I.P.?

When you support F.I.P. you become involved with international health issues. You have an opportunity to network globally. You can achieve international recognition. And you'll receive the *International Pharmacy Journal* and a newsletter for each section you join.

Joining is easy — just complete the application and mail with your dues to ASHP (ASHP will handle the conversion to Dutch currency).

To find out more about the upcoming Pharmacy World Congress '91, to be held in Washington, DC September 1 - 6, fill out return the coupon below.

F.I.P. Application Form

☐ Please register me as an associate individual member of the International Pharmaceutical Federation (F.I.P.). Dues are $47.00.

☐ In addition, I would like to become a member of the following section(s):

___ Hospital Pharmacists Section ($12.00)
___ Section for Community Pharmacists ($18.00)
___ Section for the Study of Medicinal Plants ($15.00)
___ Section for Official Laboratories and Medicines Control Services ($9.00)
___ Industrial Pharmacists' Section ($9.00)
___ Press and Documentation Section ($9.00)
___ Academic Section ($9.00)
___ Section on Clinical Biology (no fee)
___ Military Pharmacists' Section (no fee)

☐ I have totaled my fees and enclose payment of $ ____________.

Method of Payment (check one):

☐ VISA ☐ MasterCard ☐ Personal check (made payable to ASHP-F.I.P. and drawn on a U.S. bank)

Account # ____________ Exp. date ______ *month/year*

Name ____________

Address ____________ *(include name of institution if this is a business address)*

____

City ______ State ____ Zip ____ Country ______

Please return to:
ASHP Customer Service Dept.
4630 Montgomery Avenue
Bethesda, MD 20814
FAX: 301-657-1251

To process your application by phone, call ASHP Customer Service at 301-657-4383. Please have your VISA, MasterCard, or purchase order number ready.

Please send me information on the F.I.P. Pharmacy World Congress '91.

Name ____________

Address ____________

City ____________

State ______ Zip ______

Country ____________

Send to:
Pharmacy World Congress '91
P. O. Box 19384
Washington, DC 20036-0384
USA

Current Literature

Drug Reaction Alerts 644

Book Reviews

Biopharmaceutics and Clinical Pharmacokinetics, Fourth Edition 649
By Milo Gibaldi
Reviewed by Donald G. Floriddia

Drug Safety in Pregnancy 650
Edited by Peter I. Folb and M. N. Graham Dukes
Reviewed by Don Uden

Books Received 650

Drug Reaction Alerts

Drug Reaction Alerts focuses primarily on serious, unlabeled reactions to new chemical entities. The citations are compiled monthly from International Pharmaceutical Abstracts, *which covers over 800 pharmacy and health-related journals worldwide. An address for reprints (when available) follows the name of the corresponding author of each citation.*

Pharmacists may use the FDA Adverse Reaction Report form that appears in most issues of Clinical Pharmacy *for submitting reports of adverse drug reactions directly to FDA.*

Abortifacients

Byrne P, Onyekwuluje T (Department of Obstetrics and Gynecology, Walsgrave Hospital, Coventry CV2 2DX, England). Uterine rupture after termination of pregnancy with **gemeprost**. *Br Med J.* 1991; 302:852. Case. (27-year-old pregnant woman in week 22 of gestation with no risk factors for uterine rupture; received gemeprost 1 mg every hour for five doses as a vaginal suppository for abortion; developed shock, and uterine contractions ceased without vaginal bleeding; surgical removal of fetus and repair of uterine rupture led to recovery)

Antidepressants

Masand P, Gupta S, Dewan M (State University of New York Health Science Center, Syracuse, NY 13210). Suicidal ideation related to **fluoxetine** treatment. *N Engl J Med.* 1991; 324:420. Cases. (58-year-old man and 28-year-old woman who were admitted to hospital for treatment of depression; man received fluoxetine 20 mg/day for three days for treatment of depression refractory to imipramine therapy; woman received fluoxetine 20 mg/day for two months as an outpatient and increased to 60 mg/day over one week in the hospital; man attempted suicide; woman had recurrent suicidal thoughts; withdrawal of fluoxetine led to disappearance of suicidal ideation within 10 days)

Anti-inflammatory Agents

Smith DL, Wernick R (Department of Medical Education, Providence Medical Center, Oregon Health Sciences University, Portland, OR 97201). Exacerbation of psoriasis by chrysotherapy. *Arch Dermatol.* 1991; 127:268-70. Case. (54-year-old man with rheumatoid arthritis and history of psoriasis; received doses of **gold sodium thiomalate** totaling 285 mg over seven weeks by i.v. injection; led to exacerbation of psoriasis; withdrawal of gold sodium thiomalate for one week led to resolution of symptoms; positive rechallenge)

Antineoplastic Agents

Lipshultz SE (Department of Cardiology, Children's Hospital, 300 Longwood Ave., Boston, MA 02115), Colan SD, Gelber RD et al. Late cardiac effects of **doxorubicin** therapy for acute lymphoblastic leukemia in childhood. *N Engl J Med.* 1991; 324:808-15. Study. (retrospective study; 115 patients, aged 3.9–31.7 years, who received doxorubicin 1–15 years earlier for treatment of lymphoblastic leukemia and in whom the disease was in continuous remission at time of study; 18 patients received doxorubicin 45 mg/sq m one time only; 97 patients received multiple doses of doxorubicin totaling 228–550 mg/sq m; median time interval between end of treatment and cardiac evaluation, 6.4 years; cumulative dose of doxorubicin was most significant predictor of abnormal cardiac function; 17% of patients who received one dose only of doxorubicin had slightly elevated left ventricular afterload; 65% of patients who received a cumulative doxorubicin dose ≥228 mg/sq m had increased ventricular afterload or decreased contractility, or both; 10% of patients developed congestive heart failure within one year of treatment)

Wagner RF, Sanchez RL (Departments of Dermatology and Pathology, University of Texas Medical Branch, Galveston, TX 77550). Presentation of sebaceous carcinoma and dermatofibrosarcoma protuberans subsequent to intralesional **interferon alfa-2b** for the treatment of in situ squamous cell carcinoma. *Arch Dermatol.* 1991; 127:272. Cases. (two men, aged 59 and 71 years, with in situ squamous cell carcinoma; received interferon alfa-2b 1.5 million units three times weekly for three weeks by intralesional injections; 59-year-old man developed dermatofibrosarcoma protuberans of scalp, and 71-year-old man developed sebaceous carcinoma of nasal root; surgical resection of new tumors led to resolution of new malignancies)

Antituberculars

Nunn P (Wellcome Trust Research Laboratory, P.O. Box 43640, Nairobi, Kenya), Kibuga D, Gathua S et al. Cutaneous hypersensitivity reactions due to thiacetazone in HIV-1 seropositive patients treated for tuberculosis. *Lancet.* 1991; 337:627-30. Study. (227 patients, 93 of whom were seropositive for human immunodeficiency virus [HIV], who had received initial antitubercular therapy with streptomycin, isoniazid, and **amithiozone**; 60 patients of the initial 227, 17 of whom were HIV-seropositive, received streptomycin, isoniazid, rifampin, and pyrazinamide in initial phase of study and amithiozone and isoniazid in continuation phase; 20% of HIV-seropositive patients and 1% of HIV-seronegative patients developed cutaneous hypersensitivity reactions; 18 of 93 HIV-seropositive patients who received initial therapy with streptomycin, isoniazid, and amithiozone developed reactions; 0 of 17 HIV-seropositive patients who received therapy in the initial and continuation phases of the study [no amithiozone] developed reactions; negative rechallenge with isoniazid and streptomycin; positive rechallenge for amithiozone in 6 of 7 HIV-seropositive patients tested)

Antivirals

Tadini G, D'Orso M, Cusini M et al. (Cinque P, Department of Infectious Diseases, University of Milan, Via Pace 9, 20122 Milan, Italy). Oral mucosa pigmentation: a new side effect of azidothymidine therapy in patients with acquired immunodeficiency syndrome. *Arch Dermatol.* 1991; 127:267-8. Cases. (two men, aged 36 and 47 years, with human immunodeficiency virus infection; received **zidovudine** 800 mg/day; developed pigmented lesions of oral mucosa after approximately 15 days and two months, respectively; withdrawal of zidovudine led to decrease in color of lesions in one man; positive rechallenge)

Corticosteroids

Greenbaum SS (Department of Dermatology, Thomas Jefferson University, Suite 4019, 111 S. 11th St., Philadelphia, PA 19107). Corticosteroid-induced juxta-articular adiposis dolorosa. *Arch Dermatol.* 1991; 127:231-3. Case. (67-year-old woman with eosinophilia–myalgia syndrome; received **prednisone** 60 mg/day increased to 80 mg/day after six weeks; developed symptoms of adiposis dolorosa four weeks later; tapering of prednisone dose to 30 mg on alternate days led to gradual resolution of symptoms and complete disappearance of lesions after four months)

Drug Abuse

McGuire P (Maudsley Hospital, London SE5 8SJ, England), Fahy T. Chronic paranoid psychosis after misuse of MDMA (ecstasy). *Br Med J.* 1991; 302:697. Cases. (two men, aged 22 and 28 years, who abused **methylenedioxymethamphetamine** for at least 18 months; developed chronic paranoid psychosis; 22-year-old man used concomitant cannabis, cocaine, and lysergide; 28-year-old man used concomitant cocaine; treatment of 22-year-old with haloperidol led to gradual improvement and discharge from hospital; suffered two relapses during next seven months; treatment of 28-year-old man with sulpiride led to some improvement but no hospital discharge)

Immunotherapy

Horn TD, Burke PJ, Karp JE et al. Intravenous administration of recombinant human **granulocyte-macrophage colony-stimulating factor** causes a cutaneous eruption. *Arch Dermatol.* 1991; 127:49-52. Cases. (three patients, aged 25–49 years, after antileukemic therapy; received granulocyte–macrophage colony-stimulating factor; 26-year-old woman and 49-year-old man received granulocyte–macrophage colony-stimulating factor 5 μg/kg/day by continuous i.v. infusion for 13 and 15 days, respectively, and 25-year-old woman received an unstated dosage by continuous i.v. infusion for at least 10 days; developed widespread, erythematous skin eruption; skin tissue biopsies from women showed variable mixture of granulocytes and lymphocytes, increased number and size of dermal macrophages, mild-to-moderate epidermal exocytosis, intercellular edema, and rare dyskeratotic keratinocytes)

Platelet-Aggregation Inhibitors

Page Y, Tardy B (Department of Emergency Medicine, Hôpital Bellevue, Bd Pasteur, 42023 St. Etienne, France), Zeni F et al. Thrombotic thrombocytopenic purpura related to **ticlopidine**. *Lancet.* 1991; 337:774-6. Cases. (four patients, aged 47–75 years; received ticlopidine 500 mg/day for 3–8 weeks; developed thrombotic thrombocytopenic purpura [TTP]; time period for development of TTP in same range as latent period before appearance of ticlopidine-induced neutropenia; no relapse during 4–43 months of follow-up in three surviving patients)

Respiratory Smooth-Muscle Relaxants

Schlieper A (Department of Psychology, Children's Hospital of Eastern Ontario, 401 Smyth Rd., Ottawa, Ontario, Canada K1H 8L1), Alcock D, Beaudry P et al. Effect of therapeutic plasma concentrations of **theophylline** on behavior, cognitive processing, and affect in children with asthma. *J Pediatr.* 1991; 118:449-55. Study. (double-blind, randomized, crossover study; 31 children, aged 8–12 years, with moderate asthma; randomly assigned to 10-day regimen of theophylline anhydrous extended-release at dose to maintain therapeutic blood concentrations; results of parents' and schoolteachers' ratings of children's attention and activity levels showed no effect by theophylline; results of children's self-reports of mood changes showed no effect by theophylline; no significant differences for measures of cognitive processing; large individual differences in sensitivity to theophylline effects)

Toxicity

Hong R (1329 Lusitana St., Suite 306, Honolulu, HI 96813), Matsuyama E, Nur K. Cardiomyopathy associated with the smoking of crystal **methamphetamine**. *JAMA.* 1991; 265:1152-4. Cases. (two women, aged 31 and 34 years, who smoked crystalline methamphetamine; 31-year-old woman noted mal-

Continued on page 649

IN
IMMUNOCOMPETENT
PATIENTS

IT'S A
CONCERN

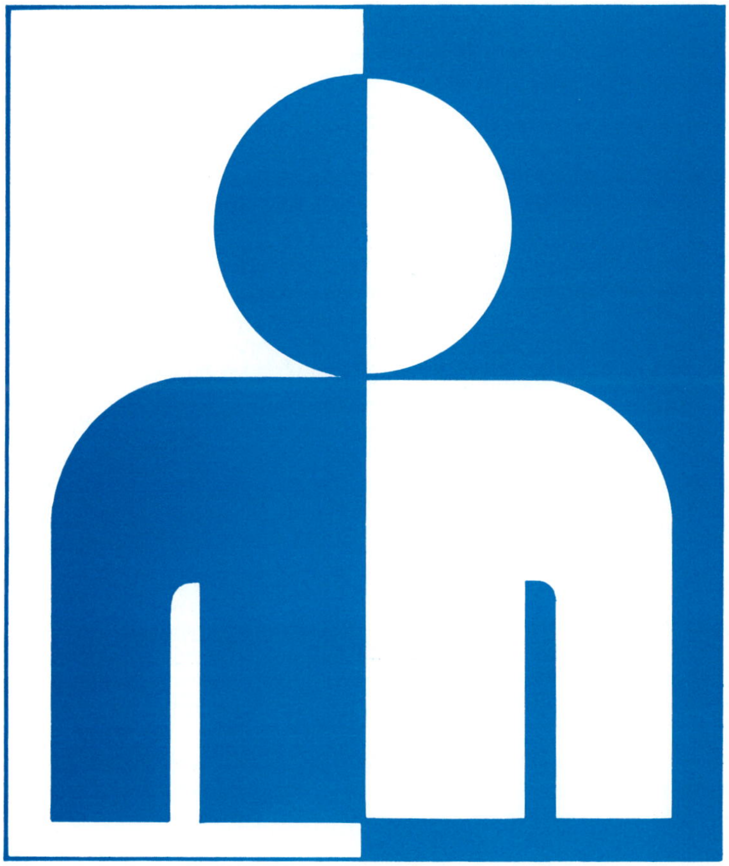

IN
IMMUNOCOMPROMISED
PATIENTS

IT'S A
MAJOR PROBLEM

Current Literature *Continued from page 645*

aise and had absent pulses in all extremities; diagnosed with diffuse peripheral vasospasm; experienced myocardial infarction and developed cardiogenic shock; therapy with methylprednisolone and sodium nitroprusside did not lead to improvement and patient died; 34-year-old woman developed severe respiratory distress; therapy with oxygen, diuretics, digoxin, sodium nitroprusside, captopril, and anticoagulants led to recovery)

Raschke R, Arnold-Capell PA (Department of Pharmacy, Good Samaritan Regional Medical Center, 1111 E. McDowell Rd., Phoenix, AZ 85006), Richeson R et al. Refractory hypoglycemia secondary to topical salicylate intoxication. *Arch Intern Med.* 1991; 151:591-3. Case. (72-year-old man with psoriasis; applied 10% **salicylic acid** cream three times daily to 80% of body surface area for approximately four weeks; developed severe, refractory hypoglycemia and appeared confused; therapy with oral fruit juices, meals, and dextrose by i.v. injection did not lead to resolution of symptoms; withdrawal of salicylic acid cream, cleansing of body surface areas, therapy with sodium bicarbonate, and hemodialysis for six hours led to decrease in blood salicylate concentration from 3.2 to 1.2 and resolution of hypoglycemia and confusion)

Book Reviews

Biopharmaceutics and Clinical Pharmacokinetics, Fourth Edition

By Milo Gibaldi.
Published by Lea & Febiger, 200 Chester Field Parkway, Malvern, PA 19355-9725, 1990. x + 406 p. Price $35.

Significant progress in the area of biopharmaceutics and clinical pharmacokinetics has occurred since the third edition of this book was published in 1984. The fourth edition of Gibaldi's *Biopharmaceutics and Clinical Pharmacokinetics* is an excellent textbook for the discipline of biopharmaceutics and pharmacokinetics; it includes material that exposes the reader to many of the advances in the discipline.

The 15 chapters discuss various aspects of drug absorption, distribution, metabolism, and excretion, including biologic and physicochemical considerations, drug concentration and clinical response, prolonged-release medication, bioavailability, and pharmacokinetic variability. Chapter 2 provides a good review of compartmental pharmacokinetics and introduces methods that permit drug analysis using noncompartmental pharmacokinetics. Figures and tables have been judiciously used throughout the book. For the most part, the chapters are essentially unchanged from the previous edition; however, I commend the author for incorporating recent advances and references into the text. Two appendixes explain some key relationships in pharmacokinetics, but the amount of information provided is limited.

In summary, this book is a valuable collection of information about the current state of the art with regard to biopharmaceutics and pharmacokinetics. Individual chapters are well documented with references, and there are ample numbers of diagrams, figures, and tables that nicely illustrate the basic concepts. Having an understanding of the basic principles of biopharmaceutics and

Continued on page 650

Continued from page 649

pharmacokinetics before reading this book would be helpful to the reader, but it is very readable and not likely to turn off any health-care professional who desires to learn about this discipline. I highly recommend this book to pharmacists, clinicians, scientists, and other individuals who are involved in the clinical evaluation and use of drugs.

Reviewed by Donald G. Floriddia, Ph.D., School of Pharmacy, University of the Pacific, 3601 Pacific Avenue, Stockton, CA 95211.

Drug Safety in Pregnancy

Edited by Peter I. Folb and M. N. Graham Dukes.

Published by Elsevier Science Publishers B.V., P.O. Box 211, 1000 AE Amsterdam, the Netherlands, 1990. xxi + 520 p. Price $243.

Hospital pharmacists are frequently asked about the potential effects and safety of drugs taken during pregnancy. The editors state that the goal of this book is "to provide a comprehensive and critical examination of the literature pertaining to the safety of medicines for the fetus and for the pregnant woman." To this end, the book meets the reader's expectations.

The chapters are organized by drug category, starting with the human teratogen thalidomide and proceeding to in-depth discussions of drugs of abuse, neurological drugs, cardiovascular drugs, antibiotics, anti-inflammatory agents, vaccines, hematologic drugs, hormonal agents, and new cytotoxic and immunosuppressive agents. An interesting and valuable aspect of this book is the critical review of studies regardless of positive or negative outcome; the studies are reviewed with respect to design and interpretation of results. The authors also briefly discuss studies that were "considered, but not included" because of flaws in study design or interpretation of results. Each chapter contains concluding or summary statements based on the author's interpretation of the data presented. This book is extensively referenced, and discussions of animal studies are included to corroborate human-derived data when appropriate.

The final 140 pages include 14 appendixes (nine in the form of tables) that are arranged by affected organ system. This classification scheme makes it very easy to focus on and locate specific fetal abnormalities, including genitourinary system abnormalities; polydactyly or syndactyly; bone abnormalities; limb-reduction deformities; anencephaly, exencephaly, or spina bifida; congenital cardiac abnormalities; hearing loss or microtia; congenital ocular abnormalities; and oral clefts. The tables are easy to use and present information from individual studies (e.g., drug of interest, number of study and control cases, description of drug-associated abnormality, concomitant drugs, statistical significance of the comparison, comments about the study).

Three appendixes address the effects of x-radiation exposure, behavioral teratology (i.e., postnatal behavioral changes that result from prenatal trauma), and prenatal attempted suicide with drugs. Two appendixes discuss the general principles of drug kinetics during pregnancy and evaluation and prediction of drug safety.

The book's index uses drug names and adverse effects, and references to *Meyler's Side Effect of Drugs* are found throughout the text.

Drug Safety in Pregnancy is well written and provides a substantial amount of information in one place. This book should be included in any medical library, hospital pharmacy, or health-care organization that serves obstetric patients.

Reviewed by Don Uden, Pharm.D., FCCP, Director of Research, Minneapolis Children's Medical Center, 2525 Chicago Avenue South, Minneapolis, MN 55404.

Books Received

Books are listed as soon as received; selected books may be reviewed in Book Reviews in subsequent issues.

The Cytotoxics Handbook, edited by Michael Allwood and Patricia Wright. Published by Radcliffe Medical Press Ltd, 15 Kings Meadow, Ferry Hinksey Road, Oxford OX2 0DP, England, 1990. x + 239 p. Price $75, £29.50.

Diseases of the Nose, Throat, Ear, Head, and Neck, Fourteenth Edition, by John Jacob Ballenger. Published by Lea & Febiger, 200 Chester Field Parkway, Malvern, PA 19355-9725, 1991. xvi + 1376 p. Price $195.

Drugs in Use: Clinical Case Studies for Pharmacists, edited by Linda J. Dodds. Published by The Pharmaceutical Press, 1 Lambeth High Street, Lone SE1 7JN, England, 1991. ix + 210 p. Price £15.00.

Hunter's Tropical Medicine, Seventh Edition, by G. Thomas Strickland. Published by W. B. Saunders, The Curtis Center, Independence Square West, Philadelphia, PA 19106-3399, 1991. xxix + 1153 p. Price $150.

A Practical Approach to Infectious Diseases, Third Edition, by Richard E. Reese and Robert F. Betts. Published by Little, Brown and Company, 34 Beacon Street, Boston, MA 02108, 1991. xvi + 1044 p. Price $55.

Regional Antineoplastic Drug Delivery in the Management of Malignant Disease, by Maurie Markman. Published by The Johns Hopkins University Press, 701 West 40th Street, Suite 275, Baltimore, MD 21211, 1991. xii + 143 p. Price $50.

Advertising Index

American Society of Hospital Pharmacists
American Journal of Hospital Pharmacy, 629
Criteria for Drug Use Evaluation, Volumes 1 and 2, 640
European Drug Index, 580
Pocket Guide to Injectable Drugs, 1991 Edition, 574
Burroughs Wellcome Company
Exosurf Neonatal, 575-579
Zovirax I.V., 646-648
International Pharmaceutical Federation (F.I.P.)
Membership, 643
Roerig, A Division of Pfizer Pharmaceuticals
Diflucan, inside front cover
Roche Laboratories, Division of Hoffmann-La Roche, Inc.
Rocephin, inside back cover, outside back cover
Toledo Hospital
Positions Available, 649
Wyeth-Ayerst Laboratories, Inc.
Ativan Injection, 570-572

News

CDC publishes guidelines for anergy testing in HIV-infected persons 653

Intravenous quinidine recommended for severe *Plasmodium falciparum* malaria; injectable quinine discontinued by CDC Drug Service 653

Single large dose of intravenous immune globulin more effective than four-day regimen in patients with Kawasaki disease, investigators report 657

News Briefs 657

Upcoming Specialty Meetings 657

CDC publishes guidelines for anergy testing in HIV-infected persons

The Centers for Disease Control has developed guidelines for evaluation and management of patients who may have tuberculous infection and anergy, caused by human immunodeficiency virus (HIV) infection, to delayed-type hypersensitivity skin-test antigens.[1]

All persons known to be infected with HIV or at increased risk of HIV infection should receive a tuberculin skin test with purified protein derivative (PPD) 5 TU administered by the Mantoux method. They should be evaluated concurrently for delayed-type hypersensitivity anergy using two of the following three skin-test antigens: mumps, tetanus toxoid, or *Candida albicans*. The antigens should be administered by the standard Mantoux method. Alternatively, a multiple-puncture device that delivers a battery of antigens may be used.

Induration should be measured 48–72 hours after the test antigens are administered. Any induration is evidence of responsiveness. Failure of the test antigens to elicit a response indicates anergy. Persons who react to PPD by developing induration of >5 mm in diameter are considered to be infected with *Mycobacterium tuberculosis* and should be evaluated for isoniazid prophylaxis once active tuberculosis is excluded. Persons who have a delayed-type hypersensitivity response but do not react to PPD are considered to not be infected with *M. tuberculosis*. Preventive therapy with isoniazid should be considered for anergic persons who are contacts of persons with infectious tuberculosis and for those who are members of groups in which the prevalence of tuberculous infection is >10% (e.g., users of intravenous drugs, prisoners, homeless persons, migrant workers, persons born in countries in Asia, Africa, and Latin America with high rates of tuberculosis).

1. Centers for Disease Control. Purified protein derivative (PPD)-tuberculin anergy and HIV infection: guidelines for anergy testing and management of anergic persons at risk of tuberculosis. *MMWR*. 1991; 40(RR-5):27-33.

Intravenous quinidine recommended for severe *Plasmodium falciparum* malaria; injectable quinine discontinued by CDC Drug Service

Intravenous quinidine gluconate is now considered by the Centers for Disease Control (CDC) to be the treatment of choice for complicated *Plasmodium falciparum* infection.[1] Injectable quinine dihydrochloride will no longer

Continued on page 657

When fear interferes . . . Ativan®

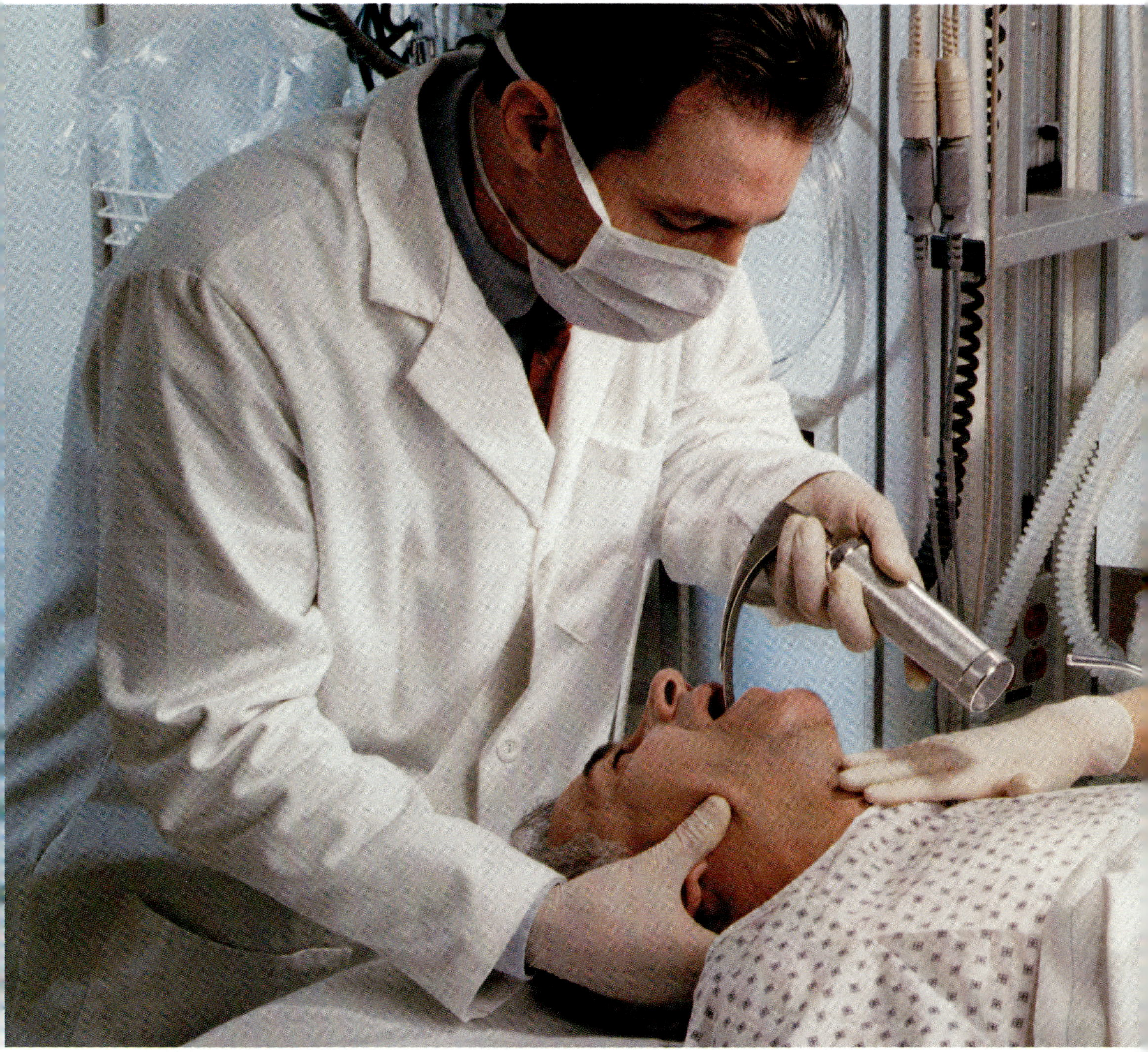

Continued from page 653

be stocked by the CDC Drug Service for emergency distribution for treatment of this condition. Intravenous therapy for malaria is indicated if vomiting is severe and oral fluids and medications are not retained, there is evidence of neurologic dysfunction, or a peripheral blood smear shows that >5% of erythrocytes are infected.

For treatment of severe *P. falciparum* malaria, a loading dose of quinidine gluconate 10 mg/kg (equivalent to quinidine base 6.2 mg/kg) is given over one to two hours, followed by continuous infusion of quinidine gluconate 0.02 mg/kg/min. The infusion rate should be slowed if the plasma quinidine concentration is >6 mg/mL, the QT interval is >0.6 seconds, or the QRS interval is >25% wider than at baseline. Hypoglycemia associated with *P. falciparum* infection may be exacerbated by quinidine-induced hyperinsulinemia; it should be treated with intravenous dextrose solutions. Quinidine therapy is continued until parasitemia is <1% and oral therapy is tolerated.

1. Centers for Disease Control. Treatment with quinidine gluconate of persons with severe *Plasmodium falciparum* infection: discontinuation of parenteral quinine from CDC Drug Service. *MMWR*. 1991; 40(RR-4):21-3.

Single large dose of intravenous immune globulin more effective than four-day regimen in patients with Kawasaki disease, investigators report

A single 2-g/kg dose of intravenous immune globulin (IVIG) is more effective than a standard four-day regimen in children with Kawasaki disease, concluded investigators conducting a multicenter, randomized, controlled trial involving 549 children with Kawasaki disease.[1]

A total of 276 children received IVIG (Immuno AG) 400 mg/kg daily for four days; 273 received a single 2-g/kg dose. All were treated within 10 days of the onset of illness, and all received aspirin (100 mg/kg/day through day 14 of illness, then 3–5 mg/kg/day). The prevalence of coronary artery abnormalities in the four-dose group relative to that in the single-dose group (after adjustment for age and sex) was 1.94 (95% confidence interval, 1.01–3.71) at two weeks and 1.84 (95% confidence interval, 0.89–3.82) at seven weeks. Those receiving the 2-g dose had lower maximal temperatures on days 2 and 3, a shorter duration of fever, and more rapid resolution of laboratory abnormalities reflecting acute inflammation. Among patients treated with the four-day regimen, a low IgG concentration on day 4 was associated with a higher prevalence of coronary artery lesions and more systemic inflammation. The frequency of adverse effects in the two groups combined was 2.7%; no significant differences were detected between groups. New or worsening congestive heart failure occurred in six patients who received a single 2-g dose of IVIG and in three patients who received the four-dose regimen.

1. Newburger JW, Takahashi M, Beiser AS et al. A single intravenous infusion of gamma globulin as compared with four infusions in the treatment of acute Kawasaki syndrome. *N Engl J Med*. 1991; 324:1633-9.

News Briefs

• A treatment IND protocol making **dideoxycytidine** (Hoffmann-La Roche) available to patients with AIDS or advanced AIDS-related complex who have not benefited from or have not tolerated therapy with zidovudine has been approved by FDA.

• Single copies of a report entitled **"Guidelines for the Assessment and Management of Iron Deficiency in Women of Childbearing Age"** can be obtained by sending a written request, along with $18, to Special Publication Office, Federation of American Societies for Experimental Biology, 9650 Rockville Pike, Bethesda, MD 20814.

• **Guidelines for the prevention and management of pelvic inflammatory disease** (PID) have been issued by the Centers for Disease Control (*MMWR*. 1991; 40(RR-5):1-25). The statement reviews the microbial etiology and pathogenesis of PID; estimates the magnitude of the problem; identifies risk factors for PID; outlines preventive strategies for use by communities, individuals, and health-care providers; and provides recommendations for diagnosis, treatment, and surveillance.

• Free, single copies of a **consensus development report on gastrointestinal surgery for severe obesity** can be obtained from William H. Hall, Director of Communications, Office of Medical Applications of Research, National Institutes of Health, Building 1, Room 259, Bethesda, MD 20892; 301-496-1143.

• The Cystic Fibrosis Foundation has awarded Leslie Hendeles, Pharm.D., University of Florida, $60,000 to conduct an **equivalency study of pancreatic enzyme supplements** administered to patients with cystic fibrosis.

Upcoming Specialty Meetings

New Directions in Nutritional Care: Nutrient Modification of the Disease Process. Chicago, IL, September 12–13; contact American Society for Parenteral and Enteral Nutrition, 8630 Fenton Street, Suite 412, Silver Spring, MD 20910; 301-587-6315.

Advances in Understanding and Treatment of Rheumatoid Arthritis. Philadelphia, PA, September 16–17; contact IBC USA Conferences Inc., 8 Pleasant Street, Building D, South Natick, MA 01760; 508-650-4700 (fax, 508-653-1627).

Therapy Consultation

The Therapy Consultation *section provides brief advice, in question-and-answer format, on how to handle specific drug-therapy problems. Readers are invited to submit questions, which will be referred to a consultant for an answer. The problems should not be highly specialized or unusual, nor should they be mundane. Questions are answered briefly, based largely on the judgment and personal experience of the consultant, although selected references may be cited to substantiate the consultant's advice.*

Assistance in identifying Therapy Consultation *topics is provided by the drug information centers at Medical College of Virginia Hospitals, Richmond; University of California Medical Center, San Diego; and University of Michigan Medical Center, Ann Arbor.*

Analgesic selection when the patient is allergic to codeine

Question: A patient is reported to be allergic to codeine. Although true allergy to codeine is rare, this patient is described as having had a "near anaphylactic" reaction. Which oral analgesics can be given safely to this patient?

Answer: It has been well established that this patient's reaction represents a true allergy to codeine. One must remember however that a very common patient complaint is "codeine allergy." Most often the patient is referring to something unexpected or unpleasant that occurred while he or she was taking codeine. That "something" is usually an extension of the pharmacologic action of codeine (e.g., nausea and vomiting); it is not an allergy.

If the reaction is a true allergy, the chances of cross-sensitivity are greatly decreased if an agent with a chemical structure different from that of the offending agent can be substituted.[1] Within the narcotic analgesic class there are at least three distinct chemical structures. Relatively simple manipulations of the morphine or thebaine molecule form many related opioids. This group of agents includes morphine, hydromorphone, oxymorphone, levorphanol, codeine, hydrocodone, oxycodone, buprenorphine, butorphanol, nalbuphine, and the related benzomorphan pentazocine.[2] Dezocine is a bridged aminotetralin that is structurally related to pentazocine.[3] Meperidine, a phenylpiperidine, and its related congeners fentanyl, sufentanil, and alfentanil are considered a second chemical group. The third chemically distinct group includes methadone and propoxyphene.[2]

This patient's acute pain might best be managed by around-the-clock administration of aspirin, acetaminophen, or a nonsteroidal anti-inflammatory drug (NSAID). If this therapy does not provide satisfactory pain relief, oral propoxyphene can be added with minimal chance of cross-sensitivity to codeine. It would be prudent, however, to continue to carefully monitor this patient for the development of sensitivity to this chemically distinct, although related, compound. Theoretically, oral methadone or meperidine could also be substituted. However, because of the high dosages of oral meperidine required for efficacy and the long duration of the sedative effects of methadone, most clinicians would not recommend these drugs for control of acute pain.

The cause of more than 80% of adverse drug reactions (ADRs) is an extension of the pharmacologic action of the drug or an abnormal threshold to the pharmacologic action of the agent.[4] A small portion of reactions occur because of a genetically determined metabolic or enzyme defect (idiosyncratic reactions).[4] The remaining ADRs (allergies) have an immunologic basis, or they appear clinically as allergies but have no demonstrated immunologic mechanism (pseudoallergies).[4] Allergies and pseudoallergies are not dose related, they require prior exposure to the compound or very similar compounds, and they are manifested as skin rashes, anaphylaxis, pulmonary reactions, hepatitis, drug fever, interstitial nephritis, and connective tissue disorders.[5]

In patients with true codeine allergies, the risk of cross-sensitivity is higher when a morphine congener is administered instead of a phenylpiperidine or a methadone-like agent.[1] Propoxyphene with aspirin, acetaminophen, or other NSAIDs appears to be an acceptable alternative to codeine in patients who are allergic to codeine or the related opioids.

1. Ginsberg GS. Managing a patient with a morphine allergy. *Drug Therapy*. 1985; 15(Jun):18-23.
2. Jaffe JH, Martin WR. Opioid analgesics and antagonists. In: Goodman and Gilman's the pharmacological basis of therapeutics. 8th ed. Gilman AG, Rall TW, Nies AS et al., eds. New York: Pergamon; 1990:485-521.
3. O'Brien JJ, Benfield P. Dezocine. *Drugs*. 1989; 38:226-48.
4. Batenhorst RL. Adverse drug reactions. In: Herfindal ET, Gourley DR, Hart LL, eds. Clinical pharmacy and therapeutics. 4th ed. Baltimore: Williams & Wilkins; 1988:1030-7.
5. DeSwarte RD. Drug allergy—problems and strategies. *J Allergy Clin Immunol*. 1984; 74:209-21.

TERRY J. BAUMANN, PHARM.D., Clinical Manager
Department of Pharmacy
Munson Medical Center
1105 Sixth Street
Traverse City, MI 49684

EXOSURF® Neonatal™

(COLFOSCERIL PALMITATE, CETYL ALCOHOL, TYLOXAPOL)

For Intratracheal Suspension / 10 mL vials

PLEASE CONSULT FULL PRODUCT INFORMATION BEFORE PRESCRIBING.

INDICATIONS AND USAGE: Exosurf Neonatal is indicated for:

1. **Prophylactic** treatment of infants with birth weights of less than 1350 grams who are at risk of developing RDS (see PRECAUTIONS),
2. **Prophylactic** treatment of infants with birth weights greater than 1350 grams who have evidence of pulmonary immaturity, and
3. **Rescue** treatment of infants who have developed RDS.

CONTRAINDICATIONS: There are no known contraindications to treatment with Exosurf Neonatal.

WARNINGS: Intratracheal Administration Only: Exosurf Neonatal should be administered only by instillation into the trachea. **General:** The use of Exosurf Neonatal requires expert clinical care by experienced neonatologists and other clinicians who are accomplished at neonatal intubation and ventilatory management. Adequate personnel, facilities, equipment, and medications are required to optimize perinatal outcome in premature infants. Instillation of Exosurf Neonatal should be performed **only** by trained medical personnel experienced in airway and clinical management of unstable premature infants. Vigilant clinical attention should be given to all infants prior to, during, and after administration of Exosurf Neonatal. **Acute Effects:** Exosurf Neonatal can rapidly affect oxygenation and lung compliance. **Lung Compliance:** If chest expansion improves substantially after dosing, peak ventilator inspiratory pressures should be reduced immediately, without waiting for confirmation of respiratory improvement by blood gas assessment. Failure to reduce inspiratory ventilator pressures rapidly in such instances can result in lung overdistention and fatal pulmonary air leak. **Hyperoxia:** If the infant becomes pink and transcutaneous oxygen saturation is in excess of 95%, FiO_2 should be reduced in small but repeated steps (until saturation is 90 to 95%) without waiting for confirmation of elevated arterial pO_2 by blood gas assessment. Failure to reduce FiO_2 in such instances can result in hyperoxia. **Hypocarbia:** If arterial or transcutaneous CO_2 measurements are <30 torr, the ventilator rate should be reduced at once. Failure to reduce ventilator rates in such instances can result in marked hypocarbia, which is known to reduce brain blood flow. **Pulmonary Hemorrhage:** In the single study conducted in infants weighing <700 grams at birth, the incidence of pulmonary hemorrhage (10% vs 2% in the placebo group) was significantly increased in the Exosurf Neonatal group. None of the five studies involving infants with birth weights >700 grams showed a significant increase in pulmonary hemorrhage in the Exosurf Neonatal group. In a cross-study analysis of these five studies, pulmonary hemorrhage was reported for 1% (14/1420) of infants in the placebo group and 2% (27/1411) of infants in the Exosurf Neonatal group. Fatal pulmonary hemorrhage occurred in three infants; two in the Exosurf Neonatal group and one in the placebo group. Mortality from all causes among infants who developed pulmonary hemorrhage was 43% in the placebo group and 37% in the Exosurf Neonatal group. Pulmonary hemorrhage in both Exosurf Neonatal and placebo infants was more frequent in infants who were younger, smaller, male, or who had a patent ductus arteriosus. Pulmonary hemorrhage typically occurred in the first 2 days of life in both treatment groups. In more than 7700 infants in the open, uncontrolled study, pulmonary hemorrhage was reported in 4%, but fatal pulmonary hemorrhage was reported rarely (0.4%). In the controlled clinical studies, Exosurf Neonatal treated infants who received steroids more than 24 hours prior to delivery or indomethacin postnatally had a lower rate of pulmonary hemorrhage than other Exosurf Neonatal treated infants. Attention should be paid to early and aggressive diagnosis and treatment (unless contraindicated) of patent ductus arteriosus during the first 2 days of life (while the ductus arteriosus is often clinically silent). Other potentially protective measures include attempting to decrease FiO_2 preferentially over ventilator pressures during the first 24 to 48 hours after dosing, and attempting to decrease PEEP minimally for at least 48 hours after dosing. **Mucous Plugs:** Infants whose ventilation becomes markedly impaired during or shortly after dosing may have mucous plugging of the endotracheal tube, particularly if pulmonary secretions were prominent prior to drug administration. Suctioning of all infants prior to dosing may lessen the chance of mucous plugs obstructing the endotracheal tube. If endotracheal tube obstruction from such plugs is suspected, and suctioning is unsuccessful in removing the obstruction, the blocked endotracheal tube should be replaced immediately.

PRECAUTIONS:

General: In the controlled clinical studies, infants known prenatally or postnatally to have major congenital anomalies, or who were suspected of having congenital infection, were excluded from entry. However, these disorders cannot be recognized early in life in all cases, and a few infants with these conditions were entered. The benefits of Exosurf Neonatal in the affected infants who received drug appeared to be similar to the benefits observed in infants without anomalies or occult infection. **Prophylactic Treatment-Infants <700 Grams:** In infants weighing 500 to 700 grams, a single prophylactic dose of Exosurf Neonatal significantly: improved FiO_2 and ventilator settings, reduced pneumothorax, and reduced death from RDS, but increased pulmonary hemorrhage (see WARNINGS). Overall mortality did not differ significantly between the placebo and Exosurf Neonatal groups (see Table 1 in full product information). Data on multiple doses in infants in this weight class are not yet available. Accordingly, clinicians should carefully evaluate the potential risks and benefits of Exosurf Neonatal administration in these infants. **Rescue Treatment-Number of Doses:** A small number of infants with RDS have received more than two doses of Exosurf Neonatal as rescue treatment. Definitive data on the safety and efficacy of these additional doses are not available. **Carcinogenesis, Mutagenesis, Impairment of Fertility:** Exosurf Neonatal at concentrations up to 10,000 μg/plate was not mutagenic in the Ames Salmonella assay. Long-term studies have not been performed in animals to evaluate the carcinogenic potential of Exosurf Neonatal. The effects of Exosurf Neonatal on fertility have not been studied.

ADVERSE REACTIONS:

General: Premature birth is associated with a high incidence of morbidity and mortality. Despite significant reductions in overall mortality associated with Exosurf Neonatal, some infants who received Exosurf Neonatal developed severe complications and either survived with permanent handicaps or died.

In controlled clinical studies evaluating the safety and efficacy of Exosurf Neonatal, numerous safety assessments were made. In infants receiving Exosurf Neonatal, pulmonary hemorrhage, apnea and use of methylxanthines were increased. A number of other adverse events were significantly reduced in the Exosurf Neonatal group, particularly various forms of pulmonary air leak and use of pancuronium. Tables 3 and 4 summarize the results of the major safety evaluations from the controlled clinical studies.

Table 3: Safety Assessments[a]—Prophylactic Treatment

Number of Doses: / Birth Weight Range:	Single Dose 500 to 700 grams		Single Dose 700 to 1350 grams		Single Dose 700 to 1100 grams		1 vs 3 Doses 700 to 1100 grams	
Treatment Group:	Placebo (Air)	EXOSURF	Placebo (Air)	EXOSURF	Placebo (Air)	EXOSURF	EXOSURF 1 Dose	EXOSURF 3 Doses
Number of Infants:	N=108	N=107	N=193	N=192	N=222	N=224	N=356	N=360
	% of Infants		% of Infants		% of Infants		% of Infants	
Intraventricular Hemorrhage (IVH)								
Overall	51	57	31	27	36	36	38	35
Severe IVH	26	25	10	8	13	14	9	9
Pulmonary Air Leak (PAL)								
Overall	52	48	16	11	32	25	29	27
Pneumothorax	23	10*	5	6	19	11*	14	12
Pneumopericardium	1	4	2	0	<1	1	1	1
Pneumomediastinum	2	1	2	3	7	1**	3	2
Pulmonary Interstitial Emphysema	43	44	13	7*	26	20	23	22
Death from PAL	4	6	<1	<1	2	1	2	1
Patent Ductus Arteriosus	49	53	66	70	50	55	59	57
Necrotizing Enterocolitis	2	4	11	13	3	4	6	2*
Pulmonary Hemorrhage	2	10**	2	4	1	4	4	6
Congenital Pneumonia	4	4	2	4	2	2	1	1
Nosocomial Pneumonia	10	10	2	4	4	7	14	15
Non-Pulmonary Infections	33	35	34	39	28	29	35	34
Sepsis	30	34	30	34	23	24	30	27
Death From Sepsis	4	4	3	3	1	2	3	2
Meningitis	4	6	3	1	2	3	1	2
Other Infections	7	4	5	3	6	10	10	11
Major Anomalies	3	1	2	4	7	4	4	4

Table 3: Safety Assessments[a]—Prophylactic Treatment (Cont.)

Number of Doses: / Birth Weight Range:	Single Dose 500 to 700 grams		Single Dose 700 to 1350 grams		Single Dose 700 to 1100 grams		1 vs 3 Doses 700 to 1100 grams	
Treatment Group:	Placebo (Air)	EXOSURF	Placebo (Air)	EXOSURF	Placebo (Air)	EXOSURF	EXOSURF 1 Dose	EXOSURF 3 Doses
Number of Infants:	N=108	N=107	N=193	N=192	N=222	N=224	N=356	N=360
	% of Infants		% of Infants		% of Infants		% of Infants	
Hypotension	70	77	52	47	59	62	54	50
Hyperbilirubinemia	22	21	63	61	27	31	20	21
Exchange Transfusion	4	3	1	2	2	2	3	1
Thrombocytopenia[b]	21	25	not available		9	8	12	10
Persistent Fetal Circulation	0	1	1	1	0	2*	1	<1
Seizures	11	8	2	2	11	9	6	5
Apnea	34	33	76	73	55	65*	62	68
Drug Therapy								
Antibiotics	96	99	98	96	98	99	>99	99
Diuretics	55	60	39	37	59	63	64	65
Anticonvulsants	14	18	23	24	20	16	9	8
Inotropes	46	40	20	20	26	20	28	27
Sedatives	62	71	65	64	63	57	52	52
Pancuronium	19	11	22	14*	19	13*	15	11
Methylxanthines	38	43	77	77	61	72*	75	82*

[a] All parameters were examined with "as-treated" analyses.
[b] Thrombocytopenia requiring platelet transfusion.
* $p<0.05$
** $p<0.01$

Table 4: Safety Assessments[a]—Rescue Treatment

Number of Doses: / Birth Weight Range:	Two Doses 700 to 1350 grams		Two Doses 1250 grams and above	
Treatment Group:	Placebo (Air)	EXOSURF	Placebo (Air)	EXOSURF
Number of Infants:	N=213	N=206	N=622	N=615
	% of Infants		% of Infants	
Intraventricular Hemorrhage (IVH)				
Overall	48	52	23	18*
Severe IVH	13	9	5	4
Pulmonary Air Leak (PAL)				
Overall	54	34***	30	18***
Pneumothorax	29	20*	20	10***
Pneumopericardium	4	1	1	2
Pneumomediastinum	8	4	5	2**
Pulmonary Interstitial Emphysema	48	25***	24	13***
Death from PAL	7	3	<1	1
Patent Ductus Arteriosus	66	57	54	45*
Necrotizing Enterocolitis	3	3	1	2
Pulmonary Hemorrhage	3	1	<1	1
Congenital Pneumonia	2	3	2	2
Nosocomial Pneumonia	5	7	2	2
Non-Pulmonary Infections	19	22	13	13
Sepsis	15	17	8	8
Death From Sepsis	<1	<1	1	<1
Meningitis	1	<1	1	<1*
Other Infections	5	8	5	6
Major Anomalies	3	3	4	4
Hypotension	62	57	50	39**
Hyperbilirubinemia	17	19	12	10
Exchange Transfusion	3	4	1	2
Thrombocytopenia[b]	10	11	4	<1**
Persistent Fetal Circulation	1	1	6	2**
Seizures	10	10	6	3*
Apnea	48	65**	37	44*
Drug Therapy				
Antibiotics	100	99	98	98
Diuretics	60	65	45	34***
Anticonvulsants	17	17	10	5**
Inotropes	36	31	27	16***
Sedatives	72	68	76	64***
Pancuronium	34	17**	33	15***
Methylxanthines	62	74**	49	53

[a] All parameters were examined with "as-treated" analyses.
[b] Thrombocytopenia requiring platelet transfusion.
* $p<0.05$
** $p<0.01$
*** $p<0.001$

Pulmonary Hemorrhage: See WARNINGS. **Abnormal Laboratory Values:** Abnormal laboratory values are common in critically ill, mechanically ventilated, premature infants. A higher incidence of abnormal laboratory values in the Exosurf Neonatal group was not reported. **Events During Dosing:** Data on events during dosing are available from more than 8800 infants in the open, uncontrolled clinical study (Table 5).

Table 5: Events During Dosing in the Open, Uncontrolled Study[a]

Treatment Type:	Prophylactic Treatment	Rescue Treatment
Number of Infants:	N=1127	N=7711
	% of Infants	% of Infants
Reflux of Exosurf	20	31
Drop in O_2 saturation ($\geq 20\%$)	6	22
Rise in O_2 saturation ($\geq 10\%$)	5	6
Drop in transcutaneous pO_2 (≥ 20 mm Hg)	1	8
Rise in transcutaneous pO_2 (≥ 20 mm Hg)	2	5
Drop in transcutaneous pCO_2 (≥ 20 mm Hg)	<1	1
Rise in transcutaneous pCO_2 (≥ 20 mm Hg)	1	3
Bradycardia (<60 beats/min)	1	3
Tachycardia (>200 beats/min)	<1	<1
Gagging	1	5
Mucous Plugs	<1	<1

[a] Infants may have experienced more than one event.
Investigators were prohibited from adjusting FiO_2 and/or ventilator settings during dosing unless significant clinical deterioration occurred.

Reflux: Reflux of Exosurf Neonatal into the endotracheal tube during dosing has been observed and may be associated with rapid drug administration. If reflux occurs, drug administration should be halted and, if necessary, peak inspiratory pressure on the ventilator should be increased by 4 to 5 cm H_2O until the endotracheal tube clears. ***>20% Drop in Transcutaneous Oxygen Saturation:*** If transcutaneous oxygen saturation declines during dosing, drug administration should be halted and, if necessary, peak inspiratory pressure on the ventilator should be increased by 4 to 5 cm H_2O for 1 to 2 minutes. In addition, increases of FiO_2 may be required for 1 to 2 minutes. ***Mucous Plugs:*** See WARNINGS.

DOSAGE AND ADMINISTRATION: See full product information.

Wellcome
BURROUGHS WELLCOME CO., Research Triangle Park, NC 27709

Printed in U.S.A. EX-Y01228

Letters

Dosage of antimycobacterial agents 664
Charles A. Peloquin

Valproic acid hepatotoxicity in adults and older children 665
Jamie T. Gilman

The Letters *column is a forum for rapid exchange of ideas among readers of* Clinical Pharmacy. *Liberal criteria are applied in the review of submissions to encourage contributions to this column.*

The Letters *column includes the following types of contributions: (1) comments, addenda, and minor updates on previously published work, (2) alerts on potential problems related to drug therapy or clinical research, (3) observations or comments on trends in drug therapy or clinical research, and (4) brief expressions of opinion about controversies in drug therapy or clinical research.*

Letters need not be submitted with the journal's manuscript checklist. The following conditions, however, must be adhered to: (1) the body of the letter must be no longer than two typewritten pages, (2) the use of references, tables, and illustrations should be minimized, (3) the authors' names, affiliations, and mailing addresses must be typed at the end of the letter in the format used by Clinical Pharmacy, *and (4) the entire letter (including references, tables, and authors' names) must be typed double-spaced on plain white paper (not letterhead). Following acceptance of a letter, the authors are required to sign an exclusive publication statement and a copyright transferal form.*

Dosage of antimycobacterial agents

I would like to supplement the information provided by Rathbun et al.[1] in *Clinical Pharmacy* on drug therapy for AIDS-associated *Mycobacterium avium* complex (MAC) disease.

The dosage regimens provided by Rathbun et al. in Table 1 are consistent with published reports, but their use is limited by the toxicities outlined in the table. The ethionamide and cycloserine dosages, in particular, should be viewed as the final dosages achieved for most patients.[2]

The dosage of ethionamide should start at 250 mg p.o. daily and be increased by 250 mg daily as tolerated, with the total given as two divided doses. Patients often achieve serum drug concentrations (SDCs) that barely exceed the minimal inhibitory concentration (MIC) for the pathogen, and SDC monitoring may indicate the need for higher dosages.

For most patients, the initial cycloserine dosage should be 250 mg p.o. daily because toxicity is very common at higher initial dosages (500–1000 mg/day). It is best to base dosage increases on SDC determinations, with samples collected 2 and 10 hours after a dose. We have noted that the serum cycloserine concentrations in some patients increase gradually over the first one or two weeks of therapy even when the dosage is constant. Although some drug accumulation is expected for a drug with an elimination half-life of 7–12 hours, it is not clear whether there are other explanations for our observations. SDC monitoring is invaluable because it is otherwise difficult to predict when a given cycloserine dosage will produce an adequate concentration.

The exact serum half-life of clofazimine is unknown, but it may be days or weeks. Therefore, unless the patient cannot tolerate a single daily dose, once-daily dosage is sufficient.

Isoniazid is frequently listed among drugs used for MAC disease, but it is essentially inactive against MAC at achievable serum concentrations.[3] Pyrazinamide, aminosalicylate sodium, and capreomycin sulfate are also generally inactive against MAC.[3]

In contrast, streptomycin and kanamycin are generally equally active and substantially less expensive than amikacin.[4,5] Therefore, in vitro testing of these agents should allow the selection of the most active and cost-effective drug. I.V. dosage of these agents may begin at 11–13 mg (as sulfate)/kg of ideal body weight (IBW) every 24 hours (typically Monday through Friday at our institution). Daily i.m. doses are generally 15 mg/kg IBW; the use of larger doses given three times weekly is being studied. Dosage should be adjusted to achieve an SDC of 35–45 μg/mL at the end of an i.v. infusion (calculated by extrapolation) or one hour after an i.m. injection.

We have noted that, in some MAC-infected patients without AIDS, rifampin 600 mg p.o. daily and ciprofloxacin 750 mg (as hydrochloride) p.o. b.i.d. fail to produce SDCs that exceed the pathogen's MIC. These patients, in whom drug absorption is apparently impaired, may require a doubling of these dosages to attain SDCs similar to those attained in patients without the absorption problem. Although most published data suggest that food does not interfere with absorption of rifampin and ciprofloxacin, we believe our experience indicates otherwise. These drugs should be given at least one hour before or two hours after a meal, and concurrent administration of antacids should be avoided. Although in vivo dose–response studies for antimycobacterial agents in MAC disease have not been completed, it seems reasonable to attempt to achieve MICs when treating the disease, especially in patients with AIDS.

Because the susceptibility of MAC to antimycobacterial agents is highly variable, attempts to establish one standard therapy may not be successful. The individualization of therapy in MAC disease has been difficult because true MIC determinations and SDC monitoring have been lacking. Radiometric techniques for susceptibility testing and high-performance liquid chromatographic assays for SDC determinations, however, are now available. Therapy for MAC disease at specialized centers such as ours succeeds only 60–70% of the time in patients without AIDS and apparently much less frequently in patients with AIDS. Given these poor results, perhaps it is time to try to maximize each patient's therapy and, hopefully, each patient's chance for survival.

1. Rathbun RC, Martin ES III, Eaton VE et al. Current and investigational therapies for AIDS-associated *Mycobacterium avium* complex disease. *Clin Pharm*. 1991; 10:280-91.
2. Peloquin CA. Antituberculosis drugs: pharmacokinetics. In: Heifets L, ed. Drug susceptibility in the chemotherapy of mycobacterial infections. Boca Raton, FL: CRC; 1991:59-88.
3. Heifets LB, Iseman MD. Choice of antimicrobial agents of *M. avium* disease based on quantitative tests of drug susceptibility. *N Engl J Med*. 1990; 323:419-20. Letter.
4. Heifets LB, Lindholm-Levy P. Comparison of bactericidal activities of streptomycin, amikacin, kanamycin, and capreomycin against *Mycobacterium avium* and *M. tuberculosis*. *Antimicrob Agents Chemother*. 1989: 33:1298-301.
5. Heifets LB, Lindholm-Levy P. In vitro activity of amikacin against *Mycobacterium avium*. *Antimicrob Agents Chemother*. 1990; 34:378-9. Letter.

Charles A. Peloquin, Pharm.D., Director
Infectious Diseases Pharmacokinetics Laboratory
National Jewish Center for Immunology and Respiratory Medicine
1400 Jackson Street
Denver, CO 80206

Valproic acid hepatotoxicity in adults and older children

Pugh and Garnett[1] recently stated in *Clinical Pharmacy* that no patient older than 10 years has died of valproic acid hepatotoxicity. There are, however, a few reports of such patients succumbing to what was believed to be this adverse drug reaction.

Dreifuss et al.,[2] in a review of the American literature, identified 37 deaths related to valproic acid hepatotoxicity. Ten of the patients were older than 10 years, but all had received valproic acid as part of a multiple-drug regimen. Scheffner et al.[3] reviewed the world literature on fatal valproic acid hepatotoxicity. Of the 95 deaths described, 8.5% occurred in patients older than 20 years. This review did not include 16 patients identified by Dreifuss et al.,[2] but did include one adult death described in more detail by Dickinson et al.[4] Egmond et al.[5] reported a possible case of late-onset fatal hepatotoxicity in a 15-year-old boy receiving valproic acid. When sufficient information is available, the reports strongly suggest that the risk of valproic acid hepatotoxicity is minimized when the drug is used as the sole antiepileptic agent.[2,4,5]

Clinicians must sometimes counsel adult patients and the families of older children for whom valproic acid therapy is being considered. These persons should be advised that, although the risk of fatal hepatotoxicity is low, it is not nonexistent.

1. Pugh CB, Garnett WR. Current issues in the treatment of epilepsy. *Clin Pharm*. 1991; 10:335-58.
2. Dreifuss FE, Santilli N, Langer DH et al. Valproic acid hepatic fatalities: a retrospective review. *Neurology*. 1987; 37:379-85.
3. Scheffner D, Konig S, Rautergerg-Ruland I et al. Fatal liver failure in 16 children with valproate therapy. *Epilepsia*. 1988; 29:530-42.
4. Dickinson RG, Bassett ML, Searle J et al. Valproate hepatotoxicity: a review and report of two instances in adults. *Exp Neurol*. 1985; 21:79-91.
5. Egmond H, Degomme P, Simpel H et al. A suspected case of late-onset sodium valproate-induced hepatic failure. *Neuropediatrics*. 1987; 18:96-8.

Jamie T. Gilman, Pharm.D., Director of Neuropharmacology
Neuroscience Center
Miami Children's Hospital
6125 SW 31st Street
Miami, FL 33155

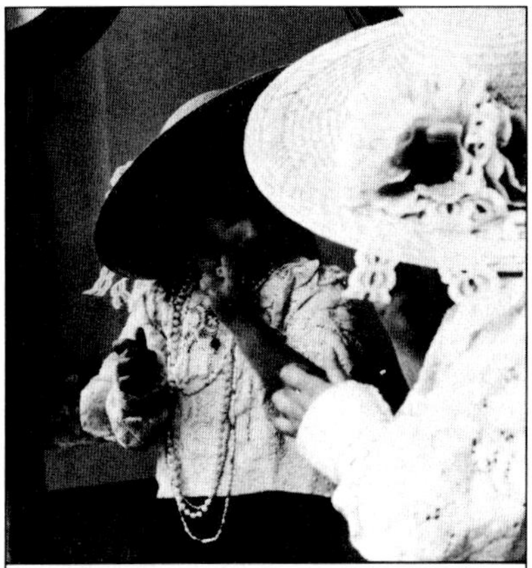

Management of acute pain in children

Varsha Bhatt-Mehta and David A. Rosen

Abstract: The pathophysiology, assessment, and pharmacologic management of acute pain in infants and children are reviewed, and the mechanism of action, pharmacokinetics, clinical efficacy, adverse effects, and dosages of opioid analgesics, nonopioid analgesics, and local anesthetics used for regional blocks are discussed.

The pathophysiology of pain and the physiologic rationale for treatment of pain are similar in children and adults. Severe pain can be controlled by i.v. or epidural administration of opioid analgesics. Neonates are more susceptible to the depressant effects of opioids, and opioid analgesia must be administered with caution in infants who are not receiving mechanical ventilation because of the associated risk of respiratory depression. Patient-controlled analgesia is a useful technique in older children. Acetaminophen and NSAIDs are useful for relieving milder pain of noninflammatory and inflammatory origin, respectively. Epidural or intrathecal administration of local anesthetics provides regional analgesia with minimal physiologic alterations. Topical application of local anesthetics is effective for many minor procedures.

A variety of pain management techniques are available for the management of acute pain in pediatric patients. The development of drugs having fewer adverse effects and noninvasive administration techniques will be important research priorities in the coming years.

Index terms: Analgesics and antipyretics; Anesthetics, local; Dosage; Mechanism of action; Opiates; Pain; Pediatrics; Pharmacokinetics; Toxicity

Clin Pharm. 1991; 10:667-85

During the past two decades numerous investigators have reported profound undertreatment of pain in infants and children. Many misconceptions regarding analgesic use and obsessive concern about addiction persist in the medical literature.

Clinical studies have documented that children's pain is far less vigorously treated than that of adults.[1,2] A survey of the incidence of pain in 170 postoperative children (mean age, eight years) revealed a high incidence of moderate and severe pain.[3] Children frequently had no analgesics prescribed, and when an analgesic was ordered, it was not administered in 40% of the cases. There was a lack of uniformity in prescription orders, and often the doses prescribed for pain relief were inadequate. Additionally, the researchers found that the nurses frequently interpreted p.r.n. to mean "as little as possible," and when given a choice, they would administer the least potent drug. Beyer et al.[4] found similar results when they compared analgesic use in 50 children and 50 adults undergoing cardiac surgery. Twelve of the 50 children did not receive any analgesia during the first three postoperative days, and the children received fewer potent analgesics than did adults. Schechter et al.[5] evaluated postoperative prescribing practices in children and adults who had similar pathophysiologic problems, such as hernia, appendectomy, burns, and fractured femurs. On the average, adults received 1.5 to 3 times as many doses of opioids per hospital day as children did, and younger children received proportionately even fewer doses.

Circumcisions and other routine care-giving procedures in newborns are stressful. However, current literature suggests that procedures are performed without analgesia or anesthesia despite availability of pain-relieving techniques for newborn infants.[6] Recent work by Anand et al.[7] has demonstrated that new-

Varsha Bhatt-Mehta, Pharm.D., is Clinical Assistant Professor, College of Pharmacy, and Clinical Pharmacist, Neonatal Intensive Care Unit, University of Michigan Medical Center, Ann Arbor, MI. David A. Rosen, M.D., is Assistant Professor, Department of Anesthesia, and Instructor, Department of Pediatrics and Communicable Diseases, University of Michigan Medical Center.

Address all reprint requests to Dr. Bhatt-Mehta at the Department of Pharmacy Services, F5203, C. S. Mott Children's Hospital, 200 East Hospital Drive, Ann Arbor, MI 48109-0008.

This is article **680-204-9119** in the **ASHP Continuing Education System**; it qualifies for 2.0 hours of continuing-education credit. See page 718 for learning objectives and test questions.

borns and infants who undergo surgery with minimal or no analgesia mount a substantial stress response, as evidenced by increased release of catecholamines, growth hormone, glucagon, and corticosteroids and by suppression of insulin. Concerns have been raised regarding the hypermetabolic state that occurs during pain and the consequent prolonged hyperglycemia and increases in blood lactate and ketone body concentrations.[8-13] The hypermetabolic response to pain may be associated with cardiac insufficiency, impaired immune response, and pulmonary insufficiency, leading to a high incidence of morbidity and mortality in critically ill infants and children.[7]

Pain has been undertreated in children for several reasons. First is the myth that infants' and children's nervous systems are immature and not capable of pain perception. Second, it is thought that because of children's cognitive limitations they will have no memory of pain; therefore, it is not necessary to offer analgesics. Finally, there is concern among pediatricians that a child might become addicted if potent opioids are used. This myth arises from the confusion between psychological and physiologic dependence. In fact, few hospitalized adults whose pain is treated with opioids become addicted.[14] Although there are no such data for pediatric patients, it should be expected that children would have a similarly low risk.

Neuroanatomy and Neurophysiology

The pathophysiology of pain and the physiologic rationale for treatment of pain are similar in children and adults.[7,15,16] These similarities mandate an aggressive approach to analgesia in children. Differences that do exist between children and adults reflect the biologic and behavioral characteristics of newborns, infants, and children in different stages of development.

There are two major types of pain receptors: mechanoreceptors and nociceptors. High-threshold mechanoreceptors are responsible for the first sharp pain experienced when tissue is injured. These receptors do not respond to heat or chemical irritation but to pressure applied to a wide area of the skin.[7] The axons leading from these receptors are myelinated and conduct in the A-delta velocity range (5–25 m/sec). Polymodal nociceptors respond to heat and analgesic substances as well as pressure. These unmyelinated axons conduct slowly in the C-fiber range (<2 m/sec) and are responsible for the dull second pain experienced on injury. Impulses are conducted to the spinal cord through primary afferent fibers with cell bodies in dorsal root ganglia. Visceral afferent fibers may be A or C fibers and, in contrast to somatic afferent fibers, reach the spinal cord through sympathetic, parasympathetic, and splanchnic nerves.[7] Acute pain in a hospitalized child typically reflects nociceptive receptor activation.

The anatomic framework for pain transmission develops during fetal life and in the first months of infancy. The density of cutaneous nociceptive nerve endings in the skin of the late fetus and newborn infant may equal or exceed that in adult skin.[17] Formation of mature dorsal horns in some regions of the spinal cord is complete by 30 weeks of gestation.[16] The partial lack of myelination has been suggested as an index of immaturity in the neonatal nervous system and has been used to support the argument that neonates and infants are not capable of pain perception.[7,16] The nociceptive nerve tracts in the spinal cord and central nervous system undergo myelination during the second and third trimesters of gestation.[16] In neonates, incomplete myelination may mean slower conduction velocity in the nerves or central nerve tracts, but this is offset by the shorter interneuron and neuromuscular distances traveled by the impulse.[16]

Evidence suggests that the complete nervous system is active during fetal development and that detrimental or developmental changes in any part would affect the entire nervous system.[18,19] There are reports of endogenous release of opiates in response to distress in the human fetus at birth.[20] Umbilical plasma concentrations of β-endorphins and β-lipoproteins from healthy, full-term, newborn infants delivered vaginally or by cesarean section have been shown to be three to five times higher than plasma concentrations in resting adults.[21,22] The high levels of β-endorphins decrease anesthetic or analgesic requirements only minimally, because the cerebrospinal fluid concentrations of β-endorphins required to produce analgesia in human adults have been found to be about 10,000 times higher than the highest concentration recorded in neonates.[23] In adults, the nociceptive impulses in the peripheral nerves are carried through unmyelinated (C-polymodal) and thinly myelinated A-delta fibers.[16]

Thus, it appears that complete myelination is not necessary for pain perception, and premature and full-term neonates who have partial myelination at birth are capable of experiencing pain. Development of the pain pathways during infancy and childhood involves the refinement of sensory modalities and intracortical connections within the limbic system and the affective and associative areas located in the frontal cortex, parietal cortex, and insula.[1]

Neuropharmacology

Acute pain due to surgery (controlled pain), trauma (uncontrolled pain), conditions such as sickle cell crisis or pancreatitis, and invasive procedures (for patients under intensive care) leads to the endogenous production of substances involved in the transmission and control of pain: substance P, serotonin, histamine, bradykinin, and potassium ions.[7,16] Compounds that can counteract the effects of these endogenous substances would be useful in the management of acute pain.

Stereospecific opiate receptors and their endogenous ligands, which have pharmacologic properties similar to those of morphine, were demonstrated to be present in the brain in the mid-1970s.[24-27] Stereospecific opiate receptors and their endogenous ligands form the endogenous opiate system, which is believed to function primarily in the control of pain. This system has been divided into enkephalinergic and endorphinergic systems; these systems may modulate pain at the spinal and supraspinal levels, respectively.[28,29] The discovery of endorphins and opiate receptors has led to reclassification of opioid analgesics into agonists, antagonists, and mixed agonist–antagonists according to their receptor-binding properties.[30-33]

A neurotransmitter is defined as an agonist; a drug that blocks the action of the neurotransmitter is an antagonist. By definition, binding of an agonist to a receptor causes alterations in the internal environment of the cell; when an antagonist binds to the receptor, cellular changes do not occur.[34] Morphine and opioids related to morphine are agonists; drugs that block the effects of opioids, such as naloxone, are antagonists.[33,34]

Opioids interact with specific receptors that are widely distributed throughout the central nervous system.[33-36] There are four major receptor groups: mu, delta, kappa, and sigma. The mu and delta receptors are related to analgesia, respiratory depression, euphoria, sedation, and physical dependence.[35] The activity of morphine at delta receptors is 50 to 100 times weaker than that at mu receptors.[33,35] Enkephalins (endogenous opiate-like neurotransmitter peptides) are more potent at delta receptors than at mu receptors. The kappa receptor, primarily related to spinal analgesia and sedation, is located in the spinal cord.[33,35,36] The sigma receptor is responsible for the psychotomimetic effects of opioids (especially mixed agonist–antagonists), such as hallucinations and dysphoria.[33]

Nonopioid peripherally acting analgesics such as nonsteroidal anti-inflammatory drugs (NSAIDs) exert their effects by interacting with the peripheral nervous system; acetaminophen affects the nonopioid receptors in the central nervous system. NSAIDs affect the generation of afferent impulses in the sensory neurons in response to tissue injury or inflammation (nociception). This interaction leads to inhibition of prostaglandin synthetase and thus inhibits the production of prostinoids such as prostaglandins, which are mediators of pain and inflammation produced de novo in response to tissue injury or other noxious stimuli.[37,38] Although central sites of action have been postulated, these agents generally do not alter sensorium or mood in therapeutic doses.[33]

Pain Assessment

Pain assessment is relatively easy in older adolescents and young adults, but decreasing age makes accurate assessment more difficult. Pain is a subjective phenomenon, and its assessment often depends on patient report.[39] In infants and young children who are unable or unwilling to report their pain, pain assessment depends on clinical judgment, much of which has not been well standardized. One of the reasons for undertreatment of pain in pediatric patients may be that the pain is difficult to assess accurately; currently, there is no universally accepted, easily administered technique for assessing pain in the pediatric population.[5,25]

Selection of the appropriate assessment tool must be based on the child's medical condition, age, sex, ethnic background, and cognitive level. For the most part, children aged three years and older are able to understand the various degrees of pain. Because young children do not have the verbal abilities of young adults, other methods have been developed to assess their pain. These methods attempt to rely on behavioral measures. The behaviors commonly associated with pain, such as facial expressions or vocalization, are placed into a scoring system to assess pain. The evaluation system developed by Grunau and Craig[40] is one of the best forms for assessing infant pain by means of facial expressions. Like most assessment tools for the infant, it is best at indicating the presence or absence of pain rather than the degree of pain.

Unlike infants, children may be able to communicate the degree of pain that they are feeling if appropriate tools are used. Children can point to pictures of children that best reflect their own experience of hurt[41-43] or quantify pain with poker chips.[44] The Children's Hospital of Eastern Ontario Pain Scale, which was developed by McGrath et al.,[45] uses behavioral assessment to evaluate pain in children aged one to seven years. This rating scale has been validated for children experiencing postoperative pain. By the time children get to school age, they are at a concrete stage of cognitive development and can begin to understand abstract phenomena. In this age group visual analogue scales of 0–100 or 0–10 may be used.

A valuable tool for assessing pain in adults is the McGill pain questionnaire.[46] Unfortunately, its 78 verbal descriptors for pain are often too complex for children to comprehend. Tessler et al.[47] have adapted this questionnaire to be effective in young adolescents. Older adolescents are at a formal stage of cognitive development and are able to abstract, quantify, and qualify phenomena; therefore, they can use adult scales.[48]

Principles of Acute Pain Management

Despite limited information, children's pain requires treatment. The clinician should have a high index of suspicion of the presence of pain in children. Depending on the severity of the pain, use of peripherally active as well as centrally active agents should be considered. Both i.v. and noninjectable routes should be considered. The i.m. route of drug administration should be avoided in the suffering child because it provides negative reinforcement for the child to report future pain.

Opioid Analgesia

Despite their adverse effects on respiration, opioids

are the most frequently used class of drugs for providing analgesia for acute pain in newborn infants, children, and adolescents. At equipotent analgesic doses, all pure agonists produce similar degrees of respiratory depression and constipation.[34] Although fentanyl is structurally related to meperidine, it has substantially less sedative and hypnotic activity than meperidine.[49] The cardiovascular response to surgery may be reduced when opioid analgesics are used in the postoperative period.[50] The increase in pulmonary vascular resistance during endotracheal suction may be blunted by opioid analgesics.[51]

Neonates are more susceptible than other age groups to the depressant effects of opioids.[52] This increased susceptibility may have a variety of causes, including altered drug metabolism and excretion resulting from immature excretory pathways. An incomplete blood–brain barrier during early neonatal life may allow greater penetration of opioids into the central nervous system receptor sites, producing a more profound effect.[53] In addition, there are changes in the proportion of mu type 1 and mu type 2 receptors during early neonatal life.[54] Theoretically, the risk of respiratory depression is increased because the proportion of mu type 1 receptors is low at birth.[55,56] One study showed that morphine depressed the respiratory rate to a greater extent in 2-day-old rats than in 14-day-old rats.[56] Should overdose occur at the mu type 1 receptors, the effects can be reversed by naloxone.[55,56]

In mechanically ventilated newborn infants, the risk of opioids causing respiratory depression may not be a major concern. Because of immature metabolic pathways, prolonged use of opioids may lead to drug accumulation in premature neonates. Infusions rates may need to be reduced before these infants are completely weaned from mechanical ventilators. When infants receive opioids for a long period of time, tolerance may develop so that complete withdrawal of the opioid may not be required before extubation. Opioid analgesia must be administered with caution in infants who are not mechanically ventilated because of the associated risk of respiratory depression.[8]

Table 1 shows the relative potency of the most commonly used agonists, antagonists, and partial agonists and their effects on mu receptors.

Morphine

Pharmacokinetics. *Neonates.* The pharmacokinetics of morphine in neonates have been investigated by several authors.[57-63] The mean elimination half-life of morphine is significantly longer in neonates (six to seven hours) than in older infants (three to four hours) and adults (two hours). The clearance is lower (6.3 versus 23.8 mL/kg/min) in neonates than in older infants, whereas the volume of distribution is the same.[58-63] Delayed excretion, possibly due to immature hepatic function, and enhanced sensitivity to morphine in this age group are clinically important because the action of a single dose of morphine sulfate may be prolonged and morphine may accumulate during infusions. Morphine concentrations in neonates receiving 20 μg/kg/hr for 24 hours have been reported to be three times higher (52 ± 31 ng/mL) than

Table 1.
Potency of Commonly Used Opioids[34,a]

Generic Name	Equipotent I.V. Dose (mg/kg)	% Bioavailability	Action on Mu Receptors[b]	Comments
Agonists				
Morphine sulfate	0.1	25	A	Vasodilator; avoid in cases of shock; seizures possible at high doses
Meperidine hydrochloride	1.0	56	A	Tachycardia, possible seizures
Codeine phosphate	1.2	60	A	I.V. administration not recommended
Methadone hydrochloride	0.1	60–80	A	Long acting
Fentanyl (as the citrate salt)	0.001	. . .	A	Chest wall rigidity, bradycardia; use muscle relaxants
Alfentanil (as the hydrochloride salt)	0.01	. . .	A	Short acting
Sufentanil (as the citrate salt)	0.0001	. . .	A	Short acting
Agonist–Antagonists[c]				
Pentazocine (as the lactate salt)	0.33	20	pAg	Ceiling effect on respiratory depression and analgesia
Buprenorphine (as the hydrochloride salt)	0.03	55	pAg	
Nalbuphine hydrochloride	0.1	20	pAg	
Antagonist				
Naloxone hydrochloride	. . .	. . .	Antg	

[a] Potency in relation to morphine.
[b] A = agonist; pAg = partial agonist; Antg = antagonist.
[c] These agents exhibit extensive first-pass metabolism.

the concentrations in older children receiving the same dose.[58] Newborn infants receiving 30–40 μg/kg/hr may develop generalized seizures.[58]

The pharmacokinetics of single doses of morphine sulfate were recently evaluated in 10 premature neonates (gestational age of <30 weeks).[59] The mean ± S.D. elimination half-life of morphine was 10 ± 3.7 hours; the mean ± S.D. total body clearance was 3.39 ± 3.28 mL/kg/min. The corresponding values in three full-term infants were 6.7 ± 4.6 hours and 15.5 ± 10 mL/kg/min, respectively. Between 18% and 22% of morphine was bound to plasma proteins. Low protein binding could increase the concentration of unbound morphine in blood and the sensitivity to morphine in neonates. Because of the apparently greater sensitivity to morphine and the lower elimination rate in the neonatal period, the infused dose of morphine sulfate usually should not exceed 15 μg/kg/hr. Neonates should receive a loading dose of 50–100 μg/kg followed by continuous infusion of 5–15 μg/kg/hr.[54,58] The infusion rate should be adjusted on the basis of patient response. Incremental doses of 50–100 μg/kg may be administered every four hours as required. Most newborn infants requiring artificial ventilatory support might tolerate morphine sulfate at a rate of 10 μg/kg/hr without developing respiratory depression.[54] In neonates, bolus administration of morphine may be acceptable because of the drug's prolonged half-life.

Infants and Children. Constant blood and cerebrospinal fluid concentrations are necessary for obtaining adequate analgesia.[62] The analgesic effect also depends on the degree of receptor occupancy.[63] In older children and adolescents, satisfactory long-term analgesia is not easily achieved with bolus administration, especially with "as-needed" i.m. and i.v. injections. Continuous infusion of morphine, which maximizes pain-free periods, has gained widespread popularity, especially for achieving postoperative pain control. The pharmacokinetics of morphine after continuous i.v. infusion in pediatric patients have been evaluated.[64–71]

In children aged 10 months to 15 years who received a 0.2-mg/kg bolus dose of morphine sulfate followed by continuous infusion of 20 μg/kg/hr, the mean plasma morphine concentration was 16–18 ng/mL approximately eight hours after the start of the infusion.[65] The authors suggest that dosing of morphine based on body weight alone produces fairly constant plasma concentrations compared with the concentrations resulting from a regimen of 0.2 mg/kg i.m. every four hours. The continuous-administration method was found to be a more acceptable technique for providing analgesia because the pain relief was continuous and the severe pain that can occur when an i.m. dose of morphine wears off was avoided.[64]

Wide variation in serum morphine concentrations (8–30 ng/mL) was observed after a 10–30 μg/kg/hr morphine sulfate infusion after cardiac surgery.[68] Infusions of 10–30 μg/kg/hr did not interfere with weaning children receiving assisted ventilation from the ventilator. For children breathing spontaneously, serum morphine concentrations lower than 30 ng/mL were not associated with hypercarbia, indicating that morphine did not interfere with spontaneous ventilation. Pain was relieved at serum morphine concentrations greater than 12 ng/mL.[68]

Olkkola et al.[70] evaluated the effects of i.v. infusions of morphine sulfate 50 μg/min in children 0.03–6 years of age. The mean steady-state plasma morphine concentration was 26.2 ng/mL. The respiratory rate decreased in children younger than four years of age, whereas no change was observed in the older children. Arterial P_{CO_2} was increased in the youngest patients only. There were no clinically important hemodynamic changes during and after morphine infusion. The dose used in this study was considerably higher than that used in other studies.[65,68] The respiratory depressant effects observed in younger children may have been due to accumulation of morphine because the mean total body clearance was 5.2 mL/kg/min in the younger children (0.03 and 0.2 year) compared with 25.8–75.6 mL/kg/min in older children. Pronounced episodic oxygen desaturation associated with obstructive apnea, paradoxic breathing, and decreased ventilation has been reported after continuous morphine infusion in adults.[71]

From the above studies it appears that infusion rates of 10–30 μg/kg/hr provide satisfactory analgesia with minimal respiratory depression while allowing a constant plasma analgesic concentration to be reached within four to eight hours.[64,65,68,69] A loading dose of morphine sulfate 0.1–0.2 mg/kg may be administered at the start of the infusion. Additionally, an incremental bolus dose of 0.05–0.1 mg/kg may be used every four hours in patients whose pain is not adequately relieved by the continuous infusion.

After five to six months of age, metabolism of morphine becomes similar to that in adults.[35,65] Patients younger than five to six months should receive the regimens recommended for neonates. Problems inherent to infusions may occur, such as equipment malfunction or errors in infusion rate settings. Careful observation of the device and patient is necessary for early detection of these errors. Adjusting the infusion rate according to the patient's response may minimize the risk of periodic desaturation.[71]

Patient-Controlled Analgesia. Patient-controlled analgesia (PCA) devices providing either bolus doses[72] or incremental bolus doses along with a continuous infusion[73] allow a patient to control the administration of analgesics according to his or her perception of pain. Pain perception after surgery is variable.[74] Allowing a patient to control the administration of analgesics reduces the problem of large interindividual variations in the response to opioids.

Studies have confirmed the effectiveness of PCA in children as young as 10 years of age.[75,76] Rodgers et al.[76] used morphine sulfate administered by PCA in 15 children 10 to 15 years of age. The average amount of morphine sulfate used on the first postoperative day by patients who had the PCA pump was 0.72 mg/kg, which was significantly higher than the dosage of 0.34 mg/kg administered i.m. to a comparable group of patients evaluated retrospectively. By the third postoperative day the amount of morphine sulfate received by the PCA group was less than that received by patients in the group evaluated retrospectively. On a visual analogue scale of 1 to 10 (0 = no pain; 10 = worst pain ever experienced), the pain relief was reported to be satisfactory, with an average score of 5 in the PCA group. The authors concluded that pain was less well controlled in the group that did not use PCA. In the authors' experience with morphine sulfate administered by PCA, optimal pain control is achieved with small doses (25–50 μg/kg) given at short lockout intervals (10–15 minutes) after a loading dose of 0.05–0.1 mg/kg. The four-hour maximum dose in this study was set at 100–200 μg/kg. Guidelines for initiating a morphine sulfate infusion administered by PCA are presented in Table 2. These guidelines are currently in place at our institution and are based on published literature[77] as well as our own experience with morphine sulfate administered by PCA.

Epidural Analgesia. Epidural administration of morphine is a novel approach to analgesia that has been shown to be highly effective.[78-82] In children, the caudal approach to the epidural space can provide analgesia from the lower extremities to the thoracic region. The advantages of this approach are a prolonged duration of profound analgesia and minimal sedation. Concerns about epidural opioid administration are related to adverse effects, which occur in 25% of patients. These include nausea, pruritus, and urinary retention.[79-81] Late respiratory depression is an infrequent but serious adverse effect of epidural morphine that is much more common in adults than in children.[79] The possibility of late respiratory depression necessitates close observation of the patient's respiratory status for up to 12 hours after administration of the drug. Morphine sulfate may be given at a dosage of 0.075 mg/kg every 8–12 hours or as a 0.04 mg/kg loading dose followed by continuous infusion of 0.125 μg/kg/min. When fentanyl is used, a loading dose generally is not given because the drug is highly lipophilic; the usual infusion rate is 1 μg/kg/hr. These guidelines are based on the current practice at our institution.

Adverse Effects. When morphine sulfate 0.1 mg/kg is administered i.v. or i.m. to otherwise unmedicated patients in pain, analgesia usually occurs without loss of consciousness. Patients may develop a sense of euphoria and a general feeling of well-being. When morphine is administered to pain-free adults, they show signs of dysphoria and anxiety[34] and a slight rise in P_{CO_2}. Morphine may cause sedation, nausea, vomiting, and, at high doses, seizures.[34,57] The nausea and vomiting are caused by stimulation of the chemoreceptor trigger zone in the brain stem. Morphine (and all other opioids at equipotent doses) inhibits intestinal smooth muscle motility and should be used with caution in patients who are at risk of biliary cholelithiasis.

Table 2.
Guidelines for Starting Patient-Controlled Analgesia (PCA) Using Morphine Sulfate in Children and Adolescents[a]

PCA Method	Intermittent Dose (mg/kg)	Lockout Interval (min)	Infusion Rate (mg/kg/hr)	Four-Hour Limit (mg/kg)
Intermittent bolus doses	0.025–0.05	8–15	0	0.24–0.5
Continuous infusion with intermittent bolus doses	0.018–0.04	8–15	0.01–0.04	0.24–0.5

[a] These guidelines are based on our current experience at the University of Michigan Medical Center.

Meperidine

Pharmacokinetics. Meperidine, which is 10 times less potent than morphine, is commonly used in children for anesthesia, sedation, or treatment of postoperative pain. However, there are few pharmacokinetic and pharmacodynamic studies of meperidine in pediatric patients. In nine infants (aged 3–18 months) who received meperidine hydrochloride 0.65–1.1 mg/kg, the elimination half-life and steady-state volume of distribution of meperidine were 2.3 ± 0.4 hours (mean ± S.D.) and 5 L/kg, respectively[83]; values in adults were 3.3 ± 0.9 hours and 4.17 L/kg. Meperidine was 85% protein bound in infants. The plasma half-life of meperidine in newborn infants after in utero exposure ranged from 6.9 to 39 hours.[84] The long half-life suggests a substantially slower elimination rate of meperidine in newborns compared with adults. Plasma meperidine concentrations of 100–200 ng/mL may be present at birth in infants of mothers who received meperidine hydrochloride 1.5–3 mg/kg at delivery.

Evaluation of the plasma concentration–effect relationship indicates that a plasma meperidine concentration of 200–400 ng/mL is required to obtain satisfactory analgesia in adults, whereas respiratory depression occurs at plasma meperidine concentrations greater than 500–600 ng/mL. Other central nervous system effects such as sedation occur at 150–300 ng/mL.[85] Although no systematic data are available for determining the plasma meperidine concentration–effect relationship in children, clinical experience suggests that the same degree of respiratory depression occurs in neonates as in adults.[86] Cyanosis and hypotonia have been associated with a plasma meperidine concentration of 560 ng/mL or a plasma normeperidine concentration of 200 ng/mL.[87]

Meperidine is metabolized to a pharmacologically active metabolite, normeperidine. The urinary excretion of meperidine and normeperidine is pH dependent, and at fluctuating urinary pH about 30% of a dose may be excreted as meperidine. The excretion of meperidine and normeperidine is limited during the first 24 hours after birth because of immature renal function. Urinary excretion of these compounds increases over the next 48 hours.[88] Normeperidine, which has half the analgesic activity of meperidine, is twice as potent as meperidine as a convulsive agent.

Adverse Effects. Adverse effects of meperidine include neurotoxicity manifested as seizures.[89] Although this is not a common occurrence at recommended dosages, high dosages of meperidine could result in substantial accumulation of normeperidine in infants and children because of immature renal function. Meperidine hydrochloride is generally used at a dosage of 1–1.5 mg/kg every three to four hours as required (8–12 mg/kg/day).[90] The seizures reported by Kyff and Rice[89] may have been due to the high dose of meperidine that the child received, leading to excessive accumulation of meperidine and normeperidine. Because of the potential for neurotoxicity with meperidine and normeperidine, meperidine should be used with caution in pediatric patients.

Comparison with Morphine. At equipotent doses (1–2 mg/kg), meperidine has few advantages over morphine. At equianalgesic doses it may produce less increase in biliary tract pressure than morphine. This finding may be of value in patients who are prone to cholelithiasis, such as those with biliary colic or sickle cell disease. However, other studies dispute this finding.[91,92] Unlike other opioids, meperidine may produce an increase in heart rate when administered intravenously. This effect is considered desirable in the pediatric population. When used in PCA, meperidine may be a good alternative to morphine in patients who are experiencing nausea or pruritus. When meperidine is administered by PCA, the dose required is about 10 times that of morphine administered by PCA. The lockout interval remains the same. Experience with meperidine administered by PCA in children is limited. Its real advantage over morphine is a higher oral bioavailability.[93,94]

Fentanyl

Fentanyl is often used in anesthesia because of its rapid onset and brief duration of action. It is also commonly used for short procedures such as bone marrow aspiration, fracture reduction, and suture of lacerations.[95] Fentanyl is 100 times more potent than morphine and has less hypnotic or sedative activity.[96] It blocks painful stimuli while maintaining hemodynamic stability even in neonates.[50] Therefore, it is ideal for trauma, cardiac, or intensive-care-unit patients. In addition to blocking the systemic and pulmonary hemodynamic responses to pain, fentanyl also prevents the endocrine stress response to painful stimuli. Although morphine has a similar effect, the drugs have not been compared at equipotent doses with respect to the intensity of the effect. Preventing the endocrine stress response may be a distinct advantage in seriously ill patients.[97]

Fentanyl (as the citrate salt) 12.5 μg/kg can blunt the cardiovascular response to surgery,[98] whereas a higher dose of 25 μg/kg is required to blunt the pulmonary response to endotracheal suction.[51] Yaster[98] observed an initial decrease in heart rate and arterial pressure in neonates irrespective of the dose administered (2.5–12.5 μg/kg).

Pharmacokinetics. The pharmacokinetic profile of fentanyl is significantly different in newborn infants than in older children or adults.[99-103] Fentanyl is highly lipophilic and penetrates the blood–brain barrier rapidly. Because of its high lipid solubility, it is removed from the plasma rapidly.[99] Pharmacokinetic studies of fentanyl in neonates, infants, and children are summarized in Table 3. The clearance and volume of distribution of fentanyl in neonates, children, and adults are compared in Figure 1. It is clear from these data that the volume of distribution and the total body clearance are greater in neonates than in children and

Table 3.
Pharmacokinetic Studies of Intravenous Fentanyl in Neonates, Infants, and Children[a]

Reference	No. Patients	Age at Treatment	Dose	V (L/kg)	CL (mL/kg/min)	$t_{1/2}$ (min)
100	14 neonates	1–14 days	10–50 μg/kg	5.1 ± 1	18 ± 4.4	317 ± 70
101	9 preterm infants	29–43 weeks postconceptional age	30 μg/kg	. . .	. . .	1062 ± 558
102	17 neonates, infants, and children	1 ± 0 days	. . .	5.94 ± 1.47	16.2 ± 2.6	294 ± 113
		7 ± 0.06 months	. . .	4.45 ± 1.64	18.1 ± 1.41	233 ± 137
		3.17 ± 0.68 years	. . .	3.06 ± 1.02	11.5 ± 4.2	244 ± 79
		12 ± 1.73 years	. . .	1.92 ± 1.04	7.05 ± 1.24	208 ± 71
104	10 children	5 months–4.5 years	50-μg/kg bolus, then 0.15–0.3 μg/kg/min	1.39 ± 0.29	12.8 ± 7.3	141 ± 98
	9 children	0.5–9 years	30 μg/kg bolus, then 0.3 μg/kg/min			
	10 adults	. . .	. . .	3.2–5.9	11.2–15.4	69–265

[a] All values are mean ± S.D. or range.

Figure 1. Age-related differences in fentanyl pharmacokinetics.[100-102,105-107]

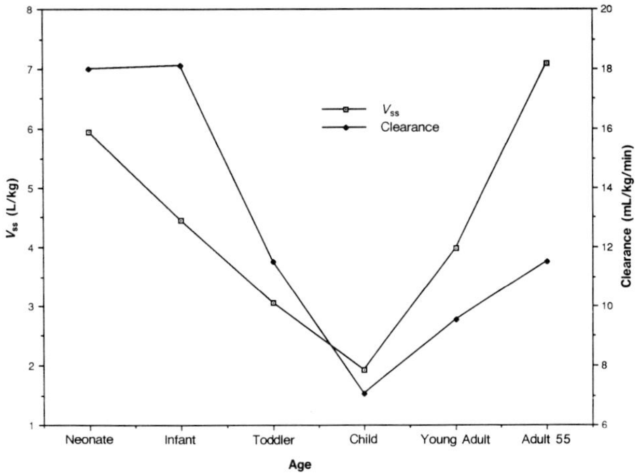

young adults. Therefore, larger initial doses may be required to achieve a given plasma concentration.

The terminal elimination half-life is prolonged in neonates (317 ± 70 minutes versus 129 minutes in adults)[100] and may be even longer (17.7 ± 9.3 hours) in preterm infants.[101] Prolongation of the fentanyl elimination half-life has important clinical implications. Repeated doses of fentanyl for maintenance analgesia will lead to the drug's accumulation and exacerbate its ventilatory depressant effects. On the other hand, infants older than three months tolerate more drug without respiratory depression.[100,108]

Adverse Effects. A serious adverse effect of fentanyl, chest wall rigidity, may occur after rapid infusions of 5 μg/kg or more. Chest wall rigidity could make ventilation difficult. Small doses of nondepolarizing neuromuscular blocking agents or midazolam may be used in conjunction with fentanyl to avoid this adverse effect. Caution should be exercised when midazolam and fentanyl are used concurrently because hypoxemia, apnea, and even respiratory arrest could be caused by an interaction between these two drugs. Frequent monitoring of vital signs and adjustment of the doses of both drugs rather than administration at regular intervals of a fixed dose based on body weight should minimize the probability of this adverse effect.[109,110]

Dosage and Administration. For sedation and analgesia in the neonatal intensive-care unit, an infusion rate of 2–4 μg/kg/hr of fentanyl (as the citrate salt) has been found to be satisfactory without causing any adverse cardiovascular effects. When maximal blunting of the stress response is indicated, infusion rates as high as 7.2 μg/kg/hr have been used with good effects. In older children in intensive-care units, infusion rates of 4–8 μg/kg/hr may be used for analgesia. At the start of therapy, a loading dose of 30–50 μg/kg of fentanyl (as the citrate salt) should be given, followed by continuous infusion of 0.3 μg/kg/min (neonates and infants), 0.25 μg/kg/min (toddlers), 0.15 μg/kg/min (children), or 0.2 μg/kg/min (adults).[99-103,108] These dosage recommendations are based on reported clearance rates and are intended to produce plasma fentanyl concentrations of about 20 ng/mL. Vital signs should be monitored at regular intervals, and the infusion rate should be slowed if adverse effects (respiratory depression, chest wall rigidity) occur.

Transdermal fentanyl has been used successfully in the treatment of postoperative pain in adults. The steady pain relief achieved through the constant blood concentrations provided by the transdermal route is preferred to the "peak and valley" effect produced by the conventional dosage forms.[111,112] Currently, there is little information on the use of transdermal fentanyl in children and adolescents. However, transdermal fentanyl appears to be a useful preparation for management of pain when i.v. access is difficult. A patch (10 sq cm) of transdermal fentanyl (Duragesic, Alza Corporation) releases fentanyl at a rate of 25 μg/hr. For a child weighing 10 kg or more, this patch would provide fentanyl at a rate of 2.5 μg/kg/hr.[113] This rate is no different from the continuous i.v. infusion rate currently being used to provide analgesia in children.

Streisand et al.[114] evaluated the oral transmucosal absorption of fentanyl by mixing it with a lollipop matrix and administering it orally. The dose that provided sedation and minimized adverse effects was 15–20 μg/kg. Oral transmucosal fentanyl citrate has been compared for safety and efficacy as a premedication with an oral solution containing meperidine hydrochloride (1.5 mg/kg), diazepam (0.2 mg/kg), and atropine sulfate (0.02 mg/kg).[115] The sedation produced by fentanyl was as effective as that produced by meperidine, but fentanyl was associated with a higher incidence of postoperative vomiting.

Fentanyl Derivatives

Experience with congeners of fentanyl (sufentanil and alfentanil) in pediatric patients is limited. Sufentanil is considered to be 5–10 times as potent as fentanyl.[116] The pharmacokinetics of sufentanil have been studied in 28 pediatric patients undergoing cardiovascular procedures.[117] Clearance was significantly lower in neonates than in infants, children, and adolescents (mean ± S.D. of 6.7 ± 6.1 mL/kg/min versus 18.1 ± 2.7, 16.9 ± 3.2, and 13.1 ± 3.6 mL/kg/min, respectively). The volume of distribution was significantly larger in neonates than in children and adolescents (mean ± S.D. of 4.15 ± 1 L/kg versus 2.73 ± 0.5 L/kg and 2.75 ± 0.5 L/kg, respectively). The mean ± S.D. elimination half-life was 783 ± 346 minutes in neonates, significantly longer than the values of 214 ± 41, 140 ± 30, and 209 ± 23 minutes observed in infants, children, and adolescents, respectively. The protein binding of sufentanil is significantly less in newborns and infants than in children and adults[118]; a higher concentration of the free drug results because of decreased protein binding.

The disposition of alfentanil in premature infants

and older children has been evaluated.[119] Compared with older children, premature infants had a significantly larger volume of distribution (mean ± S.D. of 1.0 ± 0.39 L/kg versus 0.48 ± 0.19 L/kg), a lower clearance (mean ± S.D. of 2.2 ± 2.4 L/kg/min versus 5.6 ± 2.4 L/kg/min), and a markedly prolonged elimination half-life (mean ± S.D. of 525 ± 305 minutes versus 60 ± 11 minutes). Rapid i.v. administration of alfentanil (as the hydrochloride salt) 20 μg/kg to preterm infants produced a rapid and sizeable fall in blood pressure and heart rate.[120]

Methadone

Methadone is eliminated slowly and has a long duration of action in children 1–18 years of age; the mean elimination half-life in this age group is 19 hours.[121] However, there appears to be large interpatient variation in volume of distribution and clearance. The mean bioavailability of methadone is about 80% (range, 44–99%). Methadone is eliminated mainly by metabolic clearance. At a urinary pH of <6, renal clearance is increased and becomes quantitatively important.[122] The mean serum half-life of methadone in nine infants exposed to methadone in utero was 53 hours in the postnatal period (from birth to seven weeks of age). In the first four days, these infants were significantly less sensitive to carbon dioxide compared with a control group of infants. Total ventilation, respiratory frequency, oxygen consumption, and end tidal P_{CO_2} were not significantly different in the two groups. The depressed ventilatory response to carbon dioxide persisted for an average of 15 days in most infants exposed to methadone in utero and lasted for a month in one infant.[123]

Codeine

Codeine is most commonly administered in the oral form, generally in combination with acetaminophen or aspirin because of the synergism between those agents and codeine. Codeine shares the effects of morphine on the central nervous system, including respiratory depression, stimulation of the chemoreceptor trigger zone, and sedation. At equipotent doses its efficacy as an analgesic and a respiratory suppressant approaches that of morphine. It also decreases gastric motility and can increase biliary tract pressure.[124]

Codeine is 60% bioavailable after oral administration. Analgesia occurs approximately 20 minutes after an oral dose and reaches a maximum at 60–120 minutes. The elimination half-life is approximately three hours. Codeine is completely metabolized in the liver before excretion in urine.[124]

Intramuscular administration of codeine has no advantage over intramuscular morphine or meperidine. Intravenous administration of codeine is associated with serious apnea and severe hypotension, probably because of histamine release.[124] Thus, codeine phosphate is used to treat mild to moderate pain in an outpatient setting, at a dose of 0.5–1 mg/kg along with acetaminophen (10 mg/kg).[97]

Partial-Agonist Opioids

Partial-agonist opioids such as nalbuphine, buprenorphine, pentazocine, and meptazinol produce less respiratory depression and biliary spasm than morphine.[125-127] They are also substantially less potent as analgesics and exhibit a ceiling effect of analgesia.[49,125]

Intramuscular nalbuphine effectively treats postoperative pain in children.[128-131] Nalbuphine hydrochloride 0.2–0.3 mg/kg i.m. provided satisfactory postoperative pain relief in children 3–11 years old undergoing tonsillectomy or orchidopexy.[128-130] Nalbuphine hydrochloride 0.3 mg/kg provided a longer pain-free period than morphine sulfate 0.2 mg/kg and did not cause important adverse effects such as nausea or excessive sedation. Compared with morphine sulfate 0.2 mg/kg i.m. administered to a control group,[128,129] nalbuphine hydrochloride 0.2–0.3 mg/kg provided adequate analgesia. It is thought that the 0.3-mg/kg dose should not pose any respiratory problems because of the ceiling effect of nalbuphine.[130] Jaillon et al.[131] compared the pharmacokinetics of i.v. and oral nalbuphine in infants, young adults, and elderly patients. Fourteen children (1.5–8.5 years) received nalbuphine hydrochloride 0.2 mg/kg i.v. or orally. The elimination half-life was much shorter in children (0.9 hours) than in young adults (1.9 hours) and the elderly (2.3 hours). The clearance of nalbuphine decreased substantially with age, whereas the systemic bioavailability increased with age.

Sublingual, i.v., and i.m. buprenorphine has been evaluated in children.[132-134] Intravenous buprenorphine provides good analgesia for moderate to severe pain in the immediate postoperative period. Adequate analgesia was reported in 240 children younger than 18 years of age who received a single 0.3-mg dose of buprenorphine (as the hydrochloride salt) i.v. for immediate postoperative pain relief.[134] In children aged 4 to 14 years, the i.v. dose of buprenorphine required to obtain "complete initial analgesia" after orthopedic surgery was 5.2 ± 2.8 μg/kg, while that of morphine was 166 ± 100 μg/kg.[132] The mean ± S.D. duration of action was longer with buprenorphine (248 ± 314 minutes) than morphine (114 ± 109 minutes). Sublingual administration of buprenorphine 5–7 μg/kg was also effective, but this dosage form is not available in the United States. Compared with morphine, buprenorphine appears to cause a slightly higher frequency of nausea and vomiting.[132,133]

Meptazinol (as the hydrochloride salt) 1 mg/kg i.m. has been shown to be as effective as meperidine for posttonsillectomy pain relief,[135] but it has not been investigated further.

Pentazocine has potent analgesic properties and a low potential for abuse. Its respiratory depression potential is, however, the same as that of morphine at equipotent doses.[136-138] Pentazocine (as the lactate salt) 0.2 mg/kg or 0.4 mg/kg i.v. has provided satisfactory analgesia in pediatric burn patients.[138] Pentazocine and nalbuphine were comparable when used for premedication; both drugs decreased apprehension at the time of anesthesia induction and also after surgery.[139]

As is evident from the above discussion, the literature on the use of partial agonists to treat acute pain in pediatric patients is scarce. At our institution these drugs are not used for acute pain relief in children.

Nonopioid Analgesia

Acetaminophen and NSAIDs are useful for relieving pain of noninflammatory and inflammatory origin, respectively.

Acetaminophen. Acetaminophen inhibits prostaglandin synthetase centrally. Hence, at equipotent doses, it does not appear to have the adverse effects associated with peripheral prostaglandin inhibition that are commonly seen with NSAIDs.[38] Acetaminophen 10–15 mg/kg every four hours orally or 15–20 mg/kg rectally is the most common nonnarcotic analgesic used in children today. At these doses it appears to be quite safe in children, including newborn infants.[140] In neonates acetaminophen is eliminated primarily as the sulfate conjugate. Sulfate conjugation compensates for the deficiency in glucuronide formation. No age-related differences in the overall elimination rate constant for acetaminophen have been found in neonates, infants, children, and adults.[141] Acetaminophen's weak analgesic properties make it suitable for treating minor pain and discomfort. It also is beneficial as an adjunct to opioid analgesics in patients with more severe pain.

Nonsteroidal Anti-inflammatory agents. The therapeutic effects of NSAIDs are derived from their ability to inhibit prostaglandin synthetase.[38] NSAIDs may provide adequate analgesia when used alone after minor surgery. They also can be used synergistically with opioid drugs.[38,142] Until recently, NSAIDs were available only in an oral dosage form. Peripherally acting agents have gained widespread use because of their low frequency of central nervous system adverse effects such as respiratory depression and sedation.[38] Therefore, these agents are preferred for mild to moderate pain.

NSAIDs are also useful for treating acute pain of inflammatory origin and for postoperative analgesia after minor surgery. They may provide adequate analgesia when used alone for these indications. However, there is concern about oral administration of NSAIDs in the immediate postoperative period. In addition, there may be an increased risk of NSAID-induced gastritis.

The most frequently used NSAIDs are ibuprofen, naproxen, and tolmetin; all of these agents are labeled by the FDA for use as analgesics in children 2–12 years old.[143] They also can be used synergistically with opioid drugs. As an analgesic, ibuprofen is used at a dosage of 4–10 mg/kg orally every six to eight hours.[143] A pediatric suspension of ibuprofen (PediaProfen, McNeil) is available. Ibuprofen was more effective than acetaminophen or acetaminophen with codeine for relief of pain after dental extraction.[144] A total of 154 children 5–12 years of age received single doses of acetaminophen elixir (240 or 360 mg), acetaminophen with codeine phosphate elixir (240 mg and 24 mg, respectively), ibuprofen suspension (200 mg), or placebo liquid in a randomized, double-blind trial. Ibuprofen provided relief in 30 minutes. All three active agents were effective at two hours. The overall rating of drug efficacy was significantly better for ibuprofen than for the other active agents. No adverse reactions were reported during the study.[145]

Naproxen and tolmetin (as the sodium salt) are both used at dosages of 5–7 mg/kg every 8–12 hours. Naproxen has a prolonged duration of action and has been used safely in adolescents.[37] Intravenous and oral dosage forms of indomethacin used for pain relief have been shown to decrease morphine requirements in children after tonsillectomy, although an improvement in the quality of analgesia was not detected.[144,146] Intravenous indomethacin is not labeled for use as an analgesic. Oral indomethacin 0.2–2 mg/kg every 8–12 hours may have a greater frequency of toxicity and is not recommended for use in children unless trials with ibuprofen, tolmetin, or naproxen have failed.[37]

All NSAIDs can cause gastritis and are best administered with meals. Nephrotoxicity and hepatotoxicity are uncommon with short-term use (i.e., several weeks).[37] Adverse reactions to one NSAID do not necessarily predict similar reactions to another NSAID.

Aspirin produces irreversible inhibition of prostaglandin synthetase, whereas inhibition by other NSAIDs is reversible.[38] Although aspirin is one of the most widely used analgesics in adults, its use in pediatrics is limited. This is because of (1) its association with Reye's syndrome and (2) a greater appreciation of its adverse effects, including gastritis and platelet dysfunction.[140] For routine use, acetaminophen is preferred over aspirin because of its wider safety margin and reduced number of adverse effects.

Regional Anesthesia

Regional anesthesia produces profound analgesia with minimal physiologic alterations. Certain types of pain are difficult to treat with systemic opioids, or adverse effects of systemic opioid therapy can be problematic. For example, systemic opioids can exacerbate bladder spasm after genitourinary surgery, but the postoperative pain can be treated quite easily with a caudal block.[147] Insertion of a catheter into the lumbar or caudal epidural space provides access for intermittent or continuous administration of local anesthetics for prolonged analgesia.[148] Regional anesthesia produces postoperative analgesia with a reduced risk of respiratory depression.[147] The risk of postanesthetic apnea in premature infants may be reduced by use of

Table 4.
Regional Nerve Block for Analgesia in Various Body Areas

Body Area	Sensory Dermatome Level	Possible Blocks
Head	Cranial nerve	Cranial nerve block
Eye	Cranial nerve	Retrobulbar block
Mouth	Cranial nerve	Cranial nerve block
Neck	C6	Supraclavicular brachial plexus block
Shoulder, arm, hand	C4–T1	Brachial plexus block
Thorax	T2–T6	Epidural thoracic or lumbar block
Abdomen	T5–L1	Epidural lumbar block
Pelvis	T10–L5	Caudal or lumbar epidural block
Thigh	L1–L5	Caudal or lumbar epidural block or femoral 3:1[a] block
Lower leg	L5–S5	Caudal or lumbar epidural block or femoral 3:1[a] and sciatic nerve block
Toes	S5–S1	Caudal epidural block or ankle block

[a] 3:1 block includes femoral, lateral femoral cutaneous, and obterator nerve blocks.

regional anesthesia.[149,150] Regional blocks should be directed toward the dermatomes responsible for the production of pain. Table 4 shows the specific levels of regional anesthesia needed to produce analgesia in various parts of the body.

Pharmacology of Local Anesthetics. Local anesthetic amines are tertiary amines that contain either ester or amide linkages. The esters are metabolized by plasma cholinesterases. Neonates and infants up to six months of age have about half the adult levels of this enzyme.[151] However, there is no evidence that this difference is clinically important. Amide local anesthetics are metabolized in the liver and bound by plasma proteins. Neonates and infants younger than three months of age have reduced liver blood flow and immature metabolic degradation pathways. Larger fractions of amide-type local anesthetics remain unmetabolized and hence active in the plasma of these infants compared with adults, and a larger proportion is excreted unchanged in urine.[152,153]

Circulating concentrations of α_1-acid glycoprotein and albumin, the essential proteins for drug binding, are low in neonates.[154–157] Thus, the concentration of free drug in plasma is increased.[158] Amide-type local anesthetics are mainly bound to α_1-acid glycoprotein, and considerable variation in the plasma concentration of this protein is a major source of variability in the free drug fraction.[151] Consequently, the duration of anesthesia, which depends on the free drug concentration, is variable.[159] Drugs such as lidocaine and bupivacaine may exist in large concentrations as free drugs in neonates if they are used at the same dosage as in older children. Local anesthetics with ester linkages are hydrolyzed to form *p*-aminobenzoic acid, which is capable of inducing allergic-type reactions. Allergic-type reactions are extremely rare with amide-type local anesthetics. The metabolic pathway of prilocaine, which has an amide linkage and is metabolized in the liver, is atypical for amide-type local anesthetics. Metabolism results in the production of oxidants that can lead to the development of methemoglobinemia. Because fetal hemoglobin is oxidized more easily than adult hemoglobin, neonates are more susceptible to methemoglobinemia.[160] Therefore, prilocaine is not recommended for neonates.

Several factors affect the minimum concentration of local anesthetic necessary to block impulse conduction along a nerve fiber. These factors include fiber size and degree of myelination of the nerve to be blocked, pH, local calcium ion concentration, and the rate at which a nerve is excited. The nerves of children are smaller than those of adults, and the process of myelination is not complete until 18 months of age. Thus, a much lower concentration of local anesthetic may achieve a block.[161,162] The pharmacologic activity of local anesthetics is related primarily to their physicochemical properties, although in vivo activity may be altered by such properties as the dose of the agent, addition of a vasoconstrictor, site of administration, or mixtures of local anesthetics. Systemic effects of local anesthetics are determined by the total dose administered and by the rapidity of absorption into the blood.[159]

At recommended doses, plasma levels of local anesthetics usually remain well below recognized toxic concentrations. Cardiovascular and central nervous system toxicities have rarely been seen in pediatric patients after local anesthetic administration.[163] Neonates and infants up to six months of age are at a greater risk for toxicity from local anesthetics, with twofold to threefold increases in elimination half-life because of greatly decreased microsomal enzyme metabolism[158,164,165] and decreased albumin and α_1-acid glycoprotein concentrations. A blood lidocaine concentration of 2.5 µg/mL causes central nervous system toxicity in newborns and infants, whereas the toxic threshold for adults is 5 µg/mL.[166] The classification and duration of action of the most commonly used local anesthetics are shown in Table 5.

Pharmacokinetics of Local Anesthetics. Although there are numerous studies describing the pharmacokinetics of local anesthetics in adults, such studies in pediatrics are scarce. When local anesthetics are administered into highly vascular regions, such as the caudal epidural space, the rate of absorption is more rapid in children than in adults.[168,169] The rapid rate of vascular absorption may be decreased by the addition of a vasoconstrictor to the local anesthetic solution. Adding a vasoconstrictor also lengthens and improves the intensity of local anesthesia and postoperative analgesia.[170-172] Increased cardiac output probably accounts for the faster absorption in children. Rapid elimination occurs because of the larger liver size compared with body surface area in children and also the greater number of metabolic sites for drug break-

Table 5.
Classification and Properties of Commonly Used Local Anesthetics[159,167]

Drug	Onset of Action	Duration of Action	Relative Potency
Esters			
Procaine	Slow	Short	1
Amethocaine	Slow	Long	8
Chloroprocaine	Fast	Short	1
Amides			
Prilocaine	Fast	Intermediate	2
Lidocaine	Fast	Intermediate	2
Mepivacaine	Fast	Intermediate	2
Bupivacaine	Intermediate	Long	8
Etidocaine	Fast	Long	6

down.[156] A larger volume of distribution may also contribute to the low plasma concentration seen in children. The net result is that children older than six months appear to tolerate quite high doses of local anesthetics. The prolonged elimination half-life reported in neonates is probably related to the larger volume of distribution, because clearance is similar to that in children six months of age and older.[158,171]

After epidural administration of a local anesthetic, there is a rapid redistribution phase and a slower elimination phase. When the maximum concentration of the drug (C_{max}), time to C_{max}, volume of distribution at steady state, and total body clearance are known, a maximum initial dose and allowable repeat doses can be determined. Ecoffey et al.[173] demonstrated a peak plasma bupivacaine concentration of 1.25 μg/mL at 29 minutes after caudal administration; the average half-life was 227 minutes. Similarly, peak plasma lidocaine concentrations occurred at 45 minutes after administration, with an average plasma lidocaine concentration of 2 μg/mL and an average half-life of 103 minutes.[171,174] Thus, the peak concentrations of both bupivacaine and lidocaine are considerably below the reported toxic concentrations of these drugs in adults (2–4 μg/mL and 5–10 μg/mL, respectively).[175] When a second dose of a local anesthetic is given into the epidural space, only one half to two thirds of the initial dose should be administered, so that the maximum plasma drug concentration may be kept within a safe range.[147]

Central Blocks

The level of sensory block required to obtain pain relief in specific parts of the body is shown in Table 4. Central blocks may be extradural (epidural) or spinal blocks. The extradural block includes caudal, lumbar, and thoracic epidural administration. The extradural analgesia technique is being used successfully in pediatric patients, including neonates.[176-180]

There are important practical considerations regarding the anatomic differences between adults and children. In infants the lower position of the spinal cord makes access to the extradural space and lumbar puncture safer in the more caudal interspaces of L4-L5 and L5-S1. In children the extradural fat is loosely packed and gelatinous, with distinct intercostal spaces.[181] In adults the fat between intercostal spaces becomes tightly packed and is divided by fibrous strands. Because of loosely packed fat in childhood, there is a low resistance to the longitudinal spread of local anesthetics, which may account for the better quality of blocks seen in children.[181] High local anesthetic extradural or spinal blocks in the region of T3-T5 in younger children (less than six years of age) are usually associated with minimal cardiovascular instability. Above this age range the cardiovascular complications arising from such blocks are similar to those seen in adults.[149,182,183]

Extradural Anesthesia. Caudal blocks are the most popular central blocks used to provide analgesia during and after surgery.[150,158,184--190] Caudal anesthesia is a simple, safe, and effective regional technique that is frequently used for operations below the diaphragm. The single-injection technique is widely used in children, including neonates.[184]

The most common drugs for caudal anesthesia are bupivacaine and lidocaine. Various methods based on patient's weight, age, and length have been proposed to guide the choice of drug and the dose to administer.[191-194] The scheme proposed by Takasaki et al.,[193] volume = 0.056 mL/kg/segment, takes body weight into account and is appropriate for attaining blocks at any level. Ecoffey et al.[148] used 0.75 mL/kg of 0.5% bupivacaine for lumbar epidural anesthesia to obtain motor and sensory blockade during upper abdominal surgery. The maximum blood concentration of bupivacaine was 1.35 μg/mL. Bupivacaine 0.125–0.25% provides prolonged analgesia when used with general anesthesia. Addition of epinephrine 1:200,000 increases the duration of block.[189] However, the effect of epinephrine on the peak plasma drug concentration and time to peak concentration seems to be small for the long-acting agents.[195] For surgery lasting more than two hours, Yaster and Maxwell[147] suggest repeating one half to two thirds of the original volume of 0.25% bupivacaine or an equal volume of 0.125% bupivacaine.[147] For postoperative pain relief, 0.125% bupivacaine provides adequate analgesia of equal duration to that of 0.25% bupivacaine with less motor block.[196] Caudal extradural block with bupivacaine provides satisfactory analgesia for four to eight hours. Complications of caudal extradural block include accidental intravascular or intraosseous injection, dural puncture, hypotension, possible urinary retention, and nausea and vomiting. Hypotension is rare in children.[197-201]

Although single-injection caudal epidural anesthesia is satisfactory for operations below the diaphragm, the volume of drug required to achieve high thoracic levels by the caudal route may become excessive. To overcome this problem, continuous lumbar epidural anesthesia, a technique well established in adults, has recently been used for upper thoracic surgeries in pediatric patients. The resistance to epidural blockade of nerve roots in the L5-S1 position that has been observed in adults is not a problem in children because of the smaller diameter of nerve fibers.[161] The lumbar technique has not been widely accepted because of its technical difficulty.[146-148,177] The development of 24-gauge epidural catheters has enabled thoracic and lumbar epidural spaces to be approached more safely. These catheters can even be inserted from the caudal space with their tips lying at the appropriate dermatome level, eliminating the need for a needle to be placed in the thoracic or lumbar region.[202]

Continuous infusion of local anesthetic avoids the peaks and troughs associated with intermittent injections.[203-206] The first reports of continuous lumbar extradural analgesia after abdominal surgery came from Meignier et al.[204] Bupivacaine 0.25% infused at 4 mg/kg/day resulted in good analgesia without causing cardiovascular instability. Successful lumbar extradural analgesia was obtained by Desparmet and colleagues[205] with a continuous infusion of 0.25% bupivacaine at a dosage of 0.08 mL/kg/hr.[205] For postoperative analgesia, higher concentrations of local anesthetic are not necessary. Low concentrations of local anesthetic are adequate to block the cortisol stress response to surgery in children.[206]

Local anesthetics are not the only choice for epidural analgesia. The presence of high concentrations of opiate receptors in the spinal cord makes it possible to achieve analgesia with small doses of opioids administered in the subarachnoid or epidural space. Administration of morphine via the lumbar route for postoperative analgesia has been described.[178,181] Extradural morphine sulfate 100 μg/kg provides a significantly longer duration of pain relief (8–24 hours) than caudal bupivacaine.[186,187] Attia et al.[176] and Dalen et al.[177] gave morphine sulfate 50 μg/kg in 2–5 mL via lumbar or thoracic extradural catheters.

Increasing the dose of morphine sulfate beyond 100 μg/kg does not improve the quality or duration of analgesia, but nausea, vomiting, and pruritus become more common.[178] These adverse effects occur in 30–40% of patients receiving extradural morphine. Although there is only one report of respiratory depression, the ventilatory response to P_{CO_2} may be depressed for 22 hours after extradural administration of morphine sulfate 0.05 μg/kg.[176] This depression is thought to be due to the spread of morphine to higher levels of the central nervous system via cerebrospinal fluid. One hour after epidural administration, the plasma morphine concentration was 12 μg/mL, much lower than that considered necessary for systemic analgesia in children.[176] Hemodynamic changes as a result of epidural anesthesia are minimal in infants and children.[207]

Intrathecal Anesthesia and Analgesia. Spinal blocks are useful in high-risk preterm infants who are predisposed to apnea, hypoxia, bradycardia, and cardiovascular instability.[208] In 1984 Abajian et al.[149] reported the use of spinal anesthesia in high-risk infants. Several other groups have used this method of anesthesia, with various drugs[209-211] and preparations of different baricity.[212] Hyperbaric bupivacaine and tetracaine and isobaric bupivacaine have been used. Abajian et al. used tetracaine hydrochloride 0.3 mg/kg in high-risk infants with an average weight of 3.5 kg who were undergoing heniorrhaphies and tetracaine hydrochloride 0.2 mg/kg in infants with an average weight of 4.7 kg. In another study in infants, 0.03 mg/kg of 0.5% bupivacaine hydrochloride produced surgical anesthesia for 75 minutes, after which motor activity returned.[209] An important advantage of spinal anesthesia found in this study was that analgesia was persistent for several hours after the return of motor function. Williams et al.[213] have used up to 4 mg of tetracaine hydrochloride to provide surgical anesthesia to neonates undergoing ligation of patent ductus arteriosus.

Peripheral Nerve Block

Longer-acting local anesthetics may be used to obtain peripheral nerve block for intraoperative and postoperative analgesia. Continuous intrapleural infusion of bupivacaine hydrochloride 1.25–2.5 mg/kg/hr by means of indwelling catheters provides effective analgesia in children undergoing anterior spinal fusion or repair of coarctation.[214] In this study, potentially toxic plasma concentrations of local anesthetic were reported at 16 hours after infusion despite use of epinephrine (1:200,000), but no clinical toxicity was observed. However, the authors recommend that the maximum rate of infusion should not exceed 2.5 mg/kg/hr.

Dorsal nerve block of the penis has been used widely for relief of pain after circumcision. The quality of analgesia is as good as that obtained with caudal extradural block, and the potential hazards of the latter are avoided.[215-218] Penile nerve block for circumcision has been shown to produce less physiologic stress than occurs in infants not receiving any anesthesia.[215-217] Successful analgesia with 10% lidocaine hydrochloride solution sprayed on the penis or 5% ointment or 2% jelly applied to the penis after circumcision has also been reported.[219]

Topical anesthetics are being used with increasing frequency for minor procedures such as bronchoscopy, laryngoscopy, and suturing of minor body lacerations. Tetracaine hydrochloride–epinephrine (adrenaline)–cocaine (TAC) solution has become a popular agent for these purposes.[220] TAC solution was first used by Pryor et al.[221] a decade ago. The original formulation of TAC contained tetracaine hydrochloride 5%, epinephrine 1:2000, and cocaine 11.8%.[221] Cocaine and epinephrine were used to provide local vasoconstriction and lengthen the time of local anesthesia, whereas tetracaine and cocaine provided local anesthesia and pain relief.

The anesthetic efficacy of TAC depends on the

method of application of the drug to the affected area. Bonadio[220] suggests thorough cleaning and debridement of the wound before application of the TAC solution. For deeper wounds the cavity should be filled with TAC solution and covered with a piece of gauze or cotton ball impregnated with TAC solution, whereas for superficial wounds a small cotton ball or piece of gauze impregnated with TAC solution and placed on the wound may be sufficient. In either case the TAC solution should remain in contact with the wound for at least 20 minutes before any surgical procedure is performed. The efficacy of TAC solution in providing local anesthesia during different types of minor surgical procedures has been evaluated. Bonadio[220] provides an excellent review of these studies.

Subsequent to the use of TAC, the effectiveness of other local anesthetic preparations without cocaine or tetracaine was evaluated. Schaffer[222] randomized children younger than 10 years of age with facial or scalp lacerations to receive either TAC or tetracaine–epinephrine solution. TAC was prepared as described by Pryor et al.,[221] whereas tetracaine–epinephrine contained the same amounts of tetracaine and epinephrine as TAC but no cocaine. Children in the TAC and tetracaine–epinephrine groups were evaluated for anesthetic efficacy, rate of wound infection, and adverse effects of the anesthetic agents. TAC was significantly more effective than tetracaine–epinephrine as an anesthetic agent, with fewer children in the TAC group requiring supplemental local anesthesia with lidocaine. The infection rate was greater in the TAC group; however, the difference was not clinically important. TAC solution appeared to be more effective as an anesthetic agent and was associated with a low incidence of wound infection. The authors recommend the use of TAC over injectable local anesthetics such as lidocaine.

Bonadio et al.[223] evaluated the efficacy of two local anesthetic solutions: one with tetracaine (TAC) and one without tetracaine (epinephrine–cocaine). The TAC solution was no more effective than the epinephrine–cocaine solution for local anesthesia in patients with minor dermal lacerations. Eliminating tetracaine from the TAC solution has been suggested.

Comparison of subcutaneous or intradermal injections of 1% lidocaine hydrochloride with epinephrine 1:100,000, 1% lidocaine hydrochloride, 1% procaine hydrochloride, and 0.9% sodium chloride revealed 1% procaine hydrochloride to be the most acceptable anesthetic; it was associated with minimal pain on injection.[224]

It appears that TAC has an advantage over lidocaine infiltration in that TAC is absorbed topically. The patient is spared the pain of injection associated with lidocaine infiltration. The reduced pain and improved patient acceptance of the method of anesthesia enhance patient cooperation during the surgical procedure to follow. The local anesthetic activity of TAC is comparable to that of lidocaine in adults as well as children.[221,225,226] TAC appears to be a safe local anesthetic when used appropriately. However, caution must be exercised against the use of large (generally greater than 3 mL) or repeated doses of TAC. If effective anesthesia is not obtained by proper application of an initial dose of TAC, supplemental lidocaine infiltration may be a better choice than a second dose of TAC. This would avoid patient exposure to excessive amounts of cocaine.

Conclusion

A variety of pain management techniques are appropriate for the management of acute pain in pediatric patients. Severe pain can be controlled by i.v. or epidural administration of opioid analgesics. PCA is a useful technique in older children. Epidural or intrathecal administration of local anesthetics provides regional analgesia with minimal physiologic alterations. Topical application of local anesthetics is effective for many minor procedures. Acetaminophen and nonsteroidal anti-inflammatory agents are commonly used to control mild to moderate pain. The development of drugs having fewer adverse effects and noninvasive administration techniques will be important research priorities in the coming years.

References

1. Schechter NL. The under treatment of pain in children: an overview. *Pediatr Clin North Am*. 1989; 36:781-94.
2. McGrath PA, Hiller LM. The enigma of pain in children: an overview. *Pediatrician*. 1989; 16:6-15.
3. Mather L, Mackie J. The incidence of postoperative pain in children. *Pain*. 1983; 15:271-82.
4. Beyer JE, DeGood DE, Ashley LC et al. Patterns of postoperative analgesic use with adults and children following cardiac surgery. *Pain*. 1983; 17:71-81.
5. Schechter NL, Allen DA, Hanson K. Status of pediatric pain control: a comparison of hospital analgesia usage in children and adults. *Pediatrics*. 1986; 77:11-5.
6. Marshall RE. Neonatal pain associated with caregiving procedures. *Pediatr Clin North Am*. 1989; 36:885-903.
7. Anand KJS, Carr DB. The neuroanatomy, neurophysiology and neurochemistry of pain, stress and analgesia in newborns and children. *Pediatr Clin North Am*. 1989; 36:795-827.
8. Gauntlett IS. Analgesia in the neonate. *Br J Hosp Med*. 1987; 6:518-9.
9. Hatch DJ. Analgesia in the neonate. *Br Med J*. 1987; 294:920.
10. Porter F. Pain in the newborn. *Clin Perinatol*. 1989; 16:549-64.
11. Fletcher AB. Pain in the neonate. *N Engl J Med*. 1987; 317:1347-8.
12. Yaster M. Analgesia and anesthesia in neonates. *Br J Pediatr*. 1987; 111:394-6.
13. Kaplan M. Pain, the neonate and the neonatologist. *J Perinatol*. 1988; 8:354-5.
14. Porter J, Jick H. Addiction rare in patients treated with narcotics. *N Engl J Med*. 1980; 302:123.
15. McGrath PJ, Craig KD. Development of psychological factors in children's pain. *Pediatr Clin North Am*. 1989; 36:828-36.
16. Anand KJS, Hickey R. Pain and its effects in the human neonate and fetus. *N Engl J Med*. 1987; 317:1321-9.
17. Gliess J, Stuttgen G. Morphologic and functional development of the skin. In: Stave U, ed. Physiology of the perinatal period. Vol. II. New York: Appleton-Century-Crofts; 1970:887.
18. Valman HB, Pearson JF. What the fetus feels. *Br Med J*. 1980; 280:233-4.

19. Flower MJ. Neuromaturation of the human fetus. *J Med Philos*. 1985; 10:237-51.
20. Gautry JP, Jolivet A, Vieph JP et al. Presence of immunoassayable beta-endorphin in human amniotic fluid: elevation in cases of fetal distress. *Am J Obstet Gynecol*. 1977; 129:211-2.
21. Cosontos K, Rust M, Holt V et al. Elevated plasma beta-endorphin levels in pregnant women and their neonates. *Life Sci*. 1979; 25:835-44.
22. Wardlaw SL, Stark RI, Baxi L et al. Plasma beta-endorphin and beta-lipoprotein in human fetus at delivery: correlation with arterial pH and pO2. *J Clin Endocrinol Metab*. 1979; 49:888-91.
23. Lerman J, Robinson S, Willis MM et al. Anesthetic requirements for halothane in young children 0–1 month and 1–6 months of age. *Anesthesiology*. 1983; 59:421-4.
24. Foley KM, Kourides IA, Inturrisi CE et al. Beta-endorphin: analgesic and hormonal effects in humans. *Proc Natl Acad Sci USA*. 1979; 76:5377-81.
25. Beyer J, DeGood D, Ashley L et al. Patterns of postoperative analgesic use with adults and children following cardiac surgery. *Pain*. 1983; 17:71-81.
26. Pert CB, Snyder SH. Opiate receptor: demonstration in nervous tissue. *Science*. 1973; 179:1011-4.
27. Terenius L. Stereospecific interaction between narcotic analgesics and a synaptic plasma membrane fraction of rat cerebral cortex. *Acta Pharmacol Toxicol*. 1973; 32:317-20.
28. Hughes J. Isolation of an endogenous compound from the brain with pharmacological properties similar to morphine. *Brain Res*. 1975; 88:295-308.
29. Jacob JJC, Ramabadran K. Role of opiate receptors and endogenous ligands in nociception. In: Williams NE, Wilson H, eds. Pain and its management. Oxford: Pergamon Press; 1983:13-32.
30. Jessel T, Iversen LL. Opiate analgesics inhibit substance P release from rat trigeminal nucleus. *Nature*. 1977; 268:549-51.
31. Hosobuchi Y, Li CH. The analgesic activity of human beta-endorphin in man. *Commun Psychopharmacol*. 1978; 2:33-7.
32. Snyder SH. Opiate receptors in the brain. *N Engl J Med*. 1977; 296:266-71.
33. Snyder SH. Drug and neurotransmitter receptors in the brain. *Science*. 1984; 224:22-31.
34. Jaffe JH, Martin WR. Opioid analgesics and antagonists. In: Goodman and Gilman's the pharmacological basis of therapeutics. 7th ed. Gilman AG, Goodman LS, Rall TW et al., eds. New York: Macmillan; 1985: 491-531.
35. Vaught JL, Rothman RB, Westfall TC. Mu and delta receptors: their role in analgesia and in the differential effects of op peptides on analgesia. *Life Sci*. 1982; 30:1443-55.
36. Wood PL. Multiple opiate receptors: support for unique mu, delta, and kappa sites. *Neuropharmacology*. 1982; 21:487-97.
37. Shannon M, Berde CB. Pharmacologic management of pain in children and adolescents. *Pediatr Clin North Am*. 1989; 36:855-71.
38. Amadio P Jr. Peripherally acting analgesics. *Am J Med*. 1984; 177 (Suppl 3A):17-26.
39. Beyer JE, Bournaki MC. Assessment and management of postoperative pain in children. *Pediatrician*. 1989; 16:30-8.
40. Grunau RVE, Craig KD. Pain expression in neonates: facial expression and cry. *Pain*. 1987; 28:395-410.
41. McGrath PA. An assessment of children's pain: a review of behavioral, physiological and direct scaling techniques. *Pain*. 1987; 28:147-76.
42. Beyer J. The Oucher: Auser's manual and technical report. Denver, CO: University of Colorado Health Sciences Center; 1988.
43. McGrath PA, de Veber L, Hearn M et al. Multidimensional pain assessment in children. In: Fields HL, Dubner R, Cervero F, eds. Advances in pain research and therapy. New York: Raven; 1985:387-93.
44. Hester NO. The pre-operational child's reaction to immunization. *Nurs Res*. 1979; 28:250-4.
45. McGrath PJ, Johnson G, Goodman JT et al. The Children's Hospital of Eastern Ontario Pain Scale (CHEOPS): a behavioral scale for rating postoperative pain in children. In: Fields HL, Dubner R, Cervero F, eds. Advances in pain research and therapy. New York: Raven; 1985:9:395-402.
46. Melzack R. The McGill pain questionnaire. Major properties and scoring methods. *Pain*. 1975; 1:277-99.
47. Tessler M, Savedra M, Ward J et al. Children's language of pain. In: Dubner R, Gebhart G, Bond M, eds. Pain research and clinical management. Vol. 3. Amsterdam: Elsevier; 1988:348-52.
48. Beyer JD, Wells N. The assessment of pain in children. *Pediatr Clin North Am*. 1989; 36:837-53.
49. Wood M. Narcotic analgesics and antagonists. In: Wood M, Wood AJJ, eds. Drugs and anesthesia: pharmacology for anesthesiologists. Baltimore: Williams & Wilkins; 1982:163-97.
50. Robinson S, Gregory GA. Fentanyl air oxygen anesthesia for patent ductus arteriosus in preterm infants. *Anesth Analg*. 1981; 60:331-4.
51. Hickey PR, Hansen DD, Wessel DL et al. Blunting of stress responses in the pulmonary circulation of infants by fentanyl. *Anesth Analg*. 1985; 64:1137-42.
52. Way WL, Costely EC, Way EL. Respiratory sensitivity of the newborn infant to meperidine and morphine. *Clin Pharmacol Ther*. 1965; 6:454-61.
53. Kupferberg HJ, Way EL. Pharmacologic basis for the increased sensitivity of the newborn rat to morphine. *J Pharmacol Exp Ther*. 1963; 141:105-12.
54. Lloyd-Thomas AR. Pain management in the pediatric patient. *Br J Anaesth*. 1990; 64:85-104.
55. Pasternak GW, Zhang AZ, Tecott L. Developmental differences between high and low affinity opiate binding sites: their relationship to analgesia and respiratory depression. *Life Sci*. 1980; 27:1185-90.
56. Leslie FM, Tso S, Hurlbut DE. Differential appearance of opiate receptor subtypes in neonatal brain. *Life Sci*. 1982; 31:1393-6.
57. Koren G, Butt W, Chinyanga H et al. Postoperative morphine infusion in newborn infants: assessment of disposition characteristics and safety. *J Pediatr*. 1985; 107:963-7.
58. Lynn AM, Slattery JT. Morphine pharmacokinetics in early infancy. *Anesthesiology*. 1987; 66:136-9.
59. Bhat R, Chari G, Gulati A et al. Pharmacokinetics of a single dose of morphine in preterm infants during the first week of life. *J Pediatr*. 1990; 117:477-81.
60. Vandenberghe H, Macleod S, Chinyanga H et al. Pharmacokinetics of intravenous morphine in balanced anesthesia: studies in children. *Drug Metab Rev*. 1983; 14:887-903.
61. Dahlstrom B, Bolme P, Feychting H et al. Morphine kinetics in children. *Clin Pharmacol Ther*. 1979; 26:354-65.
62. Dahlstrom BE, Paazlow LK, Segre G et al. Relation between morphine pharmacokinetics and analgesia. *J Pharmacokinet Biopharm*. 1978; 6:41-53.
63. Berkowitz BA, Ngai SH, Young JC et al. The disposition of morphine in surgical patients. *Clin Pharmacol Ther*. 1975; 17:629-35.
64. Bray RJ. Post operative analgesia provided by a morphine infusion in children. *Anesthesia*. 1983; 38:1075-8.
65. Bray RJ, Beeton C, Hinton W et al. Plasma morphine levels produced by continuous infusions in children. *Anesthesia*. 1986; 41:753-5.
66. Beasley SW, Tibbals J. Efficacy and safety of continuous morphine infusion for post operative analgesia in the pediatric surgical ward. *Aust NZ J Surg*. 1987; 57:233-7.
67. Dilworth NM, Maakeller A. Pain relief for the pediatric surgical patient. *J Paediatr Surg*. 1987; 22:264-6.
68. Lynn AM, Openheim KE, Tyler DC. Morphine infusion after pediatric cardiac surgery. *Crit Care Med*. 1984; 12:863-6.
69. Miller AJW, Rode H, Cywes S. Continuous morphine infusion for post operative pain in children. *S Afr Med J*. 1987;

72:396-8.
70. Olkkola KT, Maunuksela EL, Korpela R et al. Kinetics and dynamics of post operative intravenous morphine in children. *Clin Pharmacol Ther.* 1988; 44:128-35.
71. Catley DM, Thornton C, Jordan C et al. Pronounced episodic oxygen desaturation in the post operative period: its association with ventilatory pattern and analgesic regime. *Anesthesiology.* 1985; 63:20-8.
72. Evans JM, MacCarthy J, Rosen M et al. Apparatus for patient controlled administration of intravenous narcotics during labour. *Lancet.* 1976; 1:17-8.
73. Hull CJ, Sibbald A. Control of post operative pain by interactive demand analgesia. *Br J Anaesth.* 1981; 53:385-91.
74. Tamsen A, Hartvig P, Fagerlun C et al. Patient controlled analgesia therapy: clinical experience. *Acta Anaesthesiol Scand.* 1982; 74:157-60.
75. Brown RE, Broadman LM. Patient controlled analgesia (PCA) for postoperative pain control in adolescents. *Anesth Analg.* 1987; 66:S22.
76. Rodgers BM, Webb CJ, Stergios D et al. Patient controlled analgesia in paediatric surgery. *J Paediatr Surg.* 1988; 23:259-62.
77. Berde CB, Lehn BM, Yee JD et al. Patient-controlled analgesia in children and adolescents: a randomized, prospective comparision with intramuscular administration of morphine for post-operative analgesia. *J Pediatr.* 1991; 118:460-6.
78. Rosen KR, Rosen DA. Caudal epidural morphine for control of pain following open heart surgery in children. *Anesthesiology.* 1989; 70:418-21.
79. Attia J, Ecoffey C, Sandouk P et al. Epidural morphine in children: pharmacokinetics and CO_2 sensitivity. *Anesthesiology.* 1986; 65:590-4.
80. Dalen B, Tanguy A, Hagerer JP. Lumbar epidural anesthesia for operative and post-operative pain relief in infants and young children. *Anesth Analg.* 1986; 65:1069-73.
81. Glenski JA, Warner MA, Dawson B et al. Post-operative use of epidurally administered morphine in children. *Mayo Clin Proc.* 1984; 59:530-3.
82. Shapiro LA, Jedeikin RJ, Shalev D et al. Epidural morphine analgesia in children. *Anesthesiology.* 1984; 61:210-4.
83. Atwood GF, Evans MA, Harbison RD. Pharmacokinetics of meperidine in infants. *Pediatr Res.* 1976; 10:328.
84. Morselli PL, Rovei V. Placental transfer of pethidine and norpethidine and their pharmacokinetics in the newborn. *Eur J Clin Pharmacol.* 1980; 18:25-30.
85. Mather LE, Meffin PJ. Clinical pharmacokinetics of pethidine. *Clin Pharmacokinet.* 1978; 3:352-68.
86. Way WL, Costley EC, Way EL. Respiratory sensitivity of the newborn infant to meperidine and morphine. *Clin Pharmacol Ther.* 1965; 6:455-61.
87. Brackbill Y, Kane J, Maniello RL et al. Obstetric meperidine usage and assessment of neonatal status. *Anaesthesiology.* 1974; 40:116-20.
88. Crawford JS, Rudofsky S. The placental transmission of pethidine. *Br J Anaesth.* 1965; 37:929-33.
89. Kyff JV, Rice TL. Meperidine-associated seizures in a child. *Clin Pharm.* 1990; 9:337-8.
90. Anon. Meperidine. Drug doses. In: Green MG, ed. The Harriet Lane handbook: a manual for pediatric house officers. 12th ed. Baltimore: Mosby Yearbook; 1991:202.
91. Economou G, Ward-McQuaid JN. A cross-over comparison of the effect of morphine, pethidine, pentazocine, and phenazocine on biliary pressure. *Gut.* 1971; 12:218-21.
92. Radnay PA, Brodman E, Mankikar D et al. The effect of equianalgesic doses of fentanyl, morphine, meperidine, and pentazocine on common bile duct pressure. *Anaesthesist.* 1980; 29:26-9.
93. Hoskins PJ, Hanks GW, Aherne GW et al. The bioavailability and pharmacokinetics of morphine after intravenous, oral, and buccal administration in healthy volunteers. *Br J Clin Pharmacol.* 1989; 27:499-505.
94. Edwards DJ, Svensson CK, Visco JP et al. Clinical pharmacokinetics of pethidine: 1982. *Clin Pharmacokinet.* 1982; 7:421-33.
95. Billmore DA, Neale HW, Gregory RO. Use of I.V. fentanyl in the outpatient treatment of pediatric facial trauma. *J Trauma.* 1985; 25:1079-80.
96. Yaster M, Deshpande JK. Management of pediatric pain with opioid analgesics. *J Paediatr.* 1988; 113:421-9.
97. Anand KJS, Sippell WG, Aynsley-Green A. Randomized trial of fentanyl anesthesia in preterm babies undergoing surgery: effects on the stress response. *Lancet.* 1987; 1:243-7.
98. Yaster M. The dose response of fentanyl in neonatal anesthesia. *Anesthesiology.* 1987; 66:433-5.
99. McClain DA, Hug CC. Intravenous fentanyl kinetics. *Clin Pharmacol Ther.* 1980; 28:106-14.
100. Koehntop DE, Rodman JH, Brundage DM et al. Pharmacokinetics of fentanyl in neonates. *Anesth Analg.* 1986; 65:227-32.
101. Collins C, Koren G, Crean P et al. Fentanyl pharmacokinetics and hemodynamic effects in preterm infants during ligation of patent ductus arteriosus. *Anesth Analg.* 1985; 64:1078-80.
102. Johnson KL, Erickson JP, Holley FO et al. Fentanyl pharmacokinetics in pediatric population. *Anesthesiology.* 1984; 61:A441.
103. Singleton MA, Rosen JI, Fisher DM. Plasma concentration of fentanyl in infants, children, and adults. *Can J Anaesth.* 1987; 34:152-5.
104. Koren G, Goresky G, Crean P et al. Pediatric fentanyl dosing based on pharmacokinetics during cardiac surgery. *Anesth Analg.* 1984; 63:577-82.
105. Bentley JB, Borel JD, Nenad RE et al. Age and fentanyl pharmacokinetics. *Anesth Analg.* 1982; 61:968-71.
106. McClain DA, Hug CC. Intravenous fentanyl kinetics. *Clin Pharmacol Ther.* 1980; 28:106-14.
107. Duthie DJR, McLaren AD, Nimmo WS. Pharmacokinetics of fentanyl during constant rate IV infusion for the relief of pain after surgery. *Br J Anaesth.* 1986; 58:930-56.
108. Hertzka RE, Gauntlett IS, Fisher DM et al. Fentanyl-induced ventilatory depression: effects of age. *Anesthesiology.* 1989; 70:213-8.
109. Yaster M, Nichols DG, Deshpande JK et al. Midazolam-fentanyl intravenous sedation in children: case report of respiratory arrest. *Pediatrics.* 1990; 86:463-7.
110. Bailey PL, Pace NL, Ashburn MA et al. Frequent hypoxemia and apnea after sedation with midazolam and fentanyl. *Anesthesiology.* 1990; 73:826-30.
111. Caplan RA, Ready BL, Oden RV et al. Transdermal fentanyl for postoperative pain management. *JAMA.* 1989; 261:1036-9.
112. Holley FO, Steennis CV. Transdermal administration of fentanyl for postoperative analgesia. *Anesthesiology.* 1986; 65:3A.
113. Ivers-Lee. Duragesic product information. West Caldwell, NJ; 1990 Aug.
114. Streisand JB, Hague B, Vreeswijk HV et al. Oral transmucosal fentanyl premedication in children. *Anesth Analg.* 1987; 66:S170.
115. Nelson DS, Streisand JB, Mulder SM et al. Comparison of oral transmucosal fentanyl citrate and an oral solution of meperidine, diazepam, and atropine for premedication in children. *Anesthesiology.* 1989; 70:616-21.
116. Hilberman M, Hyer D. Potency of sufentanil. *Anesthesiology.* 1986; 64:665-6.
117. Greeley WJ, de Braijn NP, Davis DP. Sufentanil pharmacokinetics in pediatric cardiovascular patients. *Anesth Analg.* 1987; 66:1067-72.
118. Meistelman C, Benhamou D, Barre J et al. Effects of age on plasma protein binding of sufentanil. *Anesthesiology.* 1990; 72:470-3.
119. Davis PJ, Killian A, Stiller RL et al. Pharmacokinetics of alfentanil in newborn premature infants and older children. *Dev Pharmacol Ther.* 1989; 13:21-7.
120. Marlow N, Weindling AM, Cooke RWI. Hazards of analge-

sia for newborn infants. *Arch Dis Child*. 1988; 63:1293-8.
121. Berde CB, Sethna NF, Holzman RS et al. Pharmacokinetics of methadone in children and adolescents in the perioperative period. *Anesthesiology*. 1987; 67:A519.
122. Nilsson MI, Meresaar U, Anggard E. Clinical pharmacokinetics of methadone. *Acta Anaesthesiol Scand*. 1982; Suppl 74:66-9.
123. Olson GD, Lees MH. Ventilatory response to carbon dioxide of infants following chronic prenatal methadone exposure. *J Pediatr*. 1980; 96:983-9.
124. Shanahan EC, Marshall AG, Garrett CPO. Adverse reactions to intravenous codeine phosphate in children. *Anaesthesia*. 1983; 38:40-3.
125. Romagnoli A, Keats AS. Ceiling effect of respiratory depression by nalbuphine. *Clin Pharmacol Ther*. 1980; 27:478-85.
126. Holmes B, Ward A. Meptazinol: a review of its pharmacodynamics and pharmacokinetic properties and therapeutic efficacy. *Drugs*. 1985; 30:285-312.
127. Vandam LD. Drug therapy: butorphanol. *N Engl J Med*. 1980; 302:381-4.
128. Wandless JG. A comparision of nalbuphine with morphine for post-orchidopexy pain. *Eur J Anaesthesiol*. 1987; 4:127-32.
129. Krishan A, Tolhurst-Cleaver CL, Kay B. Controlled comparision of nalbuphine and morphine for post-tonsillectomy pain. *Anaesthesia*. 1985; 40:1178-81.
130. Faithful NS, Tolhurst-Cleaver OL. Nalbuphine for post-operative pain. *Eur J Anaesthesiol*. 1987; 4:450.
131. Jaillon P, Gardin ME, Lecocq B et al. Pharmacokinetics of nalbuphine in infants, healthy young volunteers, and elderly patients. *Clin Pharmacol Ther*. 1989; 46:226-33.
132. Maunuksela EL, Korpela R, Olkkola KT. Comparison of buprenorphine with morphine in the treatment of postoperative pain in children. *Anesth Analg*. 1988; 67:233-9.
133. Maunuksela EL, Korpela R, Olkkola KT. Double-blind, multiple dose comparison of buprenorphine and morphine in postoperative pain of children. *Br J Anaesth*. 1988; 60:48-55.
134. Harcus AW, Ward AE, Smith DW. The monitored release of buprenorphine: results in the young. *J Int Med Res*. 1980; 8:153-5.
135. Ridley SA, Matthews NC, Dixon J. Meptazinol vs pethidine for postoperative pain relief in children. *Anaesthesia*. 1986; 41:263-8.
136. Bellville JW, Green J. The respiratory and subjective effects of pentazocine. *Clin Pharmacol Ther*. 1965; 6:12-6.
137. Rita L, Seleny FL, Levin RM. A comparision of pentazocine and morphine for pediatric premedication. *Anesth Analg*. 1970; 49:377-82.
138. Wilson RD, Priano LL, Traber DL. Evaluation of a nonnarcotic analgesic, pentazocine, in burned children. *Plast Reconstr Surg*. 1971; 48:466-70.
139. Rita L, Seleny F, Goodrazi M. Comparison of the calming and sedative effects of nalbuphine and pentazocine for paediatric premedication. *Can Anaesth Soc J*. 1980; 27:546-9.
140. Rumack BH. Aspirin vs acetaminophen: a comparative view. *Pediatrics*. 1978; 62:943-6.
141. Miller RP, Roberts RJ, Fischer LJ. Acetaminophen elimination kinetics in neonates, children and adults. *Clin Pharmacol Ther*. 1976; 19:284-94.
142. Beaver WT. Combination analgesics. *Am J Med*. 1984; 77(Suppl 3A):38-53.
143. Stiehm ER. Nonsteroidal anti-inflammatory drugs in pediatric patients. *Am J Dis Child*. 1988; 142:1281-2.
144. Maunuksela EL, Olkkola KT, Korpela R. Does prophylactic intravenous infusion of indomethacin improve management of postoperative pain in children? *Can J Anaesth*. 1986; 65:A432.
145. Moore PA, Hargraves JA. Post-extraction pain relief in children: a clinical trial of liquid analgesics. *Int J Clin Pharmacol Ther Toxicol*. 1985; 23:573-7.
146. Maunuksela EL, Olkkola KT, Korpela R. Intravenous indomethacin as a postoperative analgesic in children: acute effects on blood pressure, heart rate, body temperature and bleeding. *Ann Clin Res*. 1987; 19:359-63.
147. Yaster M, Maxwell LG. Pediatric regional anesthesia. *Anesthesiology*. 1989; 70:324-38.
148. Ecoffey C, Dubousset AM, Samiik K. Lumbar and thoracic epidural anesthesia for urologic and upper abdominal surgery in infants and children. *Anesthesiology*. 1986; 65:87-90.
149. Abajian C, Mellish RWP, Browne AF et al. Spinal anesthesia for surgery in the high risk infant. *Anesth Analg*. 1983; 63:506-10.
150. Spear RM, Deshpande JM, Maxwell LG. Caudal anesthesia in the awake, high-risk infant. *Anesthesiology*. 1988; 69:407-9.
151. Zsigmind EK, Downs JR. Plasma cholinesterase activity in newborn and infants. *Can Anaesth Soc J*. 1971; 18:278-85.
152. Mihaly GW, Moore RG, Thomas J et al. Pharmacokinetics of anilide local anesthetics in neonates: I. Lignocaine. *Eur J Clin Pharmacol*. 1978; 13:143-52.
153. Meffin P, Long GJ, Thomas J. Clearance and metabolism of mepivacaine in the human neonate. *Clin Pharmacol Ther*. 1973; 14:218-25.
154. Lesez KM, Swartz J, Strong A et al. The effects of age on the serum concentration of alpha-1 acid glycoprotein in newborns, infants and children. *Anesthesiology*. 1986; 65:A421.
155. Wood M, Wood AJJ. Changes in plasma drug binding and alpha-1 acid glycoprotein in mothers and newborn infants. *Clin Pharmacol Ther*. 1979; 19:426-34.
156. Morselli PL, Franco-Morselli R, Borsi L. Clinical pharmacokinetics in newborns and infants: age related differences and therapeutic implications. *Clin Pharmacokinet*. 1980; 5:485-527.
157. Mather LE, Thomas J. Bupivacaine binding to plasma protein fractions. *J Pharm Pharmacol*. 1978; 30:653-4.
158. Mazoit JX, Denson OD, Samii K. Pharmacokinetics of bupivacaine in infants after caudal anesthesia. *Anesthesiology*. 1988; 68:387-91.
159. Covino BG. Pharmacology of local anesthetic agents. *Br J Anaesth*. 1986; 58:701-16.
160. Feig SA. Methemoglobinemia. In: Nathan DG, Oski FA, eds. Hematology of infancy and childhood. Philadelphia: Saunders; 1974:378-89.
161. Wildsmith JAW. Peripheral nerves and local anesthetic drugs. *Br J Anaesth*. 1986; 58:692-700.
162. Murat I, Walker J, Esteres C et al. Effect of lumbar epidural anesthesia on plasma cortisol levels on children. *Can J Anaesth*. 1988; 35:20-4.
163. Eyres RL, Brown TCK, Hastings C. Plasma level of bupivacaine during convulsions. *Anaesth Intensive Care*. 1983; 14:385.
164. Mango R, Berlin A, Karlson K et al. Anaesthesia for caesarean section: IV. Placental transfer and neonatal elimination of bupivacaine following epidural analgesia for elective caesarean section. *Acta Anaesthesiol Scand*. 1976; 20:141-7.
165. Morgan DJ, McQuillian D, Thomas J. Pharmacokinetics and metabolism of the anilide local anesthetics in neonates: II. Etidocaine. *Eur J Clin Pharmacol*. 1978; 13:359-65.
166. Ralston DH, Shnider SM. The fetal and neonatal effects of regional anesthesia in obstetrics. *Anesthesiology*. 1978; 48:34-64.
167. Ritchie JM, Greene NM. Local anesthetics. In: Goodman and Gilman's the pharmacological basis of therapeutics. 6th ed. Goodman LS, Gilman AG, eds. New York: Macmillan; 1980:300-20.
168. Eyres RL, Kidd J, Oppenheim R et al. Local anesthetic plasma levels in children. *Anaesth Intensive Care*. 1978; 6:243-7.
169. Eyres RL, Bishop W, Oppenheim RC et al. Plasma bupivacaine concentrations in children during caudal epidural analgesia. *Anaesth Intensive Care*. 1983; 11:20-2.
170. Murat I, Delleur MM, Saint-Maurice C. The effects of age and addition of adrenaline to bupivacaine for continuous lumbar epidural anesthesia in children. *Anesthesiology*. 1986; 65:A428.
171. Ecoffey C, Desparmet J, Berdeaux A et al. Pharmacokinetics

of lignocaine in children following caudal anesthesia. *Br J Anaesth.* 1984; 56:1399-1401.
172. Rothstein P, Arthur GR, Feldman H et al. Pharmacokinetics of bupivacaine following intercostal block. *Anesthesiology.* 1981; 57:A426.
173. Ecoffey C, Desparmet J, Maury M et al. Bupivacaine in children: pharmacokinetics following caudal anesthesia. *Anesthesiology.* 1985; 63:447-8.
174. Yaster M, Arnoff D, Kornhauser DM et al. The pharmacokinetics of lidocaine during caudal anesthesia in children. *Anesthesiology.* 1985; 63:A465.
175. Tucker GT. Pharmacokinetics of local anesthetics. *Br J Anaesth.* 1986; 58:717-31.
176. Attia J, Ecoffey C, Sandouk P et al. Epidural morphine in children: pharmacokinetics and CO_2 sensitivity. *Anesthesiology.* 1986; 65:590-4.
177. Dalen B, Tanguy A, Haberer JP. Lumbar epidural anesthesia for operative and postoperative pain relief in infants and young children. *Anesth Analg.* 1986; 65:1069-73.
178. Glenski JA, Warner MA, Dawson B et al. Postoperative use of epidurally administered morphine in children. *Mayo Clin Proc.* 1984; 59:530-3.
179. Ruston FG. Epidural anaesthesia in infants and children. *Can Anaesth Soc J.* 1954; 1:37-41.
180. Shapiro LA, Jedeikin RJ, Shalev D et al. Epidural morphine analgesia in children. *Anesthesiology.* 1984; 61:210-4.
181. Bosenberg AT, Bland BAR, Schulte-Steinberg O et al. Thoracic epidural anesthesia via the caudal route in infants. *Anesthesiology.* 1988; 69:265-9.
182. Arthur DS. Post operative thoracic epidural analgesia in children. *Anaesthesia.* 1980; 35:1131-6.
183. Broadman LM. Regional anaesthesia in pediatric practice. *Can J Anaesth.* 1987; 34:S34-48.
184. Broadman LM, Hannallah RS, Norden JM et al. "Kiddie caudals": experience with 1154 consecutive cases without complications. *Anesth Analg.* 1987; 66:748-54.
185. Bramwell RGB, Bullen C, Radford P. Caudal block for postoperative analgesia in children. *Anaesthesia.* 1982; 37:1024-8.
186. Jensen BH. Caudal block for post operative pain relief in children after genital operations: a comparison between bupivacaine and morphine. *Acta Anaesthesiol Scand.* 1981; 25:373-5.
187. Krane EJ, Jacobson LE, Lynn AM et al. Caudal morphine for postoperative analgesia in children: a comparison with caudal bupivacaine and intravenous morphine. *Anesth Analg.* 1987; 66:647-53.
188. McGown RG. Caudal analgesia in children. *Anaesthesia.* 1982; 37:806-18.
189. Warner MA, Kunkel SE, Offord KO et al. The effects of age, epinephrine, and operative site on duration of caudal analgesia in pediatric patients. *Anesth Analg.* 1987; 66:995-8.
190. Arthur DS. Caudal anaesthesia in neonates and children. *Anaesthesia.* 1980; 35:1136-7.
191. Hain VR. Anaesthetic doses for extradural anaesthesia in children. *Br J Anaesth.* 1978; 50:303-8.
192. Satoyoshi M, Kamiyama Y. Caudal anaesthesia for upper abdominal surgery in infants and children: a simple calculation of the volume of local anaesthetic. *Acta Anaesthesiol Scand.* 1984; 28:57-62.
193. Takasaki M, Dihi S, Hawabata Y et al. Dosage of lidocaine for caudal anesthesia in infants and children. *Anesthesiology.* 1977; 47:527-9.
194. Armitage EN. Caudal block in children. *Anaesthesia.* 1979; 34:396.
195. Sharpe TD, Gorskey GV, Sabourni MA et al. Do epinephrine containing solutions decrease the risk of using bupivacaine for caudal anaesthesia in children? *Can Anaesth Soc J.* 1986; 33:S114-S115.
196. Wolf AR, Valley RD, Fear DW et al. Bupivacaine for caudal anaesthesia in infants and children: the optimal effective concentration. *Anesthesiology.* 1988; 69:102-6.
197. Eather KF. Regional anesthesia for infants and children. *Int Anesthesiol Clin.* 1975; 12:19-48.
198. Arthur DS, McNicol LR. Local anaesthetic techniques in pediatric surgery. *Br J Anaesth.* 1986; 58:760-78.
199. Melman E, Penuelas J, Marrufo J. Regional anesthesia in children. *Anesth Analg.* 1975; 54:387-90.
200. Lunn JN. Postoperative analgesia after circumcision: a randomized comparison between caudal analgesia and intramuscular morphine in boys. *Anaesthesia.* 1979; 34:552-4.
201. May AE, Wandless J, James RH. Analgesia for circumcision in children: a comparison of caudal bupivacaine and intramuscular buprenorphine. *Acta Anaesthesiol Scand.* 1982; 26:331.
202. Desparmet J. Equipment for paediatric epidurals. *Anaesthesia.* 1986; 41:337-8.
203. Murat I, Delleur MM, Esteve C et al. Continuous extradural anaesthesia in children: clinical and hemodynamic implications. *Br J Anaesth.* 1987; 59:1441-50.
204. Meignier M, Souron R, LeNeet JC. Postoperative dorsal epidural analgesia in children with respiratory disabilities. *Anesthesiology.* 1983; 59:473-6.
205. Desparmet J, Meistelman C, Barre J et al. Continuous epidural infusion of bupivacaine for postoperative pain relief in children. *Anesthesiology.* 1987; 67:108-10.
206. Murat I, Walker J, Esteve C et al. Effect of lumbar epidural anaesthesia on plasma cortisol levels in children. *Can Anaesth Soc J.* 1988; 35:20-4.
207. Delluer MM, Murat I, Saint-Maurice C. Hemodynamic changes during lumbar epidural anesthesia in children. *Anesthesiology.* 1986; 65:A426.
208. Kurth CD, Spitzer AR, Broennle AM et al. Postoperative apnea in preterm infants. *Anesthesiology.* 1987; 66:483-8.
209. Gallaghar TM, Crean PM. Spinal anaesthesia in infants born prematurely. *Anaesthesia.* 1989; 44:434-6.
210. Harnik EV, Hoy GR, Potoliachio S et al. Spinal anesthesia in premature infants recovering from respiratory distress syndrome. *Anesthesiology.* 1986; 64:95-9.
211. Rice L, Demas P, Crooms J et al. Duration of spinal anesthesia in infants under 1 year of age: comparison of 3 drugs. *Anesth Analg.* 1987; 66:S148.
212. Mahe V, Ecoffey C. Spinal anesthesia with isobaric bupivacaine in infants. *Anesthesiology.* 1988; 68:601-3.
213. Williams RK, Abajian JC, Mazuzan JE. Total spinal anesthesia for repair of PDA in neonates. Paper presented at American Academy of Pediatrics Spring Session. San Diego, CA:1991 Mar 15–17.
214. McIlvaine WB, Knox RF, Fennessey PV et al. Continuous infusion of bupivacaine via intrapleural catheter for analgesia after thoracotomy in children. *Anesthesiology.* 1988; 69:261-4.
215. White J, Harrison B, Richmond P et al. Postoperative analgesia for circumcision. *Br Med J.* 1983; 286:1934.
216. Hove RL, Bromberger PJ, Groreman HD et al. Regional anesthesia during newborn circumcision. *Clin Pediatr.* 1983; 22:813-8.
217. Maxwell LG, Yaster M, Wetzel RC. Penile nerve block reduces the physiologic stress of newborn circumcision. *Anesthesiology.* 1986; 65:A432.
218. Williamson PS, Williamson ML. Physiologic stress reduction by a local anesthetic during newborn circumcision. *Pediatrics.* 1983; 71:36-40.
219. Tree-Trakaran T, Pirayavaraporn S. Postoperative pain relief for circumcision in children: comparison among morphine, nerve block, and topical analgesia. *Anesthesiology.* 1985; 62:519-22.
220. Bonadio WA. TAC: a review. *Pediatr Emerg Care.* 1989; 5:128-30.
221. Pryor GJ, Kilpatrick WR, Opp DR et al. Local anesthesia in minor lacerations: topical TAC vs lidocaine infiltration. *Ann Emerg Med.* 1980; 9:568-71.
222. Schaffer DJ. Clinical comparision of TAC anesthetic solutions with and without cocaine. *Ann Emerg Med.* 1985; 14:1077-80.
223. Bonadio WA, Wagner V. Efficacy of tetracaine-adrenaline-cocaine topical anesthetic without tetracaine for facial lac-

eration repair in children. *Pediatrics*. 1990; 86:856-7.
224. Morris RW, Whish KM. A controlled trial of pain on skin infiltration with local anaesthetics. *Anaesth Intensive Care*. 1984; 12:113-4.
225. Sanal SH, Weavil PD, Dell'Aria JC et al. Local anesthesia in simple facial and scalp lacerations: a randomized trial of topical tetracaine-adrenalin-cocaine versus lidocaine infiltration. *Am J Dis Child*. 1988; 142:391-2. Abstract.
226. Hegenbarth MA, Altieri MF, Hawk W et al. Topical tetracaine-adrenalin-cocaine (TAC) versus lidocaine infiltration for laceration repair in children. *Pediatr Emerg Care*. 1988; 4:296. Abstract.

Treatment of asthma in children

CHRISTINE M. MURPHY, SHANNON L. COONCE, AND PAMELA A. SIMON

Abstract: The epidemiology, etiology and pathophysiology, clinical presentation and diagnosis, and drug therapy of asthma in children are reviewed.

Recent advances in drug therapy have, for unknown reasons, been accompanied by an increase in the morbidity and mortality associated with childhood asthma. The cause of asthma is not precisely understood, but an inflammatory process and hyperactivity of airways are common findings in the disease. Asthma in children can be classified as intermittent, chronic, or indeterminate; a severe, prolonged episode not relieved by usual treatment is called status asthmaticus. The hallmark symptoms of asthma are coughing, dyspnea, and wheezing.

Beta-adrenergic agonists can be used orally for diagnostic purposes or for nocturnal asthma; i.v. or s.c. for emergency treatment; or by inhalation for relief of acute asthmatic episodes. Experience with anticholinergics in children is limited, and these agents should be used only when other options have failed. Inhalation of cromolyn sodium is very safe and is useful for the prophylactic treatment of mild to moderate asthma. Corticosteroids, which are used both for acute asthmatic episodes and for long-term treatment, can be given orally, i.v., or by inhalation. Theophylline is used for prophylactic therapy in children with chronic asthma. Selection of a drug regimen is based on knowledge of efficacy, pharmacokinetics, compliance, and toxicity.

The treatment of asthma in children requires consideration of drug properties in young patients. Drugs used to treat childhood asthma include β agonists, anticholinergics, cromolyn sodium, corticosteroids, and theophylline.

Index terms: Asthma; Bronchodilators; Cromolyn sodium; Drug administration routes; Parasympatholytic agents; Pediatrics; Respiratory smooth-muscle relaxants; Steroids, cortico-; Sympathomimetic agents; Theophylline
Clin Pharm. 1991; 10:685-703

In the past 20 years the therapeutic approach to asthma has changed more than for almost any other disease. Formerly, patients with asthma were instructed to drastically restrict their lifestyles. They were commonly ordered to restrict activities to indoor, air-conditioned areas to avoid inhaled allergens and were typically placed on strict diets to avoid food allergies.[1] Today the majority of patients with asthma can lead normal lives; some have even achieved world-class athletic status.

This dramatic shift in the approach to asthma has come about primarily through the development and use of new medications. Since 1970 the pharmaceutical industry has introduced the β_2-selective adrenergic stimulants, cromolyn sodium, and the inhaled corticosteroid preparations. During the same period, the pharmacokinetics and pharmacodynamics of theophylline were being defined, which would allow using this drug with maximum effectiveness and minimal toxicity.

Unfortunately, there have also been disturbing developments. In the past decade morbidity and mortality due to asthma have increased.[2-4] During the 1980s the number of hospitalizations due to asthma increased 4.5% per year among 0- to 17-year-old children, with the greatest annual increase (6.8%) occurring in 0- to 4-year-old black children.[2] Deaths due to asthma have increased 6.2% per year among patients aged 5 to 34 years, with the greatest increase occurring in 5-to 14-year-old patients. Also, excessive asthma-related mortality has been noted in four geographic regions, the largest being the urban areas of New York City and Chicago.[3]

The reasons for these worrisome changes are not completely clear. Originally, it was thought that they could be attributed to coding changes in the *Interna-*

CHRISTINE M. MURPHY, PHARM.D., is Specialty Pharmacy Resident in Ambulatory Care, SHANNON L. COONCE, PHARM.D., is Clinical Pharmacy Resident, and PAMELA A. SIMON, PHARM.D., is Clinical Assistant Professor, Department of Pharmacy Practice, The University of Illinois at Chicago.

Address reprint requests to Dr. Simon at the Department of Pharmacy Practice, The University of Illinois at Chicago, 833 South Wood Street, Room 244 (M/C 886), Chicago, IL 60612.

The insight, support, and encouragement of Jesse Joad, M.D., are acknowledged.

This is **article 680-204-9121** in the **ASHP Continuing Education System;** it qualifies for 1.0 hour of continuing-education credit. See page 724 for learning objectives and test questions.

tional Classification of Diseases, but the most recent data do not support this as the only explanation. Other possible explanations include an overall increase in asthma prevalence, an increase in airborne allergens or air pollution, or uneven access to health care among socioeconomic groups. Finally, and of most concern, is the possibility that the aforementioned "advances" in pharmacotherapy have contributed to the temporally related increases in morbidity and mortality.[4]

It is therefore important for health professionals to understand asthma and the use of drugs to treat it. Because of the importance of asthma's deleterious effects in young children and the unique problems of drug dosage and delivery in pediatric patients, it is appropriate to concentrate on the specific population of children with asthma.

Epidemiology

Asthma is one of the most common chronic illnesses in children. Asthma and wheezing accounted for 1.7% of all office visits to a pediatrician (over 2.2 million visits) in 1980–81.[5] The second National Health and Nutrition Examination Survey found that 7% of the 7399 children surveyed had been diagnosed as having asthma at some time and that 3.6% of children had a current diagnosis of asthma.[6] Currently diagnosed asthma or wheezing was more common in boys compared with girls, in black compared with white children, and in urban compared with rural dwellers. Socioeconomic factors did not affect asthma prevalence. In children, death from asthma is rare, ranging from 0.1 to 0.5 deaths per 100,000 children per year.[7] However, this rate appeared to increase during the 1980s.[3] Approximately half of all children with asthma will be essentially asymptomatic by the time they reach adulthood.[8]

The psychosocial costs related to asthma are also great. School absences due to illness are higher than average among children with asthma.[9] Associations have been made between chronic asthma and divorce or familial disruption.[10] Marion et al.[11] found that, among 25 families that included a child with chronic asthma, the average annual expenditure related to that child's care was $1087 (6.4% of annual income). Total expenditure included both the direct cost of physician care, medications, and hospitalization as well as the indirect cost of travel and time lost from work. These costs constituted 3.7–3.9% of total family income in high- and middle-income families but 11.9% in low-income families.

Etiology and Pathophysiology

The precise cellular abnormality in asthma is a mystery. Studies of the bronchial smooth muscle of normal and asthmatic subjects have demonstrated no difference in contractile properties. Therefore, it appears that a defect in the control of airway smooth muscle is responsible for its hyperresponsiveness.[12] Common theories propose basic dysfunction of the β-adrenergic receptor–adenylate cyclase system,[13] an inherent abnormality in the irritant or cough receptors that are mediated by acetylcholine,[14] or an ultimate dependence of the pathophysiologic pathways of the disease on calcium ions.[15] It is most likely that asthma involves a complex interrelationship among all of these defects. The inherent abnormality causing asthma may be genetically transferred and apparently occurs according to the principles of polygenic inheritance. Asthma is dependent not only on the inheritance of mutant genes but also on environmental influences that govern the expression of the disease.[16]

The pathophysiology of asthma has been better defined in recent years.[17-19] A major finding in asthma is hyperactivity of the airways. It is now thought that inflammation of the airways contributes to this increased bronchial reactivity.[18] After exposure to a precipitant, either immunologic (allergic) or nonimmunologic, the asthmatic patient may develop immediate symptoms (early asthmatic response), or the symptoms may be delayed for three to seven hours (late asthmatic response). When both reactions occur in the same patient, it is labeled a dual asthmatic response.[19] The late asthmatic response is particularly troublesome because of its tendency to be more persistent—it may last 24 hours or longer—and because of its association with more frequent and severe exacerbations of asthma.[17,19]

The cellular occurrences that lead to these reactions are best exemplified by the response of the lung to allergen exposure.[17-18] Within 30 minutes following antigen exposure in a sensitized patient, mast cells, in a process mediated by immunoglobulin E, degranulate and release numerous substances, including preformed, stored mediators (e.g., histamine, eosinophil chemotactic factor of anaphylaxis, neutrophil chemotactic factors, kininogenase) and mediators that are newly synthesized when the cells degranulate (e.g., leukotrienes C_4, D_4, and E_4; prostaglandins; monohydroxyeicosatetraenoic acids; hydroxyeicosatetraenoic acid; thromboxanes; adenosine; bradykinin; platelet-activating factor). Other mediators are by-products of degraded mast cells (e.g., heparin, tryptase, superoxide dismutase, peroxidase).[20] The immediate release of these mediators is thought to cause the edema and smooth muscle contraction that result in the early asthmatic response.[19]

The mediators also contribute to the subsequent inflammatory reaction in the airways. Mucus secretion is stimulated by histamine, prostaglandins, and leukotrienes as well as by neurogenic mechanisms that are initiated by bradykinin and mediated by neuropeptides such as substance P.[18,20] Airways are then infiltrated by a variety of granulocytic cells.[17] These cells may migrate to the area through a chemotactic response to mediators[18,20] (e.g., eosinophil chemotactic factor of anaphylaxis, neutrophil chemotactic factors, platelet activating factor), or they may be activated directly. The eosinophil is the predominant cell type involved, but macrophages, basophils, lymphocytes, and neutrophils are also present. These cells are capable of releasing substances (e.g., interleukins, granulocyte and macrophage colony-stimulating factor, lipoxygenase, and cyclooxygenase products of arachidonic acid metabolism) that further fuel the inflammatory process and may damage the epithelial cells lining the airways. Damage to the epithelial lining can further increase bronchial hyperactivity by exposing sensory nerve endings and potentiating mediator activity.[18] The precise role of each mediator substance is not yet known, but it appears that the entire process is a complex interaction between a number of cell types and their released products.[17] This cellular inflammatory process is thought to be expressed clinically as the late asthmatic response.

Definitions

Asthma is "a disease characterized by an increased responsiveness of the trachea and bronchi to various stimuli and manifested by a widespread narrowing of the airways that changes in severity either spontaneously or as a result of therapy."[21] Clinically, this definition can be modified to include the causes for the airway narrowing: bronchial smooth muscle spasm, increased secretion of mucus and inflammatory cells into the lumen of the airway, and inflammatory edema in the peribronchiolar tissues.

From a therapeutic standpoint, it is necessary to classify asthma based on the chronicity of symptoms.[22] *Intermittent asthma* is defined as the presence of symptoms during no more than five days per month with extended symptom-free periods. A typical example of a patient with intermittent asthma is the child whose two or three yearly disease exacerbations are precipitated by viral upper respiratory tract infections but who is completely free of asthmatic symptoms between exacerbations.

On the other hand, *chronic asthma* is defined as the presence of symptoms during more than five days per month for more than three months and during more than half of the days in any one month. This is illustrated by the child who very frequently (often daily) suffers symptoms of asthma (even mild symptoms such as simple coughing).

Indeterminate asthma is defined as the presence of symptoms for at least five days per month for less than three months (or less than half of the days in any one month) with extended symptom-free periods. Many patients in the indeterminate classification will eventually be considered to have chronic asthma as they become more aware of their asthma symptoms and obtain benefit from treatment. Also, some patients with indeterminate asthma may well have a seasonal pattern to their exacerbations. For example, the ragweed-sensitive patient may have symptoms chronically during the late summer and fall but only intermittently during the rest of the year.

Within the classification above, the severity of the symptoms can vary widely.[22] Both the chronicity and severity of the asthma symptoms will determine the drug therapy for the patient.

Infrequently, patients may progress to a severe, prolonged episode of asthma known as *status asthmaticus*, which is an acute, severe exacerbation of asthma that is not relieved by usual treatment.[23] Status asthmaticus is a medical emergency that requires intensive therapy and monitoring to prevent serious morbidity or death.

Clinical Presentation and Diagnosis

The hallmark symptoms of asthma are coughing, dyspnea, and wheezing. Other common signs and symptoms include tachypnea, a prolonged expiratory phase of respiration, tachycardia, pulsus paradoxus (a change of more than 10 mm Hg in systolic blood pressure with inspiration), chest pain or tightness, abdominal pain, and vomiting (often posttussive). Patients with marked symptoms commonly use the accessory muscles of breathing, and muscular retractions are most prominent in children in the intracostal, subcostal, and sternocleidomastoid regions. The patient may assume a posture, in which he or she is hunched or leaning forward, that improves the effectiveness of accessory muscle use.[16,24] If the episode is severe, the patient may develop severe dyspnea (which interferes with speech), anxiety, cyanosis, diaphoresis, and a change in mental status. Any patient may have any or all of these symptoms.

A thorough evaluation is critical to accurate diagnosis of asthma in a child. To be diagnosed as having asthma, a child must (1) have symptoms that are consistent with asthma (e.g., coughing, wheezing, or dyspnea) or a history of recurrent bronchitis or pneumonia, and (2) demonstrate reversibility of symptoms either spontaneously or with the help of medications used to treat asthma.[22]

Objective testing supports the diagnosis.[22] A child with asthma alone must have a chest roentgenogram that is normal except for showing peribronchial thickening. Spirometry (pulmonary function testing) is obtained in children, generally those at least six years old, who are able to correctly perform the necessary techniques. The required demonstration of symptom reversibility is indicated by a spontaneous or bronchodilator-induced increase of ≥25% in FEF_{25-75} (forced expiratory flow rate from 25% to 75% of vital capacity) to a value ≥75% of the predicted value, with the FVC (forced vital capacity) being ≥80% of the predicted value.[22] Although the FEV_1 (forced expiratory volume in one second) is frequently considered the standard test of reversibility, it is primarily an effort-dependent test of large (>2 mm) airway function. In contrast, the FEF_{25-75} is primarily an effort-independent test of small (<2 mm) airway function. FEF_{25-75} may be a more sensitive test than FEV_1 in some patients.[25] In children who are not able to perform spirometric techniques, other evidence of symptom reversibility must be obtained to make the diagnosis of asthma. This requires a thorough medication history and includes determining the response to medications that have been tried in the past.

Allergen sensitivity testing is frequently conducted on patients recently diagnosed as having asthma, and the results of this testing, when correlated with the patient's history, may help guide therapy. The skin test is the most commonly used allergen test because of its high sensitivity and low cost relative to an alternate, the radioallergosorbent test (RAST). In the skin test, small quantities of allergen are introduced into the skin when the skin is pricked in the immediate presence of diluted allergen extract. Formation of a wheal and flare at the site within 15 to 30 minutes of application indicates a positive test.

In the RAST, the patient's serum is tested for the presence of specific immunoglobulin E antibodies. Because it is less sensitive and more expensive than skin testing, the RAST is usually employed only when a patient consistently reacts positively to the negative control skin test (dermatographism), when antihistamine therapy cannot be discontinued (skin tests are unreliable in a patient taking antihistamines), or if extensive eczema or other skin lesions are present.

In patients who do not respond appropriately to antiasthmatic therapy, other diagnoses may be entertained.[16] These may include congenital malformations of the respiratory, cardiovascular, or gastrointestinal system; presence of foreign bodies in the respiratory system; immunodeficiency syndromes; and cystic fibrosis. In certain populations, tuberculosis may be considered likely. Also, gastroesophageal reflux can cause symptoms of bronchospasm.[26]

Interest in the relationship between chronic sinusitis and the control of asthma has recently been renewed.[27,28] The two disorders frequently coexist in the same patient and may, in fact, be related pathophysiologically. Children often do not have the typical symptoms of sinusitis (e.g., headache, fever) but rather have cough (frequently nocturnal) and nasal discharge.[27] Some investigators argue that treatment of the sinusitis with a three- to four-week course of antimicrobials directed against the common infecting organisms (*Haemophilus influenzae, Streptococcus pneumoniae, Staphylococcus aureus, Strep. viridans*) improves and even alleviates asthma.[28] A cause-and-effect relationship between chronic sinusitis and asthma has yet to be proved.

Patient History. The evaluation of a patient suspected of having asthma must include (1) characterization of symptoms (as described above), (2) definition of precipitating factors, (3) an attempt to initially characterize the chronicity of symptoms, and (4) an assessment of the severity of symptoms. The patient history includes a review of systems, which should be specific for symptoms of related atopic diseases, and a family history.

Symptoms may be precipitated by a variety of stimuli.[29] Any patient may be bothered by any or all of the following provoking factors. Asthma in children is almost uniformly exacerbated by inhaled irritants (e.g., cigarette smoke, air pollution), exercise, inhalation of cold air, and infections (usually viral upper respiratory tract infections). Asthma induced by viral illness may occur because of damage to bronchial epithelial cells, which exposes and sensitizes irritant neuroreceptors, or because the virus-infected cell produces a substance that causes dysfunction of the β-adrenergic receptor and other homeostatic mechanisms in the airway. Both theories are supported by the fact that nonasthmatic individuals can experience bronchial hyperactivity during a viral respiratory infection.[29] Emotional stress and laughing or crying may also precipitate asthmatic symptoms.

In some children, allergens may be a major precipitant of asthma exacerbation. These children typically have a seasonal pattern to their symptoms. They also frequently suffer with other allergic disorders such as allergic rhinitis, conjunctivitis, or atopic dermatitis (eczema).[30] The common allergens causing symptoms are released by plants.[31] Pollen may arise from trees, grasses, or weeds. Each of these plant groups generally pollinate at approximately the same time each year: trees in the spring, grasses in early summer to midsummer, and weeds in the late summer to fall. The onset and duration of the pollen season and the most common offending plant species vary depending on geographic location and weather. Mold spores can also give rise to allergic symptoms. The outdoor molds release their spores in the early spring through late fall. During this long season, spore counts rise and fall depending on the regional flora on which the molds grow (e.g., grains and other crops, forests, orchards). Indoor molds grow on house plants and in damp areas such as basements. Allergies to indoor molds, to house-dust mites, and to animal dander contribute to perennial asthmatic symptoms.

Drugs can also provoke asthma in some patients. These include aspirin[32,33] and other nonsteroidal anti-inflammatory agents (with the possible exception of the nonacetylated salicylates),[34,35] β-adrenergic blocking drugs,[36] the food dye tartrazine (FD&C Yellow No. 5),[34] and sulfites (preservatives found in many foods and drugs).[37]

Chronicity of symptoms is best defined by determining the level of interference with daily activities caused by asthma.[22] As thoroughly as possible, given the constraints of patient and parent memory and the ability to recognize symptoms as abnormal, the number of nighttime awakenings and the frequency of interference with play caused by asthma should be ascertained. It is easiest to approximate the weekly occurrences of such interference with activities. Also, the number of school days missed and the number of emergency room visits per month may aid in defining the chronicity of the patient's symptoms.

Nighttime awakening due to asthma, or so-called nocturnal asthma, requires further comment. Nocturnal symptoms occur frequently in asthma and have been correlated with decreases in pulmonary function.

Symptoms are typically worst between 0300 and 0700. Possible reasons for nocturnal symptoms include activation of mast cells in the asthmatic patient during the normal diurnal decrease in plasma epinephrine concentration, reflex stimulation of the parasympathetic nervous system, accumulation of airway secretions in the supine position, and increased exposure to allergens (e.g., house dust) during the night. It is likely that all of these explanations are correct to some extent.[38] A recent investigation has demonstrated that the inflammatory process is ongoing during the night in the airways of patients with nocturnal asthma but not in asthmatics without important nocturnal symptoms.[39] Nocturnal asthma is often associated with more severe disease and an increased risk of sudden asthmatic death.[38,39]

The severity of the patient's symptoms may be ascertained by questioning the child and parents about the number of emergency room visits, the number of hospitalizations, whether the child has ever required mechanical ventilation or admission to an intensive-care unit, and whether the child has ever lost consciousness during an acute exacerbation of asthma.[22]

Beta-Adrenergic Agonists

The β_2-agonists are first-line agents for the treatment of asthma because of their ease of administration, rapid onset of action, and relative safety.

Mechanism of Action. Stimulation of β-adrenoreceptors causes activation of adenylate cyclase, which results in increased production of adenosine 3',5'-cyclic phosphate (cAMP), which, in turn, activates cAMP-dependent protein kinases. These enzymes phosphorylate myosin light-chain kinase, effectively inactivating it. Myosin light-chain kinase catalyzes the phosphorylation of myosin in a reaction that is necessary for the coupling of actin and myosin during smooth muscle contraction. Therefore, inactivation of myosin light-chain kinase ultimately leads to smooth muscle relaxation.[40]

In addition, cAMP appears to disinhibit protein kinase, which, in turn, causes calcium to bind to the cell membrane and to the cytoplasmic reticulum. This results in a lowering of the intracellular calcium concentration and in smooth muscle relaxation.[41] By a similar mechanism, β_2-adrenoreceptor stimulation inhibits the release of histamine from mast cells but does not alter release of mediators from granulocytic cell types. Therefore, the β agonists reverse and prevent the early asthmatic response, but do not appreciably affect the late asthmatic response.[42]

Human peripheral lung tissue has β_1 and β_2 receptors in a ratio of approximately 1:3.[43,44] In the human lung, β_1-receptors do not appear to exert an important bronchodilating effect.[45] It would seem, therefore, that bronchodilation results directly from stimulation of β_2-receptors and that it is desirable to selectively stimulate only those receptors. One way to improve β_2 selectivity of agonist drugs is to increase the size of the alkyl substituent on the terminal amino group of the molecule.[46] Terbutaline, albuterol, and bitolterol, agents that have a tertiary butyl group in this position, are very β_2-selective[47] (Table 1). Another attempt to improve bronchoselectivity was the development of bitolterol. It differs from the other β_2-selective agents in that it is an inactive prodrug, 3,4-diester colterol.[49] It is converted in the lung to the active form, colterol, by esterase hydrolysis. In spite of this biotransformation, the onset of action with bitolterol is comparable to that with albuterol.[50]

Table 1.
Properties of β-Adrenergic Agonists Used in Asthma[48]

Drug	Relative Stimulation of Adrenergic Receptors[a] β_2	β_1	α	Duration of Action When Given by Inhalation (hr)
Albuterol	+++	+	0	4–6
Bitolterol[b]	+++	+	0	4–6
Ephedrine	++	++	+++	3–5
Epinephrine	+++	+++	+++	1–2
Isoetharine	+++	++	0	2–3
Isoproterenol	+++	+++	0	2–3
Metaproterenol	+++	++	0	3–5
Pirbuterol	+++	+	0	5
Terbulatine	+++	+	0	4–6

[a] +++ = high, ++ = medium, + = low, 0 = none.
[b] Prodrug hydrolyzed to colterol in vivo.

Toxicity. The toxicity of β agonists in patients with asthma comes from their causing adrenergic responses other than bronchodilation. The most prominent adverse effect is cardiac stimulation. The increase in heart rate may be a reflexive response to β_2-mediated peripheral vasodilation (suggesting that additional β_2 selectivity should not further reduce the prevalence of this adverse effect) or a result of direct stimulation of the β_1-adrenergic receptor. Cardiac stimulation is the dose-limiting adverse effect of some β agonists.[51,52]

Hypokalemia has also been reported, but the clinical importance of this adverse effect is controversial.[53,54] Patients with pre-existing hypokalemia (e.g., stressed individuals with high concentrations of circulating catecholamines) or those with a pathologically or pharmacologically sensitized myocardium may be at risk for adverse sequelae from the hypokalemia.[53] The muscle tremor seen with the use of β agonists appears to be β_2-mediated and is dose related.[52] Nervousness and anxiety may also occur.

The frequency of adverse effects with the β agonists also depends on their route of administration. Adverse effects are least frequently associated with drug inhalation since the drug is delivered directly to the site of action. Oral and injectable administration are associated with more adverse effects because the drugs are administered systemically.[51,55] In general, the adverse effects of the β agonists are dose dependent, regardless of the route of administration.[52]

Tolerance. In vitro studies have demonstrated that β-adrenergic receptors may become desensitized (tolerant) to stimulation by β-agonists. This may occur because (1) receptors are removed from the cell surface and stored within the cell (down-regulation), or (2) receptors are phosphorylated, which makes them unable to activate adenylate cyclase.[56]

Sears et al.[57] have brought the problem of tolerance into practical focus by describing better control of asthma when patients take β_2 agonists on an as-needed basis only rather than on a regular schedule. Although the regularly scheduled β agonist used in this study was fenoterol, the authors pointed out that these results must be generalized to all β agonists (until conflicting evidence arises) because of the potential impact of the phenomenon on asthma-related morbidity. Using the lowest effective dose only on an as-needed basis has been recommended as a way to avoid desensitization.[56,57] This recommendation may have important clinical implications for the use of the new agents salmeterol and formoterol, which are selective β_2 agonists with a duration of action of up to 12 hours.[58,59]

The clinical significance of tolerance to β agonists is questionable.[46] Clearly, tolerance to the extrapulmonary effects of the β agonists develops in most patients. In terms of bronchodilatory effects, it appears that the diminution of drug response manifests as a shortening in duration rather than a lessening of effect; thus, tolerance may influence the dosage interval in some patients.[60]

Administration by Mouth. The noncatecholamine sympathomimetic agents are generally well absorbed from the gastrointestinal tract.[47] Absence of hydroxyl groups or of other substitutions on the aromatic nucleus of the catecholamine molecule results in prolonged duration of action and increased oral effect because catechol-*O*-methyltransferase is relatively slow to degrade these drugs.[46,47]

Systemic administration of β agonists results in more adverse effects than administration by inhalation.[51] Oral agents have a role in asthma management in that they are useful for a diagnostic maneuver (Table 2). For example, a small supply of albuterol syrup could be prescribed for a young child who has not yet had a documented history of symptom reversibility and who would otherwise require a nebulizer. The parent would then keep a symptom diary for two weeks without administering the albuterol and for another two weeks while giving the drug. An improvement in symptoms during drug treatment would indicate reversibility with bronchodilators. A single, bedtime dose of an oral extended-release β agonist is used in the treatment of nocturnal asthma.[63,64]

Administration by Injection. Subcutaneous injection of epinephrine had long been the standard of therapy for the emergency management of acute asthmatic episodes in children.[24] Two recent therapeutic advances, however, have changed this approach. First, β selectivity of the aerosolized bronchodilators has improved. Second, recent data have shown aerosolized β_2 agonists to be as effective as, and safer than, subcutaneous epinephrine.[65,66] These advances have shifted first-line therapy in the emergency room toward the use of aerosolized β_2 agonists.[67]

Subcutaneous injection of epinephrine or terbutaline may still be required, on occasion, in the emergency treatment of asthma. If, for any reason, an aerosolized β agonist cannot be administered immediately, or if the child cannot tolerate or will not cooperate with a nebulized treatment, then a drug should be administered subcutaneously.[68]

Another pharmacologic maneuver, which is used to

Table 2.
Pediatric Dosages of β-Adrenergic Agonists for Asthma[61,62]

Drug	Dosage Form[a]	Dosage
Albuterol	MDI	2 puffs (90 μg/puff) q 4–6 hr p.r.n.
	Neb (0.5%, as sulfate)	0.25 mL q 4–6 hr p.r.n. if pt. < 20 kg; otherwise, 0.5 mL or 0.01–0.03 mL/kg (up to 1 mL) q 4–6 hr p.r.n. For emergency treatment, 0.06 mL/kg, then 0.03 mL/kg q 20 min
	Oral tab or soln	0.1 mg (as sulfate)/kg (up to 2 mg/dose) q 6–8 hr p.r.n.
	Ext-rel oral tab	4–8 mg (as sulfate) at bedtime
Bitolterol mesylate	MDI	2 puffs (370 μg/puff) q 4–6 hr p.r.n.
Epinephrine hydrochloride	Injection (1:1000, of epinephrine)	0.01 mL/kg (up to 0.4 mL/dose) s.c. q 15 min × 4 doses or q 4 hr p.r.n.
Isoproterenol hydrochloride[b]	Injection	0.05–0.1 μg (of isoproterenol)/kg/min initially, then adjust by 0.1 μg/kg/min q 5–10 min (up to 1.5 μg/kg/min) p.r.n. or until heart rate ≥ 180/min or arrhythmia occurs
Metaproterenol sulfate	MDI	2–3 puffs (650 μg/puff) q 3–4 hr p.r.n.
	Neb (5%)	0.2 mL q 4–6 hr p.r.n. if pt. < 5 yr; otherwise, 0.3 mL q 4–6 hr p.r.n.
	Oral tab or soln	1.3–2.6 mg/kg/day p.r.n. (divided and given q 6–8 hr) if pt. < 6 yr; 10 mg q 6–8 hr p.r.n. if 6–9 yr; 20 mg q 6–8 hr p.r.n. if > 9 yr
Pirbuterol acetate	MDI	2 puffs (pirbuterol 200 μg/puff) q 4–6 hr p.r.n.
Terbutaline sulfate	MDI	2 puffs (200 μg/puff) q 4–6 hr p.r.n.
	Oral tab	1.25–2.5 mg t.i.d. p.r.n.
	Injection	0.01 mg/kg s.c. (up to 0.25 mg); repeat once in 15–20 min p.r.n.

[a] MDI = metered-dose inhaler, Neb = solution for nebulization.
[b] Should be given only in intensive-care area with constant cardiac monitoring.

avoid endotracheal intubation in a patient with status asthmaticus or to treat a patient in respiratory failure, is the intravenous administration of isoproterenol.[69-70] This therapeutic intervention must be performed only in an intensive-care setting, where continuous cardiac monitoring is available, because of the risk of arrhythmias and myocardial ischemia. The use of intravenous terbutaline[71] and albuterol[72] has also been investigated for this purpose in children.

Administration by Inhalation. All children with asthma must have a reliable method of receiving an inhaled treatment with a β_2 agonist to treat acute asthmatic episodes. The reliability of a specific method of administration in any given patient depends on the ability of the patient to coordinate his or her breathing and to perform a breath-hold. Inhaled β agonists may be administered via a metered-dose inhaler (MDI) alone, MDI plus a spacing device, dry-powder inhaler, or compressed-air nebulizer. These methods differ in ease of use, portability, and convenience. If flawless technique is performed, there is probably no difference between them in terms of efficacy.[73] Using a nebulizer is simplest for the patient because it requires only tidal breathing. It is the most reliable drug-delivery system, especially in an acutely dyspneic patient.[55] Generally, children younger than four or five years must receive inhaled β agonists by this method to ensure delivery of the drug to the site of action.[55]

Nebulized β_2-agonists are the initial treatment of acute asthmatic episodes and status asthmaticus in children and have been shown to be more effective than aminophylline[74,75] and at least as effective as subcutaneous epinephrine.[65]

Nebulized Albuterol. Traditionally, bronchodilator treatments are administered in the emergency room setting every one to three hours.[76,77] However, a patient with very severe symptoms may require nebulized albuterol treatments more frequently and in higher doses than are traditionally used.[76-78] Robertson et al.[76] demonstrated a more rapid improvement in pulmonary function with albuterol 0.5 mg/kg (as the sulfate salt, solution for nebulization) every 20 minutes compared with an hourly dose of 0.15 mg/kg (maximum dose, 5 mg). The difference in pulmonary function between the two groups was not significant at the end of two hours. Adverse effects were comparably mild in both groups.

A follow-up study compared albuterol 0.05 and 0.15 mg/kg given every 20 minutes.[78] At the end of two hours (six doses), pulmonary function was improved to a significantly greater extent in the high-dose group compared with the low-dose group. Mild adverse effects, such as tremor and hyperactivity, occurred similarly in both groups. Serum potassium concentration decreased 20% in both groups.

In a third study, hourly administration of albuterol 0.15 mg/kg was compared with 0.30 mg/kg, also given hourly.[77] Improvement in pulmonary function was comparable after the first dose, but the group that received 0.30-mg/kg doses continued to improve, whereas pulmonary function in the group that received 0.15-mg/kg doses appeared to plateau. At the end of three hours, the 0.30-mg/kg dose group had significantly improved pulmonary function compared with the 0.15-mg/kg dose group. Once again, adverse effects were mild and comparable between the two groups.

To summarize, patients with moderate symptoms may benefit from nebulized albuterol 0.30 mg/kg administered every hour. More severely ill patients (possibly those who do not respond well to the initial nebulized treatment) may benefit from the more aggressive but time-consuming regimen of albuterol 0.15 mg/kg administered every 20 minutes. Neither of these aggressive therapies should be attempted at home.

Nebulized Terbutaline. Continuously nebulized terbutaline has recently been studied in the management of severe asthma in children. Moler et al.[79] studied 19 patients with severe asthma and impending respiratory failure during 27 separate hospital admissions. Patients were enrolled in the study only after failing standard treatment with hourly nebulized terbutaline treatments, aminophylline infusion, and intravenous methylprednisolone. Terbutaline was administered by a device that infused terbutaline sulfate (0.4 mg per mL of 0.9% sodium chloride solution) into a nebulizer at 4 mg/hr. The nebulizer delivered oxygen at 6 L/min; additional humidified, heated oxygen was also provided.

Patients were treated for an average of 15.4 hours (range, 3–37 hours). Even the most severely ill patients (i.e., those with an initial arterial carbon dioxide pressure of ≥39 mm Hg) demonstrated significant clinical improvement in the first eight hours of treatment, and none of the patients required endotracheal intubation or intravenous isoproterenol. Adverse effects of therapy were not appreciable. The authors concluded that continuously nebulized terbutaline is a safe and effective alternative to intravenous isoproterenol for the treatment of severe asthma in children. However, they cautioned that this treatment must be attempted only in pediatric intensive-care units with the capability of mechanically ventilating the child if necessary and that further study is required to evaluate the therapy in children with advanced respiratory failure (i.e., arterial carbon dioxide pressure of ≥60 mm Hg) and to determine the pharmacokinetics of the drug when administered in this fashion. A similarly designed study supports these findings.[80] Both of these studies were conducted before albuterol solution for nebulization was available in the United States.

Inhalers. When a child is about four or five years old, the drug administration device can be changed from a nebulizer to an MDI plus a spacer. Spacers theoretically improve response by increasing the amount of drug that reaches the lungs.[81] Studies support the use of these spacers for patients who have poor inhalation technique when they use an MDI alone.[82,83] The devices probably do not further benefit patients with good MDI technique.[82]

In choosing among the spacers available in the United States, the practitioner must consider the reservoir size, the inclusion of and type of incentive device in the design, and the cost. Two spacers, Inhal-aid and Inspirease (Key Pharmaceuticals), include an effective incentive device in their design. In our experience, however, the musical whistle on the Inspirease can act as a positive reinforcement for children, rather than the negative one it was designed to be, and can lead to incorrect use of the spacer.

Several studies have evaluated an MDI plus a spacer versus nebulized treatment in the emergency administration of a β_2 agonist for severe asthma.[84-86] In every study, the spacer was the Nebuhaler (A. B. Dracho, Sweden), which is not available in the United States and which has some advantages (e.g., larger reservoir) over the available spacing devices. The MDI with the spacer was at least as effective as nebulized treatments in each of these studies. In spite of the difficulties that some of the children had with using the MDI and spacer,[85,86] the combination may provide an efficacious and economical alternative to nebulized treatments for acute asthmatic episodes in some children. However, nebulization of β agonists remains the standard treatment for this indication.[86] Spacers may be useful even in very young children. Recently, symptomatic benefit was seen in 6- to 36-month-old children with reversible airways disease after administration of albuterol via an Aerochamber spacer (Monaghan Medical Corporation) with a mask.[87]

Administration of albuterol via a dry-powder inhaler is also feasible in the 4- to 8-year age group. The powder has been shown to be as effective as β_2 agonists administered via an MDI, with both dosage forms producing a comparably low frequency of adverse effects.[88,89] Notably, patients do not appear to cough after inhaling albuterol dry powder; coughing is common after inhalation of cromolyn powder.[89]

A child about eight years old can usually learn to use an MDI without a spacer. MDIs are portable and, if used correctly, tend to be a less expensive form of medication delivery than home nebulizers. However, it is often difficult for children (and most adults) to use the inhalers correctly.[82,90,91] The correct technique for the use of an MDI is as follows[92]:

1. Shake the canister well.
2. Place the mouthpiece approximately 1 inch (2 fingerbreadths) away from the mouth and open the mouth wide.[93] (Closing the lips gently around the canister is also acceptable and should be encouraged if the patient is unable to perform the open-mouth technique.)
3. Exhale to the end of a normal breath.
4. Actuate the canister at the beginning of a slow, deep inhalation.
5. Hold the breath for at least 5–10 seconds.
6. Exhale normally.
7. Wait at least one minute before repeating.

The major problems that patients have with using MDIs are taking the slow inspiratory breath after actuating the canister and holding the breath for 10 seconds.[94] Another difficulty is coordinating the timing of the actuation of the canister and the inspiratory breath. There appears to be no difference in clinical effect between a simultaneous inhalation or short delay before inhalation. Both of these, however, are better than a long delay (>two seconds).[95]

Poor technique is not only seen in the patients who use the devices, but also in the health-care professionals who prescribe and dispense them.[96,97] Also, Mickle et al.[97] found that only 27% of pharmacists, when presented with a prescription for an albuterol MDI, spontaneously offered education. An additional 33% of pharmacists provided education in response to a specific patient request. Information about spacing devices was not offered by any pharmacist.

Lee and Evans[82] found that 30% of children who previously demonstrated correct MDI technique were later unable to perform the technique correctly. Therefore, it is important to check a child's technique periodically to ensure that no bad habits develop. This is conveniently accomplished when the patient is given a medication refill or during follow-up clinic visits.

Anticholinergics

Interest in the use of anticholinergic agents has recently been renewed for the treatment of both acute and chronic asthma. Some asthmatics may demonstrate bronchoconstriction induced by the parasympathetic nervous system. It is thought that, in those patients, anticholinergic drugs can prevent bronchoconstriction. These agents antagonize the effect of acetylcholine at the cholinergic receptor site responsible for bronchoconstriction. Studies of the use of anticholinergics in chronic asthma are sparse, and their results are inconclusive.[98,99]

There are also conflicting results from studies of anticholinergic treatment of acute asthmatic episodes.[100,101] Studies that indicated a response were conducted in older children who could perform pulmonary function tests. The combination of ipratropium bromide and a β agonist significantly increased the percentage change in FEV_1 from baseline when compared with a β agonist alone.[101] There was no difference between groups in clinical score or frequency of adverse effects.

Whether this change in FEV_1 from baseline is clinically meaningful is not clear. There appears to be a subgroup of patients who respond to anticholinergic agents.[98] However, at this time, there is no way to prospectively identify those patients.

The majority of the studies that examined an anticholinergic agent in the management of acute episodes of pediatric asthma involved nebulized ipratropium bromide, a dosage form not currently available in the United States. If an anticholinergic agent is to be used, inhaled atropine is the only option for children. Because it lacks a quaternary ammonium structure, atropine may produce adverse effects (e.g., tachycardia, dry mouth, flushing) more commonly than ipratropium. The dose of atropine sulfate via nebulizer is 0.05 mg/kg (maximum, 2 mg).[102] Experience with anticholinergics in the management of acute episodes of pediatric asthma is limited, and these agents should be reserved for instances when other therapies are failing.

Cromolyn Sodium

Mechanism of Action. Cromolyn sodium's precise mechanism of action is not completely understood, but the drug's stabilizing effect on mast cells appears to play an important role.[103] The cellular mechanism for mast cell stabilization is likewise unknown, but a common theory proposes that cromolyn sodium (or simply cromolyn) interferes with calcium transport across the mast cell membrane, thereby interfering with mediator release.[104]

Based on this mechanism of action, one might expect cromolyn to be effective only for allergen-induced symptoms. In fact, it prevents the release of mediators from mast cells induced by both immunologic[103] and nonimmunologic[105-107] stimulation. Cromolyn does not have any bronchodilatory effects. It does block both early and late asthmatic responses.[108]

Administration. Cromolyn is available in three dosage forms. The solution for nebulization,[109,110] MDI,[111,112] and powder for inhalation[113,114] have all been demonstrated to be effective in the treatment of pediatric asthma. Although the drug is commonly thought to be effective only in children, beneficial effects from cromolyn have recently been demonstrated in the treatment of asthma in adults.[115] The solution for nebulization and MDI were first marketed in the United States in 1982 and 1986, respectively. Since then, the powder, which was the source of most of the adverse effects associated with cromolyn, has become obsolete for antiasthmatic therapy.

Nedocromil sodium, an investigational agent, has a mechanism of action similar to that of cromolyn and has been shown to be effective in the management of asthma.[116]

Place in Therapy. Cromolyn is used in the prophylactic treatment of mild to moderate asthma. Because cromolyn must be present before exposure to an asthma precipitant to prevent mast cell degranulation, it must be used constantly to be effective.[117] Onset of the therapeutic effect of cromolyn is usually delayed; thus, a therapeutic trial at least six weeks long is necessary to assess response.[118] The dosage of cromolyn sodium is two puffs (800 μg/puff) from the MDI or 2 mL of the solution for nebulization (10 mg/mL) four times daily. Especially during the initial period of cromolyn therapy, frequent β-agonist administration may be required for symptom control. Cromolyn sodium and β agonists are compatible when administered together in a nebulizer.[119] When symptoms are controlled with cromolyn alone, the frequency of administration may be decreased to three times daily and then twice daily.[120,121]

Toxicity. Cromolyn is considered safe, and the frequency of adverse effects is low.[113,122] The most common adverse effects are throat irritation, dryness, hoarseness, and cough associated with administration of the powder. Local adverse effects can be diminished by having the patient drink water before and after drug inhalation. Using a β-adrenergic agonist by MDI before cromolyn administration can minimize cough associated with the latter drug's use.[118] There are rare case reports of more severe cromolyn-associated reactions, including anaphylaxis.[123]

Corticosteroids

Corticosteroids have been used in the management of asthma for many years, and recently their role has shifted to that of primary therapy.[124] The precise mechanism of action of corticosteroids is not known, but their beneficial effect in the treatment of asthma, in which inflammation is an important feature,[18] is unquestionable.

Mechanism of Action. Corticosteroids are thought to exert their therapeutic effects by altering protein synthesis at multiple tissue sites.[124] Corticosteroids pass through cell membranes and bind to cytoplasmic receptors. The steroid–receptor complex is transported to the nucleus and causes an increase in the synthesis of messenger ribonucleic acid and proteins. The newly synthesized proteins enhance β-adrenergic response, inhibit arachidonic acid production, and decrease mucus production.[124] Corticosteroids also induce the production of lipocortin, a protein that inhibits the synthesis and release of mediators known to promote inflammation.[18,42] Therefore, corticosteroids initially exert their primary effect on the late asthmatic response. Only after extended administration do these agents decrease bronchial hyperactivity.[18]

Choice of Drug and Regimen. When choosing a corticosteroid agent, it is important to minimize the potential for adverse effects by selecting one with potent glucocorticoid activity, minimal mineralocorticoid activity, and a short to intermediate duration of action. Therefore, the drugs of choice are hydrocortisone or methylprednisolone for intravenous therapy, prednisone or prednisolone for oral therapy, and beclomethasone dipropionate, triamcinolone acetonide, or flunisolide for inhalation therapy.

Intravenous and oral therapy have been shown to be equally effective in the management of an acute asthmatic episode.[125] Inhaled corticosteroids, even in high dosages, have not been shown to abort an acute exacerbation of asthma.[126,127] Therefore, administration of a short course of high-dose oral corticosteroid (burst therapy) is required before initiation of long-term corticosteroid therapy.

Because corticosteroid dosage has varied among studies, it is almost impossible to identify an optimal regimen. In general, the dosage and duration of therapy must be sufficient to improve the patient's condi-

Table 3.
Pediatric Dosages of Corticosteroids for Asthma[61,62]

Drug	Dosage Form[a]	Dosage
Beclomethasone diproprionate	MDI	1–2 puffs (42 μg/puff) q 6–12 hr[b]
Flunisolide	MDI	2 puffs (25 μg/puff) q 12 hr[b]
Hydrocortisone sodium succinate	Injection	4–8 mg (of hydrocortisone)/mg/kg i.v. (up to 250 mg) once, then 2–4 mg/kg q 6 hr[c]
Methylprednisolone sodium succinate	Injection	1–2 mg (of methylprednisolone)/kg i.v. once, then 0.5–1 mg/kg q 6 hr[c]
Prednisone	Oral tablets	Burst therapy: 10 mg q 12 hr if pt. < 1 yr; 20 mg q 12 hr if 1–4 yr; 30 mg q 12 if 5–13 yr; 40 mg q 12 hr if >13 yr Long-term therapy: 10 mg q.o.d. if pt < 1 yr; 20 mg q.o.d. if 1–4 yr; 30 mg q.o.d. if 5–13 yr; 40 mg q.o.d. if >13 yr
Triamcinolone acetonide	MDI	1–2 puffs (100 μg/puff) q 6–12 hr[b]

[a] MDI = metered-dose inhaler.
[b] Initial dosage. Adjust to minimal effective dosage.
[c] Initial dosage. Convert to oral therapy within 48 hr when possible.

tion, prevent immediate recurrence of symptoms, and avoid adverse effects.[128]

The dosages of prednisone used for burst therapy (Table 3) are generally at the upper end of the commonly recommended dosage range for children (i.e., approximately 2 mg/kg/day). High doses are usually given for less than seven days and then discontinued without a taper. In the treatment of other disorders, corticosteroid dosage is generally tapered to minimize the potential for relapse or flaring of the disease state and to avoid addisonian crisis or other withdrawal phenomena. Tapering is not necessary in the treatment of acute asthma. Because asthma is a reversible disease,[21] relapse of acute symptoms is dependent on reexposure to a precipitant, not withdrawal of a drug. In fact, burst therapy has been shown to prevent relapse of asthmatic symptoms[129,130] and cause, at most, transient suppression of the hypothalamic–pituitary–adrenal (HPA) axis.[131]

Long-term administration of corticosteroids may be accomplished by inhalation or alternate-day oral therapy; the frequency of adverse effects from both methods is comparably low.[132,133] The concomitant use of inhaled and oral corticosteroids may lead to increased adrenal suppression and other adverse effects.[132,133]

Toxicity. There has been concern about the administration of corticosteroids in the treatment of childhood asthma because of the adverse effects associated with their use.[134] However, it should be remembered that asthma is potentially life threatening and that a fatal outcome due to inadequate drug therapy would be unacceptable.[135] The frequency of adverse effects with corticosteroids is dependent on duration of treatment, time of administration, corticosteroid preparation, route of administration, dose, and dosage interval.

Burst therapy rarely produces clinically important adverse effects.[128] An increase in appetite and mild cushingoid effects may occur toward the end of the burst with either no[136] or only transient[131] HPA-axis suppression (<10 days). However, four or more corticosteroid bursts per year may place some patients at greater risk for HPA-axis suppression.[137] The frequency of adverse effects increases dramatically when systemic corticosteroids are administered daily for long-term treatment of asthmatic symptoms. Even small dosages of oral corticosteroids, if administered for a long enough time, can produce growth suppression, cushingoid changes in appearance, posterior subcapsular cataracts, osteoporosis, and HPA-axis suppression.[138]

HPA-axis suppression results from the negative feedback of exogenously administered corticosteroids on the hypothalamus, pituitary, and adrenal glands. In an attempt to decrease the magnitude of suppression with maintenance therapy, patients are given oral corticosteroids every other day. The degree of HPA-axis suppression in asthmatic children is decreased when alternate-day, rather than daily, therapy is used.[139,140]

With the introduction of corticosteroid inhalers, it was believed that HPA-axis suppression would be completely avoided. Although many studies have demonstrated a lack of HPA-axis suppression in children using inhaled beclomethasone dipropionate,[126,141-144] triamcinolone acetonide,[145] and flunisolide,[146,147] HPA-axis suppression has been reported in other studies.[148,149] A dose-dependent suppression of HPA-axis function has been shown with the use of inhaled corticosteroids.[150,151]

Another concern about the use of corticosteroids in children is the risk of growth suppression. Many years ago, growth impairment with daily oral corticosteroid therapy was noted.[152] Some investigators have also attributed growth retardation to long-term inhalation[153] or alternate-day oral corticosteroid therapy.[154] This effect may be dose dependent.[154]

Others have related growth suppression to the severity of asthma.[133,155] For example, a child with asthma may have a short stature because of chronic hypoxemia, recurrent infections, long-term stress, and suppression of normal activity. Additional support for this association is the growth acceleration seen after initiation of therapy that either includes[154,156] or does not include[133] corticosteroids. Still other investigators have documented normal height in asthmatic children treated with corticosteroids[157] and no change in expected growth after the introduction of corticosteroids.[158,159]

Balfour-Lynn[158] stated that the conflicting reports of growth suppression stem from differences in age of the children who were studied. Balfour-Lynn studied 66 asthmatic children, over 60% of whom were in the 50th percentile for height before entering the study. The rate of growth was normal in all patients until the age of 10 years. At this point, 35 children continued to grow at a normal rate while 30 of the children who had delayed onset of puberty showed growth retardation. The tendency for delayed onset of puberty was independent of the severity of asthma. At the onset of puberty, all 30 children who had had delayed puberty had growth acceleration, and they were not significantly different in adult height from the children with normal onset of puberty. Twenty-six of the 66 children were treated with inhaled beclomethasone dipropionate. There was no significant suppression of growth in these steroid-treated patients, and all achieved the predicted adult height.

Other adverse effects unique to treatment with inhaled corticosteroids are primarily local and include dry or sore throat,[145,147] dysphonia,[160], and oropharyngeal candidiasis.[161] The frequency of complications has been shown to increase with larger doses in adults,[162] but this result was not reproducible in children.[161] The risk of candidal infection can be minimized by using a spacing device to decrease oropharyngeal drug deposition[163,164] or by rinsing the mouth and spitting the water out after each use.

Short-term Therapy. Corticosteroids are indicated for the treatment of acute exacerbations of childhood asthma. A number of studies have shown that corticosteroids cause clinical improvement during acute asthmatic attacks, but these trials included only patients who sought emergency medical care.[130,136,165-168] Harris et al.[129] investigated the effects of oral prednisone early in the course of an acute exacerbation of asthma before emergency care was needed. Forty-one patients (median age, 12 years) were enrolled in the study after having an incomplete response to inhaled albuterol. Patients were randomly assigned to receive high-dose oral prednisone or placebo for one week, and then therapy was discontinued without tapering. All 22 patients in the steroid-treated group responded to prednisone with an improvement in peak expiratory flow rate, a decrease in symptoms, and a decrease in the need for a β-agonist inhaler. Of the 19 patients receiving placebo, 8 required prednisone intervention because of progression of symptoms and a decline in pulmonary function. The investigators concluded that early administration of high-dose oral prednisone can prevent a serious exacerbation and the need for emergency care.

Brunette et al.[169] studied intervention even earlier in the course of acute asthma. At the onset of symptoms of upper respiratory tract infection (usually coryza) and before any signs of wheezing, all patients were treated with oral metaproterenol and theophylline. One group of patients additionally received prednisone 1 mg/kg/day for the duration of the infection followed by a dosage taper. The use of prednisone resulted in a significant reduction in metaproterenol use, prevalence of asthma attacks, and number of symptomatic days. Also, the number of emergency room visits and hospitalizations decreased significantly in the prednisone-treated group.

Long-term Therapy. Less than 10 years ago, corticosteroids were not used for the management of chronic symptoms until a child's symptoms were shown not to be controlled by β agonists, theophylline, cromolyn, or repeated bursts of corticosteroids. Some practitioners still follow this step-care approach,[170-172] but recently others have proposed inhaled corticosteroids as first-line agents in the management of asthma.[173]

Inhaled corticosteroids and cromolyn have been compared in patients with chronic, non-steroid-dependent asthma not controlled by bronchodilators alone.[174-176] Although the data conflict, most studies have shown greater improvement with corticosteroids than with cromolyn. None of the studies associated the severity of symptoms with the response to either drug, although Svendsen et al.[176] identified a subgroup of patients whose pulmonary function improved while receiving cromolyn as opposed to corticosteroids. This subgroup of patients was not further described in terms of severity of disease or any other characteristic that might assist in prospectively identifying patients who would respond to cromolyn. Nonetheless, in patients with mild to moderate asthmatic symptoms, cromolyn would probably be preferred initially over inhaled corticosteroids because it is safer. Inhaled corticosteroids, then, would be reserved for patients with more severe symptoms or those who do not respond to cromolyn. The combination of cromolyn plus inhaled corticosteroids has not been shown to be of any greater benefit than corticosteroids alone in the treatment of chronic asthma.[174,177]

Currently, beclomethasone dipropionate, triamcinolone acetonide, and flunisolide are the most commonly used inhaled corticosteroids. The use of inhaled corticosteroids has improved symptomatic control and pulmonary function in children whose symptoms were not previously controlled with other long-term therapies.[126,141,145,147] Also, the addition of inhaled corticosteroids has permitted reduction or discontinuation of oral corticosteroid therapy.[126,141,145,146]

Problems in administering inhaled corticosteroids occur in children younger than eight years, who have difficulty with MDI technique. Spacing devices have been used to improve drug delivery.[162,178] Corticosteroid solutions for nebulization and dry powder for inhalation are not available in this country. Therefore, in young children, the options are alternate-day oral dosing or inhalation with the use of an Aerochamber and mask. Administration of albuterol by the latter method in 6- to 36-month-old children resulted in a reduction of bronchospastic symptoms.[87] We have, in a few instances, administered corticosteroids in this fashion with positive results.

After initial stabilization, the dosage frequency for inhaled beclomethasone dipropionate may be reduced to twice daily.[142,179] This is accomplished by dividing the total 24-hour dosage into two equal doses given every 12 hours. This regimen improves compliance[142] without adversely affecting symptom control or pulmonary function.[142,179] None of the studies of twice-daily administration used more than 400 μg/day (eight puffs/day). Therefore, if higher doses are required, increasing the frequency to three or four times per day should be considered.

Theophylline

Place in Therapy. The use of theophylline in both short- and long-term management of asthma has come into question in recent years because of doubt regarding the drug's efficacy and concern regarding its safety relative to cromolyn or inhaled corticosteroids.[74,75] Theophylline in asthma therapy is now reserved for prophylactic treatment of chronic asthma in patients who do not respond to initial treatment with cromolyn or inhaled corticosteroids.[18]

In chronic asthma, theophylline has been shown to be more effective than inhaled albuterol at controlling symptoms and improving morning peak expiratory flow rates.[180] Oral theophylline, when used twice daily, also offers improved compliance compared with inhaled albuterol.

Numerous comparative trials of cromolyn and theophylline have been conducted.[120,121,181-183] Cromolyn has been shown to be as effective as theophylline in improving spirometric assessments in children with asthma. The data conflict as to the comparative ability of the two agents to control the symptoms of asthma; results of one study indicated superiority of theophylline,[181] and others favored cromolyn.[120,183] Cromolyn produces a markedly lower frequency of adverse effects than theophylline.[120-121,181]

Two studies have evaluated the effectiveness of concomitant therapy with cromolyn and theophylline in children. Hambleton et al.[181] found a statistically significant benefit in favor of the combination of theophylline plus cromolyn over cromolyn alone in terms of peak expiratory flow rate (81% of predicted versus 75% of predicted; $p < 0.05$) and symptom control (71% versus 59% days that were symptom-free, $p < 0.05$). There was no difference when the combination therapy was compared with theophylline alone. On the other hand, Newth et al.[183] found that the cromolyn–theophylline combination was significantly better than theophylline alone in controlling symptoms (61% versus 46.5% days that were symptom-free, $p < 0.05$) and that there was no difference between the combination and cromolyn alone. Also, patients receiving combination therapy required significantly fewer treatments with β agonists for acute symptoms than those receiving either drug alone. Although these studies demonstrate a statistical benefit for combination therapy, the actual clinical benefit obtained may not be meaningful.

A more recent study demonstrated a benefit from the addition of cromolyn to pre-existing bronchodilator therapy (including theophylline) in uncontrolled asthma in adults and children.[184] However, the response of the majority of patients to cromolyn alone is not known. Therefore, it is not clear whether or not the beneficial response was due to combination therapy or cromolyn alone.

In steroid-dependent asthmatic patients, the maintenance drug of choice, in addition to corticosteroids, is theophylline. The combination of theophylline plus corticosteroids in these patients significantly improves symptom control, pulmonary function, and exercise tolerance and reduces the need for additional medications.[185,186] Extended-release theophylline preparations have also been used for the prevention of nocturnal asthmatic symptoms.[63-64,187]

Mechanism of Action. The mechanism of action of theophylline is unknown, but there are currently a number of theories proposed. These theories include (1) adenosine antagonism, (2) indirect β-adrenergic stimulation secondary to release of catecholamines, (3) drug influences on intracellular calcium binding, and (4) inhibited production of contractile prostaglandins.[40] The previously held belief that theophylline exerts its bronchodilatory effects through inhibition of phosphodiesterase has now been discounted.[40] In fact, theophylline does not inhibit this enzyme at therapeutic concentrations. The ultimate effect of theophylline, whatever its subcellular mechanisms, is bronchodilation. In addition, theophylline exerts other pharmacologic actions, which include transient diuresis, inhibition of uterine contractions, and effects on the diaphragmatic muscles.[188] The primary effect of theophylline is on the early asthmatic response. Although theophylline does inhibit the late asthmatic response, it does not prevent the bronchial hyperactivity that follows this response even after prolonged administration. Therefore, its effects on the late asthmatic response are not appreciable clinically.[18,42]

Administration. Theophylline may be administered intravenously or orally. Intravenous administration is reserved for emergency situations (i.e., status asthmaticus) when aggressive treatment with inhaled sympathomimetics and systemic corticosteroids is not providing sufficient relief. It should be noted, however, that the routine use of intravenous theophylline in the emergency room setting has been extensively debated and is no longer recommended by most practitioners.[74,75] Another possible use of the intravenous preparation is in selected patients who are unable to take oral medications. The route of choice for maintenance use of theophylline is oral.

Choice of Formulation. There are many extended-release oral theophylline preparations on the market.

Recommended preparations for routine use in asthmatic children should demonstrate sufficient extent and rate of absorption, limited peak-to-trough fluctuation in serum concentration over a 12-hour dosing interval, and minimal effect of food on the rate and extent of absorption.[189] Since it is difficult to guarantee a fasting state at the time of drug administration in a child, preparations that are markedly influenced by food are best avoided.[190] Given these considerations, the most suitable products are Slo-bid capsules (Rorer Pharmaceuticals) and Theo-Dur tablets (Key Pharmaceuticals).[188] Extended-release theophylline products should not be generically substituted.

Capsule preparations offer a method of administering theophylline to young children who are unable to swallow tablets.[189] These capsules, which can also be swallowed whole, contain many small beads that may be emptied onto a single spoonful of food and administered orally to the child. Children often object more to the texture than the taste of the beads, and so it sometimes helps to disguise them with a food of a similar gritty texture (e.g., grits, farina, strawberry preserves).

There are liquid theophylline and aminophylline preparations available as well. Unfortunately, maintaining therapeutic serum concentrations in children with liquid theophylline preparations requires giving the medication at least as frequently as every six hours.[189] This necessitates administration of a dose in the middle of the night, which means waking both the patient and the parent. Such a regimen is unreasonable for most families. If a liquid preparation is chosen, a product that is alcohol-free and offers a concentration that allows a reasonable volume of liquid to be administered (even with higher doses) should be used.

Pharmacokinetics. Theophylline pharmacokinetics differ markedly between pediatric and adult patients. The volume of distribution of theophylline in children older than six years is about the same as in adults (0.45 L/kg; range, 0.3–0.7 L/kg),[191,192] but in term and preterm neonates it is approximately 0.6 and 0.7 L/kg, respectively.[193] Theophylline is approximately 40% bound to plasma proteins in both pediatric and adult patients[194] and is less extensively protein-bound in neonates.[193-194]

Theophylline is primarily metabolized by the cytochrome P-450 component of the hepatic microsomal oxidative enzyme system.[195] In older children, as in adults, the metabolites are generally inactive and rapidly excreted by the kidney.[195] Two important differences in the metabolism and excretion of theophylline are seen in neonates. First, methylation of theophylline to caffeine becomes a more prominent metabolic pathway, presumably because of the relative underdevelopment of other metabolic pathways and the limited ability of the neonate to eliminate caffeine.[196] Second, neonates excrete a much larger portion of a theophylline dose unchanged in the urine (50%) compared with older children and adults (15%).[195,196] Dosage must, therefore, be adjusted for renal failure in this very young age group.

The clearance of theophylline varies widely with age. Changes in clearance occur because of variations in and development of the enzymatic metabolic pathway for theophylline in the liver. Neonates eliminate the drug very slowly and therefore have a relatively long theophylline half-life[193]; this allows for a 12-hour dosing interval with liquid preparations. In the first 12 months of life, a child's theophylline clearance rapidly increases.[197] Because of this, maintaining therapeutic theophylline concentrations in infants is very difficult and requires frequent monitoring of serum concentrations and dosage adjustments.

In children who are one to nine years old, theophylline clearance remains fairly constant, but dosage must be adjusted to account for changes in the patient's weight. Between the ages of 9 and 16 years, a child's clearance gradually decreases until it approximates that of an adult.[198] In children older than one year, serum theophylline concentrations should be checked every 6 to 12 months and when clinically indicated (i.e., when the patient is experiencing symptoms of theophylline toxicity or asthma). Appropriate dosage adjustments should be made based on serum concentration data.

In all patients, numerous factors can influence the clearance of theophylline.[199,200] Among the factors that can increase theophylline clearance are smoking (which may be a factor in adolescents), diet (high protein/low carbohydrate, large quantities of charcoal-broiled beef), and drugs that induce hepatic enzymes (e.g., phenobarbital, phenytoin, carbamazepine, rifampin). Factors that can decrease clearance include diet (low protein/high carbohydrate), certain disease states (cirrhosis, cor pulmonale, congestive heart failure, fever, viral illness) and certain drugs (erythromycin, ciprofloxacin, propranolol, cimetidine, oral contraceptives).

Some of these interactions are more likely to occur in children. Fever or viral illness can decrease theophylline clearance, but whether the febrile or infectious process is responsible is not clear. The interaction may result in toxic serum theophylline concentrations.[199] Because of the use of erythromycin for common pediatric infections, such as otitis media, the erythromycin–theophylline interaction may be particularly bothersome. Serum theophylline concentrations may increase up to 25% after five or six days of concomitant treatment with erythromycin, and a dosage adjustment may be required. A general guideline is that if the patient's steady-state theophylline concentration is ≥13 μg/mL, the dosage should be empirically decreased by 25%.[199,200]

Dosage. The recommended initial pediatric dosages for theophylline (Table 4) reflect the aforementioned pharmacokinetic considerations. An individual patient's dosage should be calculated using the lesser of actual or ideal body weight if the patient is obese. The dosage should be increased gradually as follows over about one week until the calculated daily dosage is

Table 4.
Pediatric Dosages of Theophylline for Asthma[61,62,a]

Patient Age (yr)	Dosage
Oral Therapy[b]	
<1	[(0.2 × age in weeks) + 5] mg/kg/day
1–9	22 mg/kg/day
9–12	20 mg/kg/day
12–16	18 mg/kg/day
Intravenous Therapy[c]	
<1	[(0.008 × age in weeks) + 0.21] mg/kg/hr
1–9	0.8 mg/kg/hr
9–12	0.7 mg/kg/hr
12–16	0.5 mg/kg/hr (for nonsmokers)
	0.7 mg/kg/hr (for smokers)

[a] Maximum initial daily dosage = 900 mg. Dosage adjustments should be based on serum concentration data.

[b] Full initial daily dosage should be achieved gradually over about one week. See text for explanation.

[c] The i.v. loading dose is calculated by multiplying the desired change in serum theophylline concentration by the patient's estimated volume of distribution.

reached: Give one half to two thirds of the total daily dosage (not to exceed 400 mg/day) for three days, then two thirds to three quarters of the total daily dosage (not to exceed 600 mg/day) for three days, then the total dose (not to exceed 900 mg/day).[201] If the extended-release products recommended above are used, theophylline can be administered on a twice-daily schedule in children without compromising symptom control or risking adverse effects.[188]

Once the patient has received the total calculated dosage for at least three days, serum theophylline concentration should be measured to assess the appropriateness of the dosage. The peak serum concentration sample should be obtained four to six hours after the morning dose in a patient taking an extended-release preparation.[199] The therapeutic range for theophylline is 10 to 20 μg/mL.[202] Clinically stable, ambulatory patients can generally be maintained in the lower end of the therapeutic serum concentration range. Severely ill patients in the hospital may require higher serum concentrations for greater effect.[188]

Maintaining therapeutic serum theophylline concentrations in infants less than one year of age is difficult. As noted previously, clearance changes rapidly in this age group. Simultaneously, the patient grows rapidly, commonly with a 100% increase in total body weight within the first four to six months of life. Finally, liquid dosage preparations must be used in children who are not yet taking solid foods, and the necessary six-hour dosing interval is difficult to maintain. For all of these reasons, we prefer to use cromolyn instead of theophylline in this group of patients whenever possible.

If infants in this age group must be given theophylline, the dosage equation of Nassif et al.,[197] which is based on postnatal age, is commonly employed. Some investigators have found that the use of this equation in premature newborns could result in toxic serum concentrations.[203] A dosage method based on postconceptional age rather than postnatal age resulted in good correlation between measured and predicted serum concentration values.[203]

Toxicity. By incrementally increasing dosage as described above, the minor caffeine-like adverse effects of theophylline (mild headache, mild nausea) can often be avoided.[201] The gastrointestinal adverse effects of theophylline (which can often be managed by administering the drug with food) may be caused by direct irritation of the gastrointestinal mucosa or by a central mechanism (since they can occur with intravenous administration).[204] At serum theophylline concentrations higher than 20 μg/mL, patients are at greater risk for more severe adverse effects such as tachycardia, cardiac arrhythmias, and seizures.[204] Theophylline has the potential to cause fatal adverse effects[205]; although the drug is effective for the treatment of chronic asthma and usually safe (when used correctly), it is not benign.

An aspect of theophylline treatment that has received considerable media attention in recent years is its effect on behavior and school performance. Rachelefsky et al.[206] concluded that a four-week course of theophylline in school-age asthmatic children can adversely affect behavior and school performance. These results were based solely on teachers' evaluations and were not supported by parents' observations. The analytical methods used in this study have raised controversy.[207] Other investigators have found positive effects of theophylline on verbal learning but negative effects on motor performance in a three-month study.[208] They concluded that further investigation is required to determine the true effect of theophylline on academic and social abilities.

Asthma Therapeutics

Each of the drugs and drug classes discussed has a specific place in the management of asthma in children.

Intermittent asthma is usually managed by intermittent treatment with an inhaled β agonist alone. Occasionally, for more severe episodes (i.e., those that do not respond to bronchodilators alone), a corticosteroid burst is required.

Chronic asthma also requires an inhaled β agonist for treatment of acute episodes. Long-term chronic prophylactic therapy is also needed. Options for prophylactic treatment are cromolyn and inhaled corticosteroids; theophylline is an alternative to these drugs. Cromolyn, although expensive, is one of the few drugs that causes no adverse effects in the great majority of patients, and inhaled administration may be preferred by some patients. Inhaled corticosteroids are now used as first-line long-term therapy for chronic asthma. Cromolyn should probably be the first choice for chronic prophylactic therapy because of its safety. However, this decision may be tempered by the severity of the patient's symptoms.

Theophylline is relatively inexpensive (even when serum drug monitoring is included in the cost), convenient to administer on a twice-daily regimen, orally administered (which may be preferred by some patients over the inhaled route), and may be more effective than cromolyn for some patients. Adverse effects are the major disadvantage of theophylline, but with judicious use it can be given very safely.

Occasional corticosteroid burst therapy may also be required for episodes that are not controlled with bronchodilators.

Indeterminate and seasonal asthma is treated as intermittent asthma until the disorder is more firmly established as being truly intermittent or chronic. Patients with seasonal chronic symptoms are treated as intermittent asthmatics throughout the year until their predictable bothersome season arrives. Then, regular prophylactic therapy with cromolyn or inhaled corticosteroids should be started. Also, patients with chronic asthma sometimes have worsening of their symptoms during particular seasons of the year and will then require addition of inhaled corticosteroids to their existing regimen during that period. Again, corticosteroid burst therapy is occasionally needed for more severe exacerbations.

Steroid-dependent asthma is identified when the patient requires frequent steroid bursts (usually about once a month) and then demonstrates a gradually worsening course over the ensuing three to four weeks. Obviously, this type of patient is treated with long-term corticosteroid administration, usually in addition to another long-term prophylactic medication and an as-needed inhaled β agonist. Because of the lack of benefit demonstrated by the combination of cromolyn and long-term corticosteroids over corticosteroids alone (in non-steroid-dependent asthmatics), theophylline may be a better choice for the long-term prophylactic medication. Once again, steroid bursts may occasionally be required, but if they are required frequently, the dose of the long-term corticosteroid should be increased.

Status asthmaticus is treated as an emergency. Initial treatment is hydration, oxygen, and frequent (or continous) inhaled β-agonist treatments. Acute therapy with intravenous theophylline is indicated only for the very severely bronchoconstricted patient with a subtherapeutic serum theophylline concentration. As previously stated, theophylline is generally not considered to be of added benefit to aggressive therapy with β agonists and systemic corticosteroids. Intravenous corticosteroids are started immediately with the ultimate goal being conversion to oral therapy within 24 to 48 hours. Intravenous isoproterenol or terbutaline may be used in an attempt to avoid mechanical ventilation, but some patients progress to this outcome in spite of this intervention.

Conclusion

The treatment of asthma in children requires the special consideration of drug efficacy, pharmacokinetics, compliance, and toxicity in young patients. Drugs used to treat childhood asthma include β agonists, anticholinergics, cromolyn sodium, corticosteroids, and theophylline.

References

1. Speer F. The management of childhood asthma. Springfield, IL: Charles C Thomas; 1958.
2. Gergen PJ, Weiss KB. Changing patterns of asthma hospitalization among children: 1979 to 1987. *JAMA*. 1990; 264: 1688-92.
3. Weiss KB, Wagener DK. Changing patterns of asthma mortality: identifying target populations at high risk. *JAMA*. 1990; 264:1683-87.
4. Buist AS, Vollmer WM. Reflections on the rise in asthma morbidity and mortality. *JAMA*. 1990; 264:1719-20. Editorial.
5. National Center for Health Statistics. Patterns of ambulatory care in pediatrics: the National Ambulatory Medical Care Survey, United States, January 1980–December 1981. Washington, DC: U.S. Government Printing Office, 1983; DHHS publication no.(PHS)84-1736. (Vital and health statistics; series 13, no. 75).
6. Gergen PJ, Mullally DI, Evans R. National survey of prevalence of asthma among children in the United States, 1976 to 1980. *Pediatrics*. 1988; 81:1-7.
7. Evans R, Mullally DI, Wilson RW et al. National trends in the morbidity and mortality of asthma in the U.S.: prevalence, hospitalization and death from asthma over two decades: 1965-1984. *Chest*. 1987; 91:655-745.
8. Blair H. Natural history of childhood asthma: 20-year follow-up. *Arch Dis Child*. 1977; 52:613.
9. Mitchell RG, Dawson B. Educational and social characteristics of children with asthma. *Arch Dis Child*. 1973; 48:467-71.
10. NIAID Task Force. Asthma and the other allergic diseases. Bethesda, MD: National Institutes of Health, 1979; NIH publication no. 79-387.
11. Marion RJ, Creer TL, Reynolds RVC. Direct and indirect costs associated with the management of childhood asthma. *Ann Allergy*. 1985; 54:31-4.
12. Godfrey S. Functional differences between the lungs of normal and asthmatic children. In: Tinkelman DG, Falliers CJ, Naspitz CK, eds. Childhood asthma: pathophysiology and treatment. New York: Marcel Dekker; 1987:1-21.
13. Szentivanyi A. The beta adrenergic theory of the atopic abnormality in bronchial asthma. *J Allergy*. 1968; 42:203-32.
14. Nadel JA. Autonomic control of airway smooth muscle and airway secretions. *Am Rev Respir Dis*. 1977; 115:117-26.
15. Middleton E. Antiasthmatic drug therapy and calcium ions: review of pathogenesis and role of calcium. *J Pharm Sci*. 1980; 69:243-51.
16. Ellis EF. Allergic disorders: asthma. In: Behrman RE, Vaughan VC, Nelson WE, eds. Nelson textbook of pediatrics. 13th ed. Philadelphia: Saunders; 1987:495-501.
17. Larsen GL. New concepts in the pathogenesis of asthma. *Clin Immunol Immunopathol*. 1989; 53:S107-18.
18. Barnes PJ. A new approach to the treatment of asthma. *N Engl J Med*. 1989; 321:1517-27.
19. Hargreave FE. Late-phase asthmatic responses and airway inflammation. *J Allergy Clin Immunol*. 1989; 83:525-7.
20. Kaliner M. Asthma and mast cell activation. *J Allergy Clin Immunol*. 1989; 83:510-20.
21. American Thoracic Society: Committee on diagnostic standards for nontuberculous respiratory diseases. Chronic bronchitis, asthma, and pulmonary emphysema: definitions and classification of chronic bronchitis, asthma, and pulmonary emphysema. *Am Rev Respir Dis*. 1962; 84:762-8.
22. Ekwo E, Weinberger M. Evaluation of a program for the pharmacologic management of children with asthma. *J Allergy Clin Immunol*. 1978; 61:240-7.

23. Galant SP. Therapeutic approach to acute asthma in children. In: Tinkelman DG, Falliers CJ, Naspitz CK, eds. Childhood asthma: pathophysiology and treatment. New York: Marcel Dekker; 1987:231-47.
24. Siegel SC, Katz RM, Rachelefsky GS. Asthma in infancy and childhood. In: Middleton E, Reed CE, Ellis EF, eds. Allergy: principles and practice. St. Louis: Mosby; 1983:863-900.
25. Andrews JL. The clinical roles of pulmonary function testing. *Med Clin North Am.* 1979; 63:355-77.
26. Orenstein SR, Orenstein DM. Gastroesophageal reflux and respiratory disease in children. *J Pediatr.* 1988; 112:847-58.
27. Silk H. Sinusitis and asthma: a review. *J Asthma.* 1990; 27:5-9.
28. Rachelefsky GS, Spector SL. Sinusitis and asthma. *J Asthma.* 1990; 27:1-3.
29. Reed CE, Townley RG. Asthma: classification and pathogenesis. In: Middleton E, Reed CE, Ellis EF, eds. Allergy: principles and practice. St. Louis: Mosby; 1983:812-31.
30. Church JA. Allergic rhinitis: diagnosis and management. *Clin Pediatr.* 1980; 19:655-9.
31. Solomon WR, Mathews KP. Aerobiology and inhalant allergens. In: Middleton E, Reed CE, Ellis EF, eds. Allergy: principles and practice. St. Louis: Mosby; 1983:1101-17.
32. Rachelefsky GS, Coulson A, Siegel SC et al. Aspirin intolerance in chronic childhood asthma: detected by oral challenge. *Pediatrics.* 1975; 56:443-8.
33. Vedanthan PK, Menon MM, Bell TD et al. Aspirin and tartrazine oral challenge: incidence of adverse response in chronic childhood asthma. *J Allergy Clin Immunol.* 1977; 60: 8-13.
34. Samter M, Beers RF. Concerning the nature of intolerance to aspirin. *J Allergy.* 1967; 40:281-93.
35. Szczeklik A, Gryglewski RJ, Czerniawska-Mysik G. Relationship of inhibition of prostaglandin biosynthesis by analgesics to asthma attacks in aspirin-sensitive patients. *Br Med J.* 1975; 1:67-9.
36. Zaid G, Beall GN. Bronchial response to beta-adrenergic blockade. *N Engl J Med.* 1966; 275:580-4.
37. Dalton-Bunnow MF. Review of sulfite sensitivity. *Am J Hosp Pharm.* 1985; 42:2220-6.
38. Hetzel MR. The pulmonary clock. *Thorax.* 1981; 36:481-6.
39. Martin RJ, Cicutto LC, Smith HR et al. Airways inflammation in nocturnal asthma. *Am Rev Respir Dis.* 1991; 143:351-7.
40. Church MK, Featherstone RL, Cushley MJ et al. Relationships between adenosine, cyclic nucleotides, and xanthines in asthma. *J Allergy Clin Immunol.* 1986; 78:670-5.
41. Anderson RGG, Nilsson KB. Role of cyclic nucleotides metabolism and mechanical activity in smooth muscle. In: Stephens NL, ed. The biochemistry of smooth muscle. Baltimore: University Park Press; 1977:263-91.
42. Chung KF. Pharmacology of airway inflammation in asthma. *Lung.* 1990; 168(Suppl):132-41.
43. Barnes PJ, Kaliner JS, Dollery CT. Human lung adrenoceptors studied by radioligand binding. *Clin Sci.* 1980; 58:457.
44. Engel G. Subclasses of β-adrenoceptors—a quantitative estimation of β_1 and β_2-adrenoceptors in guinea pig and human lung. *Postgrad Med.* 1981; 57:77-83.
45. Lofdahl CG, Svedmyer N. Selectivity of β-adrenergic stimulating and blocking agents. *Eur J Respir Dis Suppl.* 1984; 136:101-3.
46. Lemanske RF, Joad J. Beta-2 receptor agonists in asthma: a comparison. *J Asthma.* 1990; 27:101-9.
47. Weiner N. Norepinephrine, epinephrine and the sympathomimetic amines. In: Goodman and Gilman's the pharmacological basis of therapeutics. 7th ed. Gilman AG, Goodman LS, Rall TW et al., eds. New York: Macmillan; 1985:145-80.
48. AHFS drug information 91. McEvoy GK, ed. Bethesda, MD: American Society of Hospital Pharmacists, 1991.
49. Walker SB, Kradjan WA, Bierman CW. Bitolterol mesylate: a beta-adrenergic agent. Chemistry, pharmacokinetics, pharmacodynamics, adverse effects and clinical efficacy in asthma. *Pharmacotherapy.* 1985; 5:127-37.
50. Harris JB, Ahrens RC, Milavetz G et al. Comparison of the intensity and duration of effects of inhaled bitolterol and albuterol on airway caliber and airway responsiveness to histamine. *J Allergy Clin Immunol.* 1990; 85:1043-9.
51. Kelly WH. New β_2-adrenergic agonist aerosols. *Clin Pharm.* 1985; 4:393-403.
52. Reed CE. Adrenergic bronchodilators: pharmacology and toxicology. *J Allergy Clin Immunol.* 1985; 76:335-41.
53. Scheinin M, Koulu M, Laurikainen E et al. Hypokalemia and other non-bronchial effects of inhaled fenoterol and salbutamol: a placebo-controlled dose-response study in healthy volunteers. *Br J Clin Pharmacol.* 1987; 24:645-53.
54. Crane J, Burgess C, Beasley R. Cardiovascular and hypokalaemic effects of inhaled salbutamol, fenoterol, and isoprenaline. *Thorax.* 1989; 44:136-40.
55. Johnson CE. Principles of nebulizer-delivered drug therapy for asthma. *Am J Hosp Pharm.* 1989; 46:1845-55.
56. Lefkowitz RJ, Caron MG, Stiles GL. Biochemical, physiological, and clinical insights derived from studies of the adrenergic receptors. *N Engl J Med.* 1984; 310:1570-9.
57. Sears MR, Taylor DR, Print CG et al. Regular inhaled beta-agonist treatment in bronchial asthma. *Lancet.* 1990; 336: 1391-6.
58. Ullman A, Svedmyr N. Salmeterol, a new long acting inhaled β_2 adrenoceptor agonist: comparison with salbutamol in adult asthmatic patients. *Thorax.* 1988; 43:674-8.
59. Becker AB, Simons FER, McMillan JL et al. Formoterol, a new long-acting selective β_2-adrenergic receptor agonist: double-blind comparison with salbutamol and placebo in children with asthma. *J Allergy Clin Immunol.* 1989; 84:891-5.
60. Nelson HS. Beta adrenergic agonists. *Chest.* 1982; 82:33S-38S.
61. The Harriet Lane Handbook. Greene MG, ed. St. Louis: Mosby-Year Book; 1991.
62. Anon. Drugs for asthma. *Med Lett Drugs Ther.* 1987; 29:11-6.
63. Milledge JS, Morris J. A comparison of slow-release salbutamol with slow-release aminophylline in nocturnal asthma. *J Int Med Res.* 1979; 7:106-10.
64. Heins M, Kurtin L, Oellerich M et al. Nocturnal asthma: slow-release terbutaline versus slow-release theophylline therapy. *Eur Respir J.* 1988; 1:306-10.
65. Becker AB, Nelson NA, Simons FER. Inhaled salbutamol (albuterol) vs injected epinephrine in the treatment of acute asthma in children. *J Pediatr.* 1983; 102:465-9.
66. Ruddy RM, Kolski G, Scarpa N et al. Aerosolized metaproterenol compared to subcutaneous epinephrine in the emergency treatment of acute childhood asthma. *Pediatr Pulmonol.* 1986; 2:230-6.
67. Sempler DA, Mellon M. Management of acute severe asthma. *Pediatr Clin North Am.* 1984; 31:879-90.
68. Weinberger M. Antiasthmatic therapy in children. *Pediatr Clin North Am.* 1989; 36:1251-84.
69. Wood DW, Downes JJ, Scheinkopf H et al. Intravenous isoproterenol in the management of respiratory failure in childhood status asthmaticus. *J Allergy Clin Immunol.* 1972; 50:75-81.
70. Parry WH, Martorano F, Cotton EK. Management of life-threatening asthma with intravenous isoproterenol infusions. *Am J Dis Child.* 1976; 130:39-42.
71. Fuglsang G, Pedersen S, Borgstrom L. Dose-response relationships of intravenously administered terbutaline in children with asthma. *J Pediatr.* 1989; 114:315-20.
72. Bohn D, Kalloghlian A, Jenkins J et al. Intravenous salbutamol in the treatment of status asthmaticus in children. *Crit Care Med.* 1984; 12:391-6.
73. Shim C. Inhalation aids of metered dose inhalers. *Chest.* 1987; 91:315-6.
74. Self TH, Ellis RF, Abou-Shala N et al. Is theophylline use justified in acute exacerbations of asthma? *Pharmacotherapy.* 1989; 9: 260-6.
75. Littenberg B. Aminophylline treatment in severe, acute asthma: a meta-analysis. *JAMA.* 1988; 259:1678-84.

76. Robertson CF, Smith F, Beck R, Levison H. Response to frequent low doses of nebulized salbutamol in acute asthma. *J Pediatr*. 1985; 106:672-4.
77. Schuh S, Reider MJ, Canny G et al. Nebulized albuterol in acute childhood asthma: comparison of two doses. *Pediatrics*. 1990; 86:509-13.
78. Schuh S, Parkin P, Rajan A et al. High- versus low-dose, frequently administered, nebulized albuterol in children with severe, acute asthma. *Pediatrics*. 1989; 83:513-8.
79. Moler FW, Hurwitz ME, Custer JR. Improvement in clinical asthma score and $PaCO_2$ in children with severe asthma treated with continuously nebulized terbutaline. *J Allergy Clin Immunol*. 1988; 81:1101-9.
80. Portnoy J, Aggarwal J. Continuous terbutaline nebulization for the treatment of severe exacerbations of asthma in children. *Ann Allergy*. 1988; 60:368-71.
81. Newman SP, Moren F, Pavia D et al. Deposition of pressurized suspension aerosols inhaled through extension devices. *Am Rev Respir Dis*. 1981; 124:317-20.
82. Lee H, Evans HE. Evaluation of inhalation aids of metered dose inhalers in asthmatic children. *Chest*. 1987; 91:366-9.
83. Pedersen S. Aerosol treatment of bronchoconstriction in children with or without a tube spacer. *N Engl J Med*. 1983; 308:1328-30.
84. Freelander M, Van Asperen PP. Nebuhaler vs. nebulizer in children with acute asthma. *Br Med J*. 1984; 288:1873-4.
85. Pendergast J, Hopkins J, Timms B et al. Comparative efficacy of terbutaline administered by Nebuhaler and by nebulizer in young children with acute asthma. *Med J Aust*. 1989; 151: 406-8.
86. Fuglsang G, Pedersen S. Comparison of Nebuhaler and nebulizer treatment of acute, severe asthma in children. *Eur J Respir Dis*. 1986; 69:109-13.
87. Conner WT, Dolovich MB, Frame RA et al. Reliable salbutamol administration in 6- to 36-month-old children by means of a metered dose inhaler and Aerochamber with mask. *Pediatr Pulmonol*. 1989; 6:263-7.
88. Kemp JP, Furukawa CT, Bronsky EA et al. Albuterol treatment for children with asthma: a comparison of inhaled powder and aerosol. *J Allergy Clin Immunol*. 1989; 83:697-702.
89. Towns SJ, Sharota E, Simpson SJ et al. Bronchodilator effects of salbutamol powder administered via Rotahaler and of terbutaline aerosol administered via Misthaler: a comparison study in children with asthma. *Med J Aust*. 1983; 1:633-6.
90. Epstein SW, Manning CPR, Ashley MJ et al. Survey of the clinical use of pressurized aerosol inhalers. *Can Med Assoc J*. 1979; 120:813-6.
91. Compton GK. Problems patients have using pressurized aerosol inhalers. *Eur J Respir Dis*. 1982; 63(Suppl 119):101-4.
92. Levison H, Reilly PA, Worsley GH. Spacing devices and metered-dose inhalers in childhood asthma. *J Pediatr*. 1985; 107:662-8.
93. Thomas P, Williams R, Reilly PA. Modifying delivery technique of fenoterol from a metered dose inhaler. *Ann Allergy*. 1984; 52:279-81.
94. Newman SP, Pavia D, Clarke SW. How should a pressurized beta-adrenergic bronchodilator be inhaled? *Eur J Respir Dis*. 1981; 62:3-21.
95. Rivlin J, Mindorff C, Levison H. Effect of administration technique on bronchodilator response to fenoterol in a metered-dose inhaler. *J Pediatr*. 1983; 102:47-72.
96. Burton AJ. Asthma inhalation devices: what do we know? *Br J Med*. 1984; 288:1650-1.
97. Mickle TR, Self TH, Farr GE et al. Evaluation of pharmacists' practice in patient education when dispensing a metered-dose inhaler. *DICP*. 1990; 24:927-30.
98. Freeman J, Landau LI. The effects of ipratropium bromide and fenoterol nebulizer solutions in children with asthma. *Clin Pediatr*. 1989; 28:556-60.
99. Raes M, Mulder P, Kerrebijn KF. Long-term effect of ipratropium bromide and fenoterol on the bronchial hyperresponsiveness to histamine in children with asthma. *J Allergy Clin Immunol*. 1989; 84:874-9.
100. Storr J, Lenney W. Nebulized ipratropium and salbutamol in asthma. *Arch Dis Child*. 1986; 61:602-3.
101. Watson WTA, Becker AB, Simons FER. Comparison of ipratropium solution, fenoterol solution, and their combination administered by nebulizer and face mask to children with acute asthma. *J Allergy Clin Immunol*. 1988; 82:1012-8
102. Guill MF, Maloney MJ, DuRant RH. Comparison of inhaled metaproterenol, inhaled atropine sulfate, and their combination in treatment of children with acute asthma. *Ann Allergy*. 1987; 59:367-71.
103. Holgate ST. Reflections on the mechanism(s) of action of sodium cromoglycate (Intal) and the role of mast cells in asthma. *Respir Med*. 1989; 83(Suppl):25-31.
104. Foreman JC, Garland LG. Cromoglycate and other anti-allergic drugs: possible mechanism of action. *Br Med J*. 1976; 1:820-01.
105. Bungaard A, Bach-Mortensen N, Schmidt A. The effect of sodium cromoglycate delivered by Spinhaler and by pressurized aerosol on exercise-induced asthma in children. *Clin Allergy*. 1982; 12:601-5.
106. Breslin FJ, McFadden ER, Ingram RH. The effects of cromolyn sodium on the airway response to hyperpnea and cold air in asthma. *Am Rev Respir Dis*. 1980; 122:11-6.
107. Sheppard D, Nadel JA, Boushey HA. Inhibition of sulfur dioxide induced bronchoconstriction by disodium cromoglycate in asthmatic subjects. *Am Rev Respir Dis*. 1981; 124:257-9.
108. Cockcroft DW, Murdock KY. Comparative effects of inhaled salbutamol, sodium cromoglycate, and beclomethasone dipropionate on allergen-induced early asthmatic responses, late asthmatic responses, and increased bronchial responsiveness to histamine. *J Allergy Clin Immunol*. 1987; 79:734-40.
109. Prenner BM. Safety, efficacy and bronchodilator-sparing effects of nebulized cromolyn sodium solution in the treatment of asthma in children. *Ann Allergy*. 1982; 49:186-90.
110. Cogswell JJ, Simpkiss MJ. Nebulised sodium cromoglycate in recurrently wheezing preschool children. *Arch Dis Child*. 1985; 60:736-8.
111. Geller-Bernstein C, Levin S. Sodium cromoglycate pressurized aerosol in childhood asthma. *Curr Ther Res*. 1983; 34:345-9.
112. Selcow JE, Mendelson LM, Rosen JP. Clinical benefits of cromolyn sodium aerosol (MDI) in the treatment of asthma in children. *Ann Allergy*. 1989; 62:195-9.
113. Godfrey S, Balfour-Lynn L, Konig P. The place of cromolyn sodium in the long term management of childhood asthma based on a 3 to 5 year follow-up. *J Pediatr*. 1975; 87:465-73.
114. Bernstein-Geller C, Sneh N. The management of bronchial asthma in children under the age of 3½ years using Intal administered by Spinhaler. *Clin Allergy*. 1980; 10:503-8.
115. Petty TL, Rollins DR, Christopher K et al. Cromolyn sodium is effective in adult chronic asthmatics. *Am Rev Respir Dis*. 1989; 139:694-701.
116. North American Tilade Study Group. A double-blind multicenter group comparative of the efficacy and safety of nedocromil sodium in the management of asthma. *Chest*. 1990; 97:1299-306.
117. Altouyan REC. Inhibition of experimental asthma by a new compound—disodium cromoglycate. *Acta Allergol*. 1967; 22:487-9.
118. Shapiro GG, Konig P. Cromolyn sodium: a review. *Pharmacotherapy*. 1985; 5:156-70.
119. Emm T, Metcalf JE, Lesko LJ et al. Update on the physical-chemical compatibility of cromolyn sodium nebulizer solution: bronchodilator inhalant solution admixtures. *Ann Allergy*. 1991; 66:185-9.
120. Selcow JE, Mendelson L, Rosen JP. A comparison of cromolyn and bronchodilators in patients with mild to moderately severe asthma in an office practice. *Ann Allergy*. 1983; 50:13-8.

121. Furukawa CT, Shapiro GG, Bierman CW et al. A double-blind study comparing the effectiveness of cromolyn sodium and sustained-release theophylline in childhood asthma. *Pediatrics*. 1984;74:453-9.
122. Settipane GA, Klein DE, Boyd GK et al. Adverse reactions to cromolyn. *JAMA*. 1979; 241:811-3.
123. Brown LA, Kaplan RA, Benjamin PA et al. Immunoglobulin E-mediated anaphylaxis with inhaled cromolyn sodium. *J Allergy Clin Immunol*. 1981; 68:416-20.
124. Kaliner M. Mechanisms of glucocorticosteroid action in bronchial asthma. *J Allergy Clin Immunol*. 1985; 76:321-9.
125. Ratto D, Alfaro C, Sipsey J et al. Are intravenous corticosteroids required in status asthmaticus? *JAMA*. 1988; 260:527-9.
126. Godfrey S, Konig P. Treatment of childhood asthma for 13 months and longer with beclomethasone dipropionate aerosol. *Arch Dis Child*. 1974; 49:591-6.
127. Wilson NM, Silverman M. Treatment of acute episodic asthma in preschool children using intermittent high dose inhaled steroids at home. *Arch Dis Child*. 1990; 65:407-10.
128. Kelly HW, Murphy S. Corticosteroids for acute, severe asthma. *DICP*. 1991; 25:72-9.
129. Harris JB, Weinberger MM, Nassif E et al. Early intervention with short courses of prednisone to prevent progression of asthma in ambulatory patients incompletely responsive to bronchodilators. *J Pediatr*. 1987; 110:627-33.
130. Loren ML, Chai H, Leung P et al. Corticosteroids in the treatment of acute exacerbations of asthma. *Ann Allergy*. 1980; 45:67-71.
131. Zora JA, Zimmerman D, Carey TL et al. Hypothalamic–pituitary–adrenal axis suppression after short-term, high dose glucocorticoid therapy in children with asthma. *J Allergy Clin Immunol*. 1986; 77:9-13.
132. Wyatt R, Waschek J, Weinberger M et al. Effects of inhaled beclomethasone dipropionate and alternate-day prednisone on pituitary–adrenal function in children with chronic asthma. *N Engl J Med*. 1978; 299:1387-92.
133. Nassif E, Weinberger M, Sherman B et al. Extrapulmonary effects of maintenance corticosteroid therapy with alternate-day prednisone and inhaled beclomethasone in children with chronic asthma. *J Allergy Clin Immunol*. 1987; 80:518-29.
134. Mok J, Kattan M, Levison H. Should corticosteroids be used in the treatment of acute, severe asthma? A case against the use of corticosteroids in acute, severe asthma. *Pharmacotherapy*. 1985; 5:331-5.
135. Kravis LP, Koliski GB. Unexpected death in children due to delayed steroids. *Am J Dis Child*. 1985; 139:558-63.
136. Shapiro GG, Furukawa CT, Pierson WE et al. Double-blind evaluation of methylprednisolone versus placebo for acute asthma episodes. *Pediatrics*. 1983; 71:510-4.
137. Dolan LM, Kesarwala HH, Holroyde JC et al. Short-term, high-dose, systemic steroids in children with asthma: the effect on the hypothalamic–pituitary–adrenal axis. *J Allergy Clin Immunol*. 1987; 80:81-7.
138. Swartz SL, Dluhy RG. Corticosteroids: clinical pharmacology and therapeutic use. *Drugs*. 1978; 16:238-55.
139. Morris HG, Neuman I, Ellis EF. Plasma steroid concentrations during alternate-day treatment with prednisone. *J Allergy Clin Immunol*. 1974; 54:350-8.
140. Kuzemko JA, Lines JG. Adrenal cortical function in asthmatic children on alternate day steroids. *Arch Dis Child*. 1971; 46:366-70.
141. Dickson W, Hall CE, Ellis M et al. Beclomethasone dipropionate aerosol in childhood asthma. *Arch Dis Child*. 1973; 48:671-5.
142. Meltzer EO, Kemp JP, Welch MJ et al. Effect of dosing schedule on efficacy of beclomethasone dipropionate aerosol in chronic asthma. *Am Rev Respir Dis*. 1985; 131:732-6.
143. Goldstein DE, Konig P. Effects of inhaled beclomethasone dipropionate on HPA axis function in children with asthma. *Pediatrics*. 1983; 72:60-4.
144. Freigang B, Ashford DR. Adrenal cortical function after long-term beclomethasone aerosol therapy in early childhood. *Ann Allergy*. 1990; 64:342-4.
145. Sly RM, Imseis M, Frazer M et al. Treatment of asthma in children with triamcinolone acetonide aerosol. *J Allergy Clin Immunol*. 1978; 62:76-82.
146. Shapiro GG, Izu AE, Furukawa CT et al. Short-term double-blind evaluation of flunisolide aerosol for steroid-dependent asthmatic children and adolescents. *Chest*. 1981; 80:671-5.
147. Meltzer EO, Kemp JP, Orgel HA et al. Flunisolide aerosol for treatment of severe chronic asthma in steroid-independent children. *Pediatrics*. 1982; 69:340-5.
148. Bisgaard H, Nielson MD, Anderson B et al. Adrenal function in children with bronchial asthma treated with beclomethasone dipropionate or budesonide. *J Allergy Clin Immunol*. 1988; 81:1088-95.
149. Priftis K, Milner AD, Conway E et al. Adrenal function in asthma. *Arch Dis Child*. 1990; 65:838-40.
150. Law CM, Honour JW, Marchant JL et al. Nocturnal adrenal suppression in asthmatic children taking inhaled beclomethasone dipropionate. *Lancet*. 1986; 1:942-4.
151. Prahl P, Jensen T. Decreased adreno-cortical suppression utilizing the Nebuhaler for inhalation of steroid aerosols. *Clin Allergy*. 1987; 17:393-8.
152. Blodgett FM, Burgin L, Iezzoni D et al. Effects of prolonged cortisone therapy on statural growth, skeletal maturation, and metabolic status of children. *N Engl J Med*. 1956; 254:636-41.
153. Littlewood JM, Johnson AW, Edwards PA et al. Growth retardation in asthmatic children treated with inhaled beclomethasone dipropionate. *Lancet*. 1988; 1:115-6.
154. Reimer LG, Morris HG, Ellis EF. Growth of asthmatic children during treatment with alternate-day steroids. *J Allergy Clin Immunol*. 1975; 55:224-31.
155. McNichol KN, Williams HB. Spectrum of asthma in children. I. Clinical and physiological components. *Br Med J*. 1973; 4:7-11.
156. Bacon CJ. Growth retardation in asthmatic children treated with inhaled beclomethasone dipropionate. *Lancet*. 1988; 1:475-6.
157. Godfrey S, Balfour-Lynn L, Tooley M. A three to five year follow up of the use of the aerosol steroid, beclomethasone dipropionate, in childhood asthma. *J Allergy Clin Immunol*. 1978; 62:335-9.
158. Balfour-Lynn L. Growth and childhood asthma. *Arch Dis Child*. 1986; 61:1049-55.
159. Brown DCP, Savacool AM, Letizia CM. A retrospective review of the effects of one year of triamcinolone acetonide aerosol treatment on the growth patterns of asthmatic children. *Ann Allergy*. 1989; 63:47-51.
160. Williams AJ, Baghat MS, Stableforth DE et al. Dysphonia caused by inhaled steroids: recognition of a characteristic laryngeal abnormality. *Thorax*. 1983; 38:813-21.
161. Shaw NJ, Edmunds AT. Inhaled beclomethasone and oral candidiasis. *Arch Dis Child*. 1986; 61:788-90.
162. Toogood JH, Lefcoe NM, Haines DSM et al. A graded dose assessment of the efficacy of beclomethasone dipropionate aerosol in severe chronic asthma. *J Allergy Clin Immunol*. 1977; 59:298-308.
163. Freigan B. Long term follow-up of infants and children treated with beclomethasone aerosol by a special inhalation device. *Ann Allergy*. 1980; 45:13-7.
164. Salzman GA, Pyszczynski DR. Oropharyngeal candidiasis in patients treated with beclomethasone dipropionate delivered by metered-dose inhaler alone and with Aerochamber. *J Allergy Clin Immunol*. 1988; 81:424-8.
165. Deshpande A, Mckenzie S. Short course of steroids in home treatment of children with acute asthma. *Br Med J*. 1986; 293:169-71.
166. Storr J, Barry W, Barrell E et al. Effect of a single oral dose of prednisolone in acute childhood asthma. *Lancet*. 1987; 1: 879-82.
167. Younger RE, Gerber PS, Herrod HG et al. Intravenous

methylprednisolone efficacy in status asthmaticus of childhood. *Pediatrics*. 1987; 80:225-9.
168. Tai A, Levy N, Bearman JE. Methylprednisolone therapy for acute asthma in infants and toddlers: a controlled clinical trial. *Pediatrics*. 1990; 86:350-6.
169. Brunette MG, Lands L, Thibodeau LP. Childhood asthma: prevention of attacks with short-term corticosteroid treatment of upper respiratory tract infection. *Pediatrics*. 1988; 81:624-9.
170. Ellis EF. Asthma in childhood. *J Allergy Clin Immunol*. 1983; 72:526-39.
171. Canny GJ, Levison H. Childhood asthma: a rational approach to treatment. *Ann Allergy*. 1990; 64:406-16.
172. Brenner M. Use of steroids in pediatric asthma. *Pediatr Ann*. 1989; 18:810-8.
173. Clark TJH. Inhaled corticosteroid therapy: a substitute for theophylline as well as prednisolone? *J Allergy Clin Immunol*. 1985; 76:330-4.
174. Mitchell I, Paterson IC, Cameron SJ et al. Treatment of childhood asthma with sodium cromoglycate and beclomethasone dipropionate aerosol singly and in combination. *Br Med J*. 1976; 2:457-8.
175. Francis RS, McEnery G. Disodium cromoglycate compared with beclomethasone dipropionate in juvenile asthma. *Clin Allergy*. 1984; 14:537-40.
176. Svendsen UG, Frolund L, Madsen F et al. A comparison of the effects of sodium cromoglycate and beclomethasone dipropionate on pulmonary function and bronchial hyperactivity in subjects with asthma. *J Allergy Clin Immunol*. 1987; 80:68-74.
177. Hiller EJ, Milner AD. Betamethasone 17 valerate aerosol and disodium cromoglycate in severe childhood asthma. *Br J Dis Chest*. 1975; 69:103-6.
178. Kershnar H, Klein R, Waldman D et al. Treatment of chronic childhood asthma with beclomethasone dipropionate aerosol: effect on pituitary–adrenal function after substitution for oral corticosteroids. *Pediatrics*. 1978; 62:189-97.
179. Williams H, Verrier Jones ER, Sibert JR. Twice daily versus four times daily treatment with beclomethasone dipropionate in the control of mild childhood asthma. *Thorax*. 1986; 41:602-5.
180. Joad JP, Ahrens RC, Lindgren SD et al. Relative efficacy of maintenance therapy with theophylline, inhaled albuterol, and the combination for chronic asthma. *J Allergy Clin Immunol*. 1987; 79:78-85.
181. Hambleton G, Weinberger M, Taylor J et al. Comparison of cromoglycate (cromolyn) and theophylline in controlling symptoms of chronic asthma. *Lancet*. 1977; 1:381-5.
182. Springer C, Goldenberg B, Dov IB et al. Clinical, physiologic, and psychologic comparison of treatment by cromolyn or theophylline in childhood asthma. *J Allergy Clin Immunol*. 1985; 76:64-9.
183. Newth CJL, Newth CV, Turner JAP. Comparison of nebulised sodium cromoglycate and oral theophylline in controlling symptoms of chronic asthma in pre-school children: a double blind study. *Aust NZ J Med*. 1982; 12:232-8.
184. Eigen H, Reid JJ, Dahl R et al. Evaluation of the addition of cromolyn sodium to bronchodilator maintenance therapy in the long-term management of asthma. *J Allergy Clin Immunol*. 1987; 80:612-21.
185. Nassif EG, Weinberger M, Thompson R et al. The value of maintenance theophylline in steroid-dependent asthma. *N Engl J Med*. 1981; 304:71-5.
186. Edmunds AT, McKenzie S, Baillie E et al. A comparison of oral choline theophyllinate and beclomethasone in severe perennial asthma in children. *Br J Dis Chest*. 1979; 73:149-56.
187. Barnes PJ, Greening AP, Neville L et al. Single-dose slow-release aminophylline at night prevents nocturnal asthma. *Lancet*. 1982; 1:299-301.
188. Hendeles L, Weinberger M. Theophylline: a "state of the art" review. *Pharmacotherapy*. 1983; 3:2-44.
189. Hendeles L, Weinberger M. Selection of a slow-release theophylline product. *J Allergy Clin Immunol*. 1986; 78:743-51.
190. Vaughan LM, Milavetz G, Weinberger MM et al. Oral bioavailability of slow-released theophylline from unencapsulated beads in preschool children with chronic asthma. *Ther Drug Monit*. 1988; 10:395-400.
191. Ellis EF, Koysooko R, Levy G. Pharmacokinetics of theophylline in children with asthma. *Pediatrics*. 1976; 58: 542-7.
192. Hendeles L, Weinberger M, Bighley L. Disposition of theophylline after a single intravenous infusion of aminophylline. *Am Rev Respir Dis*. 1978; 118:97-103.
193. Aranda JV, Sitar DS, Parsons WD et al. Pharmacokinetic aspects of theophylline in premature newborns. *N Engl J Med*. 1976; 295:413-6.
194. Shaw LM, Fields L, Mayock R. Factors influencing theophylline serum protein binding. *Clin Pharmacol Ther*. 1982; 32:490-6.
195. Tang-Liu DDS, Williams RL, Riegelman S. Nonlinear theophylline elimination. *Clin Pharmacol Ther*. 1982; 31:358-69.
196. Bonati M, Latini R, Marra G et al. Theophylline metabolism during the first month of life and development. *Pediatr Res*. 1981; 15:304-8.
197. Nassif EG, Weinberger MM, Shannon D et al. Theophylline disposition in infancy. *J Pediatrics*. 1981; 98:158-61.
198. Wyatt R, Weinberger M, Hendeles L. Oral theophylline dosage for the management of chronic asthma. *J Pediatrics*. 1978; 92:125-30.
199. Hendeles L, Massanari M, Weinberger M. Theophylline. In: Evans WE, Schentag JJ, Jusko WJ, eds. Applied pharmacokinetics: principles of therapeutic drug monitoring. 2nd ed. Spokane; Applied Therapeutics; 1986:1105-88.
200. Jonkman JHG, Upton RA. Pharmacokinetic drug interactions with theophylline. *Clin Pharmacokinet*. 1984; 9:309-34.
201. Hendeles L, Weinberger M, Wyatt R. Guide to oral theophylline therapy for the treatment of chronic asthma. *Am J Dis Child*. 1978; 132:876-80.
202. Weinberger MM, Bronsky EA. Evaluation of oral bronchodilator therapy in asthmatic children. *J Pediatr*. 1974; 84:421-7.
203. Hatzopoulos FK, Reitz SJ, Kraus DM et al. Evaluation of a theophylline dosing method based on postconceptional age in infants. *Pharmacotherapy*. 1988; 8:129. Abstract.
204. Hendeles L, Bighley L, Richardson RH et al. Frequent toxicity from IV aminophylline infusions in critically ill patients. *Drug Intell Clin Pharm*. 1977; 11:12-8.
205. Paloucek FP, Rodvold KA. Evaluation of theophylline overdoses and toxicities. *Ann Emerg Med*. 1988; 17:135-44.
206. Rachelefsky GS, Wo J, Adelson J et al. Behavior abnormalities and poor school performance due to oral theophylline use. *Pediatrics*. 1986; 78:1133-8.
207. Schriver RC. School performance and theophylline. *Pediatrics*. 1987; 80:123-4. Letter.
208. Joad JP, Ahrens RC, Lindgren SD et al. Extrapulmonary effects of maintenance therapy with theophylline and inhaled albuterol in patients with chronic asthma. *J Allergy Clin Immunol*. 1986; 78:1147-53.

Research Notes

Prediction of serum albumin concentration after albumin supplementation in pediatric patients receiving parenteral nutrition

EMILY B. COCHRAN AND SUSAN L. HOGUE

Clin Pharm. 1991; 10:704-6

Albumin plays an important role in regulating oncotic pressure and maintaining intravascular volume and serves as a transport protein for various plasma constituents, including bilirubin, amino acids, fatty acids, hormones, and certain drug moieties.[1-3] Because albumin is synthesized in the liver from amino acids, provision of adequate protein is a primary factor regulating albumin synthesis.[1] Thus, serum albumin concentration is used as a marker of visceral protein status and in the assessment of nutritional status. Hypoalbuminemia has been associated with morbidity and mortality in adults[4-6] and with morbidity in pediatric patients.[7,8]

Although the results of studies evaluating the effects of normalizing serum albumin concentrations on outcome are contradictory,[6,7,9] supplemental albumin is often given via parenteral nutrient solutions. Often the approach to albumin supplementation is empirical, and albumin is added to the nutrient solution until the serum albumin concentration reaches a desired level. The ability to predict the albumin dose required to achieve a desired serum albumin concentration would allow prompt normalization of albumin levels, minimize waste of an expensive product that is in short supply, and reduce the need for extensive serum albumin concentration monitoring. Two equations for calculating the dose of albumin required to increase serum albumin to a desired concentration have been derived by Hardin et al.[10] and Brown et al.[11] from data on adult patients. Although the equation described by Hardin et al.[10] has been used successfully to determine albumin replacement doses in children,[7] neither equation has been validated for infants. The objective of our study was to determine if either equation described for adults could be used to predict albumin requirements in hypoalbuminemic infants.

Methods. Pediatric patients who were receiving parenteral nutrient solutions and who had had a serum albumin concentration below the age-related normal concentration (2.3 g/dL in infants up to 12 months of age and 4.5 g/dL in patients 12–36 months of age) before they began receiving the solutions were prospectively evaluated for inclusion in the study. Patients with ongoing losses of protein due to wounds (e.g., gastroschisis, burns, and extensive debridement and grafting of lower extremities) or who did not have a serum albumin concentration determination at least 24 hours after infusion of the albumin were not included.

Human serum albumin (Alpha Therapeutic Corp., Los Angeles, CA) 1–1.5 g/kg/day was added to the parenteral nutrient solution prescribed. All solutions were infused over 24 hours. Albumin supplementation was continued for one to four days, depending on the clinical judgment of the prescriber. A follow-up serum albumin concentration measurement was performed at least 24 hours after the albumin supplementation was completed. Serum albumin concentrations were determined in the hospital's clinical laboratory by certified laboratory personnel using the bromocresol green method.

The equations that were compared for their predictive abilities were those of (1) Hardin et al.,[10] Albumin dose (in grams) = weight (in kilograms) × 3 dL/kg × change in SAC, and (2) Brown et al.,[11] Albumin dose (in grams) = (change in SAC – 0.33)/0.003, where SAC is serum albumin concentration and change in SAC is the difference between the final and initial serum albumin concentrations. Because our patients received a specific dose of albumin, the equations were rearranged to solve for final (or predicted) serum albumin concentration.

EMILY B. COCHRAN, PHARM.D., is Assistant Professor, Department of Clinical Pharmacy, College of Pharmacy, The University of Tennessee (UT), Memphis, and Clinical Pharmacist, Le Bonheur Children's Medical Center, Memphis. SUSAN L. HOGUE, PHARM.D., is Pediatric Pharmacotherapy Fellow, Department of Clinical Pharmacy, College of Pharmacy, UT.

Address reprint requests to Dr. Cochran at the Department of Clinical Pharmacy, The University of Tennessee, 26 South Dunlap Street, Memphis, TN 38163.

Supported in part by The Center for Pediatric Pharmacokinetics and Therapeutics, The University of Tennessee, Memphis, and by a grant from the Pharmacy Sciences Liaison, The Upjohn Company.

Presented in part at the 17th Annual Meeting of the Southern Society for Pediatric Research, New Orleans, LA, January 18, 1990.

Table 1.
Demographic Characteristics of the Study Patients and Their Initial and Final Serum Albumin Concentrations

Patient	Age	Weight (kg)	Gender	Diagnosis or Surgical Procedure	Albumin Concentration (g/dL) Initial	Final
1	2 mo	3.0	F	Colitis	1.6	2.5
2	1 mo	1.4	F	Small bowel resection	1.8	2.4
3	6 mo	3.3	M	Gastroesophageal reflux	1.9	4.1
4	12 mo	12.1	F	Liver transplant	2.0	3.0
5	3 mo	2.0	F	Intestinal stricture	2.1	3.6
6	3 wk	3.0	M	Tetralogy of Fallot	1.9	2.9
7	5 wk	4.4	F	Truncus arteriosus	1.8	3.6
8	28 mo	10.5	M	Perforated duodenal ulcer	1.8	2.9
9	5 mo	3.8	F	Bronchopulmonary dysplasia	2.2	3.7
10	2 wk	1.0	M	Small bowel resection	1.6	2.2
11	2 wk	2.2	M	Small bowel resection	2.1	2.9
12	3 wk	1.7	F	Small bowel resection	1.9	3.7
13	2 mo	2.7	M	Colonic stricture	1.9	2.7
14	2 wk	2.6	M	Status post Nissen fundoplication	2.0	2.8
15	7 wk	2.6	M	Colonic stricture	1.9	2.7
16	15 mo	5.8	F	Malnutrition	2.8	3.6
17	2.5 mo	3.1	M	Hepatic cystectomy	2.0	3.3
18	3 wk	2.2	M	Primary-closure gastroschisis	1.9	3.0
19	5 wk	3.5	M	Tetralogy of Fallot	1.9	3.2
20	1 wk	2.6	M	Primary-closure gastroschisis	2.1	2.8

The student's t test for paired data was used to test for differences between the albumin concentrations predicted by each equation and the actual values measured in the laboratory. Regression analysis was used to evaluate the relationship between the albumin dose infused and the absolute increase in serum albumin concentration. The a priori level of significance was set at <0.05.

Results. Twenty patients (12 males and 8 females) with a median age of 4.6 months (range, one week to 28 months) and a mean ± S.D. weight of 3.7 ± 2.8 kg were included in the analysis. Demographic data and the initial and final serum albumin concentrations are presented in Table 1. The parenteral nutrient solutions infused (either peripherally [6 patients] or centrally [14]) provided a mean ± S.D. of 2.5 ± 0.4 grams of protein per kilogram per day and 88 ± 28 kcal/kg/day and provided 40–100% of anticipated caloric needs. The mean ± S.D. initial serum albumin concentration was 2.0 ± 0.3 g/dL (range, 1.6–2.8). After albumin supplementation (mean ± S.D. dose, 3.2 ± 0.7 g/kg [range, 1.5–5 g/kg]), the serum albumin concentration increased to 3.0 ± 0.5 g/dL (range, 2.2–4.1 g/dL) 29–111 hours after the infusion was completed.

The absolute increase in serum albumin concentration was significantly correlated with the total albumin dose infused ($p < 0.01$, $r^2 = 0.55$). The measured final albumin concentrations are compared with the values predicted by the two equations in Figure 1.

The final mean ± S.D. concentration predicted with the equation of Hardin et al. was 3.0 ± 0.3 g/dL and did not differ from the value determined in the laboratory (3.0 ± 0.5 g/dL). The concentration predicted with the equation of Brown et al. was 2.3 ± 0.2 g/dL, which was significantly lower than the laboratory-measured value ($p = 0.0001$).

Figure 1. Correlation between final serum albumin concentrations predicted with the equations of Hardin et al.[10] (circles) and Brown et al.[11] (triangles) and measured final concentrations. The dashed line is the line of identity.

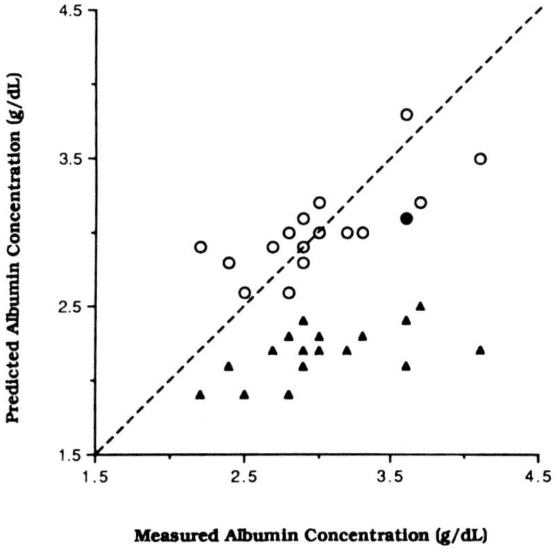

Discussion. Hypoalbuminemic patients who are receiving parenteral nutrition may have albumin added to their nutrient solutions.[6,7,10-12] The approach to albumin supplementation has been empirical and varies in both the amount of albumin infused and the rate of replacement. Albumin replacement therapy rapidly normalizes serum albumin concentration, and as long as adequate amounts of protein and calories are also provided, serum concentrations can be maintained within a desired range. A method of calculating the albumin dose necessary to achieve the desired concentration in individual patients would result in savings in product cost and savings from less frequent serum concentration monitoring.

The equation of Hardin et al.[10] was developed from data on 13 malnourished adults who received up to 150 g of albumin over a 24-hour period. Subsequently, this formula was used successfully to determine the amount of albumin required to normalize serum concentrations in hypoalbuminemic children (mean age, four years) who were intolerant of enteral feedings.[7] In our study, this equation was useful in predicting final albumin concentrations in parenterally fed infants who were younger and smaller than the pediatric patients previously studied.

The equation described by Brown et al.[11] was developed by using regression analysis of data for a heterogeneous group of hypoalbuminemic adults receiving parenteral nutrition through a central i.v. catheter; the equation was subsequently validated in a larger group of similar patients.[12] In our patients this equation underpredicted the albumin concentration that resulted from the albumin dose infused. There are several possible explanations for the inability of this equation to accurately predict the replacement doses of albumin for our patients. First, the patients studied by Brown et al.[11] were in negative nitrogen balance during the first week of the study. The unavailability of sufficient substrate to meet requirements may have resulted in utilization of the supplemented albumin for energy. While we did not perform nitrogen-balance studies in our patients, positive nitrogen balance and weight gain have been observed in a similar group of pediatric patients receiving fewer calories and lower doses of protein than were provided on average to the patients in our study.[13] Second, the patients we studied were not critically ill, nor did they have ongoing protein losses as a result of wounds or sepsis. Several of Brown et al.'s patients had septic events that would have increased the amount of albumin required to normalize serum concentrations. Finally, the amount of albumin infused was greater on a per kilogram basis in our patients; this resulted in more rapid normalization of the serum albumin concentration.

Conclusion. While hypoalbuminemia secondary to malnutrition is not an indication for the infusion of human serum albumin, there are patients who may benefit from its use. For the pediatric patients in this study, the albumin replacement dose was calculated reliably with the equation of Hardin et al.[9] Future studies evaluating the effects of normalizing the serum albumin concentration on outcome in pediatric patients are needed to further validate the efficacy of this scarce, expensive product.

References

1. Rothschild MA, Oratz M, Schreiber SS. Albumin synthesis. Part 1. *N Engl J Med*. 1972; 286:748-57.
2. Rothschild MA, Oratz M, Schreiber SS. Albumin synthesis. Part 2. *N Engl J Med*. 1972; 286:816-21.
3. Kaminski MV, Williams SD. Review of the rapid normalization of serum albumin with modified total parenteral nutrition solutions. *Crit Care Med*. 1990; 18:327-35.
4. Reinhardt GF, Myscofske JW, Wilkens DB et al. Incidence and mortality of hypoalbuminemic patients in hospitalized veterans. *J Parenter Enter Nutr*. 1980; 4:357-9.
5. Mullen JL, Buzby GP, Matthews DC et al. Reduction of operative morbidity and mortality by combined preoperative and postoperative nutritional support. *Ann Surg*. 1980; 192:604-13.
6. Brown RO, Bradley JE, Bekemeyer WB et al. Effect of albumin supplementation during parenteral nutrition on hospital morbidity. *Crit Care Med*. 1988; 16:1177-82.
7. Ford EG, Jennings LM, Andrassy RJ. Serum albumin (oncotic pressure) correlates with enteral feeding tolerance in the pediatric surgical patient. *J Pediatr Surg*. 1987; 22:597-9.
8. Atkinson SD, Tuggle DW, Tunell WP. Hypoalbuminemia may predispose infants to necrotizing enterocolitis. *J Pediatr Surg*. 1989; 24:674-6.
9. Foley EF, Borlase BC, Dzik WH et al. Albumin supplementation in the critically ill. *Arch Surg*. 1990; 125:739-42.
10. Hardin TC, Page CP, Schwesinger WH. Rapid replacement of serum albumin in patients receiving total parenteral nutrition. *Surg Gynecol Obstet*. 1986; 163:359-62.
11. Brown RO, Bradley JE, Luther RW. Response of serum albumin concentrations to albumin supplementation during central total parenteral nutrition. *Clin Pharm*. 1987; 6:222-6.
12. Reid DJ, Brown RO, Vehe KL et al. Predicting human-albumin replacement dosages in hypoalbuminemic patients receiving total parenteral nutrition. *Clin Pharm*. 1988; 7:894-7.
13. Helms RA, Johnson MR, Christensen ML et al. Altered caloric and protein requirement in neonates receiving a pediatric amino acid formulation. *Pediatr Res*. 1987; 21:429SA. Abstract.

A nonexponential, nonlogarithmic pharmacokinetic dosing method for gentamicin

Thomas E. Lackner, Weeranuj Yamreudeewong, and Peter D. Weiss

Clin Pharm. 1991; 10:706-10

Many methods of calculating aminoglycoside doses have been devised that are intended to produce serum aminoglycoside concentrations within the usual therapeutic range.[1-8] The widely used Sawchuk-Zaske (SZ) method is effective in determining dosages for individual patients on the basis of measured gentamicin concentrations.[7] However, the SZ method requires the use of logarithms and exponents, precluding rapid calculation without an electronic calculator or a computer. For this reason, less complicated methods involving empirical dosage adjustments and nomograms are often used.[1-6] These methods are less likely to achieve therapeutic gentamicin concentrations than the SZ method, however.[9] Nomograms are designed to achieve fixed peak and trough concentrations, making it difficult for the clinician to tailor the dosage according to the severity of the infection and the potential for toxicity. Furthermore, nomograms incorporate mean pharmacokinetic values that frequently differ from those for a particular patient. Finally, nomograms do not provide a way to base dosage adjustments on measured concentrations.

We developed a method for calculating gentamicin dosage regimens from measured serum gentamicin concentrations that does not involve logarithms or exponents. The purpose of this study was to determine whether our method yields a dosage regimen similar to that calculated by the SZ method. The precision and bias of the methods in achieving desired peak and trough serum gentamicin concentrations were also compared.

Methods. One hundred ten patients who were at least 18 years of age and of either gender and who were receiving gentamicin and had stable renal function were prospectively studied. Stable renal function was defined as a change in the serum creatinine concentration of no more than 0.5 mg/dL during or within five days of treatment with gentamicin. All patients for whom a gentamicin pharmacokinetic consultation was ordered over a four-month period were selected for the study; a pharmacokinetic consultation was requested for 87% of the patients whose gentamicin concentrations were measured during this period. Gentamicin was prescribed only for approved indications, either alone or in combination with other antibiotics.

Patients with a diagnosis of liver disease or who were morbidly obese (total body weight, ≥195% of lean body weight) were excluded from the study because the reliability of creatinine clearance estimates is compromised in such individuals.[10,11] Other than a history of allergy to an aminoglycoside antibiotic, no other medical condition justified exclusion.

The requirement to obtain informed consent from subjects was waived by the institutional review board, since standard procedures for patient care were followed.

Renal function was assessed by estimating creatinine clearance by the method of Cockcroft and Gault[12]; the lesser of lean body weight and actual body weight was used. The serum creatinine concentration was measured before treatment with gentamicin and at least every three days during treatment. Clinical symptoms of cochlear and vestibular toxicity (diminished hearing of spoken words, dizziness, and vertigo) noted in the patients' medical records were recorded. Audiometry was not routinely performed.

Gentamicin was administered by 60-minute intermittent intravenous infusions at constant intervals. Serum gentamicin concentrations were measured in venous blood collected one, three, and six hours after the first gentamicin dose was infused. If the patient had received gentamicin recently before the study began, a blood sample was also obtained within 20 minutes before the administration of gentamicin. The exact starting and stopping times of infusion, the sampling times, and the doses were recorded for each patient on a form with instructions that was given to the patient's primary nurse to complete.

All serum samples were frozen at –15 °C and analyzed within 18 hours to prevent in vitro inactivation by β-lactam antibiotics.[13] The samples were analyzed for gentamicin by fluorescence polarization immunoassay (TDx, Abbott Diagnostic Division, North Chicago, IL). A standard curve was constructed from results for six duplicate standards containing concentrations of 0, 0.5, 1.5, 3, 6, and 10 μg/mL and was determined to be linear within that range. Two control samples containing gentamicin 2.4 and 6.2 μg/mL were analyzed in duplicate daily. The coefficient of variation was less than 10% for gentamicin concentrations between 0 and 10 μg/mL.

The SZ method was used to adjust gentamicin doses. The serum gentamicin concentration-versus-time data for individual patients were fitted by linear regression of the logarithms of the data for a one-compartment model. The true peak and trough gentamicin concentrations were extrapolated from the measured concentrations by using the calculated first-order elimination rate constant. The true peak concentration was defined as the concentration at the end of the infusion, and the true trough concentration was defined as the concentration present immediately before the infusion. The new gentamicin dosage regimen was calculated by using the pharmacokinetic data obtained from the regression analysis.[7] Patients with gentamicin concentrations of less than the minimum measurable concentration (0.5 μg/mL) were excluded from the study. Patients whose concentration-versus-time profile resulted in a correlation coefficient of less than 0.98 based on the three initial postinfusion concentration measurements were excluded from the study. The gentamicin dosage could not be determined optimally by any method, given the uncertainty in pharmacokinetic variables associated with a large scatter of concentration-versus-time data (i.e., a correlation coefficient of less than 0.98).

All gentamicin dosages were calculated to achieve true peak concentrations of 4–10 μg/mL and true

---

THOMAS E. LACKNER, PHARM.D., FASCP, is Chief Clinical Pharmacist, Pharmacy Corporation of America, Minneapolis, MN, and Clinical Assistant Professor, College of Pharmacy, The University of Minnesota, Minneapolis; at the time of this study he was Associate Professor of Clinical Pharmacy, The St. Louis College of Pharmacy, St. Louis, MO, and Director of Pharmacokinetics Services, The Jewish Hospital of St. Louis (JHSL). WEERANUJ YAMREUDEEWONG, PHARM.D., is Assistant Professor of Clinical Pharmacy, College of Pharmacy, Northeast Louisiana University, and Clinical Pharmacist, E. A. Conway Memorial Hospital, Monroe, LA; at the time of this study she was Clinical Pharmacy Resident, JHSL. PETER D. WEISS, M.D., is Clinical Instructor in Medicine, Division of Hematology and Oncology, Washington University School of Medicine, St. Louis, MO.

Address reprint requests to Dr. Lackner at Pharmacy Corporation of America, 5155 East River Road, Suite 404, Minneapolis, MN 55421.

The assistance of Brad Wilson, M.A., Division of Biostatistics, Washington University School of Medicine, St. Louis, MO, is acknowledged.

Presented in part, at the 23rd Annual ASHP Midyear Clinical Meeting, Dallas, TX, December 8, 1988.

trough concentrations of 0.5–2 μg/mL; specific target concentrations were based on the patient's clinical condition and the location and severity of the infection. Calculated doses were rounded to the nearest 10 mg. Calculated dosage intervals were rounded to the nearest 6, 8, 12, 18, 24, 36, or 48 hours. Increments of 24 hours were used if the calculated dosage interval exceeded 48 hours. Steady-state true peak and trough concentrations were predicted from the rounded dose and dosage interval.[7]

After at least five half-lives—estimated from the initial pharmacokinetic analysis—had elapsed since the recommended gentamicin dosage regimen was instituted, single blood samples for determining the peak and trough serum gentamicin concentration were obtained within 20 minutes before the infusion and at one hour after the infusion ended. The true peak and trough gentamicin concentrations were compared with the predicted concentrations.

The dosage regimen determined by the SZ method was compared with that calculated by our four-step gentamicin-dosing method, described below.

1. The serum gentamicin concentration-versus-time data were plotted on log-linear graph paper, the best-line fit of the data was determined visually, and the gentamicin half-life for each patient was estimated.
2. The true peak gentamicin concentration (C_{max}) was determined by back-extrapolation from the serum concentration-versus-time plot to the end of the gentamicin infusion.
3. The gentamicin dosage interval (in hours) was calculated as follows: Dosage interval = $[(N)(t_{1/2})] + t'$, where $t_{1/2}$ is the elimination half-life of gentamicin (in hours), N is the number of elimination half-lives that must elapse before the gentamicin concentration decreases from the desired true peak to the desired true trough, and t' is the desired infusion duration (in hours). In this study the desired infusion duration was always one hour. The calculated dosage interval was rounded to the nearest 6, 8, 12, 18, 24, 36, or 48 hours. Increments of 24 hours were used if the calculated interval exceeded 48 hours.
4. The gentamicin dose (in milligrams) was calculated as follows: Dose = $(\Delta C_{desired})(D)/\Delta C_{measured}$, where $\Delta C_{desired}$ is the difference between the desired true peak and true trough serum concentrations and $\Delta C_{measured}$ is the difference between the measured true peak and true trough concentrations at the initial dose (D). The dose calculated was then rounded to the nearest 10 mg. Calculation of the dose is independent of calculation of the dosage interval.

The predictive performance of the two methods was determined by using the method of Sheiner and Beal[14] with SAS software.[15] The differences between the gentamicin doses and between the dosage intervals calculated by the two methods were calculated for each patient. A Wilcoxon sign-rank statistic was determined to test the hypothesis that there would be no difference between doses or between the dosage intervals calculated by the two methods (i.e., that the mean difference equals zero). The absolute and relative precision (the magnitude of the differences between the predicted and measured true peak and trough gentamicin concentrations) and bias (the extent to which the typical peak or trough concentration prediction is too low or too high) of each method were determined by calculating the mean squared prediction error and the mean prediction error. The 95% confidence intervals for precision and bias and the difference in these variables between the two methods were computed to determine their absolute and relative performance. The a priori level of significance was set at <0.05.

Results. The SZ and simplified gentamicin-dosing methods were compared in 81 patients. Of the 110 patients initially evaluated, 27 were excluded from the final analysis because the correlation coefficient for serum gentamicin concentration versus time was less than 0.98 and 2 were excluded because of an increase in their serum creatinine level during treatment. The cause of the increase in serum creatinine could not be established for either of these patients. No patients had symptoms of auditory or vestibular toxicity. Nearly two thirds of the patients were hospitalized on the general medicine ward, one fourth on the general surgery ward, and the remainder (in descending order) on the medical and surgical intensive-care units, urology unit, cardiovascular surgery unit, obstetrics unit, and coronary-care unit. The demographics, pharmacokinetic data, and diagnoses of the patients are compiled in Table 1.

There was no significant difference between the SZ method and our method in the mean ± S.D. gentamicin dose or dosage interval calculated (Table 2). In fact, the gentamicin doses calculated by the two methods were identical in 79 patients. In the two remaining patients the dose calculated by our method was no more than 8% higher than the dose calculated by the SZ method. The dosage intervals calculated by the two methods were identical in 75 patients. In the remaining six patients the dosage interval calculated by our method differed by no more than one increment. The mean ± S.D. predicted true peak concentrations (6.3 ± 1.3 μg/mL) and trough concentrations (1.0 ± 0.4 μg/mL) were identical for doses calculated by the two methods. The mean measured true peak gentamicin concentration was not significantly different from the mean predicted true peak concentration for either method because the confidence interval for the mean prediction error for both methods included zero. Both methods underestimated the true trough concentration because the lower and upper bounds of the confidence interval for the mean prediction error were negative for both. The measured trough concentration was less than 0.5 μg/mL higher than predicted in 74% of the patients. The confidence intervals for the difference in the mean squared error and mean prediction error between methods for both peak and trough concentrations indicate no significant difference in precision or bias.

Discussion. The SZ method and our method were

equally precise in determining gentamicin dosage requirements. The gentamicin dosages calculated by both methods resulted in predicted true peak concentrations that were not significantly different from those measured. Even though the mean predicted true trough concentrations for both methods were significantly different from the measured concentrations, we do not believe that the difference would be clinically meaningful in most patients. Although previous studies of the SZ method did not show a significant difference between the predicted and measured true peak or trough concentrations, underprediction of trough concentrations by the SZ method has been reported.[18,19]

The poor correlation coefficient for the three postinfusion serum gentamicin concentrations in several of our patients was associated with inaccurate recording of infusion times.

The relatively large mean volume of distribution is probably attributable to five patients with ascites, in whom individual volumes of distribution exceeded 0.43 L/kg. In addition, the gentamicin volume of distribution is directly related to its half-life,[19] and the mean half-life of gentamicin in our study was at the upper end of the normal range for patients with normal renal function.[19] The larger volume of distribution we observed may reflect this relatively long half-life in our patients.

Our method for calculating gentamicin dosages resembles a method reported by Chiou et al.[20] Their method involves back-extrapolation of the best-fit line of the logarithms of concentration-versus-time coordinates to the midpoint of the infusion period. However, the infusion period is highly variable[21]; our method does not require knowledge of both the starting and ending times. Furthermore, unlike Chiou et al.'s method, our method enables the dosage interval to be calculated.

Although our method does not directly incorporate the infusion duration in the calculation of dose, the infusion duration is reflected in the change in gentamicin concentration calculated from the true peak and trough concentrations. However, unlike the SZ method, our method does not allow the intended duration of infusion of the new dose to be selected inde-

Table 1.
Characteristics of the Study Group (n = 81)

Characteristic	Mean ± S.D. (Range) or No. Patients
Demographics	
Age (yr)	63 ± 21 (18–96)
Actual body weight (kg)	69 ± 22 (31–152)
Lean body weight (kg)[a]	59 ± 14 (27–87)
Serum creatinine concentration (mg/dL)	1.0 ± 0.4 (0.5–3.2)
Creatinine clearance (mL/min)[b]	58 ± 27 (17–125)
Pharmacokinetics	
Elimination rate constant (hr^{-1})	0.22 ± 0.09 (0.05–0.46)
Half-life (hr)	3.66 ± 1.95 (1.50–14.1)
Volume of distribution (L/kg [ABW[c]])	0.35 ± 0.14 (0.16–1.05)
Total body clearance (L/kg/hr)[d]	0.07 ± 0.03 (0.02–0.23)
Site of infection	
Blood	8
Intra-abdominal[e]	23
Pulmonary	17
Skin, soft tissue	5
Urinary tract	11[f]
Other	18

[a] Calculated by the method of Devine[16] or Hallynck et al.[17]
[b] Calculated by the method of Cockcroft and Gault.[12]
[c] ABW = actual body weight.
[d] Total body clearance equals the elimination rate constant multiplied by the volume of distribution.
[e] Intra-abdominal infections included peritonitis, diverticulitis, abscess, cholecystitis, and pancreatitis.
[f] One patient had concurrent pneumonia and urinary tract infection.

Table 2.
Results for the Two Gentamicin Dosing Methods

Variable	Sawchuk-Zaske Method	Our Method	Difference[a]
Dose (mg/kg [ABW[b]])			
Mean ± S.D.	2.07 ± 0.52	2.07 ± 0.52	0.003 ± 0.019
Range	0.99–3.42	0.99–3.42	
Dosage interval (hr)			
Mean ± S.D.	12.02 ± 5.17	11.95 ± 5.30	0.07 ± 1.43
Range	8–36	6–36	
Median (hr)	12	12	
Mean squared error (precision)[c]			
Peak	1.54 (1.08, 2.00)	1.56 (1.10, 2.02)	−0.02 (−0.07, 0.03)
Trough	0.24 (0.07, 0.42)	0.28 (0.07, 0.49)	−0.04 (−0.08, 0.01)
Mean prediction error (bias)[c]			
Peak	−0.086 (−0.36, 0.19)	−0.089 (−0.37, 0.19)	0.003 (−0.02, 0.03)
Trough	−0.20 (−0.30, −0.10)	−0.10 (−0.30, −0.08)	0.01 (−0.03, 0.02)

[a] None of the differences was significant.
[b] ABW = actual body weight.
[c] The values in parentheses are the lower and upper bounds of the 95% confidence interval for the mean value.

pendently from the infusion duration on which the calculation was based. Mathematical comparisons show that the effect of an infusion duration different from that with which the gentamicin dose is calculated depends on the ratio of the time difference between the disparate infusion durations and the patient's gentamicin half-life (i.e., the ratio of the difference between the infusion duration and the gentamicin half-life). The smallest error occurs when the gentamicin half-life is large relative to the difference between infusion durations. The estimated error in the dose calculated by our method over a range of half-lives from 0.5 to 10 hours and a change in infusion duration from 0.5 hour to 1.5 hours is 3–64%. Our experience indicates that the variation in infusion time is typically less than 0.5 hour and that gentamicin half-lives generally exceed 1 hour. Therefore, with our method the potential error in the calculated dose would be less than 25% for most patients. While the consideration of a difference in the infusion periods by the SZ method permits a more accurate estimate of the dose, undetected variation in the infusion period would compromise the accuracy of both methods.

The true peak concentration may not always have to be calculated. If the patient's rate of drug elimination is very low or the blood sample is obtained soon after the end of the infusion (especially when the infusion period is short), the true peak concentration will approximate the measured concentration.[22] Mathematically, the gentamicin concentration one hour after the end of an infusion in a patient with a gentamicin half-life of at least five hours will equal or exceed 87% of the true peak.

The validity of our method in different populations (including pediatric patients, burn patients, and patients with very short or very long gentamicin half-lives) must still be determined. We could not analyze our data with respect to renal function because we estimated creatinine clearance by using a method that may be compromised by the presence of malnutrition, a factor we did not assess.[23] The accuracy of our method for other aminoglycosides is unknown. However, the similarity among the aminoglycosides in pharmacokinetic properties and the effectiveness of the SZ method for other aminoglycosides suggest that our method would be equally effective.

As with any method, the gentamicin dosage regimen calculated should always be reviewed for appropriateness before being implemented. Furthermore, serum gentamicin concentrations should be monitored, even after the desired concentration is achieved.

Our study design did not enable a comparison of the clinical outcomes for the gentamicin dosages calculated by the two methods because all the patients received the dosages calculated by the SZ method only. However, because the calculated doses and dosage intervals were identical for nearly all the patients, we believe that any differences in clinical outcomes would have been negligible.

Conclusion. The gentamicin dosage regimen calculated by our method and its predictive performance were similar to those of the Sawchuk-Zaske method in adult patients.

References

1. McHenry MC, Gavan TL, Gifford RW et al. Gentamicin dosage for renal insufficiency. Adjustment based on endogenous creatinine clearance and serum creatinine concentration. *Ann Intern Med.* 1971; 74:192-7.
2. Barza M, Brown RB, Shen D et al. Predictability of blood levels of gentamicin in man. *J Infect Dis.* 1975; 132:165-74.
3. Dettli LC. Drug dosage in patients with renal disease. *Clin Pharmacol Ther.* 1974; 16:274-80.
4. Sarubbi FA, Hull JH. Amikacin serum concentrations: prediction of levels and dosage guidelines. *Ann Intern Med.* 1978; 89:612-8.
5. Hull JH, Sarubbi FA. Gentamicin serum concentrations: pharmacokinetic predictions. *Ann Intern Med.* 1976; 85:183-9.
6. Chan RA, Benner EJ, Hoeprich RD. Gentamicin therapy in renal failure: a nomogram for dosage. *Ann Intern Med.* 1978; 76:775-8.
7. Sawchuk RJ, Zaske DE. Pharmacokinetics of dosing regimens which utilize multiple intravenous infusions: gentamicin in burn patients. *J Pharmacokinet Biopharm.* 1976; 4:183-95.
8. Burton ME, Brater DC, Chen PS et al. A Bayesian feedback method of aminoglycoside dosing. *Clin Pharmacol Ther.* 1985; 37:349-57.
9. Lesar TS, Rotschafer JC, Strand LM et al. Gentamicin dosing errors with four commonly used nomograms. *JAMA.* 1982; 248:1190-3.
10. Hull JH, Hak LJ, Koch GG et al. Influence of range of renal function and liver disease on predictability of creatinine clearance. *Clin Pharmacol Ther.* 1981; 29:516-21.
11. Dionne RE, Bauer LA, Gibson GA et al. Estimating creatinine clearance in morbidly obese patients. *Am J Hosp Pharm.* 1981; 38:841-4.
12. Cockcroft DW, Gault MH. Prediction of creatinine clearance from serum creatinine. *Nephron.* 1976; 16:31-3.
13. Pickering LK, Gearhart P. Effect of time and concentration upon interaction between gentamicin, tobramycin, netilmicin, or amikacin and carbenicillin or ticarcillin. *Antimicrob Agents Chemother.* 1979; 15:592-6.
14. Sheiner LB, Beal SL. Some suggestions for measuring predictive performance. *J Pharmacokinet Biopharm.* 1981; 9:503-12.
15. SAS Institute. SAS-STAT guide for personal computers. Version 6. Cary, NC: SAS Institute; 1987.
16. Devine BJ. Gentamicin therapy. *Drug Intell Clin Pharm.* 1974; 8:650-5.
17. Hallynck TH, Soep HH, Thomas JA et al. Should clearance be normalised to body surface area or to lean body mass? *Br J Clin Pharmacol.* 1981; 11:523-6.
18. Sawchuk RJ, Zaske DE, Cipolle RJ et al. Kinetic model for gentamicin dosing with the use of individual patient parameters. *Clin Pharmacol Ther.* 1977; 21:362-9.
19. Zaske DE, Cipolle RJ, Rotschafer JC et al. Gentamicin pharmacokinetics in 1,640 patients: method for control of serum concentrations. *Antimicrob Agents Chemother.* 1982; 21:407-11.
20. Chiou W, Huang SM, Huang YC. Midpoint back-extrapolation method for the rapid estimation of drugs' volume of distribution and dosage adjustment exhibiting multicompartmental characteristics. *Int J Clin Pharmacol Ther Toxicol.* 1980; 18:1-4.
21. Armitstead JA, Nahata MC. Effect of variables associated with intermittent gentamicin infusions on pharmacokinetic predictions. *Clin Pharm.* 1983; 2:153-6.
22. Rodvold KA, Zokufa H, Rotschafer JC. Aminoglycoside pharmacokinetic monitoring: an integral part of patient care? *Clin Pharm.* 1988; 7:608-13.
23. Lau AH, Berk SI, Prosser T et al. Estimation of creatinine clearance in malnourished patients. *Clin Pharm.* 1988; 7:62-5.

DUE Criteria

The DUE Criteria *section of* Clinical Pharmacy *features model drug-use evaluation criteria that may be employed as a component of a comprehensive quality assurance program. The criteria sets are presented in the format used in the ASHP book* Criteria for Drug Use Evaluation. *Some of the criteria sets will have been originally published in that book; others will be presented here for the first time and published in future volumes of the ASHP book. The practitioners who developed a criteria set are acknowledged.*

In selecting drug products for coverage in DUE Criteria, *priority is given to products that have been recently marketed, those that are frequently prescribed, those that have high potential risk associated with their use, and those that are expensive. When feasible, a criteria set will be linked with a Drug Review that appears in the same issue.*

These criteria sets are a starting point for the development of DUE criteria for a specific practice setting. Readers are encouraged to modify the model criteria to fit their own circumstances.

Criteria for use of ketorolac tromethamine in adult inpatients and outpatients[a]

Element	Standard 100%	Standard 0%	Exception[b] or Critical Preventive/ Responsive Measure[c]	Sources of Information
Justification for Use				
1. Short-term management of pain (e.g., after general surgery [orthopedic, gynecologic, and abdominal] or oral surgery)[1]	X		1A. None	1. History and physical examination (H&P), physician orders, progress notes
and				
2. Patient unable to take oral medications	X		2A. None	2. H&P, physician orders, progress notes, nursing notes
and				
3. History of narcotic drug abuse	X		3A. None	3. H&P, physician orders, progress notes, nursing notes
or				
4. History of drug-seeking behavior	X		4A. None	4. H&P, physician orders, progress notes, nursing notes
or				
5. Treatment of moderate to severe pain in patient with unknown medical history seen in emergency department	X		5A. None	5. H&P, physician orders, progress notes, nursing notes
or				
6. Ileus	X		6A. None	6. H&P, physician orders, progress notes, nursing notes
or				
7. Decreased level of consciousness, respiratory depression, or oversedation with or intolerance to narcotic analgesics	X		7A. None	7. H&P, physician orders, progress notes, nursing notes
Critical (Process) Indicators				
8. Baseline serum creatinine (SCr) concentration measured within 48 hours before initial ketorolac dose	X		8A. None	8. Physician orders, laboratory reports, H&P
9. No history of hypersensitivity to ketorolac or other nonsteroidal anti-inflammatory agents (NSAIDs)[1,2]	X		9A. None	9. H&P, allergies
10. No history of complete or partial syndrome of nasal polyps, angioedema, or bronchospastic reactivity to aspirin or other NSAIDs[1,3]	X		10A. None	10. H&P, allergies, progress notes
11. No history of peptic ulcer disease or NSAID-induced gastropathy[2]	X		11A. None	11. H&P, progress notes
12. Ketorolac not used in pregnant patient[1,4,5]	X		12A. Benefit outweighs risk to fetus	12. H&P, progress notes, laboratory reports

Prepared by Michele F. Shepherd, Pharm.D., Clinical Specialist, Department of Pharmacy, Abbott Northwestern Hospital, Minneapolis, MN, and Clinical Assistant Professor, College of Pharmacy, University of Minnesota, Minneapolis.

Element	Standard 100%	Standard 0%	Exception[b] or Critical Preventive/ Responsive Measure[c]	Sources of Information
				12A. Progress notes
13. Ketorolac not used during labor and delivery[1]	X		13A. None	13. H&P, progress notes
14. Ketorolac not used during breast-feeding[1,6]	X		14A. None	14. H&P, progress notes
15. Ketorolac not used in child[1]	X		15A. None	15. H&P, physician orders
16. Appropriate ketorolac tromethamine dosage[1]: a. Loading dose: 30 or 60 mg i.m. b. Maintenance dosage: 50% of the loading dose i.m. every 6 hours on a regular schedule	X		16A. Dosing on an as-needed (p.r.n.) basis: if pain returns within 3–5 hours, increase next dose by up to 50%; if pain does not return for 8–12 hours, decrease next dose by up to 50% or allow 8–12 hours to elapse before next dose 16B. Patient >65 years of age: lower end of dosage range used[1,7] 16C. Patient weight <50 kg: lower end of dosage range used[1] 16D. Patient with renal dysfunction: lower end of dosage range used[1,8]	16, 16A–C. Physician orders, medication administration record (MAR), progress notes 16D. Physician orders, progress notes, MAR, laboratory reports
17. Maximum daily dosage: 120 mg[1]	X		17A. Maximum dosage on first day: 150 mg[1]	17, 17A. Physician orders, MAR, progress notes
18. Dose not administered intravenously	X		18A. None	18. Physician orders, MAR, progress notes, nursing notes
19. Short-term therapy[1]	X		19A. None	19. Physician orders, MAR, progress notes
20. No concomitant treatment with NSAIDs or salicylates	X		20A. Benefit outweighs risk 20B. Ketorolac dosage reduced in patient receiving high-dose salicylate therapy[1]	20. Physician orders, MAR, progress notes 20A. Progress notes 20B. Progress notes, physician orders, MAR
21. Patient receiving concomitant lithium therapy monitored for signs of lithium toxicity (tremor, nausea, diarrhea, polyuria, polydipsia, lethargy, fatigue, muscle weakness, supratherapeutic serum lithium concentration)[9]	X		21A. None	21. Physician orders, progress notes, nursing notes, laboratory reports
22. Patient receiving concomitant methotrexate therapy monitored for signs of methotrexate toxicity (blood dyscrasias, hepatic fibrosis, cirrhosis, pneumonitis, pulmonary fibrosis, fever, cough, dyspnea, chest pain, hypoxemia, pulmonary infiltrates, supratherapeutic serum methotrexate concentration)[10]	X		22A. None	22. Physician orders, progress notes, nursing notes, laboratory reports, radiologic reports
Complications				
23. Gastrointestinal effects: nausea, dyspepsia, pain, diarrhea, bleeding, peptic ulcer, perforation[1,11,12]	X		23A. Identify other drug and nondrug causes 23B. Provide symptomatic care and supportive therapy 23C. If severe reaction, discontinue ketorolac or switch to alternative analgesic therapy	23. Progress notes, nursing notes 23A–C. Progress notes, physician orders, MAR, nursing notes
24. Central nervous system effects: drowsiness, dizziness, headache, sweating[1,11–13]	X		24A. Identify other drug and nondrug causes 24B. Provide symptomatic care and supportive therapy 24C. If severe reaction, discontinue ketorolac or switch to alternative analgesic therapy	24. Progress notes, nursing notes 24A–C. Progress notes, physician orders, MAR, nursing notes
25. Renal effects: oliguria, increased SCr concentration, hematuria, proteinuria, overt renal failure evidenced by progressively increasing SCr or sus-	X		25A. Identify other drug and nondrug causes 25B. Adjust ketorolac dosage per element 16D, discontinue ke-	25. Progress notes, nursing notes, laboratory reports, nursing flowsheets 25A. Physician orders, prog-

Element	Standard 100%	Standard 0%	Exception[b] or Critical Preventive/ Responsive Measure[c]	Sources of Information
tained increase in SCr of at least 0.5 mg/dL when measured by similar analytical techniques, 50% reduction in urine output, or elevated blood urea nitrogen concentration (>50% increase over several days)[1]			torolac, or switch to alternative analgesic therapy 25C. Recheck SCr concentration and monitor daily until ≤10% above baseline or desired level 25D. If mild reaction, increase hydration and use diuretic therapy if necessary 25E. If severe reaction, discontinue ketorolac; use supportive measures if necessary, including diuretic therapy or hemodialysis	ress notes, MAR, nursing notes 25B. Physician orders, progress notes, MAR 25C. Physician orders, progress notes, laboratory reports 25D, E. Physician orders, progress notes, nursing notes, MAR
26. Hematologic effects: prolonged bleeding time[1,14–16]	X		26A. Identify other drug and nondrug causes 26B. Provide symptomatic care and supportive therapy 26C. If severe reaction, discontinue ketorolac or switch to alternative analgesic therapy	26. Progress notes, nursing notes, laboratory reports 26A–C. Physician orders, progress notes, MAR, nursing notes
27. Miscellaneous: edema, myalgia, fluid retention, pain at injection site[1,11,12]	X		27A. Identify other drug and nondrug causes 27B. Provide symptomatic care and supportive therapy 27C. If severe reaction, discontinue ketorolac or switch to alternative analgesic therapy	27. Progress notes, nursing notes 27A–C. Progress notes, physician orders, MAR, nursing notes
Outcome Measures				
28. Decrease in pain severity or increase in time until pain recurs and control of pain at tolerable level	X		28A. Patient died 28B. Ketorolac discontinued because of adverse effects	28. Progress notes, physician orders, nursing notes, MAR 28A. Progress notes 28B. Progress notes, physician orders, MAR, nursing notes

[a] Criteria address justification for use (indications), critical (process) indicators, complications of therapy, and patient outcome. Each criterion consists of an element, a standard, exceptions to the standard, and sources of information. The element is the minimum level of evidence needed to show that patient care was optimal. The standard defines the deviation from an element that is acceptable. If no deviation is acceptable, the standard is 100%. Exceptions are circumstances in which deviation is allowable. Sources of information listed are the most reliable sources. Sources pertaining to an element or exception are identified by the number assigned to the element or exception (e.g., 20, 20A).

[b] For justification for use and critical (process) indicators.

[c] For complications and outcome measures.

References

1. Syntex Laboratories, Inc. Toradol package insert. Palo Alto, CA; 1990 Mar.
2. Lanza FL, Karlin DA, Yee JP. A double-blind placebo controlled endoscopic study comparing the mucosal injury seen with an orally and parenterally administered new nonsteroidal analgesic ketorolac tromethamine at therapeutic and supratherapeutic doses. *Am J Gastroenterol.* 1987; 82:939. Abstract.
3. Settipane GA. Aspirin and allergic diseases: a review. *Am J Med.* 1983; 74(Suppl):102–9.
4. Greer IA, Johnston J, Tulloch I et al. Effect of maternal ketorolac administration on platelet function in the newborn. *Eur J Obstet Gynecol Reprod Biol.* 1988; 29:257–60.
5. Walker JJ, Johnstone J, Lloyd J et al. The transfer of ketorolac tromethamine from maternal to foetal blood. *Eur J Clin Pharmacol.* 1988; 34:509–11.
6. Wischnik A, Manth SM, Lloyd J et al. The excretion of ketorolac tromethamine into breast milk after multiple oral dosing. *Eur J Clin Pharmacol.* 1989; 36:521–4.
7. Jallad NS, Garg DC, Martinez JJ et al. Pharmacokinetics of single-dose oral and intramuscular ketorolac tromethamine in the young and elderly. *J Clin Pharmacol.* 1990; 30:76–81.
8. Martinez JJ, Garg DC, Pages LJ et al. Single dose pharmacokinetics of ketorolac in healthy young and renal impaired subjects. *J Clin Pharmacol.* 1987; 27:722. Abstract.
9. Reiman IW, Forlich JC. Effects of diclofenac on lithium kinetics. *Clin Pharmacol Ther.* 1981; 30:348–52.
10. Thyss A, Milano G, Kubar J et al. Clinical and pharmacokinetic evidence of a life-threatening interaction between methotrexate and ketoprofen. *Lancet.* 1986; 1:256–8.
11. O'Hara DA, Fragen RJ, Kinzer M et al. Ketorolac tromethamine as compared with morphine sulfate for treatment of postoperative pain. *Clin Pharmacol Ther.* 1987; 41:556–61.
12. Staquet MJ. A double-blind study with placebo control of intramuscular ketorolac tromethamine in the treatment of cancer pain. *J Clin Pharmacol.* 1989; 29:1031–6.
13. Yee JP, Koshiver JE, Allbon C et al. Comparison of intramuscular ketorolac tromethamine and morphine sulfate for analgesia of pain after major surgery. *Pharmacotherapy.* 1986; 6:253–61.
14. Conrad KA, Fagan TC, Mackie MJ et al. Effects of ketorolac tromethamine on hemostasis in volunteers. *Clin Pharmacol Ther.* 1988; 43:542–6.
15. Roe RL, Burno JJ, Ellis DJ. Effects of a new nonsteroidal anti-inflammatory agent on platelet function in male and female subjects. *Clin Pharmacol Ther.* 1981; 29:277. Abstract.
16. Spowart K, Greer IA, McLaren M et al. Haemostatic effects of ketorolac with and without concomitant heparin in normal volunteers. *Thromb Haemost.* 1988; 60:382–6.

CP Continuing Education

The ASHP Continuing Education System gives readers a self-assessment mechanism for selected articles in Clinical Pharmacy *and* AJHP. *It allows readers to obtain continuing-education credit for these articles.*

For the purpose of CE-credit enrollment, a blank answer sheet is published at the end of each installment of the column for the CE articles in that issue. An enrollee accumulates these answer sheets until the enrollment is submitted, using the form that is published in the June and December issues of Clinical Pharmacy *and in the June and December issues of* AJHP. *Any combination of tests within an 18-month period, from both* Clinical Pharmacy *and* AJHP, *may be included in an enrollment. More complete details about enrollment in the system appear in the semiannual enrollment form.*

Article 680-204-9119 (see page 667)
Qualifies for 2.0 hours of CE credit

Management of acute pain in children

Learning Objectives

After studying this article, the reader should be able to

1. Identify neurophysiologic changes that occur during late fetal development and during infancy and state how these changes relate to pain perception.
2. Recommend initial dosages of morphine and fentanyl, given by continuous intravenous infusion or by epidural administration, for infants and children.
3. Compare the adverse-effect profiles of morphine, meperidine, and fentanyl in neonates, infants, and children.
4. Differentiate between opioid agonists and partial agonists with respect to their effects on opioid receptors and their adverse-effect profiles.
5. Identify differences in the pharmacokinetics of opioid agonists in pediatric and adult patients.
6. Describe the techniques used to provide regional analgesia.
7. Identify differences in the adverse-effect profiles and pharmacokinetics of local anesthetics in pediatric and adult patients.
8. Compare tetracaine–epinephrine (adrenaline)–cocaine (TAC) solution and other local anesthetics with respect to efficacy and adverse effects in children.

Self-assessment Questions

For each question there is only one best answer.

1. Neurophysiologic and neuroanatomic findings indicate that
   a. Complete myelination of nerve tracts is not necessary for pain perception.
   b. Myelination of nociceptive pathways is completed during the first trimester of gestation.
   c. Incomplete myelination may result in faster impulse conduction.
   d. Nociceptive nerve endings in the skin may be less dense in neonates than in adults.
2. Opioid stimulation of which of the following types of receptors is responsible for analgesia?
   a. Kappa.
   b. Mu.
   c. Sigma.
   d. Theta.
3. Inadequate treatment of pain in pediatric patients has been attributed to
   a. Unfounded fears of addiction and adverse effects.
   b. Difficulties in assessing the extent of pain.
   c. As-needed (p.r.n.) medication orders being interpreted to mean as little drug as possible.
   d. All of the above alternatives are correct.
4. Compared with children and adults, neonates treated with morphine are likely to
   a. Have a substantially longer elimination half-life.
   b. Be less sensitive to the pharmacologic effects of morphine.
   c. Have a larger morphine volume of distribution.
   d. Have a higher fraction of morphine bound to plasma proteins.
5. The recommended intravenous infusion rate of mor-

Continued on page 723

now appropriate to treat the child with

a. Nebulized cromolyn sodium.
b. Nebulized β agonist.
c. Intravenous aminophylline.
d. Systemic corticosteroids.

9. A six-year-old boy requires institution of oral theophylline therapy for his asthma. He weighs 22.4 kg (75th percentile). An appropriate initial drug regimen is

a. Theo-Dur tablets 250 mg every 12 hours.
b. Slo-bid capsules 125 mg every 12 hours for three days, then 250 mg every morning and 125 mg every evening for three days, then 250 mg every 12 hours.
c. Theo-Dur Sprinkle capsules 200 mg every 12 hours for three days, then 300 mg every morning and 200 mg every evening for three days, then 300 mg every 12 hours.
d. Aminophylline solution 105 mg t.i.d.

10. A 10-year-old girl requires corticosteroid burst therapy for her asthma. She weighs 35 kg (50th percentile) and is clinically stable enough to be treated at home. An appropriate drug regimen is

a. Prednisone 30 mg p.o. b.i.d. for two days, then 15 mg b.i.d. for two days, then 15 mg daily for two days, then 10 mg daily for two days, then 5 mg daily for two days, then discontinue.
b. Prednisone 30 mg p.o. every other day.
c. Methylprednisolone 40 mg (as sodium succinate) i.v. every six hours.
d. Prednisone 30 mg p.o. every 12 hours for five to seven days, then discontinue.

Policies Regarding Personnel Advertising
Clinical Pharmacy

Personnel advertising is accepted in *Clinical Pharmacy* for Positions Open and Training Programs.

Only those employees who will not discriminate on the basis of race, sex, religion, age, color, or national origin should submit personnel advertising. Ads should include the statement "Equal Opportunity Employer." Employers are encouraged to specify salary range in their position advertising. Advertisers listing residency or fellowship positions are strongly encouraged to comply with the profession's consensus of definitions for these two types of training programs (see *AJHP*. 1987; 44:1142-4).

The deadline for receipt of final copy and for cancellations is the 15th of the month two months before the month of publication. The sizes available are: full page (7″ × 10″) at $1175, half page (vertical = 3 1/4″ × 10″; horizontal = 7″ × 4 3/4″) at $790, and quarter page (3 1/4″ × 4 9/16″) at $520. There is a $35 charge for typesetting quarter- and half-page advertisements and $55 for full-page advertisements.

Effective with the October 1991 issue and at the advertiser's option, personnel ads (maximum 100 words) will run not only in *Clinical Pharmacy* (one time) but also on PharmNet (ASHP's electronic bulletin board service, which is available to all ASHP members) for a period of 30 days, beginning shortly after advertising copy is received.

The address for insertions (which must be accompanied by payment, organizational purchase order, or advertising agency insertion order) is: Advertising Placement Manager, *Clinical Pharmacy*, 4630 Montgomery Avenue, Bethesda, MD 20814. The fax number is 301-657-1615.

For information regarding the Career Opportunities section of the *American Journal of Hospital Pharmacy*, please contact Advertising Placement Manager, 301-657-3000, ext. 288.

ASHP also offers the Personnel Placement Service, which consists of monthly listings of positions open and of brief résumés of individuals seeking positions. For more information, write to Personnel Placement Service, ASHP, 4630 Montgomery Avenue, Bethesda, MD 20814.

Current Literature

Drug Reaction Alerts 726

Book Reviews

Diseases of the Nose, Throat, Ear, Head, and Neck, Fourteenth Edition 729
Edited by John Jacob Ballenger
Reviewed by Elaine R. Green

Handbook of Psychiatric Emergencies 730
By William R. Dubin and Kenneth J. Weiss
Reviewed by Susan S. Fish

Drug Reaction Alerts

Drug Reaction Alerts focuses primarily on serious, unlabeled reactions to new chemical entities. The citations are compiled monthly from International Pharmaceutical Abstracts, *which covers over 800 pharmacy and health-related journals worldwide. An address for reprints (when available) follows the name of the corresponding author of each citation.*

Pharmacists may use the FDA Adverse Reaction Report form that appears in most issues of Clinical Pharmacy *for submitting reports of adverse drug reactions directly to FDA.*

Anticonvulsants

Kaya IS, Dilmen U, Toppare M et al. (Senses DA, Department of Pediatrics, Medical Center Hospital, Turkish Health and Therapy Foundation, Ankara, Turkey). **Valproic acid**-induced pancytopenia and Coombs test positivity. *Lancet.* 1991; 337:1227-8. Case. (16-year-old woman with petit mal epilepsy; received increasing doses of valproic acid reaching 800 mg/day after three months; complained of weakness and general malaise; hemoglobin, 2.8 g/dL; results of direct Coombs test were indicative of anemia, and bone marrow examination revealed hypocellularity with some dyserythropoietic features; withdrawal of valproic acid and transfusion of blood led to hemoglobin of 9.9 g/dL)

Drug Interactions

Blickstein D (Division of Hematology, Beilinson Medical Center, 49100 Petah Tiqva, Israel), Shaklai M, Inbal A. **Warfarin** antagonism by **avocado**. *Lancet.* 1991; 337:914-5. Cases. (two patients, aged 15 and 30 years, who were adequately anticoagulated with warfarin after parieto-occipital brain infarction and pulmonary embolism, respectively; 15-year-old patient ate at least 100 g/day of avocado for an unreported period of time; 30-year-old ate 200 g/day of avocado for two days; international normalized ratios decreased from 2.5–2.7 to 1.6–1.7; elimination of avocado from diet led to restoration of effective anticoagulation; positive rechallenge in 15-year-old patient)

Immunosuppressive Agents

Kitahara S (First Department of Surgery, Shinshu University School of Medicine, Matsumoto 390, Japan), Makuuchi M, Kawasaki S et al. Lymphoproliferative disorders after **FK 506**. *Lancet.* 1991; 337:1234. Case. (six-year-old boy after liver transplantation; received FK 506 at doses to maintain plasma concentrations at 0.4–1.0 ng/mL and prednisone starting on postoperative day 50 and continuing for approximately two months; histological specimens showed diffuse large cell malignant lymphoma; reduction of FK 506 to doses that maintained trough plasma concentrations at 0.1–0.25 ng/mL did not lead to resolution of lymphoproliferative disorder; laparotomy showed multiple, palpable tumors; surgical closure of nine lesions in jejunum led to gradual recovery and complete regression of tumors)

Continued on page 729

Continued from page 726

Liposomes

Levine SJ (Critical Care Medical Department, National Institutes of Health, Building 10, Room 10D48, 9000 Rockville Pike, Bethesda, MD 20892), Walsh TJ, Martinez A et al. Cardiopulmonary toxicity after **liposomal amphotericin B** infusion. *Ann Intern Med.* 1991; 114:664-6. Case. (22-year-old man with lymphoma; received amphotericin B 5 mg/kg/day over 50 minutes as a liposomal preparation containing 7:3 molar ratio of dimyristoylphosphatidylcholine and dimyristoylphosphatidylglycerol for a total dose of 1136 mg; developed transient hypoxemia, elevated pulmonary artery pressure, and depressed cardiac output; withdrawal of amphotericin B and therapy with furosemide, nitroglycerin, and morphine sulfate did not lead to resolution of cardiopulmonary effects; additional therapy with furosemide and nitroglycerin led to hypotension, therapy with dopamine 15 μg/kg/min for several hours, and improvement; positive rechallenge)

Pediatrics

Hengster P, Fille M, Menardi G (Department of Surgery I and Institute for Hygiene, University Hospital Innsbruck, 6020 Innsbruck, Austria). Suppurative lymphadenitis in newborn babies after change of **BCG vaccine**. *Lancet.* 1991; 337:1168-9. Cases. (77 children; received approximately 0.5 mL of Pasteur intradermal BCG vaccine containing a more virulent Calmette-Guérin strain of *Mycobacterium bovis;* developed suppurative lymphadenitis; surgical removal of suppurative lymph nodes showed signs of caseous necrosis at incision sites)

McCabe M, Sibert JR (Department of Child Health and Welsh National Poisons Unit, University of Wales College of Medicine, Llandough Hospital, Penarth, South Glamorgan CF6 1XX, Wales, UK), Routledge PA. Phosphate enemas in childhood: cause for concern. *Br Med J.* 1991; 302:1074. Case. (32-month-old girl with constipation; received 90-mL rectal enema containing **sodium phosphate monobasic** 12.8 g per 128 mL and **sodium phosphate dibasic** 10.24 g per 128 mL; became drowsy and developed gray skin color, marked abdominal tenderness, and decreased bowel sounds; serum concentrations suggested systemic absorption of enema components; therapy with appropriate replacement solutions, cefotaxime 500 mg twice daily, and metronidazole 80 mg three times daily and digital removal of large fecal mass led to improvement and discharge after seven days)

Pairaudeau PW (Southampton General Hospital, Southampton SO9 4XY, England), Wilson RG, Hall MA et al. Inhalation of **baby powder**: unappreciated hazard. *Br Med J.* 1991; 302:1220-1. Case. (12-week-old boy; inhaled talcum powder that was inadvertently spilled on face during diaper change; vomited once and refused to eat; admitted to hospital with cyanosis four hours after exposure; suffered respiratory arrest 30 minutes after admission; therapy with mechanical ventilation and corticosteroids led to recovery but with residual wheezing)

Ponnighaus JM, Fine PE, Moreno C (MRC Tuberculosis and Related Infections Unit, Hammersmith Hospital, London W12, England). Hypersensitivity to **dextran** in **BCG vaccine**. *Lancet.* 1991; 337:1039. Case. (nine-month-old girl; received dextran-only placebo as part of BCG vaccine study; developed swelling at site of injection and difficulty breathing within a few hours; received BCG vaccine with dextran six to eight months before placebo injection; high serum anti-dextran immunoglobulin G concentrations five months after placebo injection)

Prolactin Inhibitors

Blin O (Clinic for Nervous Disorders and Locomotor Apparatus, CHU Timone, 13385 Marseille, France), Schwertschlag US, Serratrice G. Painful clitoral tumescence during **bromocriptine** therapy. *Lancet.* 1991; 337:1231-2. Case. (28-year-old woman; received bromocriptine 2.5 mg twice daily for three days to suppress lactation; developed painful clitoral tumescence not related to sexual arousal but noticed overall increase in libido; withdrawal of bromocriptine led to resolution of tumescence but development of breast congestion; positive rechallenge)

Sulfonamides

Quinn AG, Ellis WR, Burn D et al. (Cartlidge N, Department of Neurology, Royal Victoria Infirmary, Newcastle upon Tyne NE1 4LP, England). Chorea precipitated by sulphasalazine. *Br Med J.* 1991; 302:1025. Case. (70-year-old woman; received **sulfasalazine** 1 g four times daily for six weeks; developed focal chorea that progressed to a general movement disorder after two more weeks of sulfasalazine therapy; withdrawal of sulfasalazine led to gradual resolution of symptoms over eight weeks)

Sympathomimetic Agents

Hatton MQ, Allen MB, Mellor EJ et al. (Cooke NJ, Department of Respiratory Medical, Leeds General Infirmary, Leeds LS1 3EX, England). **Salmeterol** rash. *Lancet.* 1991; 337:1169-70. Case. (32-year-old woman with asthma; received salmeterol two puffs (25 μg/puff) twice daily from a metered-dose inhaler for four days; developed pruritic, burning maculopapular rash that became more severe one hour after inhaling salmeterol, reached a peak at three hours, and improved gradually until the next dose; withdrawal of salmeterol led to resolution of rash but worsening of asthma; positive rechallenge with metered-dose inhaler and dry salmeterol powder without propellant)

Book Reviews

Diseases of the Nose, Throat, Ear, Head, and Neck, Fourteenth Edition

Edited by John Jacob Ballenger.
Published by Lea & Febiger, 200 Chester Field Parkway, Malvern, PA 19355-9725, 1991. 1376p. Price $195.

This classic textbook of otolaryngology, first published in 1908, contains 68 chapters organized into six parts. Many well-known otolaryngologists from across the United States contributed chapters to this edition of the book.

Part I, "The Nose and Accessory Sinuses," contains 14 chapters, including a chapter on AIDS. Part II, "Neck, Pharynx, Oro-pharynx and Nasopharynx, Maxilla, and Mandible," comprises 10 chapters, several of which concentrate on surgical aspects of treatment. Part III, "Diseases of the Larynx," contains two chapters devoted to areas of interest to pharmacists: nutritional care of the patient with head and neck cancer or trauma, and chemotherapy of head and neck cancers. The other 15 chapters in part III focus on the physiology and pathology of laryngeal problems. Part IV, "Imaging the Head and Neck," contains two chapters that describe various imaging techniques used on the head and neck. Part V, "The Ear," contains 19 chapters that cover a wide variety of topics including development and anatomy of the ear, vestibulometry, and reconstructive surgery. Part VI, "Bronchoesophagology," constitutes six chapters that describe diagnostic techniques used in specific parts of the alimentary tract.

Generally, this book provides extensive information on anatomy, physiology, pathology, clinical features of diseases related to otolaryngology, diagnostic techniques, and nonpharmacologic approaches to treatment. Very few chapters or even parts of chapters extensively discuss the pharmacotherapy of problems related to the ears, nose, and throat.

Diseases of the Nose, Throat, Ear, Head, and Neck remains a classic textbook that provides extensive information on otolaryngological problems. Because the emphasis is not on the pharmacotherapy of these problems, this book is unlikely to be of great interest to pharmacists; instead, this book belongs in the medical library as a general reference.

Reviewed by Elaine R. Green, Pharm.D., Department of Pharmacy, School of Pharmacy, State University of New York at Buffalo, Buffalo, NY 14260.

Handbook of Psychiatric Emergencies

By William R. Dubin and Kenneth J. Weiss.

Published by Springhouse Corporation, 1111 Bethlehem Pike, Springhouse, PA 19477, 1991. x + 294 p. Price $22.95.

This pocket-sized handbook describes the wide variety of psychiatric emergencies seen in a general hospital's emergency department (ED). The authors of this book, two psychiatrists, have an excellent understanding of ED situations and priorities and have consistently organized their book to be useful, a necessity for the ED setting.

In chapter 1, the review of patient assessment is very basic and probably most helpful to a medical student or other clinician unfamiliar with performing a mental status examination. Chapter 2 contains a thorough, concise discussion of medicolegal issues that pertain to psychiatric patients and many other patients. The issues include duty to care for and protect the patient, maintenance of patient confidentiality, evaluation of patient competence, duty to warn potential victims of the patient, practitioner liability, and patient rights. This chapter should be required reading for all clinical practitioners, because the principles discussed apply to almost all clinical settings.

Chapters 3 through 14 discuss various psychiatric situations that might be encountered in an ED. Some of the subjects are obvious: delirium, alcohol and other drug emergencies, schizophrenia and mania, violent and self-destructive behavior, depression, and anxiety. The authors broadly define psychiatric emergencies and include chapters on domestic abuse, sexual assault, child abuse and neglect, and abuse of elderly persons. Chapter 15 discusses a variety of situations such as homelessness, drug-seeking behavior, AIDS, and hysteria. The final chapter concisely presents psychotropic drug reactions.

The general approach taken to each subject is that the role of the ED clinician is to (1) rule out medical illness in the patient either as a cause of the emergency or as a problem masked by the emergency, (2) treat the acute emergency, (3) reduce the risk of harm to the clinician and others, and (4) determine the best setting in which to treat the patient. All the chapters are organized into brief sections. "Identifying the problem" describes mental status and physical symptoms, laboratory test abnormalities, and differential diagnosis. "Interpersonal intervention" discusses the best ways to approach and interview the patient and includes suggested questions and phrases to use during the interview. Tips on how to elicit necessary information, how to defuse a potentially violent situation, when to show empathy, when to negotiate (and when not to), and how and when to set limits with the patient are very practical. "Pharmacologic intervention" recommends specific drug regimens and, importantly, which drugs not to use and why. "Educational intervention" includes information that should be given to the patient, family, or other support persons concerning acute and chronic situations and contains suggestions on how to assess the patient's receptiveness to this information. "Disposition" considers whether the patient should be discharged to home from the ED, given an appointment with a psychiatric practitioner for the following day, admitted to a medical unit, or admitted to a psychiatric unit. "Medicolegal considerations" discusses issues specific to each patient situation and notes differences between jurisdictions.

Although the clinician can always find treatment recommendations with which to disagree (e.g., naloxone dose too low), this book's approach is generally consistent with real-life practice. The possible reactions of the clinician to the patient (e.g., anger, disgust, paternalism) are acknowledged throughout, and useful suggestions for dealing with these feelings are presented. This book is well indexed and easy to read.

The *Handbook of Psychiatric Emergencies* would be most useful to a pharmacist who is new to the ED setting, works where a large number of patients have the problems discussed in the book, or practices in a psychiatric unit and would like to understand the initial presentation and emergency treatment of these patients. Other potential users of the book include medical students, nurses new to the ED setting, and emergency medicine residents.

Reviewed by Susan S. Fish, Pharm.D., Boston City Hospital Emergency Department, Department of Health and Hospitals, 818 Harrison Avenue, Boston, MA 02118.

Advertising Index

American Society of Hospital Pharmacists
Criteria for Drug Use Evaluation, Volumes 1 and 2, 666
QARx, 725
Amgen Inc.
Epogen, inside front cover
Burroughs Wellcome Company
Exosurf Neonatal, 659-663
Roerig, A Division of Pfizer Pharmaceuticals
Diflucan, 719-722
SmithKline Beecham
Tagamet, inside back cover, outside back cover
St. Jude Children's Research Hospital
Institutional, 665
Wyeth-Ayerst Laboratories, Inc.
Ativan Injection, 654-656

News

Haemophilus b immunization recommendations updated by American Academy of Pediatrics	733
American Academy of Pediatrics issues recommendations on treatment of Lyme disease	738
Benazepril approved for treatment of hypertension	739
News Briefs	739
Upcoming Specialty Meetings	739

Haemophilus b immunization recommendations updated by American Academy of Pediatrics

According to the American Academy of Pediatrics (AAP), all infants should be immunized with *Haemophilus influenzae* type b conjugate vaccine at about two months of age.[1] The immunization series should be initiated with *Haemophilus* b oligosaccharide conjugate (diptheria CRM_{197} protein conjugate) vaccine (HbOC, HibTITER, Lederle–Praxis) or *Haemophilus* b polysaccharide conjugate (meningococcal protein conjugate) vaccine (PRP-OMP, PedvaxHIB, Merck Sharp & Dohme), the only *Haemophilus* b vaccines labeled for use in infants less than 15 months of age. The first dose can be given when other routine immunizations are given. In children 15 months or older, the safety and efficacy of the three available vaccines—HbOC, PRP-OMP, and *Haemophilus* b polysaccharide conjugate (diphtheria toxoid conjugate) vaccine (PRP-D, ProHIBit, Connaught)—are considered by the AAP to be equivalent.

Two regimens are recommended for routine immunization of children younger than seven months: (1) three doses of HbOC at two month intervals, followed by a fourth dose of vaccine (HbOC, PRP-OMP, or PRP-D) when the infant is 15 months old, and (2) two doses of PRP-OMP at two-month intervals, followed by a third dose of PRP-OMP at the age of 12 months.

If the immunization series is initiated when the infant is 7–11 months of age, recommended regimens for HbOC and PRP-OMP are identical: The first two doses are given at two-month intervals, and the third dose is given at the age of 15–18 months. The same vaccine product should be used for the first and second doses. Any of the three vaccines may be used for the third dose.

If the immunization series is delayed until the child is 12–14 months of age, two doses of HbOC or PRP-OMP are recommended. If the second dose is administered at or after 15 months, any of the three vaccines may be used.

Readers should refer to the published document for a complete discussion of the rationale for specific recommendations and for information on handling special circumstances, such as delays in the administration schedule.

1. American Academy of Pediatrics. *Haemophilus influenzae* type b conjugate vaccines: recommendations for immunization of infants and children 2 months of age and older: update. *Pediatrics*. 1991; 88:169-72.

Continued on page 738

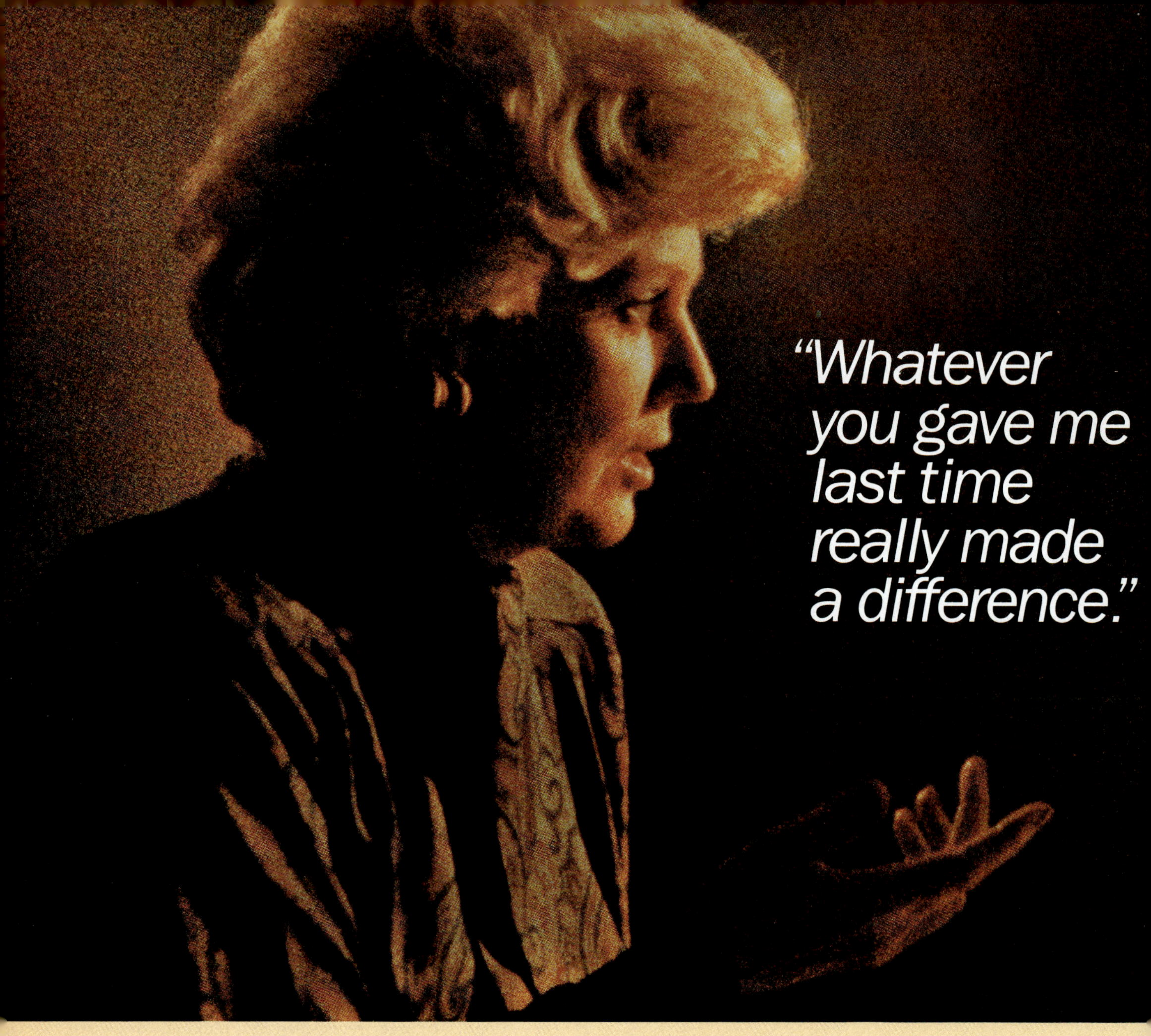

WYETH-AYERST LABORATORIES
Philadelphia, PA 19101

If outpatients are treated with ATIVAN® Injection, care must be taken on the day of treatment to prevent their undertaking any activity requiring full awareness or coordination.

days. A follow-up visit should be scheduled after 14 days of therapy. Treatment may be discontinued at that time if all symptoms have resolved; otherwise, treatment should be continued until symptoms are resolved. Penicillin-allergic patients may receive erythromycin 30 mg/kg/day in divided doses or 250 mg three times daily, but erythromycin may be less effective than other recommended antimicrobials.

The preferred treatment for late-stage Lyme disease depends on the clinical manifestations. Patients with mild carditis, arthritis, or isolated seventh nerve palsy with normal cerebrospinal fluid findings may be treated with one of the oral regimens recommended for early-stage disease. Intravenous therapy with ceftriaxone 75–100 mg/kg once daily (maximum dosage, 2 g/day) or penicillin G 300,000 units/kg/day given in divided doses every four hours (maximum dosage, 20 million units/day) is recommended for patients with severe carditis or persistent arthritis. Intravenous ceftriaxone, at the same dosage, is recommended for treatment of patients with meningitis or encephalitis. When intravenous antimicrobial therapy is required, a 14- to 21-day course is suggested.

1. American Academy of Pediatrics. Treatment of Lyme borreliosis. *Pediatrics*. 1991; 88:176-9.

Benazepril approved for treatment of hypertension

A nonsulfhydryl angiotensin-converting-enzyme inhibitor, benazepril hydrochloride (Lotensin, Ciba–Geigy) has been approved for marketing in the United States. The drug is labeled for the treatment of hypertension.

Benazepril is almostly completely converted to benazeprilat, a more active compound, and to glucuronide conjugates of benazepril and benazeprilat. Peak reductions in blood pressure are achieved two to four hours after an oral dose. Maximum effects on blood pressure are typically achieved after one to two weeks of therapy. Both benazepril and benazeprilat are more than 95% bound to plasma proteins. The half-life of benazeprilat is about 10 hours. The two compounds are eliminated primarily by renal excretion. A dosage reduction is recommended if the patient's creatinine clearance is less than 30 mL/min. Increasing age and hepatic dysfunction do not appear to alter drug disposition.

The adverse-effect profile of benazepril resembles those of other ACE inhibitors. The most commonly reported reactions are headache, dizziness, and fatigue.

An initial dosage of 10 mg once daily is recommended for patients not receiving a diuretic. The usual dosage is 20–40 mg/day, given in one or two daily doses. An initial dose of 5 mg is recommended for patients in whom diuretic therapy cannot be discontinued several days before benazepril therapy is begun.

Lotensin is available as 5-, 10-, 20-, and 40-mg tablets in bottles and unit dose packages of 100.

News Briefs

- **A treatment IND protocol for 4-hydroperoxycyclophosphamide** (Pergamid, Nova Pharmaceutical Corp.) has been approved by FDA. The drug will be used as a bone marrow purging agent for patients with acute myelogenous leukemia who have achieved a second or later remission with conventional drug therapy and need an autologous bone marrow transplant.

- Labeled indications for **ceftriaxone sodium** (Hoffmann-La Roche) have been expanded to include treatment of pharyngeal gonorrhea caused by non-penicillinase-producing strains of *Neisseria gonorrhoeae;* a single 250-mg intramuscular dose of ceftriaxone is recommended.

- An **ophthalmic solution of 0.3% norfloxacin** (Merck Sharp & Dohme) has been approved for marketing.

- Copies of **three 1991 reports on medicines under development for treatment of cancer, cerebrovascular or cardiovascular disorders, or debilitating diseases** can be obtained by writing to Editor, New Medicines in Development for Older Americans, Pharmaceutical Manufacturers Association, 1100 15th Street. N.W., Washington, DC 20005. For each drug, the manufacturer, indication, and stage of development are listed. The information is based on PMA-sponsored surveys of government and industry sources.

Upcoming Specialty Meetings

Cancer Treatment—Trends in the 90s. Skokie, IL, October 12; contact American Cancer Society, 1618 Orrington Avenue, Evanston, IL 60201; 708-328-5147.

Antibody Engineering: New Technology and Application Implications. San Diego, CA, December 16–18; contact International Business Communications USA Conferences, 8D Pleasant Street, South Natick, MA 01760; 508-650-4700, (fax) 508-653-1627.

American Society for Parenteral and Enteral Nutrition 16th Clinical Congress. Orlando, FL, January 19–22; contact A.S.P.E.N., 8630 Fenton Street, Suite 412, Silver Spring, MD 20910; 301-587-6315.

Therapy Consultation

The Therapy Consultation *section provides brief advice, in question-and-answer format, on how to handle specific drug-therapy problems. Readers are invited to submit questions, which will be referred to a consultant for an answer. The problems should not be highly specialized or unusual, nor should they be mundane. Questions are answered briefly, based largely on the judgment and personal experience of the consultant, although selected references may be cited to substantiate the consultant's advice.*

Assistance in identifying Therapy Consultation *topics is provided by the drug information centers at Medical College of Virginia Hospitals, Richmond; University of California Medical Center, San Diego; and University of Michigan Medical Center, Ann Arbor.*

Treatment options for a patient with osteoarthritis and a history of ulcer disease

Question: A 70-year-old female nursing home patient is having increasing knee pain related to osteoarthritis. Her medical history includes duodenal ulcers several years ago and mild dementia. She does not currently smoke cigarettes but has a 40-pack/year smoking history. How should her osteoarthritis be treated?

Answer: The treatment of osteoarthritis (degenerative joint disease) in patients with peptic ulcer disease is a common but frustrating situation. Treatment should be individualized. Osteoarthritis, the most common joint disease, primarily affects the elderly. It is a slowly progressive disease that principally affects the hands and large weight-bearing joints (hips, knees, vertebrae). The pathology involves cartilage destruction, subchondral sclerosis, cyst formation, and formation of large osteophytes at joint margins.[1] The symptoms are primarily pain and loss of joint motion.

Osteoarthritis is not a systemic disease; its symptoms are confined to the joints. If inflammation is present, it is typically mild and considered secondary.[1,2] Therefore, complex drug therapy is not required. Systemic corticosteroids and disease-modifying antirheumatic drugs such as gold compounds or hydroxychloroquine have no role in the treatment of osteoarthritis. Intra-articular corticosteroids may improve symptoms temporarily but can impair cartilage metabolism if overused; thus, they should be used sparingly.[1] Treatment is limited to oral analgesics and nonsteroidal anti-inflammatory drugs (NSAIDs) in conjunction with basic physical measures.

The first step is to assess the cause and nature of the pain. Pain typically occurs with use of the affected joint. Therefore, weight loss, limitation of high-impact physical exercise, or the use of a walking aid can be useful. Evidence of inflammation—heat, redness, and soft-tissue swelling around the joint—require NSAID therapy. In the absence of substantial inflammation, however, the goal is pain relief, and treatment should begin with simple analgesic therapy in the form of acetaminophen (up to 4 g/day) or low doses of an NSAID.[2] Narcotic analgesics such as propoxyphene or codeine could also be used sparingly, although the risk of habituation with long-term use should be considered.

Unfortunately, some patients do not respond well to analgesics alone, and a trial of NSAID therapy may be required. The problem of NSAID-related gastropathy has received much attention in recent years. Endoscopic studies consistently estimate that 14–31% of patients receiving long-term NSAID therapy have gastric ulcers and an even higher percentage have milder changes in the gastric mucosa.[3] These ulcers are typically asymptomatic, are relatively shallow, and heal easily on their own, even during continued treatment with NSAIDs.[3] The presence of nausea or dyspepsia correlates poorly with objective pathology. Very few of these ulcers develop serious bleeding. Estimates of the relative risk of hospitalization because of gastric bleeding for NSAID users compared with nonusers are controversial. More reliable cohort studies suggest that the relative risk is about 2.[3,4] Therefore, the risk of serious gastrointestinal complications in an individual patient is acceptable, but the use of NSAIDs by millions of Americans creates substantial morbidity in the population as a whole.

Selection of an NSAID would be simplified if one NSAID carried a lower risk. There is no strong evidence from epidemiologic data that any NSAID is safer than another, although ibuprofen is generally associated with low risk.[5,6] Endoscopic studies have shown that enteric-coated aspirin causes less damage than plain or buffered forms.[7] Nonacetylated salicylates, such as salsalate, cause a low rate of gastric damage because they do not inhibit prostaglandin synthesis and do not dissolve in the stomach.[8]

Once a decision is made to use an NSAID, another question is whether to begin prophylactic therapy against NSAID-induced gastropathy. Misoprostol was approved for this indication and is the only drug shown to prevent gastric ulcers caused by NSAIDs.[3] However, misoprostol can cause adverse effects, has not been shown to prevent major gastric bleeding, and may not prevent duodenal ulcers in patients receiving NSAID therapy.[3]

Although most attention has been placed on gastric damage caused by NSAIDs, the drugs also increase the risk of duodenal ulcer.[3,9] Ranitidine has been shown to reduce the rate of duodenal ulceration caused by NSAIDs.[9] Because any prophylactic therapy carries some cost and risk of adverse effects, prophylaxis should be reserved for patients at high risk of gastrointestinal bleeding (the elderly, smokers, patients with rheumatoid arthritis, patients with a history of gastrointestinal bleeding, or those who use corticosteroids).[3,10] In the typical elderly nursing home patient with osteoarthritis, I would use prophylactic therapy in patients with a history of ulcers only if the ulcer disease is currently or recently active or if the patient smokes, has a history of NSAID-related gastrointestinal bleeding, or has another compelling risk factor.

In summary, this patient should have a trial of acetaminophen alone to control her knee pain. If that is ineffective, I would try low-dose NSAID therapy.[2,3] The dosage may be gradually increased if necessary. The choice of NSAID is unclear, but my preferences are salsalate, enteric-coated aspirin, or ibuprofen. I would not start prophylactic anti-ulcer therapy in this patient because she does not have current risk factors for gastrointestinal bleeding. If prophylaxis were used, ranitidine might be a better choice than misoprostol for preventing activation of duodenal ulcer disease. However, neither misoprostol nor histamine H_2-receptor antagonists have been adequately tested in patients with a history of peptic ulcer disease.

1. Mankin HJ, Treadwell BJ. Osteoarthritis: a 1987 update. *Bull Rheum Dis*. 1986; 36(5):1-10.
2. Bradley JD, Brandt KD, Katz BP et al. Comparison of an anti-inflammatory dose of ibuprofen, an analgesic dose of ibuprofen, and acetaminophen in the treatment of patients with osteoarthritis of the knee. *N Engl J Med*. 1991; 325:87-91.
3. Sell AH, Weinstein WM, Kurata J et al. Nonsteroidal anti-inflammatory drugs and peptic ulcer disease. *Ann Intern Med*. 1991; 114:307-19.
4. Hawkey CJ. Nonsteroidal anti-inflammatory drugs and peptic ulcers. *Br Med J*. 1990; 300:278-85.
5. Carson JL, Strom BL, Morse ML et al. The relative gastrointestinal toxicity of the nonsteroidal anti-inflammatory drugs. *Arch Intern Med*. 1987; 147:1054-9.
6. Griffen MR, Piper JM, Daugherty JR et al. Nonsteroidal anti-inflammatory drug use and increased risk for peptic ulcer disease for elderly persons. *Ann Intern Med*. 1991; 114:257-63.
7. Silvoso GR, Ivey KJ, Butt JH et al. Incidence of gastric lesions in patients with rheumatic disease on chronic aspirin therapy. *Ann Intern Med*. 1979; 91:517-20.
8. Lanza F, Rack MF, Doucette M et al. An endoscopic comparison of the gastroduodenal injury seen with salsalate and naproxen. *J Rheumatol*. 1989; 16:1570-4.
9. Ehsanullah RS, Page MC, Tildesley G et al. Prevention of gastroduodenal damage induced by nonsteroidal anti-inflammatory drugs: controlled trial of ranitidine. *Br Med J*. 1988; 297:1017-21.
10. Fries JF, Miller SR, Spitz PW et al. Toward an epidemiology of gastropathy associated with nonsteroidal anti-inflammatory drug use. *Gastroenterology*. 1989; 96(Suppl):647-55.

DONALD R. MILLER, PHARM.D.

Associate Professor
College of Pharmacy
North Dakota State University

Clinical Pharmacist
VA Medical Center
Fargo, ND 58102

Letters

Hyperthyroidism associated with mercury poisoning 742
Michael McCann, Stuart Scheckner

Ethnicity and clozapine-induced agranulocytosis 743
Karen Overstreet Price

The Letters *column is a forum for rapid exchange of ideas among readers of* Clinical Pharmacy. *Liberal criteria are applied in the review of submissions to encourage contributions to this column.*

The Letters *column includes the following types of contributions: (1) comments, addenda, and minor updates on previously published work, (2) alerts on potential problems related to drug therapy or clinical research, (3) observations or comments on trends in drug therapy or clinical research, and (4) brief expressions of opinion about controversies in drug therapy or clinical research.*

Letters need not be submitted with the journal's manuscript checklist. The following conditions, however, must be adhered to: (1) the body of the letter must be no longer than two typewritten pages, (2) the use of references, tables, and illustrations should be minimized, (3) the authors' names, affiliations, and mailing addresses must be typed at the end of the letter in the format used by Clinical Pharmacy, *and (4) the entire letter (including references, tables, and authors' names) must be typed double-spaced on plain white paper (not letterhead). Following acceptance of a letter, the authors are required to sign an exclusive publication statement and a copyright transferal form.*

Hyperthyroidism associated with mercury poisoning

The paper on elemental mercury poisoning recently published in *Clinical Pharmacy*[1] prompts us to report a personal experience that suggests a relationship between long-term mercury exposure and certain autoimmune disorders.[2,3]

One of us, a 52-year-old man (hereafter called the patient), had practiced general dentistry from 1964 to 1984 and had a toxic mercury exposure in 1978 after mercury was spilled onto carpeting in his work area. In addition, the patient had regularly removed mercury–silver (amalgam) dental fillings with a high-speed drill, and his amalgamator was found to leak mercury.

The patient gradually developed nausea, indigestion, weight loss, tachycardia, fatigue, tremor, anxiety, and panic attacks associated with feelings of impending death. Symptoms improved when he was away from his office for prolonged periods. Finally, symptoms of peripheral numbness, cold sweats, chills, tachycardia, and recent memory loss prompted a neurologic investigation, which revealed encephalopathy. By the time mercury toxicity was suspected, the patient was disabled and had to give up his practice.

During initial chelation therapy with edetate calcium disodium, the serum thyroxine (T_4) concentration rose from 8 to 27 μg/dL (normal, 4.5–12 μg/dL). Uptake of radioactive iodine by the thyroid gland was high. The patient was treated with propylthiouracil for hyperthyroidism. Current values of thyroid function tests are serum T_4 concentration, 7.8 μg/dL; serum thyroid-stimulating hormone concentration, 1.3 μU/mL (normal, 0.5–5.0 μU/mL); and triiodothyronine uptake, 33.1% (normal, 25–35%). The titer of antithyroglobulin antibody was elevated at 1:320 (normal, up to 1:10), and the value from a second (repeat) determination was 1:80; the titer is now normal. The titer of antimicrosomal thyroid antibody was 1:400 (normal, up to 1:100) and remains at the same value. The patient is clinically euthyroid and takes no medication.

It is unlikely that this spontaneous development of and recovery from hyperthyroidism was coincidental. Studies for the presence of the following autoantibodies were negative: antinuclear, anti-double-stranded DNA, anti-RNA, anti-soluble-nuclear antigen, anti-La (La is an extractable nuclear antigen formerly called SS A), anti-RO (RO is another extractable nuclear antigen, formerly SS B), antiadrenal, and antiscleroderma. These results suggest autoimmunity specific for thyroglobulin in this patient. The concentration of circulating immune complexes, measured by two nonspecific methods, was higher than normal. The numbers of T and B cells were normal. Mercury induces immune-complex formation in rats and mice.[3] The laboratory results above suggest that mercury may have been intimately, albeit indirectly, related to the symptoms and signs of hyperthyroidism in this patient.

There is evidence in animals that mercury alters the sulfur–hydrogen bond in various molecules, including hemoglobin, immunoglobulins, thyroxine, and even insulin.[4,5] In this regard, it is notable that the patient had transient polycythemia; the hematocrit was 54.5% and is now 50%. Mercury may also alter normal hemoglobin molecules, an effect that could signal the body's immune system to recognize the altered hemoglobin as nonself.

The total body burden of mercury in cases of toxicity in humans is difficult to measure clinically, but the half-life of mercury in the central nervous system in mammals is much longer than that in other tissues.[6,7] This may account for a continued abnormal antigen drive long after the mercury concentration in extracellular fluid becomes normal.

It is also possible that the varied clinical manifestation of mercury exposure—the fact that some persons become ill and others do not—is related to the individual's specific class II HLA histocompatibility antigens that control recognition of foreign antigens.

The effects of mercury exposure should be vigorously investigated using modern immunologic techniques. Although mercury's toxic potential is now recognized—in this country, mercury can no longer be an ingredient of interior paints, and Sweden will prohibit the use of mercury-containing dental amalgams starting in 1992—exposure to the element is still widespread. The mercury–silver dental fillings used in the United States, for example, contribute heavily to Americans' total body burden of mercury.[8] Because immunoglobulins are important in fetal organogenesis, and because the fetus is particularly sensitive to maternal mercury exposure,[9] it is particularly important to study the immunologic effects of mercury in pregnancy.

Mercury exposure should be considered for more than its classic toxicological effects. Even minuscule amounts of a foreign antigen or hapten, such as mercury, can have profound clinical effects in genetically susceptible individuals. The link between autoimmune disorders, such as thyroid dysfunction, and mercury should prove to be an important and fertile topic of investigation.[2,3,10-12]

1. Florentine MJ, Sanfilippo DJ II. Elemental mercury poisoning. *Clin Pharm.* 1991; 10:213-21.
2. Hultman D, Enestrom S. Mercury induced B-cell activation and antinuclear antibodies in mice. *J Clin Lab Immunol.* 1989; 28:143-50.
3. Bellon B, Capron M, Druet E et al. Mercuric chloride induced autoimmune disease in Brown-Norway rats: sequential search for anti-basement membrane antibodies and circulating immune complexes. *Eur J Clin Invest.* 1982; 12:127-34.
4. Dailey HA. Effect of sulfhydryl group modification in the activity of bovine ferrochelatase. *J Biol Chem.* 1984; 259:2711-5.
5. Vallee BL, Ulmer DD. Biochemical effects of mercury, cadmium and lead. *Annu Rev Biochem.* 1972; 41:91-127.
6. Sugita M. The biological half-time of heavy metals: the existence of a third, "slowest" component. *Int Arch Occup Environ Health.* 1978; 41:25-40.
7. Newton D, Fry FA. The retention and distribution of radioactive mercuric oxide following accidental inhalation. *Ann Occup Hyg.* 1978; 21:21-32.
8. Clarkson TW, Friberg L, Nylander M et al. Prediction of intake of mercury vapor from amalgam. In: Clarkson TW, Friberg L, Nordberg GF et al., eds. Biological monitoring of toxic metals. New York: Plenum; 1988: 247-55.
9. Koos BJ, Longo L. Mercury toxicity in pregnant women, fetus and newborn infant. *Am J Obstet Gynecol.* 1976; 126:390-409.
10. Hirsch F, Couderc J, Sapin C et al. Polyclonal effect of $HgCl_2$ in the rat: its possible role in experimental autoimmune disease. *Eur J Immunol.* 1982; 12:620-5.
11. Nishida M, Muraoka K, Nishikawa K et al. Differential effects of methylmercury chloride and mercuric chloride on the histochemistry of rat thyroid peroxidase and the thyroid peroxidase activity of isolated pig thyroid cells. *J Histochem Cytochem.* 1989; 37:723-7.
12. Pelletier L, Pasquier R, Rossert J et al. Autoreactive T cells in mercury-induced autoimmunity: ability to induce the autoimmune disease. *J Immunol.* 1988; 140:750-5.

Michael McCann, M.D.
Department of Allergy and Immunology
Kaiser Medical Center
12301 Snow Road
Parma, OH 44130

Stuart Scheckner, D.D.S.
4854 Primrose Path
Sarasota, FL 34242

Ethnicity and clozapine-induced agranulocytosis

Bond[1] suggested in the June issue of *Clinical Pharmacy* that "the influence of ethnicity on psychotropic drug disposition and effect will become increasingly important in clinical practice." Ethnicity may also play a role in the development and severity of psychotropic-induced adverse effects, as has been reported with the new antipsychotic agent clozapine.[2-4]

The major adverse effect of clozapine is agranulocytosis, and this reaction was noted to be especially dangerous and prevalent during an "epidemic" in southwest Finland in 1975.[3-5] The frequency of agranulocytosis during this outbreak was approximately 21 times greater than that observed in other countries.[3,4] Local genetic or environmental factors may have been involved in the Finnish cases, but they have yet to be elucidated.[3,4]

More recently, it has been found that a disproportionate number of clozapine-treated patients in the United States who have developed agranulocytosis during treatment have been of eastern European Jewish heritage.[2] Results of genetic typing have indicated that a genetic factor may be associated with the susceptibility of Jewish patients to develop agranulocytosis when treated with clozapine.[2] In addition, the frequency of some phenotypes common among the Ashkenazi Jewish population is greatly increased in patients who develop clozapine-induced agranulocytosis.[2]

No studies comparing the pharmacokinetics of clozapine in different ethnic groups have been performed. In addition, there are no recommendations about dosage or about precautions, such as intensified hematologic monitoring, for Finnish or Jewish patients treated with clozapine. Nevertheless, the possible genetic factors involved in the development of agranulocytosis should be consid-

Continued on page 744

Letters *Continued from page 743*

ered when these patients are being treated with this drug. These possible ethnic differences may become even more important as more patients receive clozapine as a result of Sandoz's less restrictive clozapine-distribution policies.

1. Bond WS. Ethnicity and psychotropic drugs. *Clin Pharm*. 1991; 10:467-70.
2. Lieberman JA, Yunic J, Egea E et al. HLA-B38, DR4, DQw3 and clozapine-induced agranulocytosis in Jewish patients with schizophrenia. *Arch Gen Psychiatry*. 1990; 26:179.
3. De la Chapelle A, Kari C, Nurinen M et al. Clozapine-induced agranulocytosis: a genetic and epidemiological study. *Hum Genet*. 1977; 37:183-94.
4. Anderman B, Griffith RW. Clozapine-induced agranulocytosis: a situation report up to August 1976. *Eur J Clin Pharmacol*. 1977; 11:199-210.
5. Amsler HA, Teerenhovi L, Barth E et al. Agranulocytosis in patients treated with clozapine: a study of the Finnish epidemic. *Acta Psychiatr Scand*. 1977; 56:241-8.

Karen Overstreet Price, M.S., Editor
Adverceutics, Inc.
14502 Greenview Drive, Suite 410
Laurel, MD 20708

Therapy Reviews

Management of postoperative pain by continuous epidural infusion of analgesics

AMY L. SHAFER AND ANDREW J. DONNELLY

Abstract: The anatomy and physiology of the epidural space and the mechanism of action, sites of action, and pharmacokinetics of analgesics administered by continuous epidural infusion are reviewed, and the efficacy, adverse effects, and postoperative indications for use of analgesics administered by this route are discussed.

Narcotics selectively block pain conduction by occupying specific opiate receptors in the spinal cord. Local anesthetics provide analgesia by axonal membrane blockade; they also can produce nonselective sympathetic and somatic (sensory and motor) blockade in addition to analgesia. A narcotic–local anesthetic mixture should provide an additive analgesic effect, without an increase in the incidence of adverse effects. Comparative efficacy studies have shown that continuous epidural infusions of narcotics, local anesthetics, and narcotic–local anesthetic combinations, when used appropriately, may produce better analgesia than conventional bolus methods of pain relief. Continuous epidural infusions also offer a safety advantage over intermittent epidural injections because peak and trough levels of the analgesic agent are avoided.

Adverse effects of epidurally administered narcotics include respiratory depression, pruritus, urinary retention, nausea and vomiting, and sedation. Adverse effects of epidurally administered local anesthetics include urinary retention, hypotension, numbness, motor weakness, tachyphylaxis, and, rarely, systemic toxicity. The cost of epidurally administered drugs is substantially higher than that for i.m. or i.v. narcotic analgesia, but this cost may be offset by other benefits such as a shorter hospital stay.

Current studies suggest superior analgesia for the majority of surgical procedures with continuous epidural analgesic infusions compared with more traditional methods of providing analgesia.

Index terms: Analgesics and antipyretics; Anesthetics, local; Dosage schedules; Drug administration routes; Injections; Mechanism of action; Opiates; Pain; Pharmacokinetics; Toxicity
Clin Pharm. 1991; 10:745-64

Pain has long been recognized as a valuable indicator of a pathologic event. Postoperative pain, however, has limited utility and numerous disadvantages. Acute pain contributes to postoperative morbidity.[1] Linked to the stress response of surgery, postoperative pain can result in catecholamine release, hypercoagulability, catabolism and protein wasting, immunosuppression, and vasoconstriction.[1,2] Pain associated with upper abdominal or thoracic surgery often causes restricted pulmonary function and subsequent acute pulmonary disease resulting from decreased vital capacity and tidal volume.[1]

The standard therapy for postoperative pain has been i.m. injection of narcotics. However, it has been reported that as many as 75% of patients receiving i.m. narcotics remain in moderate to severe pain, a rate that is considered unacceptable.[3] Suboptimal pain therapy has been attributed to several factors, including inappropriate drug orders, a wide patient variability in narcotic requirements, and the fear of narcotic addiction.[1] Inappropriate prescribing practices may be attributed in part to the physician's inability to fully

AMY L. SHAFER, PHARM.D., is Clinical Pharmacist, Operating Room, New England Medical Center, Boston, MA. ANDREW J. DONNELLY, PHARM.D., M.B.A., is Assistant Director for Clinical Services and Clinical Pharmacist, Operating Room, Rush-Presbyterian-St. Luke's Medical Center, Chicago, IL.

Address reprint requests to Dr. Shafer at the Department of Pharmacy (420), New England Medical Center, 750 Washington Street, Boston, MA 02111.

The assistance of the following persons in the review of this manuscript is acknowledged: F. Michael Ferrante, M.D., Graf Hilgenhurst, M.D., Timothy Lubenow, M.D., L. Michael Newman, M.D., and Michael Spector, M.D.

This is **article 680-204-9124** in the **ASHP Continuing Education System;** it qualifies for 1.0 hour of continuing-education credit. See page 792 for learning objectives and test questions.

appreciate the pain of the patient[1] and to the fourfold to sixfold variation in short-term postoperative narcotic requirements among patients.[4] In one study, more than 85% of all injections intended for i.m. administration were actually given subcutaneously, which suggests nonuniform absorption as one explanation for the wide variation in dose–response curves among individuals.[5]

The epidural route of administration for analgesia has grown in popularity over the past 5 to 10 years. The first analgesics routinely administered by this route were local anesthetics. Sacral[6,7] and then lumbar[8] epidural cocaine injections were reported in 1901; later, agents more appropriately designed for epidural use, such as lidocaine and bupivacaine, became available. Placement of a drug in the spinal canal for postoperative analgesia was reported in 1949.[9] Most of the early reports in this field were case studies, rather than scientific research identifying drug mechanisms or pharmacokinetic profiles. Consequently, widespread clinical use of the described techniques did not occur. In the 1970s, research in this area increased as opiate receptors were identified in the spinal cord,[10] and epidural morphine was administered as a bolus injection for relief of postoperative pain.[11] Today, epidural narcotics, local anesthetics, or both are commonly administered for intraoperative anesthesia and postoperative analgesia. Continuous infusion rather than intermittent injection of these agents has been associated with less frequent adverse effects and has broadened their clinical uses.

In this article, the anatomy and physiology of the epidural space and the mechanism of action, sites of action, and pharmacokinetics of analgesics administered by continuous epidural infusion are reviewed. In addition, the efficacy, adverse effects, and indications for use of analgesics commonly administered by continuous epidural infusion for postoperative pain relief are discussed.

Anatomy and Physiology

Spinal Cord. The spinal cord is a cylindrical mass of nervous tissue occupying the upper two thirds of the spinal canal. It is enclosed by the spinal (vertebral) column, which is a segmented structure composed of 33 individual vertebrae. These are divided into five groups (from the top downward: cervical [C], thoracic [T], lumbar [L], sacral [S], and coccygeal). The spinal cord extends from the base of the skull at the foramen magnum to the superior border of the second lumbar vertebra.[12] Absence of the spinal cord below L2 makes epidural punctures in the lumbar area safer to perform. However, epidural catheterization is possible throughout the length of the spinal cord.[13-17] Figure 1 summarizes the anatomy of the spinal cord.

There are 31 pairs of spinal nerves (mixed nerves that contain afferent and efferent fibers [both somatic and autonomic]), each arising from a ventral and a dorsal root.[12] Each spinal nerve innervates specific areas of the skin, referred to as dermatomes. Knowledge of dermatomal distribution is useful in determining placement of the epidural catheter to obtain desired analgesia.

Within the spinal column, the spinal cord is surrounded by three membranes (meninges): the pia mater, arachnoid mater, and dura mater. The pia mater, the innermost membrane, is highly vascular and responsible for nourishing the cells within the spinal cord. The arachnoid mater, the middle membrane, is located immediately under the dura mater. The dura mater, the outermost membrane, is the toughest of the three sheaths surrounding the spinal cord. Cerebrospinal fluid (CSF) is contained in the space between the pia mater and the arachnoid mater. This space is referred to as the subarachnoid or intrathecal space. In the spinal root region, the arachnoid mater contains bunches of arachnoid cells that protrude through the subdural space (the space between the dura mater and the arachnoid mater), the dura mater, and the walls of veins. These bunches of cells form arachnoid granulations or "villi" and are important in drug transport in the CSF.[18,19] Both the dura mater and the arachnoid mater end at the lower border of the second sacral vertebra. The subdural space is small and contains serous fluid (lymph), but no CSF. The dura mater and the arachnoid mater are in such close proximity that if the dura mater is punctured, the arachnoid mater is usually also punctured.[12,18-20]

Epidural Space. The epidural space (also known as the extradural space or peridural space) is located between the outer surface of the dura mater and the bony and ligamentous walls of the spinal canal. Extending from the foramen magnum to the sacral hiatus, it is generally a small, conical space and is not as voluminous as the subarachnoid space. The epidural space narrows as it ascends, with the largest capacity being in the caudal canal. The smaller capacity of the space at upper levels has direct implications for epidural analgesia because a given volume of agent will affect a greater number of segments in the cervical and thoracic spinal regions compared with the lumbar spinal regions.[12,18-20] Figure 2 depicts the epidural space and surrounding anatomy.

The contents of the epidural space include nerve roots, fat, spinal arteries, lymphatic channels, and a valveless venous system.[12,18-20] These structures can influence both the location of epidural entry and the pharmacokinetics of the agents injected into the epidural space.

Fat is found in the greatest quantities in the posterior portion of the epidural space and is a loose, lobulated, semifluid areolar tissue. The quantity of fat in the epidural space varies in direct proportion to the amount of fat contained elsewhere in the body.[12] Epidural fat contains a rich network of capillaries and provides a large surface area for the uptake of agents.

Epidural veins receive blood from the basivertebral veins and the spinal cord. The epidural veins are large and valveless and form a plexus that is most dense in

Figure 1. Spinal cord anatomy. (Reprinted with permission of the National Association of Orthopedic Nurses from: Genge ML. Epidural analgesia in the orthopedic patient. *Orthop Nurs.* 1988; 7[Jul-Aug]:11-18.)

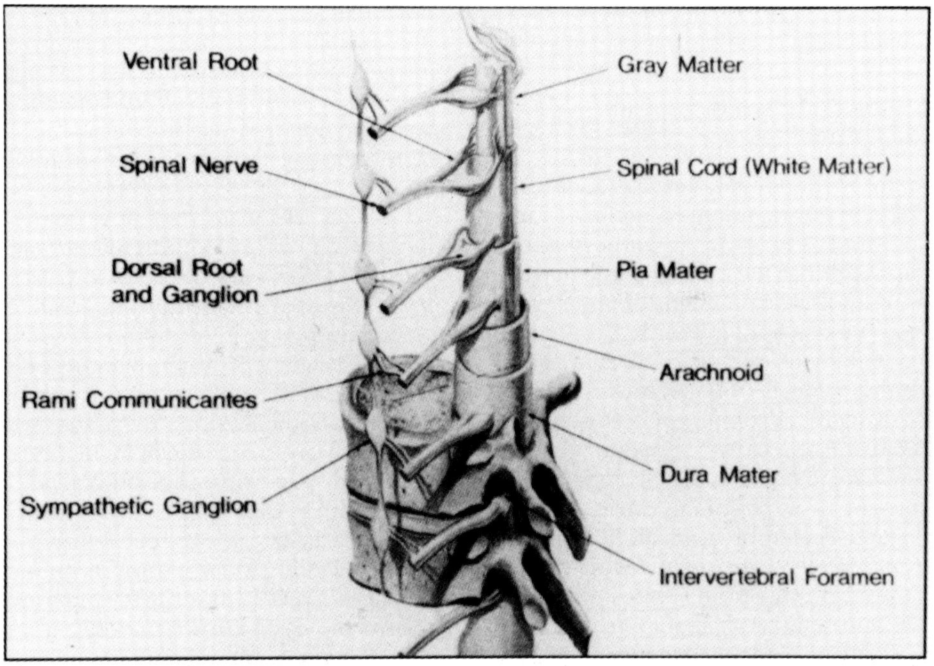

Figure 2. Epidural space and surrounding anatomy. (Reprinted with permission of the National Association of Orthopedic Nurses from: Genge ML. Epidural analgesia in the orthopedic patient. *Orthop Nurs.* 1988; 7[Jul-Aug]:11-18.)

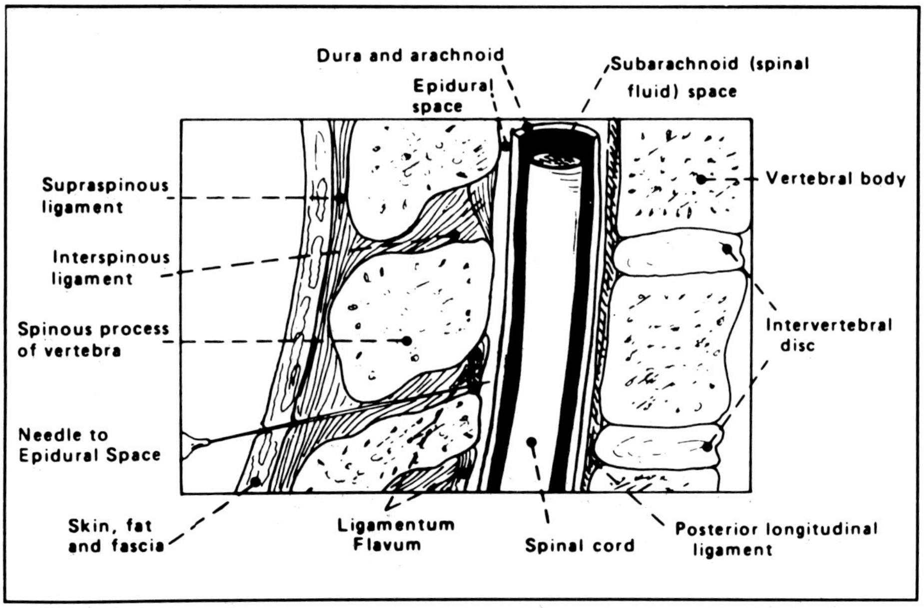

the anterolateral part of the epidural space. The epidural veins communicate superiorly with intracranial sinuses (occipital, sigmoid, and basilar venous sinuses) via the basivertebral veins, posteriorly through the azygos vein to tributaries of the inferior vena cava (iliac and uterine veins), and with thoracic and abdominal veins by way of the intervertebral foramina. Because the main longitudinal channels of the epidural plexus are valveless, a continuous vascular connection exists between the cerebral venous sinuses and the pelvis. As a result, direct access to the brain is possible for agents injected epidurally. Thus, the potential for central nervous system (CNS) toxicity exists if an agent is administered in sufficient doses. In the dural cuff region, arachnoid granulations invaginate the epidural veins. At these sites, drug passage into the CSF is facilitated.[12,18] Ventral and dorsal spinal nerve roots also pass through the epidural space. The spinal dural membrane covers the spinal nerve roots. The dural covering of the nerve roots becomes thinner as the intervertebral foramina are approached.[18] Local anesthetics are injected into the epidural space to block the spinal nerve roots and to block nerve conduction, thereby producing analgesia.

Mechanism and Sites of Action of Epidural Narcotics and Local Anesthetics

Mitigation of pain at the spinal cord level can be achieved by (1) blocking the receptors from the actions of the neurotransmitters released by the primary afferent pain fibers, (2) preventing the release of the neurotransmitters from the afferent pain fibers, (3) interrupting the transmission of nociceptive information in the dorsal horn, or (4) blocking afferent pain fiber impulse conduction (inhibition of cell depolarization secondary to sodium-channel blockade). Depending on the agent chosen for epidural administration, one or more of these effects can be realized.

Narcotics. Various areas of the spinal cord (e.g., substantia gelatinosa) and certain portions of the brain (e.g., medullary dorsal horn, periaqueductal gray matter) contain substantial numbers of opiate receptors. Agents (both endogenous and exogenous) that occupy these receptors can alter the transmission of nociceptive information in the CNS and hence modulate pain. Opiate receptors can be divided into five types: mu (types 1 and 2), kappa, delta, sigma, and epsilon. The mu, kappa, and delta receptors constitute approximately 40%, 50%, and 10%, respectively, of the spinal opiate receptors.[21] Activation of mu receptors appears to result in the relief of both somatic (body wall) and visceral (organ) pain, whereas activation of kappa and delta receptors relieves primarily visceral pain and somatic pain, respectively.[22] Table 1 presents a summary of the possible CNS effects that can be seen when these receptors are activated.[23,24]

Because narcotics act at specific spinal cord receptors, these drugs selectively block pain conduction and have no effect on motor or sensory function. Hence, the term "selective spinal analgesia" has been used to describe the pain relief obtained by epidurally administered narcotics. The two major sites of action of epidurally administered narcotics are the presynaptic and postsynaptic receptors in the substantia gelatinosa of the dorsal horn of the spinal cord.[22] Lipid-soluble narcotics are also taken up into the posterior radicular artery, which is located near the dural cuff region. Absorption into the systemic circulation (via the epidural venous plexus) can also contribute to the analgesic effects of epidurally administered narcotics.[22]

Narcotics vary in terms of their predominant sites of action in the CNS. Morphine appears to act predominantly at the spinal cord level; supraspinal migration of the drug contributes to a secondary analgesic effect.[25] Fentanyl, because of its high lipid solubility, also seems to have substantial brain activity via systemic absorption. Lofentanil (not commercially available in the United States) is a lipid-soluble agent with a high affinity for opiate receptors. Lofentanil has primarily a spinal action with little supraspinal activity. This specificity has been attributed to the drug's slow dissociation from opiate receptors and substantial storage in spinal lipid.[26]

Table 1.
Opiate Receptors and Actions[a]

Receptor Type	Activity
Mu-1	Supraspinal analgesia Miosis Euphoria Hypothermia
Mu-2	Respiratory depression Physical dependence Sedation Bradycardia
Kappa	Spinal analgesia Sedation (more than mu-2) Miosis Respiratory depression (possible)
Delta	Analgesia Alterations in affective behavior
Sigma	Psychomotor stimulation Hallucinations
Epsilon	Dysphoria Analgesia

[a] Adapted from references 23 and 24.

Local Anesthetics. Local anesthetics produce analgesia by axonal membrane blockade. Local anesthetics prevent nerve impulse conduction by penetrating the axonal membrane and attaching to a receptor site located on the internal surface of a sodium channel. Receptor attachment results in blockade of the sodium channel, inhibition of sodium conductance, and a decrease in the rate and degree of the depolarization phase of the action potential. If the necessary threshold potential level is not achieved, the action potential cannot be propagated and neural conduction is prevented.[27]

Local anesthetics can produce nonselective sympathetic and somatic (sensory and motor) blockade in addition to analgesia. These effects are directly related to the concentration of local anesthetic and the depth of nerve penetration. C fibers (pain transmission and autonomic activity) and B fibers (preganglionic sympathetic) appear to be most easily blocked by a given concentration of local anesthetic. Fibers responsible for touch and pressure sensation (A-alpha, A-beta, and A-delta) and those responsible for motor function (A-alpha and A-beta) are blocked by increasing concentrations of anesthetic. Therefore, the minimum blocking concentration (C_m) of local anesthetic is lowest for C fibers and highest for motor function fibers. This is the basis for development of what is termed "differential nerve block." Depending on the concentration of local anesthetic, analgesia can be selectively obtained. However, when the concentration of local anesthetic is sufficient, sympathetic, sensory, and motor blockade will also occur.[28] Some degree of autonomic block is unavoidable with epidural administration of local anesthetics and is discussed in the Adverse Drug Reactions section.

Figure 3 depicts the primary sites of action of epidural narcotics and local anesthetics.

Pharmacokinetics and Pharmacodynamics

Basic properties governing the movement of local anesthetics and narcotics in the epidural and subarachnoid spaces explain differences in onset of action, duration of action, achievable plasma concentrations, and the relative efficacy and toxicity of various epidurally administered analgesics. Local anesthetics and narcotics must penetrate the dura to reach their sites of action in the spinal cord, while available drug is also distributed to epidural fat or systemically absorbed via epidural veins. The amount of injected drug reaching the CSF is small; approximately 4% of an epidural bolus dose of morphine or meperidine can be found in the CSF.[29] Once in the subarachnoid space, drug molecules can interact with receptors in the spinal cord or spinal nerve roots. They can also be carried by bulk flow of CSF toward the brain and away from the site of injection, a phenomenon known as rostral spread.

Table 2 lists the physical and pharmacologic properties of narcotics and local anesthetics administered by the epidural route. Although the information presented below is useful in obtaining a baseline understanding of drug effects, it must be considered in the context of a continuous infusion for postoperative

Figure 3. Primary sites of action of epidural narcotics and local anesthetics. (Reprinted with permission of the W. B. Saunders Company from: Litwack K, Lubenow T. Practical points in the management of continuous epidural infusions. *J Post Anesth Nurs.* 1989; 4:327-30.)

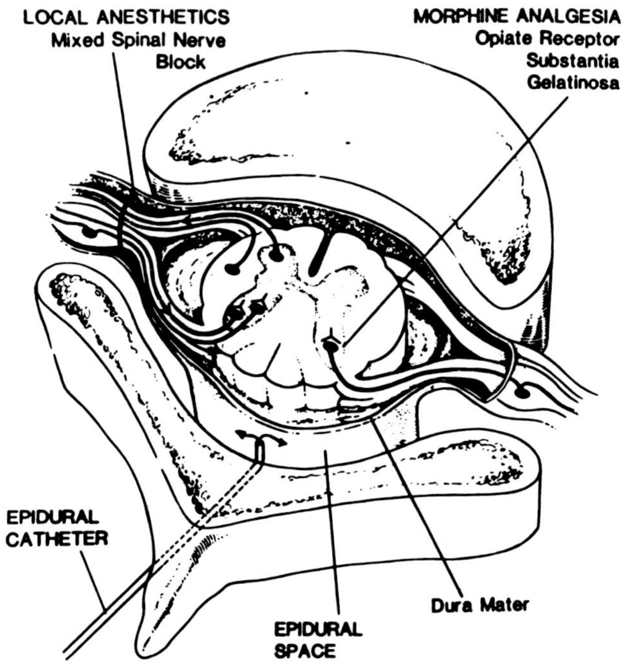

pain relief. In this situation, onset and duration are lesser factors, important primarily when infusion rates are altered or discontinued. An appreciation of catheter placement considerations, dermatomal spread, and systemic absorption is most useful in assessing the appropriateness, efficacy, and toxicities of the drugs chosen for administration. It should also be emphasized that variability among patients with respect to pain perception and dosage requirements is large, and individualized dosing of epidural narcotics or local anesthetics is necessary regardless of standard recommendations.

Narcotics. Lipid solubility appears to be the most important determinant of narcotic onset of action, dermatomal spread, and duration of effect.[28] Drugs with low lipid solubility have a slower onset of action, greater dermatomal spread, and longer duration of effect than those with high lipid solubility.

Onset. The relationship between lipid solubility and onset is explained by the more rapid penetration through the dura mater of highly lipid soluble narcotics. All drugs enter the CSF by diffusion through the arachnoid villi at the dural root cuffs, but highly lipid-soluble narcotics also gain access by uptake into the spinal arteries.[33] These arteries, which run close to the dural cuff region, are small and thus easily penetrated by lipid-soluble drugs.[21] Rapid access to the CSF is demonstrated clinically by the similarity in onset of action of lipophilic narcotics administered by epidural injection and by direct subarachnoid injection.[21] Aside from lipid solubility, onset of action is affected to a minor degree by molecular weight and shape.[34]

Morphine, a narcotic with comparatively low lipid solubility, has a relatively slow onset of action of approximately 30–40 minutes when injected as an epidural bolus. It will reach the CSF slowly (peak CSF concentrations occur in 90 minutes[35]) because of the small percentage of lipid-soluble, unionized drug that is available to diffuse across the dura mater and arachnoid villi and into spinal arteries. Epidural injection of more lipophilic drugs such as meperidine, fentanyl, or methadone will result in rapid onset (approximately 10–15 minutes for each) because more unionized drug is available to speed membrane transfer. Several studies have demonstrated the comparative onsets of opioids and their relationship to lipid solubility.[36,37]

Duration. The duration of epidural analgesia is also related to the lipid solubility of the agent.[38] Morphine has a long duration of action because drug molecules diffuse slowly away from spinal cord receptors and through lipid membranes. The durations of action of the more lipophilic agents fentanyl, meperidine, and methadone are shorter.

Duration of effect is also influenced by opiate-receptor affinity. Lofentanil and sufentanil, which have higher affinity for spinal opiate receptors,[39] have long durations of action.[31] Their duration may also be longer because of nonspecific binding to epidural fat, an effect opposite to the net effect of lipid solubility on duration.[40] Finally, duration of action depends on the

Table 2.
Physical and Pharmacologic Properties of Narcotics and Local Anesthetics during Epidural Bolus Administration[a]

Drug	pKa	Partition[b] Coefficient	Onset of Action of Bolus (min)	Duration of Action of Bolus (hr)	Typical Bolus Dose
Narcotics					
Morphine	7.9	1.4	30	12–20	1–6 mg[c]
Fentanyl	8.4	813	5	3–6	25–100 μg[d]
Meperidine	8.5	39	5–10	6–8	20–60 mg[e]
Methadone	9.3	116	10	6–10	2–6 mg[e]
Alfentanil	6.5	129	5	2–3	1 mg[f]
Sufentanil	8.0	1778	5	4–6	10–50 μg[d]
Hydromorphone	8.0	1.4	15	10–16	1–1.5 mg[e]
Lofentanil	7.8	1450	15	7–8	. . .
Buprenorphine	8.6	. . .	20	6–12	0.06–0.3 mg[f]
Butorphanol	. . .	. . .	15	5–9	4 mg[g]
Local Anesthetics					
Chloroprocaine	9.0	0.14	6–12	0.5–1	300–750 mg[e]
Bupivacaine	8.1	27.5	4–17	2–5	12.5–35 mg[e]
Lidocaine	7.9	2.9	5–15	1–2	160–300 mg[e]

[a] Adapted from references 21 and 30–32.
[b] Octanol:pH 4 buffer (for narcotics) or n-heptane:pH 4 buffer (for local anesthetics); both correlate directly with lipid solubility.
[c] Expressed as mg of sulfate salt.
[d] Expressed as μg of base drug (given as citrate salt).
[e] Expressed as mg of hydrochloride salt.
[f] Expressed as mg of base drug (given as hydrochloride salt).
[g] Expressed as mg of tartrate salt.

dose of drug, the pain stimulus, and much interpatient variation.[28]

Dermatomal Spread. This term refers to the magnitude of longitudinal area of the spinal cord (and the corresponding body dermatomes) affected by the injected drug. Hydrophilic drugs, such as morphine, will exhibit greater dermatomal spread than lipophilic narcotics. Ionized drug, which binds less readily to opiate receptors, will eventually be present in the water phase of the CSF and will freely migrate upward by rostral flow, extending the level of spinal analgesia. The clinical importance of this dermatomal or rostral spreading is evidenced by the fact that a lumbar epidural injection of morphine is as effective as a thoracic epidural injection for relief of thoracic pain.[41-43] Lipophilic drugs exhibit a lesser degree of dermatomal spread. Thus, the dermatomes affected by surgical pain are important in the determination of the site of catheter placement (lumbar or thoracic). Of equal clinical importance is the phenomenon of delayed respiratory depression, which is believed to be caused by continued rostral spread of narcotic to the fourth ventricle (see Adverse Drug Reactions).

Systemic Uptake. The pharmacodynamics and pharmacokinetics of epidural narcotics are complicated by the fact that plasma concentrations often reach the analgesic range. Drug absorption from the epidural space via the epidural venous system is responsible for this systemic uptake. Studies have demonstrated that, in general, analgesia from epidurally administered narcotics correlates well with CSF concentrations rather than plasma concentrations of drug, although plasma concentrations may reach analgesic levels via systemic uptake.[21]

The earliest study of epidural narcotic pharmacokinetics was performed with meperidine hydrochloride,[44] in which a single epidural bolus of 100 mg was injected in seven patients who had postoperative pain. Peak CSF concentrations occurred in 12–20 minutes, coinciding with complete pain relief. Peak blood concentrations occurred after 40 minutes. These blood concentrations were in the analgesic range in some patients, but they resulted in no actual increase in analgesia and a mild transitory sedative effect. Analgesia lasted well beyond the time when blood concentrations had declined below effective levels. These findings led the authors to conclude that the analgesic effect resulted from a direct spinal mechanism of action and not a central mechanism of action.

Other studies have confirmed these findings[29,35,45]; studies with morphine[35,46-48] and fentanyl[49,50] also support a spinal mechanism of action. In most cases, peak plasma concentrations decline much more rapidly than do CSF concentrations, so systemically absorbed drug could contribute to analgesia for only an initial fraction of the duration of a bolus dose, something that has been shown for morphine and meperidine.[29] With continuous infusion or repeat bolus dosing, however, the contribution of plasma concentrations may be substantial, especially with drugs such as methadone that have relatively long elimination half-lives. Recent studies comparing plasma fentanyl concentrations after epidural and i.v. infusions or injections have found concentrations to be similar within 18 hours; the authors suggest that, over time, epidural fentanyl may have no advantage over i.v. fentanyl with respect to efficacy.[51,52]

Systemic narcotic absorption after epidural administration proceeds via the epidural venous plexus, the azygos vein, and then the inferior vena cava. Partial obstruction of the inferior vena cava, which is seen during pregnancy, may distend the epidural and azygos veins, increasing the rate of systemic drug absorption. In these situations, analgesia may correlate better with plasma concentrations than with CSF concentrations of drug.[53,54] Vascular uptake does not correlate well with the lipid solubility of a drug. Although morphine achieves a more rapid peak plasma concentration (occurring 10 minutes after epidural injection[25]) than meperidine,[55] fentanyl also develops rapid peak plasma concentrations after an epidural bolus.[56] In summary, epidurally administered narcotics may exert substantial central action as a result of systemic absorption, but narcotics that are administered i.v. will not have their action enhanced by favorable partition into the CSF.[21] Finally, the pharmacokinetics of epidural narcotics may be affected by pre-existing plasma concentrations. Substantial plasma concentrations before epidural injection may decrease vascular absorption by reduction in the concentration gradient.[28] Higher CSF levels and longer duration of action may result.

Local Anesthetics. *Effect of Lipophilicity.* Lipid solubility is the primary determinant of potency for the local anesthetics.[30] Agents such as chloroprocaine hydrochloride, which has relatively low lipid solubility, have low anesthetic potency and must be injected in higher concentrations (2–3%) to achieve desired effects compared with lidocaine hydrochloride (1–2%), which has intermediate potency and lipophilicity, and bupivacaine hydrochloride (0.25–0.5%), which has high anesthetic potency and lipophilicity. Unlike the narcotics, the onset of action of local anesthetics does not correlate directly with lipophilicity in vivo. Chloroprocaine has the most rapid onset, followed by lidocaine and finally bupivacaine. Peak CSF drug concentrations occur within 10 to 20 minutes for all drugs,[33] indicating rapid penetration of the dura mater after epidural injection.

Lipid-soluble local anesthetics such as bupivacaine are sequestered in epidural fat, which prolongs the duration of action after injection. Absorption of lipid-soluble agents into the systemic circulation is slowed.[33] After a single epidural injection, the increment in peak whole blood drug concentration per 100 mg of drug is approximately 1.0 μg/mL for lidocaine hydrochloride and 0.5 μg/mL for bupivacaine hydrochloride.[57] With repeat injection or continued administration of bupivacaine, epidural fat concentrations rise but blood concentrations tend to remain the same, provided an appropriate dose is given. The administration of additional lidocaine, a more hydrophilic drug, by repeated doses or continuous infusion may result in minimal drug accumulation in epidural fat but may produce substantial increases in the plasma concentration.[18] Because of its relatively stable blood concentrations, bupivacaine is more ideally suited than lidocaine for continuous administration by infusion despite the longer duration of action and longer elimination half-life of bupivacaine.

Effect of Injection Volume. The volume of solution administered may influence the spread of the anesthetic. A 30-mL epidural injection of 1% lidocaine hydrochloride was shown to produce an anesthetic level that was 4.3 dermatomes higher than that achieved with 10 mL of 3% lidocaine hydrochloride.[58] Other than spread, however, the mass of drug administered (milligrams) is more important than the volume for onset, depth, and duration of effect.[30]

Effect of Added Vasoconstrictor. Epinephrine (e.g., as a 1:200,000 solution) is often added to local anesthetic solutions before injection to decrease, by causing vasoconstriction, the rate of vascular absorption. Local anesthetics, except cocaine, are vasodilators at concentrations commonly used for regional anesthesia. An epinephrine-induced decrease in the rate of vascular local-anesthetic distribution allows for more local-anesthetic molecules to reach the spinal site of action, which improves the depth and duration of effect. Epinephrine may also reduce systemic toxicity by reducing the vascular uptake of the local anesthetic. The clinical importance of this effect differs based on the local anesthetic; lidocaine has a markedly increased duration of action when administered with epinephrine for epidural blockade,[59] but the duration of action of bupivacaine is not affected substantially.[60] The higher lipid solubility of bupivacaine may be responsible for this diminished effect, because slow release from epidural fat contributes to the drug's usually longer duration of action.

Epinephrine may also enhance analgesia produced by local anesthetics by direct agonist effects on the α-adrenergic receptor. Research has shown that inhibitory receptors in the dorsal horn of the spinal cord are stimulated by α-receptor agonists such as epinephrine or clonidine.[18]

In practice, epinephrine is often administered with lidocaine during the initial intraoperative bolus into the epidural space to prolong the effects of this bolus and to test for appropriate initial placement of the epidural catheter. Inadvertent vascular placement of the catheter is revealed by immediate systemic effects of epinephrine on heart rate and blood pressure. Epinephrine is not commonly added to postoperative epidural continuous infusions, because prolonging the duration of action is no longer a concern.

Effect of Added Sodium Bicarbonate. Sodium bicarbonate can also be added to the local anesthetic solution immediately before injection of the initial bolus dose for intraoperative epidural anesthesia. Sodium bicarbonate reduces the onset time by raising the pH of the injection, which increases the availability of unionized local anesthetic molecules and hence the ability of the drug to diffuse across the dura to the site of action. The amount of bicarbonate added to the solution depends on the pH of the local anesthetic; a final pH of approximately 7 without precipitate formation is ideal. When postoperative continuous infusions are administered, the addition of bicarbonate is not necessary.

Effect of Injection Speed. Injection speed, again a concern only for bolus dosing, has only a minor effect on the spread of analgesia and influences plasma concentrations of lidocaine[61] but not of bupivacaine.[62] Rapid injection of over 30 mL of solution may increase intracranial pressure, causing headache, cerebral hemorrhage, or isolated hemorrhage of a small vessel.[18] Rapid injection is not useful and is potentially dangerous.

Effect of Patient Age. The exact relationship between patient age and epidural dosage requirements is complex and uncertain. The duration and spread of epidural anesthesia are directly proportional to the age of the patient. This relationship is postulated to occur because of a reduced lateral leakage of solution from a progressive sclerotic closure of the intervertebral foramina in elderly patients.[63] Age does not, however, appear to correlate with plasma concentrations. Dosage requirements for epidural blockade diminish at the extremes of age, however, and dosages should be reduced in the elderly and the very young for this reason.

Agents and Dosage

Agents. A wide spectrum of narcotic and nonnarcotic agents have been administered epidurally by continuous infusion for postoperative analgesia. Morphine has been extensively studied and has proved highly successful for pain relief.[13,36,64-72] Pruritus and a potential for delayed respiratory depression with morphine (see Adverse Drug Reactions) have resulted in the examination of alternative agents. More lipid-soluble narcotics (i.e., fentanyl, sufentanil, alfentanil, meperidine, methadone) are effective, have a more rapid onset of action, cause minimal adverse effects, and are not associated with late respiratory depression.[13,36,64,71,73-75] Hydromorphone has also been effectively administered by continuous epidural infusion.[76] In general, when narcotics are administered appropriately, no importantt differences in the quality of analgesia are seen among them.[28]

Local anesthetics have also been administered postoperatively by continuous epidural infusion. Bupivacaine, lidocaine, and chloroprocaine have been used most frequently.[15-17,64,69,77-84] Of these, bupivacaine has been most widely used. Bupivacaine's popularity can be attributed to its predilection for sensory versus motor nerve block, a lesser degree of tachyphylaxis, and its favorable safety profile (stable plasma concentrations over a wide range of epidural doses).[28,64]

Continuous epidural infusions of narcotic–local anesthetic combinations are the standard in many institutions today. Bupivacaine has been used in combination with fentanyl, morphine, meperidine, and sufentanil.[15,17,64,68,69,77,85] For several reasons, a narcotic–local anesthetic mixture is an excellent choice for postoperative pain relief. Because epidurally administered local anesthetics and narcotics have different mechanisms of action, an additive analgesic effect occurs. As a result, smaller concentrations of each agent can be used in combination than when the agents are used alone. Because most of the complications and adverse effects from these two classes of drugs are not additive, a reduction in the incidence of adverse effects (e.g., tachyphylaxis for local anesthetics, CNS depression with narcotics) is possible. A combination also provides the greatest adaptability to patient needs, because the amount of each agent can be varied to reduce specific adverse effects.

Dosage. Although dosage guidelines for continuous epidural infusions have been developed, the dosage needs to be individualized based on patient-specific characteristics. To highlight this point, Sjostrom et al.[29] found that maximum CSF concentrations of narcotics in individuals varied up to sixfold after epidural administration.

When determining the dosage of a continuous epidural infusion, factors that should be considered are the patient's previous medical history, underlying disease states, type of surgery, and position of catheter placement. A lower dosage of epidural agent is often required in older patients and those of short stature. Logas et al.[68] reduced the initial and maximal epidural infusion rates in patients older than 60 years of age or less than 1.68 meters tall, or both. Adequate analgesia was obtained in these patients. The surgical procedure performed also dictates the dosage (infusion rate) of the epidural infusion. Certain types of surgery are associated with greater pain and may necessitate a larger initial dosage. The placement of the epidural catheter in relation to the agent selected for the continuous epidural infusion can influence the dose required for adequate analgesia. Morphine is capable of producing analgesia over many dermatomes and, as mentioned previously, can be an effective agent for thoracic pain even with lumbar administration. The more lipophilic narcotics produce optimal results when they are used to treat pain of a localized nature. The analgesia produced by these agents occurs mainly at the dermatomes near the epidural catheter tip. To expand the number of dermatomes affected, the infusion rate must be increased.[28]

The relative analgesic potencies of epidural fentanyl, alfentanil, and morphine were determined by Chrubasik et al.[36] Relative to morphine sulfate (potency =1), the potencies of alfentanil and fentanyl are 1 and 10, respectively.

Table 3 lists guidelines for continuous epidural administration of narcotics and local anesthetics. Any drug injected or infused into the epidural space should be free of neurotoxic preservatives (such as methylparaben or benzyl alcohol); for example, morphine or lidocaine products should be clearly marked as appropriate for epidural administration.

General Efficacy

Several advantages of continuous epidural infusions of narcotics, local anesthetics, or both over conventional methods of postoperative analgesia have been

Table 3.
Continuous Epidural Infusion Guidelines for Narcotics and Local Anesthetics[a]

Drug[b]	Initial Bolus Dose (mg)	Infusion Concentration (mg/mL)	Infusion Rate (mg/hr)
Morphine sulfate	2	0.05–0.25	0.2–1.5
Meperidine hydrochloride	50–100	10–20	5–20
Fentanyl (as citrate)	0.05–0.1	0.005–0.025	0.02–0.15
Sufentanil (as citrate)	0.05	0.001	0.05–0.1
Alfentanil (as hydrochloride)	1	0.25	0.2
Methadone hydrochloride	4–6	0.05	0.25–1.5
Hydromorphone hydrochloride	0.5–3	0.02–0.05	0.15–0.3
Bupivacaine hydrochloride	12.5–35	1–5	15–37.5
Lidocaine hydrochloride	160–300	4	120–240

[a] Adapted from references 15, 17, 28, 36, 68, 69, 71, 76, 77, 79, 82, 83, and 85–87.

[b] Preservative-free solutions must be used for admixture and administration. A typical combination solution would contain bupivacaine hydrochloride 1 mg/mL with fentanyl 0.01 mg (as citrate)/mL, sufentanil 0.001 mg (as citrate)/mL, morphine sulfate 0.1 mg/mL, or meperidine hydrochloride 1 mg/mL and would be infused at 5–15 mL/hr.

proposed and tested. Superior pain relief at a smaller cumulative dose has been proposed and will be discussed later in this section through review of comparative efficacy trials. It is important to bear in mind that therapy with continuous epidural infusion may sometimes require supplemental i.v. or i.m. narcotic administration for relief of additional pain during patient manipulation or other stress.

Another proposed advantage of continuous epidural infusion compared with systemic narcotic therapy is less sedation and respiratory depression. Because of fewer central effects, epidural administration may result in comparatively faster return of peak expiratory flow,[88,89] higher arterial oxygen tension,[89] lower arterial carbon dioxide tension,[89] and fewer overall pulmonary complications.[88] Use of epidural analgesia may prevent prolonged postoperative intubation of patients specifically at risk for respiratory depression. Earlier extubation was also demonstrated when epidural morphine was used after cardiac surgery.[66]

When compared with either systemic or epidural bolus dosing, epidural continuous infusion allows for the achievement of steady-state conditions without wide fluctuations in drug concentration. Dosage adjustment can be easily accomplished, and adverse effects or suboptimal analgesia occur slowly over time, allowing correction before they become problematical. Tachyphylaxis, a common complication of bolus local-anesthetic therapy, is much diminished when administration is by continuous infusion. In addition, as discussed earlier, continuous epidural infusions of narcotic–local anesthetic combinations appear to be more efficacious than continuous infusions of a single agent.

Advantages to the use of epidural local anesthetics arise from the sympathetic block caused by these agents. When administered in the lumbar region, local anesthetics may reduce the incidence of deep vein thrombosis and pulmonary embolism postoperatively, possibly secondary to sympathetic block at L1 and L2 with improved lower limb blood flow.[90] Sympathetic block may also improve graft and limb blood flow after vascular surgery.[91] Similarly, local anesthetic-induced sympathetic block at T6 to L1 may decrease the risk of postoperative ileus.[92]

The effect of epidural agents on the postoperative stress response is controversial. This response, induced by surgical injury and semistarvation, typically consists of an increase in metabolic rate and cardiac output, a release of catabolic substances (e.g., cortisol, corticotrophin, antidiuretic hormone, catecholamines, glucagon), and a reduction in insulin release. The stress response may last a few days to weeks after surgery, depending on the degree of surgical trauma. Levels of cortisol, glucose, catecholamines, and other substances are used to measure the stress response; the clinical importance of changes in these levels is uncertain. Epidural block with local anesthetics has been shown to decrease plasma catecholamine levels.[93] The stress-response blocking effect of epidural local anesthetics is clinically important only when the drug is administered before surgery and lasts only for 24–48 hours or less postoperatively.[28] Excessive epidural local anesthetic block has been shown to obtund other neuroendocrine and metabolic responses to surgery.[94] It has been demonstrated that local anesthetics prevent a rise in plasma glucose and allow for only minimal changes in plasma cortisol. This evidence of a reduction in the stress response was found to be significant for lower abdominal surgery but not for the more stressful upper abdominal procedures.[94] The mechanism of reduction in the stress response by local anesthetics is thought to be blockade of afferent noxious stimuli from surgery and possibly epidural blockade of efferent impulse flow to the adrenal medulla and other organs. Epidural narcotics do not substantially affect the stress response. Epidural morphine is not effective in preventing intraoperative changes in plasma cortisol or glucose, but it may slightly modify or delay these changes postoperatively.[95]

A landmark study by Yeager et al.[96] suggests that another important advantage of epidural analgesia is decreased overall morbidity and mortality among high-risk surgical patients. Outcomes included a reduction in the overall postoperative complication rate, a shorter intensive-care-unit stay, and a shorter overall duration of hospitalization compared with patients receiving other forms of injectable narcotic therapy. Another study[77] also suggests that a shorter duration of hospitalization is possible with epidural rather than i.m. on-demand therapy.

Finally, several studies have shown that patients prefer epidural over i.m. narcotic therapy.[97-99]

Comparative Efficacy

To determine the place of continuous epidural infusion in postoperative pain management, controlled studies comparing this administration method with the standard methods of pain relief must continue to be performed. Postoperative pain relief can be provided by three general methods: (1) narcotic administration via the i.m., i.v., or epidural route by standard methods or patient-controlled analgesia (PCA) infusers; (2) local anesthetic administration via the epidural, intercostal, or intrapleural route and by direct injection into a peripheral nerve; and (3) mechanical means such as cryoanalgesia and transcutaneous electrical nerve stimulation. Trials have compared the efficacy of continuous epidural infusions of narcotics, local anesthetics, or both for the treatment of postoperative pain with epidural narcotic administration via a PCA infuser, standard i.v. PCA therapy, intermittent epidural injections of narcotics or local anesthetics, i.v. or i.m. narcotic administration, and other methods of pain relief such as cryoanalgesia. In reviewing these trials, consideration should be given to the following:

1. The method of patient randomization to a treatment group.
2. The type of pain being treated and the similarity of pain in the treatment and control groups.
3. The indicator of positive outcome (i.e., improved analgesia versus duration of analgesia).
4. The location of catheter placement and its appropriateness for the type of pain being treated and the agent chosen.
5. The definition of continuous infusion (i.e., the term is often used incorrectly to describe repeat intermittent epidural injections).

Most determinations of analgesia are subjective and rely totally or in part on a visual analog scale (VAS) or descriptive scales that measure pain intensity or severity and require patient cooperation. The VAS, for example, consists of a straight line with anchor words at each end (e.g., "no pain at all" to "pain as severe as possible"). The patient marks the line at a point that corresponds to the intensity of the pain being experienced. The scale is scored by measuring the distance from the "no pain" end of the line to the patient's mark. Also, standardized dosage equivalents for the i.v., i.m., and epidural routes of administration have not yet been determined, which makes comparisons of dosage and hence analgesic efficacy more difficult.

Table 4 presents a summary of the comparative trials examining the use of continuous epidural infusions for the treatment of postoperative pain. One general comment concerning these studies is that most investigators allowed supplementary analgesics to be administered when needed. However, a general finding in these studies was that the group receiving continuous epidural infusion required less supplementary analgesia. Several of the studies summarized in Table 4 require additional elaboration of the results.

In the study performed by Marlowe et al.,[76] several reasons were given to explain why the total hydromorphone dosage required by the group receiving epidural PCA was significantly lower than that required by the group receiving continuous infusion. The patients randomized to the infusion group appeared to have undergone more extensive and painful operations, and the adjustment of the epidural infusion appeared less than optimal in this group. Additionally, a small number of patients ($n = 8$) were studied in each group.

In a trial assessing postoperative pain relief in thoracotomy patients, Logas et al.[68] attributed the poor pain response seen in patients receiving a continuous epidural infusion of bupivacaine hydrochloride to the low infusion rate (3–6 mL/hr) and concentration (1 mg/mL) used.

The study by Loper et al.,[52] which is the only controlled trial of its type to date, examined the use of a continuous epidural infusion of fentanyl versus continuous intravenous infusion of fentanyl for postoperative (knee surgery) analgesia. No clinical advantages were seen in the epidural group; similar pain scores and adverse effect profiles were observed for both regimens. Examination of the study methodology, however, may explain why these results were obtained. The placement of the epidural catheter may not have been appropriate for the surgery performed. The catheter was placed in the L2–L3 or L3–L4 interspace, which covers the opiate receptors and dorsal horn neurons subserving the L3–L4 dermatome. However, to cover this dermatome, a more appropriate catheter placement may have been at the T11–T12 interspace. In addition, this study used a high-concentration (50 μg/mL), low-volume epidural infusion. This type of infusion would further compound the effect of an inappropriate catheter placement, because sufficient migration of the lipophilic fentanyl to the appropriate site in the spinal cord would be highly unlikely. Therefore, additional study needs to be performed, with particular attention paid to catheter placement and infusion volume.

In the study performed by Griffiths et al.,[83] two continuous epidural bupivacaine infusion were compared with intermittent epidural injections for the treatment of postoperative pain in patients undergoing thoracic surgery. Poor pain relief was seen in the group receiving the continuous epidural infusion, whereas better, but not total, pain relief was obtained in the group receiving intermittent injections. The investigators theorized that the number of thoracic segments blocked in this patient population was insufficient to afford total pain relief in either group because of the need to adjust the dose based on complications (hypotension, drowsiness). The authors attributed the greater efficacy seen in the patients receiving intermittent injections to the more frequent monitoring afforded these patients. Adverse effects were experienced by patients

Table 4.
Summary of Comparative Trials of Epidural Analgesia[a]

Reference	Type of Surgery	No. Patients	Drug and Regimen[b]	Catheter Placement	Outcome
76	Laminectomy, lower and upper abdominal, orthopedic, thoracic, thoracoabdominal	16	Cont. e.d. hydromorphone hydrochloride 0.15–0.3 mg/hr vs. intermittent e.d. PCA 0.15–0.3 mg injection (15–30 min lockout interval)	L2–L4	No difference in level of analgesia or adverse effect profiles. Total dosage for PCA less than that for cont. e.d. ($p < 0.05$).
100	Lumbar fusion	46	Cont. e.d. morphine sulfate 0.5 mg/hr vs. i.v. PCA morphine	Lumbar	Greatest decrease in VAS score for cont. e.d. morphine on postoperative day 1; however, unpredictable pain relief seen. Incidence of adverse effects greater in cont. e.d. group.
72	Upper abdominal	30	Cont. e.d. morphine sulfate 0.5 mg/hr vs. intermittent bolus e.d. morphine sulfate 2–5 mg	T9–T11	VAS and global evaluations significantly better with cont. e.d. ($p < 0.001$). Cont. e.d. avoided trough periods (chance of pain breakthrough lessened).
66	Open heart	60	Cont. e.d. morphine sulfate 0.1 mg/hr vs. intermittent i.v. bolus morphine sulfate 2 mg; no reference to supplementary analgesia	T2–T4	Better pain relief seen in cont. e.d. group. cont. e.d. reduced postoperative stress and was not detrimental to cardiovascular functions.
52[c]	Anterior cruciate ligament repair (knee)	20	Cont. e.d. fentanyl (as citrate) 100 μg/hr vs. continuous fentanyl (as citrate) i.v. infusion of 100 μg/hr	L2–L4	Similar degree of pain relief with both techniques. No significant differences in adverse effect profiles.
14[d]	Upper abdominal	20	Cont. e.d. fentanyl (as citrate) 60 μg/hr vs. intermittent i.m. injections of papaveretum 15–20 mg; no supplementary analgesia required	T7	Better analgesia ($p < 0.01$) and less sedation ($p < 0.01$) seen in cont. e.d. group. Postoperative respiratory function tests better in cont. e.d. group.
92	Colonic	60	Cont. e.d. morphine sulfate 2–6 mg/day vs. cont. e.d. bupivacaine hydrochloride 10–15 mg/hr vs. intermittent bolus e.d. morphine sulfate 2 mg (additional 1 mg/10 kg > 50 kg) vs. intermittent i.m. injection of oxycodone 0.15 mg/kg	Not stated	Pain intensity lower in cont. e.d. morphine group at 24 hours compared with oxycodone group ($p < 0.05$); lower in cont. e.d. bupivacaine and intermittent e.d. morphine groups at 3 hours compared with oxycodone ($p < 0.05$).
13[d]	Thoracic	90	Cont. e.d. morphine sulfate 0.1 mg/hr vs. intermittent bolus e.d. morphine sulfate 5 mg vs. intermittent bolus e.d. bupivacaine hydrochloride 25 mg	T4–T5	Postoperative analgesia achieved equally in all three groups. Cont. e.d. morphine resulted in avoidance of the major systemic adverse effects seen in the other two groups.
60[c]	Pulmonary resection	53	Cont. e.d. morphine sulfate 0.3–0.6 mg/hr vs. cont. e.d. bupivacaine hydrochloride 1 mg/mL and morphine sulfate 0.1 mg/mL 3–6 mL/hr vs. cont. e.d. bupivacaine hydrochloride 3–6 mg/hr vs. cont. e.d. saline vs. intermittent i.m. injections of morphine sulfate 0.1 mg/kg	Not stated	Pain relief significantly better in cont. e.d. morphine and cont. e.d. morphine and bupivacaine groups ($p < 0.05$) compared with i.m. morphine group.
77[c]	Total knee replacement	42	Cont. e.d. bupivacaine hydrochloride 15–37.5 mg/hr vs. cont. e.d. meperidine hydrochloride 1 mg/mL and bupivacaine hydrochloride 1.25 mg/mL 6–15 mL/hr vs. systemic analgesics	Lumbar	Both epidural regimens superior to systemic analgesics ($p = 0.0001$). Fewer adverse effects and shorter duration of stay in e.d. groups. Sensory and motor loss less in group receiving combination regimen.
15[c]	Cholecystectomy	20	Cont. e.d. bupivacaine hydrochloride 25 mg/hr and morphine sulfate 0.2 mg/hr vs. thoracic paravertebral block with bupivacaine hydrochloride 25 mg/hr	T7–T8	Paravertebral group had significantly higher pain scores and a greater need for systemic morphine ($p < 0.05$).

Continued on next page

Table 4 *(continued)*

Reference	Type of Surgery	No. Patients	Drug and Regimen[b]	Catheter Placement	Outcome
75	Thoracotomy	68	Cont. e.d. fentanyl (as citrate) 0.6 μg/kg/hr vs. cryoanalgesia	T6–T9	Superior analgesia produced in cont. e.d. fentanyl group ($p < 0.05$). A larger number of patients required supplemental analgesia in cryoanalgesia group ($p < 0.001$).
70	Hysterectomy	40	Cont. e.d. bupivacaine hydrochloride 20 mg/hr vs. intermittent i.m. injections of ketobemidone 5 mg	T12–L1	VAS and pain scores significantly better in cont. e.d. bupivacaine group ($p < 0.01$). Postoperative bowel movements returned earlier in cont. e.d. group.
79[e]	Total knee replacement	30	Cont. e.d. bupivacaine hydrochloride 15–37.5 mg/hr vs. systemic narcotic administration	Lumbar	Better pain relief in cont. e.d. bupivacaine group ($p < 0.05$). Fewer adverse effects seen and fewer supplementary analgesics required in cont. e.d. group. Varying degrees of motor block seen in bupivacaine group (eight patients).
80[e]	Upper abdominal, hip fracture repair	40	Cont. e.d. bupivacaine hydrochloride 7.5–25 mg/hr vs. intermittent i.m. injections of morphine sulfate 10–15 mg; no reference to supplementary analgesia	T10–L3	Cont. e.d. bupivacaine reduced postoperative convalescence time. Efficacy of pain relief not evaluated.
81	Hysterectomy	22	Cont. e.d. bupivacaine hydrochloride 20 mg/hr vs. intermittent e.d. injections of morphine sulfate 4 mg (initial dose) and 2 mg (subsequent doses)	T12–L1	Pain relief better in cont. e.d. bupivacaine group ($p < 0.05$). Bowel function restored earlier in cont. e.d. group.
83[e]	Thoracic	20	Cont. e.d. bupivacaine hydrochloride 0.25 mg/kg/hr vs. intermittent bolus e.d. bupivacaine hydrochloride 5 mg/mL with epinephrine 5 μg/mL	T2–T6	Poor pain relief seen in cont. e.d. group; adverse effects may have prevented optimal dosage from being used. Adverse effects were less of a problem in cont. e.d. group.
16	Cholecystectomy	20	Cont. e.d. bupivacaine hydrochloride 25 mg/hr vs. intrapleural bupivacaine hydrochloride 100-mg bolus followed by 50 mg/hr	T7	Both techniques provided good analgesia; no significant differences in terms of analgesia between the two groups. Greater sensory nerve blockade in cont. e.d. group.

[a] All studies were randomized and prospective unless otherwise noted. Cont. = continuous, e.d. = epidural, PCA = patient-controlled analgesia, L = lumbar, VAS = visual analog scale, T = thoracic.

[b] Supplementary analgesia required unless otherwise indicated.

[c] Double-blind.

[d] Controlled but not randomized.

[e] Not randomized.

in both treatment groups. Hypotension frequently accompanied each intermittent bupivacaine injection. Hypotension was also a problem with the continuous infusion but was more easily corrected. Drowsiness also occurred frequently. The lower concentration of the bupivacaine infusion resulted in the least incidence of drowsiness while still providing analgesia. Urinary retention, seen in all male patients receiving a continuous infusion of bupivacaine, was possibly related to a reduced sensation of fullness in the bladder secondary to interference with sympathetic inflow and to overdistension of the bladder in the early postoperative period. It was thought that the patients in the group receiving intermittent injections had periods during which the segmental block had decreased substantially to allow spontaneous micturition.

In summary, continuous epidural infusions of narcotics, local anesthetics, and narcotic–local anesthetic combinations, when used appropriately, may produce better analgesia than conventional bolus methods of pain relief. Further, continuous epidural infusions offer an advantage over intermittent epidural injections because peak and trough concentrations of the analgesic agent are avoided. With correct catheter placement, a continuous epidural infusion of an appropriate agent or agents should be effective in treating the postoperative pain produced by the majority of surgical procedures.

Complications of Catheter Placement

Epidural catheter placement is an invasive procedure and can result in serious morbidity on rare occasions. The following adverse effects of catheter placement have been described.

Inadvertent Dural Puncture on Catheter Placement. Insertion of an 18-gauge epidural needle beyond the dura mater into the subarachnoid space may cause post-dural-puncture headaches at a frequency of 70–80%.[18] Symptomatic treatment for headache may take the form of increased oral or i.v. fluid intake, systemic analgesics, maintenance of a supine posture, and placement of an epidural blood patch (an epidural injection of autologous blood at the site of the puncture injury) by anesthesia personnel. If the needle is introduced above the L2 position, damage to the spinal cord could potentially result.

Infection in the Epidural Space. The introduction of a foreign body into the epidural space may rarely result in meningitis or epidural abscess formation. Strict adherence to aseptic technique in the placement and maintenance of epidural catheters and in the preparation of epidural infusions is important for the prevention of infection.

Bleeding into the Epidural Space. Bleeding during placement of an epidural catheter may result in an epidural or subarachnoid hematoma, a potential cause of permanent neurologic damage. Such an event requires immediate medical and surgical attention. Symptoms of epidural hematoma include severe back pain, sensory and motor deficits, and urinary or fecal incontinence. Patients at high risk for the development of hematoma include those receiving anticoagulant therapy (often used during vascular or cardiac surgery) or those with pre-existing coagulation defects. The placement of epidural catheters in these patients is a subject of much controversy. Although reports of hematoma in these patients exist, several large comparative trials have revealed no increase in frequency.[101-103] Risk–benefit analysis should be considered in the decision to place an epidural catheter in any patient potentially at risk for epidural hematoma formation.

Catheter Migration after Placement. Catheters initially placed correctly may subsequently migrate out of the epidural space into the interspinous area, into a blood vessel, or across the dura. Migration into the interspinous area results in loss of analgesia (if narcotics are used) or unilateral analgesia with decreased dermatomal spread (if local anesthetics are used). Intravascular migration is an important concern if the bolus administration technique is used, but it may be of lesser importance when a continuous infusion is used. Loss of analgesia may occur, without systemic toxicity, if the epidural agent is continuously infused because subtherapeutic plasma levels from systemic absorption of an epidural infusion over time will equal i.v. infusion levels at steady state.[28] Transdural (subdural or subarachnoid) migration may cause exaggerated response and adverse effects regardless of whether the administration is by bolus injection or continuous infusion.[28] Adverse effects most commonly seen after transdural migration include sedation and respiratory depression with narcotic administration or hypotension and motor block with local anesthetic administration.[28]

Inappropriate Injection of Drugs through Epidural Catheter. Drugs intended for i.v. administration, such as total parenteral nutrient solutions, fat emulsion, potassium chloride, or diazepam have been inadvertently injected into epidural catheters. The importance of proper labeling of catheters and elimination or covering of ports for injection should be emphasized.

Adverse Drug Reactions

Respiratory Depression. Detracting from the popularity of postoperative epidural analgesia have been reports of unpredictable or delayed respiratory depression. Surgery itself, especially abdominal or thoracic procedures, can cause marked effects on respiration by restricting deep breathing or limiting the patient's ability to cough. By relieving postoperative pain, any analgesic may improve muscular movement and respiration, and thus increase vital capacity toward normal preoperative values. In one comparative trial,[104] analgesia with epidural bupivacaine was associated with a significant reduction in the incidence of pulmonary complications and chest infection compared with i.m. morphine injections or i.v. morphine infusion. However, local anesthetics are not without negative respiratory effects; if a high motor block is produced, expiratory reserve volume and intercostal and abdominal muscle activity may be reduced, making effective coughing difficult.[105]

The major cause of respiratory complications, however, is the epidural use of narcotics rather than local anesthetics. Narcotic-associated respiratory depression occurs by two proposed mechanisms, which lead to early or delayed onset of symptoms. Early respiratory depression, which usually occurs within one hour of a bolus epidural injection, is generally thought to be secondary to vascular absorption of the drug and subsequent redistribution to the brain. Most literature reports of epidural narcotic-induced respiratory depression describe early respiratory depression. Early respiratory depression has been reported with morphine, meperidine, and fentanyl and can be associated with all lipophilic narcotics. It is fairly predictable and resembles that described with i.v. or i.m. narcotic administration. After the epidural administration of 4 mg of morphine sulfate to healthy volunteers, the ventilatory response was shown to be similar to that produced by 10 mg of i.m. or i.v. morphine sulfate.[106] Another report of this early depression of ventilation describes a reduced ventilatory response to carbon dioxide after a continuous epidural infusion of fentanyl.[73] This reduced response occurred rapidly, but remained stable throughout the infusion and caused no clinically important respiratory effects. In general, bolus dosing is more frequently associated with early respiratory depression than is continuous infusion, as was shown for fentanyl in one study.[74]

Delayed respiratory depression is the most serious drug-related complication associated with the administration of epidural narcotics. First reported in 1980 with epidural morphine,[107,108] this complication typically peaks 3–12 hours after a bolus dose.[42,109] This time delay corresponds well with the time at which a substantial concentration of morphine reaches the fourth ventricle in the brain by rostral spread. Hydrophilic narcotics such as morphine are much more likely to cause delayed depression because drug molecules linger in the CSF without being taken up in large quantity by lipids. The chance for substantial migration of drug with the CSF flow is greater for morphine than for more lipophilic drugs such as fentanyl or meperidine. Most reports implicate morphine as the leading cause of this delayed respiratory depression (frequency, 0.09–3%[110]). Hydromorphone may also cause delayed respiratory depression. No reports to date have described this complication with fentanyl, sufentanil, or meperidine.

Several factors that potentially could contribute to the occurrence of either type of respiratory depression have been identified.[18] They include residual effects of i.m. or i.v. narcotics, a lack of narcotic tolerance, increased intrathoracic pressure, increased intra-abdominal pressure resulting in partial obstruction of the vena cava with increased flow through the azygos vein and increased systemic absorption of epidural drug, inadvertent dural puncture or migration of the epidural catheter, large bolus doses of morphine, and thoracic placement of an epidural catheter for morphine infusion or injection. One of the most important factors is the supplemental administration of i.m. or i.v. narcotics during epidural analgesia. It has been recommended that respiration be carefully assessed any time i.m. or i.v. narcotics are required within 24 hours of an epidural morphine bolus, and that standard i.m. or i.v. dosages be reduced when appropriate.[18]

One nationwide survey of bolus epidural morphine administration reported that the overall frequency of respiratory depression was 0.25–0.4%, which is quite low.[111] Respiratory depression is thought to be considerably less frequent in patients made tolerant to narcotics through previous long-term administration (e.g., patients being treated for chronic pain).

Management and Monitoring. Respiratory depression responds to treatment with narcotic antagonists. Because delayed respiratory depression may outlast a single dose of the short-acting agent naloxone, treatment is usually accomplished with a bolus of naloxone hydrochloride (0.1–0.4 mg) followed by an i.v. infusion (5 μg/kg/hr).[112] These doses have been shown to successfully reverse respiratory depression without affecting narcotic analgesia. Investigators have had some success in preventing respiratory depression, without affecting analgesia, by administering a single 6-mg oral dose of naltrexone hydrochloride at the time of the epidural morphine bolus,[113] whereas others have found that 9 mg of naltrexone hydrochloride was necessary.[114]

Monitoring of respiratory function during epidural narcotic therapy is important, although there is much debate as to the degree of monitoring required. Most authors agree that close monitoring of patients receiving epidural morphine is essential for 12 to 24 hours after a bolus dose or discontinuation of an infusion.[106] Some recommend confinement of high-risk patients to an intensive-care unit for this period,[115] whereas others believe that intensive-care-unit monitoring is essential for all patients receiving bolus morphine or any continuously infused narcotic.[116] In a survey of epidural monitoring conducted in 1984, 33% of respondents stated that epidural narcotics were administered outside the intensive-care unit in selected patients.[117]

Pulse oximeters, apnea monitors, or end-tidal carbon dioxide monitors have been used to detect respiratory depression. Although the measurement of end-tidal carbon dioxide concentration in expired air is recognized as the most sensitive method of detecting increases in plasma carbon dioxide concentration associated with respiratory depression, the tight-fitting mask that must be used with this technique is often objectionable to patients. Pulse oximeters can be easily applied to a patient's finger or toe and can reliably measure arterial oxygen saturation in a continuous and noninvasive manner.[118] Both pulse oximeters and apnea monitors are plagued by frequent false alarms caused by patient movement, but they are currently the most frequently used monitoring equipment. The least invasive and most reliable indicator of epidural narcotic-induced respiratory depression is thought to be the simple monitoring of respiratory rate and level of consciousness. Many institutions have discontinued requirements of intensive-care-unit admission, pulse oximetry, and apnea monitoring for patients receiving continuous epidural narcotic infusions and prefer frequent assessment by a highly trained nursing staff. The importance of clear and specific nursing orders for monitoring vital signs and administering reversal agents such as naloxone, proper education of nursing personnel, and 24-hour access to anesthesia staff for emergency medical care cannot be understated.

Pruritus. A less serious adverse effect of epidural narcotics is generalized pruritus. This problem has been reported primarily with morphine and fentanyl, but it has also been reported with meperidine, methadone, and hydromorphone.[119] The frequency of pruritus has been reported to range from 1% to100%,[120] with a multicenter survey reporting an average frequency of 2–5% after an epidural bolus of morphine.[120] Symptoms can be mild or severe; it is thought that mild pruritus probably occurs in close to 100% of patients receiving epidural narcotics, whereas severe effects occur at a frequency of 1%. The frequency of pruritus is significantly greater with epidural than with i.v. morphine injection[121] and in parturient patients.[119]

The cause of epidural-narcotic-induced pruritus is unknown. Because it can occur with administration of preservative-free preparations, it is not thought to be due to preservatives in drug products. Histamine release, once a proposed mechanism, is probably unrelated; the onset of pruritus is relatively predictable at two to three hours after an epidural narcotic bolus[121] and the effect occurs with the non-histamine-releasing opioid fentanyl. Although data are conflicting, effects are probably dose related. A current proposed mechanism is widespread alteration in sensory modulation that occurs when the drug reaches the cervical level by rostral spread.[121]

Pruritus is reliably abolished with the administration of i.v. naloxone. Subcutaneous nalbuphine hydrochloride (10 mg) has also been used to treat the problem[122] without a change in analgesia. Pruritus may diminish or disappear if another narcotic is substituted for the offending agent,[28] and it often subsides despite subsequent therapy.[21] Diphenhydramine has been used to treat pruritus, with poor response.[119] Prophylactic naltrexone hydrochloride in doses of 6 mg orally has been used to prevent pruritus with good results,[113,114] and prior use of epidural bupivacaine may reduce the incidence of pruritus.[123]

Urinary Retention. An adverse effect shared by local anesthetics and narcotics is urinary retention, with an additive frequency when both classes of drug are administered. Local anesthetics produce urinary retention by parasympathetic blockade of sacral nerves arising from the S2–S4 vertebral segments. With bolus epidural injection of a local anesthetic, effects are usually of short duration and have little to no effect on postblock bladder function. When continuous infusions of local anesthetics are used, however, bladder catheterization may be required if urinary retention becomes troublesome. The incidence of urinary retention caused by local anesthetics is high. Up to 80% of patients may experience symptoms with bolus or infusion administration.[28] The administration of local anesthetics at the thoracic rather than lumbar level may spare blockade of sacral segments and reduce the incidence of urinary retention, although the clinical importance of epidural catheter placement site has not fully been determined.

Narcotics administered by spinal routes cause urinary retention more commonly than those administered by other routes.[28,121] Retention may occur with morphine as well as with more lipophilic narcotics. Symptoms range from mild hesitancy to an inability to void to painful bladder distention. Symptoms are typically insidious in onset, occurring between 30 minutes and 10 hours after an epidural morphine sulfate bolus of 10 mg in one study.[121] Another study, however, reported a rapid onset of detrusor muscle relaxation within 15–30 minutes of epidural morphine injection.[124] Retention may last more than 15 hours after a bolus dose or presumably after discontinuation of an infusion.[124] The frequency of epidural-narcotic-induced urinary retention has been reported to range from 3% to 100%; one study of 90 patients receiving morphine reported a frequency of 22%.[125] Urinary retention appears to be more common in males than in females.[124] It is unclear whether this effect is dose related, because reviews and studies of the subject have presented conflicting conclusions.[21,119,124] The mechanism by which this effect occurs is unknown. A CNS effect, such as reduction in parasympathetic flow from the sacral cord or rostral spread of drug to the pons and micturition center, or a direct effect on opiate receptors in the bladder has been postulated.[124] An opiate-receptor effect seems most likely, because urinary retention can be reversed by administration of naloxone.[121]

Treatment is usually naloxone hydrochloride in a single i.v. dose of 0.4–0.8 mg or a bolus of 0.1–0.4 mg followed by an infusion of 5–10 μg/kg/hr, with immediate results.[121,124] Naltrexone hydrochloride, once again in a prophylactic oral dose of 6 mg, has been reported to reduce the incidence of retention.[113] Bethanechol chloride (5 mg subcutaneously), a parasympathomimetic agent, has been tried with minimal success in some patients and has actually increased discomfort in others.[121] Bladder catheterization is sometimes necessary, but it increases the risk of infection and should be reserved for patients in whom other treatment modalities have been unsuccessful. In one report, 0.3–25% of patients receiving bolus morphine required bladder catheterization[111]; this rate may be higher in patients receiving continuous infusions.

Nausea and Vomiting. As with systemic narcotic administration, epidural narcotics can cause nausea and vomiting. Pain itself can contribute to nausea in postoperative patients,[21] as can the residual effects of intraoperative narcotics and volatile anesthetics. The frequency of nausea and vomiting from epidural narcotics in postoperative patients is reported to be equal to or lower than that from systemic narcotics.[21] A 17% frequency was reported for epidural administration,[108] whereas a 30% frequency is common for systemic administration.[21] Nausea and vomiting are thought to be caused by rostral spread of epidural drug to the vomiting center and chemoreceptor trigger zone in the brain. After administration of a 10-mg bolus dose of epidural morphine sulfate, nausea begins within approximately four hours and lasts an average of three hours.[121] With repetitive bolus dosing, nausea and vomiting become less frequent, perhaps because tolerance develops[21]; patients receiving continuous infusions of narcotic may have the same reduced occurrence of nausea and vomiting over time. Nausea and vomiting are effectively treated by administration of naloxone[21] or another narcotic antagonist. Antiemetics such as droperidol, prochlorperazine, perphenazine, or metoclopramide are also effective.

Cardiovascular Effects. Epidural administration of local anesthetics almost always results in some degree of sympathetic block, which can affect peripheral vasculature and cardiac function.[18] The result of a sympathetic block depends on the level of the epidural injection. Peripheral sympathetic innervation originates between the T1 and L2 vertebral spaces; cardiac sympathetic fibers leave the cord at the T1 to T4 level. Parasympathetic fibers affecting the vasculature are usually unaffected by epidural drug administration, because they arise either from the cranial or sacral levels of the cord.

If a local anesthetic is administered at the lumbar or low thoracic level, only lower peripheral sympathetic fibers will be affected. Blockade of these fibers results in vasodilation in the pelvis and lower limbs and, if the T6 to L1 fibers are affected, pooling of blood in the abdominal organs. This effect is measurable by a substantial increase in lower limb skin temperature. Vasodilation can produce a dramatic reduction in blood pressure, venous return, and cardiac output, especially in patients in a sitting or head-up posture or in those with partial inferior vena cava obstruction (e.g., pregnant patients and those with intestinal obstruction or ascites). Hypotension is the most common cardiovascular effect of epidural local-anesthetic administration.[126] Cardiac vagal tone is increased, thereby maintaining heart rate near preblockade levels despite the reduction in blood pressure. Reflex responses to lower peripheral vasodilation include increases in peripheral vasoconstriction and cardiac sympathetic response above the level of the epidural block, resulting in a reduction in blood flow to the head, neck, and upper limbs and increased cardiac contractility. Lumbar epidural local anesthetic administration can actually improve ejection fraction and cardiac output by reducing preload and increasing contractility.[127]

A local-anesthetic epidural block in the high thoracic region can result in total sympathetic block by cutting off sympathetic outflow to both cardiac and peripheral nerve tracts. Vasodilation of the lower limbs is accompanied by similar effects in the upper limbs, head, and neck. Blood pressure and peripheral vascular resistance are reduced by approximately 20%. There is a decrease or little change in the heart rate because the parasympathetic tone is left unopposed and compensatory reduction in this tone may occur to some extent.[19] A local anesthetic block above the T4 level may actually benefit those patients with low myocardial reserve by preventing the increased myocardial oxygen consumption usually associated with various surgical procedures (e.g., coronary artery, aortic, and vascular surgery).[126] The cardiovascular system, however, has no further compensatory mechanisms to maintain cardiac output or heart rate in the face of hypovolemia or other insult.[18]

Evidence from animal data and human observation suggests that vascular autoregulation may occur in response to the effects of local anesthetics approximately 30 minutes after an epidural injection or the start of an infusion.[18] Serious hypotension is uncommon 20 to 30 minutes after a bolus of bupivacaine, and cardiovascular effects are usually less important after the start of a continuous infusion than after administration of a bolus dose.[18] Based on clinical experience, Gregg[28] believes that most patients receiving continuous epidural infusions of bupivacaine can maintain blood pressure with adjustment of the administration rate and adequate i.v. fluid administration. Pressors may also be used, if necessary. Cardiovascular effects of epidural narcotics are usually minimal; a nonsignificant reduction in blood pressure has been reported with morphine.[125]

Neurologic Effects. In addition to sympathetic block, local anesthetics can produce adverse effects by temporary blockade of motor or sensory fibers. Motor block results in complete or partial loss of motor function to the lower limbs and is assessed by the patient's ability to flex the knees and ankles. Leg weakness caused by motor block can negate the potential benefit of early ambulation that is possible with the use of epidural analgesia. Furthermore, substantial and prolonged motor block can lead to the formation of decubiti on the patient's heels, sacrum, and other pressure points.[28] Factors that determine the motor effects of epidural local anesthetic administration include the choice of drug, the dosage (higher dosages result in more motor block), the catheter site, and the method of administration (continuous infusions produce less motor block than bolus administration).[18,28] The combination of a low-dosage bupivacaine infusion with a low-dosage narcotic infusion offers good analgesia with complete preservation of motor function in most patients.[18]

Sensory block produces a loss of sensation in the lower extremities and can occur after epidural local anesthetic administration.

More severe neurologic effects are rarely seen with local anesthetic use. Reports of transient or permanent paraplegia exist, but they often involve inadvertent subdural injection of large amounts of local anesthetic or of solutions containing benzyl alcohol or other known neurotoxic preservatives.[128] Care should always be taken to avoid the use of solutions containing neurotoxic preservatives and to test for placement of the catheter in the epidural space before administration of any drug. Severe neurologic deficits are probably not a direct effect of either local anesthetics or narcotics.[21,128]

Other Adverse Effects. As mentioned previously, tachyphylaxis can occur with repeat administration of local anesthetics. Short-acting agents are associated with a higher frequency of tachyphylaxis[18]; bupivacaine has a longer duration of action than other local anesthetics and does not present a problem, especially when administered by continuous infusion in combination with a narcotic.

Systemic toxicity from local anesthetics is rare but can be serious. Most systemic toxicity occurs after inadvertent i.v. bolus injection or large epidural bolus doses of a local anesthetic that result in rapid achievement of toxic serum concentrations.[28] Adverse effects include CNS toxicity, with the possible occurrence of seizures, and cardiac toxicity resulting in arrhythmias and cardiac arrest. Cardiac toxicity is especially serious when caused by bupivacaine, as it is often refractory to resuscitation. Systemic toxicity during continuous epidural infusion of low-dose bupivacaine solutions is extremely rare.

Sedation is a common adverse effect of i.m. or i.v. narcotic administration. Sedation may also accompany epidural narcotic infusions but to a lesser degree than with systemic administration.[28] Highly lipophilic narcotics such as sufentanil may be associated with the greatest frequency of sedation when given epidurally.[31] Partial narcotic agonists may also be associated with a higher frequency of this adverse effect.[28] Sedation may be minimized by reducing the rate of narcotic infusion.

Other rare adverse effects of epidural narcotics or local anesthetics include dysphoria, euphoria, anxiety, and hallucinations after epidural narcotic administration; precipitation of narcotic withdrawal; and allergic reactions to narcotics, ester-type local anesthetics (e.g. chloroprocaine), or rarely, amide-type local anesthetics (e.g., bupivacaine, lidocaine). There has been one report of possible deliberate tampering by a patient with an epidural narcotic infusion to increase the rate of administration.[87]

Place in Therapy

The decision to provide analgesia via continuous epidural infusion of a narcotic, a local anesthetic, or both is made by examining the efficacy of the technique for a given surgical procedure and the risk-to-benefit ratio for each patient case. The localization of pain at an appropriate dermatomal level for catheter placement is essential. Several appropriate indications for postoperative epidural analgesia have been suggested.[1,28] Analgesia after major thoracic surgery (thoracotomy or lung lobectomy) or upper abdominal surgery is an appropriate indication; placement of the catheter is usually thoracic in these cases, and adequate analgesia can usually be achieved with continuous infusion of a narcotic–local anesthetic mixture. Patients undergoing major vascular surgery may benefit from epidural analgesia; the use of an epidural infusion administered at the lumbar or low thoracic level is acceptable. Patients undergoing orthopedic surgery involving the lower limbs may also benefit from epidural analgesia, especially those requiring postoperative continuous passive motion therapy. Lumbar infusions are often used in these patients. Epidural morphine analgesia has also been used after open-heart procedures. Finally, specific high-risk patients may benefit from epidural analgesia; patients with severe respiratory disease or morbid obesity are at high risk for postoperative complications, and epidural analgesia may reduce their risk of prolonged intubation. However, these patients are also at the highest risk for adverse effects from epidural drugs and require intensive monitoring.

Absolute contraindications to epidural therapy include severe systemic infection or infection in the area of catheter insertion, a major coagulation defect, uncorrected hypovolemia, and patient refusal.

Protocols for epidural analgesia should be developed. Nursing orders should include monitoring standards and thresholds for contacting anesthesia staff regarding inappropriate respiratory rate, heart rate, blood pressure, or sensory level. Anesthesia staff should be notified if thresholds are reached or if patients experience adverse effects such as somnolence, confusion, pruritus, nausea, vomiting, or urinary retention. Standard infusion solutions are adequate for most patients and allow pharmacy staff to prepare batch products. Only preservative-free products should be used to mix epidural infusions; these products often cost considerably more than standard pharmaceuticals. Occasionally, a patient with severe respiratory or cardiovascular disease may require a special solution, such as one with a reduced concentration of local anesthetic or narcotic.

The cost in materials and manpower of epidural therapy can be substantially higher than that of traditional i.m. or i.v. narcotic analgesia. Although preliminary clinical research points to a possible reduction in postoperative complications and length of hospital or intensive-care-unit stay, a conclusive overall cost benefit cannot yet be attributed to postoperative epidural analgesia.

Conclusion

Continuous epidural analgesic infusions provide effective postoperative pain relief. Current studies suggest superior analgesia for the majority of surgical procedures with this administration method compared with more traditional methods of providing analgesia.

References

1. Brown DL, Carpenter RL. Perioperative analgesia: a review of risks and benefits. *J Cardiothorac Anesth*. 1990; 4:368-83.
2. Woloski BM, Smith EM, Meyer WJ et al. Corticotropin-releasing activity of monokines. *Science*. 1985; 230:1035-7.
3. Cohen FL. Postsurgical pain relief: patient's status and nurses' medication choices. *Pain*. 1980; 9:265-74.
4. White PF. Patient-controlled analgesia: a new approach to the management of postoperative pain. *Semin Anesth*. 1985; 4:255-66.
5. Cockshott WP, Thompson GT, Howlett LJ et al. Intramuscular or intralipomatous injections? *N Engl J Med*. 1982; 307:356-8.
6. Cathelin MF. Une nouvelle voie d'injection rachidienne. Methode des injections epidurales par le procede du canal sacre. Applications a l'homme. *C R Soc Biol* (Paris). 1901; 53:452.
7. Sicard JA. Les injections medicamenteuses extra-durales par voie sacro-coccygienne. *C R Soc Biol* (Paris). 1901; 53:396.

8. Tuffier T. Analgesie cocainique par voie extradurale. *C R Soc Biol* (Paris). 1901; 53:490.
9. Cleland JG. Continuous peridural and caudal analgesia in surgery and early ambulation. *Northwest Med J*. 1949; 48:26-34.
10. Pert CB, Snyder SH. Opiate receptor: demonstration in nervous tissue. *Science*. 1973; 179:1011-4.
11. Behar M, Magora D, Olshwang D et al. Epidural morphine in the treatment of pain. *Lancet*. 1979; 1:527-9.
12. Lee JA, Atkinson RS, Watt MJ. Lumbar puncture and spinal anesthesia. New York: Churchill Livingstone; 1985.
13. El-Baz NM, Faber LP, Jensik RJ. Continuous epidural infusion of morphine for treatment of pain after thoracic surgery: a new technique. *Anesth Analg*. 1984; 63:757-64.
14. Welchew EA, Thornton JA. Continuous thoracic epidural fentanyl: a comparison of epidural fentanyl with intramuscular papaveretum for postoperative pain. *Anaesthesia*. 1982; 37:309-16
15. Bigler D, Dirkes W, Hansen R et al. Effects of thoracic paravertebral block with bupivacaine versus combined thoracic epidural block with bupivacaine and morphine on pain and pulmonary function after cholecystectomy. *Acta Anaesthesiol Scand*. 1989; 33:561-4.
16. Scott NB, Mogensen T, Bigler D et al. Comparison of the effects of continuous intrapleural vs epidural administration of 0.5% bupivacaine on pain, metabolic response and pulmonary function following cholecystectomy. *Acta Anaesthesiol Scand*. 1989; 33:535-9.
17. Scott NB, Mogensen T, Bigler D et al. Continuous thoracic extradural 0.5% bupivacaine with or without morphine: effect on quality of blockade, lung function and the surgical stress response. *Br J Anaesth*. 1989; 62:253-7.
18. Cousins MJ, Bromage PR. Epidural neural blockade. In: Cousins MJ, Bridenbaugh PO, eds. Neural blockade in clinical anesthesia and management of pain. Philadelphia: Lippincott; 1988:253-360.
19. Stanton-Hicks M. Subarachnoid and extradural analgesic techniques. In: Smith G, Covino BG, eds. Acute pain. Boston: Butterworth; 1985:228-56.
20. Murphy TM. Spinal epidural and caudal anesthesia. In: Miller RD, ed. Anesthesia. New York: Churchill Livingstone; 1986:1061-111.
21. Cousins MJ, Cherry DA, Gourlay GK. Acute and chronic pain: use of spinal opioids. In: Cousins MJ, Bridenbaugh PO, eds. Neural blockade in clinical anesthesia and management of pain. Philadelphia: Lippincott; 1988:955-1029.
22. Yaksh TL, Noueihed R. The physiology and pharmacology of spinal opiates. *Am Rev Pharmacol Toxicol*. 1985; 25:443-56.
23. Baumann TJ, Lehman ME. Pain management. In: DiPiro JT, Talbert RL, Hayes PE et al., eds. Pharmacotherapy: a pathophysiologic approach. New York: Elsevier; 1989:642-59.
24. Lipman AG. Clinically relevant differences among the opioid analgesics. *Am J Hosp Pharm*. 1990; 47:S7-S13.
25. Gourlay GK, Cherry DA, Cousins MJ. Cephalad migration of morphine in CSF following lumbar epidural administration in patients with cancer pain. *Pain*. 1985; 23:317-26.
26. Yaksh TL, Noueihed RY, Durant AC. Studies of the pharmacology and pathology of intrathecally administered 4-aminopiperidine analogues and morphine in the rat and cat. *Anesthesiology*. 1986; 64:54-66.
27. Savarese JJ, Covino BG. Basic and clinical pharmacology of local anesthetic drugs. In: Miller RD, ed. Anesthesia. New York: Churchill Livingstone; 1986:985-1013.
28. Gregg R. Spinal analgesia. In: Oden RV, ed. Anesthesiology clinics of North America: management of postoperative pain. Philadelphia: Saunders; 1989:79-100.
29. Sjostrom S, Hartvig P, Persson P et al. Pharmacokinetics of epidural morphine and meperidine in humans. *Anesthesiology*. 1987; 67:877-88.
30. Covino BG. Clinical pharmacology of local anesthetic agents. In: Cousins MJ, Bridenbaugh PO, eds. Neural blockade in clinical anesthesia and management of pain. Philadelphia: Lippincott; 1988:111-44.
31. Donadoni R, Rolly G, Noordwin H et al. Epidural sufentanil for postoperative pain relief. *Anaesthesia*. 1985; 40:634-8.
32. Lippmann M, Mok MS. Epidural butorphanol for the relief of postoperative pain. *Anesth Analg*. 1988; 67:418. Letter.
33. Tucker GT, Mather LE. Properties, absorption and disposition of local anesthetic agents. In: Cousins MJ, Bridenbaugh PO, eds. Neural blockage in clinical anesthesia and management of pain. Philadelphia: Lippincott; 1988:47-110.
34. Moore RA, Bullingham RSJ, McQuay HJ et al. Dural permeability to narcotics: in vitro determination and application to extradural administration. *Br J Anaesth*. 1982; 54:1117-28.
35. Tamsen A, Sjostrom S, Hartvig P et al. CSF and plasma kinetics of morphine and meperidine after epidural administration. *Anesthesiology*. 1983; 59:A196. Abstract.
36. Chrubasik J, Wust H, Schulte-Monting J et al. Relative analgesia potency of epidural fentanyl, alfentanil, and morphine in treatment of postoperative pain. *Anesthesiology*. 1988; 68:929-33.
37. Rosen M, Dailey P, Hughes S et al. Epidural sufentanil for postoperative analgesia after cesarean section. *Anesthesiology*. 1988; 68:448-54.
38. Torda TA, Pybus DA. Comparison of four narcotic analgesics for extradural analgesia. *Br J Anaesth*. 1982; 54:291-5.
39. Leysen JE, Gommeren W, Niemegeers CJE. Sufentanil, a superior ligand for mu-opiate receptors: binding properties and regional distribution in rat brain and spinal cord. *Eur J Pharmacol*. 1983; 87:209-25.
40. Mather LE. Clinical pharmacokinetics of fentanyl and its newer derivatives. *Clin Pharmacokinet*. 1983; 8:422-46.
41. Larsen VH, Iversen AD, Christensen P et al. Postoperative pain treatment after upper abdominal surgery with epidural morphine at thoracic or lumbar level. *Acta Anaesthesiol Scand*. 1985; 29:566-71.
42. Bromage PR, Camporesi EM, Durant PAC et al. Rostral spread of epidural morphine. *Anesthesiology*. 1982; 56:431-6.
43. Fromme GA, Steidl LJ, Danielson DR. Comparison of lumbar and thoracic epidural morphine for relief of postthoracotomy pain. *Anesth Analg*. 1985; 64:454-5.
44. Cousins MJ, Mather LE, Glynn CJ et al. Selective spinal analgesia. *Lancet*. 1979; 1:1141-2.
45. Glynn CJ, Mather LE, Cousins MJ et al. Peridural meperidine in humans: analgesic response, pharmacokinetics and transmission into CSF. *Anesthesiology*. 1981; 55:520-6.
46. Gustafsson LL, Friberg-Nielsen S, Garle M. Extradural and parenteral morphine: kinetics and effects in postoperative pain. A controlled clinical study. *Br J Anaesth*. 1982; 54:1167-74.
47. Nordberg G, Hedner T, Mellstrand T et al. Pharmacokinetic aspects of spinal morphine. *Anesthesiology*. 1983; 58:545-51.
48. Weddel SJ, Ritter RR. Serum levels following epidural administration of morphine and correlation with relief of postsurgical pain. *Anesthesiology*. 1981; 54:210-4.
49. Wolfe MJ, Davies GK. Analgesic action of extradural fentanyl. *Br J Anaesth*. 1980; 52:357-8.
50. Lomessy A, Magnin C, Viale J et al. Clinical advantages of fentanyl given epidurally for postoperative analgesia. *Anesthesiology*. 1984; 61:466-9.
51. Estok PM, Glass PCA, Goldberg JS et al. Use of patient controlled analgesia to compare intravenous to epidural administration of fentanyl in the postoperative patient. *Anesthesiology*. 1987; 67:A230. Abstract.
52. Loper KA, Ready LB, Downey M et al. Epidural and intravenous fentanyl infusions are clinically equivalent after knee surgery. *Anesth Analg*. 1990; 70:72-5.
53. Hughes SC, Rosen MA, Shnider, SM et al. Maternal and neonatal effects of epidural morphine for labor and delivery. *Anesth Analg*. 1984; 63:319-24.
54. Husemeyer RP, Cummings AJ, Rosankiewicz JR et al. A study of pethidine kinetics and analgesia in women in labour following intravenous, intramuscular and epidural administration. *Br J Clin Pharmacol*. 1982; 13:171-6.
55. Gourlay GK, Cherry DA, Plummer JL et al. The influence of

drug polarity on the absorption of opioid drugs into CSF and subsequent cephalad migration following lumbar epidural administration: application to morphine and pethidine. *Pain*. 1987; 31:297-305.

56. Justins D, Knott C, Luthman J et al. Epidural versus intramuscular fentanyl: analgesia and pharmacokinetics in labour. *Anaesthesia*. 1983; 38:937-42.
57. Tucker GT, Mather LE. Clinical pharmacokinetics of local anaesthetic agents. *Clin Pharmacokinet*. 1979; 4:241-78.
58. Erdimir HA, Soper LE, Sweet RB. Studies of factors affecting peridural anesthesia. *Anesth Analg*. 1965; 44:400-4.
59. Bromage PR. A comparison of the hydrochloride salts of lignocaine and prilocaine for epidural analgesia. *Br J Anaesth*. 1965; 37:753-61.
60. Keir L. Continuous epidural analgesia in prostatectomy: a comparison of bupivacaine with and without adrenaline. *Acta Anaesthesiol Scand*. 1974; 18:1-4.
61. Scott DB, Jebson PJR, Braid DP et al. Factors affecting plasma levels of lignocaine and prilocaine. *Br J Anaesth*. 1972; 44:1040-9.
62. Rosenberg PH, Heinonen E. Differential sensitivity of A and C nerve fibers to long-acting amide local anaesthetics. *Br J Anaesth*. 1983; 55:163-7.
63. Bromage PR. Mechanisms of action of extradural analgesia. *Br J Anaesth*. 1975; 47:199-212.
64. Schwartz BR, Gregg RV, Kessler DL et al. Continuous postoperative epidural analgesia in management of postoperative surgical pain. *Urology*. 1989; 34:349-52.
65. Chrubasik J, Wiemers K. Continuous-plus-on-demand epidural infusion of morphine for postoperative pain relief by means of a small, externally worn infusion device. *Anesthesiology*. 1985; 62:263-7.
66. El-Baz N, Goldin MD. Continuous epidural morphine infusion for pain relief after open heart surgery. *Anesthesiology*. 1983; 59:A193. Abstract.
67. Oyama T, Marakawa T, Baba S et al. Continuous vs. bolus epidural morphine. *Acta Anaesthesiol Scand*. 1987; 85:77-9.
68. Logas WG, El-Baz N, El-Ganzouri A et al. Continuous thoracic epidural analgesia for postoperative pain relief following thoracotomy: a randomized prospective study. *Anesthesiology*. 1987; 67:787-91.
69. Cullen ML, Staren ED, El-Ganzouri A et al. Continuous epidural infusion for analgesia after major abdominal operations: a randomized, prospective, double-blind study. *Surgery*. 1985; 98:718-28.
70. Planner RS, Cowie RW, Babarczy AS. Continuous epidural morphine analgesia after radical operations upon the pelvis. *Surg Gynecol Obstet*. 1988; 166:229-32.
71. Dyer RA, Anderson BJ, Michell WL. Postoperative pain control with a continuous infusion of epidural sufentanil in the intensive care unit: a comparison with epidural morphine. *Anesth Analg*. 1990; 71:130-6.
72. Rauck R, Knarr D, Denson D et al. Comparison of the efficacy of epidural morphine given by intermittent injection or continuous infusion for the management of postoperative pain. *Anesthesiology*. 1986; 65:A201. Abstract.
73. Renaud B, Brichant JF, Clergue F et al. Ventilatory effects of continuous epidural infusion of fentanyl. *Anesth Analg*. 1988; 67:971-5.
74. Ahuja BR, Strunin L. Respiratory effects of epidural fentanyl. *Anaesthesia*. 1985; 40:949-55.
75. Gough JD, Williams AB, Vaughan RS et al. The control of post-thoracotomy pain: a comparative evaluation of thoracic epidural fentanyl infusions and cryo-analgesia. *Anaesthesia*. 1988; 43:780-3.
76. Marlowe S, Engstrom R, White PF. Epidural patient-controlled analgesia (PCA): an alternative to continuous epidural infusions. *Pain*. 1989; 37:91-101.
77. Raj PP, Knarr D, Vigdorth E et al. Comparative study of continuous epidural infusions versus systemic analgesics for postoperative pain relief. *Anesthesiology*. 1985; 63:A238. Abstract.
78. Wattwil M, Thoren T, Hennerdal S et al. Epidural analgesia with bupivacaine reduces postoperative paralytic ileus after hysterectomy. *Anesth Analg*. 1989; 68:353-8.
79. Raj PP, Knarr DC, Vigdorth E et al. Comparison of continuous epidural infusion of a local anesthetic and administration of systemic narcotics in the management of pain after total knee replacement surgery. *Anesth Analg*. 1987; 66:401-6.
80. Pflug AE, Murphy TM, Butler SH et al. The effects of postoperative peridural analgesia on pulmonary therapy and pulmonary complications. *Anesthesiology*. 1974; 41:8-17.
81. Thoren T, Sundberg A, Wattwil M et al. Effects of epidural bupivacaine and epidural morphine on bowel function and pain after hysterectomy. *Acta Anaesthesiol Scand*. 1989; 33:181-5.
82. Holmdahl MH, Sjogren S, Strom G et al. Clinical aspects of continuous epidural blockade for postoperative pain relief. *Ups J Med Sci*. 1972; 77:47-56.
83. Griffiths DPG, Diamond AW, Cameron JD. Postoperative extradural analgesia following thoracic surgery: a feasibility study. *Br J Anaesth*. 1975; 47:48-55.
84. Ross RA, Clarke JE, Armitage EN. Postoperative pain prevention by continuous epidural infusion. *Anaesthesia*. 1980; 35:663-8.
85. Fischer RL, Lubenow TR, Liceaga A et al. Comparison of continuous epidural infusion of fentanyl-bupivacaine and morphine-bupivacaine in management of postoperative pain. *Anesth Analg*. 1988; 67:559-63.
86. Hord AH, Kokenes C. Postoperative pain, a review of management methods. *Hosp Formul*. 1989; 24:28-40.
87. Kreitzman TR, Samuela SI. Epidural opioid infusion: an unusual problem. *Anesthesiology*. 1990; 73:1272-3.
88. Rawal N, Sjostrand UH, Christoffersson E et al. Comparison of intramuscular and epidural morphine for postoperative analgesia in the grossly obese: influence on postoperative ambulation and pulmonary function. *Anesth Analg*. 1984; 63:583-92.
89. Rawal N, Sjostrand UH, Dahlstrom B et al. Epidural morphine for postoperative pain relief: a comparative study with intramuscular narcotic and intercostal nerve block. *Anesth Analg*. 1982; 61:93-8.
90. Modig J, Borg T, Karlstrom G et al. Thromboembolism after total hip replacement: role of epidural and general anesthesia. *Anesth Analg*. 1983; 62:174-80.
91. Cousins MJ, Wright CJ. Graft, muscle, skin blood flow after epidural block in vascular surgical procedures. *Surg Gynecol Obstet*. 1971; 133:59-64.
92. Scheinin B, Asantila R, Orko R. The effect of bupivacaine and morphine on pain and bowel function after colonic surgery. *Acta Anaesthesiol Scand*. 1987; 31:161-4.
93. Pflug AE, Halter JB. Effect of spinal anesthesia on adrenergic tone and the neuroendocrine responses to surgical stress in humans. *Anesthesiology*. 1981; 55:120-6.
94. Kehlet H. The modifying effect of general and regional anaesthesia on the endocrine metabolic response to surgery. *Reg Anaesth*. 1982; 7:S38. Abstract.
95. Christensen P, Brandt MR, Rem J et al. Influence of extradural morphine on the adrenocortical and hyperglycaemic response to surgery. *Br J Anaesth*. 1982; 54:23-7.
96. Yeager MP, Glass DD, Neff RK. Epidural anesthesia and analgesia in high-risk surgical patients. *Anesthesiology*. 1987; 66:729-36.
97. Anderson I, Thompson WR, Varkey GP et al. Lumbar epidural morphine as an effective analgesic following cholecystectomy. *Can Anaesth Soc J*. 1981; 28:523-9.
98. Brownridge P, Frewin DB. A comparative study of techniques of postoperative analgesia following cesarean section and lower abdominal surgery. *Anaesth Intensive Care*. 1985; 13:123-30.
99. Modig J, Paalzow L. A comparison of epidural morphine and epidural bupivacaine for postoperative pain relief. *Acta Anaesthesiol Scand*. 1981; 25:437-41.
100. Johnson RG, Miller M, Murphy M. Intraspinal narcotic analgesia: a comparison of two methods of postoperative pain

relief. *Spine*. 1989; 14:363-6.
101. Odoom JA, Sih IL. Epidural analgesia and anticoagulant therapy. *Anaesthesia*. 1983; 38:254-9.
102. Rao TLK, El-Etr AA. Anticoagulation following placement of epidural and subarachnoid catheters: an evaluation of neurologic sequela. *Anesthesiology*. 1981; 55:618-20.
103. Baron HC, LaRaja RD, Rossi G et al. Continuous epidural analgesia in the heparinized vascular surgery patient: a retrospective review of 912 patients. *J Vasc Surg*. 1987; 6:144-6.
104. Cuschieri RJ, Morran CG, Howie JC et al. Postoperative pain and pulmonary complications: a comparison of three analgesic regimens. *Br J Surg*. 1985; 72:495-8.
105. Freund FB, Bonica JJ, Ward RJ et al. Ventilatory reserve and the level of motor block during high spinal and epidural anesthesia. *Anesthesiology*. 1967; 28:834-7.
106. Rawal N, Wattwil M. Respiratory depression after epidural morphine—an experimental and clinical study. *Anesth Analg*. 1984; 63:8-14.
107. Boas RA. Hazards of epidural morphine. *Anaesth Intensive Care*. 1980; 8:377-8.
108. Reiz S, Westberg M. Side-effects of epidural morphine. *Lancet*. 1980; 2:203-4.
109. Camporesi EM, Nielsen CH, Bromage PR et al. Ventilatory CO_2 sensitivity after intravenous and epidural morphine in volunteers. *Anesth Analg*. 1983; 62:633-40.
110. Etches RC, Sandler AN, Daley MD. Respiratory depression and spinal opioids. *Can J Anaesth*. 1989; 36:165-85.
111. Gustafsson LL, Schildt B, Jacobsen K. Adverse effects of extradural and intrathecal opiates: a report of a nationwide survey in Sweden. *Br J Anaesth*. 1982; 54:479-85.
112. Rawal N, Schott U, Dahlstrom B et al. Influence of naloxone infusion on analgesia and respiratory depression following epidural morphine. *Anesthesiology*. 1986; 64:194-201.
113. Mok MS, Shaui SP, Lee C et al. Naltrexone pretreatment attenuates side effects of epidural morphine. *Anesthesiology*. 1986; 65:A200. Abstract.
114. Abboud TK, Afrasiabi A, Davidson J. Prophylactic oral naltrexone with epidural morphine: effect on adverse reactions and ventilatory responses to carbon dioxide. *Anesthesiology*. 1990; 72:233-7.
115. Mott JM, Eisele JH. Intraspinal opioids: implications for monitoring. Monitoring in the intensive care unit is not always necessary. *J Clin Monit*. 1989; 5:190-1. Editorial.
116. LaPorta RF, Johnson MD. Intraspinal opioids: implications for monitoring. Monitoring in the intensive care unit is essential. *J Clin Monit*. 1989; 5:186-9. Editorial.
117. Mott JM, Eisele JH. A survey of monitoring practices following spinal opiate administration. *Anesth Analg*. 1986; 65:S105. Abstract.
118. Choi HJ, Little MS, Fujita RA et al. Pulse oximetry for monitoring during ward analgesia: epidural morphine versus parenteral narcotics. *Anesthesiology*. 1986; 65:A37. Abstract.
119. Bromage PR. The price of intraspinal narcotic analgesia: basic constraints. *Anesth Analg*. 1981; 60:461-3. Editorial.
120. Bromage PR, Camporesi EM, Chestnut D. Epidural narcotics for postoperative analgesia. *Anesth Analg*. 1980; 59:473-80.
121. Bromage PR, Camporesi EM, Durant PAC et al. Nonrespiratory side effects of epidural morphine. *Anesth Analg*. 1982; 61:490-5.
122. Davies GD, From R. A blinded study using nalbuphine for prevention of pruritus induced by epidural fentanyl. *Anesthesiology*. 1988; 69:763-5.
123. Scott PV, Fisher HB. Intraspinal opiates and itching: a new reflex? *Br Med J*. 1982; 284:1015-6.
124. Rawal N, Mollefors K, Axelsson K et al. An experimental study of urodynamic effects of epidural morphine and of naloxone reversal. *Anesth Analg*. 1983; 62:641-7.
125. Rawal N, Sjostrand UH, Dahlstrom B. Postoperative pain relief by epidural morphine. *Anesth Analg*. 1981; 60:726-31.
126. Scott DB. Acute pain management. In: Cousins MJ, Bridenbaugh PO, eds. Neural blockade in clinical anesthesia and management of pain. Philadelphia: Lippincott; 1988:861-83.
127. Baron JF, Coriat P, Mundler O et al. Left ventricular global and regional function during lumbar epidural anesthesia in patients with and without angina pectoris. Influence of volume loading. *Anesthesiology*. 1987; 66:621-7.
128. Kane RE. Neurologic deficits following epidural or spinal anesthesia. *Anesth Analg*. 1981; 60:150-61.

Problems of the Randomized Clinical Trial

As medicine has become increasingly scientific and less accepting of unsupported opinion or proof by anecdote, the randomized controlled clinical trial has become the standard technique for changing diagnostic or therapeutic methods. The use of this technique creates an ethical dilemma. Researchers participating in such studies are required to modify their ethical commitments to individual patients and do serious damage to the concept of the physician as a practicing, empathetic professional who is primarily concerned with each patient as an individual. . . .

The purpose of the randomized clinical trial is to avoid the problems of observer bias and patient selection. It seems to us that techniques might be developed to deal with these issues in other ways.

—Hellman S, Hellman DS. Of mice but not men: problems of the randomized clinical trial. *N Engl J Med*. 1991; 324:1585-9.

Assessment and treatment of acetaminophen overdose

RICHARD K. LEWIS AND FRANK P. PALOUCEK

Abstract: The assessment and treatment of acute acetaminophen toxicity are reviewed, and several unresolved issues are discussed.

The drug most commonly involved in analgesic ingestions, as a single agent or in combination, is acetaminophen. Hepatotoxicity, the major manifestation of acetaminophen ingestion, is believed to result from the accumulation of a toxic metabolite, *N*-acetylimidoquinone. The clinical features of acetaminophen toxicity are divided into four stages ranging from minor symptoms, such as gastrointestinal irritation, to coma and death. The most reliable method for assessing the severity of acetaminophen ingestion is comparison of serum acetaminophen concentrations with the Rumack-Matthew nomogram. Delaying the start of antidotal therapy for more than 10 hours after the ingestion increases the risk of toxicity; no benefit is observed when antidotal therapy is initiated more than 24 hours after ingestion. Acetaminophen is often marketed in combination with other drugs; a detailed patient history and a urine toxicology screen help determine whether multiple toxic ingestions have occurred. The roles of ipecac, gastric lavage, and activated charcoal in therapy are controversial.

The mainstay of treatment for acetaminophen intoxication is a 17-dose course of acetylcysteine.

Index terms: Acetaminophen; Acetimidoquinone; Acetylcysteine; Analgesics and antipyretics; Antidotes; Blood levels; Dosage; Dosage schedules; Metabolism; Poisoning; Toxicity
Clin Pharm. 1991; 10:765-74

Analgesic ingestions are a serious problem in the United States. Since the inception of the American Association of Poison Control Centers (AAPCC) National Data Collection System, analgesics have consistently been the most commonly ingested medicinal product and the second most common cause of fatalities in reported exposures. The drug most commonly involved in analgesic ingestions, as a single agent or in combination, is acetaminophen. Data from the past six years show a consistency in the occurrence and outcome of acetaminophen exposures (Table 1). Children less than six years old account for 63% of acetaminophen ingestions, and 73% of all ingestions are accidental.[1-6] Acute acetaminophen ingestions are rarely fatal because of the availability of an antidote, acetylcysteine. This article reviews the assessment and treatment of acetaminophen ingestions and discusses several unresolved issues in patient management.

Hepatotoxic Mechanism of Acetaminophen

Acetaminophen toxicity is primarily manifested as hepatotoxicity. To understand the hepatotoxic mechanism of acetaminophen, one must understand the drug's metabolism (Figure 1). In therapeutic doses, only 2–4% of acetaminophen is excreted in the urine unchanged, with the remaining 96% metabolized in the liver.[8] Approximately 90% of hepatically eliminated acetaminophen is metabolized to a glucuronide or sulfate conjugate. In adults, the remaining 10% is metabolized by the cytochrome P-450 system to an intermediate metabolite, *N*-acetylimidoquinone. This metabolite is considered responsible for the hepatic cell death associated with acetaminophen toxicity. In usual acetaminophen doses, this metabolite is quickly metabolized to a nontoxic derivative by glutathione conjugation. Toxic doses of acetaminophen saturate the glucuronic acid or sulfate pathway. When saturation occurs, the cytochrome P-450 system may metabolize 45% of the ingested acetaminophen to the toxic intermediate. Glutathione conjugation must then increase to prevent accumulation of the toxic metabolite, but glutathione stores are limited and may become depleted. Once glutathione stores are reduced by approximately 70%, the toxic intermediate begins to accumulate and covalently binds to hepatic cells, resulting in hepatocyte necrosis and death.[7]

Clinical Features

An individual's capacity to metabolize acetaminophen in large doses cannot be assessed; therefore, pre-

RICHARD K. LEWIS, PHARM.D., is Director of Ambulatory Care Pharmacy Services, The University of Illinois Hospital and Clinics (UIH&C), and Clinical Assistant Professor, Department of Pharmacy Practice, College of Pharmacy, The University of Illinois at Chicago (UIC); at the time this manuscript was prepared, he was a Clinical/Administrative Resident and Fellow, UIC and Michael Reese Hospital and Medical Center (MRHMC). FRANK P. PALOUCEK, PHARM.D., is Clinical Assistant Professor, Department of Pharmacy Practice, College of Pharmacy, UIC, and Pharmacotherapist in Emergency Medicine, MRHMC and UIH&C.

Address reprint requests to Dr. Lewis at The University of Illinois at Chicago, College of Pharmacy, Department of Pharmacy Practice (M/C 886), 833 South Wood Street, Room 244, Chicago, IL 60612.

This is **article 680-204-9122** in the **ASHP Continuing Education System**; it qualifies for 1.0 hour of continuing-education credit. See page 793 for learning objectives and test questions.

dicting a patient's potential for developing serious toxicity is extremely difficult. The clinical features of toxicity are reasonably uniform and have been divided into four stages.

Stage 1. Stage 1 of acetaminophen toxicity occurs from the time of ingestion to 24 hours after ingestion. Symptoms, including gastrointestinal irritation, pallor, lethargy, and diaphoresis, are usually minor and not pathognomonic.[9] Metabolic acidosis and coma have been reported during stage 1 in massive ingestions associated with serum acetaminophen concentrations greater than 800 μg/mL at four hours after ingestion.[10,11] However, coma is usually attributable to a coingestant and not to acetaminophen alone.[12]

Stage 2. Stage 2 of acetaminophen toxicity typically occurs 24–48 hours after ingestion and may be characterized by a deceptive lack of symptoms. The patient may even insist on being discharged. In this stage, there may be a minimal increase in serum concentrations of hepatic enzymes, and patients may complain of right upper quadrant pain. A slight decrease in renal function is also possible, but unlikely.[9]

Stage 3. Stage 3, also known as the hepatic stage, of acetaminophen toxicity typically occurs 72–96 hours after ingestion. The patient may appear to return to stage 1 symptoms, but the symptoms are more severe. Serum aspartate aminotransferase (AST) concentrations greater than 10,000 IU/L have been reported to occur in this stage.[13] Alanine aminotransferase (ALT) concentrations 100 times normal may also be seen.[9] Nausea, vomiting, jaundice, and central nervous system (CNS) symptoms, such as lethargy, confusion, and potentially, coma, are characteristics of stage 3. Coagulation disorders have been reported and renal dysfunction may or may not be present.[14]

Stage 4. Stage 4, also known as the recovery stage, of acetaminophen toxicity occurs four days to two weeks after ingestion. During this stage, clinical symptoms subside and laboratory values return to normal. If the patient survives, permanent liver damage is rare.[14]

Normal therapeutic doses of acetaminophen in patients with underlying liver disease, e.g., alcoholic hepatitis, have led to the development of hepatic dysfunction similar in presentation to that of the acute overdose.[15] In children, chronic repeated overdoses,

Table 1.
Acetaminophen Ingestions Reported by the AAPCC National Data Collection System[1-6]

Year	Total Exposures	Major Effects	Deaths	Use of Acetylcysteine
1984	35,074	383	23	3,087
1985	32,753	319	29	2,882
1986	39,365	379	29	3,162
1987	66,634	272	35	3,447
1988	86,382	351	52	4,935
1989	97,548	369	57	4,972

Figure 1. Acetaminophen metabolism. (Adapted with permission from reference 7.)

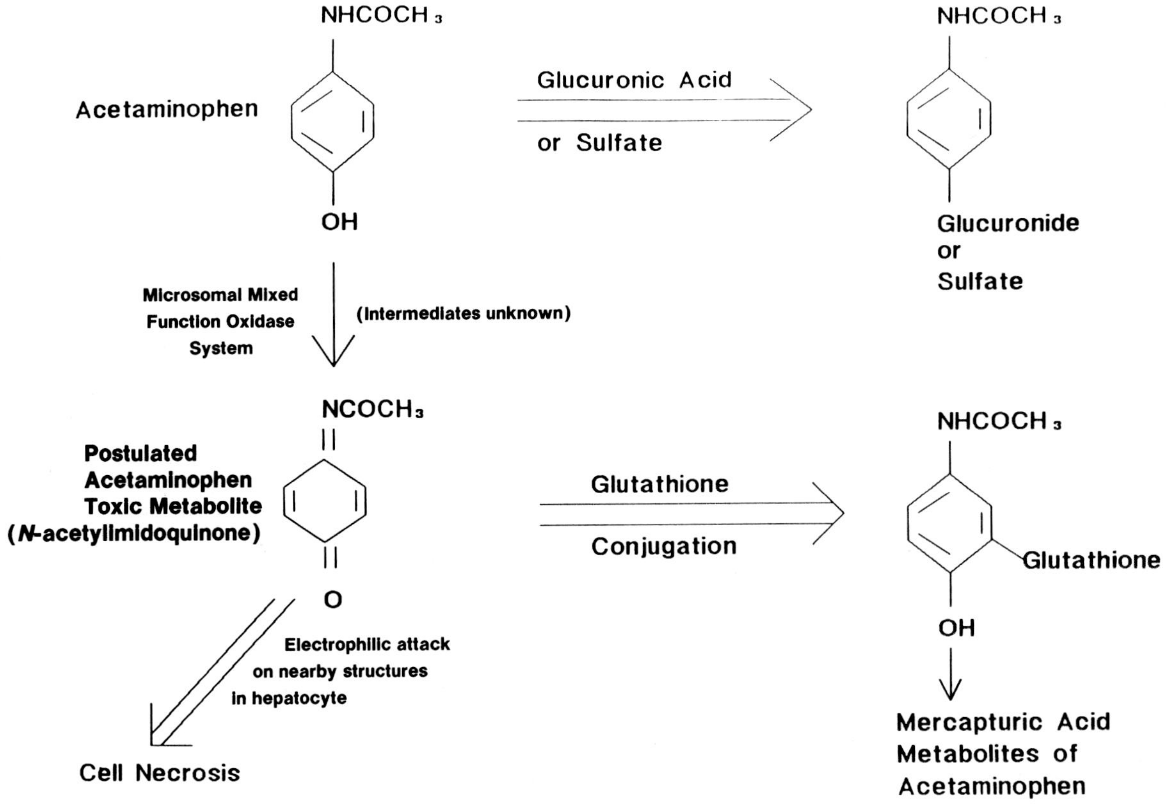

Figure 2. Rumack-Matthew nomogram. (Adapted with permission from reference 13. *Arch Intern Med.* 1981;141:380-5. Copyright 1981, American Medical Association.)

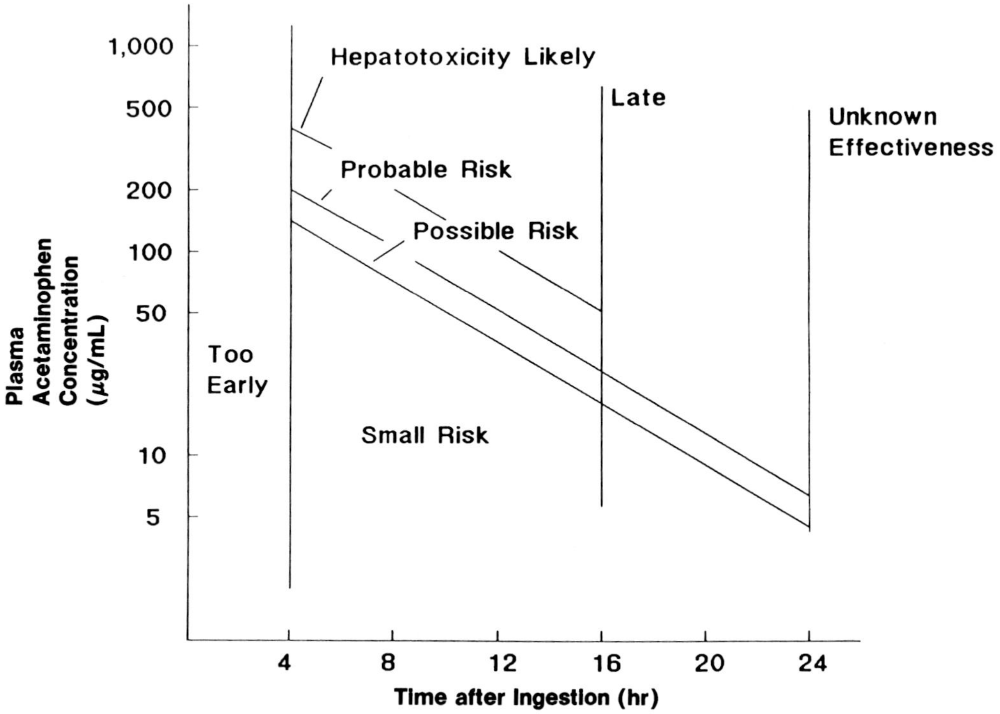

exceeding 75–150 mg/kg/day over two to four days, have been reported, and as little as two times the usual dose has been shown to lead to severe toxicity.[16,17] Fortunately, this rarely occurs. In neither circumstance, underlying liver disease or chronic ingestion, is there an identifiable predictor of toxicity.

Nonhepatic Toxicity

Acetaminophen has also caused acute nonhepatic toxicity, such as renal failure, myocardial necrosis, and pancreatic inflammation.[14,18] However, it is not entirely clear if these sequelae are a direct toxic effect or if they are secondary to hepatic failure and shock.

Assessment of Acetaminophen Toxicity

Traditionally, the assessment of any acute ingestion involves obtaining a detailed history, a thorough physical examination, and a metabolic laboratory workup, from which presumptive diagnosis and prognosis are determined. Treatment, which is usually gastric decontamination or supportive care or both, is then initiated. Laboratory determination of urine or serum drug concentrations rarely alters treatment decisions. Acetaminophen is an important exception because its toxicity is unpredictable and delayed. The decision to initiate antidotal therapy is most appropriately based on timed serum drug concentrations plotted on the widely available Rumack-Matthew nomogram (Figure 2). However, if serum acetaminophen concentrations are not available to the primary care provider within the appropriate time frame, empirical antidotal therapy should be initiated. Antidotal therapy should not affect the outcome of acetaminophen levels.

Interpretation of Patient History. When concentrations are unavailable or results will be obtained at a time after the cutoff for appropriately initiating antidotal therapy, the clinician may rely on patient history to assess the severity of ingestion. The physical examination may not be of assistance in assessing the severity of an acetaminophen ingestion because symptoms preceding fulminant hepatic dysfunction are vague or nonexistent. However, the clinician must remember that acetaminophen is often marketed in combination products, and a physical examination is often useful in identifying and directing therapy for coingestants.

The decision to initiate antidotal therapy may be based on the history of the amount of drug ingested, either as a total dose or on a milligram per kilogram basis. Toxicity is generally expected in adults with an acute acetaminophen ingestion exceeding 7.5 g; 13–25 g is considered a lethal dose. However, it may be difficult to determine how much acetaminophen was ingested. The amount claimed to have been ingested may be inaccurate or indeterminable. A recent study examining the value of rapid acetaminophen concentration screening in all overdoses found that 14.6% of patients claiming acetaminophen ingestion had insignificant serum concentrations (<10 μg/mL).[19] The false-positive history rate is 29% at our institution.[20]

Table 2.
Pharmacokinetic Profile of Acetaminophen[23]

Salt fraction	100%
Bioavailability	89%
Absorption rate constant	1.4 hr^{-1}
Volume of distribution	0.85 L/kg
Half-life	4 hr
Elimination rate constant	0.17 hr^{-1}

Two earlier studies questioned the usefulness of relying on history alone. In one report, the amount claimed to have been ingested ranged from unknown to 50 g, yet the highest serum acetaminophen concentration was 112 μg/mL.[21] In another study, reported ingestions ranged from 6 to 25 g, yet the highest serum concentration was 160 μg/mL.[22] Although the doses ingested were not reported as milligrams per kilogram of body weight in either of these studies, one can conclude that the amount of acetaminophen claimed to be ingested may not result in expected serum concentrations. Both of these studies were based on adult patients, and the reliability of ingestion history in pediatric patients has not been adequately studied.

When results of concentration determinations will not be available by the time that antidotal therapy should be initiated, use of published pharmacokinetic data (Table 2) may facilitate interpretation of the ingestion history. By assuming a one-compartment model and instantaneous absorption, one would predict that the peak serum concentration (C_{peak}) would numerically approximate the milligrams per kilogram dose. This relationship is expressed mathematically as

$$C_{peak} = \text{Dose}\,(F)/V$$

where the dose is expressed as milligrams per kilogram of body weight, the fraction absorbed (F) equals 0.89, and the volume of distribution (V) equals 0.85 L/kg. This equation is the basis for the commonly quoted indication for antidotal therapy of serum acetaminophen concentrations of 140–150 mg/kg in pediatric patients, suggesting an expected peak concentration of 140–150 mg/L, the lower value on the Rumack-Matthew nomogram (Figure 2). If one applies this calculation to the proposed 7.5-g total dose, toxicity would be expected only in individuals weighing less than 50 kg. Conversely, toxicity should be expected in children between 10 and 20 kg who have ingested total doses of 1.5–3.0 g.

Pharmacokinetic calculations may be used to predict serum acetaminophen concentrations at any time after an ingestion, but the accuracy of these predictions would be diminished by the occurrence of events such as nonlinear pharmacokinetics or saturated metabolism. Edwards and coworkers[23] retrospectively compared 80 predicted serum acetaminophen concentrations with measured values in 44 carefully selected adult patients in whom serum acetaminophen concentrations were measured within 16 hours of ingestion. Overall, the correlation coefficient was 0.73. The model predicted four-hour serum concentrations to be 59% of the historical milligrams per kilogram ingested dose. In five patients meeting ideal criteria (i.e., acetaminophen concentrations were determined at exactly four hours after ingestion, and the patient did not vomit before the blood sample was taken), the correlation between actual and calculated four-hour serum concentrations was 0.99. This model has subsequently been evaluated in 98 patients with a history of acetaminophen ingestion.[20] No patients were excluded from the study. The correlation coefficient obtained was only 0.09. This discrepancy highlights the difficulty in applying pharmacokinetic values from a normal adult population to an overdose situation.

Standard gastric decontamination has a substantial impact on resultant serum acetaminophen concentrations.[24] Children receiving ipecac within one hour of ingestion had serum acetaminophen concentrations 77% lower than predicted. Ipecac given one to four hours after ingestion resulted in observed concentrations only 40% lower than predicted.

It has also been suggested that an acetaminophen elimination half-life between 4 and 12 hours, calculated from actual serum concentrations, predicts toxicity.[25] This may be the basis of antidotal therapy. It is unknown at this time whether prolonged elimination half-lives predict toxicity, are secondary to hepatotoxicity, or are due to the effects of coingestants on absorption and elimination of acetaminophen. The need to await results of at least two serum concentration determinations during the elimination phase may also preclude timely initiation of antidotal therapy.

Thus, pharmacokinetically based methods of assessing acetaminophen toxicity may help in the initial assessment but should not be substituted for actual serum concentrations when these become available. Initiation of antidotal therapy can be based on these methods, but the decision to initiate or finish antidotal therapy must be based on acetaminophen serum concentrations whenever possible.

Use of Rumack-Matthew Nomogram. The most widely accepted approach to assessing acute acetaminophen ingestions is to plot serum concentrations obtained four or more hours after ingestion on the Rumack-Matthew nomogram (Figure 2). Serum acetaminophen concentrations must be obtained in any patient suspected of acetaminophen ingestion. The nomogram is a semilogarithmic graph of serum concentration versus time after ingestion, divided into four risk categories. Patients whose serum concentrations exceed the lowest plotted line, defined by concentrations of 150, 75, and 40 mg/L at 4, 8, and 12 hours after ingestion, respectively, are at possible risk of hepatotoxicity. The risk of hepatotoxicity increases with each subsequently higher line. Patients who have serum concentrations greater than 300 mg/L at four hours after ingestion and do not receive antidotal therapy have a 50% mortality rate.[25]

The plotted lines used in the nomogram are based on normal population pharmacokinetic values. The nomogram was evaluated in 662 patients older than 12 years who had acute ingestions of at least 7.5 g, and who received antidotal therapy only if serum acetaminophen concentrations fell within the probable or severe risk category of the nomogram.[13] Of the untreated cases below the nomogram's possible risk category, there were no fatalities and only 0.4% developed toxicity. Delaying antidotal therapy for more than 10 hours after ingestion increased the risk of toxicity (increased liver function test values), and no benefit was seen with antidotal therapy initiated more than 24 hours after ingestion.

This nomogram was not initially evaluated in children less than six years of age, who account for more than 60% of all ingestions.[1-6] However, subsequent observations in 417 pediatric cases suggested equal or superior efficacy of applying the nomogram for treatment determination.[26] To date, there have been no comparative trials employing the nomogram versus any other method for determining the need for antidotal therapy. Also, it should be noted, the nomogram is useful in acute ingestions only.

Supportive Care

A patient with suspected acute acetaminophen ingestion should receive the same supportive care as would be given in all toxic ingestions. Adequate airway, respiratory, and circulatory function must be established and maintained. If the patient is unconscious or obtunded, appropriate doses of thiamine, dextrose, and naloxone must be administered. Consideration of naloxone is critical. Although acetaminophen does not cause CNS depression, it is often coingested with narcotics.

Gastric Decontamination

The role and choice of agents used in gastric decontamination for any toxic ingestion remain controversial. Gastric decontamination, by means of lavage or ipecac-induced emesis, may be beneficial within four hours of an ingestion of potentially toxic doses of acetaminophen. The appropriate choice of ipecac, gastric lavage, or activated charcoal should be made on the basis of time since ingestion, physical findings, and presence of coingestants.

Gastric decontamination with either ipecac or lavage, as indicated by the patient's condition, is encouraged when results of acetaminophen concentration determinations will not be available within eight hours after ingestion. If serum acetaminophen concentrations will be available within eight hours, gastric decontamination may not be necessary.

The alert and oriented patient being treated at home for possible toxicity should receive syrup of ipecac if travel time to a health-care facility will exceed one hour from the time of ingestion. Activated charcoal may also be used if present at home. The obtunded patient should receive gastric lavage for diagnostic purposes at any time and for therapeutic purposes, when indicated, within one hour after ingestion.

A rapid (30-second) diagnostic technique for determining serum acetaminophen concentrations with one drop of whole blood should soon be available.[27] This test should decrease the number of gastric decontamination procedures, reduce attendant complications, and preclude unnecessary, empirical antidotal therapy.

Charcoal. The acceptance of charcoal as an effective means of treating toxic acetaminophen ingestions is increasing; however, it is still controversial. Charcoal decreases acetaminophen absorption; however, it also decreases acetylcysteine absorption and may induce nausea and vomiting, which could increase the problems of administering oral acetylcysteine.

Considerable controversy has surrounded the concomitant use of oral activated charcoal and acetylcysteine. The ability of charcoal to adsorb the antidote resulted in acetaminophen ingestions being considered a contraindication to charcoal use. Six in vitro or animal studies and six studies in humans have examined the effects of charcoal on acetaminophen and acetylcysteine absorption. The in vitro and animal studies show that oral acetaminophen is well adsorbed (50–90%) by activated charcoal at all physiologic intestinal pH values (Table 3).[28-33] The adsorption of acetaminophen is optimal with charcoal doses of 6 g per gram of acetaminophen, which is easily within the range of recommended doses of charcoal for poisonings. The degree of acetylcysteine adsorption, 10–50%, is less than that for acetaminophen and is greatly decreased in the presence of neutral physiologic solutions (e.g., in the small and large intestine). This finding suggests that delaying the administration of acetylcysteine at least one hour after a dose of charcoal should substantially decrease the amount of acetylcysteine adsorbed by charcoal. Specific regimens, such as alternating acetylcysteine and charcoal every two hours or increasing acetylcysteine doses by 20–30%, are empirical.

To date, a total of 54 volunteers have been studied in six clinical trials (Table 4).[34-39] Four studies have evaluated the effects of oral activated charcoal on inhibition of acetaminophen absorption, and two studies have evaluated its effects on inhibition of acetylcysteine absorption; however, no study has directly compared the effects of charcoal on both. When given at one hour after ingestion of acetaminophen, charcoal adsorbs approximately 25% of the acetaminophen dose and has an effect comparable to that of ipecac. The effects on acetylcysteine appear dose related, are not as great as the reduction in acetaminophen absorption, and result in absorbed doses that are well within the range of the oral and intravenous dosage regimens that have been employed to date. Toxicities associated with ipecac use, the potential delay in administering acetylcysteine secondary to ipecac-induced vomiting, the comparable efficacy of charcoal and ipecac in initial gastric decontamination in the alert patient (by definition, the patient with stage 1 toxicity), and the aforementioned

Table 3.
In Vitro or Animal Studies of the Effect of Activated Charcoal on Acetaminophen or Acetylcysteine[a]

Ref.	Dose of Activated Charcoal	Results
28	AC 0.1–1.0 g with acetaminophen 125 mg	54–99% of acetaminophen adsorbed in 1 hr, no variance with altered temperature or pH; complete adsorption of acetaminophen with dose ratio of AC:acetaminophen ≥4:1, desorption <2% with ratios of ≥5:1
29	AC (unstated dose and time) with acetaminophen 3250 or 6500 mg	23% adsorption of 3250-mg dose, 8% adsorption of 6500-mg dose
30	Various ratios of 12 AC products with acetaminophen with or without acetylcysteine in test tubes	Petroleum-based AC products exhibited greatest capacity to adsorb acetaminophen; acetylcysteine minimally affected acetaminophen adsorption by AC
	AC:acetaminophen 5:1 (toxic range of acetaminophen doses) in dogs	89% decrease in acetaminophen C_{max}, 94% decrease in acetaminophen AUC; no serious toxicity noted, mean increase in AST was 64%
	AC 3–7.5 g with acetaminophen 1 g in mice	Acetaminophen LD_{50} increased by 100% with AC; no significant differences in mortality
	Acetylcysteine 375 mg/kg with or without AC in mice	Mortality lower with AC + acetylcysteine than with acetylcysteine alone
31	AC 1–5 g with acetaminophen 3 g or acetylcysteine or both	40–97% adsorption of acetaminophen with or without acetylcysteine; 10–54% adsorption of acetylcysteine when acetaminophen was not present; 11–68% adsorption of acetylcysteine when acetaminophen was present; acetylcysteine adsorption was less in simulated intestinal fluid than in simulated gastric fluid
32	AC:acetylcysteine 0.5–7:1 in test tubes	30–60% adsorption of acetylcysteine; 84% less adsorption in simulated biologic fluids
33	AC:acetylcysteine 3–6:1 in nonbiologic fluids in test tubes (simulated clinical doses)	55–96% adsorption of acetylcysteine

[a] AC = activated charcoal, LD_{50} = dose at which 50% mortality occurs.

Table 4.
Clinical Trials of Activated Charcoal with Acetaminophen or Acetylcysteine[a]

Ref.	Study Design	No. Patients	Dose of Activated Charcoal (g)	Results
Acetaminophen				
34	XO	7	10 at 0 and 60 min	Acetaminophen AUC 63% lower at time 0 and 23% lower at 60 min; AC also compared with cholestyramine, no difference found
35	XO	5	5 or 10 at 0 min, 10 at 30 min	Acetaminophen *F* decreased by 48% for 5-g dose and 62% for 10-g dose at 0 min; *F* decreased by 50% for 10-g dose at 30 min; acetaminophen elixir, suspension, and tablets compared; suspension and tablets equivalent
36	R, XO, OD	10	50 at 0 min	AUC decreased by 25%; AC compared with ipecac, no difference in AUC found; hyperemesis noted in 2 ipecac patients
Acetylcysteine				
37	XO, OD[b]	3	50 at 0 min	No difference in acetylcysteine AUC, C_{max}, or t_{max}; AUC decreased 10% with AC
38	R, XO, OD	19	100 at 30 min before acetylcysteine	Acetylcysteine AUC decreased by 39%, C_{max} by 29%, and t_{max} by 25% with AC; wide intrapatient variation in plasma acetylcysteine concentrations noted; authors recommend 40% increase in acetylcysteine dose if AC given concomitantly
39	XO, OD	10	60 at 0 min	No difference in acetylcysteine AUC, C_{max}, t_{max}, or $t_{1/2}$ found; AUC decreased by 18%, $t_{1/2}$ decreased from 114 to 82 min[c]

[a] OD = simulated overdose, R = randomized, XO = crossover design, AC = activated charcoal.
[b] Acetylcysteine dose = 140 mg/kg.
[c] Data for six subjects only; four excluded because of vomiting after acetylcysteine dose.

data suggest that charcoal is appropriate in the initial management of these patients.

Acetylcysteine

The mainstay of treatment used in acetaminophen intoxication is acetylcysteine (Mucomyst, Mead Johnson). Acetylcysteine is believed to prevent hepatotoxicity by replacing the depleted glutathione stores necessary to prevent accumulation of *N*-acetylimidoquinone. Specifically, acetylcysteine is given to replete the sulfhydryl source for detoxification of the reactive intermediate. Indications for the use of acetylcysteine in acetaminophen intoxication are as follows: (1) serum acetaminophen concentrations in the possibly toxic range of the Rumack-Matthew nomogram, (2) an estimated ingestion of greater than 140 mg/kg, and (3) an estimated half-life of greater than four hours when the time of ingestion is unknown. The latter two indications for acetylcysteine should be considered empirical, and verification with serum concentration determinations is recommended.

The loading dose of acetylcysteine is 140 mg/kg orally, followed by a maintenance dose of 70 mg/kg orally every four hours for 17 doses. The specific dosage regimen is empirical. The dosage regimen of oral acetylcysteine initially used in the United States was 140 mg/kg followed by 70 mg/kg every eight hours for three days (48% lower than current protocol). This regimen resulted in mild increases in liver function test results during stage 3 in a single patient.[40] Current standards indicate that all patients with toxic serum concentrations should receive the entire course of 17 doses.

The major adverse effect associated with acetylcysteine therapy is nausea and vomiting, usually resulting from the strong rotten egg odor. To assist ingestion, the standard 20% solution of acetylcysteine should be diluted to 5%, using a beverage such as orange juice or soda. Acetylcysteine is available in 4-mL, 10-mL, 30-mL, and 100-mL vials of 20% solution; therefore, a large number of vials may be required to prepare the entire 17 doses, especially if the 100-mL vial is not stocked. For example, the loading dose alone for a 70-kg patient would require more than 50 mL of acetylcysteine.

Rumack and colleagues[13] at the Rocky Mountain Poison Center have been evaluating the use of acetylcysteine since 1976. By 1981, these investigators had evaluated data from 662 patients treated for acetaminophen intoxication and had published strong evidence to support the use of acetylcysteine. Their data suggested that patients treated with acetylcysteine had significantly lower serum AST concentrations during stage 3 than patients who had not received therapy.

In 1988, the results of another study from the Rocky Mountain Poison Center were published.[41] Data from 2,540 patients were used to evaluate the relationships among severity of ingestion, hepatotoxicity, and delay in treatment with acetylcysteine. Only 2,540 of 11,195 patients met the inclusion criterion of a single acute overdose documented by at least one serum acetaminophen concentration 4–24 hours after ingestion that was treated with a minimum of 17 doses of acetylcysteine. In part 1 of this study, patients who received acetylcysteine within eight hours of ingestion ($n = 729$) were analyzed. The data from these patients were divided into six groups depending on the serum concentration four hours after ingestion, which ranged from <150 μg/mL to 500 μg/mL. The median serum AST concentration (40.5 IU/L) of the group of 28 patients with four-hour serum acetaminophen concentrations ≥ 400 μg/mL was significantly higher than the median serum AST concentration of the other five groups. However, an actual serum AST concentration of 40.5 IU/L is probably not clinically important.

In part 2 of this study, the median and mean peak serum AST concentrations in 2023 patients were evaluated to determine the effect of delaying acetylcysteine treatment. The differences in these concentrations between the 0- to 4-hour and the 4- to 8-hour treatment delay groups were not significant, suggesting that a delay of up to eight hours in acetylcysteine treatment may not alter outcome. Significant increases in the percentage of patients with serum AST concentrations greater than 1000 IU/L and significant increases in the median and mean peak serum AST concentrations were found to occur in patients who did not receive acetylcysteine in an 8- to 10-hour time frame, as compared with patients who received acetylcysteine in a 4- to 8-hour time frame.

Are 17 Doses of Acetylcysteine Necessary? Although patients who did not receive 17 doses of acetylcysteine were excluded from the 1988 Rocky Mountain Poison Center study, only 2% of the 1630 patients in this group developed hepatotoxicity, suggesting that not all patients with acetaminophen intoxication need 17 doses.[41] Details on these patients were not discussed in the study; therefore, the only conclusion to be drawn is that the need for 17 doses of acetylcysteine requires further investigation.

Additional evidence questioning the current dosage protocol can be found by examining the dosage protocol for intravenous acetylcysteine. The dosage protocol for the pyrogen-free intravenous formulation is a 150-mg/kg loading dose, followed by 50 mg/kg over the next 4 hours and 100 mg/kg over the last 16 hours.[42] This total dose of 300 mg/kg over a 20-hour period is only 22% of the total oral dosage used in the United States (1330 mg/kg).

Efficacy of Intravenous Acetylcysteine. Intravenous acetylcysteine is used in Great Britain and Canada and is considered the treatment of choice for acetaminophen overdoses by some authors.[43] However, i.v. acetylcysteine is still investigational in the United States, and a pyrogen-free formulation is not available for use in this country.[a] The major advantages of i.v. administration are a shorter treatment duration and a lower incidence of nausea and vomiting. The major disadvantage is the potential for anaphylactoid reactions.[44]

In 1981, Prescott[42] compared the outcomes of 100 patients who received i.v. acetylcysteine with those of 60 patients who received i.v. cysteamine or methionine and a control group of 57 patients who received supportive care alone. Patients who received i.v. acetylcysteine within 10 hours were significantly less likely to develop severe liver damage than those patients who received supportive care alone, i.v. cysteamine or methionine, or i.v. acetylcysteine more than 10 hours after ingestion. Prescott[42] also attempted to compare oral and i.v. acetylcysteine, but only 2 of 52 patients in the oral group completed therapy without vomiting.

The results of the study by Smilkstein and coworkers[41] suggested a possible benefit of oral over i.v. acetylcysteine when treatment was delayed more than 10 hours. Only 34% of 578 high-risk patients who were treated with oral acetylcysteine within 10–24 hours of ingestion developed hepatotoxicity, as compared with 67% of 27 high-risk patients who received i.v. acetylcysteine within the same time frame as in Prescott's study. The Rocky Mountain Poison Center is currently comparing these two routes and regimens in a prospective study.

Laboratory Monitoring

Acetaminophen is often marketed in combination with other drugs, such as codeine, propoxyphene, decongestants, and antihistamines. Therefore, a urine toxicology screen is essential in acetaminophen ingestions to help rule out other potentially toxic ingestions.

Because acetaminophen toxicity is usually manifested as hepatotoxicity, liver function tests should be monitored every 24 hours for three to four days in patients who have initial acetaminophen concentrations in the possibly toxic range or higher.[45] Serum bilirubin concentrations are usually the first to change and should be closely monitored during stages 1 and 2. Serum aminotransferase concentrations usually peak at three to four days after ingestion, and values greater than 1000 IU/L indicate that some hepatic cell necrosis has occurred.[26]

Because there is a potential for renal failure, serum creatinine concentration and blood urea nitrogen (BUN) should also be monitored. However, it is important to note that BUN may not be elevated because of the liver's inability to produce urea by-products. Electrolytes and fluid balance should be monitored, especially if vomiting has occurred.

Serum acetaminophen concentrations also need to be monitored. However, once a proper diagnosis of acute acetaminophen toxicity has been established, a full course of treatment is indicated and is independent of subsequent serum acetaminophen concentrations.

Pediatric Considerations

Acetaminophen ingestions in pediatric patients are usually due to accidental exposure and are less likely to result in hepatotoxicity than are ingestions in adults.[26] Additionally, there are no well-documented cases of fatality occurring in a pediatric patient secondary to acute acetaminophen exposure. Review of AAPCC annual summaries of fatalities indicates that only 5 of 225 deaths primarily attributed to acetaminophen occurred in pediatric patients.[1-6] Of these five cases, only one was categorized as general accidental exposure; the remainder occurred in cases of chronic repeated exposures.

Reasons for the apparent resistance in children to acute acetaminophen hepatotoxicity are unclear but may be related to variations in metabolic capacity. Infants and children appear to have a greater capacity to metabolize acetaminophen to a sulfate conjugate than adults.[46] The significance of this finding is unclear because the overall elimination half-life of acetaminophen in usual therapeutic dosages does not vary with age, although it is possible that infants and children have a higher threshold for saturation of the metabolic pathway. The capacity to metabolize acetaminophen to the proposed toxic intermediary has been shown only in adults; this has never been studied in children. It has been shown, in mice, that age has an inverse relationship to glutathione synthesis; thus, children may replete glutathione stores more rapidly than adults.[47] In addition to these potential metabolic etiologies for improved outcomes in children, consideration should be given to the infrequency of toxic serum concentrations in these accidental pediatric exposures.

Health-care providers who have the potential of becoming involved in the treatment of a pediatric patient with acetaminophen ingestion should be aware of misprinted information in the 11th edition of the *Harriet Lane Handbook*.[48] The Rumack-Matthew nomogram reprinted in the book begins at two hours instead of four hours after ingestion. The book also recommends a loading dose of acetylcysteine, followed by only five maintenance doses, which is inconsistent with the current standard of practice. These misprints were brought to the attention of the editors of the handbook, and several letters were published in professional journals.[49,50] Subsequent printings of the handbook were corrected; however, copies of the 11th edition were distributed and could inadvertently be used for information on the treatment of acetaminophen toxicity.

Use of Cimetidine

Theoretically, there is a potential role for cimetidine in the treatment of acetaminophen overdose. Cimetidine has been shown to inhibit cytochrome P-450 in the liver; thus, it inhibits the metabolism of many drugs, including acetaminophen. Therefore, if acetaminophen metabolism could be inhibited by cimetidine, the toxic intermediate that causes hepatic necrosis would not be generated (Figure 1).

In animal studies, rats receiving a combination of cimetidine and acetylcysteine were found to have significantly less hepatotoxicity and a greater survival rate than rats receiving 0.9% sodium chloride solution, acetylcysteine, or cimetidine.[51] Rats receiving both cimetidine and acetylcysteine were also found to have significantly less glutathione depletion than the other groups, suggesting that the agents may have prevented accumulation of the toxic intermediate. Oxidative metabolism was chemically induced in the rats; the cimetidine and acetylcysteine were given to the rats before the acetaminophen, and a large dose of cimetidine was used (25 mg/kg).

Initial human experiences are not as promising. Thirteen volunteers receiving 1 g of acetaminophen with or without 300 mg of cimetidine every six hours had no significant differences in renal and nonrenal clearances of acetaminophen. Additionally, studies performed in human microsomal tissues suggest a need for cimetidine concentrations 5–10 times putative therapeutic concentrations.[52]

An ongoing prospective trial is comparing acetylcysteine therapy alone versus acetylcysteine and cimetidine 300 mg every six hours in patients receiving initial acetylcysteine doses more than eight hours after ingestion. The experience in the initial 80 patients shows no difference in the frequency or severity of elevations in AST.[53]

Conclusion

At present, the only proven method of initially assessing the severity of an acetaminophen ingestion involves the comparison of serum drug concentrations with the Rumack-Matthew nomogram. Gastric decontamination is considered first-line therapy for patients treated within four hours of ingestion who do not have any contraindications. However, once a possibly toxic serum concentration is documented on the Rumack-Matthew nomogram, a 17-dose course of oral acetylcysteine is considered the treatment of choice in the United States. Recent studies have indicated that treatment with acetylcysteine may be delayed up to eight hours after ingestion without substantially changing patient outcome. This allows time to obtain and interpret serum acetaminophen concentrations before active treatment measures are initiated. This treatment "window" suggests a valuable role for rapid diagnostic devices. Current standards indicate that most patients with documented toxic serum acetaminophen concentrations should receive 17 doses of acetylcysteine, but recent data suggest the possibility that fewer doses may achieve the same outcome. Although intravenous acetylcysteine may offer some minor advantages, such as less nausea and vomiting, current data suggest that both oral and i.v. acetylcysteine produce similar outcomes if administered within 10 hours of ingestion. The use of activated charcoal may be vital, particularly in mixed ingestions. Although an antidote for acetaminophen toxicity is available and ingestions are infrequently morbid events, controversies over assessment and treatment continue.

---

[a]Health-care providers should contact the Rocky Mountain Poison Center at 800-525-6115 for assistance in the care of patients who require intravenous therapy.

References

1. Litovitz TL, Schmitz BF, Bailey KM. 1989 Annual report of the American Association of Poison Control Centers National Data Collection System. *Am J Emerg Med.* 1990; 8:394-442.
2. Litovitz TL, Schmitz BF, Holm K. 1988 Annual report of the American Association of Poison Control Centers National Data Collection System. *Am J Emerg Med.* 1989; 7:495-545.
3. Litovitz TL, Schmitz BF, Matyunas N et al. 1987 Annual report of the American Association of Poison Control Centers National Data Collection System. *Am J Emerg Med.* 1988; 6:479-515.
4. Litovitz TL, Martin TG, Schmitz BF. 1986 Annual report of the American Association of Poison Control Centers National Data Collection System. *Am J Emerg Med.* 1987; 5:405-45.
5. Litovitz TL, Normann SA, Veltri JC. 1985 Annual report of the American Association of Poison Control Centers National Data Collection System. *Am J Emerg Med.* 1986; 4:427-58.
6. Litovitz TL, Veltri JC. 1984 Annual report of the American Association of Poison Control Centers National Data Collection System. *Am J Emerg Med.* 1985; 3:423-50.
7. Black M. Acetaminophen hepatotoxicity. *Gastroenterology.* 1980; 78:382-92.
8. Slattery JT, Levy G. Acetaminophen kinetics in acutely poisoned patients. *Clin Pharmacol Ther.* 1979; 25:184-95.
9. Linden CH, Rumack BH. Acetaminophenoverdose. *Emerg Med Clin North Am.* 1984; 2:103-19.
10. Flanagan RJ, Mant TGK. Coma and metabolic acidosis early in severe acute paracetamol poisoning. *Hum Toxicol.* 1986; 5:179-82.
11. Zezulka A, Wright N. Severe metabolic acidosis early in paracetamol poisoning. *Br J Med.* 1982; 285:851-2.
12. Read RB, Tredger JM, Williams R. Analysis of factors responsible for continuing mortality after paracetamol overdose. *Hum Toxicol.* 1986; 5:201-6.
13. Rumack BH, Peterson RC, Koch GG et al. Acetaminophen overdose: 662 cases with evaluation of oral acetylcysteine treatment. *Arch Intern Med.* 1981; 141:380-5.
14. Ellenhorn MJ, Barceloux DG. Medical toxicology: diagnosis and treatment of human poisoning. New York: Elsevier; 1988:156-66.
15. Seeff LB, Cuccherini BA, Zimmerman HJ et al. Acetaminophen hepatotoxicity in alcoholics: a therapeutic misadventure. *Ann Intern Med.* 1986; 104:399-404.
16. Blake KV, Bailey D, Zientek GM et al. Death of a child associated with multiple overdoses of acetaminophen. *Clin Pharm.* 1988; 7:391-7.
17. Henretig FM, Selbst SM, Forrest C et al. Repeated acetaminophen overdosing causing hepatotoxicity in children. *Clin Pediatr.* 1989; 28:525-8.
18. Jeffery WH, Lafferty WE. Acute renal failure after acetaminophen overdose: report of two cases. *Am J Hosp Pharm.* 1981; 38:1355-8.
19. Ashbourne JF, Olson KR, Khayam-Bashi H. Value of rapid screening for acetaminophen in all patients with intentional drug overdose. *Ann Emerg Med.* 1989; 18:1035-8.
20. Paloucek FP, Lafin S, Leikin JB. The use of serum acetaminophen sampling in an emergency room. *Vet Hum Toxicol.* 1989; 31:358. Abstract.
21. Ambre J, Alexander M. Liver toxicity after acetaminophen ingestion: inadequacy of the dose estimate as an index of risk. *JAMA.* 1977; 238:500-1.
22. Shnaps Y, Halkin H, Dany S et al. Inadequacy of reported intake in assessing the potential hepatotoxicity of acetaminophen overdose. *Isr J Med Sci.* 1980; 16:752-5.
23. Edwards DA, Fish SF, Lamson MJ et al. Prediction of acetaminophen level from clinical history of overdose using a pharmacokinetic model. *Ann Emerg Med.* 1986; 15:1314-9.
24. Amitai Y, Mitchell AA, McGuigan MA et al. Ipecac-induced emesis and reduction of plasma concentrations of drugs following accidental overdose in children. *Pediatrics.* 1987; 80:364-7.
25. Prescott LF, Wright N, Roscoe P et al. Plasma paracetamol half-life and hepatic necrosis in patients with paracetamol overdosage. *Lancet.* 1971; 1:519-22.
26. Rumack BH. Acetaminophen overdose in young children: treatment and effects of alcohol and other additional ingestants in 417 cases. *Am J Dis Child.* 1984; 138:428-33.
27. Shannon M, Saladino R, McCarty D et al. Clinical evaluation of an acetaminophen meter for the rapid diagnosis of acetaminophen intoxication. *Ann Emerg Med.* 1990; 19:1133-6.
28. Bainbridge CA, Kelly EL, Walkling WD. In vitro adsorption

of acetaminophen onto activated charcoal. *J Pharm Sci*. 1977; 66:480-3.
29. Corby DG, Decker WJ. Management of acute poisoning with activated charcoal. *Pediatrics*. 1974; 54:324-8.
30. Van De Graaff WB, Thompson WL, Sunshine I et al. Adsorbent and cathartic inhibition of enteral drug absorption. *J Pharmacol Exp Ther*. 1982; 221:656-63.
31. Rybolt TR, Burrell DE, Shults JM et al. In vitro coadsorption of acetaminophen and n-acetylcysteine onto activated carbon powder. *J Pharm Sci*. 1986; 75:904-6.
32. Chinouth RW, Czajka PA. N-acetylcysteine adsorption by activated charcoal. *Vet Hum Toxicol*. 1980; 22;392-4.
33. Klein-Schwartz W, Oderda GM. Adsorption of oral antidotes for acetaminophen poisoning (methionine and n-acetylcysteine) by activated charcoal. *Clin Toxicol*. 1981; 18:283-90.
34. Dordoni B, Willson RA, Thompson RPH et al. Reduction of absorption of paracetamol by activated charcoal and cholestyramine: a possible therapeutic measure. *Br Med J*. 1973; 3:86-7.
35. Levy G, Houston BJ. Effect of activated charcoal on acetaminophen absorption. *Pediatrics*. 1976; 58:432-5.
36. McNamara RM, Aaron CK, Gemborys M et al. Efficacy of charcoal cathartic versus ipecac in reducing serum acetaminophen in a simulated overdose. *Ann Emerg Med*. 1989; 18:934-8.
37. North DS, Peterson RG, Krenzelok EP. Effect of activated charcoal administration on acetylcysteine serum levels in humans. *Am J Hosp Pharm*. 1981; 38:1022-4.
38. Ekins BR, Ford DC, Thompson MIB et al. The effect of activated charcoal on n-acetylcysteine absorption in normal subjects. *Am J Emerg Med*. 1987; 5:483-7.
39. Renzi FP, Donovan JW, Martin TG et al. Concomitant use of activated charcoal and n-acetylcysteine. *Ann Emerg Med*. 1985; 14:568-72.
40. Peterson RG, Rumack BH. Treating acute acetaminophen poisoning with acetylcysteine. *JAMA*. 1977; 237:2406-7.
41. Smilkstein MJ, Knapp GL, Kulig KW et al. Efficacy of oral n-acetylcysteine in the treatment of acetaminophen overdose: analysis of the national multicenter study (1976 to 1985). *N Engl J Med*. 1988; 319:1557-62.
42. Prescott LF. Treatment of severe acetaminophen poisoning with intravenous acetylcysteine. *Arch Intern Med*. 1981; 141:386-9.
43. Prescott LF, Illingworth RN, Critchley JAJH et al. Intravenous n-acetylcysteine: the treatment of choice for paracetamol poisoning. *Br Med J*. 1979; 2:1097-100.
44. Walton NG, Mann TAN, Shaw KM. Anaphylactoid reaction to n-acetylcysteine. *Lancet*. 1979; 12:1298. Letter.
45. Goldfrank LR, Howland MA, Weisman RS et al. Acetaminophen. In: Goldfrank LR, Flomenbaum NE, Lewin NA et al., eds. Toxicologic emergencies. Norwalk, CT: Appleton-Century-Crofts; 1986:222-32.
46. Miller RP, Roberts RJ, Fischer LJ. Acetaminophen kinetics in neonates, children and adults. *Clin Pharmacol Ther*. 1976; 19:284-94.
47. Hart JG, Timbrell JA. The effect of hepatotoxicity on paracetamol hepatotoxicity in mice. *Biochem Pharmacol*. 1979; 28:3015-7.
48. Rowe PC, ed. Specific poisoning: acetaminophen. In: Harriet Lane handbook. 11th ed. Chicago: Year Book Medical Publishers; 1987:247-8.
49. Ruck B, Caraccio TR, Mofenson HC. Dosage of acetylcysteine in acetaminophen poisoning. *Pediatrics*. 1988; 82:674-5. Letter.
50. Brent J, Rumack BH, Kulig KW. Dosage of acetylcysteine in acetaminophen poisoning. *Pediatrics*. 1988; 82:675-6. Letter.
51. Speeg KV Jr, Mitchell MC, Maldonado AL. Additive protection of cimetidine and n-acetylcysteine treatment against acetaminophen-induced hepatic necrosis in the rat. *J Pharmacol Exp Ther*. 1985; 234:550-4.
52. Slattery JT, McRorie TI, Reynolds R et al. Lack of effect of cimetidine on acetaminophen disposition in humans. *Clin Pharmacol Ther*. 1989; 46:591-7.
53. Burkhart K, Janco N, Kulig K et al. Cimetidine as adjunctive treatment for acetaminophen overdose. *Vet Hum Toxicol*. 1989; 31:337. Abstract.

Scientific and Ethical Soundness of Randomized Clinical Trials

Randomized clinical trials are an important element in the spectrum of biomedical research. Not all questions can or should be addressed by this technique; feasibility, cost, and the relative importance of the issues to be addressed are weighed by investigators before they elect to proceed. Properly carried out, with informed consent, clinical equipoise, and a design adequate to answer the question posed, randomized clinical trials protect physicians and their patients from therapies that are ineffective or toxic. Physicians and their patients must be clear about the vast gulf separating promising and proved therapies. The only reliable way to make this distinction in the face of incomplete information about pathophysiology and treatment mechanism is to experiment, and this will increasingly involve randomized clinical trials. The alternative—a retreat to older methods—is unacceptable.

—Passamani E. Clinical trials—are they ethical? *N Engl J Med*. 1991; 324:1589-92.

Treatment of chronic iron overload

MARILYN H. KIRKING

Abstract: The clinical features and therapy of chronic iron overload are reviewed.

Chronic iron overload is classified as primary or secondary hemochromatosis. In primary hemochromatosis a genetic defect in iron metabolism results in increased absorption of iron from the gastrointestinal tract. The excess iron in secondary hemochromatosis may be derived from increased gastrointestinal absorption due to ineffective erythropoiesis or from medicinal, dietary, or transfusional sources.

Phlebotomy is the treatment of choice in patients with primary hemochromatosis. Iron chelation therapy is indicated in patients who are not candidates for phlebotomy. Deferoxamine mesylate, the only commercially available iron chelator, is usually administered subcutaneously or intravenously over 10–12 hours/day. Serum ferritin concentrations are measured every three to six months to monitor the effectiveness of therapy. The adverse effects of deferoxamine include local skin reactions, ototoxicity, cataracts, growth impairment, and increased susceptibility to infectious organisms. Patient compliance may be compromised by the routes of administration and cost of deferoxamine. Early detection and prompt treatment are necessary to prevent organ damage.

Phlebotomy and iron chelation therapy are effective in the treatment of chronic iron overload.

Index terms: Bloodletting; Compliance; Costs; Deferoxamine mesylate; Drug administration routes; Heavy metal antagonists; Hemochromatosis; Toxicity
Clin Pharm. 1991; 10:775-83

Iron overload occurs when there is an absolute increase in body iron stores resulting from increased gastrointestinal absorption of iron or an exogenous source of iron, such as transfused blood. The clinical importance of iron overload has become more apparent as patients with genetically determined disorders of iron metabolism or refractory anemias live longer. This article reviews the clinical manifestations and current medical management of chronic iron overload.

Classification and Incidence

Iron overload without associated tissue damage is referred to as hemosiderosis or siderosis. In hemosiderosis, little or no increase in total body iron content is seen but a redistribution of iron results in excess iron stores in the lungs, kidneys, or liver. Excess iron in these organs is termed idiopathic pulmonary siderosis, paroxysmal nocturnal hemoglobinuria, and hepatic siderosis, respectively.

Hemochromatosis is used to describe iron overload that causes tissue damage.[1] Primary or hereditary hemochromatosis is caused by a genetic defect in iron metabolism that increases the intestinal absorption of iron from a normal diet. It is inherited as an autosomal recessive trait with a gene frequency of 1 in 20 in persons of European descent[2] and is more common in men than in women. Approximately 1 in 400 persons may be homozygous for this trait and at risk of developing iron overload. Secondary or acquired hemochromatosis results from some abnormality other than a primary increase in the intestinal absorption of iron.[1] The source of excess iron can be medicinal or dietary, but the condition is more commonly the result of repeated blood transfusions or ineffective erythropoiesis.

Transfusional iron overload has generally been associated with thalassemia major. In the United States, some 1000 patients with thalassemia major currently receive regular blood transfusions.[3] Thalassemias are a group of hereditary hemoglobin synthesis disorders that occur more frequently in individuals of Mediterranean, African, or Oriental origin.[4]

The number of persons at risk for iron overload is magnified when patients with chronic anemias requiring regular blood transfusions are included. For example, sickle cell anemia affects approximately 50,000 persons in the United States.[3] Although only a small percentage of these patients receive regular transfusions, the number of persons at risk for iron overload has been estimated to exceed 4000.[3] Chronic renal-failure patients receiving dialysis are also at risk for

MARILYN H. KIRKING is Ambulatory Care Pharmacist, Department of Pharmacy Services, University of Michigan Hospitals, and Clinical Instructor, College of Pharmacy, University of Michigan, Ann Arbor.

Address reprint requests to Ms. Kirking at University of Michigan Hospitals, Ambulatory Care Pharmacy, Taubman Health Care Center, 1500 E. Medical Center Drive, Ann Arbor, MI 48109.

The assistance of Samir M. Hanash, M.D., Ph.D.; Mary B. Ross, M.B.A.; and other members of the *Michigan Drug Letter* Editorial Board in reviewing the manuscript is acknowledged.

Adapted from an article that appeared in the May 1991 issue of the *Michigan Drug Letter*, a publication of the Department of Pharmacy Services, University of Michigan Medical Center, Ann Arbor.

This is **article 680-204-9123** in the **ASHP Continuing Education System;** it qualifies for 1.0 hour of continuing-education credit. See page 794 for learning objectives and test questions.

iron overload from iron therapy or blood transfusions. However, with the use of recombinant erythropoietin therapy and the subsequent decrease in the frequency of blood transfusions, iron overload may take longer to develop.

In countries where dietary iron intake is low, such as India, liver iron concentrations are low and the clinical manifestations of iron overload are rarely seen. Countries with a heavy per capita consumption of meat and a lower incidence of iron deficiency, like Australia, have a higher incidence and earlier presentation of iron overload.[5]

Clinical Features

Symptoms of iron overload occur when body iron stores reach 15–20 g. Death commonly occurs when body iron exceeds 1 g per kilogram of body weight.[6] The rate of iron accumulation is affected by the underlying disease state and environmental factors. In primary hemochromatosis, symptoms of iron overload often are not seen until the ages of 40–60 years. In contrast, patients with thalassemia major often manifest symptoms of iron overload during the first decade of life.

Excess iron deposited in the parenchymal cells of the liver, heart, and endocrine glands eventually causes functional insufficiency of these organs. The degree of tissue damage appears to be related more to the amount of parenchymal iron than to total body iron stores.[7] Ineffective erythropoiesis and increased intestinal absorption of iron result in greater parenchymal iron loading, whereas iron derived from parenteral sources is preferentially deposited in the reticuloendothelial system. However, when plasma iron is elevated and total iron-binding capacity saturation is greater than 60%, iron is also deposited in the parenchymal cells.

The liver is usually the first organ to be affected by iron overload. Hepatomegaly is present in over 95% of symptomatic patients.[7] As the iron overload persists or increases, cirrhosis develops and slowly leads to hepatic failure. An increased incidence of hepatocellular carcinoma has been reported in patients with cirrhosis.[8] Two thirds of untreated patients with primary hemochromatosis die of hepatic failure, bleeding from esophageal varices, or hepatocellular carcinoma.[9]

In young patients, cardiac dysfunction is often the initial feature of hemochromatosis. Arrhythmias with progressive severe heart failure resistant to treatment occur in 5–15% of symptomatic patients.[10] Damage to the hypothalamic–pituitary–gonadal axis results in delayed puberty or failure of puberty, secondary amenorrhea, and secondary hypogonadism.[3] Hypothyroidism has been observed, although it may not be clinically apparent. Hormone replacement is usually not necessary if iron chelation therapy is begun.[11] Hypoparathyroidism caused by iron overload may make the maintenance of adequate calcium levels in iron-overloaded patients difficult; the result may be hypocalcemic tetany.[3]

Up to 80% of patients with hemochromatosis show symptoms of carbohydrate intolerance.[7] Hyperinsulinemia is the earliest disturbance of carbohydrate metabolism. Diabetes mellitus occurs in 30–60% of patients with advanced hemochromatosis.[7] In one report of 29 patients who had normal glucose tolerance before undergoing long-term chelation therapy, the 6 patients who developed diabetes mellitus had cirrhosis or chronic active hepatitis.[12] Although not as common as diabetes, pancreatic insufficiency may occur, resulting in diarrhea and malabsorption syndromes.[13]

A variety of other clinical effects have been observed. Some patients exhibit a slowly progressive degenerative arthritis that initially involves the hands but may include the larger joints (e.g., knees, hips, wrists, and shoulders).[7] Osteoporosis accompanied by ascorbic acid deficiency has also been observed.[13] Patients with symptomatic disease may have a generalized abnormal pigmentation of the skin (ranging from bronze to slate gray) that is more prominent in sun-exposed areas, the genital region, or scar tissue.[13] Abdominal pain has been noted in 35–40% of patients with primary hemochromatosis[13]; while the reasons for this symptom are not clear, it is more common in the elderly. Lethargy, somnolence, disorientation, stupor, and psychomotor retardation have also been reported.[4]

Laboratory Identification

Although distinguishing between primary and secondary hemochromatosis is necessary for optimal therapy, early recognition of iron overload is a more important determinant of successful treatment. Normal total body iron stores are between 3 and 4 g, depending on body weight.[13] Approximately 1 g is stored in the tissues as ferritin, the soluble diffusible form, and as hemosiderin, the insoluble aggregate.[13] Sixty to seventy percent of total body iron is contained in the hemoglobin of circulating red blood cells; smaller amounts are present in tissue enzymes.[13] Since iron is recycled for hemoglobin synthesis, the only iron that normally needs to be replaced is that lost in epithelial cells exfoliated from the gastrointestinal tract and skin and that lost in menstrual blood. Daily iron requirements are approximately 1 mg for adult males and postmenopausal females and 1.5 mg for females of childbearing age.[13]

Direct and indirect methods are used to measure iron stores. A rough estimate of iron load can be made from the patient's transfusion history. Packed red blood cells contain approximately 1 mg of iron per milliliter.[14] Patients who receive 2 units of packed red blood cells every three weeks add 7–8 g of iron each year to their body iron stores.[14] This estimate does not include the amount of iron absorbed from the gastrointestinal tract or removed by chelation therapy.

The earliest abnormalities that can be easily detected in laboratory tests are an increased serum iron concentration (greater than 170 μg/dL; normal = 50–150 μg/dL) and an increased total iron-binding capacity (TIBC) saturation (greater than 60%; normal = 30%).[15] TIBC saturation is calculated by dividing the serum iron concentration by the TIBC (normal = 200–400 μg/dL).[15] These values, along with an increased serum ferritin concentration (greater than 300 μg/L; normal = 15–200 μg/L), are the most helpful in screening for iron overload.[15]

Although these laboratory values are useful in screening for hemochromatosis, patients without iron overload may also have elevated values. For example, serum iron may be elevated in patients with alcoholic liver disease who do not have excess iron stores. Although TIBC saturation is a better predictor of iron overload than serum iron alone, serum iron and TIBC saturation may also be increased in patients with aplastic anemia, hemolytic states, or sideroblastic anemia.[13]

Serum ferritin concentration is generally considered a more reliable indicator of iron overload. It usually increases in proportion to total body iron stores in patients who have received a total of less than 100 units of blood or until ferritin concentrations exceed 4000 μg/L.[16] Each 1 μg of serum ferritin per liter is equal to approximately 8 mg of stored iron when the serum ferritin concentration is less than 500 μg/L.[17] However, increased serum ferritin does not reflect body iron stores in conditions such as hepatocellular necrosis (often seen in alcoholic liver disease) or other conditions in which inflammation or tissue damage, including hemolysis, is present. Measurement of serum ferritin may be less sensitive than serum iron and TIBC saturation measurements in detecting iron overload during the early stages of the disease. Some patients with normal serum ferritin concentrations have had excess hepatic iron.[7] In patients without ascorbic acid deficiency, a close correlation was found between serum ferritin concentrations and iron stores.[18] In patients with β thalassemia, ascorbic acid deficiency has been found to disrupt the correlation of serum ferritin with liver iron and the number of units of blood transfused.

Since increased serum ferritin and iron concentrations are not specific for iron overload, other tests to quantify the total iron load may be necessary. Direct measurements of iron stores can be obtained from biopsies of the liver and bone marrow, the main storage sites for iron. Biopsy also allows a histologic evaluation that can define the tissue iron distribution and extent of tissue damage. The presence of large amounts of iron in parenchymal cells is associated with organ damage, while the presence of iron in the reticuloendothelial cells is insignificant.[7]

The liver biopsy is used most often and is the definitive diagnostic test for hemochromatosis. Its advantages include the ability to determine iron load in patients whose transfusion history is unknown or who have had few if any transfusions. The liver biopsy also histologically documents the presence of fibrosis or cirrhosis and can be used to monitor the effectiveness of chelation therapy. Of course, biopsies are invasive and carry associated risks.[19]

A deferoxamine mesylate excretion test can be performed as an alternative to a liver biopsy. A 10-mg/kg dose of deferoxamine mesylate is administered intramuscularly and is followed by a 24-hour urine collection. Creatinine and iron levels are measured in the sample. The upper limit of the normal range for the 24-hour test is 2 mg of iron or 1.5 mg of iron per gram of creatinine.[20] In a study by Bonkovsky et al.,[20] the results of a 4-hour urine collection were closely correlated with those of a 24-hour urine collection. The upper limit of normal for the four-hour excretion test is 2.5 mg of iron per gram of creatinine. Patients with urinary iron excretions above normal may not have iron overload but rather may have active liver inflammation like that seen in chronic hepatitis or alcoholism. Although not a reliable predictor of liver iron concentration, the test result can be used to exclude iron overload in patients with normal urinary iron excretion.

Recent progress has been made with noninvasive techniques for quantifying total iron stores. Iron content estimates made with dual-energy computed tomography (CT) of the abdomen have correlated closely with estimates from a liver biopsy. Howard et al.[21] found that a normal hepatic density on CT did not exclude iron overload but that an increased density with increased serum ferritin indicated iron overload. Nuclear magnetic resonance (NMR) scanning provides a quantitative assessment of hepatic iron. Other possible applications of NMR in this area include the ability to measure iron in the heart, pancreas, and brain and to distinguish parenchymal from reticuloendothelial iron.[22]

Treatment

Although removal of excess stored iron is the mainstay in the treatment of chronic iron overload, strategies to prevent excess iron accumulation or decrease the rate of accumulation should also be considered. Treatment of secondary conditions such as hypersplenism and folate deficiency decrease the absorption of dietary iron. If a patient requires more than 200 mL of blood per kilogram per year (28 units for a 70-kg person), a splenectomy will also decrease the amount of blood required for transfusions by approximately one third.[3] Avoiding iron-rich foods (e.g., meat) and alcohol should decrease the rate of iron loading, particularly in anemias with high rates of erythropoiesis that do not require regular blood transfusions. Tea has been reported to inhibit the absorption of inorganic iron by as much as 95%.[23] Transfusion techniques and goals may also alter the rate of iron accumulation. The transfusion of young red cells increases the interval between transfusions but has not had a substantial impact on iron loading.[24] The process of separating young red cells, which have a half-life of 40–47 days (compared with 28 days for conventional red cells), from blood is time consuming and expensive. When hemoglobin concentrations are adequate to suppress erythropoiesis, the absorption of dietary iron decreases.[25] However, the need for more transfusions to maintain the higher hemoglobin level could outweigh the benefits.[3]

Phlebotomy. Phlebotomy (venesection) is the most effective means of removing iron. Approximately 250 mg of iron is removed with each 500 mL of blood withdrawn.[26] Phlebotomy is the treatment of choice in patients with primary hemochromatosis. The frequency of phlebotomy, which can be performed as often as two or three times a week, is determined by the hematocrit, hemoglobin concentration, degree of iron overload, presence of organ dysfunction, and limitations imposed by other conditions affected by blood loss, such as coronary heart disease. The absorption of iron from the gastrointestinal tract may increase after phlebotomy. Serum iron and ferritin levels should be monitored at three- to four-month intervals to determine if further phlebotomy is indicated.[13] Phlebotomy cannot be used in patients with moderate to severe iron-loading anemias who are transfusion dependent or in patients with primary hemochromatosis and severe cardiac disease, anemia, or hypoproteinemia. For these patients, chelation therapy provides the only means of effectively removing iron.

Chelation Therapy. After more than 25 years of use, deferoxamine mesylate remains the only iron chelator commercially available in the United States. Deferoxamine, a complex hydroxylamine derived from *Streptomyces pilosus,* acts as a chelating agent by binding ferric ions to the 3-hydroxamic groups of the molecule, thereby forming ferrioxamine. Ferrioxamine is water soluble and is excreted primarily by the kidneys, giving the urine a characteristic reddish color. A secondary pathway of elimination is through the feces via the bile.

Although this is not observed clinically, 1 g of deferoxamine mesylate theoretically can bind 85 mg of iron.[16] Clinically, with body iron stores of 4–5 g, a 1-g dose of deferoxamine mesylate is about 8% efficient, resulting in the excretion of approximately 7 mg of iron.[16] Subcutaneous deferoxamine reportedly has removed a maximum of 20–30 mg of iron per day.[27] The main source of iron chelated by deferoxamine is that in transit between the major functional (hemoglobin), transport (plasma transferrin), and storage (ferritin) iron-containing proteins and not the iron within the proteins.[28]

Factors that should be considered before initiating chelation therapy include the degree of iron overload, transfusion history, medical history, age, and psychosocial history. Patients with clinical signs of iron toxicity or iron loads exceeding 0.7 g/kg require aggressive chelation therapy. Hoffbrand and Wonke1[29] suggested starting deferoxamine therapy after 25–50 units of blood have been transfused if there is no excess bleeding and the patient is expected to survive for more than two or three years.

Controversy exists as to when chelation therapy should be started for transfusion-dependent pediatric patients. Some believe that deferoxamine infusions should begin when transfusions are initiated.[30] However, if chelation therapy is started while iron levels are relatively normal, there is a higher incidence of deferoxamine toxicity. One study showed a significant reduction in adverse effects on growth and bone development when deferoxamine therapy was initiated after the age of three years.[31] A more common practice is to begin chelation therapy after four or five years of regular transfusions.[3] In children with thalassemia major, iron chelation is recommended after 10–15 units of blood have been given.[23] A study involving nine patients with sickle cell anemia indicated that their iron overload was quantitatively and qualitatively similar to that seen in thalassemia major and other hematologic disorders.[32] The authors concluded that if less than five years of transfusions is expected, chelation therapy is probably unnecessary.

Chelation therapy is not always necessary in elderly patients, since the risk of tissue toxicity from iron overload may be minimal when life expectancy is considered. Another factor to consider is the ability of the patient or family to cope with chelation therapy.

Route of Administration and Dosage. Subcutaneous administration of deferoxamine is preferred for iron-overloaded patients with no substantial organ damage. Administration can be accomplished on an outpatient basis with a battery-powered portable infusion pump. The duration of subcutaneous deferoxamine infusions ranges from 6 to 12 hours/day, with 10–12 hours/day being the most frequently used interval. When the subcutaneous infusion interval is less than 12 hours, the effectiveness of deferoxamine decreases; 6-hour subcutaneous deferoxamine infusions are only 70% as effective as 24-hour intravenous infusions.[33] Iron excretion after a 12-hour subcutaneous deferoxamine infusion is comparable to that after a 24-hour subcutaneous infusion.[34]

The solubility of deferoxamine mesylate requires that the concentration not exceed 250 mg/mL; this limits the amount that can be administered subcutaneously to 2–4 g. In children less than six years of age, a subcutaneous infusion of 40–50 mg/kg/day given over 12 hours for five or six days a week is usually sufficient to balance transfusional iron overload.[35] In adults with established iron overload, 50–100 mg/kg given over 12 hours generally decreases tissue iron stores.[28] Intermittent high-dose subcutaneous therapy of 150 mg/kg given over 12–24 hours once every few weeks has been successfully used in patients with dyserythropoietic anemias associated with excessive gastrointestinal iron absorption.[36]

Intravenous administration is used for patients who are not compliant with subcutaneous therapy or have massive iron stores and extensive organ damage. The intravenous route allows the use of higher doses of deferoxamine, which results in greater iron excretion and faster depletion of excess iron stores. Intravenous deferoxamine mesylate in doses up to 16 g given over 24 hours has been used in patients who are heavily iron overloaded. Administering these higher doses over a shorter period has been associated with flushing, hypotension or hypertension, and tachycardia or bradycardia.[16] Home intravenous deferoxamine therapy involving a permanent central venous catheter and a portable infusion pump has been successful in depleting excess iron stores. A dose of 15 mg/kg/hr given over 12 hours has been used safely for 12–25 months.[37]

Intramuscular injections of deferoxamine remove only half the iron of an equivalent subcutaneous dose because of the shorter duration of action and decreased exposure to the labile iron.[28] Deferoxamine is poorly absorbed when administered orally and has a minimal effect on iron excretion.

Deferoxamine has been used in maintenance hemodialysis and continuous ambulatory peritoneal dialysis (CAPD). In one report, a patient underwent hemodialysis with deferoxamine three times a week for two years.[38] Approximately 16 mg of iron was removed per dialysis. Deferoxamine mesylate 1.5 g was diluted in 250 mL of 0.9% sodium chloride injection and infused into the venous return from the dialzyer during the first two hours of a four-hour dialysis. When the patient was switched to CAPD, a comparison was made of iron excretion obtained by giving 250 mg of deferoxamine mesylate per liter of dialysate with five exchanges each day, five exchanges every other day, and the first, third, and fifth exchanges each day. The addition of deferoxamine daily to each dialysis bag provided the greatest iron excretion (approximately 14 mg/day).

Monitoring Therapy. The effectiveness of chelation therapy can be monitored by measuring the serum ferritin concentration at three- to six-month intervals. An initial steep decline in serum ferritin in heavily iron-overloaded patients is likely because of an improvement in liver function, not because of a substantial decrease in iron stores. Thalassemia major is considered well controlled if the serum ferritin concentration is 1000–2000 μg/L.[28]

Measurements of urinary iron excretion should be used cautiously in monitoring the effectiveness of deferoxamine therapy. Urinary iron does not reflect the 30–50% of the total iron mobilized and excreted in the feces. Also, daily urinary iron excretion varies and with increasing deferoxamine doses reaches a plateau that is a function of the degree of iron loading.[39]

Adverse Effects. Most patients who receive 1 g or more of deferoxamine mesylate subcutaneously at the recommended concentration of 250 mg/mL notice local swelling, erythema, itching, and tenderness at the needle site. The tenderness usually disappears several days after the infusion. The reactions can be minimized by diluting the deferoxamine in 5–10 mL of sterile water for injection, adding 1 mg of hydrocortisone to each milliliter of deferoxamine solution,[40] rotating injection sites daily, applying topical corticosteroids, or administering oral antihistamines. Painful lumps may form under the skin, usually when the rate of deferoxamine administration exceeds the rate of absorption from the injection site or when the needle is inserted too close to the dermis.[41] Because some patients complain of pain caused by daily insertion of the needle, a topical anesthetic can be applied beforehand.[40]

Intramuscular deferoxamine mesylate injections at the maximum concentration of 250 mg/mL are painful because injection volumes exceed 2 mL. When the intramuscular dose of deferoxamine was accidentally given intravenously, flushing, lightheadedness, headache, and loss of consciousness were observed.[5]

Anaphylactic reactions have been reported in patients receiving deferoxamine by the intravenous and intramuscular routes.[3] Desensitization can be achieved by starting intravenous deferoxamine mesylate at a low dose of 0.015 mg and increasing the dose 10-fold every 30 minutes until 1.5 g is reached. The patient can then be switched to a subcutaneous infusion of the desired dose over 24 hours. The infusion duration then can be gradually decreased to 12 hours over several days.[42] Intravenous deferoxamine desensitization requires intensive monitoring and the availability of resuscitative equipment and personnel.

Cataracts have been reported in patients given intramuscular and high-dose intravenous deferoxamine injections.[37,43,44] Since higher peak levels of deferoxamine occur with intramuscular and high intravenous doses, retinal damage may be caused by the direct toxic effect of deferoxamine on the retina or inhibition of iron-dependent enzyme activity.[4] The lens opacities usually improve after therapy is stopped. Treatment can be restarted at lower doses after two to three weeks or when symptomatic recovery occurs.[41] Lens opacities are rare when subcutaneous dosages of less than 100 mg/kg/day are used. Subcutaneous deferoxamine infusions have not been associated with cataract formation in humans.[3] Even in the absence of deferoxamine therapy, subcapsular punctiform lens opacities may occur in patients with siderosis.[40]

A relationship seems to exist between retinal toxicity and the degree of iron overload. Patients without iron overload are very sensitive to deferoxamine-induced ocular toxicity. Patients with serum ferritin concentrations of over 3000 μg/L developed visual symptoms when deferoxamine mesylate dosages exceeded 150 mg/kg/day, whereas patients with ferritin concentrations averaging 1000 μg/L developed visual symptoms at dosages of 70–100 mg/kg/day.[45,46] However, in a study of 52 patients with a wide range of iron stores who received subcutaneous or intravenous deferoxamine for up to 12 years, only 1 patient had symptomatic loss of vision and hearing. Of the 51 asymptomatic patients, 1 had mild macular stippling.[47]

Ototoxicity has also been reported during deferoxamine therapy, but its significance is not clear. Several studies indicate that the risk is related to the dose of deferoxamine and the degree of iron overload.[45,48] As with ocular toxicity, ototoxicity is believed to be a greater risk with higher doses of deferoxamine and lower ferritin levels. In Cohen et al.'s[47] study of 52 patients, only 1 patient had symptomatic loss of hearing, and 1 asymptomatic patient had mild, bilateral, high-frequency sensorineural hearing loss. When audiometric abnormalities are detected, the dosage of deferoxamine can be reduced or treatment can be stopped until hearing is regained. Wonke et al.[49] reported that hearing improved in three patients with chronic audiometric abnormalities after the patients were switched from deferoxamine to another iron chelator, diethylene triaminepenta-acetic acid (DTPA).[49]

Since some patients may be left with only partial recovery of sight and hearing, patients should be encouraged to report immediately any hearing loss, night blindness, decreased visual acuity, impaired peripheral vision, or loss of color vision. Patients should undergo yearly ophthalmologic examinations. Audiometric evaluations should be made at least every year and perhaps every six months in patients whose condition is well controlled and who have serum ferritin concentrations of less than 2000 μg/L.

Growth impairment has been observed in prepubescent patients with ferritin concentrations below 1000 μg/L or in patients receiving a dosage of more than 70 mg/kg/day.[41] Increased growth occurred in 16 of 19 patients with low serum ferritin levels when the deferoxamine dosage was reduced by 50%. A study comparing the growth and sexual maturation of patients beginning deferoxamine therapy between the ages of 5 and 10 years with those beginning therapy after age 10 showed no significant difference between the groups in final height or mean parental height.[50] However, growth failure has been reported in patients treated with deferoxamine during the first 14 months of life, when iron stores would not be grossly elevated.[31] Skeletal abnormalities have been reported in the offspring of animals given deferoxamine during the early stages of pregnancy.[41] Deferoxamine should not be administered during pregnancy.

Iron-overloaded patients are more susceptible to infection. Severe infections with *Yersinia enterocolitica* have occurred when deferoxamine was given.[51-54] This organism, which has receptors for ferrioxamine, usually has low pathogenicity because of its high requirements for iron.[55] However, when deferoxamine is given, any iron in the tissues becomes more available to the organism. Severe colitis, peritonitis, septicemia, or any unusual infection should be evaluated for the presence of *Y. enterocolitica*. When such an infection is suspected, deferoxamine therapy should be stopped. Antimicrobial treatment can be initiated before culture results are obtained. Mild infections can be treated with trimethoprim–sulfamethoxazole or tetracycline. Severe infections should be treated with intravenous antimicrobials, such as gentamicin, cefotaxime, or ciprofloxacin. Trimethoprim–sulfamethoxazole should be given for one month after the clinical cure.[56] The patient should be closely monitored for reinfection when deferoxamine therapy is reinstituted.

Pneumocystis carinii pneumonia and mucormycosis have also been reported to occur in association with deferoxamine therapy.[57,58] Early diagnosis of mucormycosis is essential to prevent mortality. Signs or symptoms of sinusitis, proptosis, palatal lesions, new infarct-like pulmonary infiltrates, or necrotic skin lesions are suggestive of mucormycosis.[59] The clinical features of *Pneumocystis carinii* are similar to other pneumonias, with fever, cough, tachypnea, and shortness of breath.

High doses of intravenous deferoxamine mesylate (approximately 180 mg/kg/day) were reported to increase serum creatinine concentrations in three patients.[60]

Adjuvant Therapy. Ascorbic acid deficiency is often observed in patients with iron overload and appears to protect the target organs, particularly the heart, from the toxic effects of iron. When the ascorbate deficiency is corrected, urinary iron excretion is enhanced in response to deferoxamine.[61] However, large oral doses of ascorbic acid enhance iron toxicity by converting inert iron stores to a more labile and chelatable form. Therefore, they should not be given to heavily iron-loaded patients starting deferoxamine therapy or to iron-loaded patients who are not receiving regular chelation therapy. Toxicity can be minimized by giving lower doses (100 mg/day in children and 200 mg/day in adults) at the time of the deferoxamine infusion and by delaying ascorbic acid supplementation until cardiac abnormalities have been reversed by chelation therapy.[29] In addition, ascorbic acid should be given on an empty stomach to avoid enhanced absorption of iron from food. Periodic evaluation of the effectiveness of ascorbic acid in increasing urinary iron excretion should be made, since this effect diminishes as iron stores are lowered with regular chelation therapy.[62]

Patient Education. A major reason for failure of iron chelation therapy is noncompliance. The method of administration is inconvenient and painful, especially for children. Parents and care givers are often reluctant to insert a needle into a child who cannot understand the benefits of chelation therapy. Older patients may dislike the change in their routines. Chelation therapy programs must be designed to be acceptable to the patient and family. Some physicians allow drug holidays one or two times a week to encourage compliance, but one must keep in mind that undertreating patients puts them through the inconvenience of therapy without giving them the full benefits. Nightly infusions seem to provide the least interference with daily activities.

The patient and family must be informed about the consequences of iron overload and how chelation therapy can minimize the damage. Other patients undergoing deferoxamine therapy and health-care providers can provide support and follow-up and help improve compliance.

Adequate training of the patient or care giver must be given to ensure that the deferoxamine is administered correctly and safely. Written instructions should be provided to reinforce procedures and pump operation.

Compliance may also be affected if the cost of chelation therapy must be borne by the patient rather than an insurance plan. The average wholesale price of a 500-mg vial of Desferal (Ciba-Geigy) is $7.29.[63] A 30-day supply of Desferal 1 g/day prepared by the patient costs $437. Rental of the infusion pump costs $400–$500 per month. Annual costs of administering Desferal 1 g/day plus supplies and equipment can exceed $12,000.

Future Therapies

Numerous studies have shown that chelation therapy and phlebotomy can prolong life and reduce the incidence of cardiac, endocrine, and liver complications in patients with hemochromatosis.[9,64-66] During the 25 years since deferoxamine was introduced, efforts have been made to find a safe, less expensive, more effective, and more easily administered iron chelator. The investigational agent DTPA has been used in chelation therapy, but its lack of selectivity for iron leads to zinc depletion. Subcutaneous DTPA given twice weekly with large supplemental doses of zinc compared favorably with daily infusions of deferoxamine.[67] DTPA, which acts extracellularly, has an additive effect on iron excretion when used with deferoxamine.[67] DTPA remains an alternative for patients who cannot tolerate deferoxamine. Like deferoxamine, DTPA is not effective orally.

An oral chelating agent under investigation is isoniazid pyridoxal hydrazone, which compares favorably with deferoxamine in its ability to remove iron. After oral treatment with 30 mg/kg/day for six days, no substantial toxicity was observed, but total iron excretion was inadequate to produce a negative iron balance in patients receiving regular transfusions.[68] Another aryl hydrazone compound, pyridoxal-1-pyrimidinyl ethoxycarbonyl methbromide, has oral activity greater than that of injected deferoxamine in animal studies.[69] Derivatives of the hydroxypyridin-4-ones have also shown promise as oral chelating agents.[70]

New drug delivery systems are being examined. The intravenous administration of deferoxamine entrapped in red blood cell ghosts results in greater urinary iron excretion than a similar dose given subcutaneously.[71] Animal studies have shown that the placement of deferoxamine in liposomes can increase its half-life and allow delivery to target organs, such as the liver and spleen.[72] Intranasal deferoxamine given every one to three hours has been used, but iron excretion is only 10–15% of that obtained with a subcutaneous dose.[73] The development of a depot dosage form of deferoxamine would provide for a slow, continuous exposure of iron to the chelator.[33]

The potential role of erythropoietin in the management of patients requiring repeated blood transfusions is being explored.[74] Bone marrow transplantation may also have an impact on the management of hematologic disorders such as thalassemia major.[3]

Conclusion

Many studies have shown the beneficial impact of chelation therapy and phlebotomy on hemochromatosis. Life has been prolonged and the incidence of complications reduced. Early detection is essential, however, to prevent organ damage. The main problems with chelation therapy are patient compliance and cost. If a safe oral chelating agent can be developed, therapy will be available to a larger group of patients and compliance will be enhanced.

References

1. Bothwell TH, Charlton RW, Cook JD et al. Iron metabolism in man. Oxford, England: Blackwell Scientific; 1979:105-15.
2. Simon M, Alexandre J-L, Fauchet R et al. The genetics of hemochromatosis. *Prog Med Genet*. 1980; 4:135-68.
3. Cohen A. Management of iron overload in the pediatric patient. *Hematol Oncol Clin North Am*. 1987; 1:521-44.
4. Forget BG, Nathan DG. Thalassemia. *Annu Rev Med*. 1975; 26:345-51.
5. Powell LW, Campbell CB, Wilson E. Intestinal mucosal uptake of iron and iron retention in idiopathic haemochromatosis as evidence for a mucosal abnormality. *Gut*. 1970; 11:727-31.
6. Modell B. Advances in the use of iron chelating agents for the treatment of iron overload. *Prog Hematol*. 1979; 11:267-312.
7. Halliday CE, Halliday JW, Powell LW. The clinical manifestations of chronic iron overload. *Baillieres Clin Haematol*. 1989; 2:403-21.
8. Niederau C, Fischer R, Sonnenberg A et al. Survival and causes of death in cirrhotic and in noncirrhotic patients with primary hemochromatosis. *N Engl J Med*. 1985; 313:1256-62.
9. Bomford A, Williams R. Long-term results of venesection therapy in idiopathic haemochromatosis. *Q J Med*. 1976; 45:611-23.
10. Short EM, Winkle RA, Billingham ME. Myocardial involvement in idiopathic hemochromatosis: morphologic and clinical improvement following venesection. *Am J Med*. 1981; 70:1275-9.
11. Flynn DM, Hoffbrand AV, Politis D. Subcutaneous desferrioxamine: the effect of three years' treatment on liver iron, serum ferritin, and comments on echocardiography. *Birth Defects*. 1982; 18:347-53.
12. De Sanctis V, D'Ascola G, Wonke B. The development of diabetes mellitus in chronic liver disease in long term chelated beta thalassaemic patients. *Postgrad Med J*. 1986; 62:831-6.
13. McLaren GD, Muir WA, Kellermeyer RW. Iron overload disorders: natural history, pathogenesis, diagnosis, and therapy. *CRC Crit Rev Clin Lab Sci*. 1983; 19:205-66.
14. Cohen A. Treatment of transfusional iron overload. *Am J Pediatr Hematol Oncol*. 1990; 12:4-8.
15. Bassett ML, Halliday JW, Powell LW. Screening for hemochromatosis. *Ann N Y Acad Sci*. 1988; 526:274-89.
16. Worwood M, Cragg SJ, Jacobs A et al. Binding of serum ferritin to concanavalin A: patients with homozygous beta-thalassemia and transfusional iron overload. *Br J Haematol*. 1980; 46:409-16.
17. Finch CA, Cook JD, Labbe RF et al. Effect of blood donation

on iron stores as evaluated by serum ferritin. *Blood.* 1977; 50:441-7.
18. Chapman RW, Hussain M, Gorman A et al. Effect of ascorbic acid deficiency on serum ferritin concentration in patients with beta-thalassaemia major and iron overload. *J Clin Pathol.* 1982; 35:487-91.
19. Kaltwasser JP, Werner E. Diagnosis and clinical evaluation of iron overload. *Baillieres Clin Haematol.* 1989; 2:363-89.
20. Bonkovsky H, Weber R, Aaron L. Four-hour measurement of urinary iron excretion after deferoxine treatment: a rapid, simple method for study of iron excretion. *Am J Gastroenterol.* 1990; 85:554-7.
21. Howard JM, Ghent CN, Cavey LS et al. Diagnostic efficacy of hepatic computed tomography in the detection of body iron overload. *Gastroenterology.* 1983; 84:209-15.
22. Stark DD, Moseley ME, Bacon BR et al. Magnetic resonance imaging and spectroscopy of hepatic iron overload. *Radiology.* 1985; 154:137-42.
23. De Alarcon PA, Donovan ME, Forbes GB et al. Iron absorption in the thalassemia syndromes and its inhibition by tea. *N Engl J Med.* 1979; 300:5-8.
24. Cohen AR, Schmidt JM, Martin MB et al. Clinical trial of young red cell transfusions. *J Pediatr.* 1984; 104:865-8.
25. Erlandson ME, Walden B, Stern G et al. Studies on congenital hemolytic syndromes. IV. Gastro-intestinal absorption of iron. *Blood.* 1962; 19:359-78.
26. Finch CA, Cook JD, Labbe RF et al. Effect of blood donation on iron stores as evaluated by serum ferritin. *Blood.* 1977; 50:441-7.
27. Cumming RLC, Miller JA, Smith JA et al. Clinical and laboratory studies on the action of deferrioxamine. *Br J Haematol.* 1969; 17:257-63.
28. Pippard MJ. Desferrioxamine-induced iron excretion in humans. *Baillieres Clin Haematol.* 1989; 2:323-43.
29. Hoffbrand AV, Wonke B. Results of long-term subcutaneous desferrioxamine therapy. *Baillieres Clin Haematol.* 1989; 2:345-62.
30. Pippard M, Callender ST. The management of iron chelation therapy. *Br J Haematol.* 1983; 54:503-7.
31. De Virgiliis S, Congia M, Frau F et al. Desferrioxamine-induced growth retardation in patients with thalassemia major. *J Pediatr.* 1988; 113:661-9.
32. Cohen A, Kron E, Brittenham G. Toxicity of transfusional iron overload in sickle cell anemia. *Blood.* 1984; 64:47. Abstract.
33. Hyman CB, Ortega JA, Aftergood L. Effects of different regimens of desferrioxamine and ascorbic acid administration and of serm alpha-tocopherol level on urinary iron excretion. In: Zaino EC, Roberts RH, eds. Chelation therapy in chronic iron overload. Miami: Symposia Specialists; 1977:109-14.
34. Pippard MJ, Callender ST, Weatherall DJ. Intensive iron-chelation therapy with desferrioxamine in iron-loading anemias. *Clin Sci Mol Med.* 1978; 54:99-106.
35. Fargion S, Taddei MT, Abutti V et al. Early iron overload in beta-thalassaemia major: when to start chelation therapy? *Arch Dis Child.* 1982; 57:929-33.
36. Pippard MJ, Weatherall DJ. Iron balance and the management of iron overload in beta-thalassemia intermedia. *Birth Defects.* 1988; 23:29-33.
37. Cohen AR, Mizanin J, Schwartz E. Rapid removal of excessive iron with daily, high-dose, intravenous chelation therapy. *J Pediatr.* 1989; 115:151-5.
38. Falk RJ, Mattern WD, Lamanna RG et al. Iron removal during continuous ambulatory peritoneal dialysis using deferoxamine. *Kidney Int.* 1983; 24:110-2.
39. Propper RD, Shurin SB, Nathan DG. Reassessment of the use of desferrioxamine B in iron overload. *N Engl J Med.* 1976; 294:1421-3.
40. Propper RL, Cooper B, Rufo RR et al. Continuous subcutaneous administration of deferoxamine in patients with iron overload. *N Engl J Med.* 1977; 297:418-23.
41. Porter JB, Huehns ER. The toxic effects of desferrioxamine. *Baillieres Clin Haematol.* 1989; 2:459-74.
42. Bousquet J, Navarro M, Robert G et al. Rapid desensitization for desferrioxamine anaphylactoid reactions. *Lancet.* 1983; 2:859-60.
43. Davies MJ, Marcus RE, Hungerford JL et al. Ocular toxicity of high-dose intravenous desferrioxamine. *Lancet.* 1983; 2:181-4.
44. Waxman HS, Brown EB. Clinical usefulness of iron chelating agents. *Prog Haematol.* 1969; 6:338-73.
45. Olivieri NF, Buncie JR, Chew E et al. Visual and auditory neurotoxicity in patients receiving subcutaneous deferoxamine infusions. *N Engl J Med.* 1986; 314:869-73.
46. Borgna-Pignatti C, de Stefano P, Broglia AM. Visual loss in patient on high-dose subcutaneous desferrioxamine. *Lancet.* 1984; 1:681. Letter.
47. Cohen A, Martin M, Mizanin J et al. Vision and hearing during deferoxamine therapy. *J Pediatr.* 1990; 117:326-30.
48. Porter JB, Jaswon MS, Huehns ER et al. Desferrioxamine ototoxicity: evaluation of risk factors in thalassaemic patients and guidelines for safe dosage. *Br J Haematol.* 1989; 73:403-9.
49. Wonke B, Hoffbrand AV, Aldouri M et al. Reversal of desferrioxamine induced auditory neurotoxicity during treatment with Ca-DTPA. *Arch Dis Child.* 1989; 6:77-82.
50. Bronspiegel-Weintrob N, Olivieri NF, Tyler B et al. Effect of age at the start of iron chelation therapy on gonadal function in beta-thalassemia major. *N Engl J Med.* 1990; 323:713-9.
51. Butzler JP, Alexander M, Segers A et al. Enteritis, abscess and septicemia due to *Yersinia enterocolitica* in a child with thalassemia. *J Pediatr.* 1978; 93:619-21.
52. Boyce N, Wood C, Holdsworth S et al. Life-threatening sepsis complicating heavy metal chelation therapy with desferrioxamine. *Aust N Z J Med.* 1985; 15:654-5.
53. Chiu HY, Flynn DM, Hoffbrand AV et al. Infection with *Yersinia enterocolitica* in patients with iron overload. *Br Med J.* 1986; 292:97.
54. Gallant T, Freedman MH, Vellend H et al. Yersinia sepsis in patients with iron overload treated with deferoxamine. *N Engl J Med.* 1986; 314:1643. Letter.
55. Robins-Browne RM, Prpic JK, Stuart SJ. Yersiniae and iron. A study in host-parasite relationships. *Contrib Microbiol Immunol.* 1987; 9:254-8.
56. Hiigjano-Korstanje JAA. Antibiotics in *Yersinia enterocolitica* infections. *J Antimicrob Chemother.* 1987; 20:123-31.
57. Boelaert JR, Vergauwe PL, Vandepitte JM. Mucormycosis infections in dialysis patients. *Ann Intern Med.* 1987; 107:782-3.
58. Kouides PA, Slapak CA, Rosenwasser LJ et al. *Pneumocystis carinii* pneumonia as a complication of desferrioxamine therapy. *Br J Haematol.* 1988; 70:383-4.
59. Daly AL, Velazquez LA, Bradley SF et al. Mucormycosis: association with deferoxamine therapy. *Am J Med.* 1989; 87:468-71.
60. Koren G, Bentur Y, Strong D et al. Acute changes in renal function associated with deferoxamine therapy. *Am J Dis Child.* 1989; 143:1077-80.
61. Hussain MAM, Flynn DM, Green N et al. Effect of dose, time and ascorbate on iron excretion after subcutaneous desferrioxamine. *Lancet.* 1977; 1:977-9.
62. Cohen A, Martin M, Schwartz E. Response to long-term deferoxamine therapy in thalassemia. *J Pediatr.* 1981; 99:689-94.
63. Drug Topics red book annual pharmacists' reference. Cardinale VA, ed. Oradell, NJ: Medical Economics; 1989:269.
64. Hoffbrand AV, Gorman A, Laulicht M et al. Improvement in iron status and liver function in patients with transfusional iron overload with long-term subcutaneous desferrioxamine. *Lancet.* 1979;1:947-9.
65. Janka GE, Mohring P, Helmig M et al. Intravenous and subcutaneous desferrioxamine therapy in children with severe iron overload. *Eur J Pediatr.* 1981; 137:285-90.
66. Modell B, Letsky EA, Flynn DM et al. Survival and desferrioxamine in thalassemia major. *Br Med J.* 1982; 284:1081-4.
67. Pippard MJ, Jackson MJ, Hoffman K et al. Iron chelation using subcutaneous infusions of diethylene triamine pentaacetic acid (DPTA). *Scand J Haematol.* 1986; 36:466-72.
68. Brittenham GM. Pyridoxal isonicotinoyl hydrazone: an effec-

tive iron-chelator after oral administration. *Sem Hematol.* 1990; 27:112-6.

69. Porter JB, Huehns ER, Hider RC. The development of iron chelating drugs. *Baillieres Clin Haematol.* 1989; 2:257-92.
70. Kontoghiorghes GJ, Aldouri MA, Hoffbrand AV et al. Effective chelation of iron in beta thalassaemia with the oral chelator 1,2-dimethyl-3-hydroxypyrid-4-one. *Br Med J.* 1987; 295:1509-12.
71. Green R, Miller J, Crosby W. Enhancement of iron chelation by desferrioxamine entrapped in red blood cell ghosts. *Blood.* 1982; 57:866-72.
72. Lau EH, Cerny EA, Wright BJ et al. Improvement of iron removal from the reticulo-endothelial system by liposome encapsulation of *N,N'*-bis (2-hydroxybenzyl)-ethylenediamine-*N,N'*-diacetic acid (HBED). Comparison with desferrioxamine. *J Lab Clin Med.* 1983; 101:806-16.
73. Gordon GS, Ambruso DR, Robinson WA et al. Intranasal administration of deferoxamine to iron overloaded patients. *Am J Med Sci.* 1989; 297:280-4.
74. Rhondeau S, Christensen R, Ross M et al. Responsiveness to recombinant erythropoietin of marrow erythroid progenitors in infants of prematurity. *J Pediatr.* 1988; 112:935-40.

Research Note

Altered aminoglycoside volume of distribution in patients with acquired immunodeficiency syndrome

Joyce M. Longley, Donald G. Pittman, and F. David Newby

Clin Pharm. 1991; 10:784-6

The treatment of multiple opportunistic infections in patients with acquired immunodeficiency syndrome (AIDS) presents a challenge. Often, several organ systems are involved and patients are receiving many drugs. In addition, many patients with AIDS have poor nutritional status, as shown by decreases in body weight, total protein, and serum albumin.[1]

Altered aminoglycoside pharmacokinetic values have been reported in hospitalized patient groups including the elderly, nutritionally deficient patients, and patients in intensive-care units.[2-4] To our knowledge, it has not been demonstrated that aminoglycoside dosing and monitoring need to be handled differently for patients with AIDS than for the general population. We conducted a retrospective study to compare the aminoglycoside pharmacokinetic values of hospitalized patients with and without AIDS.

Methods. Pharmacokinetics service records for all patients who received intermittent intravenous infusions of amikacin, gentamicin, or tobramycin between October 1988 and March 1990 were reviewed retrospectively. Approximately 90% of all hospitalized patients treated with aminoglycosides are monitored by the hospital's pharmacokinetics service. Patients accepted into the study met the following criteria:

1. Blood samples for determination of peak and trough serum aminoglycoside concentrations were drawn around the patients' fourth or fifth dose, at which time the drug concentrations were estimated to be at steady state (defined as five half-lives).
2. They were not receiving penicillins.
3. They were between the ages of 20 and 65 years.
4. Serum creatinine concentration was less than 2 mg/dL.

Patients who met the criteria were divided into two groups: those infected with human immunodeficiency virus (HIV) who had had a life-threatening opportunistic infection or Kaposi's sarcoma or both, and a control group. The control group was drawn from the general hospital population, and no patient in that group was known to be infected with HIV.

The following information was recorded for each patient: age, height, actual body weight, ideal body weight, sex, blood urea nitrogen (BUN), serum creatinine, estimated creatinine clearance (calculated by Cockcroft-Gault equation),[5] total serum protein concentration, serum albumin concentration, the times that blood samples were drawn, time of aminoglycoside infusion, dosage regimen, and concurrent medications.

Serum collection times for each patient were scheduled by the pharmacokinetics service. Blood samples were drawn approximately 30 minutes before and at least 30 minutes after a 30-minute infusion. Times for serum samples and infusion times were taken from the pharmacokinetic monitoring sheets posted on the door of each patient's room. The monitoring sheet required the nursing and laboratory personnel to document the exact times when samples were drawn and doses were infused. Both patient groups received their aminoglycosides via gravity-flow infusions. Serum samples were frozen until assayed by fluorescence polarization immunoassay (TDx, Abbott Diagnostics). The within-day and between-day coefficients of variation for the gentamicin, amikacin, and tobramycin assay systems were 0.89–2.63%, 0.84–3.67%, and 1.74–3.11%, respectively.

The elimination rate constant (k, in hr^{-1}) was determined by using a one-compartment pharmacokinetic model[6]:

$$k = \ln (C_1/C_2)/\Delta t$$

where C_1 and C_2 are serum drug concentrations at times 1 and 2 and Δt = elapsed time. The volume of distribution (V, in liters) was calculated using a one-

Joyce M. Longley, Pharm.D. is Assistant Professor of Pharmacy Practice, Mercer University, Southern School of Pharmacy (MU, SSP), Atlanta, GA, and Pharmacokinetics Service Coordinator, Piedmont Hospital, Atlanta. Donald G. Pittman, Pharm.D., is Assistant Professor of Pharmacy Practice, MU, SSP, and Education and Clinical Service Coordinator, Piedmont Hospital. F. David Newby, Ph.D., is a medical student at Emory University School of Medicine, Atlanta.

Address reprint requests to Dr. Longley at the Department of Pharmacy, Piedmont Hospital, 1968 Peachtree Road N.W., Atlanta, GA 30309.

Presented at the 25th Annual ASHP Midyear Clinical Meeting, Las Vegas, NV, December 6, 1990.

Table 1.
Patient Characteristics and Pharmacokinetic Data[a]

Variable	AIDS Patients (n = 23)	Control Patients (n = 28)
Patient Characteristics		
Age (yr)	39 ± 9 (24–61)	43 ± 12 (22–61)
Ideal body weight (kg)[b]	67.0 ± 9.3 (52.3–84.5)	73.0 ± 6.4 (47–84.5)
Actual body weight (kg)[b]	63.8 ± 9.2 (49.5–83.6)	75.4 ± 14.7 (49.1–111)
Blood urea nitrogen (mg/dL)[b]	14.9 ± 8.1 (3–37)	10.0 ± 4.0 (4–19)
Serum creatinine (mg/dL)	0.9 ± 0.4 (0.4–1.9)	1.0 ± 0.2 (0.5–1.4)
Creatinine clearance (mL/min)[b,c]	104.3 ± 28.3 (43.06–140)	86.2 ± 19.9 (55.2–132)
Total serum protein concentration (mg/dL)	6.3 ± 1.1 (4.8–9.8)	6.3 ± 0.7 (4.7–7.2)
Serum albumin concentration (mg/dL)[b]	2.8 ± 0.5 (1.7–4)	3.4 ± 0.63 (2.3–4.5)
Pharmacokinetic Data[d]		
k (hr^{-1})	0.234 ± 0.085 (0.05–0.371)	0.264 ± 0.161 (0.107–0.356)
$t_{1/2}$ (hr)	3.6 ± 2.4 (1.8–12.7)	2.8 ± 0.7 (1.94–4.3)
V (L)[b]	20.2 ± 3.3 (15–26.6)	17.7 ± 3.6 (15–25.6)
V (L/kg)[b]	0.325 ± 0.075 (0.191–0.48)	0.261 ± 0.04 (0.198–0.329)
CL (L/hr)	4.71 ± 1.86 (1.21–8.88)	4.560 ± 0.924 (2.7–6.52)

[a] Values expressed as mean ± S.D. (range).
[b] Significantly different between the two groups.
[c] Calculated by modified Cockcroft-Gault equation using ideal body weight.[5]
[d] k = elimination rate constant; $t_{1/2}$ = half-life; V = volume of distribution; CL = drug clearance.

compartment pharmacokinetic model[6]:

$$V = D\,(1-e^{-kt'})\,/\,(C_{ss,\,max})\,(t')\,(k)\,(1-e^{-k\tau})$$

where D = dose in milligrams, t' = duration of drug infusion in hours, $C_{ss,\,max}$ = peak serum concentration immediately after infusion, and τ = dosage interval. Volume of distribution, in liters per kilogram, was calculated by using ideal body weight; however, if actual body weight was less than ideal body weight, the actual body weight was used.

Data were analyzed by using one-way analysis of variance (ANOVA) for independent samples. Values were considered significant at $p < 0.05$.

Results. Data were gathered for 51 patients (23 with AIDS and 28 without AIDS) who were receiving aminoglycosides and met the study criteria. Patient demographics and laboratory values are summarized in Table 1. All 23 patients in the AIDS group were men; 10 were receiving amikacin, 11 were receiving tobramycin, and 2 were receiving gentamicin. The control group consisted of 8 women and 20 men; 20 were receiving tobramycin and 8 were receiving gentamicin. The patients with AIDS had the following diagnoses upon admission: *Mycobacterium avium intracellularae* infection, *Pneumocystis carinii* pneumonia, cryptococcal meningitis, cytomegalovirus infection, and upper-respiratory-tract infection. Three patients were concurrently receiving pentamidine, two amphotericin B, six ganciclovir, and one acyclovir. The control patients were admitted with diagnoses of neoplastic diseases, diabetic complications, pneumonias, phlebitis, urinary tract infections, intra-abdominal infections, esophagitis, and eye infections. The control patients were concurrently receiving imipenem–cilastatin, metronidazole, erythromycin, vancomycin, ciprofloxacin, or cephalosporins (cefoperazone, cefazolin, ceftazidime, cefamandole, or cefuroxime). The AIDS patient group was approximately 5% below ideal body weight, and the control group was approximately 4% above ideal body weight.

There were significant differences between groups for BUN and creatinine clearance, yet there was no significant difference for serum creatinine concentration. Serum albumin values in the patients with AIDS were significantly lower than in the control patients; however, total protein was not found to be different between the two groups.

Table 1 shows the mean pharmacokinetic values for the two groups. The elimination rate constant (k) was smaller in the AIDS group than in the control group; however, this difference was not statistically significant. Likewise, there was no significant difference in the half-lives of aminoglycosides between the AIDS and control groups. Volume of distribution expressed in liters and in liters per kilogram was significantly larger in the AIDS group than in the control group. The volume of distribution of our control population compares well with the literature average of 0.25 L/kg.[7]

Discussion. For 16 of the 23 patients with AIDS, total body weight was less than ideal body weight. Since aminoglycoside dosages in patients who weigh less than their ideal body weight are determined on the basis of actual body weight, actual body weight was used to calculate volume of distribution in liters per kilogram.

The lower body weight and decreased serum albumin concentrations in patients with AIDS suggest that patients with AIDS could have increased extracellular body water. This has been observed in patients with nutritional deficiencies; for example, Barac-Nieto et al.[8] demonstrated that the percentage of weight in water may be increased in nutritionally deficient people.

Aminoglycosides are distributed to extracellular

body fluids. It has been shown that patients with a substantial decrease in serum protein and albumin concentrations may exhibit a shift in the total body water out of the intravascular space into the extravascular space because of decreased oncotic pressure. Total serum protein concentrations in our patients with AIDS were not significantly different from those in our control population, yet serum albumin concentrations were significantly lower in the patients with AIDS. Zarowitz et al.[3] showed that patients with less than ideal body weight and with serum albumin concentrations less than 3.5 g/dL have a higher volume of distribution in liters per kilogram. The average serum albumin concentration in our patients with AIDS was 2.8 ± 0.5 mg/dL.

A study by Tointon et al.[9] showed aminoglycoside volume of distribution per ideal body weight to be larger in patients who weighed less than their ideal body weight. When our patients with AIDS were compared with the control patients based on volume of distribution per ideal body weight, there was no significant difference.

One interesting point is that the patients with AIDS had a significantly greater estimated creatinine clearance (104 mL/min versus 86 mL/min) but had a longer calculated half-life, although this was not significantly different. Because of this observation, it may be helpful to use a longer dosage interval with larger doses on a milligram-per-kilogram basis in those patients. However, determinations of serum drug concentration are still the most important basis for individual patients' aminoglycoside regimens.

Conclusion. This study suggests that patients with AIDS may have an expanded aminoglycoside volume of distribution, possibly because many of these patients are nutritionally deficient. Controlled prospective studies are needed.

References

1. Kotler DF, Wang J, Pierson RN. Composition studies in patients with the acquired immunodeficiency syndrome. *Am J Clin Nutr.* 1985; 42:1255-65.
2. Zaske DE, Irvine P, Strand LM et al. Interpatient variations in gentamicin dose requirements for geriatric patients. *JAMA.* 1982; 248:3122-6.
3. Zarowitz BJ, Pilla AM, Popovich J. Expanded gentamicin volume of distribution in patients with indicators of malnutrition. *Clin Pharm.* 1990; 9:40-4.
4. Mann HJ, Fuhs DW, Awang R et al. Altered aminoglycoside pharmacokinetics in critically ill patients with sepsis. *Clin Pharm.* 1987; 6:148-53.
5. Cockroft DW, Gault MH. Prediction of creatinine clearance from serum creatinine. *Nephron.* 1976; 16:31-3.
6. Chow M, Deglin J, Hanalson A et al. Prediction of gentamicin serum levels using a one-compartment open linear pharmacokinetic model. *Am J Hosp Pharm.* 1978; 35:1078-81.
7. Hull JH, Sarrubi FA. Gentamicin serum concentrations: pharmacokinetic predictions. *Ann Intern Med.* 1976; 85:183-9.
8. Barac-Nieto M, Spurr GB, Lotero H et al. Body composition in chronic undernutrition. *Am J Clin Nutr.* 1978; 31:23-40.
9. Tointon MM, Job ML, Peltier TT et al. Alterations in aminoglycoside volume of distribution in patients below ideal body weight. *Clin Pharm.* 1987; 6:160-2.

DUE Criteria

The DUE Criteria *section of* Clinical Pharmacy *features model drug-use evaluation criteria that may be employed as a component of a comprehensive quality assurance program. The criteria sets are presented in the format used in the ASHP book* Criteria for Drug Use Evaluation. *Some of the criteria sets will have been originally published in that book; others will be presented here for the first time and published in future volumes of the ASHP book. The practitioners who developed a criteria set are acknowledged.*

In selecting drug products for coverage in DUE Criteria, *priority is given to products that have been recently marketed, those that are frequently prescribed, those that have high potential risk associated with their use, and those that are expensive. When feasible, a criteria set will be linked with a Drug Review that appears in the same issue.*

These criteria sets are a starting point for the development of DUE criteria for a specific practice setting. Readers are encouraged to modify the model criteria to fit their own circumstances.

Criteria for stress ulcer prophylaxis in intensive-care patients[a]

Element	Standard 100%	Standard 0%	Exception[b] or Critical Preventive/ Responsive Measure[c]	Sources of Information
Justification for Use				
1. Prophylaxis of stress ulcers in patient with one or more of the following risk factors[1–3]: a. Shock (e.g., cardiogenic, hypovolemic, septic, or neurogenic) b. Sepsis c. Acute renal failure or hepatic failure d. Mechanical ventilation for >24 hours e. Burns over >25% of body surface area f. Multiple trauma (injury to major visceral organs or multiple fractures) g. Closed head injury h. Major surgery, including any procedure of more than two hours' duration (e.g., neurosurgical procedures, repair of abdominal aortic aneurysm, coronary artery bypass grafting)	X		1A. None	1. History and physical examination (H&P), progress notes, culture and susceptibility reports, laboratory reports, anesthesia records
Critical (Process) Indicators				
2. No history of hypersensitivity to agent(s) prescribed	X		2A. None	2. H&P, progress notes, allergy reports
3. One of following agents selected for prophylaxis: a. Maalox TC, Mylanta II, or antacid with equivalent acid-neutralizing capacity (ANC)	X		3A. None	3. Physician orders, medication administration record (MAR)

Prepared by Mark D. Peters II, Pharm.D., Assistant Professor, Department of Pharmacy Practice and Administration, Rutgers University College of Pharmacy (RUCP), Piscataway, NJ, and Clinical Pharmacy Coordinator, Department of Pharmacy, JFK Medical Center, Edison, NJ; Katherine A. Michael, Pharm.D., Assistant Professor, Department of Hospital Pharmacy Practice and Administration, Medical University of South Carolina, Charleston, SC; Julie A. Sjolander, Pharm.D., Assistant Professor, Department of Pharmacy Practice and Administration, RUCP, and Clinical Pharmacist, Monmouth Medical Center, Long Branch, NJ; Keith A. Swanson, Pharm.D., Vice Chairman and Assistant Professor, Department of Pharmacy Practice and Administration, RUCP, and Clinical Pharmacist, Monmouth Medical Center; and Richard A. Medina, M.D., Gastroenterologist, Associate Attending Physician, Department of Internal Medicine, JFK Medical Center, Edison, NJ.

Element	Standard 100%	Standard 0%	Exception[b] or Critical Preventive/ Responsive Measure[c]	Sources of Information
b. Sucralfate c. Histamine H_2-receptor antagonist (cimetidine, famotidine, or ranitidine)				
4. Combined use of two or more agents (element 3) from different drug classes limited to the following indications: a. Documented failure to maintain gastric pH above 4.0 when maximum dosage of single agent given b. Breakthrough bleeding during single-agent therapy (overt bleeding or drop in hemoglobin concentration of 1–2 g/dL with associated guaiac-positive nasogastric [NG] tube aspirate with or without positive fecal occult blood test result)	X		4A. None	4. Physician orders, MAR, progress notes, nursing flow sheets, laboratory reports
5. Misoprostol or omeprazole not given concurrently with agent indicated for stress ulcer prophylaxis	X		5A. None	5. Physician orders, MAR
6. Appropriate dosage administered: a. Antacid: Maalox TC, Mylanta II, or other antacid with equivalent ANC 30–60 mL p.o. or per NG tube every 1–2 hr[3,4] b. Sucralfate: 1 g p.o. or per NG tube every 6 hr[5,6] c. Cimetidine: 300 mg i.v. or p.o. every 4–6 hr[1,2,7,8] or as continuous i.v. infusion of 900–1200 mg/24 hr[9–11] d. Famotidine: 20 mg i.v. or p.o. every 12 hr e. Ranitidine: 50 mg i.v. every 6–8 hr,[13,14] 150 mg p.o. every 12 hr,[15] or continuous i.v. infusion of 150 mg/24 hr[15,16]	X		6A. If pH <4.0, may increase infusion rate of cimetidine to 2400 mg/24 hr[12]; may give 300-mg i.v. bolus dose before infusion started or rate increased 6B. If pH <4.0, may increase infusion rate of ranitidine to 200 mg/24 hr[15]; may give 50-mg i.v. bolus dose before infusion started or rate increased	6. Physician orders, MAR 6A, B. Physician orders, MAR, progress notes, nursing flow sheets
7. Patient weight obtained within 24 hours of admission or at start of stress ulcer prophylaxis	X		7A. None	7. H&P, progress notes, nursing notes, nutrition notes
8. Dosage of H_2-receptor antagonist adjusted for renal impairment on basis of calculated or measured creatinine clearance (CL_{cr}) a. Cimetidine: If $CL_{cr} \leq 30$ mL/min, give 300 mg i.v. or p.o. every 12 hr[9] or continuous i.v. infusion of 600 mg/24 hr b. Famotidine: If $CL_{cr} \leq 10$ mL/min, give 20 mg i.v. or p.o. every 24 hr[17] c. Ranitidine: If $CL_{cr} \leq 50$ mL/min, give 50 mg i.v. every 12–24 hr, 150 mg p.o. every 24 hr,[15] or continuous i.v. infusion of 50–100 mg/24 hr	X		8A. None	8. Physician orders, MAR, laboratory reports
9. H_2-antagonist therapy switched from i.v. to oral route as soon as patient able to take oral medications or receiving enteral nutrition	X		9A. IV therapy continued in patient with severe nausea or vomiting, active GI bleeding, continuous NG suction, malabsorption syndrome, or questionable absorptive capacity (e.g., ileus, short bowel)	9, 9A. Physician orders, MAR, progress notes, nursing flow sheets, nursing notes
10. Stress ulcer prophylaxis regimen continued until patient discharged from intensive-care unit or until risk factors corrected	X		10A. None	10. Physician orders, MAR, progress notes, nursing flow sheets

Element	Standard 100%	Standard 0%	Exception[b] or Critical Preventive/ Responsive Measure[c]	Sources of Information
11. Gastric pH monitored via NG tube aspirates at least once each shift or every dosage interval, whichever is more frequent	X		11A. Patient receiving sucralfate alone or does not have NG tube in place	11. Progress notes, nursing notes, nursing flow sheets 11A. Physician orders, MAR, nursing notes, nursing flow sheets
12. Signs of GI bleeding (gross or occult blood in NG tube aspirate, hematochezia, melena, fecal occult blood, or decreases in hematocrit or hemoglobin concentration) monitored daily	X		12A. Patient does not have NG tube in place	12. Progress notes, nursing notes, nursing flow sheets, laboratory reports 12A. Nursing notes, nursing flow sheets
<u>Antacids</u>				
13. Antacids not given within two hours of oral doses of quinolone antimicrobials, tetracycline, iron supplements, or isoniazid[18]	X		13. None	13. Physician orders, MAR
<u>Sucralfate</u>				
14. Sucralfate not given within two hours of oral doses of quinolone antimicrobials, digoxin, or phenytoin[18]	X		14. None	14. Physician orders, MAR
15. In patient receiving sucralfate and antacids, sucralfate given at least 30 min before or after antacids[5,6]	X		15. None	15. Physician orders, MAR
<u>H_2-Receptor Antagonists</u>				
16. Serum theophylline concentration monitored in patient receiving theophylline or aminophylline and H_2-receptor antagonist, and theophylline or aminophylline dosage adjusted as needed[19]	X		16. None	16. Laboratory reports, progress notes, physician orders, MAR
17. Serum phenytoin concentration monitored in patient receiving phenytoin and H_2-receptor antagonist, and phenytoin dosage adjusted as needed[19]	X		17. None	17. Laboratory reports, progress notes, physician orders, MAR
18. Serum lidocaine concentration monitored in patient receiving i.v. lidocaine and H_2-receptor antagonist, and lidocaine dosage adjusted as needed[19]	X		18. None	18. Laboratory reports, progress notes, physician orders, MAR
19. Serum procainamide concentration monitored in patient receiving procainamide and H_2-receptor antagonist, and procainamide dosage adjusted as needed[19]	X		19. None	19. Laboratory reports, progress notes, physician orders, MAR
20. Serum quinidine concentration monitored in patient receiving quinidine and H_2-receptor antagonist, and quinidine dosage adjusted as needed[19]	X		20. None	20. Laboratory reports, progress notes, physician orders, MAR
21. Prothrombin time monitored in patient receiving warfarin and H_2-receptor antagonist, and warfarin dosage adjusted as needed[19]	X		21. None	21. Laboratory reports, progress notes, physician orders, MAR
22. Level of sedation monitored in patient receiving benzodiazepine and H_2-receptor antagonist, and benzodiazepine dosage reduced if needed[19]	X		22. None	22. Nursing notes, progress notes, physician orders, MAR
23. Pulse and blood pressure monitored in patient receiving β-blocker and H_2-receptor antagonist, and β-blocker dosage adjusted as needed[19]	X		23. None	23. Nursing flow sheets, progress notes, physician orders, MAR
Complications				
<u>Antacids[20]</u>				
24. Gastrointestinal effects: constipation or diarrhea		X	24A. Identify other drug and nondrug causes 24B. Provide symptomatic care	24. Progress notes, nursing notes 24A. Physician orders, prog-

Element	Standard 100%	Standard 0%	Exception[b] or Critical Preventive/ Responsive Measure[c]	Sources of Information
			24C. Consider alternative agent if reaction intolerable	ress notes, nursing notes 24B, C. Physician orders, progress notes, nursing notes, MAR
25. Metabolic alkalosis (pH >7.45 with serum carbon dioxide concentration of >30 meq/L)		X	25A. Identify other drug and nondrug causes 25B. Switch to alternative agent	25. Progress notes, laboratory reports, nursing flow sheets 25A. Physician orders, progress notes, nursing notes 25B. Physician orders, progress notes, MAR
26. Hypermagnesemia (serum magnesium concentration, >2.5 meq/L)		X	26A. Identify other drug and nondrug causes 26B. Avoid use of antacids for stress ulcer prophylaxis in patient with severe renal insufficiency 26C. Switch to alternative agent	26. Progress notes, laboratory reports 26A. Physician orders, progress notes, nursing notes 26B. Physician orders, progress notes, laboratory reports, MAR 26C. Physician orders, progress notes, MAR
27. Hyperaluminemia (serum aluminum concentration, >200 μg/L)		X	27A. Identify other drug and nondrug causes 27B. Switch to alternative agent	27. Progress notes, laboratory reports 27A. Physician orders, progress notes, nursing notes 27B. Physician orders, progress notes, MAR
Sucralfate[21]				
28. Constipation		X	28A. Identify other drug and nondrug causes 28B. Provide symptomatic care 28C. Consider alternative agent if adverse effect intolerable	28. Progress notes, nursing notes 28A. Physician orders, progress notes, nursing notes 28B, C. Physician orders, progress notes, nursing notes, MAR
29. Drowsiness, dizziness		X	29A. Identify other drug and nondrug causes 29B. Switch to alternative agent	29. Progress notes, nursing notes 29A. Physician orders, progress notes, nursing notes 29B. Physician orders, progress notes, MAR
30. Pruritus		X	30A. Identify other drug and nondrug causes 30B. Provide symptomatic care 30C. Switch to alternative agent if reaction intolerable	30. Progress notes, nursing notes 30A. Physician orders, progress notes, nursing notes 30B, C. Physician orders, progress notes, nursing notes, MAR
31. Hyperaluminemia (serum aluminum concentration, >200 μg/L)		X	31A. Identify other drug and nondrug causes 31B. Switch to alternative agent	31. Progress notes, laboratory reports 31A. Physician orders, progress notes, nursing notes 31B. Physician orders, progress notes, MAR
32. Hypophosphatemia (serum phosphate concentration, <2.5 mg/dL)		X	32A. Identify other drug and nondrug causes 32B. Provide supportive care 32C. Consider use of alternative agent	32. Progress notes, laboratory reports 32A. Physician orders, progress notes, nursing notes 32B, C. Physician orders, progress notes, MAR
H_2-Receptor Antagonists[9,15,17]				
33. Central nervous system effects, including mental confusion, hallucinations, disorientation, depression, headache, dizziness		X	33A. Identify other drug and nondrug causes 33B. Switch to alternative agent	33. Progress notes, nursing notes 33A. Physician orders, progress notes, nursing notes 33B. Physician orders, progress notes, MAR
34. Rash		X	34A. Identify other drug and nondrug causes 34B. Provide symptomatic care 34C. Switch to alternative agent	34. Progress notes, nursing notes 34A. Physician orders, progress notes, nursing notes

Element	Standard 100%	Standard 0%	Exception[b] or Critical Preventive/ Responsive Measure[c]	Sources of Information
				34B, C. Physician orders, progress notes, MAR
35. Gastrointestinal effects: constipation or diarrhea		X	35A. Identify other drug and nondrug causes 35B. Provide symptomatic care 35C. Consider alternative agent if adverse effect intolerable	35. Progress notes, nursing notes 35A. Physician orders, progress notes, nursing notes 35B, C. Physician orders, progress notes, nursing notes, MAR
36. Hematologic effects, including thrombocytopenia (platelet count, <100,000/cu mm) and neutropenia (leukocyte count, <4000/cu mm)		X	36A. Identify other drug and nondrug causes 36B. Switch to alternative agent	36. Progress notes, laboratory reports 36A. Physician orders, progress notes, nursing notes 36B. Physician orders, progress notes, MAR
37. Elevated serum aminotransferase concentrations (aspartate aminotransferase, >40 IU/dL; alanine aminotransferase, >35 IU/dL; γ-glutamyltransferase, >85 IU/L in men and >55 IU/L in women)		X	37A. Identify other drug and nondrug causes 37B. Switch to alternative agent if elevated levels persist	37. Progress notes, laboratory reports 37A. Physician orders, progress notes, nursing notes 37B. Physician orders, progress notes, laboratory reports, MAR
Outcome Measure				
38. Stress ulceration prevented	X		38A. Patient died 38B. Patient unable to tolerate therapy	38. Progress notes, nursing notes 38A. Progress notes 38B. Progress notes, nursing notes, laboratory reports

[a] Criteria address justification for use (indications), critical (process) indicators, complications of therapy, and patient outcome. Each criterion consists of an element, a standard, exceptions to the standard, and sources of information. The element is the minimum level of evidence needed to show that patient care was optimal. The standard defines the deviation from an element that is acceptable. If no deviation is acceptable, the standard is 100%. Exceptions are circumstances in which deviation is allowable. Sources of information listed are the most reliable sources. Sources pertaining to an element or exception are identified by the number assigned to the element or exception (e.g., 6, 6A).

[b] For justification for use and critical (process) indicators.

[c] For complications and outcome measures.

References

1. Wilcox CM, Spenney JG. Stress ulcer prophylaxis in medical patients: who, what, and how much. *Am J Gastroenterol.* 1988; 83:1199–211.
2. Kleiman RL, Adair CG, Ephgrave KS. Stress: current understanding of pathogenesis and prophylaxis. *Drug Intell Clin Pharm.* 1988; 22:452–60.
3. Hastings PR, Skillman JJ, Bushnell LS et al. Antacid titration in the prevention of acute gastrointestinal bleeding: a controlled randomized trial in 200 critically ill patients. *N Engl J Med.* 1978; 298:1041–5.
4. Gonzalez ER, Morkunas AR. Prophylaxis of stress ulcers: antacid titration vs. histamine-2 receptor blockade. *Drug Intell Clin Pharm.* 1985; 19:807–11.
5. Laggner AN, Lenz K, Base W et al. Prevention of upper gastrointestinal bleeding in long-term ventilated patients. *Am J Med.* 1989; 86(Suppl 6A):81–4.
6. Bresalier RS, Grendell JH, Cello JP et al. Sucralfate suspension versus titrated antacid for the prevention of acute stress-related gastrointestinal hemorrhage in critically ill patients. *Am J Med.* 1987; 83(Suppl 3B):110–6.
7. Poleski MH, Spanier AH. Cimetidine versus antacids in the prevention of stress erosions in critically ill patients. *Am J Gastroenterol.* 1986; 81:107–11.
8. Weigelt JA, Aurbakker CM, Gewetz BL et al. Cimetidine versus antacids in prophylaxis for stress ulceration. *Arch Surg.* 1981; 116:597–601.
9. SmithKline Beecham. Tagamet package insert. Philadelphia, PA; 1990 Aug.
10. Frank W, Kalstadt R, Rockhold F et al. Comparison between continuous and intermittent infusion regimens of cimetidine in ulcer patients. *Clin Pharmacol Ther.* 1989; 46:234–9.
11. Rovers JP, Souney PF. A critical review of continuous infusion H_2 receptor therapy. *Crit Care Med.* 1989; 17:814–21.
12. Tome G, Fiasse R, Reynaert P et al. Effect of a 2g cimetidine infusion on twenty-four hour intragastric pH in critically ill patients. *Intensive Care Med.* 1988; 14:379–83.
13. Noseworthy TW, Shustack A, Johnston RG et al. A randomized trial comparing ranitidine and antacids in critically ill patients. *Crit Care Med.* 1987; 15:817–9.
14. More DG, Raper RF, Munro IA et al. Randomized, prospective trial of cimetidine and ranitidine for control of intragastric pH in the critically ill. *Surgery.* 1985; 97:215.
15. Glaxo Inc. Zantac package insert. Research Triangle Park, NC; 1989 Sep.
16. Morris DL, Markham SJ, Beechey A et al. Ranitidine bolus or infusion prophylaxis for stress ulcer. *Crit Care Med.* 1988; 16:229–32.
17. AHFS drug information 91. McEvoy GK, ed. Famotidine. Bethesda, MD: American Society of Hospital Pharmacists; 1991:1756–61.
18. Hansten PD, Horn JR, eds. Drug interactions. 6th ed. Philadelphia, PA: Lea & Febiger; 1989: 193, 291, 331.
19. Tatro DS, ed. Drug interaction facts. St. Louis, MO: Lippincott; 1990: 55, 124, 145, 380, 451, 594, 604, 702.
20. AHFS drug information 91. McEvoy GK, ed. Antacids and adsorbents. Bethesda, MD: American Society of Hospital Pharmacists; 1991:1706–11.
21. AHFS drug information 91. McEvoy GK, ed. Sucralfate. Bethesda, MD: American Society of Hospital Pharmacists; 1991:1782–84.

CP Continuing Education

The ASHP Continuing-Education System gives readers a self-assessment mechanism for selected articles in Clinical Pharmacy *and* AJHP. *It allows readers to obtain continuing-education credit for these articles.*

For the purpose of CE-credit enrollment, a blank answer sheet is published at the end of each installment of the column for the CE articles in that issue. An enrollee accumulates these answer sheets until the enrollment is submitted, using the form that is published in the June and December issues of Clinical Pharmacy *and in the June and December issues of* AJHP. *Any combination of tests within an 18-month period, from both* Clinical Pharmacy *and* AJHP, *may be included in an enrollment. More complete details about enrollment in the system appear in the semiannual enrollment form.*

Article 680-204-9124 (see page 745)
Qualifies for 1.0 hour of CE credit

Management of postoperative pain by continuous epidural infusion of analgesics

Learning Objectives

After studying this article, the reader should be able to

1. Describe the anatomy of the epidural space.
2. Describe and compare the mechanisms of action of epidurally administered narcotics and local anesthetics.
3. Discuss the pharmacokinetic principles affecting the onset, duration, and dermatomal spread of epidurally administered narcotics and local anesthetics.
4. List the proposed advantages of epidural continuous infusion of narcotic--local anesthetic combinations for postoperative pain relief compared with (1) bolus epidural injection or continuous epidural infusion of single agents and (2) intermittent intramuscular narcotic therapy.
5. Identify and discuss the five most common adverse effects associated with the epidural infusion of narcotics, local anesthetics, or both.

Self-assessment Questions

For each question there is only one best answer.

1. Which of the following structures, contained in the epidural space, may influence the location of epidural entry and the pharmacokinetics of the agent(s) injected into the epidural space?
   a. Fat.
   b. Nerve roots.
   c. Valveless venous system.
   d. All of the above alternatives are correct.

2. Which of the following is not true concerning the mechanisms and sites of action of epidurally administered narcotics and local anesthetics?
   a. Narcotics selectively block pain conduction but may produce some sensory and motor blockade.
   b. The major sites of action of epidurally administered narcotics are the presynaptic and postsynaptic opiate receptors in the substantia gelatinosa of the dorsal horn of the spinal cord.
   c. Local anesthetics produce analgesia by axonal membrane blockade of type C nerve fibers.
   d. The concentration of the local anesthetic and depth of nerve penetration will determine whether analgesia is selectively obtained with local anesthetics.

3. The most important determinant of the onset of action, dermatomal spread, and duration of effect of an epidurally administered narcotic is
   a. The lipid solubility of the agent.
   b. The agent's affinity for opiate receptors.
   c. The dose of the agent.
   d. The location of the epidural injection.

4. Which of the following is not true concerning the use of bupivacaine in continuous epidural infusions?
   a. It has a predilection to produce sensory versus motor nerve block.
   b. It produces less tachyphylaxis than other local anesthetics.
   c. It has low lipid solubility, which prolongs its duration of action.
   d. It has a favorable safety profile.

5. Combinations of narcotics and local anesthetics are commonly used in postoperative continuous epidural infusions to take advantage of

Current Literature

Drug Reaction Alerts 803

Book Reviews

Drug Interactions & Updates, 1991 805
By Philip D. Hansten and John R. Horn
Reviewed by Mary Lea Gora

Infections in Intravenous Drug Abusers 805
Edited by Donald P. Levine and Jack D. Sobel
Reviewed by Stephen Mendel

Books Received 806

Drug Reaction Alerts

Drug Reaction Alerts focuses primarily on serious, unlabeled reactions to new chemical entities. The citations are compiled monthly from International Pharmaceutical Abstracts, *which covers over 800 pharmacy and health-related journals worldwide. An address for reprints (when available) follows the name of the corresponding author of each citation.*

Pharmacists may use the FDA Adverse Reaction Report form that appears in most issues of Clinical Pharmacy *for submitting reports of adverse drug reactions directly to FDA.*

Antibiotics

Ostlere LS, Langtry JA, Staughton RC (Westminster Hospital, London SW1P 2AP, England). Allergy to **spiramycin** during prophylactic treatment of fetal toxoplasmosis. *Br Med J.* 1991; 302:970. Case. (38-year-old pregnant woman; received spiramycin 1.5 g twice daily for eight weeks as chemoprophylaxis for congenital toxoplasmosis; developed allergic skin reaction; therapy with 0.025% beclomethasone dipropionate ointment led to resolution of rash; withdrawal of beclomethasone dipropionate ointment led to reappearance of rash; withdrawal of spiramycin led to resolution of symptoms; pregnancy progressed normally; no signs of toxoplasmosis in neonate)

Anticoagulants

Eichinger S (First Department of Internal Medicine, University of Vienna, A7090 Vienna, Austria), Kyrle PA, Brenner B et al. Thrombocytopenia associated with low-molecular-weight heparin. *Lancet.* 1991; 337:1425-6. Case. (72-year-old man with rib fractures; received **low molecular weight heparin** 3000 anti-Xa units; days 9 to 12, platelet count gradually decreased to 23,000/μL; platelet count remained less than 30,000/μL until day 19; therapy with 10 platelet transfusions did not lead to increased platelet count; replacement of heparin with epoprostenol on day 21 led to platelet count of 93,000/μL; patient died two days later because of respiratory failure; results of examinations at autopsy showed bilateral pulmonary embolism, thrombosis of both iliac and jugular veins, and right adrenal bleeding)

Antihistamines

MacConnell TJ, Stanners AJ (Bristol Royal Infirmary, Bristol BS2 8HW, England). Torsades de pointes complicating treatment with **terfenadine**. *Br Med J.* 1991; 302:1469. Case. (45-year-old woman with urticaria; received terfenadine 120 mg/day initially and increased to 360 mg/day for two weeks; developed torsades de pointes; withdrawal of terfenadine and therapy with temporary ventricular pacing led to complete recovery)

Anti-inflammatory Agents

Le Gros V, Saveuse H, Lesur G et al. (Brion N, Center Hospital de Versailles, 78157 Le Chesnay Cedex, France). Lung and skin hypersensitivity to 5-aminosalicylic acid. *Br Med J.* 1991; 302:970. Case. (54-year-old woman with ulcerative colitis; received oral **mesalamine** 250 mg three times daily for five days; developed lung opacities, bronchospasm, and erythematous skin rash; withdrawal of mesalamine after 17 days led to gradual resolution of symptoms over three weeks)

Antimalarial Agents

Singh K, Shanks GD, Wild H (Chulalongkorn University, 10400 Bangkok, Thailand). Seizures after **mefloquine**. *Ann Intern Med.* 1991; 114:994. Case. (57-year-old man; received mefloquine hydrochloride 250 mg once weekly for three weeks as chemoprophylaxis for malaria; experienced a single grand mal seizure three days after third dose; serum mefloquine concentration, 491 ng/mL [reported mean for prophylactic regimen, 450 ng/mL]; recovery without specific therapy)

Antimanic Agents

Winter R (Department of Medicine, Hammersmith Hospital, London W12 OHS, England). **Lithium** intoxication. *Br Med J.* 1991; 302:1267-9. Case. (41-year-old woman with bipolar disorder; received lithium 2.1 g/day as maintenance therapy; developed diarrhea and vomiting for five days while traveling, and subsequently had a change in behavior; husband increased lithium dosage to 2.7 g/day; patient developed acute renal failure; on hospitalization, serum lithium concentration was 4.8 mM; therapy with hemodialysis, replacement fluids, and total parenteral nutrition led eventually to improved consciousness and polyuria; patient required ongoing hospitalization)

Antivirals

Klutman NE, Hinthorn DR (University of Kansas Medical Center, Kansas City, KS 66103). Excessive growth of eyelashes in a patient with AIDS being treated with **zidovudine**. *N Engl J Med.* 1991; 324:1896. Case. (20-year-old man with AIDS; received zidovudine 200 mg every four hours for approximately two weeks; developed abnormal eyelash growth; eyelashes measured 1.5–2.0 cm four weeks after initiation of zidovudine therapy; other body hair was not affected)

Drugs, Adverse Reactions

Vale JA, Kirby RS, Lees W (Department of Urology and Radiology, St. Bartholomew's and Middlesex Hospital, London EC1A 7BE, England). **Papaverine**, benzodiazepines, and prolonged erections. *Lancet.* 1991; 337:1552. Cases. (two men, aged 30 and 47 years, with histories of erectile failure; received test dose of papaverine 60 mg by intracavernosal injection and antianxiety dose of **diazepam** 5–10 mg by i.v. injection; developed full erection that persisted 5–6 hours after papaverine injection; therapy with local application of ice packs to one man and norepinephrine by intracavernosal injection to other man led to reduction of erection)

Drug Interactions

Win N, Mitchell DC, Jones PA et al. (French EA, University Hospital, Nottingham NG7 2UH, England). Azapropazone and **warfarin**. *Br Med J.* 1991; 302:969-970 Cases. (four patients, aged 38–81 years, who were maintained on long-term warfarin therapy; received **apazone** for three to seven days; developed increased anticoagulation; withdrawal of apazone or apazone and warfarin and therapy with various combinations of vitamin K, blood, and plasma led to recovery of three patients and death of fourth patient)

Gastrointestinal Drugs

Ahmad S (Cardio-Diagnostic Clinic, 1000 Brookside Drive, Fairmont, WV 26554). **Famotidine** and cardiac arrhythmia. *DICP.* 1991; 25:315. Case. (40-year-old man with duodenal ulcer; received famotidine 40 mg/day for three weeks; complained of dizziness and malaise; electrocardiogram showed second-degree atrioventricular block and heart rate of 38 beats/min; withdrawal of famotidine led to recovery within two days; positive rechallenge)

Gloves

Sussman GL (202 St. Clair Avenue W., Toronto, Ontario M4V 1R2, Canada), Tarlo S, Dolovich J. The spectrum of IgE-mediated responses to **latex**. *JAMA.* 1991; 265:2844-7. Cases. (nine females and five males, aged 3–45 years; exposed to latex gloves as a result of skin contact, latex in air, or intraoperative contact; developed allergic reactions, including three women and one man who developed intraoperative anaphylaxis; all patients had positive reactions to latex skin test; serum IgE antibody to latex detected by radioallergosorbent test in all but one tested patient)

Hemorheologic Agents

Oren R, Yishar O, Lysy J et al. (Ligumsky M, Gastroenterology Unit, Hadassah University Hospital, 91120 Jerusalem, Israel). **Pentoxifylline**-induced gastrointestinal bleeding. *DICP.* 1991; 25:315-6. Case. (67-year-old woman; received a single dose of pentoxifylline 400 mg; developed bleeding duodenal ulcer; treatment of bleeding vessel with bipolar hemostatic probe led to cessation of bleeding; therapy with blood transfusion and cimetidine led to uneventful recovery)

Parasympatholytic Agents

McLeod AA, Thorogood S, Barnett S (Cardiac Department, Poole General Hospital, Dorset BH15 2JB, England). Torsades de pointes complicating treatment with **terodiline**. *Br Med J.* 1991; 302:1469. Case. (83-year-old woman; received terodiline hydrochloride 37.5 mg/day for two years; developed torsades de pointes; withdrawal of terodiline hydrochloride and therapy with magnesium 5 g [as the sulfate salt] led to resolution of arrhythmia; positive rechallenge)

Pediatrics

Brock PR, De Zegher F, Casteels-Van Deale M et al. (Vanderschueren-Lodeweyckx M, Department of Pediatrics, University Hospital Gasthuisberg, 3000 Louvain, Belgium). Malignant disease in Bloom's syndrome children treated with growth hormone. *Lancet.* 1991; 337:1345-6. Cases. (four children with Bloom's syndrome; received **somatropin** 0.1 unit/kg/day by s.c. injection for 5–44 months; 5.5-year-old child developed B-cell non-Hodgkin's lymphoma with widespread abdominal disease after five months; 13-year-old child developed stem cell leukemia after 44 months; both children who developed tumors had humoral and cellular immunodeficiencies; mean height velocity increased from 2.4 to 5.8 cm/yr during treatment with somatropin)

Burtin P, Daoud P, Jacqz-Aigrain E et al. (Moriette G, Intensive Care Unit, Hôpital Port-Royal, Paris, France). Hypotension with **midazolam** and **fentanyl** in the newborn. *Lancet.* 1991; 337:1545-6. Cases. (six newborn infants, gestational age 30–37 weeks, with respiratory distress syndrome who received fentanyl 1.5 or 2.5 μg/kg by i.v. bolus injection or 1 or 2 μg/kg/hr by continuous i.v. infusion; received midazolam 200 μg/kg as i.v. bolus injection or 60 μg/kg/hr by continuous i.v. infusion or both; developed hypotension; therapy with albumin by i.v. infusion led to recovery in four to eight hours)

Thyroid Drugs

Kung AW (Department of Medicine, University of Hong Kong, Queen Mary Hospital, Hong Kong), Pun KK. Bone mineral density in premenopausal women receiving long-term physiological doses of **levothyroxine**. *JAMA.* 1991; 265:2688-91. Study. (retrospective controlled study; 26 premenopausal women, aged 18–42 years, with Hashimoto's thyroiditis who received levothyroxine at a mean dose of 111 µg/day for a mean duration of 7.5 years and 26 age-matched controls; women who received levothyroxine had total bone mineral densities in normal range but had significantly lower regional bone mineral densities at femoral neck, trochanter, Ward's triangle, both arms, and pelvis compared with control group; no correlation between total or regional bone mineral densities and [1] levothyroxine dosage or therapy duration or [2] thyroid function test results)

Uricosuric Agents

Collins CE, Thomas DJ, Gumpel JM (Mount Vernon Hospital, Northwood, Middlesex HA6 2RN, England). Catatonia in the **allopurinol** hypersensitivity syndrome. *Br Med J.* 1991; 302:970. Case. (67-year-old woman with gout; received allopurinol 100 mg three times daily for six weeks; developed vague affect, widespread maculopapular rash, fever, and decreased renal function; withdrawal of allopurinol and therapy with hydrocortisone 200 mg by i.v. injection every 6 hours for 48 hours followed by oral prednisolone 40 mg/day for two weeks led to rapid improvement of catatonia, rash, and temperature and resumption of normal renal function)

Book Reviews

Drug Interactions & Updates, 1991

By Philip D. Hansten and John R. Horn.
Published by Lea & Febiger, 100 Washington Square, Philadelphia, PA 19355-9725, 1990. xi + 522 p. Available directly from Applied Therapeutics, Inc., P.O. Box 5077, Vancouver, WA 98668-5077. Price $65 (U.S.), $75 plus 7% general sales tax (Canada), $75 (elsewhere).

Twenty years ago, the first edition of *Drug Interactions* was one of the first textbooks containing a collection of the primary literature on adverse experiences secondary to coadministration of two drugs. Since then, Hansten and Horn have revised and updated the book several times; it now contains concise, clinically relevant information on drug–food and drug–ethanol interactions in humans, in addition to drug–drug interactions. Reports of drug interactions with tobacco and marijuana are also included.

The book has improved since the sixth edition, published in 1989. The seventh edition is published as a three-ring binder with 8- × 11-inch looseleaf pages; quarterly updates of monographs are to be inserted in a separate section. A tab index, a new feature, provides quick access to these updates. Every two years, the updates are integrated into the new edition. Incorporation of *Drug Interaction Newsletter*, which at one time was published separately, into the book means that each monograph update also includes an article covering a drug interaction topic. The first *Newsletter* in the 1991 edition contains an interesting article entitled "The Top 40 Drug Interactions," which lists the interactions that the authors consider to be most relevant to the clinician; the information appears in tabular form and could serve as a quick reference in a hospital pharmacy.

The book begins with a brief instruction to users and an introductory chapter on mechanisms and clinical characteristics of drug interactions; this chapter, not available in the previous edition, provides a concise, yet comprehensive, overview of the subject. Reading the chapter would aid the young professional or serve as a brief review for the senior pharmacist.

The next 17 chapters provide drug interaction information based on drug category (e.g., antihypertensive drug interactions). Each chapter is divided into individual drugs (e.g., clonidine interactions) or pharmacologic class (e.g., angiotensin-converting-enzyme inhibitor interactions) followed by a monograph describing an interaction with the coadministered agent. Approximately 200 new monographs have been added since 1989, and the previously published monographs have been revised. As in the previous edition, each monograph is divided into four sections: a summary, and descriptions of the mechanism, clinical significance, and management of the interaction.

The references appear at the end of each monograph instead of at the end of each chapter, allowing for easy referral. The index is important for identifying potentially interacting drugs, as the format of the chapters does not allow for easy, at-a-glance identification of interactions. However, not all the drug names are listed individually in the index; some are listed by pharmacologic class. Because of this inconsistency, the potential for a clinically relevant interaction to be missed is a concern.

The levels of clinical significance (major, moderate, and minor) are defined at the beginning of the book, and each interaction has a rating assigned to it. The estimated clinical significance of each interaction is denoted by typeface: bold (major), italic (moderate), and roman (minor). The definition of the level of clinical significance now appears at the bottom of each page as a reminder.

Drug Interactions & Updates serves as an important tool for identifying potential adverse interactions and as an adjunct to the skills and knowledge of the professional. However, the book contributes little to assessing the risk of adverse drug reactions in patients receiving the interacting drugs; more research needs to be conducted in this area. Hansten and Horn have made various improvements, both in format and content, to their book that heighten its worth. *Drug Interactions & Updates* continues to serve as a valuable source of drug interaction information.

Reviewed by Mary Lea Gora, Pharm.D., Pharmacy Drug Information Service, University of Cincinnati Hospital, 234 Goodman Street, Cincinnati, OH 45267.

Infections in Intravenous Drug Abusers

Edited by Donald P. Levine and Jack D. Sobel.
Published by Oxford University Press, 200 Madison Avenue, New York, NY 10016, 1990. x + 395 p. Price $75.

Hospital admissions caused by complications of intravenous drug abuse (IVDA) are increasing daily; i.v. drug abusers constitute the second largest group of patients infected by the human immunodeficiency virus (HIV) and diagnosed with AIDS. Consequently, infections in patients with HIV who abuse drugs run the gamut from common infectious diseases to more serious, life-threatening infectious complications of IVDA, in addition to the infectious diseases to which AIDS patients are susceptible.

Although health-care personnel who care for IVDA patients and treat infectious complications of IVDA could obtain most of the data found in this textbook on their own, the process would be tedious and time-consuming. The editors have compiled review articles, studies, and case reports in the area of IVDA and added the wisdom of many experts in this field.

The first few chapters of the book provide the reader with a brief history of the epidemiology of IVDA, a review of host defenses and how they are altered in IVDA, and a quick review of the microbiology and immunology of the infectious complications that accompany IVDA. The rest of the text explains the diagnosis and management of infectious complications as it follows potential patients from the emergency department to the radiology suite and then to the hospital bed. A very long chapter 7 is devoted entirely to the radiological evaluation and diagnosis of infections in i.v. drug abusers. Chapters 8 through 14 discuss infectious manifestations of IVDA in specific organ systems (e.g., eye, brain, heart). Chapter 15 discusses diagnosis, management, and complications of mycotic aneurysm. The final chapter looks at AIDS and its relationship to IVDA in terms of disease transmission, as well as infectious complications caused by the combination of HIV infection and IVDA.

The editors and chapter authors have done a great service by compiling a massive amount of literature and presenting it in a concise, easy-to-read, well-referenced manner. There are only two deficiencies to mention. First, each author emphasizes the diagnosis, not the treatment, of IVDA-associated infections; there are perhaps only two or three paragraphs per chapter devoted to treatment. Second, almost all the chapter authors are from Detroit-area hospitals; although each author does discuss the myriad infections reported in the literature, there is a definite bias toward the problems of IVDA patients in Detroit.

This book is an excellent reference on the infectious problems of IVDA patients. It would be a valuable asset to all physicians and pharmacists but primarily to those involved in the care of i.v. drug abusers.

Reviewed by Stephen Mendel, Pharm.D., University Hospitals of Cleveland, 2074 Abington Road, Cleveland, OH 44106.

Books Received

Books are listed as soon as received; selected books may be reviewed in Book Reviews in subsequent issues.

Casarett and Doull's Toxicology: The Basic Science of Poisons, Fourth Edition, edited by Mary O. Amdur, John Doull, and Curtis D. Klaassen. Published by Pergamon Press, Inc., Maxwell House, Fairview Park, Elmsford, NY 10523, 1991. xiii + 1033 p. Price $62.50.

USAN and the USP Dictionary of Drug Names, edited by Carolyn A. Fleeger. Published by the United States Pharmacopeial Convention, Inc., 12601 Twinbrook Parkway, Rockville, MD 20852, 1991. 824 p. Price $90; airmail shipments outside the U.S. and Canada, $130.

Advertising Index

American Society of Hospital Pharmacists
ASHP Membership, 783
Clinical Pharmacy, 738
Concepts in Clinical Pharmacokinetics, 741
Medication Errors: A Closer Look, 744
MedTeach, 806
Position Available, 744
Amgen Inc
Epogen, inside front cover
Burroughs Wellcome Company
Exosurf, 795-799
Roche Laboratories, Division of Hoffmann-La Roche, Inc.
Rocephin, inside back cover, outside back cover
Ross Laboratories
Survanta, 737-738
Wyeth-Ayerst Laboratories, Inc.
Ativan Injection, 734-36

News

Highlights of the Seventh International Conference on AIDS 809
Roberta J. Wong

Study raises safety questions about β-agonist inhaler overuse 822

News Briefs 822

Upcoming Specialty Meetings 822

Highlights of the Seventh International Conference on AIDS

The Seventh International Conference on AIDS, held in Florence, Italy, June 16–21, was the venue for some 8000 scientists from more than 70 countries. New and refined scientific theories, study results, and treatment advances for opportunistic infections, AIDS-related neoplasms, and early human immunodeficiency virus (HIV) disease were reported. Novel educational strategies were described, and statistics on cases diagnosed were presented. More than 3000 posters and almost 500 oral presentations highlighted the scientific and clinical advances against HIV infection and underscored the conference theme—Science Challenging AIDS. Protests over the restrictive United States immigration policy continued. As a result, the eighth international conference, scheduled in Boston, Massachusetts, in May 1992, will be held in Amsterdam, the Netherlands. In 1993 the Conference will be held in Berlin, Germany; thereafter, it will be scheduled every two years.

Since resistance emerges only after several mutations in the viral gene sequence, patients with late-stage disease may already have a variety of viral strains present in sufficient numbers to overcome therapy. Early intervention and the use of other antiviral therapies may help minimize the clinical effects of resistance.

Basic Research. Robin Weiss, Ph.D., Director of Research, Chester Beatty Laboratories, Institute of Cancer Research, London, England, reviewed the life cycle of HIV. Although the basic steps are well known, the precise mechanism of the interaction between HIV and cell membranes still needs clarification. In addition to CD4, which binds to gp120, other cells may be crucial for HIV to successfully infect a target cell. It has been proposed that another molecule or cell must be present to alter the membrane of the target cell and to allow HIV to penetrate the cell surface. These components may include leukocyte function associated antigen-1 (LFA-1) lymphocytes, the Fc receptor on macrophages, galactocerebroside, or proteinases. Translating these theories regarding mechanisms of infection into new clinical therapies will remain one of the biggest challenges for the 1990s.

Continued on page 814

A change to Zefazone is no small change

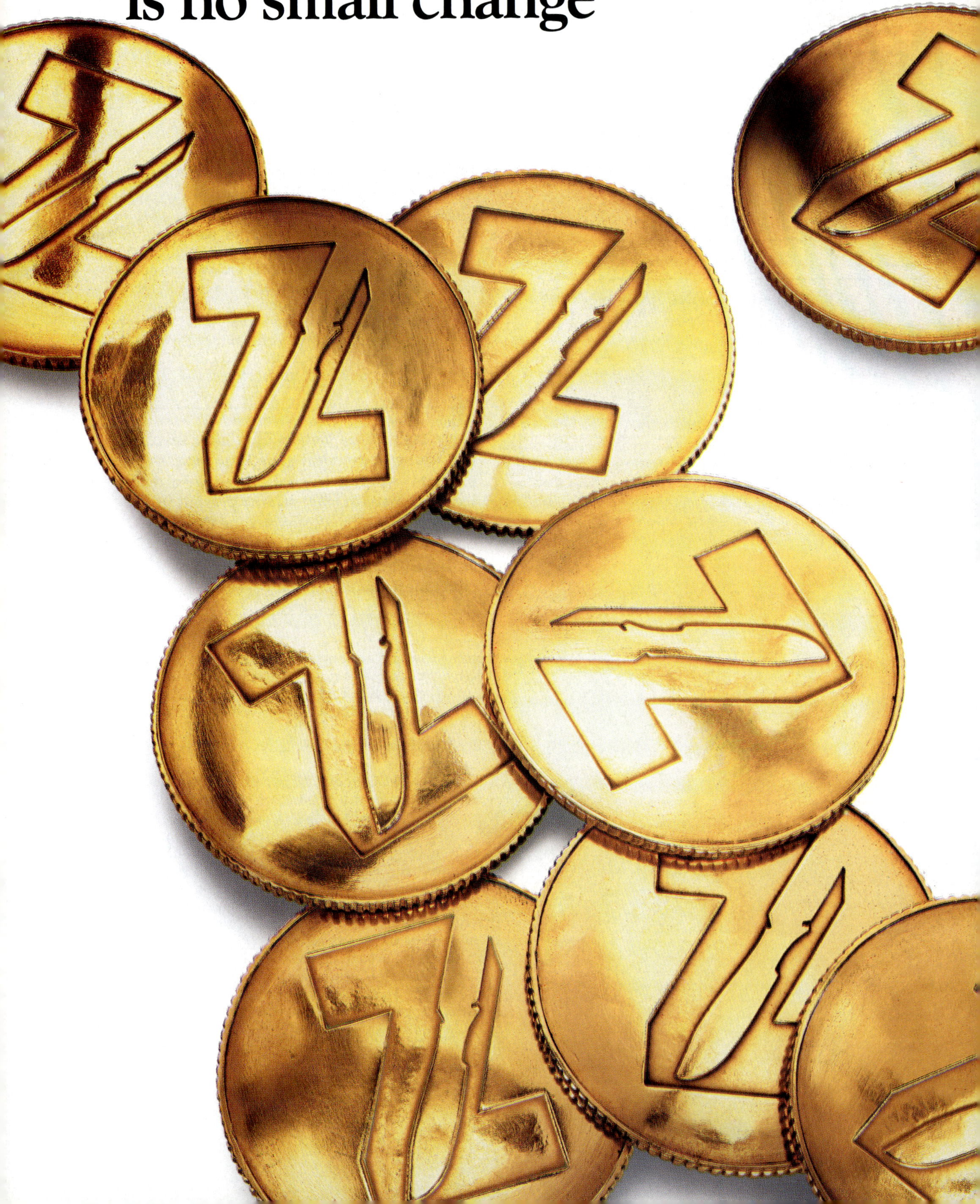

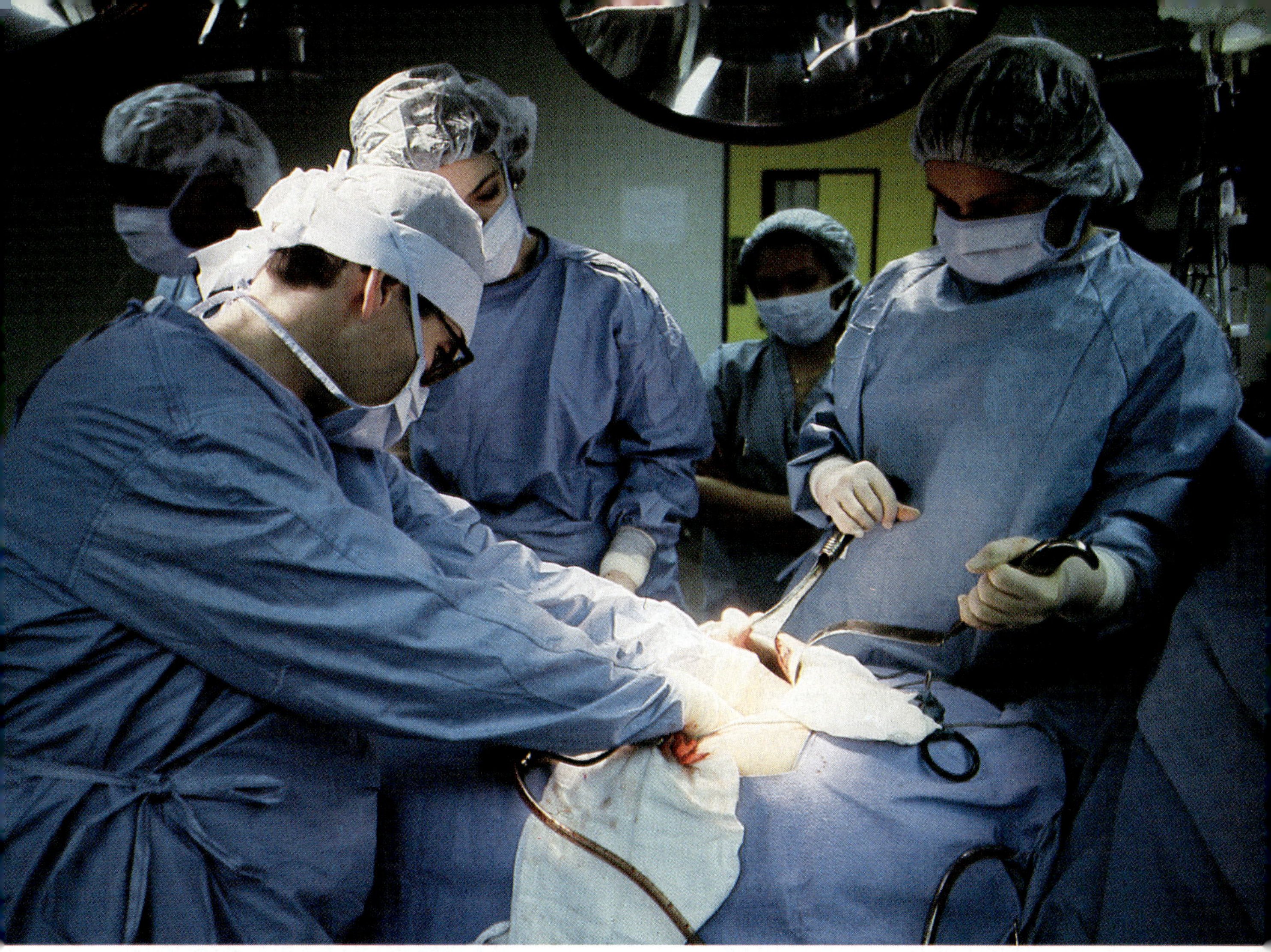

Continued from page 809

Structural similarity of gp120 and part of MHC Class II protein has been studied by Angus Dalgleish, MRC Clinical Research Centre, Harrow, United Kingdom. MHC binds antigens, and this complex then binds T cells to induce antibody production specific to the antigen. The structural similarity of gp120 and major histocompatibility complex (MHC)Class II proteins was explored by investigators who entered various chemical sequences of gp120 into a computer and created a three-dimensional representation of the protein. The importance of the structural similarity between gp120 and MHC may become apparent as scientists elucidate the specific interaction of gp120 with the immune system.

According to Thomas Schulz, Clinical Research Scientist, Institute for Cancer Research, London, gp120 may be a pivotal protein for successful infection. It may be cleaved at the V3 loop of the envelope protein to allow penetration of viral RNA into target cells. A mutation at the V3 loop or the addition of antibodies that neutralize enzymatic cleavage prevents HIV infection of target cells. Once gp120 is cleaved, infection by other HIV strains appears inhibited. Further laboratory study will delineate which proteins are essential for HIV infection.

William Haseltine, M.D., Chief, Division of Human Retrovirology, Dana-Farber Cancer Institute, Boston, reported on progress in gene regulation. The *tat* gene is instrumental in successful HIV replication. In vitro studies have shown that inhibition or removal of the *tat* gene from viral genome halts HIV replication. To date, seven regulatory genes have been discovered; all act at different stages of the life cycle. Mike Poznansky, also of the Dana-Farber Cancer Institute, discussed theoretical applications of gene therapy. In one application, HIV-infected peripheral lymphocytes would be harvested from a patient, and a defective virus (one that is unable to replicate) would be injected into the lymphocytes. If these treated lymphocytes were then reinjected into the patient, the defective virus would be spread throughout the immune system. This defective virus would render lymphocytes immune to future infection with virulent HIV strains. This postulated model may someday allow specific treatment of a patient's disease to reduce the rate of HIV replication.

Combining portions of an IgE antibody and a partial CD4 receptor may trigger the immune system into attacking HIV particles, said Susanne Krauss, M.D., University of Munich, Munich, Germany. Basophils attach to IgE, while HIV particles bind to the CD4 receptor. Presenting HIV to the basophil promotes recognition and subsequent release of toxins that cause destruction of HIV in vitro. This technique may produce a new type of therapy against HIV infection.

Concentrations of HIV particles are 10–15 times higher in lymph nodes, adenoids, and tonsils than in peripheral blood, and these tissues may be a major reservoir of infection, said Cecilia Graziosi, M.D., National Institute of Allergy and Infectious Diseases of work performed in conjunction with St. Luke's Hospital, New York. The total amount of virus in an infected individual appears to be much greater than earlier studies had indicated. Previous estimates were based on the amount of virus found in T cells of infected individuals. The higher number of viral particles found in other tissues may explain how HIV is able to infect CD4+ cells over time, inducing severe immunodeficiency. The use of animal models to explore these areas may offer a better understanding of the progression of HIV disease.

The clinical relevance of resistance is still unclear, said Douglas Richman, M.D., Ph.D., University of California, San Diego. As expected, the incidence of drug resistance is higher in treated individuals with late-stage disease than in patients with early HIV infection who receive treatment. "The amount of virus replication is inversely proportional to the CD4 cell count. The opportunity for emergence of resistant viruses increases as the replication events increase," said Richman. Since resistance emerges only after several mutations in the viral gene sequence, patients with late-stage disease may already have a variety of viral strains present in sufficient numbers to overcome therapy. Early intervention and the use of other antiviral therapies may help minimize the clinical effects of resistance.

Robert Bollinger, M.D., Johns Hopkins University, Baltimore, and Edward Winger, M.D., Immunodiagnostics Laboratories, San Francisco, independently concluded that p24 antigen is the most reliable marker for monitoring progression of HIV disease. Both investigators presented findings indicating that p24 antigens are detected in more than 90% of asymptomatic patients. Bollinger further claimed that zidovudine 1500 mg/day caused a marked decrease in p24 antigen levels after 16 or 24 weeks of therapy. CD4 cell counts and p24 antigen levels can predict progression in up to 67% of HIV-infected patients. Neil Bodsworth, M.D., University of New South Wales, Sydney, Australia, also reported that p24 antigen is a good indicator of survival. His review of data from 113 patients demonstrated a shorter survival in patients with p24 antigen concentrations greater than 1000 ng/mL at the start of zidovudine therapy than in those with lower p24 antigen concentrations.

Advances in Treatment of HIV Infection. According to Terri Creagh-Kirk, Clinical Research Scientist, Burroughs Wellcome Company, zidovudine was well tolerated by 92% of 540 HIV-infected children less than 12 years of age who received zidovudine therapy for a median of 80 days. The dosage was decreased from 180 mg/sq m given orally every six hours to 120 mg/sq m because of adverse effects in only 5% of patients; 3% of patients were unable to tolerate zidovudine, and therapy was discontinued temporarily during the study. Zidovudine therapy resulted in weight gain and height increases during the study. Immunologic improvements were also documented.

Didanosine (dideoxyinosine, ddI) appears to maintain cognitive function in up to 83% of children treated for 6–12 months, said Pamela Wolters, Medical Illness Counseling Center, Bethesda, of work performed in collaboration with the Pediatric Branch of National Cancer Institute (NCI). Ninety-five patients 9 months to 18.8 years of age who had symptomatic HIV infection were enrolled in this open study. Children who were infected via perinatal transmission and exhibited neurologic complications at enrollment generally stopped responding after six months of therapy; patients who were infected by other modes of transmission experienced more prolonged benefit. Overall, improvements were seen in the first six months of therapy in most patients and are not expected to appear after this period.

Continued on page 820

EXOSURF® Neonatal™

(COLFOSCERIL PALMITATE, CETYL ALCOHOL, TYLOXAPOL) For Intratracheal Suspension / 10 mL vials

PLEASE CONSULT FULL PRODUCT INFORMATION BEFORE PRESCRIBING.

INDICATIONS AND USAGE: Exosurf Neonatal is indicated for:

1. **Prophylactic** treatment of infants with birth weights of less than 1350 grams who are at risk of developing RDS (see PRECAUTIONS),
2. **Prophylactic** treatment of infants with birth weights greater than 1350 grams who have evidence of pulmonary immaturity, and
3. **Rescue** treatment of infants who have developed RDS.

CONTRAINDICATIONS: There are no known contraindications to treatment with Exosurf Neonatal.

WARNINGS: Intratracheal Administration Only: Exosurf Neonatal should be administered only by instillation into the trachea. **General:** The use of Exosurf Neonatal requires expert clinical care by experienced neonatologists and other clinicians who are accomplished at neonatal intubation and ventilatory management. Adequate personnel, facilities, equipment, and medications are required to optimize perinatal outcome in premature infants. Instillation of Exosurf Neonatal should be performed **only** by trained medical personnel experienced in airway and clinical management of unstable premature infants. Vigilant clinical attention should be given to all infants prior to, during, and after administration of Exosurf Neonatal. **Acute Effects:** Exosurf Neonatal can rapidly affect oxygenation and lung compliance. **Lung Compliance:** If chest expansion improves substantially after dosing, peak ventilator inspiratory pressures should be reduced immediately, without waiting for confirmation of respiratory improvement by blood gas assessment. Failure to reduce inspiratory ventilator pressures rapidly in such instances can result in lung overdistention and fatal pulmonary air leak. **Hyperoxia:** If the infant becomes pink and transcutaneous oxygen saturation is in excess of 95%, FiO_2 should be reduced in small but repeated steps (until saturation is 90 to 95%) without waiting for confirmation of elevated arterial pO_2 by blood gas assessment. Failure to reduce FiO_2 in such instances can result in hyperoxia. **Hypocarbia:** If arterial or transcutaneous CO_2 measurements are <30 torr, the ventilator rate should be reduced at once. Failure to reduce ventilator rates in such instances can result in marked hypocarbia, which is known to reduce brain blood flow. **Pulmonary Hemorrhage:** In the single study conducted in infants weighing <700 grams at birth, the incidence of pulmonary hemorrhage (10% vs 2% in the placebo group) was significantly increased in the Exosurf Neonatal group. None of the five studies involving infants with birth weights >700 grams showed a significant increase in pulmonary hemorrhage in the Exosurf Neonatal group. In a cross-study analysis of these five studies, pulmonary hemorrhage was reported for 1% (14/1420) of infants in the placebo group and 2% (27/1411) of infants in the Exosurf Neonatal group. Fatal pulmonary hemorrhage occurred in three infants; two in the Exosurf Neonatal group and one in the placebo group. Mortality from all causes among infants who developed pulmonary hemorrhage was 43% in the placebo group and 37% in the Exosurf Neonatal group. Pulmonary hemorrhage in both Exosurf Neonatal and placebo infants was more frequent in infants who were younger, smaller, male, or who had a patent ductus arteriosus. Pulmonary hemorrhage typically occurred in the first 2 days of life in both treatment groups. In more than 7700 infants in the open, uncontrolled study, pulmonary hemorrhage was reported in 4%, but fatal pulmonary hemorrhage was reported rarely (0.4%). In the controlled clinical studies, Exosurf Neonatal treated infants who received steroids more than 24 hours prior to delivery or indomethacin postnatally had a lower rate of pulmonary hemorrhage than other Exosurf Neonatal treated infants. Attention should be paid to early and aggressive diagnosis and treatment (unless contraindicated) of patent ductus arteriosus during the first 2 days of life (while the ductus arteriosus is often clinically silent). Other potentially protective measures include attempting to decrease FiO_2 preferentially over ventilator pressures during the first 24 to 48 hours after dosing, and attempting to decrease PEEP minimally for at least 48 hours after dosing. **Mucous Plugs:** Infants whose ventilation becomes markedly impaired during or shortly after dosing may have mucous plugging of the endotracheal tube, particularly if pulmonary secretions were prominent prior to drug administration. Suctioning of all infants prior to dosing may lessen the chance of mucous plugs obstructing the endotracheal tube. If endotracheal tube obstruction from such plugs is suspected, and suctioning is unsuccessful in removing the obstruction, the blocked endotracheal tube should be replaced immediately.

PRECAUTIONS:

General: In the controlled clinical studies, infants known prenatally or postnatally to have major congenital anomalies, or who were suspected of having congenital infection, were excluded from entry. However, these disorders cannot be recognized early in life in all cases, and a few infants with these conditions were entered. The benefits of Exosurf Neonatal in the affected infants who received drug appeared to be similar to the benefits observed in infants without anomalies or occult infection. **Prophylactic Treatment-Infants <700 Grams:** In infants weighing 500 to 700 grams, a single prophylactic dose of Exosurf Neonatal significantly: improved FiO_2 and ventilator settings, reduced pneumothorax, and reduced death from RDS, but increased pulmonary hemorrhage (see WARNINGS). Overall mortality did not differ significantly between the placebo and Exosurf Neonatal groups (see Table 1 in full product information). Data on multiple doses in infants in this weight class are not yet available. Accordingly, clinicians should carefully evaluate the potential risks and benefits of Exosurf Neonatal administration in these infants. **Rescue Treatment-Number of Doses:** A small number of infants with RDS have received more than two doses of Exosurf Neonatal as rescue treatment. Definitive data on the safety and efficacy of these additional doses are not available. **Carcinogenesis, Mutagenesis, Impairment of Fertility:** Exosurf Neonatal at concentrations up to 10,000 μg/plate was not mutagenic in the Ames Salmonella assay. Long-term studies have not been performed in animals to evaluate the carcinogenic potential of Exosurf Neonatal. The effects of Exosurf Neonatal on fertility have not been studied.

ADVERSE REACTIONS:

General: Premature birth is associated with a high incidence of morbidity and mortality. Despite significant reductions in overall mortality associated with Exosurf Neonatal, some infants who received Exosurf Neonatal developed severe complications and either survived with permanent handicaps or died.

In controlled clinical studies evaluating the safety and efficacy of Exosurf Neonatal, numerous safety assessments were made. In infants receiving Exosurf Neonatal, pulmonary hemorrhage, apnea and use of methylxanthines were increased. A number of other adverse events were significantly reduced in the Exosurf Neonatal group, particularly various forms of pulmonary air leak and use of pancuronium. Tables 3 and 4 summarize the results of the major safety evaluations from the controlled clinical studies.

Table 3: Safety Assessments[a]—Prophylactic Treatment

Number of Doses: Birth Weight Range:	Single Dose 500 to 700 grams		Single Dose 700 to 1350 grams		Single Dose 700 to 1100 grams		1 vs 3 Doses 700 to 1100 grams	
Treatment Group: Number of Infants:	Placebo (Air) N=108	EXOSURF N=107	Placebo (Air) N=193	EXOSURF N=192	Placebo (Air) N=222	EXOSURF N=224	EXOSURF 1 Dose N=356	EXOSURF 3 Doses N=360
	% of Infants		% of Infants		% of Infants		% of Infants	
Intraventricular Hemorrhage (IVH)								
Overall	51	57	31	27	36	36	38	35
Severe IVH	26	25	10	8	13	14	9	9
Pulmonary Air Leak (PAL)								
Overall	52	48	16	11	32	25	29	27
Pneumothorax	23	10*	5	6	19	11*	14	12
Pneumopericardium	1	4	2	0	<1	1	1	1
Pneumomediastinum	2	1	2	3	7	1**	3	2
Pulmonary Interstitial Emphysema	43	44	13	7*	26	20	23	22
Death from PAL	4	8	<1	<1	2	1	2	1
Patent Ductus Arteriosus	49	53	66	70	50	55	59	57
Necrotizing Enterocolitis	2	4	11	13	3	4	6	2*
Pulmonary Hemorrhage	2	10**	2	4	1	4	4	6
Congenital Pneumonia	4	4	2	4	2	2	1	1
Nosocomial Pneumonia	10	10	2	4	4	7	14	15
Non-Pulmonary Infections	33	35	34	39	28	29	35	34
Sepsis	30	34	30	34	23	24	30	27
Death From Sepsis	4	4	3	3	1	2	3	2
Meningitis	4	6	3	1	2	3	1	2
Other Infections	7	4	5	3	6	10	10	11
Major Anomalies	3	1	2	4	7	4	4	4

Table 3: Safety Assessments[a]—Prophylactic Treatment (Cont.)

Number of Doses: Birth Weight Range:	Single Dose 500 to 700 grams		Single Dose 700 to 1350 grams		Single Dose 700 to 1100 grams		1 vs 3 Doses 700 to 1100 grams	
Treatment Group: Number of Infants:	Placebo (Air) N=108	EXOSURF N=107	Placebo (Air) N=193	EXOSURF N=192	Placebo (Air) N=222	EXOSURF N=224	EXOSURF 1 Dose N=356	EXOSURF 3 Doses N=360
	% of Infants		% of Infants		% of Infants		% of Infants	
Hypotension	70	77	52	47	59	62	54	50
Hyperbilirubinemia	22	21	63	61	27	31	20	21
Exchange Transfusion	4	3	1	2	2	2	3	1
Thrombocytopenia[b]	21	25	not available		9	8	12	10
Persistent Fetal Circulation	0	1	1	1	0	2*	1	<1
Seizures	11	8	2	2	11	9	6	5
Apnea	34	33	76	73	55	65*	62	68
Drug Therapy								
Antibiotics	96	99	98	96	98	99	>99	99
Diuretics	55	60	39	37	59	63	64	65
Anticonvulsants	14	18	23	24	20	16	9	8
Inotropes	46	40	20	20	26	20	28	27
Sedatives	62	71	65	64	63	57	52	52
Pancuronium	19	11	22	14*	19	13*	15	11
Methylxanthines	38	43	77	77	61	72*	75	82*

[a] All parameters were examined with "as-treated" analyses. * $p<0.05$

[b] Thrombocytopenia requiring platelet transfusion. ** $p<0.01$

Table 4: Safety Assessments[a]—Rescue Treatment

Number of Doses: Birth Weight Range:	Two Doses 700 to 1350 grams		Two Doses 1250 grams and above	
Treatment Group: Number of Infants:	Placebo (Air) N=213	EXOSURF N=206	Placebo (Air) N=622	EXOSURF N=615
	% of Infants		% of Infants	
Intraventricular Hemorrhage (IVH)				
Overall	48	52	23	18*
Severe IVH	13	9	5	4
Pulmonary Air Leak (PAL)				
Overall	54	34***	30	18***
Pneumothorax	29	20*	20	10***
Pneumopericardium	4	1	1	2
Pneumomediastinum	8	4	5	2**
Pulmonary Interstitial Emphysema	48	25***	24	13***
Death from PAL	7	3	<1	1
Patent Ductus Arteriosus	66	57	54	45*
Necrotizing Enterocolitis	3	3	1	2
Pulmonary Hemorrhage	3	1	<1	1
Congenital Pneumonia	2	3	2	2
Nosocomial Pneumonia	5	7	2	2
Non-Pulmonary Infections	19	22	13	13
Sepsis	15	17	8	8
Death From Sepsis	<1	<1	1	<1
Meningitis	1	<1	1	<1*
Other Infections	5	8	5	6
Major Anomalies	3	3	4	4
Hypotension	62	57	50	39**
Hyperbilirubinemia	17	19	12	10
Exchange Transfusion	3	4	1	2
Thrombocytopenia[b]	10	11	4	<1**
Persistent Fetal Circulation	1	1	6	2**
Seizures	10	10	6	3*
Apnea	48	65**	37	44*
Drug Therapy				
Antibiotics	100	99	98	98
Diuretics	60	65	45	34***
Anticonvulsants	17	17	10	5**
Inotropes	36	31	27	16***
Sedatives	72	68	76	64***
Pancuronium	34	17**	33	15***
Methylxanthines	62	74**	49	53

[a] All parameters were examined with "as-treated" analyses. * $p<0.05$ *** $p<0.001$

[b] Thrombocytopenia requiring platelet transfusion. ** $p<0.01$

Pulmonary Hemorrhage: See WARNINGS. **Abnormal Laboratory Values:** Abnormal laboratory values are common in critically ill, mechanically ventilated, premature infants. A higher incidence of abnormal laboratory values in the Exosurf Neonatal group was not reported. **Events During Dosing:** Data on events during dosing are available from more than 8800 infants in the open, uncontrolled clinical study (Table 5).

Table 5: Events During Dosing in the Open, Uncontrolled Study[a]

Treatment Type: Number of Infants:	Prophylactic Treatment N=1127	Rescue Treatment N=7711
	% of Infants	% of Infants
Reflux of Exosurf	20	31
Drop in O_2 saturation (≥20%)	6	22
Rise in O_2 saturation (≥10%)	5	6
Drop in transcutaneous pO_2 (≥20 mm Hg)	1	8
Rise in transcutaneous pO_2 (≥20 mm Hg)	2	5
Drop in transcutaneous pCO_2 (≥20 mm Hg)	<1	1
Rise in transcutaneous pCO_2 (≥20 mm Hg)	1	3
Bradycardia (<60 beats/min)	1	3
Tachycardia (>200 beats/min)	<1	<1
Gagging	1	5
Mucous Plugs	<1	<1

[a] Infants may have experienced more than one event. Investigators were prohibited from adjusting FiO_2 and/or ventilator settings during dosing unless significant clinical deterioration occurred.

Reflux: Reflux of Exosurf Neonatal into the endotracheal tube during dosing has been observed and may be associated with rapid drug administration. If reflux occurs, drug administration should be halted and, if necessary, peak inspiratory pressure on the ventilator should be increased by 4 to 5 cm H_2O until the endotracheal tube clears. ***>20% Drop in Transcutaneous Oxygen Saturation:*** If transcutaneous oxygen saturation declines during dosing, drug administration should be halted and, if necessary, peak inspiratory pressure on the ventilator should be increased by 4 to 5 cm H_2O for 1 to 2 minutes. In addition, increases of FiO_2 may be required for 1 to 2 minutes. ***Mucous Plugs:*** See WARNINGS.

DOSAGE AND ADMINISTRATION: See full product information.

Wellcome

BURROUGHS WELLCOME CO., Research Triangle Park, NC 27709

Printed in U.S.A. EX-Y01228

Continued from page 814

Early use of zidovudine in asymptomatic HIV-infected patients or patients with generalized lymphadenopathy reduces the rate of disease progression, said Paul Volberding, M.D., Chief of the AIDS Program, San Francisco General Hospital, San Francisco. For the AIDS Clinical Trials Group (ACTG) protocol 016, Kaplan-Meier curves showed a reduced rate of progression in patients treated within three months of study enrollment compared with patients who started therapy at least one year after study enrollment. ACTG protocol 019 demonstrated a significant reduction in progression to AIDS or AIDS-related complex in symptomatic and asymptomatic patients with CD4 cell counts of less than 500/cu mm. Anemia was the most frequently occurring adverse effect, appearing within six to nine months of the start of therapy.

Zidovudine and dideoxycytidine appear to be well tolerated when administered together, according to Margaret Fischl, M.D., Director of AIDS Comprehensive Program, University of Miami School of Medicine, Miami. Fifty-six patients were enrolled in the ACTG 106 Phase I–II trial, which evaluated dosage levels. Patients were diagnosed as having AIDS-related complex (52%) or AIDS (48%). The mean CD4 cell count was 60–70/cu mm. Adverse effects included peripheral neuropathy (two patients), anemia (five), neutropenia (eight), and hepatotoxicity (four). The combination of oral zidovudine 600 mg and dideoxycytidine 0.03 mg/kg daily was associated with a sustained increase in the CD4 cell count, along with a persistent decrease in p24 antigen levels.

Interim data from a Phase I trial of zidovudine and didanosine were presented by Ann Collier, M.D., University of Washington, Seattle. Fifty-two patients were enrolled in this trial and were assigned to one of five treatment groups: group 1, zidovudine 150 mg and didanosine 90 mg daily; group 2, zidovudine 300 mg and didanosine 334 mg daily; group 3, zidovudine 600 mg and didanosine 334 mg daily; group 4, zidovudine 300 mg and didanosine 500 mg daily; group 5, zidovudine 600 mg and didanosine 500 mg daily. "No unexpected toxicities were reported . . . and no pharmacokinetic interactions between zidovudine and [didanosine] were noted . . . . All groups showed a rise in CD4 counts during this [24-week] period," said Collier. Adverse effects included peripheral neuropathy (five patients), elevated liver-function test results (two), and lethargy and fatigue (one). No patient in group 1 exhibited toxicity. Zidovudine 600 mg daily will be compared with the five combination regimens.

Drug holidays to zidovudine may reverse zidovudine resistance, said Michael Bach, M.D., Maine Medical Center, Portland. Six patients with documented resistance to zidovudine were treated with didanosine for up to 1.5 years. Resistance to zidovudine decreased while resistance to didanosine increased over the study period. Bach postulated that reversal of resistance to zidovudine may be due to a mutation at the Leu-74 codon. A mutation at the Thr-215 codon was apparent in isolates resistant to both drugs. The relevance of this mutation is still being explored. Richard Reichman, M.D., AIDS Clinical Trials Unit, University of Rochester, Rochester, Minnesota, also reported similar findings. Of 15 patients treated with didanosine, 50% displayed a fourfold increase in didanosine-resistant isolates. Simultaneously, the mean sensitivity to zidovudine increased from 0.13 to 0.01 μM ($p = 0.01$).

R82913 appears to be well tolerated in humans, according to Mike Youle, former Registrar of the Kobler Institute, London. R82913 is a tetrahydroimidazo-benzodiazepinone (TIBO) derivative, a compound structurally similar to the benzodiazepines. In a pilot study of 22 patients with AIDS or severe AIDS-related complex, no severe adverse effects or bone marrow toxicities were reported. The daily dosage was increased over four months from 10 mg to 120 or 300 mg. A reduction in p24 antigen levels was seen over the study period. R82913 is a reverse transcriptase inhibitor but appears to be active against HIV-1 only, not HIV-2 or animal retroviruses. Although the exact mechanism is not known, R82913 is thought to inhibit reverse transcriptase in a manner different from that of zidovudine and other nucleoside analogues.

Although the number of cases is expected to stabilize in North America and Europe, in the sub-Saharan region of Africa up to six million people are thought to be infected, suggesting a dismal outlook for this region.

Vaccines. Daniel Zagury, M.D., Universite Pierre et Marie Curie, Paris, has been forced to halt his vaccine trials after more than three years of study. Zagury gained international attention when he told the scientific community in 1987 that he had self-injected his vaccine product, a vaccinia-based product that incorporates part of HIV into the vaccine. Since 1987, several other trials involving patients have been conducted. The question of improper inactivation of HIV recently arose after three patients died while participating in the study. A full investigation into the laboratory preparation of the vaccine and the conduct of the trial will be conducted by the French Ministry of Health.

Spectrum of Disease. More than 9.5 million people worldwide are estimated to be infected with HIV, reported James Chin, M.D., World Health Organization, Geneva. The main route of exposure is overwhelmingly sexual transmission. "It's unlikely that a new spurt of infections in the heterosexual population will occur," said Chin. "It's possible that the number of new cases has peaked, unless studies document sharp increases in the heterosexual population." Transmission via blood transfusions and injectable drug use accounts for a small percentage of cases. Although the number of cases is expected to stabilize in North America and Europe, in the sub-Saharan region of Africa up to six million people are thought to be infected, suggesting a dismal outlook for this region. Blood transfusions hold the highest degree of risk of infection after a single exposure, with more than 90% of patients becoming infected after receiving infected blood. The risk of infection from perinatal transmission of HIV is 30%, probably because of the protective effect of the placenta. Sexual intercourse, injectable drug use, and accidental injections account for fewer than 2.5% of the total number of cases.

Maxime Ankrah, Senior Lecturer, Department of Social Work and Social Administration, Makerere University, Kampala, Uganda, forecasts a bleak picture for families of central and eastern Africa. Up to six million children may become orphans in the next decade as a direct result of AIDS. In addition to treating infected individuals the health-care system must recognize the impact on patients' families or other care givers. All these persons may require emotional support and education. Families should be the target of educational interventions and be used to promote behavioral changes.

An update on cases diagnosed in San Francisco and identified by the San Francisco Public Health department was reported by George Lemp, M.D., San Francisco Public Health Department. Between July 1981 and December 1990, 9872 patients were diagnosed as having AIDS. The data show an improvement in survival, which coincides with the widespread use of prophylaxis for *Pneumocystis carinii* pneumonia (PCP) and the availability of zidovudine during 1986 and 1987. Patients diagnosed after 1985 had a longer survival period and a better quality of life than those who did not receive zidovudine therapy or PCP prophylaxis. Patients with AIDS-related lymphoma, however, had no change in survival rates. Among patients with Kaposi's sarcoma, a modest improvement in long-term survival was evident if the diagnosis was made after 1985.

A CD4 cell count of less than 50/cu mm is indicative of only 12 months' survival, Robert Yarchoan, M.D., Senior Investigator, NCI, told scientists. Forty-one patients were studied retrospectively. Patients with CD4 cell counts of less than 50/cu mm were more likely than patients with higher CD4 cell counts to develop *Mycobacterium avium–intracellulare* infection or non-Hodgkin's lymphoma. As a result of this study, Yarchoan suggested that a CD4 cell count of less than 50/cu mm be used instead of death as a study endpoint in future studies.

Dementia may destroy up to 38% of brain cells, concluded Ian Everall, Senior Registrar in Psychiatry, Institute of Psychiatry, London. Neuronal loss occurs in the absence of inflammation. Although the mechanism is not known, a possible theory is that gp120 binds to vasoactive intestinal peptide, which releases calcium and destroys the neuron. Future research may more precisely delineate the mechanism of destruction, enabling scientists to explore therapies to prevent gp120 binding or to inhibit calcium release.

Treatment of Opportunistic Infections. A new antiprotozoal agent is currently under investigation for the treatment of PCP and cerebral toxoplasmosis, said Henry Masur, M.D., National Institutes of Health (NIH), Bethesda, Maryland. After a 42-day course of 566C80 2-[*trans*-4(4-chlorophenyl)cyclohexyl]-3-hydroxy-1,4-naphthoquinone, Burroughs Wellcome), five of eight patients with cerebral toxoplasmosis had a reduction in clinical symptoms, while six of eight patients showed radiologic improvement. Long-term follow-up indicated that five of seven patients maintained clinical and radiologic improvements while on maintenance therapy. One patient relapsed during therapy, and one patient stopped therapy because of toxicity. More than 80% of patients with PCP responded to 566C80 given twice daily, three times daily, or four times daily. Twenty-two patients were treated in these pilot studies; only one patient failed to respond to therapy. Three patients experienced hypoxemia because of the severity of their disease and could not complete the treatment regimen. Trials comparing 566C80 with standard therapies for PCP and toxoplasmosis are ongoing.

Thirty-four patients with mild or moderate PCP participated in a dose-ranging study of 566C80, reported Judith Falloon, M.D., NIH. Dosages were 750 mg three times daily for five days, followed by 750 mg twice daily for 16 days; 750 mg three times daily for 21 days; or 750 mg four times daily for 21 days. 566C80 effectively treated 79% of patients. At six-months' follow-up, 9 (90%) of 10 patients, 13 (87%) of 15 patients, and 5 (56%) of 9 patients who received therapy two, three, or four times daily, respectively, remained free of relapse.

Lynne Mofenson of the Pediatric, Adolescent, and Maternal AIDS Branch, National Institute of Child Health and Human Development, Bethesda, presented data showing that periodic infusions of intravenous immune globulin (IVIG) are associated with a 30% decrease in the incidence of bacterial infections. A total of 370 patients with symptomatic HIV infection or AIDS who were 2 months to 12 years of age were randomized to receive IVIG or placebo infusions every 28 days. Patients were allowed to receive zidovudine and PCP prophylaxis concurrently in accordance with FDA-approved labeled indications. IVIG therapy reduced the incidence of bacterial infections and subsequent hospital admissions but did not seem to delay death compared with a placebo group. This use of IVIG is not a labeled indication.

Sparfloxacin appears to be active against *Mycobacterium avium* in vitro, said C. Perrone, Inserm U. 13, Hôpital Claude-Bernard, Paris. Two strains, MO-1 and LV-2, were used. The minimum inhibitory concentrations of sparfloxacin for 99% of isolates of MO-1 and LV-2, respectively, were 0.5 mg/L and 2.0 mg/L. Sparfloxacin displayed much higher MICs than did other agents that are active against *M. avium*. Preclinical and clinical trials with this agent are planned.

Cost of Care. Zidovudine therapy prolongs life and is cost-effective, reported Michael Drummond, Centre for Health Economics, University of York, United Kingdom. Zidovudine-treated patients had a median survival of 46% over a two-year period, compared with a median survival of 21% over the same period for patients not treated with zidovudine. Untreated patients spent almost 50% of their time hospitalized, compared with only 20% for patients receiving zidovudine therapy. The number of days spent in the hospital was similar for the two groups, but patients treated with zidovudine lived longer and therefore spent a lower percentage of their remaining lives in the hospital. Zidovudine treatment significantly improves quality of life. The addition of zidovudine therapy was calculated to increase the cost of medical care by $11,187 per year of life.

Approximately $32,000 is spent per year for the medical care of one AIDS patient, concluded Fred Hellinger, Agency for Health Care Policy and Research, U.S. Department of Health and Human Services. The yearly treatment cost for HIV-infected patients is approximately $5150. Total expenditures in 1991 are estimated at $5.8 billion for AIDS patients and $1.4 billion for HIV-infected patients. These expenditures represent approximately 1.3% of the annual U.S. health budget. If the current projection of a 21% increase each year in the number of newly diagnosed cases of HIV infection is correct, the cost of care for HIV-infected persons may increase to more than $10.4 billion in 1994.

Summary. HIV infection continues to challenge and perplex scientists. Although advances are unraveling the mystery of HIV infection, vaccine therapy and long-term effective antiretroviral therapy remain distant prospects. Educational interventions have resulted in only modest reductions in HIV transmission rates in selected areas of the United States and Europe. Rates of transmission in Asia and Africa continue to escalate. AIDS continues to be a multicultural and increasingly heterosexual problem worldwide. Continued research and consistent educational interventions provide the greatest hope for the 1990s.

ROBERTA J. WONG, PHARM.D., FASHP
Clinical Pharmacy Correspondent

Study raises safety questions about β-agonist inhaler overuse

A Canadian study showing an association between increased use of β agonists administered by metered-dose inhaler and risk of death from asthma has attracted considerable debate. At question is whether β-agonist use increases the risk of death or serves as a marker for severe disease. A report of the study has not yet been published. Boehringer Ingelheim, the study sponsor, has provided the findings to FDA and drug regulatory agencies of other countries.

The findings are from a case–control study taken from a cohort of some 12,300 patients with asthma. *The Lancet*, in a brief account of the primary study findings, noted that all 44 patients who died from asthma had used β agonists in the preceding 12 months.[1] An additional 85 patients experienced a "near-death" episode in which they experienced hypercapnia or required intubation. The likelihood of death or near death was associated with the number of drug canisters used each month; the relative risk was 2.0 per canister per month (95% confidence interval = 1.6–2.4). The likelihood of death was increased by 2.6 per canister per month (95% confidence interval = 1.9–3.9).

1. Anon. Warning on β-agonists. *Lancet*. 1991; 388:307.

News Briefs

• Eli Lilly and Company is discontinuing production and distribution of **U-100 protamine zinc insulins and all U-40 insulins,** effective December 1, 1991.

• The Centers for Disease Control has updated its recommendations for **prevention and control of influenza** (*MMWR*. 1991; 40(RR-6):1–15). The primary changes in the statement relate to the inclusion of different influenza strains in the trivalent vaccine prepared for the 1991–1992 season.

• The American College of Clinical Pharmacy is preparing six home-study modules for its **Pharmacotherapy Self-Assessment Program**; the first module, on cardiovascular therapy, was released in August. A grant from Sandoz Pharmaceuticals supported development of the program. Further information can be obtained from ACCP Associate Director Toni Host, 3101 Broadway, Suite 380, Kansas City, MO 64111; 816-531-2177.

• The American Academy of Pediatrics has issued a report titled **"The U.S. Immunization Crisis."** Single copies can be obtained free of charge by calling Leslee Williams at 708-981-7389 or Carolyn Kolbaba at 708-981-7945.

• **"Guidelines for the Care of Children and Adolescents with HIV Infection,"** a report of the New York State Department of Health AIDS Institute Criteria Committee for the Care of HIV-Infected Children, has been published as a supplement to the July 1991 issue of *The Journal of Pediatrics*.

Upcoming Specialty Meetings

American College of Rheumatology. Boston, MA, November 17–21; contact ACR, 60 Executive Park South, Suite 150, Atlanta, GA 30329; 404-633-3777.

Gerontological Society of America. San Francisco, CA, November 22–26; contact GSA, 1275 K Street, N.W., Suite 350, Washington, DC 20005; 202-842-1275.

American Association for Cancer Education. Baltimore, MD, December 5–8; contact C. M. Brooks, Office of Educational Development, University of Alabama at Birmingham, UAB Station, 401 CH19, Birmingham, AL 35294; 205-934-3054.

American Society of Hematology. Denver, CO, December 7–10; contact J. D. McGreevey, Jr., ASH, 6900 Grove Road, Thorofare, NJ 08086; 202-857-1118.

American Academy of Dermatology. Dallas, TX, December 7–12; contact AAD, P.O. Box 3116, Evanston, IL 60204; 708-869-3954.

American Epilepsy Society. Philadelphia, PA, December 10–15; contact P. S. Bourgeois, AES, 638 Prospect Avenue, Hartford, CT 06105; 203-232-4825.

Southern Society for Pediatric Research. New Orleans, LA, January 29–31; contact R. F. Jacobs, M.D., Arkansas Children's Hospital, 800 Marshall Street, Little Rock, AR 72202; 501-370-1416.

American Association for Geriatric Psychiatry. San Francisco, CA, February 14–17; contact AAGP, P.O. Box 376, Greenbelt, MD 20768; 301-220-0952.

International Symposium on Intensive Care and Emergency Medicine (12th), sponsored by the European Society of Intensive Care Medicine, the Society of Critical Care Medicine, and the World Federation of Societies of Intensive Care. Brussels, Belgium, March 23–27; contact Professor J. L. Vincent, Department of Intensive Care, Erasme University Hospital, Route de Lennik 808, B-1070 Bruxelles, Belgium; 32 2 526 33 80.

Second European Symposium on Controlled Drug Delivery. Noordwijk aan Zee, the Netherlands, April 1–3; contact Secretariat, Second European Symposium on Controlled Drug Delivery, Dr. ir. J. A. van Alsté, Mrs. A. D. Kamphuis, University of Twente/CCBMT, P.O. Box 217, 7500 AE Enschede, the Netherlands; 31-53-89.33.67, (fax) 31-53-33.42.57.

Letters

Retreatment with digoxin immune Fab 823
Nancy M. Allen

Laboratory monitoring of heparin therapy 824
Ann K. Wittkowsky

Correction 824

The Letters *column is a forum for rapid exchange of ideas among readers of* Clinical Pharmacy. *Liberal criteria are applied in the review of submissions to encourage contributions to this column.*

The Letters *column includes the following types of contributions: (1) comments, addenda, and minor updates on previously published work, (2) alerts on potential problems related to drug therapy or clinical research, (3) observations or comments on trends in drug therapy or clinical research, and (4) brief expressions of opinion about controversies in drug therapy or clinical research.*

Letters need not be submitted with the journal's manuscript checklist. The following conditions, however, must be adhered to: (1) the body of the letter must be no longer than two typewritten pages, (2) the use of references, tables, and illustrations should be minimized, (3) the authors' names, affiliations, and mailing addresses must be typed at the end of the letter in the format used by Clinical Pharmacy, *and (4) the entire letter (including references, tables, and authors' names) must be typed double-spaced on plain white paper (not letterhead). Following acceptance of a letter, the authors are required to sign an exclusive publication statement and a copyright transferal form.*

Retreatment with digoxin immune Fab

Digoxin immune Fab is composed of the isolated and purified Fab fragments produced from digoxin-specific ovine antibodies. From the time of the drug's development the immunogenic potential of digoxin immune Fab has been a concern. Clinically, digoxin immune Fab has been found to be safe and effective.[1,2] In one paper, possible allergic responses were reported in only six patients (0.8% of those evaluated).[2] Only one report of retreatment with digoxin immune Fab has been published.[2] We had a patient who was retreated with digoxin immune Fab 87 days after her first treatment.

A 67-year-old, 59-kg black woman who had a long history of sarcoidosis and end-stage pulmonary fibrosis was admitted to the hospital with atrial flutter. She was treated with digoxin and quinidine. Several days after sinus rhythm had been restored, the patient was found to have a junctional rhythm (rate, 40–50 beats/min). Her serum digoxin concentration at that time was 6.2 ng/mL. She was given digoxin immune Fab 120 mg, and sinus rhythm was restored. A day later, she had a six-second sinus pause for which she received no treatment. She was not noted to have more sinus pauses or further episodes of atrial flutter or junctional rhythm and was discharged taking digoxin and quinidine.

Approximately three months later, the patient was admitted with complaints of recurrent syncope. She was still taking digoxin and quinidine, and her electrocardiogram (ECG) showed ventricular bigeminy. Her serum digoxin concentration was 1.5 ng/mL, and her serum quinidine concentration was 2.1 μg/mL. Several days later she had an episode of complete heart block accompanied by hypotension and syncope. Her digoxin dosage had been increased and her renal function had decreased; her serum digoxin concentration was now 2.7 ng/mL. Digoxin was discontinued, and no further treatment was required. The following day the patient became hypotensive and had a cardiopulmonary arrest. She was intubated and given atropine, and sinus rhythm returned.

The patient was transferred to another hospital for management of presumed digoxin toxicity. Her serum digoxin concentration on arrival was 2.5 ng/mL, and her ECG showed a junctional rhythm (heart rate, 70–80 beats/min). She was given digoxin immune Fab 80 mg, after which the ECG showed sinus rhythm. Approximately 18 hours after administration of digoxin immune Fab, the patient became hypotensive and had a junctional rhythm (heart rate was not recorded). Treatment with an external cardiac pacemaker and atropine was unsuccessful, and the patient died. She had no apparent allergic reaction to the digoxin immune Fab.

It is impossible to tell if the patient's rhythm disturbances were caused by digoxin toxicity. The recurrence of junctional rhythm may have been caused by a rebound in the free digoxin concentration (i.e., release of digoxin from digoxin–antibody complexes), but it is more likely that the patient's arrhythmias were due to her underlying chronic disease. We were unable to measure the free serum digoxin concentration just before the patient died.

There are only three previous accounts of retreatment with digoxin immune Fab—two unpublished reports (Carpenter V, Burroughs Wellcome Co. Personal communication. 1991 Jan) and one published report.[2] Little information is available about these cases except that there were no apparent adverse reactions or allergic responses. The immunogenic potential of digoxin immune Fab and the clinical significance of that potential are still unknown.

The case presented here is only the second published account of retreatment with digoxin immune Fab. More data are needed to completely evaluate the immunogenic potential of repeated doses of this drug.

1. Antman EM, Wenger TL, Butler VP et al. Treatment of 150 cases of life-threatening digitalis intoxication with digoxin-specific Fab antibody fragments. *Circulation.* 1990; 81:1744-52.
2. Hickey AR, Wenger TL, Carpenter VP et al. Digoxin immune Fab therapy in the management of digitalis intoxication: safety and efficacy results of an observational surveillance study. *J Am Coll Cardiol.* 1991; 17:590-8.

Nancy M. Allen, Pharm. D., Clinical Pharmacist in Cardiology
Department of Medicine
Division of Cardiology
Duke University Medical Center
Box 31123
Durham, NC 27710

Laboratory monitoring of heparin therapy

Carter[1] presented in the July issue of *Clinical Pharmacy* a heparin dosage algorithm based on prolonging the activated partial thromboplastin time (APTT) to 1.5–2.0 times a control value. The clinical application of this range of APTT ratios is complicated by the fact that APTT values depend in part on the reagent used to perform the test. The sensitivity of a given reagent to detect the clotting defect induced by heparin is influenced by the phospholipid and activator-substance makeup of the reagent as well as by laboratory instrumentation and procedures. Wide variations in APTT results have been observed between reagents produced by different manufacturers[2] and between different batches of reagent produced by the same manufacturer.[3] This variability is not corrected by using APTT ratios. Inconsistent results between laboratories—and within laboratories when reagents are changed—affect not only the dosage and monitoring of individual heparin regimens but also the reliability, reproducibility, and application of the results of clinical trials involving anticoagulation with heparin.

To overcome these limitations, a more consistent method for heparin monitoring must be employed. A practical approach is to determine reagent-specific therapeutic ranges by preparing in vitro heparin response curves for each new batch of APTT reagent.[3,4] This method is based on the observation that the therapeutic range for heparin serum concentrations is 0.2–0.4 units/mL by protamine titration.[4] Heparin is added in increasing concentrations to pooled normal plasma, and APTT values are determined using a single reagent. The APTT range (in seconds) between which heparin concentrations correspond to 0.2–0.4 units/mL becomes the therapeutic range for that reagent.

The in vitro effect of heparin on the APTT of normal pooled plasma may not be comparable to the in vivo sensitivity of individual patients. However, in clinical application, the use of reagent-specific APTT therapeutic ranges has resulted in adequate heparin dosage without thromboembolic complications in patients with deep venous thrombosis, pulmonary embolism, or both.[5] This method offers a practical alternative for heparin monitoring that considers the sensitivity of the specific APTT reagent in use in any clinical laboratory. The heparin dosage algorithm presented by Carter can be adjusted for each successive APTT reagent in use in a clinical setting by applying the reagent-specific therapeutic range.

1. Carter BL. Therapy of acute thromboembolism with heparin and warfarin. *Clin Pharm.* 1991; 10:503-18.
2. Brandt JT, Triplett DA. Laboratory monitoring of heparin: effect of reagents and instrumentation on the activated partial thromboplastin time. *Am J Clin Pathol.* 1981; 76:530-7.
3. Shojania AM, Tetreault J, Turnbull G. The variations between heparin sensitivity of different lots of activated partial thromboplastin time reagents produced by the same manufacturer. *Am J Clin Pathol.* 1988; 89:19-23.
4. Hirsh J. Heparin. *N Engl J Med.* 1991; 22:1565-74.
5. Zanke B, Shojania AM. Comparison of two aPTT methods for monitoring heparin therapy: aPTT ratio and heparin response of pooled normal plasma. *Am J Clin Pathol.* 1990; 93:684-9.

Ann K. Wittkowsky, Pharm.D., Clinical Pharmacist, Cardiology
Department of Pharmacy
University of Washington Medical Center, RC-32
Seattle, WA 98195

Correction

Management of postoperative pain by continuous epidural infusion of analgesics (October 1991, Therapy Review). On page 753, Table 3 should indicate that the infusion concentration of meperidine hydrochloride is 1–2 mg/mL.

Advances in the treatment of unstable angina pectoris

Sarah A. Spinler and Lisa E. Davis

Abstract: The pathogenesis, clinical manifestations and diagnosis, and drug and nondrug therapies of unstable angina pectoris are reviewed.

Coronary-artery plaque fissure and rupture, with subsequent platelet aggregation and thrombosis, are the primary underlying stimuli for unstable angina. Unstable angina has been defined as consisting of new-onset angina; angina that is increasing in frequency, intensity, or duration (crescendo angina); or angina at rest. The diagnosis of unstable angina is based on the clinical presentation, electrocardiographic findings, the lack of evidence of myocardial infarction (MI), exercise testing, and coronary angiography. I.V. nitroglycerin is the cornerstone of medical therapy for unstable angina; it relieves chest pain and has a short onset of action. I.V. nitroglycerin, however, has not been shown to reduce the occurrence of MI or death, and its beneficial effects may decrease over time. Aspirin reduces the occurrence of MI and death in patients with unstable angina, but the ideal dosage has not been established. Heparin may reduce the frequency of angina and MI, but its effect on mortality is unknown. Nifedipine has produced beneficial effects in small trials, whereas larger trials have suggested that the drug has deleterious effects when used in the treatment of unstable angina. Verapamil and diltiazem may be effective in relieving chest pain. Calcium-channel blockers have generally not been proved to reduce the risk of MI and death. Data evaluating the efficacy of β-adrenergic blockers as monotherapy for unstable angina are lacking; these drugs should not be used in patients with vasospastic or Prinzmetal's angina. Thrombolytic therapy has produced mixed results when used in the treatment of unstable angina. Nondrug therapies for unstable angina include intra-aortic balloon counterpulsation, percutaneous transluminal coronary angioplasty, and coronary-artery bypass surgery.

Numerous drug and nondrug therapies may be employed in the treatment of unstable angina pectoris.

Index terms: Angina pectoris; Aspirin; Cardiac drugs; Diltiazem; Heparin; Nifedipine; Nitroglycerin; Verapamil
Clin Pharm. 1991; 10:825-38

Symptomatic ischemic heart disease is a continuum that includes stable angina pectoris, unstable angina, and myocardial infarction (MI). Angina may occur in patients with underlying atherosclerosis when there is an imbalance between myocardial oxygen supply and demand. The stimulus for unstable angina is primarily a decrease in myocardial oxygen supply. Pathological causes of diminished myocardial blood flow in unstable angina have been elucidated over the past decade.[1] The major drugs used to improve myocardial blood flow and decrease oxygen demand in unstable angina are nitrates, aspirin, heparin, β-adrenergic blockers and calcium-channel blockers. Nondrug strategies for treatment of refractory unstable angina include intra-aortic balloon counterpulsation, percutaneous transluminal coronary angioplasty, and aortocoronary bypass graft surgery. This article reviews the pathophysiology, clinical manifestations, and treatment approach to unstable angina.

Pathogenesis

Plaque Fissure and Rupture. Rupture or hemorrhage of an atherosclerotic plaque is the initiating event of acute myocardial ischemia.[2] Endothelial injury, such as plaque rupture or hemorrhage, and subsequent exposure of subendothelial tissue lead to coronary thrombus formation through activation of platelets and the coagulation system. Fibrin thrombi, which entrap platelet aggregates, can partially occlude coronary arteries. In addition, vasoconstriction may occur at sites of atherosclerotic plaques and at sites of endo-

Sarah A. Spinler, Pharm.D., is Assistant Professor of Clinical Pharmacy, Philadelphia College of Pharmacy and Science (PCPS), and Adjunct Assistant Professor of Pharmacy in Medicine, University of Pennsylvania, Cardiovascular Section, Hospital of The University of Pennsylvania, Philadelphia. Lisa E. Davis, Pharm.D., is Assistant Professor of Clinical Pharmacy, PCPS.

Address reprint requests to Dr. Spinler at the Philadelphia College of Pharmacy and Science, Woodland Avenue at 43rd Street, Philadelphia, PA 19104.

This is **article 680-204-9127** in the **ASHP Continuing Education System**; it qualifies for 1.0 hour of continuing-education credit. See page 876 for learning objectives and test questions.

Figure 1. Constituents involved in platelet adhesion and aggregation (see text for details). vWF = von Willebrand factor; PDGF = platelet-derived growth factor; BTG = beta thromboglobulin; PF4 = platelet factor 4; Arach. Acid = arachidonic acid; ADP = adenosine diphosphate; 5HT = serotonin; Va and Xa = activated clotting factors; Tx A_2 = thromboxane A_2; 1a, 1b, 1c, IIa, IIb, IIIa, and IIIb = glycoprotein receptor sites. Adapted and reprinted from reference 8, with permission of Health Management Publications, Inc.

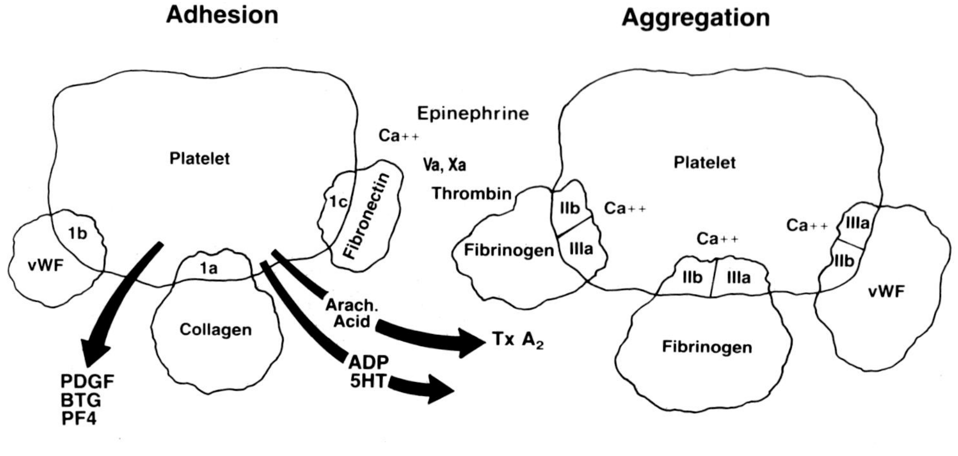

thelial injury that result from plaque fissure or ulceration.[3] Intracoronary thrombus formation and, less commonly, coronary vasoconstriction, lead to periods of decreased coronary blood flow, transiently reduce regional myocardial perfusion, and consequently cause symptoms of myocardial ischemia.[4] Factors that may aggravate ischemia in patients with severe coronary stenoses include hypertension, tachycardia, thyrotoxicosis, anemia, sympathomimetic drug therapy, and abrupt discontinuation of antianginal agents such as β blockers.[5,6]

Platelet Activation. Coronary-artery plaque fissure and rupture, with subsequent platelet aggregation and thrombosis, are the primary underlying stimuli for unstable angina. Rupture and fissure may occur in severely occlusive and less occlusive plaques as well. Fissure follows thinning of the fibrous cap that overlies the lipid core of a soft plaque.[7] Macrophages are then believed to infiltrate the site of fissure and release collagenases and elastinases, which eventually weaken the fibrous cap and trigger plaque rupture.[2] Exposure of collagen within the necrotic plaque core activates platelets, which begin to adhere, aggregate, and possibly decrease coronary blood flow. Shear forces caused by turbulent blood flow across the ruptured plaque can also stimulate platelet activation. Platelet adhesion occurs through binding of collagen to the platelet glycoprotein 1a-receptor complex and is supported through bridging of von Willebrand factor to the glycoprotein 1b-receptor and of fibronectin to the 1c-receptor (Figure 1).[8] Secretion of adenosine diphosphate (ADP), von Willebrand factor, fibrinogen, and calcium ions from platelet storage granules further supports this activation. Recruitment of adjacent platelets (platelet aggregation) is facilitated by the release of serotonin, epinephrine, beta thromboglobulin, platelet-derived growth factor, and platelet factor 4, a potent platelet activator, from either platelet storage granules or disrupted endothelium. In addition, the stimulation of phospholipase A_2 in the platelet membrane leads to the release of arachidonic acid and its subsequent metabolism to thromboxane A_2, a potent platelet aggregator and vasoconstrictor.[8] Other stimulants for platelet aggregation include thrombin, ADP, epinephrine, and collagen. The final common pathway for platelet aggregation is the binding of fibrinogen to the glycoprotein IIb–IIIa-receptor complex, located on the platelet surface, which links adjacent platelets. Additional proteins such as von Willebrand factor, fibronectin, and vitronectin act as adhesive proteins for aggregated platelets.[3,9]

Activation of Coagulation. Activation of the extrinsic pathway of coagulation also occurs at the time of endothelial injury in patients with unstable angina (Figure 2).[10] Tissue factor is exposed in the disrupted subendothelium and forms a complex with factor VIIa.[1] This complex then activates factor X, either directly or indirectly, through activation of factor IX. Activated factor X (factor Xa) binds to a cofactor, factor Va; in the presence of calcium ions, this complex stimulates the conversion of prothrombin to thrombin. Thrombin triggers the conversion of fibrinogen to fibrin, the latter of which forms a thrombus at the site of the ruptured plaque. Thrombin also promotes coagulation by activating factors V and VIII.[11]

Antithrombogenic Mechanisms. Homeostatic mechanisms that balance the above thrombogenic stimuli include release of adenylate cyclase by intact endothelium adjacent to the injury, which causes degradation of ADP and subsequent accumulation of intracellular adenosine 3',5'-cyclic phosphate (cyclic AMP). Cyclic AMP serves to dampen platelet responsiveness by decreasing thromboxane A_2 formation through inhibition of phospholipase A_2.[8]

Several other mediators oppose thrombus formation. Antithrombin III, which circulates as a complex with endothelial-derived heparin-like molecules, inhibits thrombin and activated clotting factors VII, IX,

Figure 2. Activation of the coagulation system in response to endothelial injury (see text for details). HMW = high molecular weight. Reprinted, with permission, from reference 10.

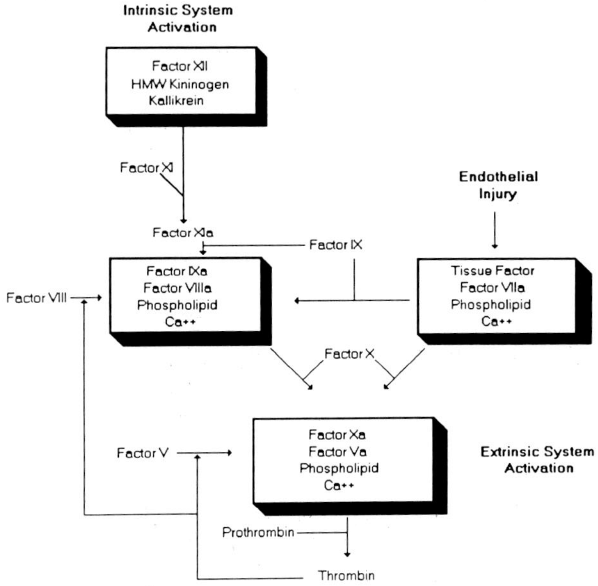

and X. In addition, endothelial cells release tissue plasminogen activator, which promotes lysis of fibrin clots, and prostaglandin I_2, a potent vasodilator and inhibitor of platelet aggregation.[12] Formation and release of nitric oxide from endothelium, which causes vasodilation and inhibits platelet aggregation, is also stimulated by the presence of thrombin.[8]

Despite these intrinsic antithrombotic processes, plaque rupture may result in overwhelming platelet aggregation, which promotes thrombus formation and growth, narrows the coronary-artery lumen, and manifests as symptoms of unstable angina. Development of new drug therapies in the treatment of unstable angina centers on decreasing platelet aggregation and thrombus formation as well as promoting thrombus dissolution.

Clinical Manifestations and Diagnosis

Unstable angina has traditionally been defined as (1) new-onset angina pectoris that is severe and occurs frequently, (2) crescendo angina pectoris, or (3) angina at rest.[6,13,14] Alternatively, some authors have recommended a clinical classification that subdivides new-onset angina, crescendo angina, and postinfarction angina based on precipitating factors (such as effort, effort and rest, or rest only) and on the intensity of antianginal treatment when angina occurred.[6,15] Discussion of postinfarction angina, a subset of unstable angina in which ischemic symptoms recur within a few weeks following MI, is beyond the scope of this review.[16]

New-onset angina is classified as unstable when angina first occurs with minimal effort or at rest and is of a duration of less than two months. Patients with a history of stable angina on effort who display a changing pattern of angina, such as increased frequency, intensity, or duration, are classified as experiencing crescendo angina. Patients in whom angina occurs spontaneously at rest frequently have recent progression of coronary atherosclerosis with associated intracoronary thrombus and are at high risk to fail medical therapy and progress to MI.[6]

The diagnosis of unstable angina is based on the characteristic qualities of anginal chest discomfort, associated electrocardiographic (ECG) findings, and absence of pathognomonic laboratory findings of MI and significant necrosis. ECG findings in patients with unstable angina may include S–T segment depression or elevation and T wave inversion. Rarely, patients will have no demonstrable ECG changes.[6,13] Since patients with unstable angina may have symptoms and ECG changes similar to those of patients with MI, myocardial enzyme laboratory analyses (creatine kinase and MB isoenzyme) are performed to exclude the diagnosis of MI.

Treatment of unstable angina is aimed at reducing the progression to MI and death. In medically treated patients, in-hospital mortality is 3% to 5%, and one-year mortality is 7% to 8%. In the first two weeks, the frequency of nonfatal MI is 8% to 10%. Patients at increased risk of death include those who fail to respond to initial therapy and those with severe left ventricular function, multivessel coronary artery disease, or disease of the left main coronary artery.[17]

High-risk patients can be identified using submaximal exercise testing, coronary angiography, or both. The use of exercise testing, which increases myocardial oxygen demand when there already may be diminished myocardial oxygen supply, is controversial. Following a three-day pain-free period of medical therapy, patients have exercised safely using a submaximal treadmill exercise protocol. Positive findings of S–T segment depression, hypotension, or ventricular arrhythmias occur in approximately 50% of such patients. A positive exercise test is associated with the presence of multivessel coronary-artery disease and subsequent occurrence of MI or cardiac death.[13]

Despite the documented safety of submaximal exercise testing, coronary angiography remains the "gold standard" to which other diagnostic tests are compared, since it allows determination of the extent and location of coronary-artery disease. Coronary angiography has demonstrated that, in patients with unstable angina, approximately 10% have coronary arteries without significant stenoses, and 13% have a stenosis of the left main coronary artery. The frequency of one-, two-, and three-vessel coronary-artery disease is equally divided between the remaining patients.[18]

Diagnosis-Based Therapy. A treatment strategy for unstable angina may be based on ECG changes, hemodynamic stability, left ventricular function, severity of coronary artery disease as determined by coronary angiography, and the response to medical therapy. Medical therapy for unstable angina includes administration of i.v. nitrates, antiplatelet agents, heparin, calcium-channel blockers, and β blockers. Percutaneous transluminal coronary angioplasty is a nonsurgical procedure that involves coronary arteriography and balloon dilation of a single-vessel stenosis that is believed to be causing ischemia.[19,20] Finally, aortocoronary bypass surgery has been successful in selected patient groups with unstable angina.[21-23] A description of the efficacy of each strategy in the treatment of unstable angina follows.

Nitrates

Acute myocardial ischemia has been treated with nitrates for more than 100 years, and i.v. nitroglycerin remains the cornerstone of medical therapy for unstable angina. Although both oral[24,25] and topical nitrates[26-28] have demonstrated benefit at reducing episodes of chest pain at rest, i.v. administration remains the route of choice because the onset of action is short and the dosage can be rapidly adjusted if symptoms or adverse effects occur.[6]

Mechanism of Action. Nitroglycerin both relieves and prevents recurrent rest pain through several possible mechanisms. Nitrates primarily decrease myocardial oxygen demand through venodilation and reduction in left ventricular filling pressure, effects that decrease left ventricular wall tension. At larger dosages, nitrates also dilate peripheral arteries and consequently reduce systolic blood pressure and, thus, myocardial oxygen demand. Nitrates induce vasodilation through activation of guanylate cyclase with the resultant generation of cyclic guanine monophosphate.[28,29] This process apparently requires the presence of free sulfhydryl groups.[28] Nitrates appear to activate guanylate cyclase through formation of nitric oxide,[30] a compound that has also been linked to the vasodilatory actions of endothelium-derived relaxing factor.[31,32]

Nitrates could potentially improve myocardial oxygen supply through coronary artery vasodilation. Intracoronary nitroglycerin has been shown to dilate large epicardial coronary arteries, stenotic coronary-artery sections, and collateral coronary arteries and to redistribute coronary blood flow from epicardial to endocardial tissue.[28] However, controversy exists as to whether or not nitrates actually increase blood flow to ischemic myocardium when coronary arteries may already be maximally dilated.[19,29,33,34] Other potential mechanisms by which nitrates may increase myocardial oxygen supply include prevention and reversal of coronary-artery spasm and inhibition of platelet aggregation. Diodati et al.[20] have documented the ability of i.v. nitroglycerin to inhibit platelet aggregation in patients with unstable angina or acute MI. Further work in a larger patient population is necessary to confirm nitroglycerin's antiplatelet effects in patients with unstable angina and to investigate the contribution of this action to relief of clinical symptoms.

Clinical Efficacy. Many investigators have reported the beneficial effects of i.v. nitroglycerin in patients with refractory unstable angina (Table 1).[25,26,35-42] Since these patients were experiencing angina at rest despite therapy with oral or topical nitrates, β blockers, or calcium-channel blockers, all reports, except one, were observational, nonrandomized, and nonblinded. In the majority of studies, the dose of nitroglycerin was adjusted to achieve relief of chest pain while maintaining a systolic blood pressure greater than 90–100 mm Hg.[35,38-40,42]

Lin and Flaherty[26] described relief of angina at rest in 88% of patients who prospectively received i.v. nitroglycerin with the dosage adjusted to decrease the mean arterial pressure by 10%. The route of nitroglycerin administration was then changed to transdermal after a mean of 36 hours. The dosage of transdermal nitroglycerin was 5–40 mg/day and was adjusted to maintain the 10% reduction in mean arterial pressure. Retrospective analysis showed that recurrent chest pain occurred in 3 of 10 crossover patients and that blood pressure was increased in two of those three patients.

In the only randomized trial, Curfman et al.[25] compared i.v. nitroglycerin with combined oral–topical nitrate therapy in patients with unstable angina.[25] The dosage of both regimens was increased until the systolic blood pressure was reduced by 20% or a predetermined maximal dosage was reached (200 μg/min for i.v. nitroglycerin). I.V. nitroglycerin reduced the frequency of rest pain from an average of 3.3 episodes per 24 hours during a 48-hour control period to 1.0 episode per 24 hours; this was comparable to the effect of the oral and topical nitrate regimen. However, the authors reported that i.v. nitroglycerin therapy produced more rapid and consistent relief of chest pain during the first 24 hours.

The observational studies detailed in Table 1 document nitroglycerin's effectiveness in relieving ischemic chest pain, decreasing the frequency of angina recurrence, and diminishing ischemic S–T segment changes in patients with unstable angina. However, there is a lack of well designed research with i.v. nitroglycerin in unstable angina. No randomized clinical trials have been conducted to document the effect of i.v. nitroglycerin on occurrence of MI and death in patients with unstable angina.

Some of the beneficial effects of nitrates in patients with unstable angina may be reduced through reflex activation of the sympathetic nervous system or the development of nitrate tolerance. A nitrate-induced decrease in systolic blood pressure may cause reflex tachycardia and vasoconstriction, responses that would diminish the benefits of nitrates on myocardial oxygen supply and demand.[19,28]

Tolerance to the hemodynamic and clinical effects of nitroglycerin has been demonstrated in 24% of patients with acute MI enrolled in a placebo-controlled study of prolonged nitroglycerin infusions.[43] Since depletion of sulfhydryl groups appears to be associated with the development of nitrate tolerance,[44] Hor-

Table 1.
Clinical Trials of Intravenous Nitroglycerin (NTG) in Unstable Angina Pectoris (AP)[a]

Ref.	*n*	NTG Dosage Range (mean) (μg/min)	Duration of NTG Infusion (mean) (days)	Concomitant Drugs	Results (*p*)[b]
35	14	9–180 (47)	2–12 (6.7)	BB	86% relieved of AP; decr. AP freq. (<0.0005)
36	14	30–350 (138)	1–16 (4.7)	BB	36% relieved of AP
37	45	5–267 (54)	NR	NR	89% relieved of AP; decr. morphine use
38	67	12–50 (30)	2–29 (7.4)	BB, CCB	63% relieved of AP; decr. S–T segment changes
39	16	85–1020	1–8 (3.2)	BB, CCB	38% relieved of AP; decr. AP freq.; decr. S–T segment changes
40	20	15–226 (72)	NR	BB, CCB	70% relieved of AP; decr. AP freq.
41	42	NR	(4.3)	BB	Decr. AP freq.; decr. MI freq. in pts. with AP relief (<0.01)
25	40	10–200 (82)	3	BB	Decr. AP freq. (<0.01)
42	35	50–350 (140)	NR	BB	Decr. AP freq.; decr. SL NTG, morphine use (all <0.001)
26	17	10–200 (84)	(1.5)	BB, CCB	88% relieved of AP

[a] BB = β-adrenergic blockers, NR = not reported, CCB = calcium-channel blockers, MI = myocardial infarction, SL = sublingual.
[b] Statistical significance not reported for results without a *p* value.

Table 2.
Randomized Clinical Trials of Aspirin in Unstable Angina Pectoris (AP)[a]

Ref.	*n* Aspirin/ *n* Placebo	Aspirin Dosage (mg/day)	Duration of Therapy (wk)	Concomitant Drugs	Results (*p*)
50	625/641	325	12	BB, N	51% decr. in cardiac death at 12 wk (0.059), 43% decr. at 1 yr (0.008); 55% decr. in MI (0.001)
49	276/139	1300	78	BB, CCB	51% decr. in cardiac death or MI (0.008)
51	121/118	650	1	BB, N, CCB, ±H	Without H: 33% decr. in refract. AP (NS), 71% decr. in MI (0.012), 44% decr. in combined endpoint (refract. AP, cardiac death, and MI) (NS) With H: 60% decr. in refract. AP (0.011), 88% decr. in MI (0.001), 64% decr. in combined endpoint (0.003)
52	399/397	75	12	BB, N, CCB, ±H	Without H: 38% decr. in MI or cardiac death at 5 days (NS), 66% decr. at 30 days (0.004), 60% decr. at 90 days (0.004) With H: 77% decr. in MI or cardiac death at 5 days (0.03), 73% decr. at 30 days (0.0005), 67% decr. at 90 days (0.0003)

[a] BB = β-adrenergic blockers, N = nitrates, MI = myocardial infarction, CCB = calcium-channel blockers, H = heparin, NS = not significant.

owitz et al.[45] investigated the potential for the sulfhydryl donor acetylcysteine to restore nitrate responsiveness in patients with unstable angina. Their double-blind, randomized trial of i.v. nitroglycerin with or without acetylcysteine investigated the ability of acetylcysteine to reverse nitroglycerin tolerance in patients with refractory unstable angina who were receiving topical nitrates and calcium-channel blockers. The frequency of rest pain was similar in each group but significantly fewer acetylcysteine-treated patients progressed to MI. Symptomatic hypotension occurred frequently in the acetylcysteine-treated patients; this effect appears to limit the clinical utility of this therapy. Additional work is necessary to determine the role of nitrate tolerance and methods to reverse or prevent nitrate tolerance in unstable angina.

Antiplatelet Agents

Aspirin. *Mechanism of Action.* Because platelet activation, platelet aggregation, and release of vasoconstrictive substances are primary pathological processes in unstable angina,[8] antiplatelet agents play an important role in management of patients with this disorder. Aspirin acetylates the enzyme cyclo-oxygenase and consequently inhibits the formation of thromboxane A_2. Although the effect of aspirin on platelet cyclo-oxygenase lasts for the life of the platelet, the effect of aspirin on endothelial cyclo-oxygenase is reversible. Aspirin inhibits secondary platelet aggregation induced by ADP, epinephrine, and small amounts of collagen. Aspirin does not inhibit platelet adhesion and, therefore, does not prevent the release of serotonin, ADP, or platelet-derived growth factor.[46-48]

Clinical Efficacy. Four large, randomized, placebo-controlled trials have confirmed the efficacy of aspirin in unstable angina (Table 2).[49-52] In the largest trial, Lewis et al.[50] enrolled 1266 men with symptoms of unstable angina at 12 university-affiliated Veterans

Administration medical centers within 48 hours of admission. Patients were randomized to receive aspirin 325 mg per day (in the form of Alka-Seltzer) or matching placebo. At 12 weeks, the aspirin group had 55% fewer acute MIs (p = 0.001) and 51% fewer cardiac deaths (p = 0.059). There was no difference in gastrointestinal (GI) adverse effects or bleeding. At 12 weeks, the study drugs were discontinued and subsequent medical care was not controlled. At the one-year follow-up, however, the mortality rate of patients who had originally been randomized to receive aspirin was 43% less than that of the placebo group (p = 0.008). Compared with the aspirin group, placebo-treated patients had more than twice as many nonfatal MIs during the 12-week study period and had double the mortality during the year compared with patients without MI.

The Canadian Multicenter Trial enrolled men and women with symptoms of unstable angina within eight days of hospitalization.[49] Patients were randomized into four treatment arms: aspirin 325 mg four times daily, sulfinpyrazone 200 mg four times daily, aspirin plus sulfinpyrazone, and placebo. Patients were followed for up to two years (mean, 18 months). The combined endpoint of cardiac death and nonfatal MI was reduced by 51% in all aspirin-treated patients (p = 0.008), with a reduction of 71% in cardiac death alone (p = 0.004). Sulfinpyrazone demonstrated neither a significant benefit on the occurrence of cardiac death or MI nor an interaction when combined with aspirin. Although GI bleeding was infrequent, GI adverse effects occurred at a greater frequency in aspirin-treated patients.

In another comparative trial, Theroux et al.[51] enrolled 479 patients with unstable angina who had at least one episode of rest pain within the last 24 hours. Patients were randomized to four treatment arms: aspirin 325 mg twice daily, heparin 5000 units i.v. followed by 1000 units/hr, both aspirin and heparin, and placebo. The heparin dosage was adjusted to maintain a partial thromboplastin time (PTT) of 1.5 to 2 times the control value. Patients were followed until definitive treatment was selected by the medical staff (average, six days). Because no deaths occurred in drug-treated groups and only two occurred in the placebo group, statistical analysis of this endpoint was not possible. Aspirin significantly reduced the frequency of MI, and aspirin in combination with heparin reduced the frequency of both MI and refractory angina. Since event rates were low in all drug-treated groups, the study lacked statistical power to detect a significant difference in MI or refractory angina between aspirin- and heparin-treated patients. However, a trend toward increased efficacy and increased bleeding was noted in patients treated with heparin alone or with aspirin plus heparin, compared with those treated with aspirin alone. Bleeding was noted in 8.3% of heparin-treated patients, 3.3% of aspirin-treated patients, and 5.1% of placebo-treated patients and occurred mainly at arterial puncture sites.

The Research Group on Instability in Coronary Artery Disease (RISC group) randomized 796 men with unstable angina within 33 hours of hospital admission into groups receiving placebo, aspirin 75 mg daily, i.v. heparin, or aspirin plus heparin.[52] Aspirin-treated patients experienced significantly lower MI or cardiac death rates at five-day, one-month, and three-month follow-ups compared with the placebo group. Treatment with heparin alone did not alter event rates. However, five-day event rates only were reduced in patients treated with the combination of aspirin and heparin. In patients treated with aspirin and heparin, there was a 75% reduction in risk of MI or cardiac death during the initial 5 days. The reason for lack of benefit in patients treated with heparin alone may be related to the fixed dose of heparin (5000 units every six hours for the first 24 hours followed by 3750 units every six hours for four days), the fact that no PTTs were monitored to ensure adequate anticoagulation, and the delay before treatment initiation. In contrast with the findings of Theroux et al.,[51] the RISC group noted only one episode of GI bleeding, which occurred in a heparin-treated patient, and a 5% frequency of GI upset in aspirin-treated patients. The reason for fewer bleeding episodes in this trial may be due to the lower dose of aspirin, lack of therapeutic anticoagulation, or to the fact that cardiac catheterization, which was performed in more than 90% of patients in the study of Theroux et al.,[51] was only performed in the RISC study if patients had refractory chest pain.

In a meta-analysis of the randomized aspirin trials, Yusuf et al.[53] estimated a 40% reduction in the rate of nonfatal MI and death (p <0.001) in patients treated with aspirin. The precise dosage of aspirin that should be used in treatment of unstable angina remains to be determined. Additional studies are necessary to clarify the role of low-dose aspirin alone or in combination with i.v. heparin during the acute phase of unstable angina.

Ticlopidine. Ticlopidine, an investigational antiplatelet agent, has also recently proved beneficial in patients with unstable angina.[54] One randomized, uncontrolled trial has compared conventional treatment with nitrates, calcium-channel blockers, and β blockers with and without ticlopidine 250 mg twice daily in patients with unstable angina who were enrolled within 48 hours of hospital admission. Patients receiving aspirin were excluded. Patients treated with ticlopidine demonstrated a 46% reduction in the combined endpoint of six-month vascular mortality and nonfatal MI (p = 0.009). Minor GI complaints were described by 5% of ticlopidine-treated patients. Ticlopidine does not block cyclo-oxygenase, but it still inhibits ADP-mediated platelet aggregation and interferes with fibrinogen binding to the glycoprotein IIb–IIIa-receptor. Whether or not the added expense of ticlopidine will be worth the benefit remains to be answered in comparative trials with aspirin. Other trials of investigational antiplatelet agents in unstable angina are planned. These drugs include thromboxane

Table 3.
Randomized Clinical Trials of Intravenous Heparin in Unstable Angina Pectoris (AP)[a]

Ref.	*n* Heparin/ *n* Control[b]	Duration of Heparin Therapy (days)	PTT Monitored	Results (*p*)
59	100/54	7	No	80% decr. in MI (*p* not applicable)
51	118/118	6	Yes	63% decr. in refractory AP (0.002); 93% decr. in MI (<0.001)
60	51/51	2[c]	No	65% decr. in refractory AP, cardiac death, or MI (<0.05)
62	33/29	≤8	NR	24% decr. in AP freq., 20% incr. in MI freq., 33% incr. in cardiac death (all NS)
52	198/199	5	No	1% incr. in MI or cardiac death at 5 days, 11% decr. at 30 days, 6% decr. at 90 days (all NS)

[a] PTT = activated partial thromboplastin time, MI = myocardial infarction, NR = not reported, NS = not significant.
[b] Heparin group received heparin plus standard therapy. Control group received placebo or standard therapy alone.
[c] Oral anticoagulation therapy started simultaneously and maintained for six months with dosage adjusted to maintain prothrombin time > twice the control value.

synthetase inhibitors, which selectively inhibit the conversion of prostaglandin H_2 to thromboxane A_2 in the arachidonic acid metabolic pathway, thromboxane A_2-receptor antagonists, and glycoprotein IIb–IIIa-receptor antagonists.

Heparin

Heparin exerts its anticoagulant effect by binding to and activating antithrombin III. Antithrombin III inhibits activated coagulation factors of the intrinsic and common pathways including thrombin; factors Xa, IXa, XIa, and XIIa; and kallikrein.[55]

A few clinical studies of heparin in patients with unstable angina were published in the early 1960s and suggested that early heparin therapy could reduce mortality and MI.[56,57] However, the importance of thrombosis in the pathogenesis of unstable angina was not recognized until the early 1980s, and heparin's potential for causing bleeding, as well as the poor design of the early trials, restricted heparin's use in acute ischemia for over two decades.[58]

Subsequently, completion of several randomized trials has further defined heparin's role in patients with unstable angina.[51,52,59,60] The results of these studies have recently been reviewed by Teshima and Hart[61] and are summarized in Table 3.[61,62] We have already described the data from the most current trials comparing aspirin and heparin.[51,52] Recently, an additional study comparing intermittent-bolus heparin with continuous infusion demonstrated the clinical superiority of a continuous infusion.[63] Chest pain and recurrent ischemia occurred less frequently in patients receiving heparin by infusion (at a dosage adjusted to maintain a PTT of 1.5 to 2 times the control value), compared with intermittent i.v. bolus injection of 5000–6000 units every six hours (with the dosing interval adjusted to maintain a PTT of ≤ 1.5 times the control value when checked once daily, one hour before administration of a dose).

Heparin appears to decrease the occurrence of MI in patients with unstable angina when administered as a continuous i.v. infusion adjusted to maintain a PTT of 1.5 to 2 times control values for 3 to 10 days,[51,52] but all studies have lacked a sample size sufficient to test the effect of heparin on mortality.[51,59,60] Comparative trials of aspirin (at a daily dosage of either 325 mg[51] or 75 mg[52]) versus i.v. heparin have failed to support the use of heparin therapy alone in patients with unstable angina. The combination of heparin and aspirin needs further evaluation to assess the potential for additive benefit versus the potential for an increase in bleeding complications. Clinical investigations with hirudin, a new, potent thrombin inhibitor that is more specific than heparin and inhibits activation of coagulation factors V, VII, and XIII, may prove beneficial at inhibiting platelet aggregation and thrombus formation in patients with acute myocardial ischemia.[64]

Calcium-Channel Blockers

During the past decade, the use of calcium-channel blockers in the treatment of acute myocardial ischemia has dramatically increased. Through vasodilation and reversal of coronary-artery spasm, calcium-channel blockers may decrease blood pressure and increase coronary-artery blood flow and favorably affect both myocardial oxygen demand and supply in patients with unstable angina. Verapamil and diltiazem may reduce myocardial oxygen demand by slowing the heart rate at rest and at exercise, whereas nifedipine may cause a slight tachycardia.[65] Limited data suggest that some calcium-channel blockers also possess antiplatelet activity as well.[66]

Numerous clinical trials have evaluated the use of verapamil, nifedipine, and diltiazem in the treatment of unstable angina in patients with underlying coronary-artery disease (Table 4).[67-81] All oral agents were administered as immediate-release formulations.

Results with nifedipine, a dihydropyridine, have been mixed. Nifedipine as monotherapy, at dosages of 60 to 120 mg per day, has been associated with less frequent episodes of rest pain, compared with a control period.[67] Other trials have assessed the use of nifedipine with other antianginals, particularly β blockers.[68,70,71,78] Addition of nifedipine to a regimen of

Table 4.
Clinical Trials of Calcium-Channel Blockers in Unstable Angina Pectoris (AP)[a]

Ref.	*n*	Drug and Dosage[b]	Concomitant Drugs	Results (*p*)
67	14	Nf 60–120 mg/day	None	Decr. AP or ischemia freq. (<0.002)
68	68	Nf 40–80 mg/day	BB, N	Decr. cardiac death, MI, or bypass surgery (0.03)
78	89	Nf 80 mg/day	BB	No change in MI or cardiac death
70	63	Nf 80–120 mg/day	BB, N	No change in AP or MI freq.
71	271	Nf 60 mg/day	N, H, W, ±BB	No change in recurrent ischemia or MI
79	12	Nf 30–90 mg/day	N	Incr. recurrent ischemia and MI compared with propranolol (0.025)
76	12	V 0.002 mg/kg/min i.v.	N, H	Decr. in recurrent ischemia (0.001)
73	9	V 320–480 mg/day	N, BB	Decr. AP freq. (*p* not reported)
80	12	V 400 mg/day	None	Decr. AP or ischemia freq. (0.006)
75	10	Nf 80 mg/day	None	Decr. AP (0.01) and ischemia (0.003) freq. in each group
	10	V 360 mg/day		
74	10	D 2.5–4.3 μg/kg/min i.v.	N	Decr. AP freq. (0.001)
81	50	D 180–360 mg/day	N	Decr. AP freq. (<0.05); no change in cardiac death or MI

[a] Nf = nifedipine, BB = β-adrenergic blockers, N = nitrates, MI = myocardial infarction, H = heparin, W = warfarin, V = verapamil hydrochloride, D = diltiazem hydrochloride.

[b] Drugs given orally unless otherwise noted.

nitrates and β blockers was superior to placebo plus conventional treatment in a randomized, placebo-controlled, double-blind study performed by Gerstenblith et al.[68]

In contrast, results from four randomized, controlled trials suggest that monotherapy with a β blocker is superior to monotherapy with nifedipine or that a benefit with nifedipine is achieved only in patients treated with concomitant β blockers.[70,71,78,79] In fact, two of these studies suggested an increase in mortality or infarction in patients treated with nifedipine, which may be associated with a tachycardia-induced increase in myocardial oxygen demand.[71,78] Treatment with nifedipine has been associated with frequent vasodilatory adverse effects, such as headache.[67] Therefore the combination of nifedipine and a β blocker, which blunts reflex tachycardia, appears preferable to nifedipine alone.[71,77]

Limited data indicate that oral verapamil hydrochloride 360–480 mg/day effectively decreases the frequency of rest pain.[80,73] Small comparative trials have suggested that oral or i.v. verapamil is at least as effective as nifedipine or propranolol in relieving chest pain and reversing S–T segment changes in patients with unstable angina and coronary disease.[75,80] Verapamil has also prolonged the P–R interval and occasionally caused heart block.[73,75] In a comparative trial, verapamil decreased the heart rate and blood pressure to a similar degree as propranolol.[80]

Only one trial has assessed the efficacy of oral diltiazem hydrochloride (up to 360 mg per day) for the treatment of unstable angina in patients with underlying coronary artery disease.[81] In a randomized study comparing diltiazem and propranolol, both drugs decreased blood pressure and heart rate similarly and reduced the occurrence of angina significantly, compared with a baseline control period. I.V. diltiazem has also been used to achieve rapid relief of chest pain in patients admitted with acute myocardial ischemia.[74,76]

Overall, studies with calcium-channel blockers have failed to document a reduction in risk of MI and death in patients with unstable angina. The largest clinical trials have been performed with nifedipine and have suggested deleterious effects on MI occurrence and mortality. Larger trials with verapamil and diltiazem, which decrease heart rate and blood pressure to a similar degree as β blockers, should be conducted to evaluate the effectiveness of these calcium-channel blockers in decreasing cardiac death or progression to MI in patients with unstable angina. Additional safety data are necessary regarding the use of verapamil and diltiazem in combination with β blockers.

Beta-Adrenergic Blockers

The initial use of β-adrenergic blockers in unstable angina was based on the clinical experience compiled in patients with stable angina pectoris[82] and acute MI.[83] These drugs decrease myocardial oxygen demand by blunting catecholamine-induced increases in heart rate and blood pressure as well as decreasing myocardial contractility. They may also benefit patients with myocardial ischemia through their antiarrhythmic properties and antiplatelet effects.[84] However, concern has been raised regarding the use of β blockers in patients with unstable angina who may have coronary vasospasm as a factor contributing to their symptoms. Theoretically, β blockade, with unopposed α-adrenergic vasoconstriction, could promote coronary vasoconstriction.[85] Indeed, β blockers have not proved effective, and should be avoided, in patients with vasospastic or Prinzmetal's angina.[80,86-88]

Since atherosclerosis and plaque rupture with thrombosis, rather than vasospasm, are the primary underlying causes of unstable angina, the effectiveness of β blockers added to concomitant therapy with vasodilating nitrates or calcium-channel blockers in patients with unstable angina has been explored in sev-

Table 5.
Clinical Trials of β-Adrenergic Blockers in Unstable Angina Pectoris (AP)[a]

Ref.	*n*	Drug and Dosage[b]	Concomitant Drugs	Results (*p*)
70	NR	P (dosage NR)	N, CCB	NR
79	14	P 60–240 mg/day	N	Decr. in recurrent ischemia or MI, compared with nifedipine (0.025)
77	42	P 160–320 mg/day	N, CCB	Decr. AP or ischemia freq. (0.03); no change in cardiac death or MI
81	50	P 120–240 mg/day	N	Decr. AP freq. (0.05); no change in cardiac death or MI, compared with diltiazem
71	165	M 200 mg/day	N, H, W, ±CCB	NR
59	214	A 100 mg/day	N, +H	Without H: 24% decr. in MI (NS) With H: 76% in MI (0.024)
95	76	A 5 mg i.v., then 100 mg/day	NR	Decr. MI (0.02)
96	20	P 0.1 mg/kg i.v., then 320 mg/27 hr	None	Decr. MI (<0.05)
90	12 11	E 44–282 μg/kg/min i.v. P (dosage NR)	N, CCB	Decr. AP freq. (0.02) in each group
92	59	E (dosage NR)	NR	No change in AP or ischemia
91	21	E 8–24 mg/min i.v.	N, BB, As, H	86% relieved of AP (*p* NR)
94	23	F 4.7 μg/kg/min i.v. (mean)	N	No change in AP or ischemia

[a] NR = not reported, P = propranolol hydrochloride, N = nitrates, CCB = calcium-channel blockers, MI = myocardial infarction, M = metoprolol tartrate, H = heparin, W = warfarin, A = atenolol, E = esmolol hydrochloride, BB = β-adrenergic blockers, As = aspirin, F = flestolol.
[b] Drugs given orally unless otherwise noted.

eral trials (Table 5).[59,70,71,77,79,81,89-94] Therapy with propranolol appears to be superior to nifedipine in patients not previously receiving a β blocker.[70,79] Compared with the addition of placebo, the addition of propranolol or metoprolol to therapy with nitrates and nifedipine further decreases the frequency of anginal episodes and myocardial ischemia.[71,77] Diltiazem and propranolol appear equally effective at reducing the frequency of chest pain when added to nitrates.[81] In the only large, randomized, placebo-controlled study, Telford and Wilson[59] found atenolol to be ineffective at decreasing the occurrence of MI in patients treated with nitrates or heparin during the first week after hospital admission. In many other trials evaluating the effectiveness of calcium-channel blockers and nitrates in unstable angina, β blockers were coadministered (Tables 1 and 4). Pooled analysis of two randomized trials of patients believed to have "threatened myocardial infarction" who received β blockers suggests a risk reduction in development of MI of less than 13%.[53,95,96]

More recently, the short-acting i.v. β blockers esmolol and flestolol have been evaluated as additions to treatment with nitrates, calcium-channel blockers, and oral β blockers (Table 5).[90-94] When the dosage was adjusted to reduce the resting rate–pressure product (heart rate × systolic blood pressure) by 20% to 30%, esmolol relieved rest pain and decreased the frequency of angina in two small open studies.[90,91] A randomized, multicenter, placebo-controlled study comparing the addition of esmolol or placebo to conventional therapy indicated a nonsignificant trend favoring esmolol over placebo.[92] Preliminary work with flestolol, an investigational nonselective short-acting β blocker, suggests favorable hemodynamic effects but no additional reduction in frequency of rest pain or myocardial ischemia compared with nitrate therapy alone.[93,94] One advantage of using short-acting agents is the rapid reversibility of adverse reactions such as hypotension, heart block, or congestive heart failure.[90,91]

Overall, data evaluating the efficacy of β blockers as monotherapy for patients with unstable angina are lacking, and results of studies evaluating the addition of β blockers to nitrates or calcium-channel blockers have been mixed. At this time, a specific β blocker for treatment of refractory patients with unstable angina cannot be recommended. Because of their documented antianginal efficacy, it is unlikely that additional well-designed trials in unstable angina will be performed with FDA-approved β blockers.[53]

Thrombolytic Therapy

The potential role of thrombolytic therapy as a treatment alternative for patients with unstable angina is currently under investigation. Thrombolytic therapy has the potential to lyse intracoronary thrombi associated with unstable angina but may pose an unacceptable bleeding risk. Results from numerous small, open studies have been mixed with regard to the ability of i.v. or intracoronary streptokinase, i.v. or intracoronary urokinase, or i.v. alteplase to decrease progression to MI or cardiac death.[97-114] Results from studies in which the presence of intracoronary thrombus was documented before thrombolytic administration have been more favorable.[98-100,104,106] Several small, placebo-controlled trials of alteplase, which have had neutral results, have lacked sufficient statistical power to demonstrate the superiority of thrombolytic therapy followed by heparin to heparin alone.[103,106,107,109,111,113,114] Ambrose and Alexopoulos[115] have postulated that the reason for the limited success of thrombolytic agents in patients with unstable angina, despite dramatic thrombolytic-associated reductions in mortality in patients with MI, may be related to a difference in the causes of the two syndromes. Patients with MI often have a large amount of fresh coronary thrombus and less severe atherosclerotic stenosis of the affected artery, whereas patients with unstable angina probably have more atherosclerosis and less thrombus. Larger, randomized, double-blind trials, including the Thrombolysis in Myocardial Ischemia (TIMI-III) trial, are in progress and will assist in defining the role of thrombolytic therapy in patients with unstable angina.[116]

Intra-aortic Balloon Counterpulsation

The intra-aortic balloon pump (IABP) may be used as a temporary measure in patients with unstable angina who fail to respond to drug therapy.[11] A large-bore, balloon-tipped catheter is inserted into the femoral artery and positioned in the descending thoracic aorta. Following insertion, the balloon catheter is connected to a pump that inflates and deflates the balloon in conjunction with the cardiac cycle. Intra-aortic balloon counterpulsation relieves ischemia by mechanically decreasing left ventricular end-diastolic pressure and increasing intra-aortic diastolic pressure; these effects decrease myocardial oxygen demand and increase coronary-artery blood flow. Concomitant i.v. heparin therapy is necessary to prevent thrombosis induced by the catheter and balloon. Complications of the IABP include insertion-site hemorrhage, infection, thrombocytopenia, and thromboembolism.[117] In addition to use in unstable angina as a bridge between medical therapy and interventional therapy such as percutaneous transluminal coronary angioplasty (PTCA) and coronary-artery bypass grafting, the IABP is also used as adjunctive therapy during angioplasty and following bypass grafting.[13]

Percutaneous Transluminal Coronary Angioplasty

PTCA is indicated in patients with unstable angina and single-vessel coronary-artery disease of suitable anatomy (that does not involve the left main coronary artery) who are refractory to medical therapy or who have been stabilized for at least three days on medical therapy and also have evidence of myocardial ischemia during exercise testing.[118] It is estimated that almost one-half of patients undergoing PTCA have unstable angina. The popularity of PTCA in patients with unstable angina stems from the concept that a single atherosclerotic coronary-artery stenosis, or "culprit lesion," can be identified as the cause of the patient's symptoms and that the symptoms can be relieved by balloon dilation of the stenosis.[119] Although PTCA can be performed safely in patients with unstable angina, the presence of intracoronary thrombus increases the risk of acute reocclusion. Often, if coronary thrombosis is identified, i.v. heparin is administered and PTCA is delayed for several days to allow for resolution of thrombi and a resulting decreased risk of acute reocclusion.[119]

The long-term outcome of patients with unstable angina and single-vessel coronary-artery disease who undergo PTCA appears similar to that of patients with stable angina who undergo PTCA and to patients who undergo coronary bypass grafting.[119] The role of PTCA in patients with unstable angina and multi-vessel coronary artery disease remains unclear.[119]

Coronary-Artery Bypass Grafting

In two large, randomized trials conducted before the utilization of PTCA or calcium-channel blockers, comparison of medical versus surgical therapy (bypass grafting) for initial treatment of unstable angina demonstrated reduced repeat hospitalizations and improved survival in a subset of surgical patients with left ventricular dysfunction (ejection fraction < 50%).[22,23] However, frequent crossover from the medical to the surgical treatment group (approximately 30% at two years and 40% at five years) limits clinical application of these results.[22]

For patients with unstable angina and multivessel disease who remain symptomatic despite medical therapy, aortocoronary bypass surgery is usually the revascularization treatment of choice. However, the presence of unstable angina significantly increases the risk of perioperative mortality. Large, randomized trials comparing outcomes of PTCA and surgery in patients with multivessel coronary-artery disease are currently underway. According to Hammermeister and Morrison,[21] patients with unstable angina most likely to benefit from bypass grafting include patients with stenosis of the left main coronary artery, triple-vessel coronary-artery disease, left ventricular dysfunction, or two-vessel disease with involvement of the left anterior descending coronary artery.[21]

Treatment Strategy

Based on the data described above for various drug and nondrug treatments, we propose the following approach in patients with unstable angina; this strategy has been adapted from that described by Munger and Oh[13] (Figure 3). The goals of therapy are to increase myocardial oxygen supply, decrease myocardial oxygen demand, relieve chest pain, decrease the frequency of recurrent angina and myocardial ischemia, prevent progression to infarction, and decrease cardiac death.

Patients with unstable angina require hospitalization and continuous ECG monitoring. Sublingual nitroglycerin is the initial treatment of choice in patients

Figure 3. Treatment strategy for unstable angina. ASA = aspirin, IV = intravenous; IABP = intra-aortic balloon pump; ECG = electrocardiographic; CAD = coronary-artery disease; 1VD, 2VD, and 3VD = one-vessel, two-vessel, and three-vessel disease, respectively; LM = left main coronary-artery disease; PTCA = percutaneous transluminal coronary angioplasty; CABG = coronary artery bypass grafting. Adapted, with permission, from reference 13.

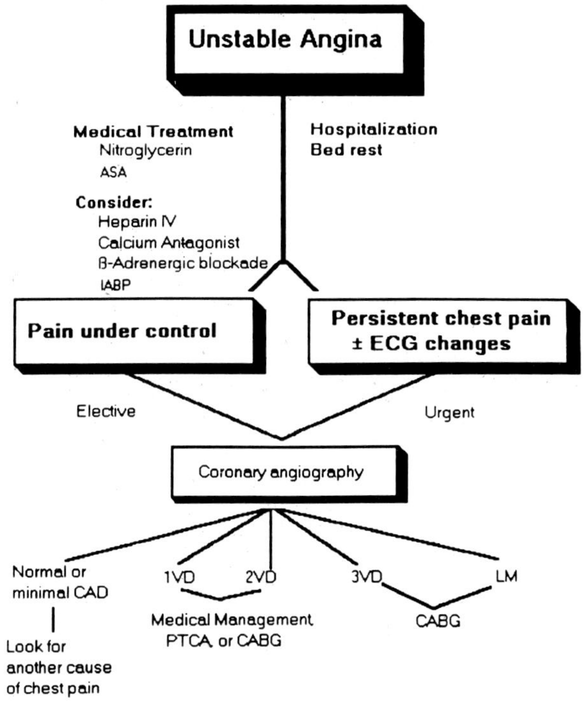

who have new-onset angina, crescendo angina, or rest angina. If angina is unrelieved with sublingual nitroglycerin, i.v. nitroglycerin should be administered. A starting dose of 5 μg/min should be increased in 5- to 10-μg/min increments every five minutes until chest pain is relieved; systolic blood pressure should be maintained at greater than 100 mm Hg. The most frequent adverse effects are hypotension and headache, which may be relieved with downward dosage adjustment. If increasingly larger doses of i.v. nitroglycerin are required to prevent angina or ischemia, the development of nitrate tolerance should be suspected and alternative antianginals administered. Future advances in the treatment of unstable angina with nitrates may include therapy with sulfhydryl donor agents, such as acetylcysteine or methionine, to prevent nitrate tolerance. Heparin resistance, manifested as decreased PTTs, has been reported to occur in a few patients receiving i.v. nitroglycerin.[120-122] Most cases have involved patients receiving high doses of i.v. nitroglycerin (>350 μg/min).[121,122] Although the exact mechanism is unclear,[123] the PTT should be monitored closely in patients receiving concomitant i.v. nitroglycerin and heparin.

All patients with unstable angina should receive antiplatelet therapy with aspirin unless this drug is contraindicated. The most effective dose of aspirin with the lowest frequency of adverse GI effects remains to be established. Typically, the dosage of aspirin administered in the United States is 325 mg once daily. Currently, if lower dosages of aspirin are administered during the first five days of treatment, the drug should be accompanied by i.v. heparin therapy.[52] Unless precluded by adverse effects, aspirin therapy should be continued indefinitely in patients with unstable angina and coronary artery disease. Future advances in knowledge about the treatment of unstable angina with antiplatelet agents will include elucidation of the optimal dosage of aspirin and comparative trials with newer, more specific agents, such as thromboxane-receptor antagonists or glycoprotein IIb–IIIa-receptor antagonists.

In patients with unstable angina that is refractory to aspirin and nitrate therapy, or in those with known intracoronary thrombus, an i.v. bolus of heparin 5000 units should be given and followed by an infusion of 1000 units/hr; the infusion should be adjusted to maintain the PTT at 1.5 to 2 times the control value. Heparin therapy should be continued for 3 to 10 days or until revascularization (PTCA or bypass grafting) is performed. Additional trials are necessary to confirm an additional benefit of heparin combined with aspirin over aspirin alone and to further evaluate the risk of bleeding.

Selection of antianginal therapy, other than nitrates and aspirin, is less well established. In patients with refractory angina and tachycardia or hypertension, reduction of the rate–pressure product with diltiazem, verapamil, or a β blocker is indicated. Because of their negative chronotropic and inotropic properties, the use of diltiazem, verapamil, or β blockers is contraindicated in patients with second- or third-degree heart block, poor left ventricular function, or congestive heart failure. Calcium-channel blockers, but not β blockers, can be safely administered in patients with bronchospasm or vasospastic angina. Nifedipine, which lacks significant conduction-system effects, should be reserved for patients with contraindications to diltiazem, verapamil, and β blockers or should be used in combination with β blockers. Caution should be exercised when combining diltiazem or verapamil with β blockers, and patients should be monitored closely for symptoms of additive bradycardia and negative inotropic effects.

Patients with persistent chest pain despite medical therapy or patients stabilized on medical therapy who manifest ischemia during exercise testing should undergo coronary arteriography. Patients with normal or minimal coronary-artery disease should be evaluated for vasospastic angina or noncardiac causes of chest pain. Patients with one- or two-vessel disease should be evaluated for medical therapy, PTCA, or bypass grafting based on the presence of symptoms, coronary anatomy, left ventricular function, and ability to define the "culprit lesion." Patients with triple-vessel or left main coronary-artery disease probably benefit the greatest from bypass grafting.

Conclusion

Advances in medical and surgical therapy for unstable angina have paralleled the expansion of understanding of the pathophysiological basis of the disease. Therapy with nitrates, aspirin, heparin, calcium-channel blockers, or β blockers has led to a low in-hospital and first-year mortality rate and a low rate of progression to MI. Future investigations will center on combination therapies and on new antiplatelet or anticoagulant drugs.

References

1. Shah PK. Pathophysiology of unstable angina. *Cardiol Clin.* 1991; 9:11-26.
2. Fuster V, Badimon L, Ambrose JA et al. Insights into the pathogenesis of acute ischemic syndromes. *Circulation.* 1988; 77:1213-20.
3. Willerson JT, Golino P, Eidt J et al. Specific platelet mediators and unstable coronary artery lesions: experimental evidence and potential clinical implications. *Circulation.* 1989; 80:198-205.
4. Capone G, Wolf NM, Meyer B et al. Frequency of intracoronary filling defects by angiography in angina pectoris at rest. *Am J Cardiol.* 1985; 56:403-6.
5. Conti CR. Unstable angina before and after infarction: thoughts on pathogenesis and therapeutic strategies. *Heart Lung.* 1986; 15:361-7.
6. Conti CR, Hill JA, Mayfield WR. Unstable angina pectoris: pathogenesis and management. *Curr Probl Cardiol.* 1989; 14:549-624.
7. Davies MJ, Thomas AC. Plaque fissuring: the cause of acute myocardial infarction, sudden ischaemic death, and crescendo angina. *Br Heart J.* 1985; 53:363-73.
8. Myler RK, Frink RJ, Shaw RE et al. The unstable plaque: pathophysiology and therapeutic implications. *J Invasive Cardiol.* 1990; 2:117-28.
9. Becker RC, Gore JM. Adjuvant antiplatelet strategies in coronary thrombolysis. *Circulation.* 1991; 83:1115-7.
10. Eisenberg PR. Preventing reocclusion after MI reperfusion therapy. *Cardio.* 1989; 6:48-56.
11. Furie B, Furie BC. The molecular basis of blood coagulation. In: Hoffman R, Benz EJ Jr, Shattil SJ et al., eds. Hematology: basic principles and practice. New York: Churchill Livingstone; 1991:1213-31.
12. Dinerman JL, Mehta J. Endothelial, platelet and leukocyte interactions in ischemic heart disease: insights into potential mechanisms and their clinical relevance. *J Am Coll Cardiol.* 1990; 16:207-22.
13. Munger TM, Oh JK. Unstable angina. *Mayo Clin Proc.* 1990; 65:384-406.
14. Beller GA. Calcium antagonists in the treatment of Prinzmetal's angina and unstable angina pectoris. *Circulation.* 1989; 80(Suppl IV):78–87.
15. Braunwald E. Unstable angina: a classification. *Circulation.* 1989; 80:410-4.
16. Gore JM, Becker RC. Management of post-infarction angina. *Cardiol Clin.* 1988; 6:165-72.
17. Hilton TC, Chaitman BR. The prognosis in stable and unstable angina. *Cardiol Clin.* 1991; 9:27-38.
18. Alison HW, Russel RO Jr, Mantle JA et al. Coronary anatomy and arteriography in patients with unstable angina. *Am J Cardiol.* 1978; 41:204-9.
19. Kimball BP, Bui S, Dafopoulos N. Changes in diameter of coronary narrowings and translesional hemodynamics after intracoronary nitroglycerin. *Am J Cardiol.* 1990; 66:705-9.
20. Diodati J, Theroux P, Latour J-G et al. Effects of nitroglycerin at therapeutic doses on platelet aggregation in unstable angina and acute myocardial infarction. *Am J Cardiol.* 1990; 66:683-8.
21. Hammermeister KE, Morrison DA. Coronary bypass surgery for stable angina and unstable angina pectoris. *Cardiol Clin.* 1991; 9:135-55.
22. Parisi AF, Khuri S, Deupree RH et al. Medical compared with surgical management of unstable angina: 5-year mortality and morbidity in the Veterans Administration Study. *Circulation.* 1989; 80:1176-89.
23. Luchi RJ, Scott SM, Parisi AF et al. Comparison of medical and surgical treatment for unstable angina pectoris. *N Engl J Med.* 1987; 316:977-84.
24. Rackley CE. Role of isosorbide dinitrate in patients with unstable angina pectoris. *Am Heart J.* 1985; 110:269-72.
25. Curfman GD, Heisimer JA, Lozner EC et al. Intravenous nitroglycerin in the treatment of spontaneous angina pectoris: a prospective, randomized trial. *Circulation.* 1983; 67:276-82.
26. Lin SG, Flaherty JT. Crossover from intravenous to transdermal nitroglycerin therapy in unstable angina pectoris. *Am J Cardiol.* 1985; 56:742-8.
27. Flaherty JT. Usefulness of intravenous and transdermal nitroglycerin therapy in patients with unstable angina. *Am Heart J.* 1986; 112:220-1.
28. Abrams J. Nitrates. Cardiovascular pharmacotherapy I. *Med Clin North Am.* 1988; 72:1-35.
29. Norlander R. Use of nitrates in the treatment of unstable and variant angina. *Drugs.* 1987; 33(Suppl 4):131-9.
30. Ahlner J, Axelsson KL. Nitrates: mode of action at a cellular level. *Drugs.* 1987; 33:32-8.
31. Palmer RMJ, Ferige AG, Moncada S. Nitric oxide release accounts for the biological activity of endothelium-derived relaxing factor. *Nature.* 1987; 327:524-6.
32. Dinerman JL, Mehta JL. Endothelial, platelet and leukocyte interactions in ischemic heart disease: insights into potential mechanisms and their clinical relevance. *J Am Coll Cardiol.* 1990; 207-22.
33. Pucillo AL, Reison DS, Cannon PJ et al. Systemic and coronary hemodynamics during intravenous nitroglycerin infusion in unstable angina. *J Am Coll Cardiol.* 1985; 5:505. Abstract.
34. Amtorp O. Hemodynamic effects of nitrates, with special reference to the coronary circulation. *Drugs.* 1987; 33:(Suppl 4):39-42.
35. Dauwe F, Affaki G, Waters DD et al. Intravenous nitroglycerin in refractory unstable angina. *Am J Cardiol.* 1979; 43:416. Abstract.
36. Brodsky SJ, Halperin JL, Klein MD et al. Intravenous nitroglycerin infusion in unstable angina. *Clin Res.* 1980; 28:608A. Abstract.
37. Mikolich JR, Nicoloff NB, Robinson PH et al. Relief of refractory angina with continuous intravenous infusion of nitroglycerin. *Chest.* 1980; 77:375-9.
38. Page A, Gateau P, Ohayon J et al. Intravenous nitroglycerin in unstable angina. In: Lichtlen PR, Engel HJ, Schrey A et al., eds. Nitrate III, cardiovascular effects. New York: Springer Verlag, 1981; 371-6.
39. Roubin GS, Harris PJ, Eckhardt I et al. Intravenous nitroglycerin in refractory unstable angina pectoris. *Aust NZ J Med.* 1982; 12:598-602.
40. DePace NL, Herling IM, Kotler MN et al. Intravenous nitroglycerin for rest angina: potential pathophysiologic mechanisms of action. *Arch Intern Med.* 1982; 142:1806-9.
41. Squire A, Cantor R, Packer M. Limitations of continuous intravenous nitroglycerin prophylaxis in patients with refractory angina pectoris. *Circulation.* 1982; 66(Suppl II):120. Abstract.
42. Kaplan K, Davison R, Parker M et al. Intravenous nitroglycerin for the treatment of angina at rest unresponsive to standard nitrate therapy. *Am J Cardiol.* 1983; 51:694-8.
43. Jugdutt BI, Warnica JW. Tolerance with low dose intravenous nitroglycerin therapy in acute myocardial infarction. *Am J Cardiol.* 1989; 64:581-7.
44. Flaherty JT. Nitrate tolerance: a review of the evidence. *Drugs.* 1989; 37:523-50.

45. Horowitz JD, Henry CA, Syrjanen ML et al. Combined use of nitroglycerin and N-acetylcysteine in the management of unstable angina pectoris. *Circulation*. 1988; 77:787-94.
46. Webster MWI, Chesebro JH, Fuster V. Platelet inhibitor therapy: agents and clinical implications. *Hematol Oncol Clin North Am*. 1990; 4:265-88.
47. Stein B, Fuster V, Israel DH et al. Platelet inhibitor agents in cardiovascular disease. *J Am Coll Cardiol*. 1989; 14:813-36.
48. Rutherford JD. Unstable angina and thrombolysis. *Chest*. 1990; 97(Suppl):156S-160S.
49. Cairns JA, Gent M, Singer J et al. Aspirin, sulfinpyrazone, or both in unstable angina. *N Engl J Med*. 1985; 313:1369-75.
50. Lewis HD, Davis JW. Archibald DG et al. Protective effects of aspirin against acute myocardial infarction and death in men with unstable angina. *N Engl J Med*. 1983; 309:396-403.
51. Theroux P, Ouimet H, McCans J et al. Aspirin, heparin, or both to treat acute unstable angina. *N Engl J Med*. 1988; 319:1105-11.
52. RISC Group. Risk of myocardial infarction and death during treatment with low dose aspirin and intravenous heparin in men with unstable coronary artery disease. *Lancet*. 1990; 336:827-30.
53. Yusuf S, Wittes J, Freidman L. Overview of results of randomized clinical trials in heart disease. II. Unstable angina, heart failure, primary prevention with aspirin, and risk factor modification. *JAMA*. 1988; 260:2259-63.
54. Balsano F, Rizzon P, Violi F et al. Antiplatelet treatment with ticlopidine in unstable angina: a controlled multicenter clinical trial. *Circulation*. 1990; 82:17-26.
55. Tollefsen DM. Heparin: basic and clinical pharmacology. In: Hoffman R, Benz EJ Jr, Shattil SJ et al., eds. Hematology: basic principles and practice. New York: Churchill Livingstone; 1991:1436-45.
56. Nichol ES, Phillips WS, Caster GG. Virtue of prompt anticoagulation therapy in impending myocardial infarction: experiences with 318 patients during a 10 year period. *Ann Intern Med*. 1959; 50:1158-73.
57. Wood P. Acute and subacute coronary insufficiency. *Br Med J*. 1961; 1:1779-89.
58. Lopez LM, Mehta JL. Anticoagulation in coronary heart disease: heparin and warfarin trials. *Cardiovasc Clin*. 1987; 18:215-29.
59. Telford AM, Wilson C. Trial of heparin versus atenolol in prevention of myocardial infarction in intermediate coronary syndrome. *Lancet*. 1981; 1:1225-8.
60. Williams DO, Kirby MG, McPherson K et al. Anticoagulant treatment in unstable angina. *Br J Clin Pract*. 1986; 40:114-6.
61. Teshima JY. Hart LL. Heparin in unstable angina. *DICP*. 1990; 24:385-6.
62. Zwerner PL, Gore JM, Corrao JM et al. Heparin in the treatment of unstable angina: a randomized prospective trial. *Circulation*. 1987; 76:(Suppl IV):180. Abstract.
63. Neri Seneri GG, Gensini GF, Poggesi L et al. Effect of heparin, aspirin, or alteplase in reduction of myocardial ischemia in refractory unstable angina. *Lancet*. 1990; 335:615-8.
64. Fuster V, Stein B, Ambrose JA et al. Atherosclerotic plaque rupture and thrombosis: evolving concepts. *Circulation*. 1990; 82(Suppl II):47–59.
65. Follath F. The role of calcium antagonists in the treatment of myocardial ischemia. *Am Heart J*. 1989; 118:1093-7.
66. Johnson GJ, Leis LA, Francis GS. Disparate effects of the calcium channel blockers, nifedipine and verapamil on α_2-adrenergic receptors and thromboxane A_2-induced aggregation of human platelets. *Circulation*. 1986; 73:847-54.
67. Previtali M, Salerno JA, Tavazzi L et al. Treatment of angina at rest with nifedipine: a short-term controlled study. *Am J Cardiol*. 1980; 45:825-30.
68. Gerstenblith G, Ouyang P, Achuff SC et al. Nifedipine in unstable angina: a double-blind, randomized trial. *N Engl J Med*. 1982; 306:885-9.
69. Sellers TD, Gibson RS, Taylor GJ et al. Relation of therapeutic response to nifedipine to coronary anatomy and motion of S–T segment during unstable angina pectoris. *Am J Med*. 1983; 75:57-64.
70. Muller JE, Turi ZG, Pearle DL et al. Nifedipine and conventional therapy for unstable angina pectoris: a randomized, double-blind comparison. *Circulation*. 1984; 69:728-39.
71. Lubsen J, Tijssen JGP for the HINT Research Group. *Am J Cardiol*. 1987; 60:18A-25A.
72. Parodi O, Maseri A, Simonetti I. Management of unstable angina by verapamil: a double-blind crossover study in the CCU. *Br Heart J*. 1979; 41:167-74.
73. Mehta J, Pepine CJ, Day M et al. Short-term efficacy of oral verapamil in rest angina: a double-blind placebo controlled trial in CCU patients. *Am J Med*. 1981; 71:977-82.
74. Colombo G, Zucchella G, Planca E et al. Intravenous diltiazem in the treatment of unstable angina: a study of efficacy and tolerance. *Clin Ther*. 1987; 9:536-47.
75. Maresta MA, Marzocchi A, Capucci A et al. Nifedipine compared with verapamil in unstable angina pectoris. *Int J Clin Pharmacol Res*. 1986; 6:291-301.
76. Mauri F, Mafrici M, Biraghi P et al. Effectiveness of calcium antagonist drugs in patients with unstable angina and proven coronary artery disease. *Eur Heart J*. 1988; 9(Suppl N):158-63.
77. Gottlieb SO, Weisfeldt ML, Ouyang P et al. Effect of the addition of propranolol to therapy with nifedipine for unstable angina pectoris: a randomized, double-blind, placebo-controlled trial. *Circulation*. 1986; 73:331-7.
78. Muller JE, Morrison J, Stone PH et al. Nifedipine for patients with threatened and acute myocardial infarction: a randomized, placebo-controlled comparison. *Circulation*. 1984; 69:740-7.
79. Myers MG, Baigrie RS, Dubbin JD. Nifedipine versus propranolol treatment for unstable angina in the elderly. *Can J Cardiol*. 1988; 4:402-6.
80. Parodi O, Simonetti I, Michelassi C et al. Comparison of verapamil and propranolol therapy for angina pectoris at rest: a randomized, multiple-crossover, controlled trial in the coronary care unit. *Am J Cardiol*. 1986; 57:899-906.
81. Theroux P, Taeymans Y, Morissette D et al. A randomized study comparing propranolol and diltiazem in the treatment of unstable angina. *J Am Coll Cardiol*. 1985; 5:717-22.
82. Prichard BNC. β-Adrenergic blocking drugs in angina pectoris. In: Avery GS, ed. Cardiovascular drugs. Vol. 2: β-Adrenoceptor blocking drugs. Baltimore: University Park Press, 1978:85-118.
83. Cruickshank JM. β-Blockade in acute myocardial infarction. *J Cardiovasc Pharmacol*. 1988; 12(Suppl 1):S59-70.
84. Cohen LS. Medical prophylaxis for the post myocardial infarct patients. *Cardiol Clin*. 1988; 6:173-8.
85. Gottlieb SO, Flaherty JT. Medical therapy of unstable angina pectoris. *Cardiol Clin*. 1991; 9:89-98.
86. Andre-Fouet X, Usdin JP, Gayet CH et al. Comparison of short-term efficacy of diltiazem and propranolol in unstable angina at rest. *Eur Heart J*. 1983; 4:691-8.
87. Robertson RM, Wood AJJ, Vaughn WK et al. Exacerbation of vasotonic angina pectoris by propranolol. *Circulation*. 1982; 65:281-5.
88. Tilmant PY, LaBlance JM, Thieuleux FA et al. Detrimental effect of propranolol in patients with coronary artery spasm countered by diltiazem. *Am J Cardiol*. 1983; 52:230-33.
89. Cohen M, Adams PC, Hawkins L et al. Usefulness of antithrombotic therapy in resting angina pectoris or non-Q-wave myocardial infarction: a pilot study from the Antithrombotic Therapy in Acute Coronary Syndromes Study Group. *Am J Cardiol*. 1990; 1287-92.
90. Wallis DE, Pope C, Littman WJ et al. Safety and efficacy of esmolol for unstable angina pectoris. *Am J Cardiol*. 1988; 62:1033-7.
91. Barth C, Ojile M, Pearson AC et al. Ultra short-acting intravenous β-adrenergic blockade as add-on therapy in acute unstable angina. *Am Heart J*. 1991; 121:782-8.
92. Hohnloser SH, Meinhertz T, Klingenheben T et al. Usefulness of esmolol in unstable angina pectoris. *Am J Cardiol*.

1991; 67:1319-23.
93. Strom J, Josephson M, Frishman WH et al. Hemodynamic effects of flestolol, a titratable short-acting intravenous beta-adrenergic receptor blocker. *J Clin Pharmacol.* 1988; 28:276-82.
94. Conti R, Somberg J, Keefe D et al. Flestolol, a titratable, short-acting beta adrenergic antagonist in the management of unstable angina. *J Am Coll Cardiol.* 1988; 11:233A. Abstract.
95. Yusuf S, Sleight P, Rossi P et al. Reduction in infarct size, arrhythmias and chest pain by early intravenous beta blockade in suspected acute myocardial infarction. *Circulation.* 1983; 67(Suppl I):32–41.
96. Norris RM, Clarke ED, Sammel NL et al. Protective effect of propranolol in threatened myocardial infarction. *Lancet.* 1978; 2:907-9.
97. Lawrence JR, Bone SI, Rogen AS et al. Fibrinolytic therapy in unstable angina pectoris: a controlled clinical trial. *Thromb Res.* 1980; 17:767-77.
98. Rentrop P, Blanke H, Karsch KR et al. Selective intracoronary thrombolysis in acute myocardial infarction and unstable angina pectoris. *Circulation.* 1981; 63:307-17.
99. Vetrovec GW, Leinbach RC, Gold H et al. Intracoronary thrombolysis in syndromes of unstable ischemia: angiographic and clinical results. *Am Heart J.* 1982; 104:946-52.
100. Ambrose JA, Hjemdahl-Monsen C, Borrico S et al. Quantitative and qualitative effects of intracoronary streptokinase in unstable angina and non-Q-wave infarction. *J Am Coll Cardiol.* 1987; 9:1156-65.
101. Gold HK, Johns JA, Leinbach RC et al. A randomized, blinded, placebo-controlled trial of recombinant human tissue-type plasminogen activator in patients with unstable angina pectoris. *Circulation.* 1987; 75:1192-99.
102. Gold HK, Johns JA, Leinbach RC et al. Thrombolytic therapy for unstable angina pectoris: rationale and results. *J Am Coll Cardiol.* 1987; 10:91B-95B.
103. Topol EJ, Nicklas JM, Kander NH et al. Coronary revascularization after intravenous tissue plasminogen activator for unstable angina pectoris: results of a randomized, double-blind, placebo-controlled trial. *Am J Cardiol.* 1988; 62:368-71.
104. Gotoh K, Minamino T, Katoh O et al. The role of intracoronary thrombus in unstable angina: angiographic assessment and thrombolytic therapy during ongoing anginal attacks. *Circulation.* 1988; 77:526-34.
105. Schreiber TL, Macina G, McNulty A et al. Urokinase plus heparin versus aspirin in unstable angina and non-Q-wave myocardial infarction. *Am J Cardiol.* 1989; 64:840-4.
106. Nicklas JM, Topol EJ, Kander N et al. Randomized, double-blind, placebo-controlled trial of tissue plasminogen activator in unstable angina. *J Am Coll Cardiol.* 1989; 13:434-41.
107. Ardissino D, Barberis P, De Servi S et al. Recombinant tissue-type plasminogen activator followed by heparin compared to heparin alone for refractory unstable angina pectoris. *Am J Cardiol.* 1990; 66:910-14.
108. Saran RK, Bhandari K, Narain VS et al. Intravenous streptokinase in the management of a subset of patients with unstable angina: a randomized controlled trial. *Int J Cardiol.* 1990; 28:209-13.
109. Williams DO, Topol EJ, Califf RM et al. Intravenous recombinant tissue-type plasminogen activator in patients with unstable angina pectoris: results of a placebo-controlled, randomized trial. *Circulation.* 1990; 82:376-83.
110. Serneri GGN, Genisini GF, Poggesi L et al. Effect of heparin, aspirin, or alteplase in reduction of myocardial ischaemia in refractory unstable angina. *Lancet.* 1990; 335:615-8.
111. Villa FP, Betriu A, Sanz G et al. Does thrombolysis improve outcome in unstable angina? A 1-year follow-up study. *Circulation.* 1990; 82(Suppl III):85. Abstract.
112. Brunelli C, Spallarossa P, Ghigliotti G et al. Thrombolysis in patients with unstable angina refractory to maximal medical therapy. *J Am Coll Cardiol.* 1988; 233A. Abstract.
113. Freeman MR, Langer A, Wilson RF et al. Randomized double blind placebo controlled trial of TPA vs heparin in unstable angina. *Circulation.* 1990; (Suppl III):84. Abstract.
114. Bar F, Vermeer F, Verheugt F et al. Thrombolytic therapy has no clinical benefit in patients with unstable angina: a placebo-controlled study in 159 patients. *J Am Coll Cardiol.* 1990; 17:45A. Abstract.
115. Ambrose JA, Alexopoulos D. Thrombolysis in unstable angina: will the beneficial effects of thrombolytic therapy in myocardial infarction apply to patients with unstable angina? *J Am Coll Cardiol.* 1989; 13:1666-71.
116. Rutherford JB. Unstable angina and thrombolysis. *Chest.* 1990; 97:156S-160S.
117. Maccioli GA, Lucas WJ, Norfleet EA. The intra-aortic balloon pump: a review. *J Cardiothorac Anesth.* 1988; 2:365-73.
118. Ryan TJ, Loop FD, Faxon DP et al. Guidelines for percutaneous transluminal coronary angioplasty: a report from the American College of Cardiology/American Heart Association Task Force on Assessment of Diagnostic and Therapeutic Procedures (Subcommittee on Percutaneous Transluminal Coronary Angioplasty). *J Am Coll Cardiol.* 1988; 12:529-45.
119. Faxon DP. Percutaneous coronary angioplasty in stable and unstable angina. *Cardiol Clin.* 1991; 9:99-113.
120. Habbab M, Haft J. Heparin resistance induced by intravenous nitroglycerine: a word of caution when both drugs are used concomitantly. *Arch Intern Med.* 1987; 147:857-60.
121. Lepor N, Amin D, Berberian M et al. Does nitroglycerin induce heparin resistance? *Clin Cardiol.* 1989; 12:432-4.
122. Becker RC, Carrao JM, Bovill EG et al. Intravenous nitroglycerin-induced heparin resistance: a qualitative antithrombin III abnormality. *Am Heart J.* 1990; 119:1254-61.
123. Stanek EJ, Nair RN, Munger MA. Nitroglycerin-induced heparin resistance. *Am Heart J.* 1991;121:1848-9. Letter.

Pathophysiology and treatment of Wilson's disease

Roberta M. Tankanow

Abstract: The pathophysiology, symptomatology, and treatment of Wilson's disease are reviewed, and new approaches to drug management are discussed.

Wilson's disease is a rare, autosomal recessive disorder that occurs between the ages of 6 and 60 years. Disturbances in copper metabolism may result in the accumulation of excess copper in the liver, the basal ganglia of the brain (lenticular degeneration), the kidneys, the cornea (Kayser-Fleischer rings), and other tissues. The diagnosis of Wilson's disease is frequently overlooked; nonspecific symptoms and multisystem involvement may mimic other disease states, such as neurologic and psychiatric disorders, and hemolytic anemia. Screening tests for Wilson's disease include 24-hour urinary copper levels, serum ceruloplasmin and copper assays, radioactive uptake of ^{64}Cu, and liver biopsy.

Current methods of therapy include the use of a chelating agent—penicillamine or trientine—for initial rapid decoppering. Penicillamine therapy has been associated with many adverse reactions, including worsening of the neurologic symptoms of the patient. Zinc is a useful agent for maintenance therapy. Investigational studies exploring the use of ammonium tetrathiomolybdate for initial rapid decoppering have shown promising results.

Unless it is recognized and treated, Wilson's disease can cause severe symptoms and, ultimately, death. Initial rapid decoppering with chelating agents, such as penicillamine and trientine, followed by lifelong maintenance therapy with zinc is the current method of treatment.

Index terms: Heavy metal antagonists; Hepatolenticular degeneration; Penicillamine; Trientine; Zinc
Clin Pharm. 1991; 10:839-49

Progressive lenticular degeneration was first described by Samuel A. Kinnier Wilson in 1912 as a rare, genetic, progressive, invariably fatal disease in young people. Wilson further described it as being manifested by spasticity, involuntary movements, dysphagia, dysarthria, and mental changes (depression, emotional lability) as well as softening of the lenticular nucleus, and finally, by cirrhosis of the liver.[1]

It is now known that hepatolenticular degeneration (disease affecting the liver and lenticular nucleus of the gray matter), or Wilson's disease, is an autosomal recessive metabolic disorder in which excessive copper accumulates primarily in the liver, the basal ganglia of the brain, and the kidneys. Because other systems are also involved, the disease may manifest as hemolytic anemia, arthritis, coagulopathies, amenorrhea, rickets, parathyroid disease, cardiac disease, and the classic Kayser-Fleischer rings in the cornea.[2-6]

The purpose of this article is to describe this complicated disease, to review current standards of therapy, and to examine new approaches in drug management.

Epidemiology

Wilson's disease typically occurs between the ages of 6 and 60 years, with the majority of patients becoming symptomatic during adolescence through the second and third decades of life. This disease is rare, affecting approximately 1 in 20,000 to 40,000 (as homozygotes). There is no propensity for gender, race, or geographic region. However, the carrier frequency (heterozygotes) may be 1 in 100.[7,8] Both parents of a patient are obligatory carriers of the abnormal gene, but they are not affected by the disease. The patient who is affected is homozygous abnormal.[9]

Pathophysiology

The disturbance of copper metabolism in Wilson's disease is caused by two mechanisms: (1) a reduction in biliary excretion of copper, and (2) a reduction in the rate of incorporation of copper into ceruloplasmin, a plasma protein and enzyme.[3] Excessive copper accumulates in the liver either chronically, causing few symptoms, or acutely, causing severe liver damage that often results in death. Levels of circulating non-ceruloplasmin-bound copper in the plasma are elevated, causing increased copper excretion through the kidneys and creating deposits of copper in various extrahepatic tissues. Copper deposition may be noted in the cornea (Kayser-Fleischer rings), the brain (especially the basal ganglia, manifested as lenticular degeneration), the kidneys (renal tubular damage), and muscles, bones, and joints.

The basic biochemical defect of the disease is still unknown. It has been demonstrated that the gene for

Roberta M. Tankanow, M.S., is Clinical Pharmacist, Investigational Drug Service, University of Michigan Hospitals, and Clinical Assistant Professor, College of Pharmacy, University of Michigan.

Address reprint requests to Ms. Tankanow at the University of Michigan Hospitals, Department of Pharmacy Services, 1500 East Medical Center Drive, Room B2D301/0008, Ann Arbor, MI 48109-0008.

Adapted from an article that appeared in the December 1990 issue of the *Michigan Drug Letter,* a publication of the Department of Pharmacy Services, University of Michigan Medical Center, Ann Arbor.

This is **article 680-204-9128** in the **ASHP Continuing Education System**; it qualifies for 1.0 hour of continuing-education credit. See page 877 for learning objectives and test questions.

Wilson's disease is assigned to chromosome 13. Several chromosome 13 DNA markers have been linked with the locus for the red blood cell enzyme esterase D. This discovery could be useful in detecting heterozygous individuals and in making prenatal and presymptomatic diagnoses.[10-12]

Normally, the body contains 70–100 mg of copper, with a balance between intestinal absorption and biliary excretion. On a daily basis, approximately 50% of the usual copper intake of 1 ± 0.4 mg is absorbed and 50% is excreted through the biliary pathway.[3,13,14] Minute amounts are detected in the urine.

Most of the copper that is intestinally absorbed is initially bound to albumin, transported through the portal blood, and stored in the liver. Smaller amounts of copper are bound to amino acids. In plasma, more than 90% of the copper is bound to ceruloplasmin, a blue α_2-globulin glycoprotein, which contains 0.3% copper. Ceruloplasmin is synthesized in the liver and incorporates copper after the metal ion permeates the hepatic cells. The mechanism of transfer of copper from the liver to other tissues is unclear. Ceruloplasmin or albumin may assume this role. Copper is distributed throughout the body in the liver, brain, heart, kidneys, lungs, intestine, spleen, endocrine glands, muscle, and bone.[15] Bile is the major pathway for excretion of copper.[1,3,15] In healthy individuals, only small amounts of copper (about 0.04 mg/day) are excreted in the urine.

In about 95% of patients with Wilson's disease, ceruloplasmin levels are low, causing a decrease in the rate of incorporation of copper into ceruloplasmin; therefore, copper is mainly bound to albumin. Excess unbound copper in the body combines with cellular or molecular sulfhydryl, carboxyl, or amino groups, causing an interference with the structure or function of these molecules. As a result, the copper becomes a toxin that can (1) cause profound morphologic changes in mitochondria and peroxisomes in the hepatocytes, (2) affect the integrity of the plasma membrane, and (3) damage lysosomal membranes, causing leakage of copper and enzymes into the cytosol where further destruction occurs.[1]

Additionally, excess copper adversely affects many other cellular elements of the liver, erythrocytes, and compounds of the central nervous system, including enzymes, polysomes, cell membranes, and mitochondria. Copper may suddenly be released from the liver in large amounts as a result of copper-induced hepatic necrosis. Rapid entry of this quantity of copper ions into the bloodstream results in hemolytic anemia.[1]

Symptomatology

The diagnosis of Wilson's disease is frequently overlooked because the symptoms are often nonspecific and can mimic other disease states.[11] The disease can simulate neurologic disorders, psychiatric disorders, viral hepatitis, chronic active hepatitis, cirrhosis of the liver, hemolytic anemia, and renal osteodystrophy.[16-19] Since the disease affects so many different organ systems and has many modes of presentation, diagnosis is often difficult. Because of the hepatic involvement, older patients (>20 years) are often misdiagnosed as having subacute viral hepatitis, postnecrotic cirrhosis, juvenile cirrhosis, or cryptogenic cirrhosis.[9] If Wilson's disease is treated early, its course can be diminished and reversed; if it is left untreated, death may occur.

Hepatic Changes. In the prepubertal patient, the most common symptoms of Wilson's disease are related to the liver and include jaundice, anorexia, nausea, lassitude, abdominal pain, weight loss, fluid retention, bruising and bleeding, and hemolytic crises. It is important to rule out Wilson's disease if these early hepatic symptoms occur in children because it is the most frequent cause of acute liver disease in this age group.[3,20,21] In children, hemolytic anemia may accompany liver failure, producing a mortality of 60–80%.[9,22,23]

Acute and chronic symptoms of liver disease caused by Wilson's disease may initially be jaundice, vomiting, malaise, and hypersplenism.[3,6,7] Nazer and coworkers[6] analyzed 27 symptomatic patients to determine the early manifestations of Wilson's disease. The mean age of the patients was 15 years (range, 6–33 years). Lethargy and anorexia (70%), jaundice (56%), and abdominal pain (48%) were the most common symptoms noted. Other physical signs included hepatomegaly (81%), splenomegaly (70%), Kayser-Fleischer rings (74%), ascites (48%), and spider nevi (30%). Twenty-two percent of the patients had a history of progressive intellectual deterioration. The duration of symptoms preceding diagnosis ranged from 5 days to 3 years (mean, 10.5 months). Biochemical evidence of hepatic involvement included anemia; 39% of patients had a hemoglobin concentration of <10 g/dL. All patients had an elevated bilirubin concentration, >506 μmol/L; an elevated aspartate aminotransferase concentration, >710 IU/L; and an increased prothrombin time, 49 seconds. Serum ceruloplasmin levels were low in 84% of the patients but normal in the other 16%.

Spontaneous remissions of liver disease may occur during the course of this disease, along with exacerbations and infections.[9] Heterotopic or orthotopic liver transplantation may be an option for those patients with fulminant hepatic failure.[18] This procedure should correct the hepatic-based metabolic defect of Wilson's disease. Transplantation allows for rapid cupriuresis, which results in correction of biochemical abnormalities and relief of symptoms.

Neurologic Changes. Neurologic symptoms of Wilson's disease occur in about one third of patients, with some overlapping hepatic and psychiatric histories.[8,24-26] Neurologic symptoms are more prevalent after puberty and may initially include a speech defect, drooling, and movement disorders, such as tremors, ataxia, rigidity, ballistic movements, dystonia, bradykinesia, and hypokinesia.[2] Occasionally, Babinski's sign is observed and abdominal reflexes are absent. Personality or mood changes and depression often accompany the neurologic signs.[24] Patients may be misdiagnosed and treated for depression, panic attacks, personality disorders, psychiatric episodes, multiple sclerosis, and basal ganglia disorders.[26] Seizures have rarely been reported.[27]

Thirty-one patients (mean age at onset, 21 ± 5 years) with Wilson's disease initially manifested symptoms of dysarthria (97%), dystonia (65%), dysdiadochokinesia (impairment of the power to perform rapidly alternating movements) (58%), rigidity (52%), gait and postural abnormalities (42%), and tremor (32%).[26] Magnetic resonance imaging (MRI) confirmed lesions in the caudate, putamen, subcortical white matter, midbrain, and pons. Some of these patients were treated initially for "psychiatric disturbances."[26]

Of particular interest is a report of late-onset neurologic involvement in a patient at the age of 51 years; the diagnosis of Wilson's disease was made at age 58 years.[25] Kayser-Fleischer rings, which are usually present with neurologic signs, were absent in this patient. Initially, the patient developed hand tremor, hepatosplenomegaly (age 51 years), loss of finger dexterity (age 52 years), gradual dysphagia (age 57 to 58 years), gait impairment, urinary incontinence, irritability, and mood lability. The serum ceruloplasmin concentration was low (14 mg/dL; normal range, 25–35 mg/dL), and the urinary copper excretion rate was high (703 μg/24 hours; normal rate, <40 μg/24 hours).

Hemolytic Anemia. Hemolytic anemia in Wilson's disease results from oxidative damage to the erythrocytes by copper released from tissues into the plasma.[22,28] In Wilson's disease, copper accumulates and is trapped in the liver; this causes cellular necrosis and a release of the ceruloplasmin-unbound copper into the circulation. This unbound copper enters the erythrocyte membrane and generates oxygen radicals and lipid peroxidases. Finally, hemolysis and methemoglobinemia ensue.

Clinical features of hemolytic anemia include diarrhea, weakness, malaise, nausea, anorexia, weight loss, abdominal pain, and rapid onset of jaundice.[22,28] Patients with Wilson's disease who have hemolysis tend to have low ceruloplasmin levels and extremely high urine and serum copper levels. In those patients without hemolysis, the ceruloplasmin level may be low, urinary copper levels are high, and serum copper values are low to normal.[23,28]

Ocular Changes. The eye is an important target organ for deposits of excess copper, resulting in sunflower cataracts (multicolor, spoke-like deposits) (15–20% of patients) and Kayser-Fleischer rings.[1,3,29] These two ocular signs rarely affect vision. Kayser-Fleischer rings may initially appear as a crescent in the superior corneal quadrant, with progression to completely circumferential, opaque, granular deposits of golden or greenish-brown. The deposits are localized in the Descemet's membrane at the limbus of the cornea.

Kayser-Fleischer rings are present in nearly all patients with neurologic symptoms and in most patients with hepatic involvement. However, they are not unique to patients with Wilson's disease; they have also been reported in patients with primary biliary cirrhosis and in patients with other liver diseases associated with massive hepatic copper accumulation.[3] Visualization with the naked eye is sometimes possible; however, most of the confirmations must be made with a slit-lamp examination. Chelation therapy with penicillamine causes the Kayser-Fleischer rings to disappear or decrease in size or intensity.[3]

Diagnostic Tests

Screening for Wilson's disease involves several laboratory tests, such as the 24-hour urinary copper. The presence of large amounts of copper in the urine (>100 μg/24 hours) can aid in the diagnosis of Wilson's disease. It is important to collect the urine in copper-free containers and to perform accurate measurements.[7] Another test involves serum ceruloplasmin assays. However, not every patient with Wilson's disease has a low ceruloplasmin level (children may have normal levels), so the diagnostic value of this test is limited. Additionally, ceruloplasmin levels may be elevated secondary to hepatitis, inflammation, neoplastic disease, acute infection, estrogen administration (oral contraceptives), or pregnancy.[1] Wilson's disease cannot be excluded if the serum ceruloplasmin concentration is >20 mg/dL (noted in 5% of patients). It is uncommon, though, for a patient with Wilson's disease to have a serum ceruloplasmin concentration >30 mg/dL.

Because liver function test results can be variable and are generally not diagnostic, a liver biopsy to assay copper content may be more useful. Copper distribution in the liver is uneven; thus, an appropriate sample size of parenchymal tissue (>5 mg or 5–10 mm of needle biopsy core) must be obtained.[3] However, not all patients with a high liver copper content (>300 μg/g dry weight) have Wilson's disease. The copper accumulation may be caused by another hepatic disease. When liver disease is present in the patient with Wilson's disease, serum copper and ceruloplasmin levels, 24-hour urinary copper measurements, and a slit-lamp examination of the eyes are standard diagnostic procedures.

Another test for the diagnosis of Wilson's disease is the demonstration of negligible incorporation of radioactive copper (^{64}Cu) into ceruloplasmin. The radioactive copper may be administered either orally or intravenously. Blood samples are then drawn at various intervals during the first 24 hours, at 24 hours, and at 48 hours. Healthy volunteers show a steady secondary rise in radioactive copper counts in the plasma from 4 to 48 hours as the radioactive copper appears in the newly synthesized ceruloplasmin. In patients with Wilson's disease, after the initial peak, the counts progressively decline over 48 hours.[30]

When a patient is diagnosed as having Wilson's disease, all family members should be screened so that prophylactic treatment can be started at once, if necessary.[3,6] If serum ceruloplasmin and urine copper levels are normal and Kayser-Fleischer rings are absent, the patient probably does not have Wilson's disease. However, an occasional affected sibling may still be missed. Serial 24-hour urine studies every two years may be one method of detecting that occasional patient. Table 1 shows a comparison in copper measurements between healthy individuals and patients with Wilson's disease.[3,7]

Therapeutic Management

Therapy for Wilson's disease may be divided into four main categories: initial decoppering, maintenance therapy, treatment during pregnancy, and treatment of the asymptomatic sibling.

Initial Decoppering

For symptomatic patients, the initial decoppering process is critical. The goal of initial decoppering therapy is to quickly lower plasma copper levels and to produce a negative copper balance (more negative than –0.15 mg/day) without inducing serious adverse effects. The agent that has FDA-approved labeling for this purpose is penicillamine.

Table 1.
Copper Laboratory Values in Adults[3,7]

Laboratory Test	Normal	Presymptomatic	Symptomatic
Serum ceruloplasmin (mg/dL)	25–35	1–5	1–5[a]
Non-ceruloplasmin-bound plasma copper (μg/dL)	10–15	15–25	25–100
Urinary copper (μg/24 hours)			
Untreated	<40	40–500	100–1000
On penicillamine	100–600	?	1500–3000
Liver copper (μg/g dry weight)	20–50	>150 (?)	200–3000
Incorporation of ^{64}Cu into ceruloplasmin at 24 hours[b]			
Oral ^{64}Cu: ratio of radioactivity in ceruloplasmin at 24 hours and peak serum radioactivity at 1–2 hours	0.8–1.2	0.1–0.3	0.1–0.3
IV ^{64}Cu: % of dose incorporated	>4	<1	<1

[a] 10% of patients with Wilson's disease have a low to normal value.

[b] ^{64}Cu into ceruloplasmin test: Normal patients show a steady secondary rise in counts in the plasma as the ^{64}Cu is incorporated into ceruloplasmin. In patients with Wilson's disease, the counts progressively fall, with no secondary rise. This value is the fraction of ^{64}Cu per milliliter of serum, multiplied by 10^6. The height of the initial peak is proportional to the rate and extent of the intestinal absorption of copper, and is inversely related to the volume of distribution of the administered copper and its rate of uptake by the liver.

Penicillamine. Penicillamine, a penicillin derivative, was first introduced in 1956 by John Walshe as a chelating agent for patients with Wilson's disease.[3] It is a sulfhydryl-containing amino acid (D-β,β-dimethylcysteine), which is produced by the hydrolytic degradation of penicillin. Penicillamine chelates many heavy metals, such as copper, iron, lead, and mercury, to form stable complexes, which are then renally excreted. The chelation of copper occurs with the combination of two molecules of penicillamine with one atom of the metal. One gram of penicillamine will result in the elimination of about 2 mg of copper. Penicillamine is an excellent chelating agent that possesses many key properties: (1) it is water soluble and resistant to metabolic degradation; (2) it easily binds to metals and their storage sites; (3) it is active at the pH of body fluids; and (4) when it forms complexes with other metals, the complex of penicillamine and the metal is less toxic than the free metallic ion.[31,32]

Chelated copper is then excreted in the urine.[7] In some patients, however, the nontoxic copper complex is stored in the liver. Liver biopsies of patients after long-term penicillamine use may reveal liver copper levels that are low, high, or unchanged from initial therapy. However, the chelated or complexed copper is a less toxic compound than the unbound copper ion, so the patient's clinical course improves.[33-37]

In addition to the chelation process, penicillamine has reduction–oxidation potential, thereby reducing the affinity of copper for proteins and polypeptides and more effectively removing copper from tissues. Penicillamine also induces the synthesis of the protein metallothionein in the liver. The combination of this protein with copper is nontoxic.[7]

The efficacy of penicillamine in treating Wilson's disease is well established. Deiss et al.[38] reported five patients with Wilson's disease (age range, 8–18 years) who were treated with penicillamine (dosage, 1.5 g daily) for up to 13 years. Four of the five patients were neurologically incapacitated before therapy. Tremors progressively lessened over 18–24 months and completely disappeared after three years of therapy. All five patients showed a decrease in serum copper levels (from a mean concentration of 58 μg/dL to 13 μg/dL), and four of five patients showed an increase in urine copper levels (from a mean value of 662 μg/24 hours to 783 μg/24 hours) during the first few weeks of therapy. Sensitivity reactions to penicillamine (fever, rash, leukopenia) were noted during the first month of therapy in three of five patients. Penicillamine was temporarily withdrawn, and corticosteroids were given for one to two weeks. Penicillamine was restarted without a recurrence of these symptoms.

Penicillamine therapy was instituted in 33 patients (age range, 10–46 years) with Wilson's disease (eight were asymptomatic) at a dosage of 1–4 g daily.[39] Twenty-three of the patients showed some form of neurologic symptoms (tremors, rigidity, choreoathetoid movements, drooling). In five patients, neurologic improvements did not always begin immediately. In four patients, the tremors actually worsened. Two patients showed hepatic manifestations (cirrhosis). Liver copper concentrations were initially high (range, 463–1561 μg/g) in two patients. A significant decrease in liver copper levels was noted in five patients, and Kayser-Fleischer rings disappeared in seven patients. Total serum copper levels erratically decreased in most patients. Adverse drug reactions were common and included rashes, leukopenia, thrombocytopenia, nausea, and fever. Fourteen patients eventually died. Death was attributed to a number of causes, including noncompliance, subtherapeutic doses, infection, and hepatic insufficiency.

Penicillamine is given orally and is well absorbed by the gastrointestinal tract. Peak plasma concentrations occur between 60 and 130 minutes after oral administration. Approximately 80% of penicillamine is protein bound; 6% is unbound drug. The remainder is present as two inactive hepatic metabolites, D-penicillamine disulfide and penicillamine cysteine disulfide.[31,32]

The recommended starting dosage of penicillamine in adults is 250 mg orally four times a day. Penicillamine should be taken on an empty stomach (30 minutes before or at least two hours after a meal), because food has been shown to decrease its absorption.[1,31,32] This dose may produce a large cupriuresis of about 2–10 mg/24 hours. With continued therapy, the urine copper levels slowly decrease; after six months of therapy, urinary excretion may be as low as 0.5 mg/day. Treatment with penicillamine or some other anticopper agent continues indefinitely.[7] It has been hypothesized that the dosage of penicillamine should be gradually increased to achieve a less dramatic initial cupriuresis.[40] This approach may prevent the neurologic worsening (possibly due to an elevation in brain copper levels) that is sometimes seen after initial penicillamine therapy. Suggested dosages are 250 mg daily, increased by 250 mg/day every four days until a 24-hour urinary copper level of about 2 mg is reached. When therapy is initiated, urinary copper excretion must be monitored weekly and the dosage of penicillamine adjusted according to copper losses.[3,7] When the desired cupriuresis is achieved, monitoring can be less frequent. Unfortunately, in patients with severe neurologic symptoms or in patients with liver failure, it may take from one to six months for the beneficial clinical effects of penicillamine to appear.[3]

The dosage of penicillamine in children has not been thoroughly studied, but a dosage of 500 mg/day in two to four divided doses for children 5–11 years of age has been suggested.[9] A dosage of 20 mg/kg/day in two to four divided doses has been recommended for children less than five years of age.[1,9]

It has been suggested that many of the penicillamine-related adverse reactions are due to the chemical structure of penicillamine, specifically the active sulfhydryl group.[41] Penicillamine also has FDA-approved labeling for use in patients with rheumatoid arthritis, and most experience with its use is in this patient population. The overall frequency of adverse reactions in 259 patients with rheumatoid arthritis who were treated with penicillamine was 58%; 27% of patients discontinued therapy because of adverse effects.[42]

Hypersensitivity reactions, manifested by skin rash, hives, and fever, occur in about 20% of patients receiving penicillamine. These reactions are commonly seen in the first 7–21 days of therapy.[1] They can occur even at low dosages of 250 mg/day. The skin eruptions subside when the drug is discontinued. If skin eruptions occur, penicillamine therapy can be reinstituted at a reduced dose and gradually increased as therapeutically indicated to prevent recurrence. Corticosteroids (prednisone 20–30 mg/day) may be given concurrently with penicillamine for one to two weeks to prevent these types of reactions.[1,42,43] Penicillamine should be administered cautiously to patients who are allergic to penicillin, although cross-sensitivity is rare.[44]

Penicillamine appears to interact with connective tissue constituents, causing an inability of the soluble collagen precursors to form insoluble collagen fibers. This reaction causes a decrease in collagen production, thus increasing the fragility of subcutaneous tissue.[1,42,43] The cutaneous lesions that occur may take months or years to become apparent. Additional cutaneous lesions that are seen with penicillamine therapy are outlined in Table 2.[1,7,41-51]

Some adverse effects that occur with penicillamine therapy are life threatening (especially the autoimmune disorders, such as lupus and Goodpasture's syndrome) and require prompt discontinuation of the drug. Others (such as the gastrointestinal and some of the cutaneous effects) subside with continued treatment or with a decreased penicillamine dosage. Penicillamine induces the formation of antinuclear factor with or without a lupus-like syndrome. It is a potent inducer of autoantibodies and autoimmune disease.[50] Table 2 provides a more comprehensive list of adverse reactions.

The adverse effects of penicillamine are often the cause of dosage reduction or discontinuation of therapy. Worsening of the neurologic syndrome occurs in 10–50% of neurologically affected patients on initial therapy.[1,7,40] Brewer and colleagues[40] reported a 22-year-old, newly diagnosed patient with Wilson's disease whose neurologic manifestations became worse after treatment with penicillamine 250 mg four times a day for six weeks.[40] His drooling worsened, and he was unable to speak or sit. Penicillamine therapy was continued because the patient had a substantial negative copper balance. The patient developed a severe seizure disorder over the next few months, which required treatment with antiepileptic medications. Penicillamine therapy was discontinued and zinc acetate therapy was started. Twenty months after diagnosis (after about nine months of zinc therapy), the patient was able to walk and his speech improved; however, his neurologic status was not substantially changed from when he was first diagnosed.

Table 2.
Adverse Effects of Penicillamine[1,7,41–51]

Organ System	Effect
Hematologic	Thrombocytopenia
	Leukopenia
	Aplastic anemia
	Agranulocytosis
Renal	Proteinuria
	Nephrotic syndrome
	Goodpasture's syndrome
Gastrointestinal	Nausea, vomiting
	Anorexia
	Diarrhea
	Dyspepsia
Ocular	Retinal hemorrhages
	Conjunctival inflammation
	Follicular conjunctivitis
	Optic neuritis
Pulmonary	Bronchoalveolitis
	Dyspnea
Taste	Dysgeusia
Autoimmune and allergic	Myasthenia gravis
	Thyroiditis
	Sjögren's syndrome
	Thrombotic thrombocytopenic purpura
	Lupus erythematosus or lupus-like syndrome
	Pemphigus
	Dermatomyositis
Rheumatologic	Acute polyarthritis
Skin	Dermatrophy
	Elastosis perforans serpiginosa
	Macular or papular rash
	Urticaria
	Lichen planus
	Aphthous stomatitis
	Psoriasiform dermatitis
	Alopecia
	Dry skin/scaling
	Nail changes
	Hypertrichosis

Of 25 patients with pretherapy neurologic symptoms, about 50% reported that some of their symptoms worsened after initial treatment with penicillamine (therapy ranged from 6 months to 26 years).[7] Penicillamine did effectively decopper patients, but the mobilization of hepatic copper may have temporarily increased metal levels in the brain and blood.[7,40] Penicillamine causes pyridoxine deficiency, which may mimic some of the neurologic manifestations of Wilson's disease; thus, it is important to provide supplementary oral pyridoxine hydrochloride 25 mg/day in adults and 12.5 mg/day in children. The mechanism appears to be that penicillamine forms a thiazolidine with pyridoxine. This reaction may be precipitated by infection, pregnancy, or a growth spurt.[50]

Trientine. If penicillamine therapy is discontinued because of serious adverse reactions, the chelating agent trientine hydrochloride (triethylenetetramine dihydrochloride, or trien; Syprine, formerly Cuprid, Merck Sharp & Dohme) may be used for initial decoppering. Although the mechanism of action for trientine is not completely elucidated, it appears to be different from that for penicillamine.[1] Sarkar et al.[52] demonstrated that trientine competes for copper that is bound to serum albumin. Penicillamine mobilizes copper in the liver, whereas trientine does not enter the liver. Both agents can mobilize copper in the kidneys, resulting in increased urinary excretion. Trientine seems to have a better ability to mobilize copper in untreated patients than in those who have been previously treated with penicillamine.[53] The urinary copper excretion induced by penicillamine is associated with a decline in the concentration of copper and radiolabeled copper in the serum. Alternatively, trientine causes the serum copper concentration to rise; the concentration returns to baseline after five hours.[54]

Only a few reports describe efficacy and toxicities of trientine therapy for Wilson's disease. Walshe[55] studied 20 patients with Wilson's disease; 11 of them had developed penicillamine intolerance (rash, severe neutropenia, arthropathy, and immune complex nephritis). Three patients with immune complex nephritis were changed to trientine therapy and recovered. Nine patients with neurologic symptoms were treated with trientine hydrochloride 1600 mg daily. Seven of the nine showed considerable improvement, including the disappearance of Kayser-Fleischer rings and the disappearance of lesions in the anterior brain. Long-term treatment with trientine predisposed patients to an iron deficiency anemia. The mean serum iron concentration before treatment was 17 μmol/L; it fell to a mean concentration of 11 μmol/L at follow-up. Eight patients on trientine therapy were treated with iron, and the serum iron concentration rose from a mean value of 8.6 to 17.6 μmol/L. Two patients who developed lupus-like syndromes after penicillamine therapy showed a similar toxicity after trientine therapy.[55]

Trientine is not useful for patients who fail to respond to penicillamine therapy.[50] It is used in patients who cannot tolerate the adverse effects of penicillamine. The recommended dosage of trientine hydrochloride for the management of Wilson's disease is 250 mg taken four times a day on an empty stomach; however, dosages of 1.6–2.4 g/day have also been safely used. In children less than 10 years old, the initial dosage is 250 mg twice daily.[1] Pyridoxine supplementation is not needed with trientine therapy.

The lupus-like syndrome seen with penicillamine may recur when patients are switched to trientine.[56] Because clinical experience with trientine is limited, little information is available about adverse reactions. Hypersensitivity reactions have not yet been reported with trientine. Iron deficiency anemia has been reported with its use, and iron supplements may be required. However, iron supplements should not be administered at the same time as the trientine dose because of the ability of iron to decrease the absorption of trientine.[53,57] Other adverse events associated with trientine therapy that were reported in four patients with biliary cirrhosis were anorexia, abdominal pain, skin rash, and rhabdomyolysis. In addition, Scheinberg and coworkers[57] noted moderate sideroblastic anemia in one patient.

Ammonium Tetrathiomolybdate. Patients who are intolerant to penicillamine or trientine still require therapy for rapid decoppering if they are symptomatic. Ammonium tetrathiomolybdate has been used to treat copper poisoning in sheep. Ammonium tetrathiomolybdate appears to block the intestinal absorption of copper by forming a tight, insoluble complex with the metal. This binding occurs immediately, causing a moderate negative copper balance.[7,58] Ammonium tetrathiomolybdate combines with albumin- and ceruloplasmin-bound copper, inactivating the toxic metal.[7,59] Patients have been treated with oral ammonium tetrathiomolybdate in dosages of 60–150 mg/day. Walshe[58] studied 12 patients who received ammonium tetrathiomolybdate 30 mg twice a day and reported responses (rise in total plasma copper concentrations) within hours of administration. Peak effects were reached in two to three days. In seven of eight previously untreated patients, a moderate rise occurred in the 24-hour urinary copper excretion. In the other four patients (concurrently treated with trientine or penicillamine), a 50% decline occurred in the rate of copper excretion. Radiolabeled copper measurements showed a delayed clearance of copper from the plasma and a delayed uptake of copper into the liver in the two patients who were studied using ^{64}Cu assays.[58]

Brewer and coworkers[60] proposed the use of ammonium tetrathiomolybdate as initial decoppering therapy for neurologically affected patients for eight weeks, with a transition to zinc acetate, penicillamine, or trientine at lower doses for maintenance therapy.[60] Pilot studies in six patients have shown no toxic effects, neurologic worsening, or lack of efficacy. Ammonium tetrathiomolybdate was initiated in the first patient at 10 mg orally three times daily with meals and escalated every three to four days until a daily dosage of 150 mg (divided into six doses per day, three with meals and three without) was attained. Three patients received higher dosages (180 mg/day) to quickly achieve a higher plasma copper level.

After six weeks of initial decoppering with ammonium tetrathiomolybdate, patients were concomitantly treated with zinc acetate for two weeks. Ammonium tetrathiomolybdate was then discontinued while zinc acetate therapy was continued.[60] The blockade of copper absorption was immediate, and it took a mean of 16.7 days to obtain complete neutralization of plasma non-ceruloplasmin-bound copper (total plasma copper minus ceruloplasmin-bound copper). No patients exhibited neurologic worsening or adverse reactions. All patients exhibited a significant decrease in 24-hour urinary copper levels with a mean decrease from 285 to 169 μg/24 hours by the end of the ammonium tetrathiomolybdate therapy. Animal studies demonstrated adverse effects on epiphyseal fusion[58,61]; however, this finding was probably due to copper deficiency because the animals were not supplemented with copper. Copper-supplemented animals have shown no adverse effects from ammonium tetrathiomolybdate. Therefore, ammonium tetrathiomolybdate should be used with some caution in children until further experience is gained.

Zinc. Zinc may also be considered for initial therapy of symptomatic patients. Its advantage is that it is nontoxic and does not produce the neurologic worsening frequently seen with penicillamine.[62] However, because of its slow onset of action, the disease can worsen before a therapeutic effect is seen, and it is not an optimal agent for use in patients who may benefit from more rapid decoppering, such as neurologically affected patients.[40] This disadvantage must be weighed against the syndrome of neurologic worsening induced by penicillamine.

Maintenance Therapy

The decoppering effects of oral zinc therapy were first noted in 1977 by Brewer and colleagues[63] in patients who were treated for sickle cell anemia. Treated patients had evidence of a copper deficiency with decreased serum ceruloplasmin levels.[63] This discovery led to clinical trials of oral zinc acetate in patients with Wilson's disease.[64,65] Interest in pursuing studies with zinc was enhanced by the agent's low potential for toxicity and the numerous adverse reactions to penicillamine therapy.[40-51]

Zinc appears to induce the synthesis of metallothionein in the intestine. This protein has a higher affinity for copper than for zinc, so it blocks the gastrointestinal absorption of copper (endogenous or exogenous). The metallothionein–copper complex is excreted mainly in the stool. The onset of zinc in producing a negative copper balance is slow; one to three weeks may be necessary for full induction of intestinal metallothionein.[7,64,65]

Zinc is useful as maintenance therapy in all patients with Wilson's disease. It is also useful in patients who have been decoppered with other agents but have had adverse reactions that prevent further treatment with the agent.[66,67] In three studies, maintenance zinc therapy produced control of the patients' symptoms with no worsening of the disease and no known adverse reactions.[68-70] Some of these patients have been treated for as long as eight years.[70]

The effective dose of zinc acetate to control copper balance was established by Hill and coworkers[14] in a study of 14 patients with Wilson's disease. The goal of therapy was to control copper balance so that patients were maintained in a neutral to negative copper balance state (from net absorption of 0.25 mg to net elimination of more than 0.15 mg/day). The dose of zinc acetate that most effectively achieved this goal was 50 mg of elemental zinc three times a day on an empty stomach (the effectiveness of zinc is decreased when taken with food). All patients who were evaluated had a negative or neutral copper balance; there was an overall mean negative balance of -0.23 ± 0.26 mg copper/day with the duration of therapy ranging from 1 month to 18 months.[14]

Further work by Brewer and colleagues[71] on 34 patients confirmed that 50 mg three times per day is effective for maintenance therapy. To date, 45 patients have been treated with this dosage and 22 of 45 have remained on zinc therapy for five years or longer. Five of these patients experienced gastric irritation, which later subsided when zinc was taken an hour after breakfast rather than an hour before breakfast. No patient has had a recurrence or worsening of symptoms of the disease. Brewer and colleagues[71] also studied the efficacy of zinc at lower daily dosages (100 mg/day and 75 mg/day) and found them to be effective. However, they concluded that the higher dosage of 150 mg/day provided more uniform zinc levels and would safeguard against occasional noncompliance (or a missed dose) that could result in subtherapeutic zinc levels.

The monitoring procedures for patients on zinc maintenance therapy include 24-hour urinary copper, non-ceruloplasmin-bound plasma copper, oral ^{64}Cu uptake (1.2% or less of the administered dose defines adequate effective therapy), and other appropriate clinical studies. A copper balance of more than +0.25 mg/day indicates inadequate control. After zinc doses are stabilized, the 24-hour urinary zinc determination averages 5–6 mg/24 hours. Noncompliance with therapy is suspected if the 24-hour urinary zinc value is <3.0 mg/dL. The non-ceruloplasmin-bound copper level is an important measurement because unbound plasma copper appears to cause most of the symptomatology of Wilson's disease. The normal range of non-ceruloplasmin-bound plasma copper is 10–15 µg/dL. The goal of zinc therapy is to reduce non-ceruloplasmin-bound copper to at least 25 µg/dL.[68,71]

Zinc is considered to be relatively nontoxic in low doses. The adult daily intake of elemental zinc in a normal diet is 10 to 15 mg. The ingestion of larger amounts (>2 g/day) may produce vomiting, abdominal cramps, and diarrhea. Zinc acetate (36% elemental zinc) is used more often than zinc sulfate (23% elemental zinc) because it is less irritating to the stomach when taken without food. Additional symptoms of elemental zinc toxicity after ingestion of 45 g include dehydration, electrolyte imbalance, lethargy, dizziness, and muscular incoordination.[72,73] However, dosages of elemental zinc 250 mg per day for six weeks in healthy volunteers have resulted in mild impairment of lymphocyte and neutrophil functions and a potentially harmful increase in the low-density lipoprotein (LDL)/high-density lipoprotein (HDL) cholesterol ratio.[73,74] A transitory effect on reducing HDL cholesterol has also been seen in male (but not female) patients with Wilson's disease who were treated with zinc acetate. Transient decreases in HDL cholesterol levels occur initially at dosages of 150 mg of elemental zinc per day, but levels return to normal after six months.[73,75]

Mild elevations of serum amylase and lipase have also been noted.[73] Pancreatic function does not appear to be affected, and the clinical importance of these alterations remains unclear. In rats, zinc administration caused hypocalcemia and possible bone resorption in the femoral epiphysis. Again, these results may have been due to copper deficiency, because the rats were not given copper supplements. Further research is needed to evaluate the clinical importance of these animal studies.[76,77]

Treatment during Pregnancy

Drug therapy with penicillamine or trientine during pregnancy has usually resulted in few to no adverse effects. Walshe[78] reported the treatment of 34 pregnant women who had Wilson's disease with either penicillamine or trientine. No fetal abnormalities were discovered, and the miscarriage rate was low.[78] However, reports describe two infants with unusual connective tissue changes (lax skin, hyperflexibility of the joints, vein fragility, varicosities, and impaired wound healing) born to women receiving penicillamine for cysteinuria (2 g/day) or rheumatoid arthritis (0.9 g/day).[79,80] Both infants subsequently died, one from septicemia and the other from unknown causes (although the infant had meconium peritonitis). The fetal abnormalities in these cases may have been linked to fetal copper deficiency caused by the penicillamine. Patients with rheumatoid arthritis or cysteinuria do not have large amounts of unbound copper to chelate. The penicillamine will cause a copper deficiency in patients who do not have Wilson's disease.[80] A case of reversible cutis laxa was reported in an infant born to a patient with Wilson's disease who was taking penicillamine 1.5 g/day. After two months of age, the child's skin appeared normal and physical and neurologic development improved.[81]

More recently, Walshe[82] reported 11 pregnancies in seven patients with Wilson's disease who were receiving trientine therapy. Eight of the 11 pregnancies resulted in normal deliveries. One infant was born with a chromosomal defect (isochromosome X); one pregnancy was therapeutically terminated because of noncompliance with trientine therapy, which resulted in severe tremors; and the third resulted in a miscarriage that was associated with a contraceptive coil. The children have been followed from three months to nine years with no adverse sequelae noted.[82] Because of the effect on human collagen tissue and potential teratogenicity, penicillamine and trientine should be used with extreme caution during pregnancy.[73,79,80]

Zinc acetate therapy (25 mg of elemental zinc twice daily, then 50 mg three times daily) has been continued in six pregnant patients who later delivered normal babies.[73] Data are continuing to accumulate to allow a more definitive conclusion as to whether zinc is completely safe during pregnancy.[73]

Pregnancy is not contraindicated in women with Wilson's disease unless there is severe hepatic dysfunction or hemolytic anemia. Women treated with penicillamine or trientine before pregnancy should remain on the medication at the lowest maintenance dosage that will control their copper balance.[1,73] Higher dosages of penicillamine (>1 g/day) may be associated with a greater incidence of fetal abnormalities.[1]

Treatment of the Presymptomatic Patient

The presymptomatic sibling of a symptomatic patient should be screened for Wilson's disease with the appropriate laboratory tests: 24-hour urinary copper levels, serum ceruloplasmin assays, slit-lamp examinations for Kayser-Fleischer rings, radiolabeled copper studies, and liver biopsy in any questionable case. The asymptomatic or presymptomatic patient may have only some of the signs and laboratory abnormalities of Wilson's disease. In a study by Walshe,[83] 90 families with at least one proven case of Wilson's disease were screened. Presymptomatic disease was diagnosed in 30 of the family members. Of 30, 11 had one or more abnormal findings, including Kayser-Fleischer rings, impaired uptake of ^{64}Cu in ceruloplasmin, and impaired copper metabolism. The diagnosis of Wilson's disease was finally made in 29 of 30 patients.[83]

Once diagnosed, prophylactic anticopper therapy can be initiated to prevent the patient from becoming symptomatic. This therapy must be continued for the rest of the patient's life.[1,7,83,84] The decoppering agents used to treat this patient population have included penicillamine, trientine, and zinc. Penicillamine or trientine hydrochloride can be used at a dosage of 250 mg four times daily on an empty stomach. The patient should be closely monitored for adverse effects. The neurologic worsening due to rapid decoppering with penicillamine is uncommon in the presymptomatic patient but has recently been reported in one patient.[85] Zinc acetate therapy can also be considered at a dosage of 50 mg (elemental zinc) three times daily taken on an empty stomach. In a study by Brewer and coworkers,[62] eight presymptomatic patients were successfully treated with zinc as the sole anticopper agent. Treatment duration ranged from 12 to 37 months.

Regardless of the drug being used, compliance should be carefully monitored. Discontinuation of medication may cause an increase in serum copper levels and can cause the patient to become symptomatic.[1,7]

A summary of the treatment of Wilson's disease is provided in Table 3.

Table 3.
Treatment of Wilson's Disease

Clinical Situation	Drug	Advantages	Disadvantages
Initial treatment			
Neurologic symptoms	Penicillamine	Rapid action	Neurologic worsening Toxicity
	Trientine	Rapid action	Lack of experience
	Zinc	Safety	Slow onset of action
Hepatic disease	Penicillamine	Rapid action	Toxicity
	Trientine	Rapid action	Lack of experience
	Zinc	Induction of hepatic metallothionein synthesis (toxic copper sequestration) Safety	Slow onset of action
Maintenance treatment	Zinc	Safety Large amount of data on copper balance and control	None so far
	Trientine		Lack of experience
	Penicillamine	Large amount of longitudinal experience	Toxicity
Presymptomatic	Zinc	Safety Large amount of data on copper balance and control	None so far
	Trientine		Lack of experience
	Penicillamine	Large amount of longitudinal experience	Toxicity Occasional induction of neurologic symptoms
Pregnancy	Penicillamine	Largest amount of experience	Toxicity Fetal penicillamine syndrome Teratogenic in animals
	Trientine		Lack of experience Teratogenic in animals
	Zinc	Safety	Limited experience

Derived from references 7, 8, 14, 38–40, 53, and 57.

Conclusion

Wilson's disease was once thought to be an invariably fatal disease affecting only a small portion of the population. It is now known that the progression of the disease can be halted if patients are diagnosed early and appropriate therapy is instituted. Once a case of Wilson's disease is identified, all members of that family should be screened for the disease with serum ceruloplasmin assays, 24-hour urinary copper excretion, liver biopsy, and ^{64}Cu uptake studies. Treatment for those individuals diagnosed as having Wilson's disease can then be initiated before symptoms occur. Appropriate initial decoppering therapy for symptomatic patients includes penicillamine, or trientine in patients who do not tolerate penicillamine. Zinc acetate should be considered as an alternative in patients for whom there is a concern of neurologic worsening or in patients who have experienced toxicity to penicillamine. Ongoing studies with ammonium tetrathiomolybdate have also shown promising results in rapidly lowering copper levels with minimal toxicity.

Zinc acetate therapy has been chosen by some physicians for maintaining a long-term negative copper balance once initial decoppering has been accomplished. The presymptomatic and the pregnant patient are two additional patient populations for which zinc therapy is useful because of its effectiveness and low toxicity profile. A key issue in all patients is compliance, because discontinuation of the treatment causes the patient to become symptomatic.

References

1. Scheinberg IH, Sternlieb I. Wilson's disease. In: Major problems in internal medicine. Vol 23. Philadelphia: Saunders; 1984:1-163.
2. Walshe JM. Wilson's disease: genetics and biochemistry: their relevance to therapy. *J Inherit Metab Dis.* 1983; Suppl 6:51-8.
3. Danks DM. Hereditary disorders of copper metabolism in Wilson's disease and Menke's disease. In: Stanbury JB, Wyngaarden JB, Frederickson DS et al., eds. The metabolic basis of inherited diseases. 5th ed. New York: McGraw-Hill; 1983:251-68.
4. Carpenter TO, Carnes DL, Anast CS. Hypothyroidism in Wilson's disease. *N Engl J Med.* 1983; 309:873-7.
5. Kuan P. Cardiac Wilson's disease. *Chest.* 1987; 4:579-83.
6. Nazer H, Ede RJ, Mowat AP et al. Wilson's disease: clinical presentation and use of prognostic index. *Gut.* 1986; 27:1377-81.
7. Brewer GJ, Yuzbasiyan-Gurkan V. Wilson's disease: an update with emphasis on new approaches to treatment. *Dig Dis.* 1989; 7:178-93.
8. Brewer GJ, Yuzbasiyan-Gurkan VA, Young AB. The treatment and diagnosis of Wilson's disease. *Curr Opin Neurol.* 1988; 1:302-6.
9. Sass-Kortsak A. Wilson's disease: a treatable liver disease in children. *Pediatr Clin North Am.* 1975; 22:963-84.
10. Bowcock AM, Farrer LA, Cavalli-Sforza LL et al. Mapping the WD locus to a cluster of linked polymorphic markers on chromosome 13. *Am J Hum Genet.* 1987; 41:27-35.
11. Frydman M, Bonne-Tamir B, Farrer LA et al. Assignment of the gene for WD to chromosome B: linkage to the esterase D locus. *Proc Natl Acad Sci.* 1985; 82:1819-21.
12. Yuzbasiyan-Gurkan VA, Brewer GJ, Boerwinkle E. Linkage of the Wilson's disease gene and polymorphic loci on chromosome 13 in N. American pedigrees. *Am J Hum Genet.* 1987: 41:A193.
13. Sternlieb I. Copper and the liver. *Gastroenterology.* 1980; 78:1615-28.
14. Hill GM, Brewer GJ, Prasad AS et al. Treatment of Wilson's disease with zinc. I. Oral zinc therapy regimens. *Hepatology.* 1987; 7:522-8.
15. Evans GW. Copper homeostasis in the mammalian system. *Physiol Rev.* 1973; 53:535-70.
16. Cartwright GE. Diagnosis of treatable Wilson's disease. *N Engl J Med.* 1978; 298:1347-50.
17. Spechler SJ, Koff RS. Wilson's disease: diagnostic difficulties in the patient with chronic hepatitis and hypoceruloplasminemia. *Gastroenterology.* 1980; 78:803-6.
18. Gur H, Aderka D, Finkelstein A et al. Fulminant Wilsonian hepatitis: difficulties in diagnosis and treatment. *Am J Gastroenterol.* 1988; 83:679-81.
19. McCullough A, Fleming CR, Thistle JL et al. Diagnosis of Wilson's disease presenting as fulminant hepatic failure. *Gastroenterology.* 1983; 84:161-7.
20. Perman JA, Werlin SL, Grand RJ et al. Laboratory measures of copper metabolism in the differentiation of chronic active hepatitis and Wilson's disease in children. *J Pediatr.* 1979; 94:564-8.
21. Nazer H, Ede RJ, Mowat AP et al. Wilson's disease in childhood. *Clin Pediatr.* 1983; 22:755-7.
22. Roche-Sicot J, Benhamou JP. Acute intravascular hemolysis and acute liver failure associated as a first manifestation of Wilson's disease. *Ann Intern Med.* 1977; 86:301-3.
23. Saito T. Presenting symptoms and natural history of Wilson's disease. *Eur J Pediatr.* 1987; 146:261-5.
24. Goldstein NP, Ewert JC, Randall RV et al. Psychiatric aspects of Wilson's disease: results of psychometric tests during long-term therapy. *Am J Psychiatry.* 1968; 124:1555-61.
25. Ross ME, Jacobson IM, Dienstag JL et al. Late-onset Wilson's disease with neurological involvement in the absence of Kayser-Fleischer rings. *Ann Neurol.* 1985; 17:411-3.
26. Starosta-Rubinstein S, Young AB, Kluink K et al. Clinical assessment of 31 patients with Wilson's disease. *Arch Neurol.* 1987; 44:365-70.
27. Smith CK, Mattson RH. Seizures in Wilson's disease. *Neurology.* 1967; 17:1121-3.
28. Forman SJ, Kumar KS, Redeker AG et al. Hemolytic anemia in Wilson's disease: clinical findings and biochemical mechanisms. *Am J Hematol.* 1980; 9:269-75.
29. Wiebers DO, Hollenhorst RW, Goldstein NP. The ophthalmologic manifestations of Wilson's disease. *Mayo Clin Proc.* 1977; 52:409-16.
30. Sternleib I, Scheinberg IH. The role of radiocopper in the diagnosis of Wilson's disease. *Gastroenterology.* 1979; 77:138-42.
31. Perrett D. The metabolism and pharmacology of D-penicillamine in man. *J Rheumatol.* 1981; 8(Suppl 7):41-50.
32. Wiesner RH, Dickson ER, Carlson GL et al. The pharmacokinetics of D-penicillamine in man. *J Rheumatol.* 1981; 8(Suppl 7):51-5.
33. Scheinberg IH, Sternlieb I, Schilsky M et al. Penicillamine may detoxify copper in Wilson's disease. *Lancet.* 1987; 2:95.
34. Mason J, McQuaid A, Pheiffer H. Can Wilson's disease patients be decoppered? *Lancet.* 1989; 1:1455.
35. Walshe JM. Wilson's disease patients can be decoppered. *Lancet.* 1989; 2:228.
36. Van den Hamer CJA, Hoogenraad TU. Copper deficiency in Wilson's disease. *Lancet.* 1989; 2:442.
37. Gibbs K, Walshe JM, Dening TR. Liver copper concentrations in Wilson's disease: effect of treatment with anti-copper agents. *J Gastroenterol Hepatol.* 1990; 5:420-4.
38. Deiss A, Lynch RE, Lee GR et al. Long-term therapy of Wilson's disease. *Ann Intern Med.* 1971; 75:57-65.
39. Sternlieb I, Scheinberg IH. Penicillamine therapy for hepatolenticular degeneration. *JAMA.* 1964; 189:748-54.
40. Brewer GJ, Terry CA, Aisen AM et al. Worsening of neurologic syndrome in patients with Wilson's disease with initial penicillamine therapy. *Arch Neurol.* 1987; 44:490-3.
41. Jaffe IA. Adverse effects profile of sulfhydryl compounds in man. *Am J Med.* 1986; 80:471-6.
42. Stein HB, Chalmers A, Schroeder ML et al. Selected adverse reactions of D-penicillamine. *Clin Invest Med.* 1984; 7:73-6.
43. Levy RS, Fisher M, Alter JN. Penicillamine: review and cutaneous manifestations. *J Am Acad Dermatol.* 1983; 8:548-58.
44. Bell CL, Graziano FM. The safety of administration of penicillamine to penicillin-sensitive individuals. *Arthritis Rheum.* 1983; 26:801-3.
45. Huskisson EC. The side effects of penicillamine therapy in rheumatoid arthritis. *J Rheumatol.* 1981; 8(Suppl 7):146-8.
46. Sternlieb I, Fisher M, Scheinberg IH. Penicillamine-induced skin lesions. *J Rheumatol.* 1981; 8(Suppl 7):149-53.
47. Lund HI, Nielsen M. Penicillamine-induced dermatomyositis. *Scand J Rheumatol.* 1983; 12:350-2.
48. Turner-Warwick M. Adverse reactions affecting the lung: possible association with D-penicillamine. *J Rheumatol.* 1981; 8(Suppl 7):166-8.
49. Dawkins RL, Garlepp MJ, McDonald BL et al. Myasthenia gravis and D-penicillamine. *J Rheumatol.* 1981; 8(Suppl 7):168-72.

50. Walshe JM. Penicillamine and the SLE syndrome. *J Rheumatol.* 1981; 8(Suppl 7):155-60.
51. Pool KD, Feit H, Kirkpatrick J. Penicillamine-induced neuropathy in rheumatoid arthritis. *Ann Intern Med.* 1981; 95:457-8
52. Sarkar B, Sass-Korstak A, Clarke R et al. A comparative study of in vitro and in vivo interaction of D-penicillamine and triethylenetetramine with copper. *Proc R Soc Med.* 1977; 70(Suppl 3):13-8.
53. Walshe JM. Treatment of Wilson's disease with trientine dihydrochloride. *Lancet.* 1982; 1:643-7.
54. Walshe JM. Copper chelation in patients with Wilson's disease. *Q J Med.* 1973; 42:441-52.
55. Walshe JM. Assessment of treatment of Wilson's disease with triethylene tetramine. In: Sarkar B, ed. Biological aspects of metals and metal-related diseases. New York: Raven; 1983:243-61.
56. Anon. A review of trientine for Wilson's disease. *Med Lett Drugs Ther.* 1986; 28:67.
57. Scheinberg IH, Jaffe ME, Sternlieb I. The use of trientine in preventing the effects of interrupting penicillamine therapy in Wilson's disease. *N Engl J Med.* 1987; 317:209-13.
58. Walshe JM. TM (MoS_4) as an "anti-copper" agent in man. In: Scheinberg IH, Walshe JM, eds. Orphan diseases and orphan drugs. London: Manchester University Press; 1986:76-85.
59. Gooneratne SR, McChowell J, Gawthorne JM. An investigation of the effects of IV administration of thiomolybdate in copper metabolism in chronic copper-poisoned sheep. *Br J Nutr.* 1981; 46:469-80.
60. Brewer GJ, Dick RD, Yuzbasiyan-Gurkan V et al. Initial therapy of Wilson's disease patients with tetrathiomolybdate. *Arch Neurol.* 1991; 48:42-7.
61. Spence JA, Suttle NF. A sequential study of the skeletal abnormalities which develop in rats given a small dietary supplement of ammonium tetrathiomolybdate. *J Comp Pathol.* 1980; 90:139-53.
62. Brewer GJ, Yuzbasiyan-Gurkan V, Lee DY et al. Treatment of Wilson's disease with zinc. VI. Initial treatment studies. *J Lab Clin Med.* 1989; 114:663-8.
63. Brewer GJ, Schoomaker EB, Leichtman DA et al. The use of pharmacologic doses of zinc in the treatment of sickle cell anemia. In: Brewer GJ, Prasad AS, eds. Zinc metabolism: current aspects in health and disease. New York: Liss; 1977:241-58.
64. Brewer GJ, Hill GM, Prasad AS et al. Zinc therapy for Wilson's disease. *Ann Intern Med.* 1983; 99:314-20.
65. Hoogenraad TU, Koevoet R, deRuyter Korver EGWM. Oral zinc sulphate as long-term treatment in Wilson's disease (hepatolenticular degeneration). *Eur Neurol.* 1979; 18:205-11.
66. Hoogenraad TU, Vanden Hamer CJA. Three years of continuous oral zinc therapy in 4 patients with Wilson's disease. *Acta Neurol Scand.* 1983; 67:356-64.
67. Brewer GJ, Scheinberg IH. Zinc therapy of Wilson's disease: two views. *Hepatology.* 1986; 6:1047-9.
68. Brewer GJ, Hill G, Prasad A et al. The treatment of Wilson's disease with zinc. IV. Efficacy monitoring using urine and plasma copper. *Proc Soc Exp Biol Med.* 1987; 184:446-55.
69. Hill GM, Brewer GJ, Juni JE et al. Treatment of Wilson's disease with zinc. II. Validation of oral ^{64}copper with copper balance. *Am J Med Sci.* 1986; 292:344-9.
70. Brewer GJ, Hill GM, Dick RD et al. Treatment of Wilson's disease with zinc. III. Prevention of reaccumulation of hepatic copper. *J Lab Clin Med.* 1987; 109:526-31.
71. Brewer GJ, Yuzbasiyan-Gurkan V, Dick R. Zinc therapy in Wilson's disease. VIII. Dose response studies. *J Trace Elem Exp Med.* 1990; 3:227-34.
72. Prasad AS. Deficiency of zinc in man and its toxicity. In: Trace elements in human health and disease. New York: Academic Press; 1976:16.
73. Brewer GJ, Yuzbasiyan-Gurkan V, Young AB. Treatment of Wilson's disease. *Semin Neurol.* 1987; 7:209-20.
74. Chandra RK. Excessive intake of zinc impairs immune responses. *JAMA.* 1984; 252:1443-6.
75. Hill GM, Brewer GJ, Block WD et al. Lipid parameters in Wilson's disease patients on zinc therapy. *Fed Proc.* 1986; 45:355.
76. Allen JG, Masters HG, Peet RL et al. Zinc toxicity in ruminants. *J Comp Pathol.* 1983; 93:363-77.
77. Yamaguchi M, Takahashi K, Okada S. Zinc-induced hypocalcemia bone resorption in rats. *Toxicol Appl Pharmacol.* 1983; 67:224-8.
78. Walshe JM. Wilson's disease (hepatolenticular degeneration). In: Berk JE, ed. Bockus: Gastroenterology. 4th ed. Vol 5. Philadelphia: Saunders; 1985:3222-35.
79. Mjolnerod OK, Dommerud SA, Rasmussen K et al. Congenital connective-tissue defect probably due to D-penicillamine treatment in pregnancy. *Lancet.* 1971; 1:673-5.
80. Solomon L, Abrams G, Dinner M et al. Neonatal abnormalities associated with D-penicillamine treatment during pregnancy. *N Engl J Med.* 1977; 296:54-5.
81. Linares A, Zarranz JJ, Rodriguez-Alarcon J et al. Reversible cutis laxa due to maternal D-penicillamine treatment. *Lancet.* 1979; 1:143.
82. Walshe JM. The management of pregnancy in Wilson's disease treated with trientine. *Q J Med.* 1986; 225:81-7.
83. Walshe JM. Diagnosis and treatment of presymptomatic Wilson's disease. *Lancet.* 1988; 1:435-7.
84. Sternleib I, Scheinberg IH. Prevention of Wilson's disease in asymptomatic patients. *N Engl J Med.* 1968; 278:353-9.
85. Glass JD, Reich SG, De Long MR. Wilson's disease: development of neurological disease after beginning therapy. *Arch Neurol.* 1990; 47:595-6.

Clinical Frontiers

Diastolic dysfunction in congestive heart failure

JULIE A. JOHNSON

Abstract: The available literature on the evaluation of diastolic function, the importance of diastolic dysfunction in congestive heart failure (CHF), and the effects of therapeutic agents on diastolic dysfunction are summarized.

The normal cardiac cycle consists of two components: systole (contraction; ventricular emptying) and diastole (dilation; ventricular filling). Recent studies have shown that 30–40% of patients with CHF have normal systolic function; the majority of these patients have diastolic dysfunction as the underlying disorder. As a result, the role of diastolic dysfunction in CHF is currently an area of interest for researchers. The two primary causes of diastolic dysfunction are left ventricular hypertrophy and ischemic heart disease. Patients with CHF caused by diastolic dysfunction and patients with CHF caused by systolic dysfunction have nearly identical clinical presentations.

Therapy with diuretics, vasodilators, angiotensin-converting-enzyme inhibitors, β-agonists, the partial β-agonist xamoterol, phosphodiesterase III inhibitors, or calcium-channel blockers may be beneficial in patients with diastolic dysfunction. Therapy with digitalis glycosides would be of no benefit, and could theoretically be detrimental, in patients with predominant diastolic dysfunction. Available data indicate that β blockers have neither an important beneficial effect nor an important detrimental effect on diastolic function.

Continued studies into diastolic dysfunction and the diastolic properties of agents that are used in the treatment of CHF should enhance the understanding of this clinical syndrome and the drugs used to treat it.

Index terms: Angiotensin-converting enzyme inhibitors; Calcium antagonists; Diuretics; Sympathomimetic agents; Vasodilating agents
Clin Pharm. 1991; 10:850-61

The traditional view of congestive heart failure (CHF) is that it is due to abnormalities in the systolic (or contractile) function of the heart. However, recent studies have shown that 30–40% of patients who have the clinical syndrome of CHF have normal systolic function[1-3]; the majority of these patients have diastolic dysfunction as the underlying pathophysiology. This fact has heightened interest in exploring techniques to assess diastolic function in patients with CHF and in defining the effects of therapeutic agents on diastolic function. As research in these areas evolves, our understanding of the pathophysiology and appropriate drug therapy of CHF should be enhanced. The purpose of this review is to summarize the available literature on the evaluation of diastolic function, the importance of diastolic dysfunction in CHF, and the effects of therapeutic agents on diastolic function. When necessary, systolic function and dysfunction will be discussed for completeness.

The Cardiac Cycle

The normal heart is able to meet the metabolic needs of the body by pumping blood at a rate that delivers sufficient amounts of oxygen to tissues. The performance of the heart, in terms of cardiac output, is determined by the volume of blood ejected with each contraction (stroke volume) and the number of cardiac cycles per unit of time (heart rate). Stroke volume is the difference between the volume of blood in the left ventricle at the end of diastole (end-diastolic volume) and that in the left ventricle at the end of systole (end-systolic volume); its determinants are preload, afterload, and contractility. The ability of the ventricle to fill during diastole—which is determined by the relaxation or lusitropic properties of the ventricle—and the ability of the ventricle to empty during systole—which is determined by the contractile or inotropic properties of the ventricle and by the forces impeding

JULIE A. JOHNSON, PHARM.D., is Assistant Professor of Pharmacy, Department of Clinical Pharmacy, University of Tennessee, 26 South Dunlap, Suite 200, Memphis, TN 38163.

This is **article 680-204-9126** in the **ASHP Continuing-Education System**; it qualifies for 1.0 hour of continuing-education credit.

ventricular emptying (afterload)—determine stroke volume. Therefore, abnormalities in either ventricular filling or ventricular emptying can lead to clinical symptoms of CHF due to elevated ventricular filling pressures or reduced cardiac output.[4]

Ventricular Systole. Figure 1 shows left ventricular pressure and volume during the various phases of systole and diastole. There are two phases in ventricular systole: (1) isovolumic contraction and (2) ejection.[6] Isovolumic contraction is initiated on mitral valve closure. During this period there is a rapid rise in ventricular pressure, although aortic pressure remains higher than left ventricular pressure and the aortic valve remains closed; thus, there is no change in ventricular volume. As ventricular pressure exceeds aortic pressure, the aortic valve opens and ejection is initiated. During the early ejection phase there is a rapid drop in ventricular volume, coincident with a continued rise in ventricular pressure. As ventricular pressure declines, ventricular emptying is slowed until ventricular pressure drops below aortic pressure and the aortic valve closes, initiating diastole.

Ventricular Diastole. Diastole is composed of four phases: (1) isovolumic relaxation, (2) rapid filling, (3) diastasis, and (4) atrial systole.[5,6] Isovolumic relaxation begins with closure of the aortic valve and ends

Figure 1. Cardiac and aortic pressures during ventricular systole and diastole (time proceeds from left to right). Phases of systole include isovolumic contraction (IC) and ejection. Phases of diastole include: (1) isovolumic relaxation (IR); (2) rapid-filling phase (RFP); (3) diastasis, or passive filling; and (4) atrial contraction. LV = left ventricular, LA = left atrial. (Adapted, with permission, from reference 5, © 1988, American Medical Association).

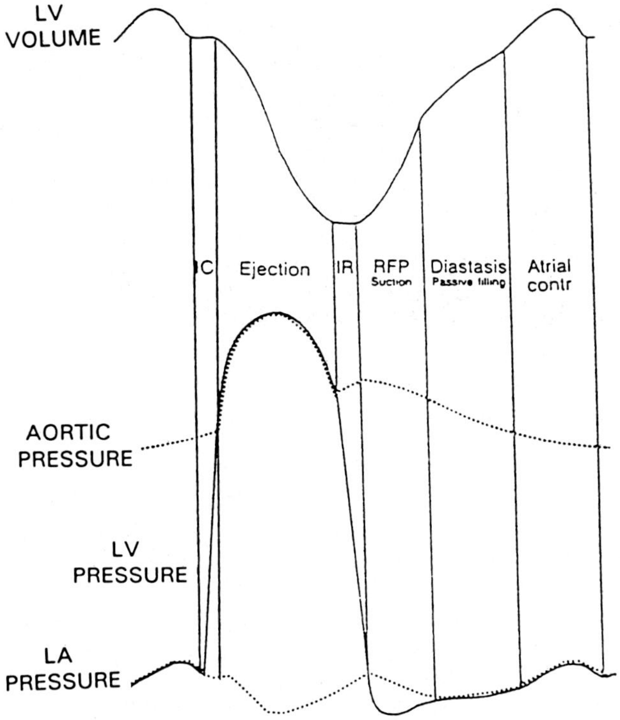

Reviews in the Clinical Frontiers *section summarize recent research advances, such as those that contribute to the understanding of a disease process or the mechanism of drug action, describe new technologies or medical procedures that are likely to affect drug therapy, or describe likely new modes of drug therapy. Preference is given to articles that assess directions of ongoing research and critically evaluate therapeutic implications in new and rapidly changing areas.*

when ventricular pressure falls below atrial pressure and allows the mitral valve to open.[5,7] As shown in Figure 1, there is a dramatic drop in ventricular pressure and no change in ventricular volume during this period. Initiation of rapid filling is marked by opening of the mitral valve and the onset of ventricular filling. Although this phase constitutes less than one third of diastole, approximately 80% of ventricular filling occurs during this phase.[5,7] There is a sharp increase in ventricular volume during this phase, with a minimal increase in ventricular pressure. Early in this phase, ventricular pressure declines as ventricular volume increases; this suggests the presence of ventricular "suction" that is accounted for in part by the chamber's elastic recoil. The isovolumic relaxation and rapid-filling phases constitute the calcium ion- (Ca^{++}) and energy-dependent phases of relaxation of the ventricular myocardium (described below).

Diastasis begins as ventricular inflow slows, and a plateau is reached on the ventricular volume curve. This phase is also called the passive-filling phase, during which approximately 5% of ventricular filling occurs. The duration of diastasis varies with heart rate, almost disappearing during tachycardia. Increases in ventricular pressure and volume are similar during this phase. The ventricular pressure–volume relationship during diastasis depends primarily on the compliance of the ventricle.

Atrial systole, the final phase of diastole, contributes about 15% to the end-diastolic volume. Because the majority of blood enters the ventricle during the rapid filling phase, atrial systole is not essential for ventricular filling in most circumstances. For example, patients with atrial fibrillation or flutter generally maintain adequate cardiac output during the arrhythmia. However, patients with diastolic dysfunction may have impaired ventricular filling during diastole and may be more dependent on atrial contraction for ventricular filling. Atrial fibrillation may be life threatening in patients with mitral valve stenosis or hypertrophic cardiomyopathy because of the loss of the atrial systole's contribution to ventricular filling.

Diastolic function of the heart is controlled by active, passive, and mechanical factors. Ventricular relaxation is an active (energy-consuming) process, which occurs on removal of Ca^{++} from the cytosol. Active relaxation of the ventricular myocardium takes place during the isovolumic relaxation and rapid-filling phases of diastole. The cellular mechanisms of active relaxation are described below.

Passive properties include (1) elastic recoil of the myocardium and (2) chamber compliance. The elastic recoil of the myocardium may play a small (but probably unimportant) role in drawing blood into the ventricle during the rapid-filling phase.[6] Chamber compliance and distensibility are the inverse of chamber stiffness. Chamber stiffness is described as the tendency of the myocardium to resist stretching in the presence of increased tension.[4,8] It is defined as the ratio of change in pressure to change in volume (dP/dV). Chamber stiffness depends on the thickness and composition of the myocardial wall. For example, an increase in wall thickness due to ventricular hypertrophy will increase chamber stiffness (decrease compliance) as will fibrous scar formation or infiltration of the myocardium with amyloid or sarcoid.

Finally, extrinsic factors influence diastolic function. The pericardium surrounds the heart and under normal conditions does not have a restrictive effect. However, as the heart enlarges and the limits of pericardial distensibility are reached, the pericardium restricts the normal compliance of the myocardium.[5,8,9] The right and left ventricle share a common wall, the interventricular septum, which may also influence diastolic function. Normally, the septum bows toward the right ventricle. Alterations in either right or left ventricular pressure or volume that shift the normal positioning of the septum will alter the geometry of the opposite ventricle and reduce its distensibility.[8,9]

Cellular Mechanisms of Myocardial Contraction and Relaxation. An appreciation of the cellular mechanisms of myocardial contraction and relaxation is necessary to understand diastolic dysfunction and the role drugs may play in treating it. A general overview of these mechanisms is provided here, but more detailed descriptions are available.[6,8,10] Myocardial contraction occurs during systole and is controlled by excitation–contraction coupling, in which Ca^{++} plays a central role. Ca^{++} enters the cytosol through calcium channels in the sarcolemma during the plateau phase of the action potential.[6,8,10] It is thought that this "trigger" Ca^{++} then stimulates the release of much larger quantities of Ca^{++} from the sarcoplasmic reticulum. The Ca^{++} that enters the cell then binds to troponin C and allows the cross-bridge formation between actin and myosin that results in the energy-consuming process of myocardial contraction.

Relaxation of the myocardium occurs during diastole, and like contraction, it is an energy-dependent process in which Ca^{++} plays a critical role. Removal of Ca^{++} from troponin C leads to relaxation; thus, the rate and extent of ventricular relaxation depend on the rate of removal of Ca^{++} from the cytosol.[8,10] Several mechanisms are responsible for ventricular relaxation, all of which require energy and are enhanced by adenosine 3',5'-cyclic phosphate (cAMP). During systole, cAMP-dependent protein kinases phosphorylate troponin I, a regulatory protein that causes Ca^{++} to dissociate more rapidly from contractile proteins during diastole and thus promotes relaxation. Ca^{++} released from the sarcoplasmic reticulum during systole undergoes reuptake into this membrane via an active-transport Ca^{++} pump. The rate of pump turnover (and therefore the rate of relaxation) is enhanced by cAMP-dependent phosphorylation of the regulatory protein phospholamban. The sodium–calcium pump and an active (adenosine 5'-triphosphate- [ATP] consuming) Ca^{++} pump are primarily responsible for extrusion of Ca^{++} that entered the cell via sarcolemmal calcium channels during the action potential. Efflux of Ca^{++} by these pumps is also enhanced by cAMP.

Assessment of Diastolic Function

A variety of methods are available to evaluate myocardial function during the phases of systole and diastole. Only a brief description of the diastolic indices will be provided in this review, and the reader is referred to other sources for detailed descriptions of tests that assess systolic and diastolic function.[4,5,9,11,12] Systolic function can be assessed by isovolumetric-phase indices and by ejection-phase indices. The most commonly used index of systolic function is ejection fraction, an ejection-phase index that is the percentage of blood ejected during systole ([stroke volume/end-diastolic volume] × 100).

Many measures are available for assessing diastolic function; however, they all have certain limitations, and many of the tests are technically difficult to perform.[4,5,9,11,12] Most of the indices are affected by heart rate, age, preload, afterload, and ejection fraction.[5] There is no index that provides a global assessment of diastolic function, nor is there an index that is considered a "gold standard."[5] The exponential isovolumic left ventricular pressure decline (–dP/dt) and the time constant for pressure decay (T) have been used to assess the isovolumic relaxation period. T reflects the rate of Ca^{++} removal from contractile proteins; thus, it is an accurate measure of the active relaxation properties of the ventricle.[4] Impaired relaxation will result in a decrease in peak –dP/dt and an increase in T.[12] Measurement of T and –dP/dt requires cardiac catheterization, which makes serial studies difficult and thereby limits the clinical usefulness of these measures.[4,5] The time from closure of the aortic valve to opening of the mitral valve can be measured with simultaneous echocardiography and phonocardiography, which provide a noninvasive measure of the isovolumic relaxation period.

Peak filling rate or +dV/dt (where dV/dt is the filling rate) is the peak rate of left ventricular filling during the rapid-filling phase. The time to peak filling rate is the time from the onset of the rapid-filling phase to peak dV/dt. The peak filling rate and time to peak filling rate are indices of the rapid-filling phase, and like T, they reflect the rate of Ca^{++} removal from contractile proteins (under most circumstances).[4,5,12] Impaired relaxation causes a decrease in the peak filling rate and a prolongation of the time to peak filling rate.[12] Both values can be measured by contrast ventriculography, radionuclide ventriculography, echocardiography, or Doppler echocardiography.[4,5] The noninvasive nature of some of these measures makes them more useful in the clinical environment. The distensibility or compliance of the ventricle is best determined during diastasis, when the relationship between ventricular pressure and ventricular volume can be determined.[5] As myocardial compliance decreases, a given ventricular volume will be associated with an increase in ventricular pressure. This measure will be affected not only by the chamber stiffness but also by pericardial restraint and ventricular interdependence. Compliance is determined in the cardiac catheterization laboratory by simultaneous measurement of ventricular pressures and volumes.[5]

Diastolic Dysfunction

Clinical States Associated with Diastolic Dysfunction. *Left Ventricular Hypertrophy.* The two primary causes of diastolic dysfunction are left ventricular hypertrophy (LVH) and ischemic heart disease. LVH is most commonly observed in patients with hypertension, although most patients with systolic dysfunction will also have some degree of compensatory LVH. In addition, patients with hypertrophic cardiomyopathy uniformly have asymmetric (septal) LVH, and patients with aortic stenosis have LVH similar to that observed in patients with hypertension.

LVH in any of these settings appears to impair diastolic function of the heart.[13-19] The increased wall thickness reduces ventricular compliance and therefore affects passive diastolic properties. However, the primary abnormality appears to be in the active phases of diastole; these patients have significantly prolonged isovolumic relaxation and reduction in filling during the rapid-filling phase.[13-19] Several studies have documented that the degree of diastolic dysfunction is positively correlated with the degree of LVH.[14,16,17,20] Interestingly, the physiologic LVH seen in endurance athletes is not associated with abnormalities in diastolic function.[20,21]

Ischemic Heart Disease. It has been recognized for many years that left ventricular filling pressures increase substantially during episodes of angina.[22] This phenomenon is believed to be due to abnormalities in systolic and diastolic function. During ischemic episodes, there may be decreased compliance of the left ventricle. However, significant impairments of the isovolumic relaxation period and rapid-filling phase also have been documented.[23,24] These diastolic abnormalities have been documented during ischemic episodes, but they also have been documented at rest in patients with ischemic heart disease.[23,24] One study showed that 91% of all patients with ischemic heart disease had abnormalities in diastolic filling.[24] The impairment of diastolic function was observed in patients with and without systolic dysfunction, although the degree of diastolic dysfunction was greater in patients with concomitant systolic dysfunction. The prevalence of diastolic dysfunction also increased with increasing coronary artery involvement (e.g., three-vessel disease versus one-vessel disease). Regional impairment of diastolic function in ischemic areas also has been documented.[25] These regional differences in diastolic function may create asynchrony in ventricular relaxation, which may impair the dissipation of ventricular pressure during diastole and result in global impairment of ventricular relaxation.[26] Regional and global improvements in diastolic function have been documented after coronary artery revascularization with percutaneous transluminal coronary angioplasty and support the underlying pathophysiological importance of ischemia.[27,28] In summary, patients with ischemic heart disease have impairments in ventricular relaxation and in passive ventricular compliance at rest and during ischemia. Diastolic function abnormalities are observed in nearly all patients with ischemic heart disease and concomitant systolic dysfunction, but these abnormalities are also seen in 86% of those with ischemia and normal systolic function.[24]

Mechanisms of Diastolic Dysfunction. Possible mechanisms of impaired diastolic function are shown in Table 1. It is thought that diastolic dysfunction may occur with both LVH and ischemic heart disease because of imbalances in energy supply and demand.

Table 1.
Possible Pathogenesis of Impaired Diastolic Function[a]

Defect	Cause and Contributing Factors
Impaired isovolumic relaxation	Prolongation of contractile state
	Increased affinity of Ca^{++} for troponin
	Decreased rate of actin–myosin cross-bridge dissociation
	Impaired removal of cytosolic Ca^{++}
	Reduced active transport of Ca^{++} into sarcoplasmic reticulum
	Reduced activity of Na^{+}–Ca^{++} pump
	Reduced activity of ATP-dependent Ca^{++} pump
	Decreased elastic recoil of myocardium
Impaired ventricular filling	Impaired isovolumic relaxation
	Impaired systolic function
	Loss of myocardial mass (e.g., myocardial infarction)
	Dilated cardiomyopathies
	Ventricular hypertrophy
	Decreased compliance of ventricular myocardium
	Ventricular hypertrophy
	Myocardial fibrosis
	Infiltrative disease
	Mechanical factors
	Pericardial restraint (e.g., pericardial tamponade, constrictive pericarditis)
	Mitral stenosis
	Changes in geometry of interventricular septum (interventricular dependence)

[a] Adapted from reference 4.

Although the exact cellular mechanisms for relaxation abnormalities have not been well defined, it is clear that diastolic dysfunction frequently precedes systolic dysfunction,[1-3] possibly because diastolic function may be more sensitive to imbalances in energy supply and demand. This phenomenon may be explained in part by Ca^{++} fluxes during systole and diastole.[4,29] During systole, Ca^{++} diffuses down a 10,000-fold concentration gradient from the sarcoplasmic reticulum and extracellular space into the cytosol. Ca^{++} transport during systole is, therefore, a rapid, passive process that does not require consumption of energy.[4,29] Conversely, during diastole high-energy phosphates are necessary for active transport of Ca^{++} against a concentration gradient. This causes Ca^{++} flux during diastole to be intrinsically slower than that during systole, and the energy dependence of Ca^{++} flux during diastole may make diastole more susceptible than systole to imbalances in energy supply and demand.

The imbalance of energy supply and demand in the myocardium during ischemia is obvious, and regional diastolic abnormalities may be present at rest in areas of chronically underperfused myocardium.[30] The energy imbalance that may lead to relaxation abnormalities in cases of hypertrophy is less obvious. Although hypertrophy decreases the energy expenditure of overloaded sarcomeres, it may also result in architectural changes that produce an imbalance between energy production and energy expenditure. These changes may include an increased intercapillary distance, which results in relative underperfusion of subendocardial regions, and a decreased ratio of mitochondria to myofibrils, which results in reduced ATP production.[30,31]

Because all the mechanisms of Ca^{++} removal from the cytosol are energy dependent, imbalances in energy supply and demand associated with ischemia or hypertrophy may result in slowed removal of Ca^{++} from the cytosol and in prolonged or incomplete relaxation.[31] (See Table 1.) This concept is supported by studies that show that ischemic heart disease and LVH are associated with impairment of the active (Ca^{++}-dependent) phases of diastole.

Filling abnormalities can be manifested by a decreased rate or extent of ventricular filling. Examples of mechanisms of impaired ventricular filling are shown in Table 1, the first of which is the impact of isovolumic relaxation abnormalities on ventricular filling. Prolongation of the rate of cytosolic Ca^{++} removal would be expected to slow ventricular filling, whereas incomplete removal of Ca^{++} would result in incomplete ventricular filling.[4] Therefore, isovolumic relaxation and ventricular filling both depend on the rate and extent of Ca^{++} removal from the cytosol.

Ventricular filling can be influenced by systolic dysfunction because it leads to an increase in end-systolic volume, thus limiting the amount of blood that may enter the ventricle during diastole. The load dependence of ventricular relaxation suggests that it also may be impaired by increased end-systolic volume. Along with these factors, most patients with systolic dysfunction will have some degree of ventricular hypertrophy or myocardial fibrosis, or both. It is for all these reasons that patients with systolic dysfunction typically have some degree of concomitant diastolic dysfunction.

Changes in the passive compliance of the ventricle will also impair ventricular filling. Ventricular hypertrophy impairs the compliance of the ventricle because a larger myocardial tissue mass must be stretched by the entering volume of blood. Myocardial fibrosis, which is commonly associated with processes causing systolic dysfunction, and infiltrative processes also reduce ventricular compliance and impair ventricular filling.

Finally, mechanical factors such as pericardial restraint may impair ventricular filling. Pericardial restraint has no effect on isovolumic relaxation. However, in the enlarged heart, the distensibility of the ventricles (and thus ventricular filling) is limited by the pericardium. Pericardial restraint leads to an increase in ventricular pressures throughout diastole. The influence of these various diastolic abnormalities on ventricular pressure and volume is shown in Figure 2.

Diastolic Dysfunction and CHF. The most common causes of CHF due to diastolic dysfunction are hypertension, ischemic heart disease, or a combination of the two.[1-3] Figure 3 shows the prevalence of the various causes from one study.[1] Although some clinicians may suggest that a diagnosis of predominantly systolic dysfunction versus predominantly diastolic dysfunction can be made at the bedside,[33] this suggestion is probably inaccurate because the clinical presentations of these patients are nearly identical (Figure 4).[1-3] Signs and symptoms of right-sided heart failure (i.e., edema, jugular venous distension, hepatomegaly), signs and symptoms of left-sided heart failure (i.e., dyspnea on exertion, orthopnea, paroxysmal nocturnal dyspnea, rales), and nonspecific findings (i.e., exercise intolerance, third or fourth heart sounds, displaced point of maximal impulse, cardiomegaly) are so similarly prevalent as to make the clinical syndromes indistinguishable. Therefore, the diagnosis must be based primarily on tests that evaluate systolic or diastolic function.

Some CHF patients have pure diastolic dysfunction, but it appears that a certain degree of concomitant diastolic dysfunction is also present in nearly all patients with systolic dysfunction.[1,5,24,34] Although the contribution of systolic dysfunction versus diastolic dysfunction to the overall syndrome of CHF is not well understood, there is some information on the role systolic dysfunction and diastolic dysfunction play in exercise intolerance. Reduced exercise tolerance is a cardinal feature of CHF, and classification of the patient's functional status is frequently based on exercise capacity. In patients with systolic dysfunction, the reduction in exercise capacity is typically believed to be due to underlying contractile abnormalities that

Figure 2. Schematic representation of diastolic pressure–volume relations that may occur in patients with congestive heart failure. Most patients have a combination of these diastolic abnormalities. In these graphs, the solid line represents the normal pressure–volume relationship, and the dashed line represents the general pressure–volume relationship observed with the various conditions. For both dashed and solid lines, the right vertical line represents isovolumic contraction, the left vertical line represents isovolumic relaxation, and the horizontal line represents the filling phases of diastole. *Abnormal pressure decay* shows the pressure–volume relationships that may be observed in patients with impaired relaxation during diastole. During isovolumic relaxation, ventricular pressure declines slowly, and unlike the normal setting, pressure decay continues during the filling phases of diastole. Although ventricular filling may be complete in the setting of abnormal relaxation (as is depicted in this graph), ventricular pressures throughout diastole are higher than normal, which may produce congestive symptoms. *Decreased passive chamber compliance* does not directly affect the calcium-dependent phases of diastole (isovolumic relaxation and rapid filling). Therefore, their phases are depicted as normal in the figure. During diastasis (right portion of horizontal line), a given ventricular volume is associated with an increased ventricular pressure; if normal end-diastolic volumes are attained, ventricular pressure will be markedly elevated, again possibly causing symptoms of congestion. *Pericardial restraint* does not affect isovolumic relaxation but restrains ventricular filling throughout diastole, producing elevated ventricular pressures throughout diastole. *Chamber dilitation* is commonly seen in patients with systolic dysfunction. It is not discussed in this review. (Reprinted from reference 32, with permission of the American Heart Association, Inc.)

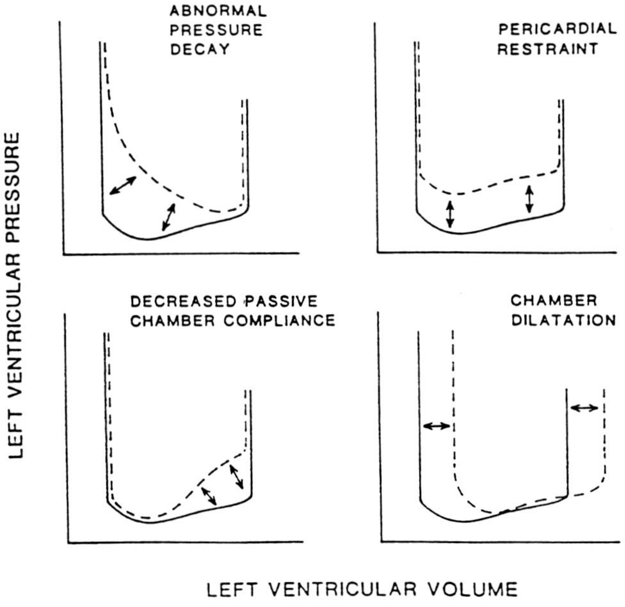

reduce cardiac output and limit blood supply to exercising muscles. Although the mechanism may be different, exercise intolerance in patients with diastolic dysfunction may also be due to reduced cardiac output. In a recent study, patients with pure diastolic dysfunction experienced exercise intolerance as a result of decreased cardiac output and stroke volume compared with that observed in controls.[35] In the patient group, the inability to enhance stroke volume during exercise was due to impaired ventricular filling during diastole.

Figure 3. Clinically suspected cause of congestive heart failure (CHF) in patients with ejection fraction ≤45% (white bars) and >45% (black bars). NS = not significant, IHD = ischemic heart disease, HCVD = hypertensive cardiovascular disease. (Reprinted, with permission, from reference 1.)

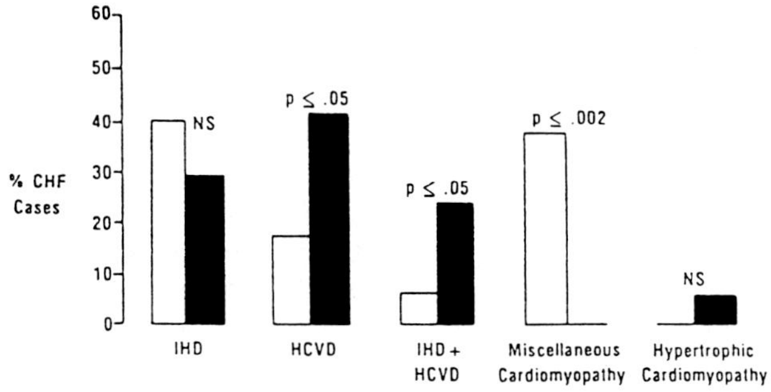

Figure 4. Prevalence of clinical findings in patients (n = 30) with clinical congestive heart failure and abnormal ejection fraction (<50%) and in patients (n = 20) with normal ejection fraction (≥ 50%). DOE = dyspnea on exertion, PND = paroxysmal nocturnal dyspnea, ORTH = orthopnea, JVD = jugular venous distension, dPMI = laterally displaced point of maximal impulse, S_4 and S_3 = fourth and third heart sounds, respectively. (Reprinted, with permission, from reference 3.)

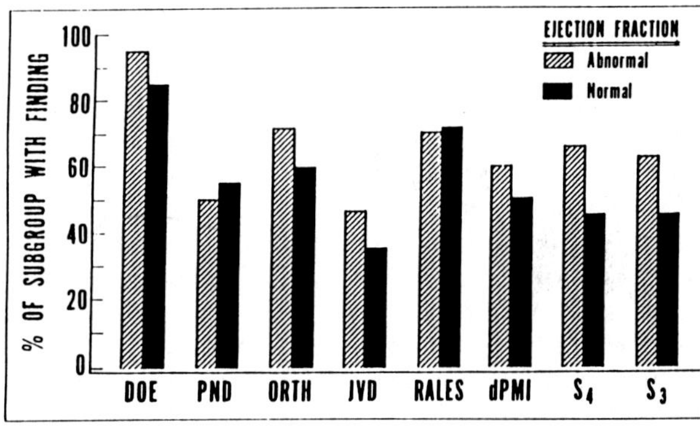

It is possible that diastolic abnormalities also play a role in the exercise intolerance of patients with predominantly systolic dysfunction. Although it is thought that exercise is limited in these patients because of contractile abnormalities, numerous investigators have shown a lack of correlation between exercise duration (or maximum oxygen consumption during exercise) and indices of left ventricular systolic function (e.g., resting left ventricular ejection fraction).[36-39] However, significant correlations between peak filling rate and exercise tolerance have been shown and suggest that diastolic function may play an important role in determining exercise tolerance.[35,40] A word of caution is in order, though, because the correlation coefficients in the two studies correlating exercise tolerance and peak filling rate were markedly different (i.e., 0.40 in one study and 0.93 in the other),[36,40] making it difficult to accurately assess the role of diastolic dysfunction in exercise intolerance. Further investigation is necessary to clarify the cause of CHF signs and symptoms in patients with diastolic dysfunction, as well as the role of diastolic dysfunction in the symptomatology of patients with predominant systolic dysfunction.

The prognosis of patients with normal ejection fraction and heart failure (presumably due to diastolic dysfunction in most cases) has not been evaluated systematically. However, these patients' prognoses appear to be better than those of their counterparts with reduced ejection fraction. The Veterans Administration Cooperative Study was a placebo-controlled trial evaluating the effects of isosorbide dinitrate plus hydralazine and those of prazosin on survival in patients with CHF.[41] This study included a subset of patients with normal ejection fraction. Although the sample size was small and the study was not designed to evaluate mortality in this subset, patients with normal ejection fraction had an 8% annual mortality rate compared with 19% in the group with low ejection fraction ($p = 0.0001$).[42] Thus, survival may be better in patients with CHF due to diastolic dysfunction, even if the symptom complex is similar to that in patients with CHF due to systolic dysfunction.

Diastolic Effects of Drugs Used in CHF

Because nearly all patients with CHF have some degree of diastolic dysfunction and 30–40% of patients with CHF may have isolated diastolic dysfunction, investigation into the diastolic properties of agents used in the management of CHF is warranted. The diastolic properties of some drug classes have been evaluated, whereas those of other drug classes have not. The following discussion will revolve around the drugs used in CHF, their documented or theoretical diastolic effects, and the appropriateness of therapy in a patient with systolic dysfunction versus diastolic dysfunction. The documented or suspected diastolic properties of the drugs will be related to the appropriate diagram in Figure 2. When this figure is referred to, the drug causes the pressure–volume relationship to shift from abnormal (dotted line) toward normal (solid line).

Diuretics. The diastolic properties of diuretic agents have not been investigated[43]; however, some data suggest that their beneficial effects in patients with CHF may be related to their effects on diastolic function. For example, diuretics have been shown to improve exercise tolerance without producing beneficial effects on systolic function.[44] Improved exercise tolerance appears to be better correlated with diastolic function than with systolic function; thus, exercise improvements associated with diuretic therapy may be due to beneficial diastolic effects. The predominant hemodynamic effect of diuretics is to reduce preload, primarily because of a reduction in ventricular pressure and not ventricular volume.[45] This effect suggests that diuretics produce a beneficial downward shift in the pressure–volume curve (Figure 2, Pericardial Restraint) that may be the result of a reduction in right ventricular filling pressures and reduced pericardial restraint on the left ventricle. Theoretically, diuretics should be useful in patients with systolic or diastolic dysfunction.

Digitalis Glycosides. Although there are no studies directly evaluating lusitropic properties of digitalis glycosides in humans, several lines of evidence suggest that they have no beneficial effects on diastolic function. The primary mechanism of digitalis glycosides is to increase intracellular Ca^{++}; if this increase is not coupled with a mechanism of increased Ca^{++} removal during diastole, digitalis glycosides would theoretically impair relaxation. In fact, diastolic contracture in response to digitalis toxicity has been documented in isolated heart models.[34] Additionally, dog studies with digoxin[46] and oubain[47] have shown that neither agent improves relaxation. Finally, clinical studies with digoxin suggest that the greatest therapeutic efficacy is seen in patients with severe heart failure. For example, Lee et al.[48] showed that digoxin was most effective in patients with severe impairment of left ventricular ejection fraction and severe chronic heart failure. None of the patients in the study with a left ventricular ejection fraction greater than 45% (suggesting predominantly diastolic dysfunction) responded to digoxin therapy.

In general, the literature suggests that digitalis glycosides would be of no benefit, and could theoretically be detrimental, in patients with predominant diastolic dysfunction. These agents should probably be reserved for patients with marked systolic dysfunction.

Vasodilators. Nitroglycerin and nitroprusside cause a downward shift in the diastolic pressure–volume curve. The reduction in pressure is not adequately explained by the change in volume; this suggests that the increased venous capacitance reduces right ventricular filling pressure and that this effect reduces pericardial pressure (Figure 2, Pericardial Restraint).[32,49-51] The proposed effect of these agents on pericardial restraint is supported by data that show that patients with the greatest elevations in right atrial pressure have the most dramatic pressure–volume shift,[32,49] and that removal of the pericardium eliminates the downward shift associated with nitroprusside therapy.[52]

The rate of pressure decay during diastole is load dependent. Therefore, a reduction in end systolic volume or afterload could indirectly enhance ventricular relaxation, and studies have shown that afterload reduction with nitroprusside may result in slight improvements in isovolumic relaxation (typically assessed by the time constant for pressure decay T).[32,49,50] Although changes in afterload may indirectly enhance relaxation, nitrates and nitroprusside do not appear to have any direct effects on ventricular relaxation properties during diastole.[32,49,50] It appears that their predominant effect is to reduce ventricular filling pressure and to thus reduce pericardial restraint. Nitrates and nitroprusside should improve symptoms in any patient with elevated right atrial pressure, whether the heart failure is due to predominantly systolic dysfunction or diastolic dysfunction.

The effects of other vasodilators on diastolic function have not been evaluated; however, some insight can be gained from the vasodilators that have been studied and from clinical trials. The data on nitrates and nitroprusside suggest that the predominant beneficial effect of these agents on diastolic function is preload reduction. Therefore, arterial vasodilators (e.g., hydralazine, minoxidil) would theoretically have minimal effects on diastolic properties and congestive symptoms. This hypothesis is supported by clinical trials suggesting that arterial vasodilators are associated with minimal improvements in symptoms and exercise tolerance.[53-55] However, combination isosorbide dinitrate–hydralazine therapy in the subset of patients in the Veterans Administration Cooperative Study[41] who had normal systolic function produced trends in mortality reduction (not significant because of sample size) similar to those observed in the entire study population.[42] Overall, the data suggest that vasodilators with venodilating properties may be beneficial in patients with isolated diastolic dysfunction, whereas arterial vasodilators may be of less benefit in this subset of patients.

Angiotensin-Converting-Enzyme Inhibitors. Limited data are available on the diastolic effects of angiotensin-converting-enzyme (ACE) inhibitors. Like the vasodilators previously discussed, ACE inhibitors cause a downward shift in the pressure–volume relationship (Figure 2, Pericardial Restraint), thereby reducing filling pressure at a given diastolic volume.[56,57] This effect appears to be due to reduced pericardial pressure. Although they reduce afterload, ACE inhibitors have not been shown to enhance isovolumic relaxation, nor do they appear to have any direct myocardial effects on diastolic function.[56,57]

Recent studies have suggested that ACE inhibitors may alter the natural progression of heart failure by slowing left ventricular dilatation.[58,59] Large, multicenter studies are currently under way to evaluate the role of ACE inhibitor therapy in altering disease progression in patients with CHF.[60,61] Because increased filling pressures play a role in stimulating ventricular dilatation and hypertrophy in patients with CHF, it has been suggested that the beneficial effects of ACE inhibitors on disease progression may be related in part to their effects on diastolic function.[57] ACE inhibitors are an exciting form of therapy for CHF because of their documented beneficial effects on symptoms, exercise tolerance, and survival. Their ability to reduce preload may make them useful in the management of patients with predominant diastolic dysfunction as well as those with systolic dysfunction.

Beta-Adrenergic-Agonists and Partial Agonists. The mechanisms responsible for removal of Ca^{++} from the cytosol are enhanced by cAMP; therefore, agents that increase intracellular cAMP should theoretically enhance relaxation.[10,62] Beta agonists fall into this category because they increase intracellular cAMP through stimulation of the β-receptor. Isoproterenol, dopamine, and dobutamine, which have positive inotropic effects that produce an increase in peak +dP/dt, have all been shown to enhance pressure decay during isovolumic relaxation, as assessed by variables such as –dP/dt and T.[48,63] Beneficial diastolic properties of the agents discussed thus far have been attributed primarily to reduced pericardial restraint as a result of reduced right ventricular filling pressures. Because dP/dt and T are load dependent, the effects observed with β agonists could also be due to reduced pericardial restraint. However, in the study by Carroll et al.,[32] the effects of dopamine and dobutamine on relaxation indices were similar in spite of the fact that dobutamine produced a significant reduction in filling pressures whereas dopamine tended to increase ventricular filling pressure (although the increase was not significant). This suggests that the effects of β agonists on diastolic function are related to direct myocardial effects, presumably enhanced removal of cytosolic Ca^{++} during diastole (Figure 2, Enhanced Pressure Decay). Intracoronary administration of drugs has been used to minimize alterations in loading conditions and heart rate, and preliminary studies with intracoronary dobutamine support the concept that the positive lusitropic properties of this agent are due to direct effects on myocardial relaxation.[64]

Long-term β-agonist therapy in patients with CHF has typically been associated with the development of tachyphylaxis, which is thought to be due to downregulation of β-receptors by β agonists.[65-67] However, prolonged therapy with the partial β agonist xamoterol has been associated with sustained symptomatic and hemodynamic improvements.[68,69] Studies investigating the diastolic properties of xamoterol have shown enhanced pressure decay during diastole and significant reductions in left ventricular filling pressures.[63,70,71] A downward and leftward shift in the pressure–volume curve has been documented during xamoterol therapy,[70] and enhanced pressure decay has been documented in the absence of a substantial effect on ventricular filling pressures.[71] Although the exact mechanism of xamoterol's diastolic properties is not known, the data suggest that it may be a combination of reduced pericardial restraint and enhanced pressure decay during diastole (Figure 2). It appears that xamoterol may be beneficial in treatment of CHF patients who have isolated diastolic dysfunction or predominant systolic dysfunction; however, its place in CHF therapy remains to be defined because a recent trial revealed that xamoterol therapy was associated with significantly higher mortality than placebo.[72]

Phosphodiesterase III Inhibitors. Phosphodiesterase III inhibitors increase intracellular cAMP concentrations by inhibiting the breakdown of cAMP. Thus, these agents would also be of theoretical benefit in enhancing relaxation during diastole. Phosphodiesterase III inhibitors possess vasodilator as well as positive inotropic properties, and studies with milrinone[73] and enoximone[49] have shown that they also have beneficial effects during diastole. Milrinone and enoximone have been shown to enhance pressure decay and peak filling rate, and they produce a downward and leftward shift in the diastolic pressure–volume curve.[49,73] Although –dP/dt is load dependent, enoximone significantly enhanced peak –dP/dt with minimal change in mean arterial pressure or peak left ventricular pressure. This result suggests that the increase in peak –dP/dt was probably due to a direct effect on myocardial relaxation (Figure 2, Enhanced Pressure Decay), which is consistent with the theoretical expectations of increased intracellular cAMP.[49]

Therapy with phosphodiesterase III inhibitors would be expected to have a beneficial effect in patients with isolated diastolic dysfunction, although this has not been investigated. Like the role of β agonists, the exact role of phosphodiesterase III inhibitors in CHF therapy remains to be established, both for systolic and diastolic dysfunction. Recent trials have suggested that both milrinone and enoximone therapy may be associated with increased mortality.[74,75]

Beta-Adrenergic Antagonists. Beta-receptor antagonists block sympathetically mediated increases in intracellular cAMP. Because cAMP enhances relaxation, β blockers may theoretically be expected to impair diastolic function. Limited data are available regarding the effect of β-adrenergic receptor blockade on the diastolic properties of the heart. A study in patients with ischemic heart disease, the majority of whom had normal systolic function and abnormal diastolic function, showed that propranolol had no significant effect on indices of diastolic filling, either at rest or during exercise.[76] In a small study of hypertensive patients receiving one month of β-blocker therapy (with metoprolol or nadolol), a significant reduction in early diastolic filling was seen in those patients who failed to respond to therapy.[77] The authors conclude that β blockers impair filling during diastole, but this impairment is counterbalanced in some patients by the reduction in blood pressure.[77]

Beta blockers have been more extensively studied in hypertrophic cardiomyopathy and for many years formed the cornerstone of medical therapy for this condition.[78,79] Symptomatic relief that is seen with β-blocker therapy may include improvements in exertional angina and dyspnea, lightheadedness, and syncope. Hypertrophic cardiomyopathy is associated with the diastolic abnormalities previously described, but it is also commonly associated with hypercontractile function and subaortic outflow obstruction. It is believed that most of the symptomatic improvements caused by β-blocker therapy in patients with hypertrophic cardiomyopathy are due to decreased heart rate and contractility, with the resultant reductions in myocardial oxygen demand and ouflow tract obstruction. The effects of β blockade on diastolic function in patients with hypertrophic cardiomyopathy are less clear. Some studies have shown that β-blocker therapy improves diastolic function by shortening isovolumic relaxation time,[80,81] whereas other studies have shown that β blockers either have no effect or a negative effect on diastolic-phase indices.[82,83] However, it does appear the reduction in heart rate associated with β blockade may indirectly enhance diastolic filling by prolonging the duration of diastole.[78,80,82,83]

The exact effects of β-blocker therapy on diastolic function are unclear. However, based on the available data, it seems most likely that β blockers have neither an important beneficial effect nor an important detrimental effect on diastolic function.

Calcium-Channel Blockers. Relative to the other drugs discussed in this review, there is a wealth of data regarding the effects of calcium-channel blockers on diastolic function. The beneficial effects of calcium-channel blockers on diastolic properties of the heart were first recognized in patients with hypertrophic cardiomyopathy. Numerous studies have documented that the calcium-channel blockers (e.g., verapamil, nifedipine, diltiazem) shorten the isovolumic relaxation time, enhance posterior wall thinning, enhance peak filling rate, shorten the time to peak filling rate, and increase filling during the rapid-filling phase.[18,19,84-87] These beneficial diastolic effects have been documented during concomitant reductions in blood pressure (nifedipine)[85] and with no change in blood pressure (nifedipine, diltiazem, verapamil).[50,84,86] Variable effects on heart rate have been reported. Nifedipine consistently causes increased heart rate,[50,85] whereas no significant change in heart rate (with diltiazem and verapamil)[18,84,86] and decreased heart rate (with verapamil)[19,87] have been reported. Therapy with calcium-channel blockers has been associated with a significant reduction in left ventricular end-diastolic pressure.[50,85]

It has been reported that patients with hypertrophic cardiomyopathy have an increased number of "calcium-antagonist receptors," and this suggests that diastolic dysfunction in such patients may be pathophysiologically different from other forms of diastolic dysfunction.[88] If this were the case, calcium-channel blockers might be less efficacious in patients with other forms of diastolic dysfunction. However, this suggestion does not appear to be true, because calcium-channel blockers have similar diastolic effects in patients with other forms of diastolic dysfunction. Studies conducted primarily in patients with ischemic heart disease have shown that calcium-channel blockers (i.e., verapamil, nicardipine, nisoldipine) shorten the time of isovolumic relaxation, enhance peak filling rate, shorten the time to peak filling rate, and enhance filling during the rapid-filling phase.[76,89-92] Reported changes in heart rate, blood pressure, and left ventricular end-diastolic pressure have been similar to those in patients with hypertrophic cardiomyopathy.[76,89-92]

Although there are numerous studies demonstrating the beneficial effects of calcium-channel blockers on diastolic function, the mechanism of this effect is controversial. A widely cited study in dogs showed that intracoronary injection of diltiazem, verapamil, and nifedipine resulted in impaired relaxation properties of the heart, whereas equipotent hypotensive intravenous doses, associated with marked increases in heart rate, resulted in no overall effect on relaxation.[93] The authors concluded that any effect on diastolic function observed with calcium-channel blockers is not due to direct myocardial relaxant effects but rather to changes in loading conditions and sympathetically mediated increases in heart rate (reductions in blood pressure and increases in heart rate would be expected to indirectly enhance ventricular relaxation). Whereas verapamil and diltiazem produced significant increases in heart rate in this study, clinical studies, which have shown that the drugs either have no effect on heart rate or decrease heart rate, raise some questions about whether the results of the dog study can be translated into the clinical environment. Because the dihydropyridines (e.g., nifedipine, nicardipine, nisoldipine) frequently increase heart rate or decrease blood pressure, or both, it is difficult to determine whether these agents have any direct myocardial relaxant effects. However, verapamil and diltiazem have been shown to enhance myocardial relaxation with no apparent changes in loading conditions or heart rate.[84,86,91] It is possible that the various classes of calcium-channel blockers may have different mechanisms for their diastolic properties. Although further investigations are necessary to elucidate the exact mechanism of diastolic effects observed with calcium-channel blockers, it is clear that these agents have beneficial properties for the management of diastolic dysfunction.

Several studies have documented that, in patients with CHF due to diastolic dysfunction, calcium-channel blockers are associated with long-term improvements in symptoms and exercise tolerance.[87,89,91] One study documented that improvement in exercise capacity was closely related to the change in peak filling rate associated with verapamil therapy.[87] In this same study, withdrawal of verapamil therapy after one to two years resulted in a reduction in peak filling rate and exercise capacity in the majority of patients. In general, the available literature suggest that calcium-channel blockers may be valuable agents for treatment of patients with CHF due to diastolic dysfunction. Use of these agents in patients with concomitant systolic dysfunction may be more problematical because of the negative inotropic properties. Therapy with calcium-channel blockers in patients with predominant systolic dysfunction has generally not been associated with prolonged hemodynamic or symptomatic improvements and may precipitate exacerbation of CHF.[55,94-97]

Conclusion

Diastolic dysfunction may play an important role in CHF. Many of the signs and symptoms associated with CHF are the result of elevated left ventricular filling pressures, and there is a reasonable amount of data to suggest that filling pressures are commonly elevated as a result of diastolic abnormalities. Diastolic function is difficult to measure accurately because it depends on so many variables. Nonetheless, continued studies into diastolic dysfunction and the diastolic properties of agents that are used in the treatment of CHF should enhance the understanding of this clinical syndrome and the drugs used to treat it.

References

1. Dougherty AH, Naccerelli GV, Gray EL et al. Congestive heart failure with normal systolic function. *Am J Cardiol*. 1984; 54:778-82.
2. Soufer R, Wohlgelernter D, Vita NA et al. Intact systolic function in clinical congestive heart failure. *Am J Cardiol*. 1985; 55:1032-6.
3. Echeverria HH, Bilsker MS, Myerburg RJ et al. Congestive heart failure: echocardiographic insights. *Am J Med*. 1983; 75:750-5.
4. Smith VE, Weisfeldt ML, Katz AM. Relaxation and diastolic properties of the heart. In: Fozzard HA, Haber E, Katz AM et al., eds. The heart and cardiovascular system. New York: Raven; 1986:803-17.
5. Harizi RC, Bianco JA, Alpert JS. Diastolic function of the heart in clinical cardiology. *Arch Intern Med*. 1988; 148:99-109.
6. Berne RM, Levy MN, eds. The cardiac pump. In: Cardiovascular physiology. St. Louis: Mosby; 1986:50-75.
7. Shub C. Heart failure and abnormal ventricular function. Pathophysiology and clinical correlation (part 2). *Chest*. 1989; 96:906-14.
8. Braunwald E, Sonnenblick EH, Ross J. Mechanisms of cardiac contraction and relaxation. In: Braunwald E, ed. Heart disease. Philadelphia: Saunders; 1988:383-425.
9. Weber KT, Janicki JS, Shroff SG. Measurement of ventricular function in the experimental laboratory. In: Fozzard HA, Haber E, Katz AM et al., eds. The heart and cardiovascular system. New York: Raven; 1986:865-86.
10. Katz AM. Interplay between inotropic and lusitropic effects of cyclic adenosine monophosphate on the myocardial cell. *Circulation*. 1990; 82(Suppl I):7-11.
11. Braunwald E. Assessment of cardiac function. In: Braunwald E, ed. Heart disease. Philadelphia: Saunders; 1988:449-70.
12. Brutsaert DL, Rademakers FE, Sys SU et al. Analysis of relaxation in the evaluation of ventricular function of the heart. *Prog Cardiovasc Dis*. 1985; 28:143-63.
13. Inouye I, Massie B, Loge D et al. Abnormal left ventricular filling: an early finding in mild to moderate systemic hypertension. *Am J Cardiol*. 1984; 53:120-6.
14. Fouad FM, Slominski JM, Tarazi RC. Left ventricular diastolic function in hypertension: relation to left ventricular mass and systolic function. *J Am Coll Cardiol*. 1984; 3:1500-6.
15. Smith VE, Schulman P, Karimeddini MK et al. Rapid ventricular filling in left ventricular hypertrophy: II. Pathologic hypertrophy. *J Am Coll Cardiol*. 1985; 5:869-74.
16. Fifer MA, Borow KM, Colan SD et al. Early diastolic left ventricular function in children and adults with aortic stenosis. *J Am Coll Cardiol*. 1985; 5:1147-54.
17. Spirito P, Maron BJ, Chiarella F et al. Diastolic abnormalities in patients with hypertrophic cardiomyopathy: relation to magnitude of left ventricular hypertrophy. *Circulation*. 1985; 72:310-6.
18. Betocchi S, Bonow RO, Bacharach SL et al. Isovolumic relaxation period in hypertrophic cardiomyopathy: assessment by radionuclide angiography. *J Am Coll Cardiol*. 1986; 7:74-81.
19. Bonow RO, Frederick TM, Bacharach SL et al. Atrial systole and left ventricular filling in hypertrophic cardiomyopathy: effect of verapamil. *Am J Cardiol*. 1983; 51:1386-91.
20. Shapiro LM, McKenna WJ. Left ventricular hypertrophy. Re-

lation of structure to diastolic function in hypertension. *Br Heart J*. 1984; 51:637-42.
21. Granger CB, Karimeddini MK, Smith VE et al. Rapid ventricular filling in left ventricular hypertrophy: I. Physiologic hypertrophy. *J Am Coll Cardiol*. 1985; 5:862-8.
22. Muller O, Rorvik K. Hemodynamic consequences of coronary heart disease with observations during anginal pain and on the effect of nitroglycerin. *Br Heart J*. 1958; 20:302-10.
23. Mann T, Goldberg S, Mudge GH et al. Factors contributing to altered left ventricular diastolic properties during angina pectoris. *Circulation*. 1979; 59:14-20.
24. Bonow RO, Bacharach SL, Green MV et al. Impaired left ventricular diastolic filling in patients with coronary artery disease: assessment with radionuclide angiography. *Circulation*. 1981; 64:315-23.
25. Sasayama S, Nonogi H, Miyazaki S et al. Changes in diastolic properties of the regional myocardium during pacing-induced ischemia in human subjects. *J Am Coll Cardiol*. 1985; 5:599-606.
26. Bonow RO. Regional left ventricular nonuniformity. *Circulation*. 1990; 81(Suppl III):54-65.
27. Bonow RO, Vitale DF, Bacharach SL et al. Asynchronous left ventricular regional function and impaired global diastolic filling in patients with coronary artery disease: reversal after coronary angioplasty. *Circulation*. 1985; 71:297-307.
28. Melchior JP, Doriot PA, Chatelain P et al. Improvement of left ventricular contraction and relaxation synchronism after recanalization of chronic coronary occlusion by angioplasty. *J Am Coll Cardiol*. 1987; 763-78.
29. Katz AM. Potential deleterious effects of inotropic agents in the therapy of chronic heart failure. *Circulation*. 1986; 73(Suppl III):184-90.
30. Pouleur H. Diastolic dysfunction and myocardial energetics. *Eur Heart J*. 1990; 11(Suppl C):30-4.
31. Katz AM. Cardiomyopathy of overload. *N Engl J Med*. 1990; 322:100-10.
32. Carroll JD, Lang RM, Neumann AL et al. The differential effects of positive inotropic and vasodilator therapy on diastolic properties in patients with congestive cardiomyopathy. *Circulation*. 1986; 74:815-25.
33. Kessler KM. Heart failure with normal systolic function. *Arch Intern Med*. 1988; 148:2109-11. Editorial.
34. Pouleur H, Hanet C, Gurne O et al. Focus on diastolic dysfunction: a new approach to heart failure therapy. *Br J Clin Pharmacol*. 1989; 28:41S-52S.
35. Kitzman DW, Higginbotham MB, Cobb FR et al. Exercise intolerance in patients with heart failure and preserved left ventricular systolic function: failure of the Frank-Starling mechanism. *J Am Coll Cardiol*. 1991; 17:1065-72.
36. Heo J, Iskandrian AS, Hakki AH. Relation between left ventricular diastolic function and exercise tolerance in patients with left ventricular dysfunction. *Cathet Cardiovasc Diagn*. 1986; 12:311-6.
37. Szlachcic J, Massie BM, Kramer BL et al. Correlates and prognostic implication of exercise capacity in chronic congestive heart failure. *Am J Cardiol*. 1985; 55:1037-42.
38. Baker BJ, Wilen MM, Boyd CM et al. Relation of right ventricular ejection fraction to exercise capacity in chronic left ventricular failure. *Am J Cardiol*. 1984; 54:5965-99.
39. Franciosa JA, Park M, Levine TB. Lack of correlation between exercise capacity and indexes of resting left ventricular performance in heart failure. *Am J Cardiol*. 1981; 47:33-9.
40. Soufer R, Lindo C, Kanakis J et al. The relationship of baseline peak filling rate to exercise capacity in congestive heart failure. *Circulation*. 1986; 74(Suppl II):138. Abstract.
41. Cohn JN, Archibald DG, Ziesche S et al. Effect of vasodilator therapy on mortality in chronic congestive heart failure. *N Engl J Med*. 1986; 314:1547-52.
42. Cohn JN, Johnson G. Heart failure with normal ejection fraction. The VHeFT study. *Circulation*. 1990; 81(Suppl III):48-53.
43. Packer M. Abnormalities of diastolic function as a potential cause of exercise intolerance in chronic heart failure. *Circulation*. 1990; 81(Suppl III):78-86.
44. Stamper M, Epstein SE, Beiser GD et al. Hemodynamic effects of diuretics at rest and during intense upright exercise in patients with impaired cardiac function. *Circulation*. 1968; 37:900-11.
45. Wilson JR, Reichek N, Dunkman WB et al. Effect of diuresis on the performance of the failing ventricle in man. *Am J Med*. 1981; 70:234-9.
46. Pouleur H, Van Mechelen H, Habib B et al. Comparisons of the inotropic effects of the β1-adrenoceptor partial agonists SL 75.177.10 and ICI 188,587 with digoxin on the intact canine heart. *J Cardiovasc Pharmacol*. 1984; 6:720-6.
47. Little WC, Rassi A, Freeman GL. Comparison of effects of dobutamine and ouabain on left ventricular contraction and relaxation in close-chest dogs. *J Clin Invest*. 1987; 80:613-20.
48. Lee DCS, Johnson RA, Bingham JB et al. Heart failure in outpatients. A randomized trial of digoxin and placebo. *N Engl J Med*. 1982; 306:699-705.
49. Herrmann HC, Ruddy TD, Dec GW et al. Diastolic function in patients with severe heart failure: comparison of the effects of enoximone and nitroprusside. *Circulation*. 1987; 75:1214-21.
50. Paulus WJ, Lorrell BH, Craig WE et al. Comparison of the effects of nitroprusside and nifedipine on diastolic properties in patients with hypertrophic cardiomyopathy: altered left ventricular loading or improved muscle inactivation? *J Am Coll Cardiol*. 1983; 2:879-86.
51. Kingma I, Smiseth OA, Belenkie I et al. A mechanism for the nitroglycerin-induced downward shift of the left ventricular diastolic pressure-diameter relation. *Am J Cardiol*. 1986; 57:673-7.
52. Shirato K, Shabetai R, Bhargava V et al. Alteration of the left ventricular diastolic pressure-segment length relation produced by the pericardium. Effects of cardiac distension and afterload reduction in conscious dogs. *Circulation*. 1978; 57:1191-8.
53. Franciosa JA, Weber KT, Levine TB et al. Hydralazine in the long-term treatment of chronic heart failure: lack of difference from placebo. *Am Heart J*. 1982; 104:587-94.
54. Franciosa JA, Jordan RA, Wilen MW et al. Minoxidil in patients with chronic left heart failure: contrasting hemodynamic and clinical effects in a controlled trial. *Circulation*. 1984; 70:63-8.
55. Agostoni PG, DeCesare N, Doria E et al. Afterload reduction: a comparison of captopril and nifedipine in dilated cardiomyopathy. *Br Heart J*. 1986; 55:391-9.
56. Konstam MA, Kronenberg MW, Udelson JE et al. Effect of acute angiotensin converting enzyme inhibition on left ventricular filling in patients with congestive heart failure. *Circulation*. 1990; 81(Suppl III):115-22.
57. Rousseau MF, Gurne O, van Eyll C et al. Effects of benazepril at on left ventricular systolic and diastolic function and neurohumoral status in patients with ischemic heart disease. *Circulation*. 1990; 81(Suppl III):123-9.
58. Pfeffer MA, Pfeffer JM, Steinberg C et al. Survival after an experimental myocardial infarction: beneficial effects of long-term therapy with captopril. *Circulation*. 1985; 72:406-12.
59. Pfeffer MA, Gervasio GA, Vaughan DE et al. Effect of captopril on progressive ventricular dilatation after anterior myocardial infarction. *N Engl J Med*. 1988; 319:80-6.
60. The SOLVD Investigators. Studies of left ventricular dysfunction (SOLVD)—rationale, design and methods: two trials that evaluate the effect of enalapril in patients with reduced ejection fraction. *Am J Cardiol*. 1990; 66:315-21.
61. Francis GS. Heart failure management: the impact of drug therapy on survival. *Am Heart J*. 1988; 115:699-702.
62. Walsh RA. Sympathetic control of diastolic function in congestive heart failure. *Circulation*. 1990; 82(Suppl I):52-8.
63. Pouleur H, Rousseau MF, Hanet C et al. Left ventricular sensitivity to β-adrenoceptor-stimulating drugs in patients with ischemic heart disease and varying degrees of ventricular dysfunction. *Circ Res*. 1987; 61(Suppl I):91-5.
64. Colucci WS, Parker JD. Effects of -adrenergic agents on systolic and diastolic myocardial function in patients with and without heart failure. *J Cardiovasc Pharmacol*. 1989; 14(Suppl

5):S28-S37.
65. Lambertz H, Meyer J, Erbel R. Long-term effects of prenalterol in patients with severe congestive heart failure. *Circulation*. 1984; 69:298-305.
66. Roubin GS, Choong CY, Devenish-Meares S et al. β-adrenergic stimulation of the failing ventricle: a double-blind, randomized trial of sustained oral therapy with prenalterol. *Circulation*. 1984; 69:955-62.
67. Colucci WS, Alexander RW, Williams GH et al. Decreased lymphocyte β-adrenergic receptor density in patients with heart failure and tolerance to the β-adrenergic agonist pirbuterol. *N Engl J Med*. 1981; 305:185-90.
68. The German and Austrian Xamoterol Study Group. Double-blind placebo-controlled comparison of digoxin and xamoterol in chronic heart failure. *Lancet*. 1988; 1;489-93.
69. Pouleur H, Etienne J, Van Mechelen H et al. Effects of the β1-adrenergic receptor partial agonist xamoterol on left-ventricular function. *Circulation*. 1990; 81(Suppl III):87-92.
70. Pouleur H, Hanet C, Rousseau MF et al. Relation of diastolic function and exercise capacity in ischemic left ventricular dysfunction. *Circulation*. 1990; 82(Suppl I):89-96.
71. de Feyter PJ, Serruys PW, Suryapranata H. Improvement of left ventricular contractility and relaxation with the β_1-adrenergic receptor partial agonist xamoterol at rest and during exercise in patients with postinfarction left ventricular dysfunction. *Circulation*. 1990; 81(Suppl III):99-106.
72. The Xamoterol in Severe Heart Failure Study Group. Xamoterol in severe heart failure. *Lancet*. 1990; 336:1-6.
73. Monrad ES, McKay RG, Bain DS et al. Improvement in indexes of diastolic performance in patients with congestive heart failure treated with milrinone. *Circulation*. 1984; 70:1030-7.
74. DiBianco R, Shabertai R, Kostuk W et al. A comparison of oral milrinone, digoxin, and their combination in the treatment of patients with chronic heart failure. *N Engl J Med*. 1989; 320:677-83.
75. Uretsky BF, Jessup M, Konstam MA et al. Multicenter trial of oral enoximone in patients with moderate to moderately severe congestive heart failure. Lack of benefit compared with placebo. *Circulation*. 1990; 82:774-80.
76. Bonow RO, Leon MB, Rosing DR et al. Effects of verapamil and propranolol on left ventricular systolic function and diastolic filling in patients with coronary artery disease: radionuclide angiographic studies at rest and during exercise. *Circulation*. 1981; 65:1337-50.
77. Fouad FM, Slominski MJ, Tarazi RC et al. Alterations in left ventricular filling with beta-adrenergic blockade. *Am J Cardiol*. 1983; 51:161-4.
78. Maron BJ, Bonow RO, Cannon RO et al. Hypertrophic cardiomyopathy: interrelations of clinical manifestations, pathophysiology and therapy. *N Engl J Med*. 1987; 316:844-52.
79. Wynne J, Braunwald E. The cardiomyopathies and myocarditides. In Braunwald E, ed. Heart disease. Philadelphia: Saunders; 1988:1410-69.
80. Bourmayan C, Razavi A, Fournier C et al. Effect of propranolol on left ventricular relaxation in hypertrophic cardiomyopathy: an echocardiographic study. *Am Heart J*. 1985; 109:1311-6.
81. Swanton RH, Brooksby IAB, Jenkins BS et al. Hemodynamic studies of β-blockade in hypertrophic obstructive cardiomyopathy. *Eur J Cardiol*. 1977; 5:327-41.
82. Bonow RO, Rosing DR, Bachrach SL et al. Effects of verapamil on left ventricular systolic function and diastolic filling in patients with hypertrophic cardiomyopathy. *Circulation*. 1981; 64:787-96.
83. Alvares RF, Goodwin JF. Noninvasive assessment of diastolic function in hypertrophic cardiomyopathy on and off β-blocking drugs. *Br Heart J*. 1982; 48:204-12.
84. Hanrath P, Mathey DG, Kremer P et al. Effect of verapamil on left ventricular isovolumic relaxation time and regional left ventricular filling in hypertrophic cardiomyopathy. *Am J Cardiol*. 1980; 45:1258-64.
85. Lorrell BH, Paulus WJ, Grossman W et al. Modification of abnormal left ventricular diastolic properties by nifedipine in patients with hypertrophic cardiomyopathy. *Circulation*. 1982; 65:499-507.
86. Suwa M, Hirota Y, Kawamura K. Improvement in left ventricular diastolic function during intravenous and oral diltiazem therapy in patients with hypertrophic cardiomyopathy: an echocardiographic study. *Am J Cardiol*. 1984; 54:1047-53.
87. Bonow RO, Dilsizian V, Rosing DR et al. Verapamil-induced improvement in left ventricular diastolic filling and increased exercise tolerance in patients with hypertrophic cardiomyopathy: short and long-term effects. *Circulation*. 1985; 72:853-64.
88. Wagner JA, Sax FL, Weisman HF et al. Calcium-antagonist receptors in the atrial tissue of patients with hypertrophic cardiomyopathy. *N Engl J Med*. 1989; 320:755-61.
89. Lahiri A, Rodrigues EA, Carboni GP et al. Effects of long-term treatment with calcium antagonists on left ventricular diastolic function in stable angina and heart failure. *Circulation*. 1990; 81(Suppl III):130-8.
90. Hanet C, Rousseau MF, van Eyll C et al. Effects of nicardipine on regional diastolic left ventricular function in patients with angina pectoris. *Circulation*. 1990; 81(Suppl III):148-54.
91. Setaro JF, Zaret BL, Schulman DS et al. Usefulness of verapamil for congestive heart failure associated with abnormal left ventricular diastolic filling and normal left ventricular systolic performance. *Am J Cardiol*. 1990; 66:981-6.
92. Lewis BS, Shefer A, Flugelman MY et al. Effect of the second-generation calcium channel blocking drug nisoldipine on diastolic left ventricular dysfunction in heart failure. *Am Heart J*. 1989; 118:505-11.
93. Walsh RA, O'Rourke RA. Direct and indirect effects of calcium entry blocking agents on isovolumic left ventricular relaxation in conscious dogs. *J Clin Invest*. 1985; 75:1426-34.
94. Tan LB, Murray RG, Littler WA. Felodipine in patients with chronic heart failure: discrepant hemodynamic and clinical effects. *Br Heart J*. 1987; 58:122-8.
95. The Multicenter Diltiazem Postinfarction Trial Research Group. The effect of diltiazem on mortality and reinfarction after myocardial infarction. *N Engl J Med*. 1988; 319:385-92.
96. Goldstein RE, Boccuzzi SJ, Cruess D et al. Diltiazem increases late-onset congestive heart failure in postinfarction patients with early reduction in ejection fraction. *Circulation*. 1991; 83:52-60.
97. Elkayam U, Amin J, Mehra A et al. A prospective, randomized, double-blind, crossover study to compare the efficacy and safety of chronic nifedipine therapy with that of isosorbide dinitrate and their combination in the treatment of chronic congestive heart failure. *Circulation*. 1990; 82:1954-61.

Therapy Update

Calcium-channel blockers for treatment of diabetic nephropathy

Kim M. Murray

Abstract: The use of calcium-channel blockers (CCBs) to reduce proteinuria associated with nephropathy in patients with diabetes mellitus is discussed.

Metabolically induced damage to the nephrons in diabetic nephropathy decreases the filtration rate and increases the glomerular plasma flow rate and transcapillary hydraulic pressure. Microalbuminuria, which is predictive of nephropathy in patients with insulin-dependent diabetes mellitus, is associated with the development of clinical proteinuria and increased mortality. Microalbuminuria should be evaluated periodically in diabetic patients, and antihypertensive therapy should be initiated when proteinuria is present or blood pressure control is needed. CCBs lower blood pressure because they prevent the action of angiotensin II by blocking the entry of calcium into renal vascular smooth muscle. Some CCBs, such as diltiazem and nicardipine, decrease glomerular pressure by increasing efferent arteriolar dilation. Others, such as nifedipine, may dilate both the afferent and efferent arterioles, thus causing increased excretion of protein. Studies in patients with diabetic nephropathy have shown that individual CCBs vary in their effects on proteinuria; this variation is attributable to their different sites of action and different effects on intrarenal activity. The choice of a CCB or an angiotensin-converting-enzyme inhibitor should be based on concomitant disease states and adverse-effect profiles.

For control of hypertension in patients with diabetic nephropathy, diltiazem should be considered initially. Nicardipine is effective for short-term use but has not been tested in long-term studies; it should be considered a reasonable alternative.

Index terms: Diltiazem; Calcium antagonists; Diabetes mellitus; Diabetic nephropathies; Hypertension; Mechanism of action; Nicardipine; Proteinuria
Clin Pharm. 1991; 10:862-5

Diabetic nephropathy is a major complication in patients with insulin-dependent diabetes mellitus (IDDM)[1]; usually it leads to death within seven years of the onset of proteinuria.[2] Because hypertension is associated with the development of diabetic nephropathy, treatment is aimed at reducing both blood pressure and proteinuria. The treatment of hypertension in the diabetic patient,[2-5] diabetic nephropathy, and the use of angiotensin-converting-enzyme (ACE) inhibitors to decrease proteinuria have been reviewed.[3,6] This paper discusses the use of calcium-channel blockers to reduce proteinuria associated with diabetic nephropathy and the selection of a specific agent.

Diabetic Nephropathy

Diabetic nephropathy is initially caused by metabolic changes, such as altered glucoregulatory or vasoregulatory hormone action, hyperglycemia-induced expansion of intracellular fluid volume, and hypertrophy of renal structures.[7] Damage to the nephrons decreases filtration rate[8-10] and increases the glomerular plasma flow rate and transcapillary hydraulic pressure.[1] As a compensatory mechanism, filtration in the best-preserved nephrons may increase; therefore, overall filtration may appear normal or enhanced.[8-10] Angiotensin II may be involved as both a systemic and a local intrarenal hormone.[11] Increases in renal vascular tone and alterations in renal blood flow, glomerular dynamics, and filtration coefficient may be influenced by angiotensin II.[11] ACE inhibitors are thought to be effective in reducing the production of angiotensin II and thus reducing intraglomerular hypertension and alterations in renal hemodynamics.

In IDDM, the onset of nephropathy usually occurs 15 to 20 years after diabetes is diagnosed, with a decline in glomerular filtration rate of 2.4 mL/min/yr.[12]

Kim M. Murray, Pharm.D., is Clinical Assistant Professor, College of Pharmacy, and Adjunct Assistant Professor, School of Medicine, University of South Carolina, Columbia.

Address reprint requests to Dr. Murray at the Department of Pharmaceutical Services, Richland Memorial Hospital, 5 Richland Medical Park, Columbia, SC 29203.

In non-insulin-dependent diabetes mellitus (NIDDM), the onset of nephropathy usually occurs sooner (5 to 10 years after diabetes is diagnosed), but the decrease in glomerular filtration rate is slower (1.1 mL/min/yr).[12] Diabetic nephropathy progresses to end-stage renal disease in 30–40% of IDDM patients and 3–8% of NIDDM patients.[12]

Detection of microalbuminuria assists in predicting the development of diabetic nephropathy in IDDM patients.[13] Microalbuminuria is also common in NIDDM patients[5,14] and is associated with the development of clinical proteinuria and increased mortality.[15] Thus, as a marker for the risk of developing proteinuria, microalbuminuria should be periodically evaluated in diabetic patients.[13,15]

No long-term studies of the effects of antihypertensive therapy on reducing mortality and morbidity in diabetic nephropathy have been reported. Further, it has not been demonstrated that decreased proteinuria is associated with reductions in mortality or morbidity, although reductions in the deterioration of renal function have been documented. Antihypertensive therapy can significantly decrease blood pressure and urinary albumin excretion and can impede the progressive deterioration of kidney function[2]; treatment should be initiated when proteinuria is present or blood pressure control is needed. Patients with severe nephropathy are less likely to respond to antihypertensive therapy.[6,16]

The Therapy Update *section provides concise analytical reviews of narrowly defined, important topics in pharmacotherapy. Priority is given to articles that focus on new or emerging standards in drug therapy. Articles are not intended to be comprehensive reviews of drugs or of disease states and their treatment.*

Effects of Calcium-Channel Blockers on Renal Function

Transmembrane calcium ion transport is necessary for angiotensin II to cause vasoconstriction, especially in the efferent arteriole.[17] Calcium-channel blockers block the entry of calcium into renal vascular smooth muscle, thus altering hormonal influence on renal blood flow and glomerular filtration rate.[18] Calcium-channel blockers may decrease glomerular pressure by increasing efferent arteriolar dilation; diltiazem and nicardipine act in this way. Other calcium-channel blockers, such as nifedipine, may further compromise the compensatory autoregulation adaptation[18] in patients with chronic renal failure by dilating both afferent and efferent arterioles and thus causing increased excretion of protein (Figure 1).

Calcium-channel blockers have been reported to cause natriuresis and diuresis.[18] Nifedipine, a dihydropyridine, displays the greatest effect. Other renal effects of calcium-channel blockers include decreased potassium excretion with no significant changes in creatinine clearance, free water clearance, or peripheral renin activity.[18] These effects are observed consistently among all classes of calcium-channel blockers, despite their various receptor sites and activity within the kidney.

Renal dysfunction induced by calcium-channel blockers has been reported in patients experiencing hypotensive episodes. Diamond et al.[17] reported four cases of nifedipine-induced acute, reversible deterioration in renal function in patients with chronic underlying mild-to-moderate renal dysfunction but without systemic hypotension. By exclusion of other causes of acute renal dysfunction, the authors concluded that the changes were due to intrarenal hemodynamic alterations. Possible explanations for the alterations include hormonal changes affecting angiotensin II and norepinephrine. An alternative mechanism may involve alterations in renal prostaglandin metabolism. Prostaglandin E_2 is protective during periods of reduced perfusion pressure and is responsible for main-

Figure 1. Effects of dilation of afferent and efferent glomerular arterioles. UAE = urinary albumin excretion.

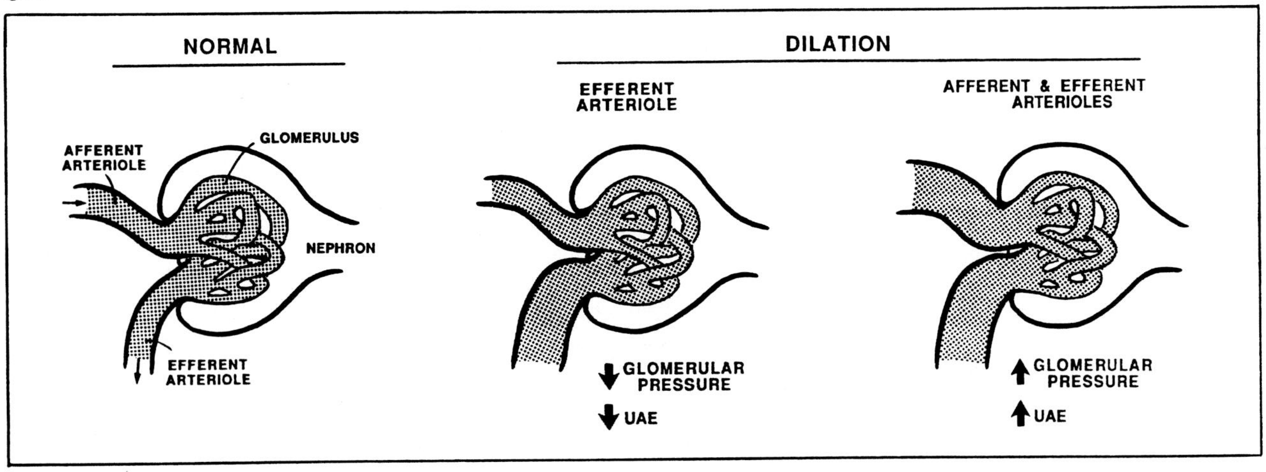

taining autoregulation of glomerular filtration.

Effects of Calcium-Channel Blockers on Proteinuria in Diabetic Nephropathy

Five studies evaluating the effects of calcium-channel blockers on proteinuria and renal function in patients with diabetic nephropathy are summarized in Table 1. All patients enrolled in the studies had proteinuric or nephrotic-range urinary albumin excretion (UAE); in four of the five studies the patients had documented systemic hypertension.

In normotensive patients given nifedipine or captopril, Mimran et al.[19] found no significant changes in serum creatinine concentration or diabetes control and similar decreases in blood pressure in the two treatment groups. After six weeks of treatment with captopril, urinary albumin excretion decreased from 86 ± 37 to 51 ± 19 μg/min (mean ± S.E.; $p < 0.05$). Surprisingly, however, nifedipine treatment resulted in a significant increase in UAE, from 86 ± 70 μg/min to 122 ± 96 μg/min (mean ± S.E.; $p < 0.05$). Because these alterations could not be explained by differences in systemic arterial blood pressure control, the difference was thought to be dependent on intrarenal hemodynamics. Whereas ACE inhibitors appear to act by selectively dilating the efferent arteriole and decreasing glomerular filtration pressure, nifedipine may cause nonselective dilation of both the afferent and efferent arterioles, which leads to increased glomerular filtration pressure and increased urinary albumin excretion.

Data from a 20-week study[20] confirmed an increase in proteinuria produced by long-acting nifedipine (from 2.8 g/day to 5.3 g/day at 6 weeks, $p = 0.022$). This study also demonstrated that treatment with extended-release diltiazem, another calcium-channel blocker, did not increase urinary protein excretion but decreased proteinuria (from 2.7 g/day to 1.3 g/day at 6 weeks, $p = 0.02$). Similar data were found during the crossover period. This study demonstrated that individual calcium-channel blockers have different sites of activity.

Bakris[21] similarly demonstrated the long-term beneficial effects of extended-release diltiazem and lisinopril in controlling systemic hypertension and decreasing nephrotic-range proteinuria. The initial six weeks of treatment with lisinopril decreased UAE by 36 ± 14% (mean ± S.E.); after crossover at six weeks, the decrease was 34 ± 12%. Diltiazem initially decreased UAE by 30 ± 12% (mean ± S.E.) from baseline; after crossover the decrease was 32 ± 11%. Persistent declines in UAE were seen with both agents at the 20-week follow-up. Both of these agents appear to selectively reduce efferent arteriolar resistance and thus decrease intraglomerular capillary pressure.

Two studies compared the effects of nicardipine and ACE inhibitors on UAE. Stornello et al.[22] compared the effects of nicardipine, captopril, and the combination of these two agents on blood pressure and renal hemodynamics during a four-week trial. Patients in all three study groups had decreases in mean blood pressure; the greatest decline was in the combination therapy group. UAE was similarly and significantly ($p < 0.05$) decreased in each treatment phase and did not corre-

Table 1.
Effects of Calcium-Channel Blockers on Proteinuria and Renal Function in Patients with Diabetic Nephropathy

Ref.	Diagnosis[a]	Antihypertensive Therapy	Study Design	Effect of Therapy[b]							
				UAE	BP	SCr	CL_{CR}	GFR	TRR	RBF	FF
19	IDDM and normal BP (n = 22)	Nifedipine (n = 7)	6 wk	+30	Dec	Unc					
		Captopril (n = 8)		−41	Dec	Unc					
		Placebo (n = 7)									
20	NIDDM and HTN (n = 14)	Nifedipine (er)[c]	6 wk with	+47		Inc					
		Diltiazem (er)	2-way crossover,	−52			Unc				
			then 2-mo								
		Nifedipine (er)	follow-up			Inc					
		Diltiazem (er)					Unc				
21	NIDDM and HTN (n = 8)	Diltiazem (er)	6 wk with	−30		Unc	Unc				
		Lisinopril	2-way crossover,	−36		Unc	Unc				
			then 18-wk								
		Diltiazem (er)	follow-up	−38							
		Lisinopril		−43							
22	NIDDM and HTN (n = 12)	Nicardipine	4 wk with	−61	Dec			Unc	Dec		Unc
		Captopril	2 × 2 factorial design	−48	Dec			Dec	Dec		Dec
		Nicardipine plus captopril		−75	Dec			Unc	Dec		Unc
		Placebo			Unc			Unc			
23	NIDDM and HTN (n = 7)	Nicardipine	4 wk with	−43	Dec			Var	Dec	Var	Unc
		Enalapril	2-way crossover,	−32	Dec			Var	Unc	Var	Unc
			no follow-up								

[a] IDDM = insulin-dependent diabetes mellitus, BP = blood pressure, NIDDM = non-insulin-dependent diabetes mellitus, HTN = hypertension.

[b] Reported as increased (Inc) or decreased (Dec) if mean values before and after drug therapy were significantly different; Unc = unchanged (or not significantly changed); or Var = variable. UAE = urinary albumin excretion, SCr = serum creatinine concentration, CL_{CR} = creatinine clearance, GFR = glomerular filtration rate, TRR = total renal vascular resistance, RBF = renal blood flow, FF = filtration fraction. UAE is reported as percentage change (increased or decreased) of mean UAE.

[c] er = Extended-release.

late with alterations in blood pressure. The decrease in UAE is attributed to the decrease or normalization of glomerular pressure.

Baba and colleagues[23] evaluated nicardipine and enalapril during a short-term trial. Similar significant reductions in blood pressure were demonstrated ($p < 0.01$). Mean UAE decreased significantly, from 32.6 µg/min at baseline to 18.5 µg/min with nicardipine ($p < 0.01$) and 22.1 µg/min with enalapril ($p < 0.05$).

Calcium-Channel Blockers versus ACE Inhibitors

Both the ACE inhibitors and the calcium-channel blockers diltiazem and nicardipine have demonstrated beneficial effects on UAE and blood pressure control in patients with diabetic nephropathy.[19-23] A number of studies comparing calcium-channel blockers with ACE inhibitors have shown similar effects[21-23]; therefore, drug selection should be based on concomitant disease states and adverse-effect profiles. Calcium-channel blockers would be indicated in patients with concurrent coronary artery disease, whereas ACE inhibitors would be more appropriate in patients with congestive heart failure.[14] In all the studies discussed here, the reported adverse effects of the different calcium-channel blockers were mild and did not cause patients to withdraw from the studies. Flushing, progressive pedal and ankle edema, and headache were reported with nifedipine.[19,20] Diltiazem was associated with mild pedal edema and headache.[20,21] Palpitations were reported by one patient receiving nicardipine; these lessened with continued therapy.[23] Because ACE inhibitors can cause hyperkalemia, they should be used with caution in patients who have end-stage renal disease or are receiving other medications that can increase serum potassium concentrations.[14]

Conclusion

Individual calcium-channel blockers act at different sites within the kidney and have different effects on intrarenal hemodynamic activity; these differences may help to explain the varying effects on proteinuria seen in patients with diabetic nephropathy who are receiving calcium-channel blockers. Because nifedipine has been shown to control blood pressure at the expense of increased UAE, other agents may be more appropriate. Nicardipine has been shown to be effective for short-term use, but long-term studies are needed. Diltiazem has been shown to have beneficial effects for the long-term decrease of proteinuria in patients with diabetic nephropathy. Therefore, if a calcium-channel blocker is required for the control of hypertension in a patient with diabetic nephropathy, diltiazem should be considered initially, with nicardipine as a reasonable alternative. Further studies are needed to evaluate the long-term effects of these agents and of new calcium-channel blockers on proteinuria in this patient population.

References

1. Reddi AS, Camerini-Davalos RA. Diabetic nephropathy, an update. *Arch Intern Med*. 1990; 150:31-43.
2. Parving HH, Smidt UM, Anderson AR et al. Early aggressive antihypertensive treatment reduces rate of decline in kidney function in diabetic nephropathy. *Lancet*. 1983; 1:1175-8.
3. Joseph JC, Schuna AA. Management of hypertension in the diabetic patient. *Clin Pharm*. 1990; 9:864-73.
4. Christlieb AR. Treatment selection considerations for the hypertensive diabetic patient. *Arch Intern Med*. 1990; 150; 1167-74.
5. Noth RH, Krolewski AS, Kaysen GA et al. Diabetic nephropathy: hemodynamic basis and implications for disease management. *Ann Intern Med*. 1989; 110:795-813.
6. Asher JP, Murray KM. Use of angiotensin-converting-enzyme inhibitors in the management of renal disease. *Clin Pharm*. 1991; 10:25-31.
7. Taguma Y, Kitamoto Y, Futaki G et al. Effect of captopril on heavy proteinuria in azotemic diabetics. *N Engl J Med*. 1985; 313:1617-20.
8. Mogensen CE. Long-term antihypertensive treatment inhibiting progression of diabetic nephropathy. *Br Med J*. 1982; 285:685-8.
9. Heeg JE, de Jong PE, van der Hem GK et al. Reduction of proteinuria by angiotensin converting enzyme inhibition. *Kidney Int*. 1987; 32:78-83.
10. Ledingham JCG. Effects of angiotensin II and of angiotensin converting enzyme inhibition in chronic renal failure. *Kidney Int*. 1987; 31(Suppl 20):112-6.
11. Johnston CI, Jackson B. Overview: angiotensin converting enzyme inhibition in renovascular hypertension. *Kidney Int*. 1987; 31(Suppl 20):154-6.
12. Tung P, Levin SR. Nephropathy in non-insulin dependent diabetes mellitus. *Am J Med*. 1988; 85(Suppl 5A):131-6.
13. Mogensen CE, Christensen CK. Predicting diabetic nephropathy in insulin-dependent patients. *N Engl J Med*. 1984; 311:89-93.
14. Dere WH, Groggel GC. Update on diabetic nephropathy in NIDDM. *Geriatrics*. 1990; 45:48-56.
15. Mogensen CE. Microalbuminuria predicts clinical proteinuria and early mortality in maturity onset diabetes. *N Engl J Med*. 1984; 310:356-60.
16. Baba T, Ishizaki T, Ido Y et al. Renal effects of nicardipine, a calcium entry blocker, in hypertensive type II diabetic patients with nephropathy. *Diabetes*. 1986; 35:1206-14.
17. Diamond JR, Cheung JY, Fang LST. Nifedipine induced renal dysfunction, alterations in renal hemodynamics. *Am J Med*. 1984; 77:905-9.
18. Chellingsworth MC, Kendall MJ. Effects of nifedipine, verapamil and diltiazem on renal function. *Br J Pharmacol*. 1988; 25:599-602.
19. Mimran A, Insua A, Ribstein J et al. Comparative effect of captopril and nifedipine in normotensive patients with incipient diabetic nephropathy. *Diabetes Care*. 1988; 11:850-3.
20 Demarie BK, Bakris GL. Effects of different calcium antagonists on proteinuria associated with diabetes mellitus. *Ann Intern Med*. 1990; 113:987-8.
21. Bakris GL. Effects of diltiazem or lisinopril on massive proteinuria associated with diabetes mellitus. *Ann Intern Med*. 1990; 112:707-8.
22. Stornello M, Valvo EV, Scapellato L. Hemodynamic, renal, and humoral effects of the calcium entry blocker nicardipine and converting enzyme inhibitor captopril in hypertensive type II diabetic patients with nephropathy. *J Cardiovasc Pharmacol*. 1989; 14:851-5.
23. Baba T, Murabayashi S, Takebe K. Comparison of the renal effects of angiotensin converting enzyme inhibitor and calcium antagonist in hypertensive type 2 (non-insulin dependent) diabetic patients with microalbuminuria: a randomised controlled trial. *Diabetologia*. 1989; 32:40-4.

Research

Modification of gastric pH with oral glutamic acid hydrochloride

MARGARET J. KNAPP, ROSEMARY R. BERARDI, JENNIFER B. DRESSMAN, JOAN M. RIDER, AND PEGGY L. CARVER

Abstract: The extent to which oral glutamic acid hydrochloride decreases mean gastric pH in fasting persons with and without simulated hypochlorhydria was studied.

Healthy nonsmoking men were randomly assigned to one of two drug regimens followed by the other regimen after a one-week washout period. In regimen 1 the fasting subjects received two 680-mg doses of glutamic acid hydrochloride given 10 minutes apart. Regimen 2 was the same, except that an oral dose of ranitidine 300 mg (as the hydrochloride salt) was administered one to two hours before the first dose of glutamic acid hydrochloride to simulate hypochlorhydria. Gastric pH was monitored radiotelemetrically before and after glutamic acid hydrochloride administration by using the Heidelberg capsule technique.

Six men 20 to 28 years of age participated in the study. For regimen 1, the gastric pH before glutamic acid hydrochloride was given was not significantly different from that after administration (grand medians, 1.4 and 1.3, respectively). In regimen 2, the median gastric pH increased to >4.0 within two hours after ranitidine treatment. Median gastric pH after the second dose of glutamic acid hydrochloride was significantly lower than before the first dose (grand medians, 1.6 and 6.2, respectively). The time to minimum pH was 2 to 15 minutes, and pH remained <3.0 for a mean of 45 minutes.

Glutamic acid hydrochloride alone did not decrease fasting gastric pH, but it significantly reduced pH in subjects with simulated hypochlorhydria produced by orally administered ranitidine.

Index terms: Achlorhydria; Gastrointestinal drugs; Glutamic acid hydrochloride
Clin Pharm. 1991; 10:866-9

Hypochlorhydria, the physiologically or pharmacologically induced decrease in gastric acid secretion, may alter the dissolution and absorption of certain drugs and dosage forms that have pH-dependent release characteristics. An elevated gastric pH resulting from an impaired ability to secrete gastric acid has been reported in several populations, including the elderly,[1-3] patients with AIDS,[4] individuals with common variable immunodeficiency,[5] and those with pernicious anemia.[6] Increased gastric pH has been associated with a decrease in the bioavailability of ketoconazole,[7] vitamin B_{12},[8] and dietary minerals such as iron and calcium.[9,10]

Oral administration of dilute hydrochloric acid has been used in an attempt to facilitate the absorption of drugs such as ketoconazole.[11] However, the administration of oral hydrochloric acid is undesirable because of its unpalatability, detrimental effects on tooth enamel, and potential for causing esophageal irritation.[1,12] Glutamic acid hydrochloride capsules (Acid-

MARGARET J. KNAPP, PHARM.D., is Assistant Clinical Scientist, Clinical Development—Central Nervous System, Parke-Davis Pharmaceutical Research Division of Warner-Lambert, Ann Arbor, MI, and Clinical Assistant Professor of Pharmacy, College of Pharmacy, The University of Michigan (UM), Ann Arbor; at the time of this study she was Clinical Pharmacy Resident, University of Michigan Medical Center (UMMC), Ann Arbor, and Clinical Instructor of Pharmacy, College of Pharmacy, UM. ROSEMARY R. BERARDI, PHARM.D., FASHP, is Associate Professor of Pharmacy, College of Pharmacy, UM, and Clinical Pharmacist, Gastroenterology, UMMC. JENNIFER B. DRESSMAN, PH.D., is Associate Professor of Pharmaceutics, College of Pharmacy, UM. JOAN M. RIDER, PHARM.D., is Assistant Professor of Clinical Pharmacy, Ferris State University, Big Rapids, MI, and Clinical Pharmacist, St. Mary's Hospital, Grand Rapids, MI; at the time of this study she was a doctor of pharmacy degree student, College of Pharmacy, UM. PEGGY L. CARVER, PHARM.D., is Assistant Professor of Pharmacy, College of Pharmacy, UM, and Clinical Pharmacist, Infectious Diseases, UMMC.

Address reprint requests to Dr. Berardi at the College of Pharmacy, The University of Michigan, Ann Arbor, MI 48109-1065.

Supported by grant M01-RR-00042 through the NIH Clinical Research Center of The University of Michigan and by the College of Pharmacy, The University of Michigan.

Presented at the 47th ASHP Annual Meeting, Boston, MA, June 6, 1990.

ulin, Eli Lilly & Co., Indianapolis, IN) have been used as a more palatable and less irritating alternative to hydrochloric acid in those patients requiring the effect of a gastric pH-lowering agent.[1,13-15] Each Acidulin capsule contains 340 mg of glutamic acid hydrochloride, which is equivalent to 0.6 mL of 10% hydrochloric acid (1.8 meq of hydrochloric acid).[12,a]

Various doses and regimens of oral glutamic acid hydrochloride have been used to lower gastric pH and enhance drug absorption. Lelawongs et al.[15] studied the effect of concurrent administration of glutamic acid hydrochloride 680 mg on the absorption of ketoconazole in healthy subjects. Although ketoconazole absorption was improved, the extent to which glutamic acid hydrochloride altered gastric pH was not determined. The in vivo effect of a specific dose and regimen of glutamic acid hydrochloride on the magnitude and duration of decreases in gastric pH has not been established.

The purpose of this study was to determine the extent to which oral glutamic acid hydrochloride decreases mean gastric pH in fasting persons with and without simulated hypochlorhydria.

Methods

The study was conducted in the clinical research center at The University of Michigan Hospital.

Subjects. Healthy, nonsmoking men were recruited for the study, which was approved by the institution's human subject review committee. Informed consent was obtained in advance in writing from all the participants. Potential subjects were screened for pre-existing clinical or laboratory evidence of gastrointestinal, renal, hepatic, or cardiac disease by physical examination and laboratory measurements. The subjects were instructed to fast for 12 hours before and during the study period. All were required to have taken no drugs (including nonprescription medications) for at least 48 hours before the first study day and throughout the study period. They were also to discontinue ingestion of alcohol and caffeine 24 hours before each study day.

Drug Regimens. The subjects were randomly assigned to receive one of two drug regimens, followed by the other regimen after a one-week washout period. In regimen 1 the subjects received two 680-mg doses of glutamic acid hydrochloride (two 340-mg capsules of Acidulin per dose), each with 120 mL of water at 25 °C. The doses were given 10 minutes apart. (Preliminary studies in our laboratory indicated that a single 680-mg dose is not sufficient to consistently lower gastric pH.) Regimen 2 was identical, except that an oral dose of 300 mg of ranitidine (as the hydrochloride salt; Zantac, two 150-mg tablets, Glaxo Inc., Research Triangle Park, NC) was administered one to two hours before the first dose of glutamic acid hydrochloride to simulate hypochlorhydria.

Measurements of pH. Gastric pH was monitored continuously before and after glutamic acid hydrochloride administration by using the Heidelberg capsule (HBC) technique.[16-18] The HBC is a radiotelemetric device consisting of a miniature pH electrode and battery-operated transmitter housed in an acrylic base 7 mm in diameter and 20 mm long. Immersion in 0.9% sodium chloride solution activates the battery, and the transmitter's output frequency is calibrated with pH 1 and 7 buffers warmed to 37 °C (body temperature). Once activated and calibrated, the capsule is attached to a 70-cm tether of surgical thread and swallowed by the subject. The tether is then affixed to the cheek with surgical tape; this maintains the position of the capsule in the stomach. The tether is also used to recover the HBC. The subject wears an antenna, strapped about the midriff, that detects the signal emitted by the capsule. Output signals are converted to pH values, which are permanently recorded on a strip chart recorder (Heidelberg International, Inc., Atlanta, GA). The HBC has a detection range of pH 1 to 8 and is accurate to within 0.5 pH unit.[19] The capsule maintains accuracy of transmission for six to eight hours.[17] On the completion of each experiment the capsule is recovered orally, the transmitter's output frequency is compared with prestudy calibration values, and the capsule is discarded.

Data Collection. *Regimen 1.* At approximately 0800 on the study day, each subject swallowed a newly activated and calibrated HBC (Heidelberg, lot 0145) with 120 mL of water at 25 °C. The tether was affixed to the cheek at a tether length of 45 to 55 cm, which corresponds approximately to a midgastric location of the HBC.[20] Baseline fasting gastric pH was determined for one to two hours after the subject swallowed the capsule.

Each subject was given the first dose of glutamic acid hydrochloride approximately two hours after swallowing the HBC. Gastric pH was monitored for an additional two hours after the second dose was given.

Regimen 2. The single oral dose of ranitidine was administered 15 to 30 minutes after subjects swallowed the HBC. The first dose of glutamic acid hydrochloride was given when the gastric pH had reached a value of ≥4 for 15 minutes. Gastric pH was monitored for an additional two hours after the second dose was given.

Data Analysis. Gastric pH was recorded digitally at 15-second intervals with an Apple IIe computer (Apple Computer Corporation, Cupertino, CA). The pH values at one-minute intervals were then sampled, and the data were analyzed by using appropriate tests. Sampling pH data at one-minute intervals has been shown to accurately describe the gastric pH profile.[20] Since pH data are not normally distributed in all cases,[20] nonparametric statistical techniques were used to describe and analyze the data. The pH data are reported as median values with interquartile ranges. The Wilcoxon signed-rank test (two-tailed) was used to determine the significance of differences between pH values obtained before and after doses of glutamic acid hydrochloride. The a priori level of significance was set at ≤0.05. The magnitude of pH change is reported in pH units. The cumulative time that gastric pH remained below 2.0, 2.5, and 3.0 over a period of one hour was also recorded, and the duration of this change is reported in minutes.

Results

Six men 20 to 28 years of age (mean age, 23.5 years) participated in the study. None had evidence of gastrointestinal, renal, hepatic, or cardiac disease. The results for regimen 1 are presented in Table 1. The median gastric pH before administration of glutamic acid hydrochloride ranged from 0.9 to 2.3 (grand median, 1.4). After glutamic acid hydrochloride administration, the median gastric pH ranged from 0.8 to 1.8 (grand median, 1.3). The difference was not significant ($p = 0.3126$).

The results for regimen 2 are summarized in Tables 1 and 2. The median gastric pH increased to >4.0 within one to two hours after oral administration of ranitidine. Median gastric pH over the 15-minute period immediately before the first dose of glutamic acid hydrochloride was given ranged from 4.7 to 6.9 (grand median, 6.2); after the second dose, the median gastric pH decreased to 0.9 to 2.2 (grand median, 1.6). The decrease was significant ($p = 0.0312$). After the second dose the median minimum gastric pH ranged from 0.6 to 1.8, representing a significant maximum decrease in gastric pH ($p = 0.0312$). The time to minimum gastric pH ranged from 2 to 15 minutes.

The cumulative duration of gastric pH change was determined for the first hour after the second dose of glutamic acid hydrochloride (Table 3). Overall, gastric pH remained <2.0 for a mean ± S.D. of 40 ± 12 minutes in all the subjects. Gastric pH remained <2.5 for 44 ± 12 minutes and <3.0 for 45 ± 11 minutes after the second dose.

Discussion

Patients with hypochlorhydria may experience inadequate dissolution and absorption of drugs and dosage forms that have pH-dependent release characteristics. Elevations in gastric pH have been associated with a decrease in the bioavailability of vitamin B_{12} and dietary minerals such as iron and calcium.[8-10] Impaired absorption of ketoconazole has been observed in patients with hypochlorhydria.[11] Although ketoconazole is generally well absorbed after oral administration, the dissolution and subsequent absorption of ketoconazole depend on an acidic gastric pH. At a pH of 2 to 3, more than 85% of a ketoconazole dose is in solution within five minutes, but at a pH of 6 only 10%

Table 1.
Effect of Glutamic Acid Hydrochloride on Gastric pH[a]

Subject	pH before Glutamic Acid			pH after Glutamic Acid		
	Q_L	Q_U	Median	Q_L	Q_U	Median
Regimen 1 (without Ranitidine)[b]						
1	1.4	1.5	1.4	1.4	1.7	1.4
2	1.0	1.6	1.2	0.8	1.1	0.8
3	0.7	1.3	0.9	0.9	1.2	1.0
4	1.9	2.4	2.3	1.3	1.8	1.5
5	1.4	1.8	1.6	1.1	1.3	1.2
6	1.2	1.9	1.6	1.6	2.0	1.8
Grand median			1.4			1.3
Regimen 2 (with Ranitidine)[c]						
1	6.4	6.6	6.5	1.9	4.8	2.2
2	5.1	6.1	5.9	0.7	1.0	0.9
3	3.2	5.2	4.7	1.8	2.0	1.9
4	6.8	7.0	6.9	1.0	1.1	1.1
5	5.9	6.2	6.1	1.1	1.5	1.2
6	5.0	5.4	5.3	1.8	2.1	2.0
Grand median			6.2			1.6

[a] Q_L and Q_U are the lower and upper quartiles, respectively, of pH values. Although pH was recorded every 15 seconds, values at one-minute intervals were used in the statistical analysis. Median values pertain to pH measured during the 15 minutes immediately before the first dose and the 15 minutes immediately after the second dose of glutamic acid hydrochloride.

[b] $p = 0.3126$ for change in pH associated with glutamic acid hydrochloride administration (two-tailed Wilcoxon signed-rank test).

[c] $p = 0.0312$ for change in pH associated with glutamic acid hydrochloride administration.

Table 2.
Magnitude of pH Change after Ranitidine Pretreatment and Glutamic Acid Hydrochloride Administration

Subject	Lowest pH after Glutamic Acid Hydrochloride Administration[a]	Change in pH[b]	Time to Lowest pH (min)[c]
1	1.7	−4.8	15
2	0.6	−5.3	15
3	1.8	−2.9	5
4	0.9	−6.0	2
5	1.0	−5.1	9
6	1.6	−3.7	13

[a] Lowest value among those that were recorded every minute for the 15 minutes after the second dose of glutamic acid hydrochloride.

[b] Difference between the lowest pH during the 15 minutes after the second dose of glutamic acid hydrochloride and the median pH during the 15 minutes before the first dose (Table 1).

[c] Time to achieve lowest pH during the 15 minutes after the second dose of glutamic acid hydrochloride.

Table 3.
Duration of Gastric pH Change after Oral Glutamic Acid Hydrochloride Administration in Subjects Pretreated with Oral Ranitidine

Subject	Time at Indicated pH (min)[a]		
	<2	<2.5	<3
1	50	54	55
2	48	49	49
3	23	31	33
4	36	36	37
5	30	34	38
6	50	59	60
Mean ± S.D.	40 ± 12	44 ± 12	45 ± 11

[a] Cumulative duration of pH change over the hour after the second dose of glutamic acid hydrochloride.

is in solution after one hour.[7,21] Ketoconazole is usually administered to fasting patients with a small amount of fluid; under these conditions gastric emptying should be complete within 30 minutes.[22] Therefore, in patients who are hypochlorhydric, if a normal (low) gastric pH is achieved and sustained for 30 minutes after the administration of ketoconazole, the drug will be exposed to approximately the same pH conditions as observed under the usual conditions of administration.

The results of this study indicate that gastric pH values of 0.9 to 2.3 in healthy fasting subjects were not significantly decreased after two oral 680-mg doses of glutamic acid hydrochloride given 10 minutes apart with 120 mL of water. In regimen 2 the gastric pH was intentionally elevated by pretreating subjects with oral ranitidine and thus simulating hypochlorhydria. After ranitidine pretreatment, the administration of two oral 680-mg doses of glutamic acid hydrochloride 10 minutes apart resulted in a significant decrease in gastric pH. The reduction in pH was maintained at <3.0 for an average of 45 minutes after the second dose of the acid.

Administration of dilute hydrochloric acid has been the method commonly used for decreasing gastric pH; however, this treatment is undesirable because of its detrimental effects on tooth enamel.[1,12] Oral capsules of glutamic acid hydrochloride have previously been used in an attempt to lower gastric pH,[1,13-15] but the magnitude and duration of the resulting decrease in pH have not been established. The results of this study suggest that the glutamic acid hydrochloride dosage regimen used would be useful in decreasing gastric pH in hypochlorhydric individuals.

Although none of the subjects in this study complained of gastrointestinal discomfort, one participant in a previous study in this laboratory experienced dyspepsia and heartburn when given similar oral doses of glutamic acid hydrochloride.

Conclusion

Glutamic acid hydrochloride by itself did not significantly decrease gastric pH in healthy fasting young adults. However, the agent did significantly reduce gastric pH in subjects with simulated hypochlorhydria produced by the oral administration of ranitidine. The results suggest that glutamic acid hydrochloride may be an alternative to dilute hydrochloric acid for the purpose of lowering gastric pH in hypochlorhydric patients receiving oral drugs, such as ketoconazole, that require an acidic pH for maximum dissolution and absorption.

[a]Eli Lilly & Co. Acidulin standard information letter. Indianapolis, IN: 1990.

References

1. Slanger A. Management of gastric achlorhydria and hypochlorhydria. *Geriatrics.* 1966; 21:193-8.
2. Holt PR, Rosenberg IH, Russell RM. Causes and consequences of hypochlorhydria in the elderly. *Dig Dis Sci.* 1989; 34:933-7.
3. Sharp GS, Fister HW. The diagnosis and treatment of achlorhydria: ten-year study. *J Am Geriatr Soc.* 1967; 15:786-91.
4. Lake-Bakaar G, Quadros E, Beidas S et al. Gastric secretory failure in patients with the acquired immunodeficiency syndrome (AIDS). *Ann Intern Med.* 1988; 109:502-4.
5. Hermans PE, Diaz-Buxo JA, Stobo JD. Idiopathic late-onset immunoglobulin deficiency. *Am J Med.* 1976; 61:221-37.
6. Weinstein WM. Gastritis. In: Sleisenger MH, Fordtran JS, eds. Gastrointestinal disease. 4th ed. Philadelphia: Saunders; 1989:792-813.
7. Carlson JA, Mann HJ, Canafax DM. Effect of pH on disintegration and dissolution of ketoconazole tablets. *Am J Hosp Pharm.* 1983; 40:1334-6.
8. Toskes PP. Current concepts of cobalamin (vitamin B_{12}) absorption and malabsorption. *J Clin Gastroenterol.* 1980; 2:287-97.
9. Schade SG, Cohen RJ, Conrad ME. Effect of hydrochloric acid on iron absorption. *N Engl J Med.* 1968; 279:672-4.
10. Recker RR. Calcium absorption and achlorhydria. *N Engl J Med.* 1985; 313:70-3.
11. Lake-Bakaar G, Tom W, Lake-Bakaar D et al. Gastropathy and ketoconazole malabsorption in the acquired immunodeficiency syndrome (AIDS). *Ann Intern Med.* 1988; 109:471-3.
12. Remington's pharmaceutical sciences. 17th ed. Gennaro AR, ed. Easton, PA: Mack; 1985:799.
13. Shay H, Gershon-Cohen J. A comparison of the effectiveness of glutamic acid hydrochloride and dilute hydrochloric acid as the replacement therapy in anacidity measured by fractional gastric acid titration and hydrogen-ion concentration curves. *Ann Intern Med.* 1936; 9:1628-38.
14. Wosika PH. Glutamic acid hydrochloride as a substitute for dilute hydrochloric acid in achlorhydria. *Am J Dig Dis Nutr.* 1936; 3:335-7.
15. Lelawongs P, Barone JA, Colaizzi JL et al. Effect of food and gastric acidity on absorption of orally administered ketoconazole. *Clin Pharm.* 1988; 7:228-35.
16. Connell AM, Waters TE. Assessment of gastric function by pH telemetering capsule. *Lancet.* 1964; 2:227-30.
17. Steinberg WH, Mina FA, Pick PG et al. Heidelberg capsule. I. In vitro evaluation of a new instrument of measuring intragastric pH. *J Pharm Sci.* 1965; 54:772-6.
18. Watson WC, Paton E. Studies on intestinal pH by radiotelemetering. *Gut.* 1965; 6:606-12.
19. Youngberg CA, Berardi RR, Howatt WF et al. Comparison of gastrointestinal pH in cystic fibrosis and healthy subjects. *Dig Dis Sci.* 1987; 32:472-80.
20. Dressman JB, Berardi RR, Dermentzoglou LC et al. Upper gastrointestinal (GI) pH in young, healthy men and women. *Pharm Res.* 1990; 7:756-61.
21. Hume AL, Kerkering TM. Ketoconazole. *Drug Intell Clin Pharm.* 1983; 17:169-74.
22. Brener W, Hendrix TR, McHugh PR. Regulation of the gastric emptying of glucose. *Gastroenterology.* 1983; 85:76-82.

Research Note

Effects of misoprostol or ranitidine on ibuprofen pharmacokinetics

RALPH E. SMALL, MELODY G. WILMOT-PATER, BARBARA A. MCGEE, AND HAYES E. WILLIS

Clin Pharm. 1991; 10:870-72

Ibuprofen is a nonsteroidal anti-inflammatory drug (NSAID) widely prescribed for the treatment of pain and inflammatory disorders.[1] The analgesic action of ibuprofen is thought to be mediated by the inhibition of cyclo-oxygenase and, consequently, the production of prostaglandin E_2 (PGE_2).[2,3] In addition to the therapeutic effects caused by a decrease in PGE_2 production, the protective effect of PGE_2 on the gastrointestinal tract is lost and can result in various degrees of gastric mucosal damage and bleeding.[4] Treatment or prevention of these deleterious effects often requires concomitant administration of a histamine H_2-receptor antagonist, sucralfate, or the synthetic prostaglandin E_1 analogue misoprostol. Therefore, it is important to evaluate the effects of these medications on the pharmacokinetic profile of ibuprofen.

The purpose of this study was to determine whether misoprostol or ranitidine therapy affects the pharmacokinetic profile of ibuprofen at steady state.

Methods. *Eligibility.* Volunteers between the ages of 18 and 40 years, in good health as determined by history, physical examination, and clinical laboratory evaluation, were recruited for the open-label, randomized, three-way crossover study. The nature of the study was explained to the subjects, and informed, written consent was obtained. Each subject provided a medical history and underwent a physical examination and clinical laboratory testing (blood chemistry, complete blood cell count, and urinalysis). Subjects were excluded from the study if they had a history of hypersensitivity to any of the study drugs; a history of gastrointestinal, renal, or hepatic disease; a known history of a blood dyscrasia; use of illicit drugs within the previous six months or an investigational drug within the past 30 days; an increase of greater than or equal to three times the normal alanine aminotransferase (ALT) value; a creatinine clearance less than 75 mL/min as estimated by the Cockcroft-Gault equation[5]; any unstable medical problem; mental impairment; or inability or refusal to follow directions.

Subjects were instructed not to ingest ethanol for one week before or during the study to avoid gastrointestinal irritation and hepatic enzyme induction. Subjects were also told not to take any prescription or nonprescription medications with the exception of oral contraceptives during the study period. Women of childbearing potential were required to have a negative serum pregnancy test within a 72-hour period preceding the initiation of therapy. Adequate contraception, by abstinence or by use of oral contraceptives one month before and throughout the study, was required because of misoprostol's abortifacient properties. The protocol was approved by the committee on the conduct of human research.

Study Design. Subjects meeting the inclusion criteria were randomly assigned to receive each of three treatments—misoprostol 200 μg plus ibuprofen 600 mg, ranitidine 150 mg (as the hydrochloride salt) plus ibuprofen 600 mg, and ibuprofen 600 mg alone—in a specified order based on a Latin square design, with an equal number of patients receiving each of the six potential administration sequences. The subjects took misoprostol and ibuprofen four times daily and ranitidine twice daily. Each regimen was taken for three full days. The last dose on the third day was taken at 2200. The fourth day was the study day during which the final dose of the regimen was taken and blood samples were collected.

The study drugs were ibuprofen 600-mg tablets (Motrin, Upjohn, Kalamazoo, MI, lot 0824WA); ranitidine 150-mg tablets (as hydrochloride, Zantac, Glaxo, Research Triangle Park, NC, lot Z10879EP); and misoprostol 200-μg tablets (Cytotec, Searle, Chi-

RALPH E. SMALL, PHARM.D., is Professor of Pharmacy and Pharmaceutics and Professor of Medicine (Rheumatology, Allergy, and Immunology), Medical College of Virginia (MCV)/Virginia Commonwealth University (VCU), Richmond. MELODY G. WILMOT-PATER, PHARM.D., is Clinical Pharmacist, MCV Hospitals. BARBARA A. MCGEE, PHARM.D., is Clinical Pharmacy Fellow in Rheumatology, Allergy, and Immunology, School of Pharmacy, MCV/VCU. HAYES E. WILLIS, M.D., is Assistant Professor of Internal Medicine, MCV/VCU.

Address reprint requests to Dr. Small at Box 533, MCV Station, Medical College of Virginia/VCU, Richmond, VA 23298-0533.

The contributions of Neal Baker, Pharm.D., in protocol preparation and data collection are acknowledged.

Supported by a grant from Glaxo, Inc., Research Triangle Park, NC.

Presented at the 48th ASHP Annual Meeting, San Diego, CA, June 4, 1991.

cago, IL, lot 1289-090). The total duration of the study was three weeks. This included a three-day washout period between treatment phases.

Each week, the subjects fasted from midnight of the night before blood drawing until three hours after receiving the study medication. On study days, the test medications were administered with approximately 100 mL of water between 0600 and 0700. Blood samples were drawn through heparinized indwelling catheters located in the forearm or by direct venipuncture. All samples were collected in red-top Vacutainer blood tubes. Samples were collected just before administration of test medications and then 0.25, 0.50, 0.75, 1.00, 1.25, 1.50, 1.75, 2.0, 2.5, 3.0, 4.0, 5.0, 6.0, 8.0, 12.0, and 16.0 hours afterward. After clot formation, the blood samples were centrifuged at 2500 rpm for 10 minutes, and the serum was collected. All samples were stored at –20 to –25 °C until the time of assay.

Analysis of Serum Samples. Serum samples were assayed for ibuprofen concentration by the biopharmaceutical analysis laboratory at Medical College of Virginia, Virginia Commonwealth University, using a high-performance liquid chromatographic method.[6] The sensitivity of this method is reported as 0.5 μg/mL. All samples from a subject's set of three trials were extracted and analyzed by the same investigator using the same calibration standards. The error in the precision of measurement of control samples from run to run was <3%.

Pharmacokinetic Calculations. The apparent peak serum ibuprofen concentration (C_{max}) and the time required to reach that concentration (t_{max}) were determined directly (without extrapolation) from the collected data. Serum concentration–time plots were constructed for each subject and treatment. From these curves, dosage-interval area under the curve (AUC_{0-6}) was calculated by applying the trapezoidal rule.

Linear regression analysis was used to determine the slope of the terminal phase of the curve when the logarithm of the serum ibuprofen concentration was plotted against time. The mean elimination rate constant (k) for each treatment was calculated from individual values, each of which was determined as the slope of the best-fit least-squares regression line. The half-life ($t_{1/2}$) was estimated from the calculated k values ($t_{1/2} = 0.693/k$).

Statistical Analysis. Analysis of variance (ANOVA) was used to evaluate the differences in t_{max}, C_{max}, AUC_{0-6}, k, and $t_{1/2}$ among treatments. ANOVA was also performed to detect a difference between men and women in the pharmacokinetic values. The level of significance for all statistical tests was <0.05. SAS software (SAS Institute, Cary, NC) was used to perform all statistical analyses.

Results. Demographic data for the 12 subjects who participated are reported in Table 1. Table 2 summarizes the pharmacokinetic values for each treatment. A comparison of the mean serum concentration curves for each treatment is shown in Figure 1.

No significant difference was detected among the treatments for any of the pharmacokinetic values, and no significant difference was found between the pharmacokinetic values of men and women.

Most subjects tolerated the test medications without adverse effects. Three subjects complained of nausea during the misoprostol treatment phase. All adverse reactions resolved without consequence.

Discussion. Misoprostol has been shown to have a gastrointestinal protective effect and has FDA-ap-

Table 1.
Characteristics of Study Participants[a]

Subject	Sex	Age (yr)	Weight (kg)	Height (in)	Alcohol Intake[b] (oz/day)
1	F	28	51	61.0	0
2	F	19	77	66.0	0
3	M	27	78	69.0	<2
4	F	26	66	67.5	<2
5	F	26	75	72.0	<2
6	F	18	50	60.0	0
7	M	24	85	71.0	0
8	F	24	97	66.0	0
9	M	22	84	71.0	<2
10	F	24	74	67.5	<2
11	M	22	61	70.0	0
12	M	20	66	71.0	<2
Mean ± S.D.		23 ± 3	72 ± 14	67.7 ± 3.9	

[a] All subjects were white, and none smoked tobacco.
[b] Intake before study, expressed as equivalent of 80-proof liquor.

Table 2.
Effect of Ranitidine or Misoprostol on Ibuprofen Pharmacokinetics[a]

Variable	Mean ± S.D. Ibuprofen Pharmacokinetic Value during Indicated Treatment		
	Ibuprofen Alone	Ibuprofen + Ranitidine	Ibuprofen + Misoprostol
AUC_{0-6} (μg·hr/mL)	190.83 ± 29.77	182.45 ± 29.53	200.42 ± 28.67
C_{max} (μg/mL)	64.15 ± 10.24	61.63 ± 10.49	66.97 ± 9.76
t_{max} (hr)	1.15 ± 0.79	0.93 ± 0.39	1.42 ± 0.82
k (hr^{-1})	0.398 ± 0.064	0.375 ± 0.053	0.382 ± 0.056
$t_{1/2}$ (hr)	1.77 ± 0.32	1.78 ± 0.49	1.85 ± 0.29

[a] AUC_{0-6} = area under the serum concentration–time curve for a six-hour ibuprofen dosage interval, C_{max} = apparent maximum serum concentration, t_{max} = time after ibuprofen dose to reach C_{max}, k = elimination rate constant, $t_{1/2}$ = half-life.

Figure 1. Mean serum ibuprofen concentrations (n = 12 for each curve) for the eight hours after the final ibuprofen dose. Mean concentrations 12 and 16 hours after the ibuprofen dose could not be calculated because many individual values were undetectable. (Black rectangles = ibuprofen alone, black triangles = ibuprofen plus ranitidine, white rectangles = ibuprofen plus misoprostol.)

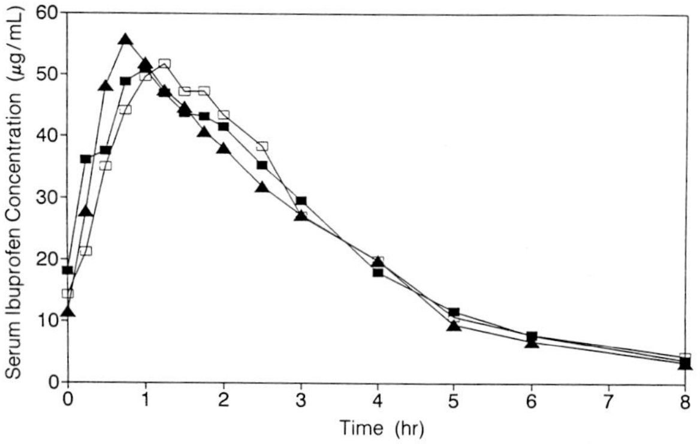

proved labeling for the prevention of NSAID-induced gastric bleeding; thus, a potential pharmacokinetic interaction of NSAIDs with this synthetic prostaglandin is of considerable importance.[7]

Two previous studies have examined the effect of ranitidine on the pharmacokinetics of ibuprofen. Stephenson and coworkers[8] examined the effects of daily doses of ranitidine and cimetidine on the steady-state pharmacokinetics of ibuprofen in a randomized, three-way crossover study with 12 healthy subjects. Ibuprofen 600 mg was given alone or with cimetidine 800 mg or ranitidine 300 mg (as the hydrochloride salt) every morning. Ranitidine and cimetidine were administered two hours before the morning ibuprofen dose. Plasma concentrations of ibuprofen were assessed over a 16-hour period, and t_{max}, C_{max}, $AUC_{0-\infty}$, and $t_{1/2}$ were compared using ANOVA. No significant differences were found among the three treatment groups. The authors concluded that the studied dosages of ranitidine and cimetidine do not significantly affect ibuprofen pharmacokinetics.

Ochs[9] evaluated the effect of ranitidine and cimetidine on ibuprofen pharmacokinetics in a single-dose, crossover comparison. Thirteen healthy subjects took a single dose of ibuprofen 600 mg alone or with ranitidine 150 mg (as the hydrochloride salt) twice daily or cimetidine 400 mg three times daily. Ranitidine and cimetidine dosing began 48 hours before the single dose of ibuprofen was taken and continued throughout the 15-hour ibuprofen pharmacokinetic study. Plasma concentrations of ibuprofen were assessed, and t_{max}, C_{max}, AUC, $t_{1/2}$, and clearance were determined. Pharmacokinetic values in the ranitidine–ibuprofen treatment group did not differ significantly from those in the ibuprofen control group. Significant increases in ibuprofen AUC and C_{max} values and a significant decrease in ibuprofen clearance were reported in the cimetidine–ibuprofen treatment group. The changes were so small (<10%) that the authors considered them to be of no clinical importance. The authors concluded that a clinically significant pharmacokinetic interaction between single doses of ibuprofen and either cimetidine or ranitidine is unlikely.

In a single-dose, randomized, three-way crossover study, Nicholson and associates[10] assessed the pharmacokinetics of misoprostol when administered with aspirin, diclofenac, ibuprofen, indomethacin, or piroxicam. Eighteen healthy volunteers received a single dose of ibuprofen 800 mg, a single dose of misoprostol 200 μg, or a single dose of ibuprofen 800 mg plus misoprostol 200 μg. Detailed information about the collected data was not provided, but the authors reported no significant difference in the misoprostol or ibuprofen concentrations when the drugs were given individually versus concomitantly. They reported similar results when misoprostol was administered with the other NSAIDs.

Based on the data reviewed and the results of our study, misoprostol has no apparent effect on the pharmacokinetics of ibuprofen.

Conclusion. Ranitidine and misoprostol, in the dosages used in this study, do not affect the pharmacokinetics of ibuprofen.

References

1. Kantor TG. Ibuprofen. *Ann Intern Med*. 1979; 91:877-82.
2. Simon LS, Mills JA. Non-steroidal anti-inflammatory drugs (part one). *N Engl J Med*. 1980; 30:1179-85.
3. Simon LS, Mills JA. Non-steroidal anti-inflammatory drugs (part two). *N Engl J Med*. 1980; 30:1237-43.
4. Cohn MM. Mucosal cytoprotection by prostaglandin E_2. *Lancet*. 1978; 1253-4.
5. Cockcroft DW, Gault MH. Prediction of creatinine clearance from serum creatinine. *Nephron*. 1976; 16:31-41.
6. Lockwood GF, Wagner JF. High-performance liquid chromatographic determination of ibuprofen and its major metabolites in biological fluids. *J Chromatogr*. 1982; 232:335-43.
7. G.D. Searle & Co. Cytotec package insert. Chicago, IL; 1988 Dec.
8. Stephenson DW, Small RE, Wood JH et al. Effect of ranitidine and cimetidine on ibuprofen pharmacokinetics. *Clin Pharm*. 1988; 7:317-21.
9. Ochs HR. Interaction of ibuprofen with the H_2-receptor antagonists ranitidine and cimetidine. *Clin Pharmacol Ther*. 1985; 38:648-51.
10. Nicholson PA, Karim A, Smith M. Pharmacokinetics of misoprostol in the elderly, in patients with renal failure and when co-administered with NSAID or antipyrine, propranolol or diazepam. *J Rheumatol*. 1990; 20S:S33-7.

DUE Criteria

The DUE Criteria *section of* Clinical Pharmacy *features model drug-use evaluation criteria that may be employed as a component of a comprehensive quality assurance program. The criteria sets are presented in the format used in the ASHP book* Criteria for Drug Use Evaluation. *Some of the criteria sets will have been originally published in that book; others will be presented here for the first time and published in future volumes of the ASHP book. The practitioners who developed a criteria set are acknowledged.*

These criteria sets are a starting point for the development of DUE criteria for a specific practice setting. Readers are encouraged to modify the model criteria to fit their own circumstances.

Criteria for use of moricizine in adult inpatients and outpatients[a]

Element	Standard 100%	Standard 0%	Exception[b] or Critical Preventive/ Responsive Measure[c]	Sources of Information
Justification for Use				
1. Management of life-threatening ventricular arrhythmias[1-4] as determined by a cardiologist, including the following: a. Sustained ventricular tachycardia (VT) defined by >100 beats/min lasting ≥30 seconds or <30 seconds when therapeutic intervention required to restore hemodynamic stability[5,6] or b. First-line drug therapy for nonsustained ventricular tachycardia (NSVT), defined by >100 beats/min lasting <30 seconds, in patient with history of hemodynamic symptoms, such as syncope, cardiovascular collapse, and cardiac arrest[1-4] or c. Second-line drug therapy for NSVT that is refractory to β-adrenergic-blocker therapy in patient with nonhemodynamic symptoms, such as dizziness and palpitations[1-3,5,6]	X		1A. Patient with severe hepatic disease	1. Progress notes, Holter monitor readings, electrocardiographic (ECG) reports, cardiology consultation, nursing notes, history and physical examination (H&P) 1A. H&P, progress notes, laboratory reports
Critical (Process) Indicators				
2. No history of pre-existing second- or third-degree atrioventricular block, or right bundle branch block associated with left hemiblock[3]	X		2A. Properly functioning pacemaker present	2, 2A. Progress notes, Holter monitor readings, H&P, ECG reports
3. In patient receiving moricizine and theophylline, serum theophylline concentration monitored regularly (when either drug started or stopped, when moricizine dosage changed, or when serum theophylline concentration unstable and at least every 3–6 months thereafter)[3,7]	X		3A. None	3. Laboratory reports, progress notes, physician orders, medication administration record (MAR)

Prepared by Teresa A. Bennett, Pharm.D., Division Head, Drug Information, Department of Pharmacy, University Medical Center, and Clinical Assistant Professor, College of Pharmacy, University of Florida Health Science Center/Jacksonville; J. Mark Trotter, Pharm.D., Clinical Pharmacy Resident, Department of Pharmacy, University Medical Center; and Alan B. Miller, M.D., Associate Professor of Medicine and Chief, Division of Cardiology, University of Florida Health Science Center/Jacksonville at University Medical Center.

Element	Standard 100%	Standard 0%	Exception[b] or Critical Preventive/ Responsive Measure[c]	Sources of Information
4. In patient receiving cimetidine, initial moricizine dosage ≤600 mg/day and therapeutic effect of moricizine monitored (ECG intervals, exercise testing, electrophysiologic [EP] testing, or Holter monitoring) regularly (when either drug started or stopped or when either dosage changed and at least every 3–6 months thereafter)[1,3,7]	X		4A. None	4. Physician orders, progress notes, ECG reports, Holter monitor readings, EP reports, MAR
5. Appropriate initial moricizine dosage: 600–900 mg/day given in three equally divided doses every eight hours[1,3]	X		5A. Hepatic or renal impairment[3] 5B. Dosing interval increased to 12 hours in patient who does not exhibit dizziness or nausea when dosed at 8-hour interval[1,7,8] 5C. Patient receiving cimetidine	5. Physician orders, progress notes, MAR 5A. Laboratory reports, progress notes 5B. Physician orders, progress notes, MAR, nursing notes 5C. Physician orders, progress notes, MAR
6. Initial moricizine dosage ≤600 mg/day in patient with hepatic or renal impairment[3]	X		6A. None	6. Physician orders, laboratory reports, progress notes, MAR
7. Moricizine therapy initiated in hospital setting[3]	X		7A. None	7. Physician orders, progress notes
8. Dosage titrated in increments of 150 mg/day at intervals of at least three days[3]	X		8A. None	8. Physician orders, progress notes, MAR
9. Therapeutic effect closely monitored (ECG intervals, exercise testing, EP testing, or Holter monitoring) in patient with hepatic impairment or congestive heart failure (CHF)[3]	X		9A. None	9. Progress notes, laboratory reports
10. No history of hypersensitivity to moricizine[3]	X		10A. None	10. H&P, allergy reports
Complications				
11. Proarrhythmia,[3,9] including new onset of VT or NSVT, ventricular flutter or fibrillation, or torsade de pointes, with or without hemodynamic compromise		X	11A. Identify other drug and nondrug causes 11B. Consider discontinuing moricizine in patients at high risk of proarrhythmia, including those with coronary artery disease, CHF, myocardial infarction, coronary-artery bypass surgery, pacemakers, or conduction abnormalities, and the elderly[1,10]	11. Progress notes, Holter monitor readings, ECG reports 11A. Physician orders, nursing notes, MAR, progress notes 11B. H&P, progress notes
12. Palpitations, dyspnea, chest pain, or CHF[3,11]		X	12A. Identify other drug and nondrug causes 12B. Consider alternative therapy if side effect persists or is intolerable	12. Progress notes, nursing notes 12A. MAR, progress notes, physician orders, nursing notes 12B. Progress notes, nursing notes
13. Dizziness[3,11]		X	13A. Identify other drug and nondrug causes 13B. Determine whether dizziness is postural and measure blood pressure 13C. Give lowest effective daily dosage in equally divided doses at 8-hour intervals[1,3,9,10] 13D. Consider alternative therapy if adverse effect persists or is intolerable	13. Progress notes, nursing notes 13A. Physician orders, progress notes, MAR, nursing notes 13B. Progress notes, nursing notes, nursing flow sheets 13C. Progress notes, physician orders, MAR 13D. Progress notes, nursing notes
14. Gastrointestinal effects[3,11]: nausea, vomiting, abdominal pain, dyspepsia, diarrhea, constipation, or dry mouth		X	14A. Identify other drug and nondrug causes 14B. Consider alternative therapy if adverse effect persists or is intolerable	14. Progress notes, nursing notes, physician orders, MAR 14A. MAR, progress notes, nursing notes, physician orders

Element	Standard 100%	Standard 0%	Exception[b] or Critical Preventive/ Responsive Measure[c]	Sources of Information
				14B. Progress notes, physician orders, nursing notes, MAR
15. Central nervous system effects[3,11]: headache, hypesthesia, asthenia, nervousness, paresthesia, anxiety, sleep disorders, blurred vision		X	15A. Identify other drug and nondrug causes 15B. Consider alternative therapy if adverse effect persists or is intolerable	15. Progress notes, nursing notes 15A. Physician orders, MAR, progress notes, nursing notes 15B. Progress notes, physician orders, MAR, nursing notes
16. Drug fever[3,9,11,12]		X	16A. Identify other drug and nondrug causes 16B. Evaluate creatine kinase, serum alanine aminotransferase and aspartate aminotransferase, erythrocyte sedimentation rate, and presence of antinuclear antibodies;[1,10] monitor white blood cell (WBC) count with differential and temperature 16C. Discontinue drug if fever persists	16. Progress notes, nursing notes, nursing flow sheets 16A. Progress notes, physician orders, nursing notes, MAR 16B. Laboratory reports, progress notes, nursing notes, nursing flow sheets 16C. Progress notes, physician orders, MAR
17. Hepatotoxicity: elevated liver function (serum bilirubin, aspartate aminotransferase, alanine aminotransferase) test results[3,11]		X	17A. Identify other drug and nondrug causes 17B. Monitor liver function test results 17C. Discontinue moricizine if elevation of liver function test results persists	17. Laboratory reports 17A. Progress notes, physician orders, MAR 17B. Laboratory reports, physician orders 17C. Laboratory reports, progress notes, physician orders, MAR
Outcome Measure				
18. Absence of VT or NSVT confirmed by Holter monitor, exercise testing, or EP testing	X		18A. Moricizine discontinued because of adverse effects 18B. Patient died	18. Progress notes, Holter monitor readings, exercise testing, or EP report 18A. Progress notes, physician orders, MAR, nursing notes 18B. Progress notes

[a] Criteria address justification for use (indications), critical (process) indicators, complications of therapy, and patient outcome. Each criterion consists of an element, a standard, exceptions to the standard, and sources of information. The element is the minimum level of evidence needed to show that patient care was optimal. The standard defines the deviation from an element that is acceptable. If no deviation is acceptable, the standard is 100%. Exceptions are circumstances in which deviation is allowable. Sources of information listed are the most reliable sources. Sources pertaining to an element or exception are identified by the number assigned to the element or exception (e.g., 5, 5A).

[b] For justification for use and critical (process) indicators.

[c] For complications and outcome measures.

References

1. Mann HJ. Moricizine: a new class I antiarrhythmic. *Clin Pharm.* 1990; 9:842–52.
2. Morganroth J. Placement of moricizine in the selection of antiarrhythmic drug therapy. *Am J Cardiol.* 1990; 65:D65–7.
3. Dupont Pharmaceuticals. Ethmozine package insert. Wilmington, DE; 1990 Jun.
4. Fitton A, Buckley MMT. Moricizine, a review of its pharmacological properties, and therapeutic efficacy in cardiac arrhythmias. *Drugs.* 1990; 40:138–67.
5. McCollam PL, Parker RB. Evaluation and treatment of ventricular arrhythmias: an update. *Clin Pharm.* 1991; 10:195–205.
6. Zipes DP. Specific arrhythmias: diagnosis and treatment. In: Braunwald E, ed. Heart disease. Philadelphia: Saunders; 1988:658–716.
7. Siddoway LA, Schwartz SL, Barbey JT et al. Clinical pharmacokinetics of moricizine. *Am J Cardiol.* 1990; 65:D21–5.
8. Morganroth J, Pratt CM. Safety and efficacy of a twice-daily dosing regimen for moricizine (Ethmozine). *Am Heart J.* 1985; 110:1188–92.
9. Morganroth J, Pratt CM. Prevalence and characteristics of proarrhythmia from moricizine (Ethmozine). *Am J Cardiol.* 1989; 63:172–6.
10. Carnes CA, Coyle JD. Moricizine: a novel antiarrhythmic agent. *DICP.* 1990; 24:745–53.
11. Kennedy HL. Noncardiac adverse effects and organ toxicity of moricizine during short- and long-term studies. *Am J Cardiol.* 1990; 65:D47–50.
12. Miura DS, Wynn J, Laitman R et al. Ethmozine toxicity: fever of unknown origin. *J Clin Pharmacol.* 1986; 26:153–5.

CP Continuing Education

The ASHP Continuing-Education System gives readers a self-assessment mechanism for selected articles in Clinical Pharmacy *and* AJHP. *It allows readers to obtain continuing-education credit for these articles.*

For the purpose of CE-credit enrollment, a blank answer sheet is published at the end of each installment of the column for the CE articles in that issue. An enrollee accumulates these answer sheets until the enrollment is submitted, using the form that is published in the June and December issues of Clinical Pharmacy *and in the June and December issues of* AJHP. *Any combination of tests within an 18-month period, from both* Clinical Pharmacy *and* AJHP, *may be included in an enrollment. More complete details about enrollment in the system appear in the semiannual enrollment form.*

Article 680-204-9127 (see page 825)
Qualifies for 1.0 hour of CE credit

Advances in the treatment of unstable angina pectoris

Learning Objectives

After studying this article, the reader should be able to

1. Describe the pathophysiological factors that cause acute myocardial ischemia.
2. Describe the clinical manifestations and diagnostic characteristics of unstable angina.
3. List seven drug or nondrug therapies used in the treatment of unstable angina.
4. Design a treatment strategy for a patient with unstable angina.
5. Critique the various drug therapies for unstable angina based on a summary of studies published in the primary literature.

Self-assessment Questions

For each question there is only one best answer.

1. The final common pathway for platelet aggregation is
   a. Platelet adhesion.
   b. The binding of fibrinogen to the glycoprotein IIb–IIIa-receptor complex on the platelet surface.
   c. The release of arachidonic acid and its subsequent metabolism to thromboxane A_2.
   d. The conversion of fibrinogen to fibrin.
   e. None of the above alternatives is correct.

2. Platelet aggregation or thrombosis is promoted by
   a. Adenosine 3',5'-cyclic phosphate (cyclic AMP) and thromboxane A_2.
   b. Antithrombin III and activated clotting factors VII, IX, and X.
   c. Epinephrine and cyclic AMP.
   d. Adenosine diphosphate and collagen.
   e. All of the above alternatives are correct.

3. The electrocardiogram of a patient suffering from unstable angina may show
   a. S–T segment depression.
   b. S–T segment elevation.
   c. T wave inversion.
   d. No changes.
   e. All of the above alternatives are correct.

4. Drugs shown to reduce the occurrence of cardiac death and myocardial infarction in unstable angina include
   a. Intravenous nitroglycerin.
   b. Aspirin.
   c. Heparin.
   d. Calcium-channel blockers.
   e. β-adrenergic blockers.

5. Which of the following statements regarding the drug treatment of unstable angina is false?
   a. β blockers should be avoided in patients with vasospastic or Prinzmetal's angina.
   b. Nifedipine has been associated with an increase in myocardial infarction in some studies.
   c. Esmolol is the β blocker of choice because of its short half-life and documented efficacy in decreasing the occurrence of infarction and recurrent ischemia.
   d. Therapy with propranolol appears to be superior to nifedipine in patients not previously receiving a β blocker.
   e. All of the above alternatives are correct.

6. Intra-aortic balloon counterpulsation
   a. Is considered first-line therapy for unstable angina.
   b. Requires concomitant heparin therapy.
   c. Relieves ischemia by increasing systolic intra-aortic pressure.
   d. Is associated with complications that are relatively uncommon and easy to manage.
   e. None of the above alternatives is correct.

7. Data regarding interventional therapy for unstable angina have not shown that
   a. The long-term outcome of patients with unstable angina and single-vessel coronary disease who undergo percutaneous transluminal coronary angioplasty (PTCA) is similar to that of patients

Answer Sheet

November 1991 *Clinical Pharmacy*

Note: An enrollment form for the ASHP Continuing Education System appears in the June and December issues. Please accumulate all the answer sheets you wish to use in one enrollment and submit them at one time with a completed enrollment form.

The American Society of Hospital Pharmacists is approved by the American Council on Pharmaceutical Education as a provider of continuing pharmaceutical education.

Place an X in the box(es) at the top of the column(s) corresponding to the test(s) you are taking. Darken the boxes corresponding to the correct answers.

❑ ACPE 680-204-9127
1.0 hour

	a	b	c	d	e
1.	❑	❑	❑	❑	❑
2.	❑	❑	❑	❑	❑
3.	❑	❑	❑	❑	❑
4.	❑	❑	❑	❑	❑
5.	❑	❑	❑	❑	❑
6.	❑	❑	❑	❑	❑
7.	❑	❑	❑	❑	❑
8.	❑	❑	❑	❑	❑
9.	❑	❑	❑	❑	❑
10.	❑	❑	❑	❑	❑

❑ ACPE 680-204-9128
1.0 hour

	a	b	c	d
1.	❑	❑	❑	❑
2.	❑	❑	❑	❑
3.	❑	❑	❑	❑
4.	❑	❑	❑	❑
5.	❑	❑	❑	❑
6.	❑	❑	❑	❑
7.	❑	❑	❑	❑
8.	❑	❑	❑	❑
9.	❑	❑	❑	❑
10.	❑	❑	❑	❑

❑ ACPE 680-204-9126
1.0 hour

	a	b	c	d	e		a	b	c	d	e
1.	❑	❑	❑	❑	❑	6.	❑	❑	❑	❑	❑
2.	❑	❑	❑	❑	❑	7.	❑	❑	❑	❑	❑
3.	❑	❑	❑	❑	❑	8.	❑	❑	❑	❑	❑
4.	❑	❑	❑	❑	❑	9.	❑	❑	❑	❑	❑
5.	❑	❑	❑	❑	❑	10.	❑	❑	❑	❑	❑

ASHP Use Only
(1.0)9127_____(3)
(1.0)9128_____(3)
(1.0)9126_____(3)

8. With respect to their use in CHF, digitalis glycosides
   a. Have been shown in numerous investigations to be useful in patients with diastolic dysfunction.
   b. Produce a benefit in patients with diastolic dysfunction by increasing intracellular calcium concentrations.
   c. May theoretically impair ventricular relaxation.
   d. Appear to be most effective in patients with mild symptoms and an ejection fraction of more than 45%.
   e. Alternatives a and b only are correct.

9. The predominant diastolic effect of nitrate and nitroprusside appears to be
   a. Preload reduction and a resultant decrease in pericardial restraint.
   b. Afterload reduction and a resultant enhancement of relaxation.
   c. A direct relaxation of myocardium.
   d. Unknown, because no diastolic effects have been documented.
   e. Alternatives a and c only are correct.

10. Beta-adrenergic agonists and phosphodiesterase inhibitors
    a. Increase intracellular cAMP concentrations by the same mechanism.
    b. Both increase intracellular cAMP concentrations but by different mechanisms.
    c. Have direct myocardial relaxant effects.
    d. Are clearly indicated in patients with diastolic dysfunction because of their proven ability to reduce mortality.
    e. Alternatives b and c only are correct.

Current Literature

Drug Reaction Alerts 880

Book Reviews

Handbook of Drug Therapy in Liver and Kidney Disease 885
Edited by Robert W. Schrier and John G. Gambertoglio
Reviewed by J. Russell May

Manual of Clinical Microbiology, Fifth Edition 885
Edited by Albert Balows, William J. Hausler, Jr., Kenneth L. Herrmann et al.
Reviewed by Patricia L. Orlando

Pharmacological Treatment of Endocrinopathies: Bone Disease, Kidney Stones and Related Disorders 890
By Charles Y. C. Pak
Reviewed by Thomas J. Comstock

Books Received 890

Drug Reaction Alerts

Drug Reaction Alerts focuses primarily on serious, unlabeled reactions to new chemical entities. The citations are compiled monthly from International Pharmaceutical Abstracts, *which covers over 800 pharmacy and health-related journals worldwide. An address for reprints (when available) follows the name of the corresponding author of each citation.*

Pharmacists may use the FDA Adverse Reaction Report form that appears in most issues of Clinical Pharmacy *for submitting reports of adverse drug reactions directly to FDA.*

Abortifacients

Fonseca W (Maternal and Child Epidemiology Unit, London School of Hygiene and Tropical Medicine, London WC1E 7HT, England), Alencar AJ, Mota FS et al. **Misoprostol** and congenital malformations. *Lancet.* 1991; 338:56. Case. (five infants whose mothers received misoprostol 400–600 μg orally or vaginally, or both, during first trimester of pregnancy as abortifacient; developed unusual congenital malformation of frontal or temporal region of skull, or both; of three mothers interviewed, none had made another attempt during her pregnancy to abort her fetus)

Antifungals

Gussenhoven MJ, Haak A, Peereboom-Wynia JD et al. (Van't Wout JW, Department of Infectious Diseases, University Hospital, 2300 RC Leiden, the Netherlands). Stevens-Johnson syndrome after **fluconazole**. *Lancet.* 1991; 338:120. Case. (30-year-old patient who was seropositive for human immunodeficiency virus; received fluconazole 150 mg/day for approximately two weeks for oral candidiasis; developed skin abnormalities; withdrawal of fluconazole for at least three days, then reinstitution of fluconazole at a dose of 100 mg/day led to severe bullae on trunk and limbs; withdrawal of fluconazole led to general improvement and no progression of skin lesions in two days)

Anti-infective Agents

Chen JP, Braham RL, Squires KE (The New York Hospital–Cornell Medical Center, New York, NY 10021). Diabetes after aerosolized **pentamidine**. *Ann Intern Med.* 1991; 114:913-4. Case. (28-year-old man who was seropositive for human immunodeficiency virus and formerly abused alcohol; received pentamidine isethionate 300 mg monthly by oral inhalation for three months as chemoprophylaxis for *Pneumocystis carinii* pneumonia; developed polydipsia and polyuria; serum glucose concentration, 641 mg/dL; therapy with insulin led to control of blood glucose concentration; positive rechallenge)

Continued on page 884

New!

Now Available!

SURVANTA®
beractant
intratracheal suspension

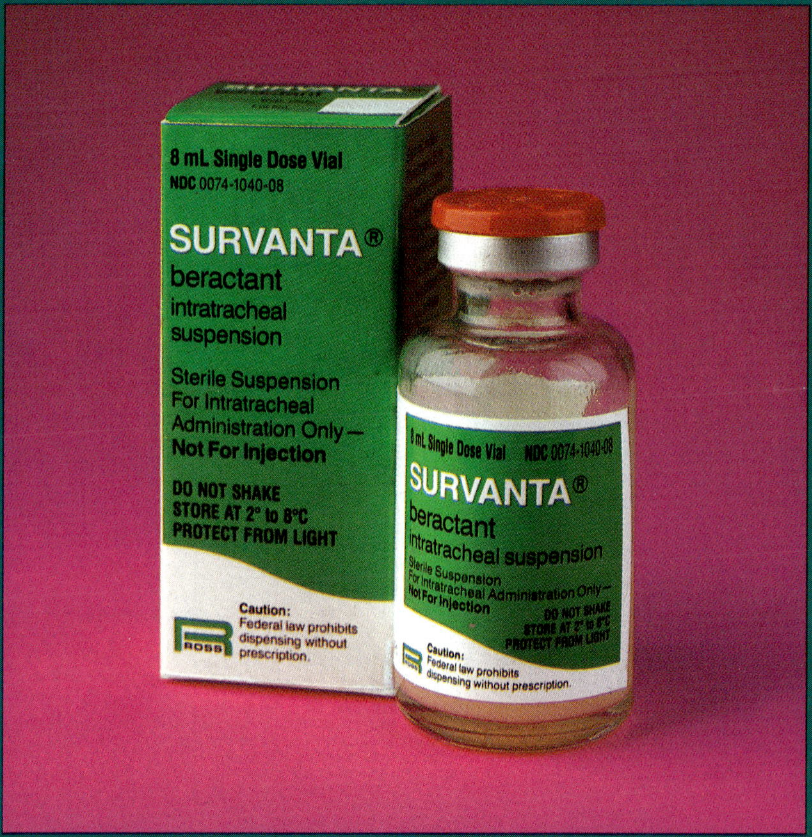

From Ross Laboratories—
Helping Premature Babies Survive™

Please see adjacent column for Brief Summary of prescribing information.

A8688/1970

ROSS LABORATORIES
COLUMBUS, OHIO 43216
Division of Abbott Laboratories, USA

LITHO IN USA

Current Literature *Continued from page 880*

Anti-inflammatory Agents

Chan JCN (Department of Clinical Pharmacology, The Chinese University of Hong Kong, Prince of Wales Hospital, Shatin NT, Hong Kong), Lai FM, Critchley JAJH. A case of Stevens-Johnson syndrome, cholestatic hepatitis and haemolytic anaemia associated with use of **mefenamic acid.** *Drug Saf.* 1991; 6:230-4. Case. (44-year-old woman with myalgia and mild ankle edema; received mefenamic acid 250 mg four times daily for four weeks; developed hemolytic anemia, Stevens-Johnson syndrome, and severe cholestatic hepatitis; concomitant acetaminophen and furosemide; therapy with methylprednisone 1 g/day for three days by i.v. injection followed by oral prednisone 30 mg/day led to resolution of rash, although renal and liver functions continued to deteriorate; therapy with prednisone 10 mg/day, furosemide 80 mg/day by i.v. injection, and albumin daily by i.v. infusion did not lead to improvement in renal and liver functions; patient died)

Antilipemic Agents

Frost PH (University of California, San Francisco, CA 94143-0326). All niacin is not the same. *Ann Intern Med.* 1991; 114:1065. Case. (56-year-old man with hypercholesterolemia; received **niacin** 4.5 g/day as Crystalline Pure Niacin, then as Nature's Plus Niacin-500; developed nausea, elevated serum alanine aminotransferase concentration, and hypolipidemia after change in niacin products; withdrawal of all niacin preparations and four days of bed rest led to complete recovery)

Drug Interactions

Khan IH (Renal Unit, Ninewells Hospital and Medical School, Dundee DD1 9SY, Scotland). **Lithium** and nonsteroidal anti-inflammatory drugs. *Br Med J.* 1991; 302:1537-8. Case. (60-year-old woman who was receiving long-term therapy with lithium; received ibuprofen 400 mg four times daily for one week for shoulder pain; developed confusion, ataxia, and stupor behavior; serum lithium concentration, 4.2 mM; serum creatinine concentration, 500 µM; withdrawal of ibuprofen and therapy with replacement fluids led to serum lithium concentration in normal range and normal renal function)

Fluorides

Duell PB (Department of Medicine, RG-26, Division of Metabolism, Endocrinology, and Nutrition, University of Washington, Seattle, WA 98195), Chesnut CH. Exacerbation of rheumatoid arthritis by **sodium fluoride** treatment of osteoporosis. *Arch Intern Med.* 1991; 151:783-4. Case (68-year-old woman with osteoporosis and rheumatoid arthritis; received fluorine 22 mg [as sodium fluoride] three times daily; developed exacerbation of rheumatoid arthritis; withdrawal of sodium fluoride for one week led to improvement in arthritic symptoms; positive rechallenge)

Hormones

Fredenrich A, Sosset C, Bernard JL et al. (Freychet P, Department of Internal Medicine, Diabetology, and Endocrinology, and Department of Surgery, Hôpital Pasteur, 06002 Nice, France). Acute pancreatitis after short-term **octreotide**. *Lancet.* 1991; 338:52-3. Case (55-year-old man with acromegaly; received octreotide 100 µg as s.c. injection for three injections; developed severe diarrhea; change to octreotide 300 µg/24 hr by continuous s.c. infusion led to complaints of abdominal pain and nausea within 24 hours; computed tomography scan revealed edema of pancreas; serum amylase concentration, 2355 IU/L; serum lipase concentration, 6174 IU/L; therapy with conventional medical treatment led to subsiding of symptoms and decreases in serum concentrations of pancreatic enzymes)

Pediatrics

Kelly K, Setlock M, Davis JP et al. Anaphylactic reactions during general anesthesia among pediatric patients—United States, January 1990–January 1991. *MMWR*. 1991; 40:437, 443. Study (case control study; 11 children, aged 3–14 years [mean, 6.9 years], who developed anaphylactic reactions within 30 minutes after start of **general anesthesia** from January 1989 through January 1991, and 64 children with meningomyelocele who did not develop anaphylactic reactions during general anesthesia from January 1990 through January 1991; 10 of 11 case patients had meningomyelocele; case children were more likely than control children to have history of allergy [odds ratio, 4.8; 95% confidence interval, 1.1–23.3], asthma [odds ratio, 7.6; 95% confidence interval, 1.0–61.7], or multiple surgical procedures [$p = 0.04$]; 10 of 11 case children tested had skin, radioallergosorbent, or enzyme-linked immunosorbent assay test results that suggested latex allergy; risk for anaphylactic reaction was higher among children with meningomyelocele or congenital genitourinary abnormality than among all other children who underwent surgery [$p < 0.001$])

Thrombolytic Agents

Brenot F (Department of Respiratory Medicine, Hôpital Antoine Beclere, 92141 Clamart, France), Pacouret G, Meyer G et al. Adverse reactions with **anistreplase**. *Lancet*. 1991; 338:114-5. Cases (three patients, aged 35–69 years, with massive pulmonary embolism but with no pre-existing cardiopulmonary disease and no previous exposure to a thrombolytic drug; received anistreplase 30 units as i.v. infusion over five minutes; developed severe hypotension; subsequently recovered, and pulmonary artery pressure and cardiac index returned to pretreatment values)

Book Reviews

Handbook of Drug Therapy in Liver and Kidney Disease

Edited by Robert W. Schrier and John G. Gambertoglio.
Published by Little, Brown and Company, 34 Beacon Street, Boston, MA 02108, 1991. xi + 388 p. $34.50.

For pharmacists who want to work actively to prevent drug-related problems in their patients, one of the most important steps should be to appropriately adjust drug dosages in patients with renal or hepatic impairment. This activity goes far beyond routine pharmacokinetic monitoring, for many more drugs are involved. Although information on this subject is available in many drug information references (including, occasionally, manufacturers' prescribing information), a practical handbook would be a useful tool for increasing efficiency in this endeavor; that handbook would be concise, well referenced, accurate, and most important, easy to use. The *Handbook of Drug Therapy in Liver and Kidney Disease* goes a long way toward meeting this need.

The handbook has three components: four general overview chapters, 10 drug class chapters, and a comprehensive drug reference table. Some limitations do exist, but each component adds to the overall usefulness of the handbook.

The general overview chapters are entitled "Altering Drug Dose," "Drug-Induced Kidney Disease," "Drug-Induced Liver Disease," and "Drug-Induced Electrolyte Disorders." Chapter 1, "Altering Drug Dose," offers a practical, straightforward review of some pharmacokinetic principles and serves as a useful introduction to the handbook; most of this chapter deals with the effect of kidney disease on these principles and includes comments on drugs and dialysis. Unfortunately, the information on liver disease is relatively brief. Although less is known about the impact of liver disease on pharmacokinetic characteristics, more attention would seem appropriate, given the purpose of the handbook. The other overview chapters appear at the end of the book; each is concise and well written. Particularly useful is the differential diagnosis section that appears after the description of each type of potential drug-induced hepatotoxic reaction.

The drug class reviews provide background documentation on dosage-adjustment logic and recommendations for adjustments. These reviews are well written with up-to-date references, several with more than 100 citations. The focus of these chapters varies. Some authors approach their topics from a disease-oriented view, emphasizing specific conditions and describing how the dosages of drugs in the class should be adjusted. Other authors take a drug-oriented approach, placing attention on drug characteristics and then discussing how specific conditions may affect them. Both approaches work, but readers would benefit from more consistency.

The final section is a comprehensive drug reference table that will likely be the most-used component of the handbook. More than 200 commonly prescribed drugs are listed. Pharmacokinetic characteristics are listed with serum half-lives for patients with liver disease, normal renal function, or no kidneys. Also listed are suggested dosage changes for patients in stages of renal impairment, with liver disease, or on dialysis. The drugs are presented in alphabetical order, regardless of class; I consider this format to be the most efficient arrangement possible, though some of my coworkers prefer that the drugs be grouped by class.

One major flaw in this handbook needs immediate attention: The index contains page number errors. The problems begin near chapter 3, with indexed topics listed about one page from where they appear in the text. The problem grows as the book continues, with the index page designations for drugs in the last chapters differing from the text by about four pages. This flaw greatly affects the intended goal of offering a handbook with easily accessible information.

I found the *Handbook of Drug Therapy in Liver and Kidney Disease* to be concise, well written, and, with the exception of the indexing error, easy to use. This handbook would serve as a useful tool for pharmacists who want to play a major role in the prevention of drug-related problems.

Reviewed by J. Russell May, Pharm.D., FASHP, Pharmacy Department, The Medical College of Georgia Hospital and Clinics, 1120 15th Street, Augusta, GA 30912-5600.

Manual of Clinical Microbiology, Fifth Edition

Edited by Albert Balows, William J. Hausler, Jr., Kenneth L. Herrmann et al.
Published by the American Society for Microbiology, 1325 Massachusetts Avenue, N.W., Washington, DC 20005, 1991. xix + 1364 p. Price $64 (ASM member), $84 (nonmember), hardbound; $56 (ASM member), $73 (nonmember), softbound.

Continued on page 889

When anxiety occurs. . .   Ativan

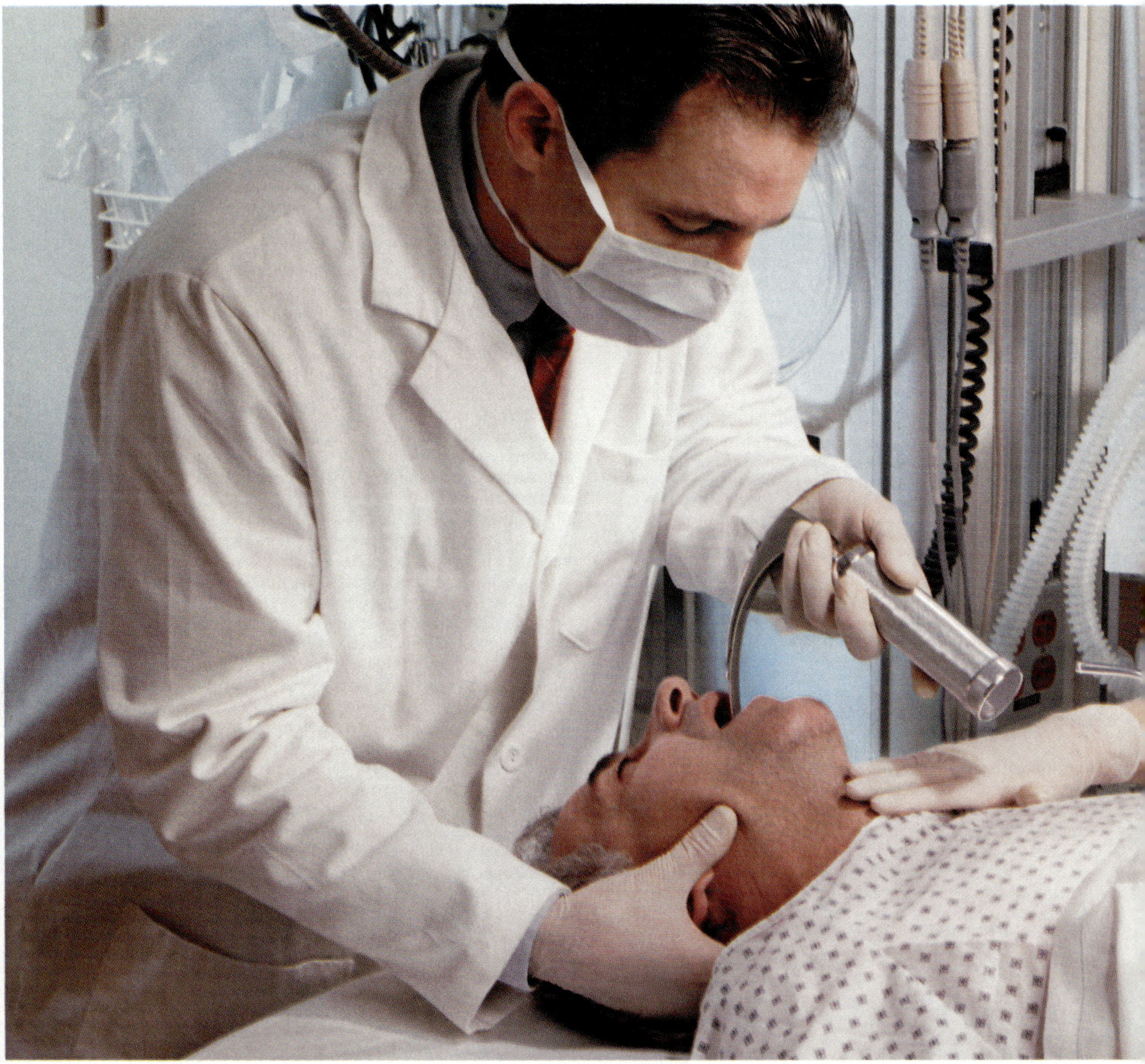

Continued from page 885

The *Manual of Clinical Microbiology* documents current practices used in clinical microbiology for detection, isolation, and identification of infectious diseases. The book discusses conceptual and practical information for the laboratory, various methods for identifying an important microbial isolate, descriptions of various pathogens and clinical relevance, and general considerations for antimicrobial susceptibility testing. This new edition includes useful tables, illustrations, color plates, and indexes. It may be viewed as a reference, a textbook, or a laboratory procedure manual, depending on the needs of its user.

The book is divided into 10 sections with 122 chapters. Section I addresses general issues in clinical microbiology, including a detailed review of microorganisms indigenous or pathogenic to humans, practical guidelines for proper collection and handling of specimens for analysis in the microbiology laboratory, a discussion of laboratory microscopy, and quality assurance and cost-control considerations that contribute to high quality health-care outcomes. The 11 chapters in Section II describe various techniques used in bacterial, mycobacterial, fungal, viral, and diagnostic immunological spectrums. Section III discusses the microbiology laboratory and nosocomial and community-acquired infections; attention is given to the epidemiology of hospital-acquired infections, with emphasis on investigating outbreaks and identifying nosocomial pathogens.

Sections IV–VIII comprise 80 chapters that address taxonomy, classification, and nomenclature of bacteria, fungi, parasites, viruses, rickettsiae, and chlamydiae. These sections compose the bulk of the book and include characterization, detection, isolation, transportation, and recovery techniques of these pathogens. Chapter 60 describes yeasts associated with overuse of broad-spectrum antimicrobials, transplantation, immunosuppressive therapy, and AIDS. Section VI, "Parasites," provides details of blood, tissue, and intestinal protozoa and helminths, with many color plates. A special chapter describes arthropods that serve as biological vectors for transmission of bacterial, viral, protozoal and metazoal diseases to humans. Section VII, "Viruses," contains current classifications of RNA- or DNA-containing viruses of vertebrates, especially viruses that infect humans.

Section IX deals exclusively with antimicrobial agents and susceptibility testing. One of the chapters provides an overview of currently marketed antibacterial and antimycobacterial agents, including mechanism of action, spectra of activity, important pharmacologic considerations, and adverse effects. Primary and alternative mechanisms of resistance to various antimicrobial agents are explained. The chapter "Assays for Antimicrobial Agents in Body Fluids" details specimen collection, processing, storage, and interpretation of results. The functions of various assay methods (bioassays, chemical assays, immunoassays, and chromatographic assays) are explained, and chromatographic assay procedures for selected antimicrobials are outlined. Two appendixes follow Section IX: preparation and storage of standard or reference antimicrobial solutions, and approximate concentrations of antimicrobial agents achieved in blood. Section X outlines quality control of media, including formulas for preparing these media.

This book is a consistent, reliable, and valuable refer-

Continued on page 890

Continued from page 889

ence for pharmacists who specialize in infectious disease pharmacotherapy or conduct antimicrobial research. It is intended for persons who know the fundamentals of microbiology and have basic laboratory skills.

Reviewed by Patricia L. Orlando, Pharm.D., Department of Pharmacy Practice, College of Pharmacy, University of Utah, Salt Lake City, UT 84112.

Pharmacological Treatment of Endocrinopathies: Bone Disease, Kidney Stones and Related Disorders

By Charles Y. C. Pak.

Published by S. Karger AG, P.O. Box CH-4009, Basel, Switzerland, 1991. viii + 141 p. Price $116; Sw.fr.145; DM174; £63.10.

This book is volume 5 of the series "Progress in Basic and Clinical Pharmacology," edited by Lomax and Vesell, and contains 9 chapters, 31 figures, 18 tables, and an index. Each chapter is a review of a pharmacologic agent used for the treatment of nephrolithiasis or osteoporosis, including sodium cellulose, phosphate salts, allopurinol, potassium citrate, tiopronin (α-mercaptopropionylglycine), thiazides, calcium citrate, estrogens, calcitonin, and diphosphonate salts. The chapters are organized into sections on historical perspective, pathophysiology of the treated condition, mechanism of action, indication and treatment guidelines, response to treatment, and adverse effects. Each chapter is independent of the others and includes a brief discussion of concomitant therapy for the indication being addressed; however, this leads to some overlap in the discussions on pathophysiology.

The first five chapters address the prevention and pharmacologic management of kidney stones, including those caused by absorptive hypercalciuria, uric acid, cystinuria, and primary hypercalciuria. The clinical data supporting use of the agent for specific conditions are summarized, and the expected outcomes of therapy are discussed. References for the clinical trials presented in these chapters are as recent as 1988.

The last four chapters of the book address osteoporosis and current therapies available for its management. References for these chapters are as recent as 1989, with a single 1990 citation for diphosphonate salts. A consensus chapter for the management of osteoporosis would have been useful as a comparison of the different therapies and their respective roles in treatment.

Most of the book was written by Pak, and there is good continuity of organization among the chapters. Other contributors are Bruce Ettinger ("Allopurinol for the Treatment of Uric Acid and Calcium Calculi"), Clare D. Edman ("Estrogens for Prevention of Postmenopausal Osteoporosis"), and Stanley Wallach ("Calcitonin Treatment of Osteoporosis"). This book serves as a single reference for the pharmacologic management of stone and bone diseases and would serve as a useful supplement to other books that address the pathophysiology of these diseases.

This book is written for medical students and persons who care for patients with kidney stones or osteoporosis. Pharmacists involved in the management of these patients or the education of students in the areas of nephrology and endocrinology will find the book useful. The book would also serve as a useful addition to the drug information library.

Reviewed by Thomas J. Comstock, Pharm.D., Department of Pharmacy and Pharmaceutics, School of Pharmacy, Virginia Commonwealth University, Medical College of Virginia Campus, Box 533, Richmond, VA 23298-0533.

Books Received

Books are listed as soon as received; selected books are reviewed in Book Reviews in subsequent issues.

Counseling Patients on Their Medications: One of the Principal Responsibilities of the Health Care Practitioner, by Arnold W. Karig and Edward A. Hartshorn. Published by Drug Intelligence Publications, Inc., 1241 Broadway, Hamilton, IL 62341, 1991. xvi + 564 p. Price $59, plus $4 shipping and handling.

Data Collection Forms in Clinical Trials, by Bert Spilker and John Schoenfelder. Published by Raven Press, 1185 Avenue of the Americas, New York, NY 10036, 1990. xv + 672 p. Price $90.

Advertising Index

Burroughs Wellcome Company
Exosurf, 815-819
Eli Lilly and Company
Hospital Division, 813
National Easter Seal Society
Institutional, 879
Ross Laboratories
Survanta, 883-884
SmithKline Beecham
Tagamet, inside back cover, outside back cover
The Upjohn Company
Zefazone, 810-812
Wyeth-Ayerst Laboratories, Inc.
Ativan Injection, 886-888
Tubex, inside front cover

News

Consensus panel stresses need for greater awareness of panic disorder and its treatment 893

E5 antiendotoxin antibody reduces mortality among subset of patients with gram-negative sepsis, study finds 897

CAST II halted because of mortality trends 897

Bristol discontinues sales of encainide 897

Study shows effect of postmenopausal estrogen therapy on cardiovascular risk 897

CDC offers recommendations for folic acid prevention of neural tube defects 898

News Briefs 898

Upcoming Specialty Meetings 898

Consensus panel stresses need for greater awareness of panic disorder and its treatment

Effective therapy is available for panic disorder, but only one in four patients with the disorder receive appropriate treatment, concluded panelists of the National Institutes of Health Consensus Development Conference on the Treatment of Panic Disorder, held in Bethesda, Maryland, September 25–27. The panel called for an aggressive educational campaign to make clinicians, patients and their families, the media, and the general public more aware of panic disorder.

One in 75 persons is affected by panic disorder. The age of onset is typically in the teenage years or during early adulthood, and the disorder is more common in women than in men. The diagnosis of panic disorder must include a medical workup to exclude other conditions causing similar symptoms. Clinicians must guard against misdiagnoses leading to costly medical investigations and delays in the provision of effective therapy. Patients with panic disorder often have associated disorders (e.g., depression, anxiety, personality disorders, alcohol or drug abuse) that require treatment.

Both pharmacologic and cognitive–behavioral therapies are effective for panic disorder. Behavioral approaches (e.g., graduated exposure) are aimed at reducing avoidance and anticipatory anxiety. Cognitive–behavioral approaches directly target panic attacks. The treatments typically involve 8–12 weekly sessions. Patients may show improvement in three to six weeks. Dropout rates range from 5–8% for cognitive–behavioral therapies to 12–16% for relaxation and exposure-based treatments. The efficacy of other forms of psychotherapy has not been proved.

Pharmacologic therapies include tricyclic antidepressants, monoamine oxidase inhibitors, and high-potency benzodiazepines. Treatment duration ranges from two to eight months. Potential risks and benefits of each drug class must be weighed when treatment decisions are made. The benzodiazepines have a rapid onset of action, and the drug-induced reduction in anxiety between attacks may be beneficial. Therapeutic effects of tricyclic

Continued on page 897

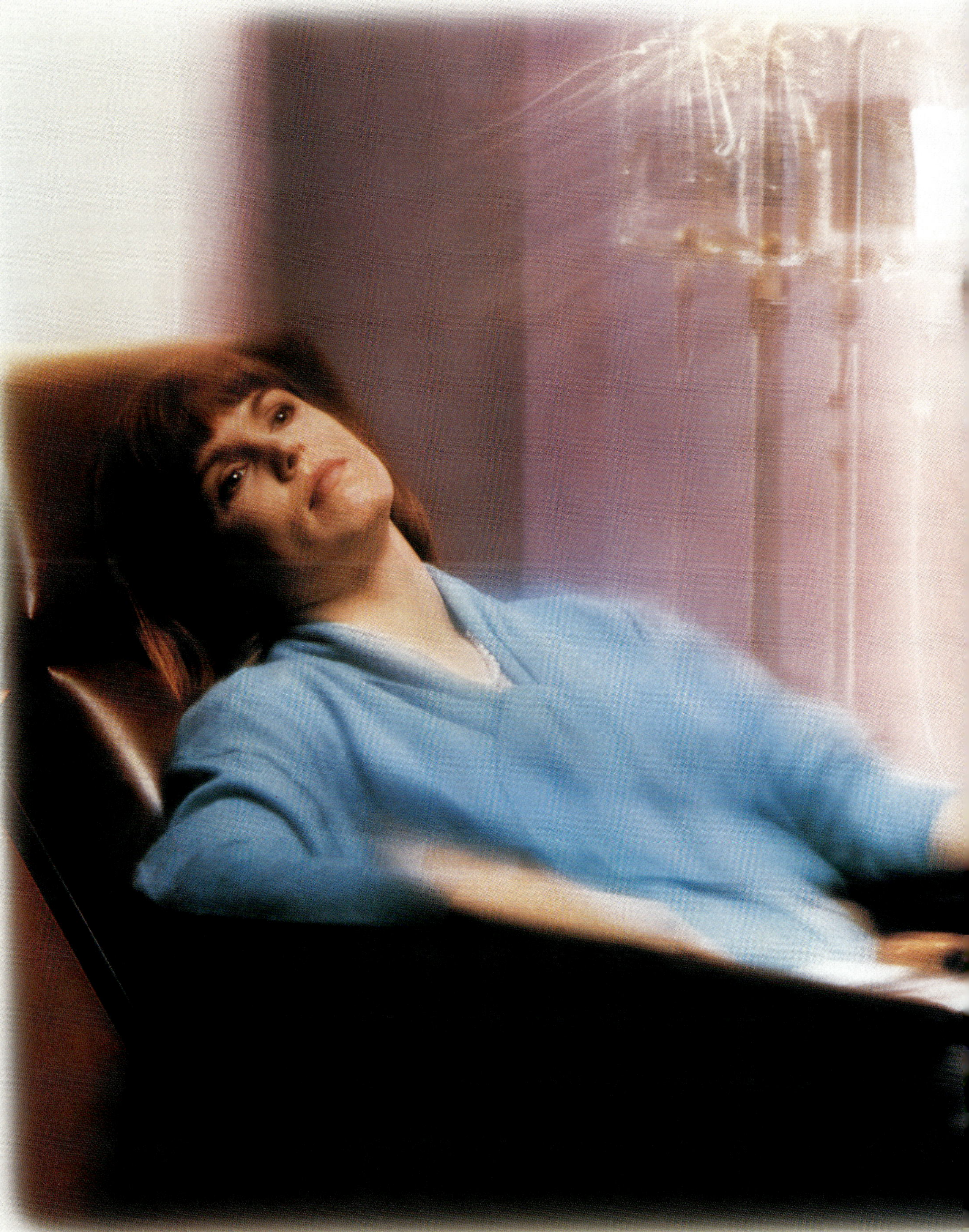

Continued from page 893

antidepressants may not be evident for three to six weeks. Attrition rates in studies involving pharmacotherapy for panic disorder were 30–35% for tricyclic antidepressants, slightly lower for monoamine oxidase inhibitors, and 15–20% for benzodiazepines. Gradually increasing the dosage to therapeutic levels may improve patient acceptance of therapy, particularly when tricyclic antidepressants are used. Relapse rates after discontinuation of therapy are moderate for antidepressants and highest for the benzodiazepines. Treatment should be withdrawn gradually. Risks during tapering of long-term benzodiazepine therapy include withdrawal syndromes and rebound of panic symptoms.

Information on the efficacy of combined pharmacologic therapy and behavioral or cognitive therapy is limited.

In selecting a therapeutic approach, clinicians must consider the degree of urgency, the patient's history, concurrent medication use and medical or psychiatric conditions that may affect the safety or efficacy of the therapy selected, the patient's attitudes toward treatment options, and compliance issues. With either pharmacologic or cognitive–behavioral approaches, treatment should be reassessed if it fails to produce a response within six to eight weeks.

Critical research needs identified by the panel included the development of reliable measures for assessment, basic research to better define the disorder, and identification of optimal treatment approaches for individual patients.

E5 antiendotoxin antibody reduces mortality among subset of patients with gram-negative sepsis, study finds

Treatment with E5 murine monoclonal IgM antibody to endotoxin reduces mortality and increases resolution of organ failure in patients with gram-negative sepsis who are not in refractory shock, according to a multicenter, double-blind, placebo-controlled trial.[1]

All patients were adults who met the study definition of gram-negative infection with a systemic septic response. Treatment consisted of a 2-mg/kg dose of E5 administered intravenously over one hour. A second dose was administered 24 hours later.

Of the 486 patients enrolled in the study, 316 (164, E5 group; 152, placebo group) had confirmed gram-negative sepsis. Among those 316 patients, no overall difference in survival was detected between the E5 and placebo groups. A treatment-related difference in survival was apparent among the 137 patients with gram-negative sepsis with or without bacteremia who were not in shock refractory to fluid resuscitation and inotrope support at study entry: The E5 group had a 2.3-fold survival advantage. E5 did not confer a survival advantage to patients with gram-negative sepsis who were in shock or to patients in whom gram-negative sepsis was not documented. Among the 137 patients with gram-negative sepsis who were not in shock, those treated with E5 experienced greater resolution of organ failure (19 [54%] of 35, E5 group; 8 [30%] of 27, placebo group); no treatment-related effect on organ dysfunction was detected in those with shock. Adverse events were similar in the E5 and placebo groups, with the exception of four apparent allergic reactions to E5.

1. Greenman RL, Schein RMH, Martin MA et al. A controlled clinical trial of E5 murine monoclonal IgM antibody to endotoxin in the treatment of gram-negative sepsis. *JAMA*. 1991; 266:1097-102.

CAST II halted because of mortality trends

The phase of the Cardiac Arrhythmia Suppression Trial comparing moricizine with placebo (CAST II) was halted by the National Heart, Lung, and Blood Institute in August because data showed a trend of decreased survival among patients receiving moricizine. The study was designed to assess whether suppression of ventricular ectopy after myocardial infarction improves long-term survival. When the trial was stopped, 1346 study patients had been followed for an average of 18 months. A total of 97 patients in the moricizine group had died, compared with 74 in the placebo group.

Bristol discontinues sales of encainide

Bristol Laboratories has announced that it will discontinue sales and commercial distribution of encainide hydrochloride (Enkaid) effective December 16, 1991. According to the company, the decision was based on continuing uncertainty over the implications of the Cardiac Arrhythmia Suppression Trial and the availability of alternative agents. A program has been established that will enable patients to receive the drug at no charge if they are receiving the drug for a labeled indication and cannot be switched to another antiarrhythmic agent. The program is open to patients who were receiving encainide for a labeled indication on or before September 16. For more information, call Bristol Laboratories at 800-527-6741.

Study shows effect of postmenopausal estrogen therapy on cardiovascular risk

Postmenopausal estrogen therapy is associated with a reduction in the incidence of coronary heart disease and in mortality from cardiovascular disease, but it does not alter the risk of stroke; these were the major findings after 10-year follow-up of the Nurses' Health Study.[1]

A total of 48,470 postmenopausal women who participated in the Nurses' Health Study and had no history of cancer or cardiovascular disease at study enrollment were followed by questionnaire every 2 years for up to 10 years. The study began in 1976.

During the follow-up period, 224 strokes, 405 cases of major coronary disease (nonfatal myocardial infarction or death from coronary causes), and 1263 deaths from all causes were documented. The relative risk of major coronary disease among current estrogen users, compared with those who had never received postmenopausal estrogen therapy, was 0.56 (after adjustment for age and other risk factors; 95% confidence interval, 0.40 to 0.80). The relative risk of stroke among current users was 0.97 (95% confidence interval, 0.65 to 1.45). When current and former users of postmenopausal estrogen therapy were compared with nonusers, the relative risk of mortality was 0.89 (95% confidence interval, 0.78 to 1.00) and the relative risk of mortality from cardiovascular disease was 0.72 (95% confidence interval, 0.55 to 0.95).

1. Stampfer MJ, Colditz GA, Willett WC et al. Postmenopausal estrogen therapy and cardiovascular disease: ten-year follow-up from the Nurses' Health Study. *N Engl J Med*. 1991; 325:756-62.

CDC offers recommendations for folic acid prevention of neural tube defects

The Centers for Disease Control (CDC) has issued interim recommendations for folic acid supplementation for women who have had an infant or fetus with spina bifida, anencephaly, or encephalocele and are planning a subsequent pregnancy.[1] The risk of neural tube defects in subsequent pregnancies is 2–3%. Supplementation with folic acid 4 mg/day from the time the woman plans to become pregnant (at least four weeks before conception) through the first three months of pregnancy is recommended. The recommendations are based on a study reported by the British Medical Research Council Vitamin Study Group showing that supplementation with folic acid 4 mg/day with or without multivitamins had a protective effect in women who had previously had infants or fetuses with neural tube defects.[2] Neural tube defects occurred in 6 (1%) of 593 infants or fetuses of women who received folic acid compared with 21 (3.5%) of 602 infants or fetuses of women who did not receive folic acid. Multivitamins without folic acid did not protect against neural tube defects.

1. Centers for Disease Control. Use of folic acid for prevention of spina bifida and other neural tube defects—1983–1991. *MMWR*. 1991; 40:513-6.
2. MRC Vitamin Study Research Group. Prevention of neural tube defects; results of the Medical Research Council Vitamin Study. *Lancet*. 1991; 338:131-7.

News Briefs

• FDA has established a toll-free telephone service (800-238-7332) to handle questions from health professionals about **FDA policies on medical advertising, marketing, and promotion** and to discuss promotional activities for health-care products that may require FDA attention. The service covers drugs, biologicals, medical devices, and veterinary products. Documents may be transmitted by fax (800-344-3332).

• **A concentrated (10-mg/mL and 25-mg/mL) preservative-free formulation of morphine sulfate** (Infumorph, Elkins-Sinn) has been approved by FDA; it is labeled for use in microinfusion devices for intrathecal or epidural injection.

• Labeled indications for **topical minoxidil solution** (Rogaine, Upjohn) have been expanded to include androgenetic alopecia in women.

• **"Innovations for Infection Control Practices" teleconferences** are scheduled for 1430–1530 Eastern time on the third Tuesday of each month through September 1992; to register, contact Teleconference Network of Texas, The University of Texas Health Science Center at San Antonio, 7703 Floyd Curl Drive, San Antonio, TX 78284, or call 512-567-2700.

• **The newsletter "Rosacea Review" and a brochure entitled "Rosacea: A Conspicuous Condition . . . A Treatable Condition"** are available free of charge to the public and to pharmacists and physicians for distribution to patients; for more information, contact The National Rosacea Society, 18-3 East Dundee Road, Suite 206, Barrington, IL 60010.

Upcoming Specialty Meetings

Alzheimer's Disease: New Approaches to Treatment, sponsored by the University of California at San Diego Alzheimer's Disease Research Center. San Diego, CA, January 24–25; contact Cass Jones, Professional Conference Management, Inc., 7916 Convoy Court, San Diego, CA 92111; 619-565-9921.

American Academy of Allergy and Immunology. Orlando, FL, March 6–11; contact AAAI, 611 East Wells Street, Milwaukee, WI 53202; 414-272-6071.

American Society for Clinical Pharmacology and Therapeutics. Orlando, FL, March 18–20; contact E. Galasso, 1718 Gallagher Road, Norristown, PA 19401; 215-825-3838.

Society for Adolescent Medicine. Washington, DC, March 19–22; contact E. Moore, 19401 East U.S. Highway 40, Suite 120, Independence, MO 64055; 816-795-8336.

American College of Preventive Medicine. Baltimore, MD, March 21–24; contact ACPM, 1015 15th Street N.W., Suite 403, Washington, DC 20005; 202-789-0003.

Bio International '92, conference on bioavailability, bioequivalence, and pharmacokinetics studies. Bad Homburg–Frankfurt, Germany, May 20–22; contact International Pharmaceutical Federation, Congress Department, Alexanderstraat 11, 2514 JL The Hague, the Netherlands.

Therapy Consultation

The Therapy Consultation *section provides brief advice, in question-and-answer format, on how to handle specific drug-therapy problems. Readers are invited to submit questions, which will be referred to a consultant for an answer. The problems should not be highly specialized or unusual, nor should they be mundane. Questions are answered briefly, based largely on the judgment and personal experience of the consultant, although selected references may be cited to substantiate the consultant's advice.*

Assistance in identifying Therapy Consultation *topics is provided by the drug information centers at Medical College of Virginia Hospitals, Richmond; University of California Medical Center, San Diego; and University of Michigan Medical Center, Ann Arbor.*

Comparing surfactant products

Question: Two surfactant products are now approved by the FDA for use in the treatment or prevention of neonatal respiratory distress syndrome. Are the products equivalent? What criteria should be used for comparison?

Answer: There are four categories of surfactant products: natural (human or bovine), modified natural, synthetic, and synthetic natural. The two products approved by FDA are Survanta, a modified natural product by Ross Laboratories, and Exosurf, a synthetic product by Burroughs Wellcome. Modified natural products such as Survanta (bovine), Infasurf (bovine) (Ony, Inc., Amherst, NY), and Curosurf (porcine) (Chiesi Farmaceutici, Parma, Italy) are derived from lung fluid lavage or minced lung extract. Some components, such as surfactant-specific protein A (SPA), have been selectively removed. Survanta contains less than 2% by weight of surfactant-specific proteins B (SPB) and C (SPC). In comparison, human surfactant is 11% protein. These proteins allow surfactant to form a stable monolayer over the alveolar air–liquid interface. Although SPA is the most abundant protein in natural surfactant, it is selectively removed from modified natural products because it does not aid in the formation of a monolayer. Concern exists over the antigenicity of bovine or porcine protein; however, antibody formation has not been identified in infants treated with products of animal origin.[1] Synthetic products such as Exosurf are completely artificial; they contain no mammalian proteins. The alcohol hexadecanol functions in lieu of SPB and SPC to enhance surface spreading.

The difference in product origin results in different dosage recommendations. The recommended 5-mL/kg dose of Exosurf delivers 67.5 mg of dipalmitylphosphatidylcholine (DPPC, also known as lecithin or colfosceril) per kilogram of body weight. The recommended 4-mL/kg dose of Survanta delivers 100 mg of mixed phospholipids per kilogram of body weight; approximately 80% of the phospholipids are natural DPPC. The products also differ with respect to packaging and storage requirements, dosing protocols, and administration techniques (see table).

Survanta and Exosurf are both labeled for prevention of neonatal respiratory distress syndrome (RDS) and for rescue therapy after RDS is established. In clinical trials, the primary difference between the two products has been rapidity of response.[2,3] Compared with Exosurf, Survanta produces a more dramatic decrease in oxygen requirements and ventilator pressures immediately after administration. The mechanism for this difference is not known. The difference does not appear to affect long-term outcome. In infants remaining ventilator dependent at 7 and 28 days after surfactant administration, ventilator settings and oxygen requirements, compared with those of placebo-treated infants, do not differ between the two products. With both products, improvement in oxygenation is usually the first sign of pharmacologic success. Hypoxia and bradycardia can occur during treatment and are directly related to the dosing procedure. Acute changes in respiratory function and the need for immediate adjustments in ventilator settings should be anticipated.

Efficacy comparisons are difficult because studies have differed in enrollment criteria, number of doses, monitoring, and outcome measures. Many practitioners believe that the optimal dosage is yet to be determined. However, it is clear that neonatal mortality is reduced by surfactant therapy. Compared with placebo-treated patients, surfactant-treated patients have mortality rates that are 5–10% lower in prophylaxis studies and 10–12% lower in rescue studies, independent of surfactant product.[3,4] Prevention studies with Survanta have shown a significantly lower incidence of RDS,[5] while prevention studies with Exosurf have not.[6] With both products, early rescue (within four hours of the onset of respiratory distress) is associated with a better clinical outcome than late rescue. Complications of prematurity, such as patent ductus arteriosus, severe intracranial bleeding, and chronic lung disease are not decreased by the use of either surfactant product.

Continued on page 911

Continued from page 909

Comparison of Currently Marketed Surfactant Products[a]

Variable	Colfosceril (Exosurf)	Beractant (Survanta)
Components	Synthetic DPPC (hexadecanol and DPPC)	Calf lung extract (<2% protein with natural DPPC and mixed phospholipids)
Dose (mg/kg)	DPPC 67.5	Phospholipids 100
Volume of dose (mL/kg)	5	4
Criterion for use	$FiO_2 > 0.3$ at arterial $Po_2 < 80$ mm Hg	$FiO_2 > 0.3$ at aterial $Po_2 < 80$ mm Hg
Indications	Rescue therapy or prophylaxis	Rescue therapy or prophylaxis
Recommended dosage for rescue therapy	Give two doses 12 hours apart, re-evaluate to determine need for third dose	Give one dose, re-evaluate to determine need for doses 2–4
Administration technique	Administer through ETT adapter via ventilator, divide dose into two aliquots with position change	Administer through disconnected ETT, divide dose into four aliquots with position change
Storage	Lyophilized powder	Refrigerated suspension
Vial size (mL)	8	8
Special instructions	Reconstitute with 8 mL of preservative-free sterile water for injection, follow mixing procedures carefully, do not shake	Warm to room temperature, do not shake
Cost per vial ($)[b]	594	594

[a] DPPC = dipalmitylphosphatidylcholine, FiO_2 = fractional inspired oxygen, Po_2 = oxygen pressure, ETT = endotracheal tube.
[b] Average wholesale price in September 1991.

Many surfactant trials have yet to be published. A comparison of Survanta and Exosurf rescue therapy is currently under way at nine medical centers. Neonates are stratified into three weight categories and receive the product assigned by a central randomization process. Each medication is administered according to its package insert guidelines, except that four doses of Exosurf are allowed if the infant is still ventilator dependent 12 hours after the third dose. At our center, 71 infants have thus far been enrolled. There has been no difference between the two medications in the mean number of doses required.

Surfactant products are very expensive. The hospital cost for one multidose course is approximately $2400. It is anticipated that all marketed products will be competitively priced. Neonatal intensive-care costs are approximately $3000/day. Unfortunately, a decreased length of hospitalization has not yet been documented with surfactant therapy. In fact, a reduction in mortality may actually increase hospital costs.

At this time, Survanta and Exosurf are considered therapeutically equivalent. Mortality is reduced by their administration. Prevention studies with Survanta show a lower incidence of RDS in the surfactant group compared with the placebo group. Survanta produces a more rapid increase in lung compliance than does Exosurf. The two products are competitively priced. It is hoped that any major differences in efficacy and long-term outcome, if present, will be identified by the comparison trial currently under way.

1. Whitsett JA, Hull WM, Luse S. Failure to detect surfactant protein-specific antibodies in sera of premature infants treated with Survanta, a modified bovine surfactant. *Pediatrics*. 1991; 87:505-10.
2. Horbar JD, Soll RF, Sutherland JM et al. A multicenter randomized placebo-controlled trial of surfactant therapy for respiratory distress syndrome. *N Engl J Med*. 1989; 320:959-65.
3. Phibbs RH, Ballard RA, Clements JA. Initial clinical trial of Exosurf, a protein-free synthetic surfactant, for the prophylaxis and early treatment of hyaline membrane disease. *Pediatrics*. 1991; 88:1-9.
4. Hoekstra RE, Jackson JC, Myers TF. Improved neonatal survival following multiple doses of bovine surfactant in very premature neonates at risk for respiratory distress syndrome. *Pediatrics*. 1991; 88:10-8.
5. Ross Laboratories. Survanta package insert. Columbus, OH; 1991 Mar.
6. Burroughs Wellcome Company. Exosurf package insert. Research Triangle Park, NC; 1990 Aug.

Rebecca Rogers Prevost, Pharm.D.
Clinical Pharmacist for Obstetrics-Gynecology-Neonatology
Regional Medical Center
877 Jefferson Avenue
Memphis, TN 38103

Letters

Inverse relationship between desmopressin dosage and antidiuresis 912
Robert E. Ariano, Beverly Seymour

Correction to *AHFS Drug Information 91* 913
Stephanie L. Scholten

Corrections 913

The Letters *column is a forum for rapid exchange of ideas among readers of* Clinical Pharmacy. *Liberal criteria are applied in the review of submissions to encourage contributions to this column.*

The Letters *column includes the following types of contributions: (1) comments, addenda, and minor updates on previously published work, (2) alerts on potential problems related to drug therapy or clinical research, (3) observations or comments on trends in drug therapy or clinical research, and (4) brief expressions of opinion about controversies in drug therapy or clinical research.*

Letters need not be submitted with the journal's manuscript checklist. The following conditions, however, must be adhered to: (1) the body of the letter must be no longer than two typewritten pages, (2) the use of references, tables, and illustrations should be minimized, (3) the authors' names, affiliations, and mailing addresses must be typed at the end of the letter in the format used by Clinical Pharmacy, *and (4) the entire letter (including references, tables, and authors' names) must be typed double-spaced on plain white paper (not letterhead). Following acceptance of a letter, the authors are required to sign an exclusive publication statement and a copyright transferal form.*

Inverse relationship between desmopressin dosage and antidiuresis

Desmopressin is the drug of choice for the treatment of postoperative diabetes insipidus and is also an important adjuvant in the management of a variety of bleeding disorders. We have observed in our surgical intensive-care unit that the relatively large i.v. doses of desmopressin acetate used in the management of postoperative bleeding disorders (e.g., 20 μg or 10 μg/sq m) have no appreciable effect on hourly urine output. In patients with postoperative diabetes insipidus, however, smaller i.v. doses of desmopressin acetate (e.g., 2 μg) result in substantial reductions in hourly urine output.

There seems to be some form of inverse relationship between the size of the desmopressin dose and the degree of antidiuresis. We do not believe that the existence of diabetes insipidus or of bleeding disorders is a primary influencing factor in this relationship. The inverse relationship has been reported in clinical trials examining the effectiveness of desmopressin in the management of bleeding disorders.[1-5] That the phenomenon is misunderstood is illustrated by a statement in a recent review article that "the doses [of desmopressin] used to induce hemostasis are not large enough to produce a clinical effect on the renal system."[6] In fact, the i.v. dose of desmopressin used for hemostasis is much larger than the dose used to affect the kidneys in patients with diabetes insipidus.

We have found no explanation in the literature for the inverse relationship between desmopressin's dosage and its antidiuretic effects, but we have postulated a mechanism. Prostacyclin, an endogenous prostaglandin, can increase renal blood flow and provoke diuresis.[7] Desmopressin stimulates the release of prostacyclin,[8] but whether this is a dose-related phenomenon is unknown. High doses of desmopressin may increase the release of prostacyclin and thereby blunt or antagonize desmopressin's antidiuretic effect. Consistent with this mechanism is the possibility that prostacyclin release is responsible for the vasodilatation (flushing and hypotension) that occurs after the rapid infusion of larger doses of desmopressin acetate (e.g., 20 μg); smaller doses (e.g., 1–4 μg) do not produce this adverse effect. (Prostacyclin may also interfere to some extent with desmopressin's platelet-aggregating properties.)

It would be interesting to measure the diuresis after a large dose of desmopressin in a patient also receiving an inhibitor of prostacyclin production (e.g., indomethacin). A prompt desmopressin-associated reduction in urine output would support our suggested mechanism. We would like to alert clinicians to monitor diuresis in patients who are treated with desmopressin for bleeding disorders related to nonsteroidal anti-inflammatory drugs.

1. Mannucci PM, Remuzzi G, Pusineri F et al. Deamino-8-D-arginine vasopressin shortens the bleeding time in uremia. *N Engl J Med*. 1983; 308:8-12.
2. Kobrinsky NL, Israels ED, Gerrard JM et al. Shortening of bleeding time by 1-deamino-8-D-arginine vasopressin in various bleeding disorders. *Lancet*. 1984; 1:1145-8.
3. Salzman EW, Weinstein MJ, Weintraub RM et al. Treatment with desmopressin acetate to reduce blood loss after cardiac surgery. *N Engl J Med*. 1986; 314:1402-6.
4. Rocha E, Llorens R, Paramo JA et al. Does desmopressin acetate reduce blood loss after surgery in patients on cardiopulmonary bypass? *Circulation*. 1988; 77:1319-23.
5. Seear MD, Wadsworth LD, Rogers PC et al. The effect of desmopressin acetate (DDAVP) on postoperative blood loss after cardiac operations in children. *J Thorac Cardiovasc Surg*. 1989; 98:217-9.
6. Salva KM, Kim HC, Nahum K et al. DDAVP in the treatment of bleeding disorders. *Pharmacotherapy*. 1988; 8:94-9.
7. Campbell WB. Lipid-derived autacoids: eicosanoids and platelet activating factor. In: Goodman and Gilman's the pharmacological basis of therapeutics. 8th ed. Gilman AG, Rall TW, Nies AS et al., eds. New York: Pergamon; 1990:607-17.
8. Belch JJF, Small M, McKenzie F et al. DDAVP stimulates prostacyclin production. *Thromb Haemost*. 1982; 47:122-3.

ROBERT E. ARIANO, PHARM.D., Clinical Pharmacist in Intensive Care
Department of Pharmacy
St. Boniface General Hospital
Winnipeg, Manitoba R2H 2A6
Canada

BEVERLY SEYMOUR
Penner Foods Pharmacy
Winnipeg, Manitoba
Canada

Correction to *AHFS Drug Information 91*

This is to inform users of *AHFS Drug Information 91*[1] that an error exists on page 86 in the ketoconazole monograph. The fourth sentence in the Dosage section should state, "For example, increasing the dosage to 600–800 mg daily may be considered for patients with blastomycosis that progresses or establishes a new focus of infection at 400 mg daily."

1. AHFS drug information 91. McEvoy GK, ed. Bethesda, MD: American Society of Hospital Pharmacists; 1991.

STEPHANIE L. SCHOLTEN, Pharmacy Resident
Pharmacy Department
University of Iowa Hospital and Clinics
Iowa City, IA 52242

Editor's note: The corrected dosage appears in Supplement A, AHFS Drug Information 91.

Corrections

Intravenous quinidine recommended for severe *Plasmodium falciparum* malaria; injectable quinine discontinued by CDC Drug Service (September 1991, News). On page 657, the article should state that the infusion rate should be slowed if the plasma quinidine concentration is >6 μg/mL, not >6 mg/mL.

Criteria for use of ketorolac tromethamine in adult inpatients and outpatients (September 1991, DUE Criteria). On pages 716 and 717, the standard for elements 23–27 should be 0%, not 100%.

Drug Review

Succimer, an oral lead chelator

Katherine V. Mann and John D. Travers

Abstract: The pharmacology, pharmacokinetics, clinical efficacy, adverse effects, and dosage and administration of succimer when used for the treatment of lead poisoning are reviewed.

Succimer is an orally active, heavy-metal chelating agent that forms stable, water-soluble complexes with lead; it also chelates other toxic heavy metals, such as arsenic and mercury. It is a designated orphan drug that is indicated for the treatment of lead poisoning, specifically in children with blood lead concentrations higher than 45 μg/dL. Succimer reverses the adverse metabolic effects of lead on heme synthesis while increasing urinary lead output without adversely affecting essential mineral excretion at the recommended dosage regimen. The rebound in lead concentrations that can occur after short courses of chelating therapies (caused by redistribution of lead from bone stores) may require frequent and multiple courses of chelation therapy.

The most common adverse effects reported in clinical trials of succimer in children and adults were nausea, vomiting, diarrhea, appetite loss, and loose stools; these effects may be related to the drug's unpleasant mercaptan odor. There are no known drug interactions between succimer and other drugs, including iron supplements, although data are limited. The recommended initial dosage in children is 10 mg/kg or 350 mg/sq m every eight hours for five days. The dosage is then reduced to 10 mg/kg or 350 mg/sq m every 12 hours for an additional two weeks.

Clinical studies indicate that succimer is relatively selective for lead and effectively lowers blood lead concentrations. Although clinical experience is limited, an oral lead chelator may offer advantages over currently available agents.

Index terms: Dosage; Drug administration; Heavy metal antagonists; Lead; Pharmacokinetics; Poisoning; Succimer; Toxicity
Clin Pharm. 1991; 10:914-22

Lead toxicity in children is an entirely preventable disease; however, lead toxicity remains an important health problem of U.S. children. Prevention of exposure to environmental lead is essential, and abatement of environmental lead is of primary importance. The 1985 Centers for Disease Control statement on prevention of lead poisoning in young children[1] is currently being updated. The revised document will provide practitioners with current recommendations regarding prevention of, screening for, and degrees of intervention in childhood lead poisoning.

Of importance to many children who already have lead intoxication is access to safe, effective therapy to reduce their body burden of lead. Chelation treatment for lead poisoning decreases the body burden of lead far more rapidly than normal excretory processes can and enhances the removal of the readily mobile soft-tissue fraction of body lead, which is potentially the most toxic fraction of body lead.[2,3]

Succimer (Chemet, McNeil Consumer Products Company) is an orally active chelating agent that was marketed in January 1991 for the treatment of lead poisoning, specifically in children with blood lead concentrations higher than 45 μg/dL. Succimer is a designated orphan drug. Although some clinicians have advocated the use of oral penicillamine for the treatment of lead poisoning, that remains an unlabeled use for penicillamine. The relative lack of specificity of penicillamine for lead, along with the incidence of adverse effects (which approached 33% of treated patients in one recent study[4]), tends to limit the usefulness of penicillamine for the treatment of lead poison-

Katherine V. Mann, Pharm.D., is Assistant Director, Medical Affairs, McNeil Consumer Products Company, Fort Washington, PA; Certified Poison Information Specialist, The Poison Control Center, Philadelphia, PA; and Lecturer in Clinical Pharmacy, Philadelphia College of Pharmacy and Science. John D. Travers M.D., M.P.H., is Assistant Director, Clinical Research, McNeil Consumer Products Company.

Address reprint requests to Dr. Mann at the McNeil Consumer Products Company, Camp Hill Road, Fort Washington, PA 19034.

This is **article 680-204-9130** in the **ASHP Continuing Education System**; it qualifies for 1.0 hour of continuing-education credit. See page 953 for learning objectives and test questions.

ing. Thus, succimer is the first oral medication indicated for the treatment of lead poisoning and the first new chelating agent for lead toxicity in the more than 40 years since the approval of edetate calcium disodium.

This review focuses on the pharmacology, pharmacokinetics, clinical efficacy, adverse effects, and dosage and administration of succimer when used for the treatment of lead poisoning.

Chemistry and Stability

The succimer molecule was first used by Friedheim and colleagues,[5] who incorporated the molecule into compounds for the treatment of schistosomiasis and trypanosomiasis. Succimer is the stable *meso* isomer of 2,3-dimercaptosuccinic acid; it also has been known as DMSA. The chemical structure of succimer is shown in Figure 1. The empirical formula for succimer is $C_4H_6O_4S_2$; the molecular weight is 182.2.[6] Succimer is a white crystalline powder with a characteristic mercaptan (sulfur) odor and taste; it is practically insoluble in water, very slightly soluble in acetone and ethanol, and very soluble in aqueous alkaline solutions. Succimer has a pKa_1 of 3.0 and a pKa_2 of 3.9. Succimer should be stored at controlled room temperature (15–30 °C).[a]

Pharmacology

Succimer is an orally active, heavy-metal chelating agent that forms stable, water-soluble complexes with lead in vitro (Figure 2)[7] and consequently increases the urinary excretion of lead.[8-14] Succimer also has been found to chelate other toxic heavy metals, such as arsenic[15] and mercury.[9,16,17]

Controlled trials of succimer,[11,12] as well as earlier animal studies,[18,a] have examined the effect of succimer administration on urinary excretion of the essential trace minerals calcium, copper, iron, and magnesium. The studies are consistent in that they find succimer specific for lead without clinically important elevations in trace mineral excretion at the doses and durations studied. In one of these trials,[11] a significant increase (1.6-fold to 1.8-fold higher than the pretreatment values) in zinc excretion was observed, and data with respect to copper excretion were conflicting. The effect of succimer on the excretion of essential minerals is small compared with that of edetate calcium disodium, which can induce a more than 10-fold increase in urinary excretion of zinc and a twofold increase in urinary excretion of copper and iron.[19,20] The potential for substantial wasting of the essential mineral zinc is a factor in limiting the course of edetate calcium disodium therapy, but not succimer therapy, to five days. Monitoring of essential minerals is not required during succimer therapy.

Although human clinical data are not available, rat data suggest that intraperitoneal edetate calcium disodium and dimercaprol (British Anti-Lewisite, BAL) may enhance gastrointestinal absorption of lead.[21] In contrast, gastrointestinal absorption of lead and whole body lead retention were markedly reduced by oral administration of succimer in rats.[21] Rat data suggest that therapy with oral succimer, unlike conventional therapy with edetate calcium disodium[22] does not result in redistribution of lead to the brain or other target organs.[23]

Figure 1. Succimer is the stable *meso* isomer of 2,3-dimercaptosuccinic acid, also known as DMSA.

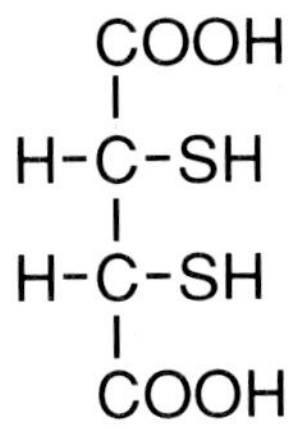

Figure 2. The in vitro succimer–lead complex is a stable five-member heterocyclic ring.[7]

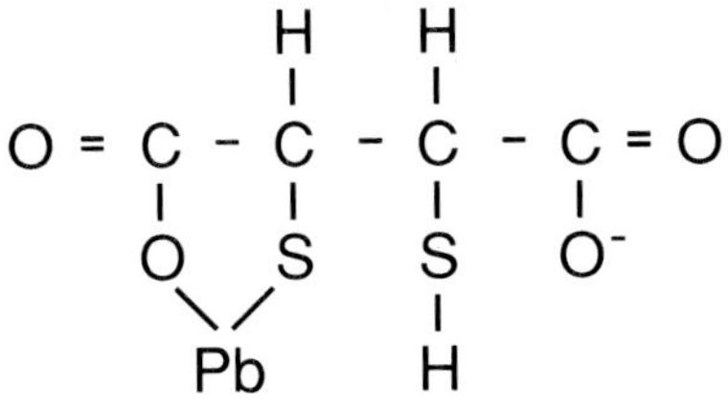

In addition to lead, succimer appears to be effective in chelating the toxic heavy metals arsenic and mercury. In various animal studies, succimer has been successful in decreasing the body burden of mercury and increasing its urinary excretion[24-27] and was more effective than equivalent molar doses of *N*-acetyl-D,L-penicillamine[24] or penicillamine.[25] With respect to arsenic, comparative efficacy studies in rodents indicated that succimer provided effective protection against the lethal effects of sodium arsenite and Lewisite.[28-31] In mice, succimer was more effective in providing protection against the lethal effects of sodium arsenite than either penicillamine or *N*-acetyl-D,L-penicillamine at equivalent molar doses[28,29,31] and was more effective than dimercaprol against the lethal effects of Lewisite in rabbits.[28,30] These comparative data have not been confirmed by controlled clinical trials in humans.

Pharmacokinetics

In a preliminary pharmacokinetic study involving 11 healthy adult male volunteers who received a single 16-, 32-, or 48-mg/kg dose of succimer labeled with carbon 14, absorption was rapid but variable, with peak absorption occurring between one and two hours.[a] Both whole blood and plasma concentration data fit a two-compartment model. The apparent elimination half-life was approximately 48 hours. Preliminary human data from this study indicate that succimer has a small volume of distribution, with the majority of drug remaining in the plasma.[a] It is not known whether succimer passes through the human placental barrier or whether it can cause fetal harm when administered to a pregnant woman or affect reproductive capacity. It is not known whether succimer is excreted in human milk. Because many drugs and heavy metals are excreted in human milk, women receiving succimer therapy should be discouraged from nursing their infants. The exact site of succimer biotransformation has not been determined. Recently, the structures of the major succimer metabolites in humans have been identified as mixed disulfides of L-cysteine.[32] Succimer appears to be rapidly and extensively metabolized, as indicated by the proportion of succimer excreted in the urine as mixed disulfides rather than as unchanged drug.[33]

The complete fate of succimer after oral administration has not been fully elucidated. Preliminary data indicate that renal elimination accounts for the majority of total clearance. Minimal amounts are eliminated by the lungs. Fecal excretion probably represents nonabsorbed drug. Succimer is rapidly excreted by the kidneys; approximately 75% of renal elimination occurs in the first 24 hours.[a] Of the total amount of drug eliminated in the urine, approximately 90% is eliminated in altered form as mixed succimer–cysteine disulfides, with the remaining 10% eliminated as unaltered drug. The majority of mixed disulfides consist of succimer in disulfide linkages with two molecules of L-cysteine; the remaining disulfides contained one L-cysteine molecule per succimer molecule. Peak excretion of altered succimer occurs between two and four hours after ingestion.[33,a]

Lead Poisoning

Succimer has been used safely and effectively outside of the United States (primarily in China) as a treatment modality for heavy-metal poisoning in more than 300 adult patients during the past 25 years.[34] In the United States, information on succimer is available from clinical pharmacology studies, clinical trials, and compassionate-use cases involving more than 300 adults and children, primarily patients with lead toxicity. Succimer has been available in the United States only as an orphan investigational drug; therefore, published literature is limited. Described herein are the results of published controlled clinical trials of succimer in children and adults, as well as clinical data establishing the duration of the treatment course. In addition to controlled studies, approximately 250 patients with lead poisoning have been treated with succimer either orally or by injection in open domestic and foreign studies, and similar results have been reported.[8-10,14,a]

Clinical studies indicate that succimer is a relatively selective and highly effective medication that lowers blood lead concentrations.[8-12,14,a] Succimer reverses the adverse metabolic effects of lead on heme synthesis while increasing urinary lead output without adversely affecting essential mineral excretion at the recommended dosage regimen. The primary indicators of drug efficacy in the controlled trials of oral succimer were lowered blood lead concentrations and increased urinary lead excretion. Secondary indicators of efficacy included restoration of red blood cell aminolevulinic acid dehydratase (ALA-D) activity, an enzyme necessary for heme synthesis, and a reduction in urinary aminolevulinic acid (ALA) and coproporphyrin.[11,12,a] Measurement of coproporphyrin and ALA-D provides clinical investigators with an indication of the effects of lead on heme biosynthetic pathways and the degree to which these effects are reversed during chelation therapy. ALA-D activity and urinary excretion of ALA are sensitive indicators of exposure to lead.

Studies Establishing Effective Dosage Level. The dose-ranging studies described below evaluated the efficacy of five days of succimer therapy in both children and adults. Graziano et al.[12] described their experience with 21 children aged two to seven years who had blood lead concentrations of 31–49 μg/dL and who also had a positive edetate calcium disodium mobilization test result (defined as urinary excretion of >0.6 μg of lead per milligram of edetate calcium disodium administered). Of the 21 patients (14 Hispanic, six black, and one white), six children were treated with edetate calcium disodium and 15 received succimer therapy. Succimer-treated children were randomly assigned to receive succimer 350, 700, or 1050 mg/sq m/day orally in three divided doses (every eight hours) for five days . These doses correspond to approximately 3.3, 6.7, and 10.0 mg/kg/dose or 10, 20, and 30 mg/kg/day, respectively. Succimer was administered orally by emptying the contents of the succimer capsules into either a fruit drink or ice cream. Edetate calcium disodium (1000 mg/sq m/day) was administered intravenously in two divided doses, also for five days.

In each treatment group, blood lead concentrations declined during the five-day treatment period. Treatment with succimer 10.0, 6.7, and 3.3 mg/kg/dose resulted in a 78%, 63%, and 42% decline in blood lead concentrations, respectively. The decline in blood lead concentrations in the edetate calcium disodium control group was 47%. As shown in Figure 3, succimer 1050 mg/sq m/day (approximately 30 mg/kg/day) was significantly more effective in reducing blood lead concentrations (78% decrease) than either conventional intravenous edetate calcium disodium therapy (47% decrease) or lower dosages of succimer. The decline in blood lead concentrations in response to succimer 700 and 350 mg/sq m/day (63% and 42% decrease, respectively) did not differ significantly from the decline in response to conventional edetate calcium disodium therapy.

Rebound in blood lead concentrations often occurs after short courses of all chelating therapies because of

Figure 3. Mean blood lead concentrations of children receiving succimer at approximately 10, 20, or 30 mg/kg/day or edetate calcium disodium ($CaNa_2EDTA$) 1000 mg/sq m/day for five days as a function of time. (Reprinted with permission from reference 12.)

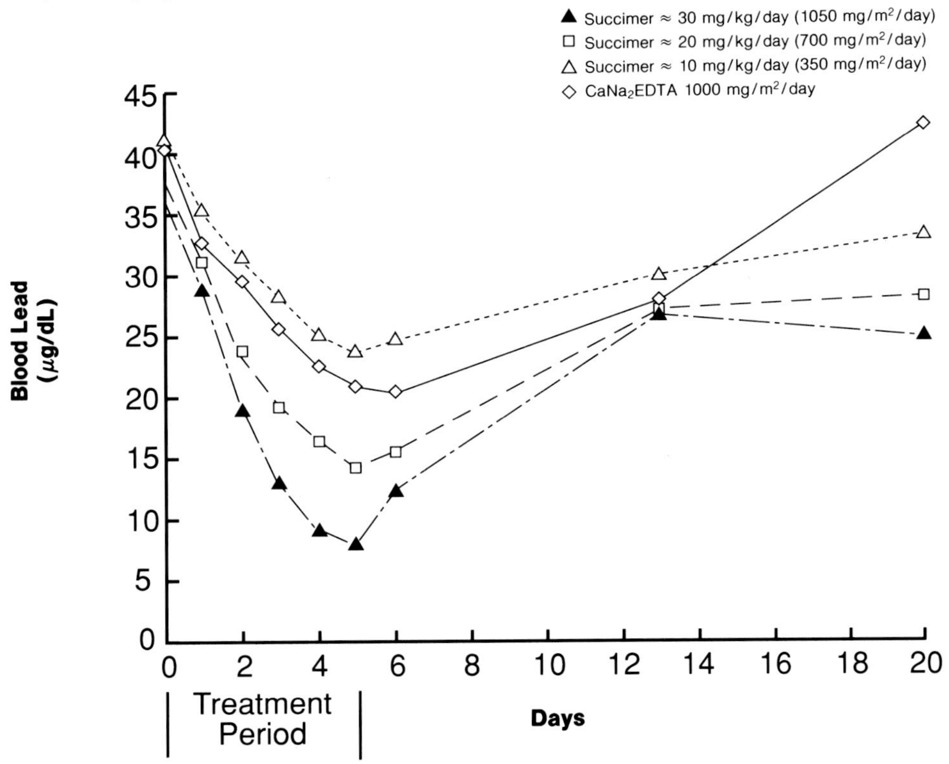

the relatively large lead burden associated with chronic lead ingestion and the subsequent re-equilibration phenomenon.[35] This rebound is thought to be caused by lead mobilization from the skeleton and re-equilibration into blood and soft tissues. As expected, blood lead concentrations rebounded after cessation of drug therapy in all treatment groups.

A significant increase in ALA-D activity occurred in all treatment groups; succimer 30 mg/kg/day was significantly more effective in restoring ALA-D activity than either lower dosages of succimer or conventional therapy with edetate calcium disodium (Figure 4).[12] No adverse reactions or changes in essential mineral excretion were reported in the succimer treatment groups. In the edetate calcium disodium treatment group, the urinary excretion of copper, iron, zinc, and calcium was significantly increased, the last perhaps because the drug contains calcium. As described by the authors, the mean urinary mineral excretion per milligram of creatinine was low for copper (from a baseline pretreatment value of 0.65 µg to a high of 1.16 µg during therapy) and iron (from a baseline pretreatment value of 1.8 µg to a high of 2.5 µg) but was large and clinically important for zinc (from a baseline pretreatment value of 3.8 µg to a high of 13.5 µg).

The results of this pediatric study are in accordance with a study in adult patients (aged 24–58 years) who had occupational lead poisoning from exposures to lead sources such as house and bridge painting and pigment mixing.[11] This multiple-dose, single-blind, randomized trial evaluated 18 men with blood lead concentrations between 44 and 96 µg/dL. Patients were randomly assigned to receive succimer 30, 20, or 10 mg/kg/day orally in three divided doses (every eight hours) for five days. In each patient, a linear decline in blood lead concentrations was observed over time (Figure 5). After five days, the mean blood concentrations of the three groups decreased by 72.5%, 58.3%, and 35.5%, respectively. The mean urinary lead excretions in the initial 24 hours were 28.6-fold, 18.6-fold, and 12.3-fold, respectively, higher than the pretreatment 24-hour urinary lead excretion. As the amount of lead available for chelation was reduced during therapy, urinary lead output decreased. Symptoms such as headache and colic improved. Metabolic indexes of lead toxicity also responded favorably to succimer treatment; red blood cell ALA-D activity, which was markedly depressed before treatment, increased in a linear, dose-dependent manner, which paralleled a decrease in urinary ALA excretion in each dosage group. Additionally, urinary excretion of coproporphyrin also decreased during succimer treatment, indicating rejuvenation of coproporphyrinogen oxidase, an enzyme necessary for heme synthesis. After cessation of therapy, blood lead concentrations rebounded, again probably indicating mobilization of lead from bone. There was no significant effect on the urinary elimination of calcium, iron, or magnesium.

Figure 4. Mean erythrocyte aminolevulinic acid dehydratase (ALA-D) activities measured as nanomoles of porphobilinogen per gram of hemoglobin per hour (nm PBG/g Hgb/hr) of children receiving oral succimer or intravenous edetate calcium disodium ($CaNa_2EDTA$) 1000 mg/sq m/day as a function of time. (Reprinted with permission from reference 12.)

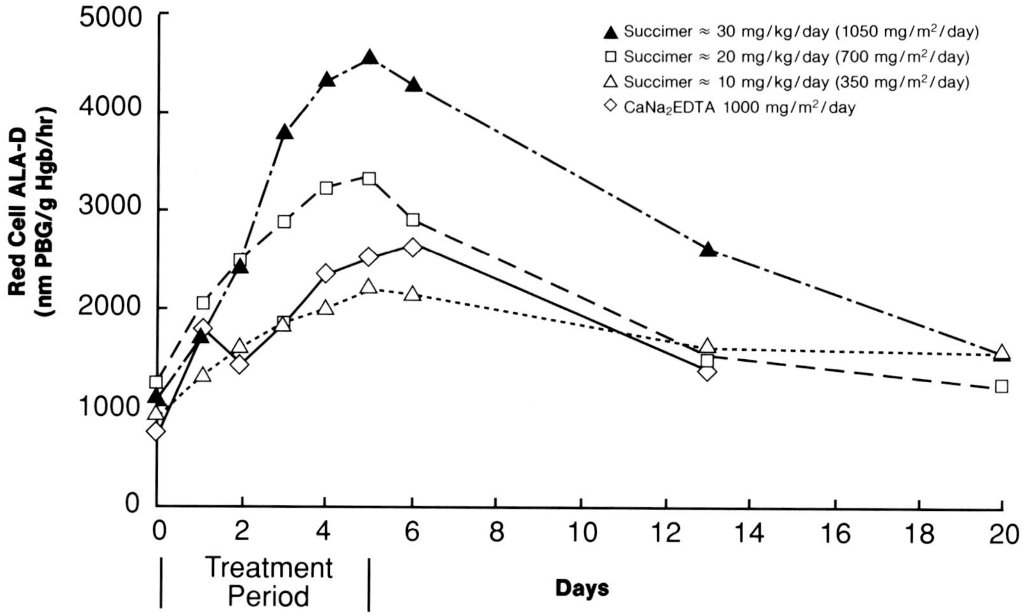

Figure 5. Mean blood lead concentrations expressed as a percentage of pretreatment values in adult male patients receiving five days of succimer therapy at 10, 20, or 30 mg/kg/day. (Reprinted with permission from reference 11.)

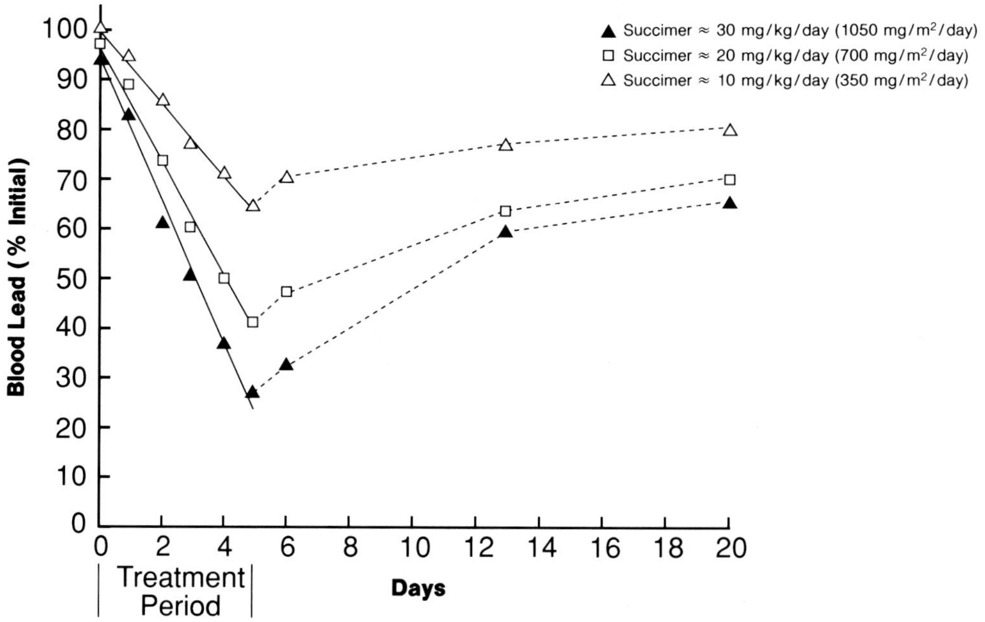

Urinary zinc excretion increased significantly ($p \leq 0.01$) in a dose-dependent fashion, but was clinically unimportant in the groups receiving 20 and 30 mg/kg/day (1.6-fold to 1.8-fold higher than the pretreatment values).

Data Establishing Treatment Course. The blood lead concentration declines in response to chelation therapy for lead intoxication and then rises, or rebounds, after the cessation of chelation therapy because of the redistribution of lead from bone stores. This phenomenon, due to the compartmental kinetics of lead, is primarily a function of body lead burden. In some patients, the rebound can be steep, requiring frequent and multiple courses of chelation therapy before the blood lead concentration stabilizes in a clinically acceptable range. The possibility of re-exposure to a lead-containing environment should be considered in a child who does not respond with an appropriate decline or has an excessive rebound in blood lead concentrations, and further efforts should be taken to ensure abatement. Further studies were conducted to determine the optimal therapeutic course of succimer, with the goal of minimizing or reducing the rebound in blood lead concentrations caused by the reequilibration phenomenon.

A multiple-dose, open-label study evaluated succimer treatment regimens for the control of rebound in blood lead concentrations.[a] Nineteen children, aged one to seven years, with blood lead concentrations of 42–67 μg/dL, were treated for five days with succimer 1050 mg/sq m/day (30 mg/kg/day) and then randomly assigned to one of three groups. Group one was followed for two weeks with no further therapy; group two was treated for two weeks with succimer 350 mg/sq m/day (once daily); and group three was treated for two weeks with succimer 700 mg/sq m/day (in two divided doses). After the initial five days, the mean percent decline in blood lead concentration in all groups was 61%. The untreated group and the group receiving 350 mg/sq m/day had a rebound in blood lead concentrations during the ensuing two weeks of treatment. In contrast, the group that received 700 mg/sq m/day had no such rebound during treatment and had less severe rebound after cessation of therapy.

Montalvan and colleagues[14] described 24 patients with lead poisoning who were treated with succimer on an ambulatory basis. This open-label study of eight adults (aged 17–53 years) and 16 children (aged 19 months to 8 years) included all patients with blood lead concentrations in excess of 41 μg/dL, as well as symptomatic patients (e.g., polyuria, abdominal colic, hyperactivity, a learning disability) with blood lead concentrations higher than 25 μg/dL. Succimer was administered at a dosage of 30 mg/kg/day for five days; patients then received a 16-day course of succimer 20 mg/kg/day. Succimer therapy resulted in a decline in blood lead concentrations in all patients; this decline was most dramatic in patients with pretreatment concentrations between 40 and 60 μg/dL. At the end of therapy, the average decline from pretreatment blood lead concentrations was reported as 40 μg/dL. Urinary lead excretion averaged 2–4 mg/24 hours in cases in which adequate urine was collected.

Lead Encephalopathy. Three adults with lead encephalopathy were reported to have improved in response to succimer therapy.[9] However, data are not available regarding the use of succimer for the treatment of this rare and sometimes fatal complication of lead poisoning in children.

Other Heavy-Metal Poisoning

No controlled, randomized clinical studies of succimer have been conducted in cases of poisoning with other heavy metals. A limited number of patients have received succimer for mercury poisoning[16,17,a] or arsenic poisoning[15,a] through compassionate-use protocols. These patients showed increased urinary excretion of the heavy metal and various degrees of symptomatic improvement. Bluhm et al.[16] compared succimer (30 mg/kg/day) and *N*-acetyl-D,L-penicillamine (250 mg every six hours) for four days in 12 patients exposed to elemental mercury vapor during an industrial accident. Therapy was initiated between 73 and 116 days after exposure. With both drugs, the increase in the urinary excretion rate of mercury depended on the pretreatment mercury levels. Succimer induced a threefold increase in mercury excretion compared with a twofold increase induced by *N*-acetyl-D,L-penicillamine.

Adverse Effects

Few adverse events have been observed in clinical trials and compassionate-use cases, and those that have been observed have generally been mild and transient.[8-12,a] However, clinical experience with succimer has been limited. Consequently, the full spectrum and incidence of adverse reactions, including the possibility of hypersensitivity or idiosyncratic reactions, have not been determined.

The most common adverse effects reported in clinical trials in children and adults were primarily gastrointestinal and included nausea, vomiting, diarrhea, appetite loss, and loose stools.[36] At times, these events have been believed to be related to the unpleasant mercaptan odor of succimer; administration in such a way as to minimize the odor may overcome some of these reactions. Rashes, some necessitating discontinuation of therapy, have been reported in about 4% of patients, primarily adults. If rash occurs, other causes (e.g., measles) should be considered before ascribing the reaction to succimer. Rechallenge with succimer may be considered when blood lead concentrations are high enough to warrant retreatment. Mild, transient elevations of serum aminotransferase concentrations have been observed in 6–10% of patients, primarily adults, receiving succimer therapy. The importance of these increases is currently unknown.[36]

Drug–Disease Interactions

A small number of children with glucose-6-phosphate dehydrogenase deficiency and sickle-cell anemia have been successfully treated with succimer without incident. Dimercaprol has reportedly caused hemolysis in patients with glucose-6-phosphate dehydrogenase deficiency.[37] A small number of patients receiving hemodialysis for renal failure have been treated with succimer. All patients tolerated the drug treatment.

Drug–Drug Interactions

There are no known drug interactions between succimer and other drugs, including iron supplements[38,a]; however, data on concomitant drug use are limited and drug combinations have not been systematically studied. Many children with elevated lead concentrations are also iron deficient, and some data suggest that iron deficiency results in increased gastrointestinal absorption of lead[39]; therefore, iron supplementation is often considered in these children. Dimercaprol reportedly forms a toxic (emetogenic) complex with iron, and concurrent therapy is not recommended.[37] In the small number of children who have been treated with succimer and iron supplements, there has been no evidence of the formation of a similar toxic chelate. In the children who have been so treated, oral iron and succimer were not administered simultaneously but were separated by two to three hours. Because there are data suggesting that the bioavailability of oral penicillamine may be decreased by concomitant administration of iron and antacids,[40,41] it may be prudent to avoid concomitant administration of succimer with these agents pending definitive studies. Data are not available on the concomitant use of succimer with edetate calcium disodium, with or without dimercaprol, and such use is not recommended.[36] Currently, after therapeutic courses of edetate calcium disodium (with or without dimercaprol), an interval of four weeks is recommended before initiation of a subsequent course of therapy with succimer, because of the lack of data regarding the sequential use of these agents.

Drug–Laboratory Test Interactions

In vitro studies indicate that succimer may cause false-positive results of ketone urinalysis that uses nitroprusside reagents (e.g., Ketostix). Succimer also may falsely decrease measurements of serum uric acid and creatine phosphokinase.[a]

Recommended Monitoring Variables

As with any drug used to treat a serious illness such as lead toxicity, monitoring for therapeutic efficacy as well as safety is recommended in patients receiving succimer. A diagnostic blood lead concentration should be determined before therapy is begun, and patients should be monitored for rebound in blood lead concentrations after therapy. Severity of the toxicity (as measured by the pretreatment blood lead concentration and the exposure history) should be used as a guide to the frequency of blood lead monitoring after a therapeutic course, but monitoring should be done at least once weekly until blood lead concentrations are stable. Reinstitution of therapy should be considered when blood lead concentrations rebound secondary to lead redistribution from bone stores. It is recommended that two weeks elapse between courses of chelation therapy unless blood lead concentrations indicate that more rapid retreatment is necessary.

Succimer heavy-metal chelates are excreted in the urine; therefore, all patients undergoing treatment should be adequately hydrated. Caution should be exercised when succimer therapy is considered in patients who have compromised renal function. Limited data suggest that succimer is dialyzable but that the lead chelates are not.[a]

Because transient elevations of serum aminotransferase levels have been observed in 6–10% of patients, primarily adults, during the course of succimer therapy, serum aminotransferases should be monitored before the initiation of therapy and at least weekly during therapy, particularly in patients with a history of liver disease. No data are available regarding the metabolism of succimer in patients with liver disease.

The possibility of allergic or other mucocutaneous reactions to the drug should be considered when succimer is readministered (as well as during initial courses). Patients requiring repeated courses of succimer should be monitored during each treatment course. One adult patient treated in Europe had a recurrent mucocutaneous reaction during the third, fourth, and fifth courses of succimer therapy; it is unclear whether this was an allergic, fixed drug reaction.[42] If rash occurs, patients should consult their physician; rechallenge with succimer may be considered when lead levels are high enough to warrant retreatment. One adult patient may have had a febrile reaction to succimer with a maximum temperature reached at two hours (39.2 °C oral); the patient's temperature returned to normal over the ensuing seven hours. This reaction was associated with chills, diaphoresis, hypertension, and slight tachycardia that resolved within one hour.[a]

FDA-Approved Labeling and Availability

Succimer is indicated for the treatment of lead poisoning in children with blood lead concentrations above 45 μg/dL. There is no clinical experience with the use of succimer in children less than one year of age. As with any type of chelation therapy, succimer is not indicated for the prophylaxis of lead poisoning in a lead-containing environment; the use of succimer should always be accompanied by identification and removal of the source of the lead exposure. Identification of the source of lead in the child's environment and its abatement are critical to a successful therapy outcome.

Chemet (succimer) is supplied as opaque white gelatin capsules of medicated beads containing 100 mg of succimer. The average wholesale cost of a bottle of 100 capsules is $230.

Dosage and Administration

The recommended initial dosage in children is 10 mg/kg or 350 mg/sq m every eight hours for five days (Table 1 provides a dosage schedule based on weight). After the initial five days of therapy, the dosage is reduced to 10 mg/kg or 350 mg/sq m every 12 hours (two thirds of initial daily dosage) for an additional

Table 1.
Succimer Pediatric Dosage Schedule

Weight		Dose (mg)[a]	No. Capsules[a]
Pounds	Kilograms		
18–35	8–15	100	1
36–55	16–23	200	2
56–75	24–34	300	3
76–100	35–44	400	4
≥100	≥45	500	5

[a] To be administered every eight hours for five days followed by doses every 12 hours for 14 days.

two weeks of therapy. A course of treatment lasts 19 days. Repeated courses may be necessary when indicated by weekly monitoring of blood lead concentrations after each course. A minimum of two weeks between courses is recommended unless blood lead concentrations indicate the need for more prompt treatment. Clinical experience with repeated courses is limited. The safety of uninterrupted therapy for longer than three weeks has not been established and it is not recommended.

For young children who cannot swallow capsules, succimer can be given by separating the capsule and administering it immediately by sprinkling the beads on soft food or by putting them in a spoon and following with a fruit drink, which may help to mask the characteristic sulfur odor. The drug should be mixed with soft food immediately before administration; stability data are not available and stability cannot be ensured when the beads are mixed in various foods over a longer period of time. Parents should be discouraged from premixing doses of succimer hours or days in advance.

Use in Pregnancy

Succimer is classified as a category C agent, indicating that animal studies have demonstrated adverse effects on the fetus; there are no controlled studies in pregnant women. Succimer should not be administered to women who are pregnant or who may become pregnant during therapy unless the potential benefit outweighs the potential risk to the fetus.[36] A disodium salt of dimercaptosuccinic acid was shown to be teratogenic and fetotoxic in pregnant mice when given subcutaneously in a dose range of 410–1640 mg/kg during the period of organogenesis.[43] A more recent study reported the absence of observed teratogenicity of succimer in fetal rats exposed to oral maternal doses of succimer up to 1000 mg/kg/day during the period of organogenesis.[44]

Toxicology

A number of animal studies evaluating acute, subacute, and chronic toxicity demonstrate that the toxic effects of succimer appear only at doses well in excess of the recommended doses. Single doses of 2300 mg/kg in rats and 2400 mg/kg in mice produced ataxia, convulsions, labored respiration, and frequently death. The median lethal single dose of succimer in mice and rats is more than 3000 mg/kg.[a]

In dogs, only minimal signs of toxicity (e.g., diarrhea, emesis, or weakness) were observed with single oral (up to 300 mg/kg) or intravenous (100 mg/kg) doses of succimer. Six-day and 28-day oral toxicity studies in dogs have shown that doses of 300 mg/kg/day or higher were toxic and lethal to some dogs; the kidneys and gastrointestinal tract were the major target organs for toxicity, and deaths were due to renal failure.[a] In one ongoing, six-month chronic toxicity study of oral succimer in dogs, thrombocytopenia was observed in animals receiving succimer at 80 or 140 mg/kg/day after three months of dosing. Ecchymoses were noted on pathology of affected animals. Depressed platelet counts were not observed in dogs receiving 10 mg/kg/day for three months.[a]

Succimer has been evaluated by various methods, and no mutagenic activity has been observed.[a]

Overdosage Management

No case of overdosage has been reported in humans. Limited data indicate that succimer is dialyzable. In case of acute overdosage, induction of vomiting or gastric lavage followed by administration of an activated charcoal slurry and appropriate supportive therapy is recommended.[36]

Conclusion

Succimer represents innovative drug therapy for the treatment of lead poisoning. Clinical studies indicate that succimer is relatively selective for lead and effectively lowers blood lead concentrations. Succimer reverses the adverse metabolic effects of lead on heme synthesis while increasing urinary lead output without adversely affecting essential mineral excretion. In addition to selectivity, efficacy, and safety benefits, as an oral agent succimer offers ease of administration and may permit physicians the option of treating children as outpatients. Although clinical experience is limited, the benefit of an oral lead chelator may offer advantages over currently available agents.

[a]Data on file, McNeil Consumer Products Company, Fort Washington, PA. 1991 Feb.

References

1. Centers for Disease Control. Preventing lead poisoning in young children: a statement by the Centers for Disease Control. Atlanta, GA: Centers for Disease Control, 1985; DHHS publication no. 99-2230.
2. American Academy of Pediatrics. Statement on childhood lead poisoning. *Pediatrics*. 1987; 79:457-65.
3. Piomelli S, Rosen JF, Chisolm JJ Jr et al. Management of childhood lead poisoning. *J Pediatr*. 1984; 105:523-32.
4. Shannon M, Graef J, Lovejoy FH. Efficacy and toxicity of D-penicillamine in low-level lead poisoning. *J Pediatr*. 1988;

112:799-804.
5. Friedheim E, DaSilva JR, Martins AV. Treatment of schistosomiasis mansoni with antimony a,a'-dimercapto-potassium succinate (TWSb). *Am J Trop Med Hyg*. 1954; 3:714-27.
6. The Merck index. 11th ed. Budavari S, O'Neil MJ, Smith A, eds. Rahway, NJ: Merck; 1989:1398.
7. Rivera M, Zheng W, Aposhian HV et al. Determination and metabolism of dithiol chelating agents: VIII. Metal complexes of meso-dimercaptosuccinic acid. *Toxicol Appl Pharmacol*. 1989; 100:96-106.
8. Bentur Y, Brook JG, Behar R et al. Meso-2,3-dimercaptosuccinic acid (DMSA) in the diagnosis and treatment of lead poisoning. *Clin Toxicol*. 1987; 25:39-51.
9. Fournier L, Garnier TR, Buisine A et al. 2,3-Dimercaptosuccinic acid treatment of heavy metal poisoning in humans. *Med Toxicol*. 1988; 3:499-504.
10. Friedheim E, Graziano JH, Popovac D et al. Treatment of lead poisoning by 2,3-dimercaptosuccinic acid (DMSA). *Lancet*. 1978; 2:1234-6.
11. Graziano JH, Siris ES, LoIacono N et al. 2,3-Dimercaptosuccinic acid as an antidote for lead intoxication. *Clin Pharmacol Ther*. 1985; 37:431-38.
12. Graziano JH, LoIacono NJ, Meyer P. Dose-response study of oral 2,3-dimercaptosuccinic acid in children vith elevated blood lead concentrations. *J Pediatr*. 1988; 113:751-7.
13. Kuntzelman DR, England KE, Angle CR. Urine lead (UPb) in outpatient treatment of lead poisoning with dimercaptosuccinic acid (DMSA). *Vet Hum Toxicol*. 1990; 4:364. Abstract.
14. Montalvan J, Okose P, Marcus S. Outpatient chelation therapy of 24 patients with lead intoxication by dimercaptosuccinic acid. *Vet Hum Toxicol*. 1990; 4:343. Abstract.
15. Lenz R, Hruby K, Druml W et al. 2,3-Dimercaptosuccinic acid in human arsenic poisoning. *Arch Toxicol*. 1981; 47:241-3.
16. Bluhm R, Bobbitt RG, Bonfiglio JF et al. 2,3-Dimercaptosuccinic acid (DMSA) versus n-acetyl-penicillamine (NAP) for the treatment of elemental mercury toxicity. *Ann Emerg Med*. 1990; 19:631. Abstract.
17. Mortensen ME, Valenzuela PM. 2,3-Dimercaptosuccinic acid (DMSA) chelation in mercury (Hg) vapor poisoning. *Vet Hum Toxicol*. 1990; 4:362. Abstract.
18. Cantilena LR Jr, Klaassen CD. The effect of chelating agents on the excretion of endogenous metals. *Toxicol Appl Pharmacol*. 1982; 63:344-50.
19. Perry HM Jr, Perry EF. Normal concentrations of some trace metals in human urine: changes produced by ethylenediaminetetracetate. *J Clin Invest*. 1959; 38:1452-63.
20. Thomas DJ, Chisolm JJ Jr. Lead, zinc and copper decorporation during calcium disodium ethylenediaminetetraacetate treatment of lead-poisoned children. *J Pharmacol Exp Ther*. 1986; 239:829-35.
21. Kapoor SC, Wielopolski L, Graziano JH et al. Influence of 2,3-dimercaptosuccinic acid on gastrointestinal lead absorption and whole-body lead retention. *Toxicol Appl Pharmacol*. 1989; 97:525-9.
22. Cory-Slechta DA, Weiss B, Cox C. Mobilization and redistribution of lead over the course of calcium disodium ethylenediamine tetraacetate therapy. *J Pharmacol Exp Ther*. 1987; 243:804-13.
23. Cory-Slechta DA. Mobilization of lead over the course of DMSA chelation therapy and long-term efficacy. *J Pharmacol Exp Ther*. 1988; 246:84-91.
24. Aaseth J, Friedheim EAH. Treatment of methylmercury poisoning in mice with 2,3-dimercaptosuccinic acid and other complexing thiols. *Acta Pharmacol Toxicol*. 1978; 42:248-52.
25. Friedheim E, Corvi C. Meso-dimercaptosuccinic acid, a chelating agent for the treatment of mercury poisoning. *J Pharm Pharmacol*. 1975; 27:624-6.
26. Magos L. The effects of dimercaptosuccinic acid on the excretion and distribution of mercury in rats and mice treated with mercuric chloride and methylmercury chloride. *Br J Pharmacol*. 1976; 56:479-84.
27. Planas-Bohne F. The influence of chelating agents on the distribution and biotransformation of methylmercuric chloride in rats. *J Pharmacol Exp Ther*. 1981; 217:500-4.
28. Aposhian HV. Biological chelation: 2,3-dimercaptopropanesulfonic acid and meso-dimercaptosuccinic acid. *Adv Enzyme Regul*. 1982; 20:301-19.
29. Aposhian HV, Tadlock CH, Moon TE. Protection of mice against the lethal effects of sodium arsenite—a quantitative comparison of a number of chelating agents. *Toxicol Appl Pharmacol*. 1981; 61:385-92.
30. Aposhian HV, Mershon MM, Brinkley FB et al. Anti-lewisite activity and stability of meso-dimercaptosuccinic acid and 2,3-dimercapto-1-propane-sulfonic acid. *Life Sci*. 1982; 31:2149-56.
31. Tadlock CH, Aposhian HV. Protection of mice against the lethal effects of sodium arsenite by 2,3-dimercapto-1-propane-sulfonic acid and dimercaptosuccinic acid. *Biochem Biophys Res Commun*. 1980; 94:501-7.
32. Maiorino RM, Bruce DC, Aposhian HV. Determination of dithiol chelating agents. VI. Isolation and identification of the mixed disulfides of meso-2,3-dimercaptosuccinic acid with L-cysteine in human urine. *Toxicol Appl Pharmacol*. 1989; 97:338-49.
33. Aposhian HV, Maiorino RM, Dart RC et al. Urinary excretion of meso-2,3-dimercaptosuccinic acid in human subjects. *Clin Pharmacol Ther*. 1989; 45:520-6.
34. Aposhian HV. DMSA and DMPS-water soluble antidotes for heavy metal intoxication. *Annu Rev Pharmacol Toxicol*. 1983; 23:193-215.
35. Chisolm JJ Jr. Evaluation of the potential role of chelation therapy in treatment of low to moderate lead exposures. *Environ Health Perspect*. 1990; 89 67-74.
36. McNeil Consumer Products Company. CHEMET product information. Fort Washington, PA; 1991 Feb.
37. AHFS drug information 91. McEvoy GK, ed. Dimercaprol. Bethesda, MD: American Society of Hospital Pharmacists; 1991:1799-1801.
38. Haust HL, Inwood M, Spence JD et al. Intramuscular administration of iron during long-term chelation therapy with 2,3-dimercaptosuccinic acid in a man with severe lead poisoning. *Clin Biochem*. 1989; 22:189-96.
39. Mahaffey KR. Nutritional factors in lead poisoning. *Nutr Rev*. 1981; 39:353-62.
40. Ifan A, Welling PG. Pharmacokinetics of oral 500-mg penicillamine: effect of antacids on absorption. *Biopharm Drug Dispos*. 1986; 7:401-5.
41. Osman MA, Patel RB, Schuna A et al. Reduction in oral penicillamine absorption by food, antacid, and ferrous sulfate. *Clin Pharmacol Ther*. 1983; 33 465-70.
42. Grandjean P, Jacobsen IA, Jorgensen PJ. Chronic lead poisoning treated with dimercaptosuccinic acid. *Pharmacol Toxicol*. 1991; 68:266-9.
43. Domingo JL, Paternain JL, Llobet JM et al. Developmental toxicity of subcutaneously administered meso-2,3-dimercaptosuccinic acid in mice. *Fundam Appl Toxicol*. 1988; 11:715-22.
44. Domingo JL, Ortega A, Paternain JL et al. Oral meso-2,3-dimercaptosuccinic acid in pregnant Sprague-Dawley rats: teratogenicity and alteration in mineral metabolism. I. Teratological evaluation. *J Toxicol Environ Health*. 1990; 30:181-90.

Research

Nomogram for dosing warfarin at steady state

DEAN A. FREDRIKS AND ROBERT W. COLEMAN

Abstract: The predictive performance of a nomogram for dosing warfarin was compared with that of a computer program.

The nomogram and the computer program were developed from the log-linear model describing warfarin pharmacodynamics at steady state. The nomogram's dose–response curves were generated by using previously reported pharmacodynamic and pharmacokinetic values for an outpatient population receiving warfarin. The series of dose–response curves were plotted by altering the pharmacodynamic values over a range of 3 standard deviations. The ability of the nomogram to predict the steady-state prothrombin time ratio (PTR) after an adjustment in the dosage of warfarin was evaluated, and the results were compared with those of a commercially available program involving Bayesian regression.

Data for 65 outpatients were evaluated. The mean ± S.D. nomogram-predicted, computer-predicted, and measured PTRs were 1.63 ± 0.27, 1.64 ± 0.24, and 1.66 ± 0.23, respectively. The mean prediction errors for the nomogram and the computer program were –0.037 and –0.026, respectively, and the mean percent absolute prediction errors were 11.6% and 11.0%, respectively. Neither method was biased, and differences between the results for the two methods were not significant.

The predictive performance of the warfarin dosing nomogram was comparable to that of the computer program.

Index terms: Anticoagulants; Computers; Dosage; Methodology; Nomograms; Warfarin
Clin Pharm. 1991; 10:923-7

Oral anticoagulants are effective in the treatment of deep venous thrombosis and pulmonary embolism. These agents are also used to prevent thromboembolic events in patients with prosthetic heart valves, chronic atrial fibrillation, dilated cardiomyopathy, and other conditions associated with a risk of thromboembolism.[1] Warfarin is the most widely prescribed oral anticoagulant, with approximately 4 million patients receiving the drug each year in the United States.[2,3] Warfarin has a narrow therapeutic index; there is a delicate balance between the thrombosis associated with underdosage and the hemorrhage associated with overdosage. Accurate dosing and frequent monitoring are crucial for maximizing efficacy and minimizing toxicity.

Warfarin therapy is generally begun in the hospital and maintained in the outpatient setting. The duration of warfarin therapy ranges from a few weeks to life[1]; patients frequently require long-term management. Although computational methods for initiating warfarin treatment are well documented,[4-12] the adjustment of dosages in outpatients undergoing maintenance therapy is usually based on trial and error. Computer programs for adjusting warfarin dosages are available to clinicians, but access to these programs and to computers is often limited.

We have developed a nomogram from the population-based relationship between warfarin dosage and prothrombin response.[8] The nomogram is designed to provide guidance to clinicians in selecting a new warfarin dosage when given a steady-state dosage and a prothrombin time. In this study we evaluated the predictive performance of the nomogram and compared its performance with that of a pharmacodynamic modeling program involving Bayesian regression (WarfCalc, Biotrack, Inc., Sunnyvale, CA).

Methods

Pharmacodynamic Model. The nomogram and the computer program are based on the log-linear pharmacodynamic model for warfarin proposed by Theofanous and Barile.[9] The model describes the effect of the warfarin-induced reduction in clotting factor synthesis on prothrombin complex activity after multiple warfarin doses have been given (when the con-

DEAN A. FREDRIKS, PHARM.D., is Assistant Professor in Clinical Pharmacy, School of Pharmacy, University of the Pacific, Stockton, CA. ROBERT W. COLEMAN, M.S., is Clinical Pharmacy Coordinator, Pharmacy Service, Veteran Affairs Medical Center, Palo Alto, CA.
Address reprint requests to Dr. Fredriks at VA Medical Center, 150 Muir Road (119), Martinez, CA 94553.

Presented at the Annual Meeting of the American College of Clinical Pharmacy, San Francisco, CA, August 7, 1990.

centration in plasma is at steady state) as a function of three pharmacodynamic variables and two pharmacokinetic variables. Steady-state prothrombin complex activity (PCA_{ss}) after multiple daily warfarin doses (D) is given by

$$PCA_{ss} = [(-m\,CL/V)/k^2][1 - (k\tau/1 - e^{-k\tau})] \quad (1)$$
$$(-m/k)\ \ln\,[(D/V)/C_{max}(1 - e^{-(CL/V)\tau})]$$

where m is the slope of the logarithmic dose–response curve, CL is the total body clearance of warfarin, V is the apparent warfarin volume of distribution, k is the first-order rate constant for intrinsic clotting factor degradation, τ is the dosage interval for warfarin, and C_{max} is the warfarin concentration above which clotting factor synthesis is maximally suppressed. PCA_{ss} was related to prothrombin time with the following relationship:

$$PCA_{ss}\ (\%) = 100\%/[(3.636 \times PTR) - 2.636] \quad (2)$$

where PTR is the prothrombin time ratio, defined as the measured prothrombin time divided by the population-based control prothrombin time.[13]

The Bayesian regression program for this model has been described previously.[10-12] The use of this model to develop a dosing nomogram is presented below.

Nomogram. Affixing the log-linear model's pharmacokinetic variables (CL and V) and pharmacodynamic variables (m, k, C_{max}) while altering the daily dose of warfarin results in a steady-state dose–response curve. The nomogram comprises a series of steady-state warfarin dose–prothrombin time response curves created by using a computer implementation of the log-linear pharmacodynamic model (DrugCalc, MediFore, Inc., Lansing, MI). The range of doses used included 0, 0.25, and 0.5 mg and increments of 0.5 mg thereafter until a PTR of greater than 3 was generated. The "normal response" curve (Figure 1, bold curve) was plotted by using literature-derived, population-based warfarin pharmacokinetic and pharmacodynamic values for a 55-year-old, 70-kg, 68-inch man (CL = 2.19 L/hr, V = 0.11 L/kg, mean ± S.D. C_{max} = 5.49 ± 1.63 mg/L, mean ± S.D. k = 0.98 ± 0.17 day^{-1}, and mean ± S.D. m = 42.16 ± 10.43%).[8,14] The series of dose–response curves (Figure 1) were then plotted by altering the pharmacodynamic values while holding the pharmacokinetic values constant.

Covariance of the pharmacodynamic variables was assumed. The standard deviations of the pharmacodynamic values provided the basis for the alterations of the dose–response curves. Response curves to the right of the normal curve were created by serially increasing the mean value of the pharmacodynamic variables (m, k, and C_{max}) by 25% of their standard deviations until eight curves (2 standard deviations) were plotted. The two outermost curves to the right of the normal curve define 2.5 and 3.0 standard deviations from normal. Response curves to the left of the

Figure 1. Warfarin dosing nomogram. PTR = prothrombin time ratio, INR = international normalized ratio, ISI = international sensitivity ratio.

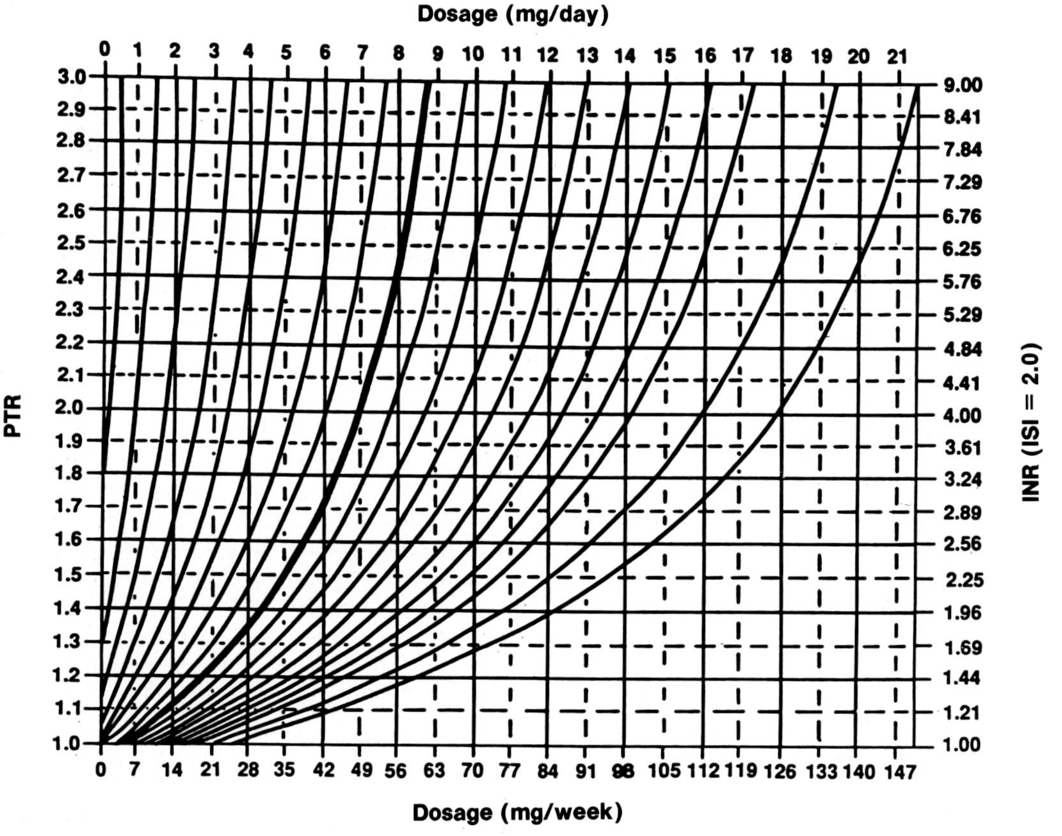

normal curve were plotted by reducing the mean values for *m*, *k*, and C_{max} by 25% of their standard deviations until eight curves (2 standard deviations) were created.

Study Design. *Patient Population.* Patient data sets from a previously conducted unpublished prospective trial comparing the performances of clinicians and a computer program (WarfCalc) in managing outpatients receiving oral anticoagulants were included in the validation and comparison analysis of the warfarin dosing nomogram. The patient population consisted of outpatients requiring warfarin dosage adjustment who were identified in the anticoagulation clinic at either the Veterans Administration Medical Center in Palo Alto, California, or the University of California at Davis Medical Center, Sacramento, between November 1984 and August 1985. The patients were between 18 and 90 years of age and were receiving warfarin for thromboembolic disorders including deep venous thrombosis, pulmonary embolism, cerebrovascular thrombosis, or arterial graft occlusion or for prevention of thrombosis due to cardiac valve replacement or atrial fibrillation. Patients excluded had taken a drug known to induce or inhibit warfarin metabolism within the previous month, were taking drugs that displace warfarin from protein-binding sites, had unstable hepatic disease or malignancy, had recent-onset New York Heart Association class III or IV congestive heart failure, or were noncompliant. Informed consent was obtained from all patients.

In the previous trial, patients with excessive or inadequate PTRs were randomized to receive either computer-assisted dosing or clinician-directed dosing. Dosing and compliance histories were collected during interviews at the clinics. A PTR of 1.7 was targeted in all dosage adjustments unless the patient's primary physician requested otherwise. PTR determinations were repeated at a second clinic visit 16 ± 6.4 days (mean ± S.D.) after the dosage adjustment. Patient compliance was again assessed during an interview.

All blood was collected by the laboratory, and prothrombin time was determined by using Dade reagent C (rabbit brain thromboplastin) in a photo-optical clot sensor (Electra 700, MLA Inc., Mount Vernon, NY 10550).

Excluded from our analysis were data outside the range of the nomogram or data sets for which the PTR changed inversely after a change in the warfarin dosage. For example, after the warfarin dosage was decreased, the follow-up PTR increased over the initial PTR.

Using the patient information and dose–response data, the computer and the nomogram predicted the PTR at the second visit on the basis of the newly prescribed dosage. The Bayesian regression program used each patient's age, weight, height, and sex, in addition to the initial warfarin dosage and associated PTR, to revise pharmacodynamic and pharmacokinetic estimates. With the new estimates and newly prescribed dosage, the computer predicted the PTR. The nomogram required the initial warfarin dosage and corresponding PTR in order to identify a dose–response curve for each patient. This "patient-specific" curve was the curve closest to the intersection of perpendicular lines drawn from the initial dosage (*x*-axis) and PTR response (*y*-axis). Then, by moving along the patient-specific curve to the intersection of that curve and the new warfarin dosage (*x*-axis), the predicted PTR was determined by a line perpendicular to the *y*-axis. An example of the use of the nomogram is given in the appendix.

Analysis. Prediction error and percent absolute prediction error were calculated for each predictive method. Prediction error was defined as the predicted PTR minus the actual PTR. The prediction error was used to assess whether the nomogram or the computer tended to consistently overpredict or underpredict the actual PTR (biased predictions). The mean prediction error was compared with zero by using the independent Student's *t* test for each method. The percent absolute prediction error was determined by multiplying the absolute value of the prediction error by 100 and dividing the product by the actual PTR. The percent absolute prediction error was a determination of the precision of the predictions. Mean percent absolute prediction errors for the computer and nomogram predictions were compared by using the Wilcoxon signed-rank test.[15] The a priori level of significance was set at <0.05.

Results

Seventy-five patients were entered into the 1984–1985 trial. Six patients were excluded from the trial: four because of documented noncompliance, one because cimetidine therapy was discontinued during the study, and one because of a malignancy discovered after the study began. We excluded four other patients: one because the dose–response curve defined by the warfarin dosage and PTR was outside the dosing nomogram and three because their warfarin dosage was decreased but their PTR increased. The patients' demographic characteristics are shown in Table 1.

Data for 65 patients were used for making predictions. The average warfarin dosage was increased slightly between the first and second clinic visits, while the average PTR showed a slight decrease. PTRs predicted by the nomogram and the computer program were similar (Table 2). Neither method resulted in biased predictions, and the precision of the predictions was similar for both. Mean prediction errors for the nomogram and the computer program were –0.037 ± 0.279 ($p = 0.29$) and –0.026 ± 0.254 ($p = 0.40$), respectively. Mean percent absolute prediction errors were 11.6 ± 11.5 (nomogram) and 11.0 ± 10.1 (program) ($p = 0.41$). The percent absolute prediction error was the greatest for the nomogram and the computer program when the initial PTRs were less than 1.3. The performances of the nomogram and the computer program were comparable across a range of initial PTRs (Table 3). The average difference in percent absolute prediction error between the methods was 0.1% (range, −10.3% to 7.0%).

Discussion

We developed the dosing nomogram for warfarin after realizing that a simple yet more scientific method was needed to aid decisions about outpatient dosing. Potential advantages of the nomogram are that it could be readily accessible in a variety of settings, it could provide guidance in otherwise empirical decisions, and it could be a unique teaching instrument, enabling practitioners to visualize the warfarin dose–PTR response curve.

Comparing the nomogram with the computer program was an important initial evaluation of its performance because the nomogram incorporates two major assumptions not made in the Bayesian regression program. The nomogram fixes the pharmacokinetic variables of the model on the basis of a standard sex, age, height, and weight, while the computer program adjusts these estimates based on the demographic characteristics of the study participants. The program also does not assume covariance of all three pharmacodynamic variables, as does the nomogram. Both the computer and the nomogram probably assume covariance of m and k, since both pharmacodynamic variables appear in the steady-state warfarin response equation as a ratio. The similarities in the performances of the nomogram and the computer program suggest that the nomogram captures enough information about the shape of the warfarin dose–response curve to be a useful tool.

Two features of the nomogram axes merit further explanation. While the y-axes plot both PTR and international normalized ratio (INR) scales, the nomogram was developed with PTR data and is designed to be used with PTRs. The nomogram's INR axis may be applicable if the international sensitivity index (ISI) of the thromboplastin used is 2.0. Also, the INR axis may be modified for different thromboplastin ISIs by using the relationship INR = PTR^{ISI}. The usefulness of this modification and the use of INR input have not been evaluated. The x-axes contain warfarin dosages in both milligrams per day and milligrams per week to aid practitioners, particularly when patients are receiving different daily doses. Given the long half-lives of warfarin and most of the vitamin K-dependent clotting factors, the use of total weekly doses seems reasonable.

There are several limitations to consider when using the nomogram. First, steady-state conditions must ex-

Table 1.
Demographic Characteristics of the Study Patients

No. patients	65
Mean age(yr)	60.7
Males/females	55/10
Weight (kg)	85.1
Height (inches)	68.8
Smokers/nonsmokers	18/47
Drinkers/nondrinkers	45/20
Primary diagnosis	
Pulmonary embolus	10
Deep venous thrombosis	9
Recurrent deep venous thrombosis	1
Atrial fibrillation	11
Transient ischemic attack	3
Cardiac valve replacement	16
Mural thrombus	3
Arterial thrombus	1
Cardiovascular accident	4
Other	7

Table 2.
Summary of Dosing and Prothrombin Time Ratio (PTR) Results

Clinic Visit	Mean ± S.D. Dosage in mg/wk (Range)	Mean ± S.D. PTR (Range)
First	45.6 ± 23.5 (14–126)	1.73 ± 0.50 (1.08–2.92)
Second	46.6 ± 22.3 (9.31–112)	
Actual value		1.66 ± 0.23 (1.35–2.30)
Nomogram prediction		1.63 ± 0.27 (1.17–2.30)
Computer program prediction		1.64 ± 0.24 (1.18–2.24)

Table 3.
Influence of Initial Prothrombin Time Ratio (PTR) on Predictive Performance

Item	Initial PTR Range			
	1.00–1.30	1.31–1.50	1.51–2.00	2.01–3.00
No. of patients	19	12	13	21
Mean ± S.D. % absolute prediction error				
Nomogram	15.3 ± 10.7	8.3 ± 8.6	10.3 ± 13.7	10.9 ± 12.0
Computer program	14.1 ± 10.6	8.5 ± 8.3	9.3 ± 10.1	10.7 ± 10.6

ist (generally at least 10 days of therapy with the same dosage regimen). Second, noncompliance, recent drug–drug or drug–disease state interactions, and changes in lifestyle (e.g., in diet and alcohol use) are not accounted for by the nomogram. Third, since the nomogram's design accounts for responses over a limited range, some patients' responses may not fall on the nomogram. This should occur only rarely, as evidenced by the one patient in our analysis who was not evaluable for this reason. This patient's dosage response data identified a curve off the nomogram to the right. Last, when a practitioner uses multiple sets of data that identify the same patient-specific curve, the practitioner should feel confident in the predictions; however, if the data sets do not identify the same patient-specific curve, it is not clear whether the nomogram failed or a change has occurred in the patient's response to warfarin.

Trends were noted in our evaluation of the nomogram that may serve as precautions. The nomogram appears to be less accurate when the initial PTR is 1.30 or less (Table 3). Convergence of the response curves in that range may explain this, since placing patient data on the most appropriate response curve is more difficult in that region. We also observed an average percent absolute prediction error of 23.6% for the five predictions that were based on curves located on the outer regions (>2.5 standard deviations) of the nomogram. Caution should be used when making predictions with those curves.

Conclusion

The warfarin dosing nomogram was comparable to the computer program in predicting the response to warfarin therapy with feedback from one set of patient-specific data. This approach to dosing warfarin in the outpatient setting appears promising; however, prospective studies are needed to validate the nomogram.

References

1. Dalen JE, Hirsh J, eds. Antithrombotic therapy—ACCP–NHLBI Consensus Conference. *Arch Intern Med*. 1986; 146:463-72.
2. Hirsh J, Levine MN. The optimal intensity of oral anticoagulant therapy. *JAMA*. 1987; 258:2723-6.
3. National Center for Health Statistics. Patterns of ambulatory care in internal medicine, United States, January 1980–December 1981. Washington, DC: U.S. Government Printing Office, 1981; DHHS publication no. 84-1741. (Vital and health statistics; series 13, no. 80.)
4. Routledge PA, Bell SM, Davies DM et al. Predicting patients' warfarin requirements. *Lancet*. 1977; 2:854-5.
5. Fennerty A, Dolben J, Thomas P et al. Flexible induction dose regimen for warfarin and prediction of maintenance dose. *Br Med J*. 1984; 288:1268-70.
6. Williams DB, Karl RC. A simple technic for predicting daily maintenance dose of warfarin. *Am J Surg*. 1979; 137:572-6.
7. Miller DR, Brown MA. Predicting warfarin maintenance dosage based on initial response. *Am J Hosp Pharm*. 1979; 36:1351-5.
8. Murray B, Coleman R, McWaters D et al. Pharmacodynamics of warfarin at steady state. *Ther Drug Monit*. 1987; 9:1-5.
9. Theofanous TG, Barile RG. Multiple-dose kinetics of oral anticoagulants: methods of analysis and optimized dosing. *J Pharm Sci*. 1973; 62:261-6.
10. Svec JM, Coleman RW, Mungall DR et al. Bayesian pharmacokinetic/pharmacodynamic forecasting of prothrombin response to warfarin therapy: preliminary evaluation. *Ther Drug Monit*. 1985; 7:174-80.
11. Lee C, Coleman RW, Mungall DR. Effect of using warfarin plasma concentrations in Bayesian forecasting of prothrombin-time response. *Clin Pharm*. 1987; 6:406-12.
12. White RH, Hong R, Venook AP et al. Initiation of warfarin therapy: comparison of physician dosing with computer-assisted dosing. *J Gen Intern Med*. 1987; 2:141-8.
13. Sheiner LB. Computer-aided long term anticoagulation therapy. *Comput Biomed Res*. 1969; 2:519-36.
14. Mungall DR, Ludden TM, Marshall J et al. Population pharmacokinetics of racemic warfarin. *J Pharmacokinet Biopharm*. 1985; 13:213-27.
15. Sheiner LB, Beal SL. Some suggestions for measuring predictive performance. *J Pharmacokinet Biopharm*. 1981; 9:503-12.

Appendix—Example of the Use of the Warfarin Dosing Nomogram

The patient has been taking warfarin sodium 5 mg/day for one month. He has taken all his doses, and today he has a prothrombin time of 24 seconds with a control value of 12 seconds. The therapeutic goal is a prothrombin time ratio (PTR) of 1.4.

Refer to the figure below and do the following:

1. Find the current dosage (A) on the top *x*-axis.
2. Find the measured PTR (B) on the left *y*-axis.
3. Place a dot (C) on the nomogram where perpendicular lines from the current dosage (A) and PTR (B) intersect.
4. Move to the population-based steady-state response curve nearest to the dot (D).
5. Follow this curve until it intersects a perpendicular line from the desired steady-state ratio and place a slash (E).
6. The recommended dosage is determined by the perpendicular line connecting the slash and the dosage axis of the graph (F).
7. The recommended dosage would be 3 mg/day or 21 mg/week.

The dosing nomogram may be used to assist the practitioner in determining the desired dosage; it cannot replace good clinical judgment.

Example of the use of the warfarin dosing nomogram (see appendix). PTR = prothrombin time ratio, INR = international normalized ratio, ISI = international sensitivity index.

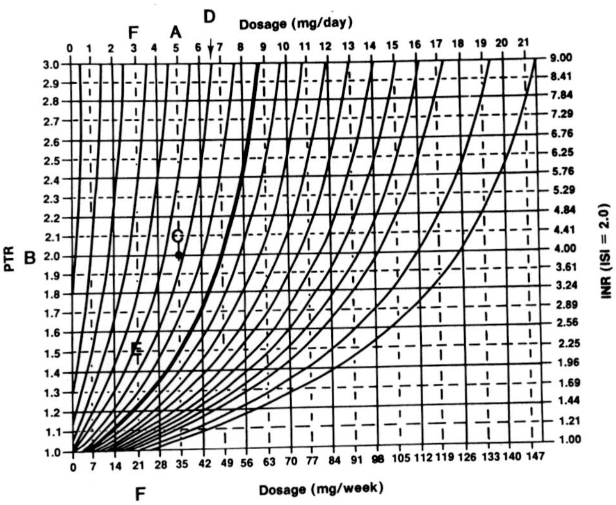

Research Notes

Estimating phenytoin dosages in black African and Indian children

JULIA H. BOTHA, RAYMOND MILLER, AND MANIKUM MOODLEY

Clin Pharm. 1991; 10:928-31

The determination of optimal dosage regimens for phenytoin is often difficult. This is largely because the metabolism of this drug at therapeutic serum concentrations approaches the upper limit of an enzyme-mediated reaction that is presumed to follow Michaelis-Menten pharmacokinetics[1-3] and that is described by the following equation:

$$\text{Dosage (mg/day)} = V_{max}\,(C_{av})/(K_m + C_{av}) \qquad (1)$$

where V_{max} is the maximum rate of metabolism (in milligrams per day), C_{av} is the average serum phenytoin concentration at steady state (in micrograms per milliliter), and K_m is the Michaelis-Menten constant (in micrograms per milliliter).

To estimate a suitable dosage of phenytoin, V_{max} and K_m values—ideally for an individual patient, or at least for the appropriate population—are required. While such values are available for adults,[4] pediatric information is more limited, and no estimates of these values for black African and Indian children have been published. It is possible that the metabolic capacity of these children may differ from that of other children; in adults, lower V_{max} and K_m values have been reported for black Africans.[5]

One objective of this study was to test which published values of V_{max} and K_m can best be used to estimate the phenytoin dosages required in black African and Indian children. The actual dosage required to produce a particular serum concentration was compared with dosages estimated to give this concentration by substituting V_{max} and K_m values from the literature[6-10] in equation 1. Because of interpatient variation, the best results with phenytoin are most likely to be achieved if the dosage is individualized by using one reliable pair of dosage and steady-state serum concentration values for a particular patient. In view of this, when two pairs of concentration and dosage values were available, the second dosage was estimated by using the first dosage–concentration pair and a nomogram. Dosage estimates made with two such feedback methods[11,12] were compared with the best estimates made from the published values alone.

Methods. The subjects were afebrile, epileptic black African and Indian children 1–16 years of age who had been receiving phenytoin and attending the pediatric epilepsy clinic at King Edward VIII Hospital in Durban, South Africa, for two years. All patients who were known to be compliant with therapy and whose average serum phenytoin concentration was at steady state were included in the study. Compliance was determined by parent interviews and capsule or tablet counts. Steady state was assumed if the same phenytoin dosage had been maintained for at least one month. Venous blood was drawn for the measurement of serum phenytoin concentrations when requested by the pediatrician as part of routine patient care. Concentrations were measured with the Abbott TDx System[13] in the hospital laboratory. Since 88% of the serum concentration measurements were for patients receiving phenytoin every 12 hours (the balance being every 24 hours), they were assumed to represent average concentrations, even though blood was not drawn at any fixed time in relation to the doses.

Naive Dosage Estimation Methods. Thirty-seven pairs of steady-state concentration and dosage values for 13 patients receiving phenytoin alone were used in this evaluation. The actual daily dosage of phenytoin sodium required to give the measured concentration was compared with the dosage estimated by substituting literature V_{max} and K_m values in equation 1. In all 37 cases, 10 sets of estimates based on published population values (Table 1) were used to estimate phenytoin dosages.

Estimates 1–5 were based on V_{max} and K_m values published by Chiba et al.[6] for 104 Japanese children between 0.5 and 16 years of age. Estimates 1–4 in-

JULIA H. BOTHA, PH.D., is Senior Lecturer, Department of Pharmacology, University of Natal (UN), Durban, South Africa. RAYMOND MILLER, D.SC., is Professor and Head, Department of Pharmacology, University of Durban–Westville, Durban. MANIKUM MOODLEY, FCP, is Senior Specialist and Senior Lecturer, Department of Paediatrics, UN.

Address reprint requests to Dr. Botha at the Department of Clinical and Experimental Pharmacology, P.O. Box 17039, Congella, 4013, South Africa.

Presented in part at the Annual Congress of the Southern African Pharmacological Society, Stellenbosch, South Africa, October 1989.

Table 1.
Published Michaelis-Menten Constants (K_m) and Maximum Rates of Metabolism (V_{max}) Used in Naive Dosage Estimates 1–10

Estimate	No. Patients	Age Range (yr)	K_m (µg/mL)	V_{max} (mg/kg/day)	Reference
1	34	0.5–3	4.1	13.8	6
2	24	4–6	4.1	11.2	6
3	24	7–9	3.6	9.5	6
4	22	10–16	3.0	8.0	6
5	104	0.5–16	3.7	10.6[a]	6
6	Not stated	"Children"	3.7	15.0	7
7	4	6–11	2.7	5.3	8
8	40	<15	3.2	$415\ (wt/70)^{0.6}$ [b]	9
9	104	0.5–16	2.2	$415\ (wt/70)^{0.6}$	9
10	37	11–60	3.4	6.5	10

[a] Because a V_{max} value for all their patients was not presented by Chiba et al.,[6] V_{max} values for individual age groups were used to derive this approximate figure.
[b] wt = weight.

volved values obtained by division into particular age groups, and estimate 5 involved values derived for the whole group. Estimate 6 was based on mean values of the ranges quoted for children by Bruni,[7] namely, K_m = 3.5–3.9 µg/mL and V_{max} = 5–25 mg/kg/day. Means of data for four overdosed children were used in estimate 7.[8] Values of K_m and V_{max} computed by Grasela et al.[9] in analyzing previously reported data for European[14] and Japanese[6] children were used in estimates 8 and 9, respectively. Grasela et al. obtained their population values by using NONMEM, a computer program designed for population pharmacokinetic analysis. They found that V_{max} was not influenced by age but was a nonlinear function of weight (i.e., weight$^{0.6}$). Finally, estimate 10 involved values derived for black patients in Johannesburg, South Africa, even though these patients were adults.[10]

Feedback Methods for Estimating Dosage. In nine patients for whom more than one pair of dosage and concentration values were available, the first pair and a nomogram were used to estimate the dosage required to give the other concentrations. The estimated dosage was then compared with the actual dosage required to give that concentration. Twenty data pairs were evaluated in this way, of which 14 were for patients taking phenytoin alone and the balance were for patients receiving phenytoin plus one other drug (carbamazepine, phenobarbital, or sodium valproate). Two nomograms were used:

1. *A Bayesian nomogram* generated by Vozeh et al.[11] from V_{max} and K_m values determined in a Swiss population and based on a Bayesian approach in which these mean values are used with the patient's dosage–concentration pair such that account is taken of variation within and among individuals.
2. *A population clearance nomogram* proposed by Graves et al.[12] and based on an exponential relationship for 177 pairs of phenytoin clearance and steady-state serum concentrations for 59 American adults. The relationship is described by the following equation:

$$D_{new} = D_{initial}\,(C_{av,\,desired})^{0.2}\,(C_{av,\,achieved})^{-0.2} \qquad (2)$$

where D_{new} is the new dosage, $D_{initial}$ is the initial dosage, and $C_{av,\,desired}$ and $C_{av,\,achieved}$ are the desired and achieved average serum phenytoin concentrations at steady state, respectively.

Dosages were also estimated by using the two best estimates of V_{max} and K_m determined in the evaluation of naive dosage estimation methods.

Statistical Analysis. For each method of dosage estimation, prediction errors were calculated by subtracting the actual daily dosage of phenytoin sodium from the estimated daily dosage. The mean prediction error for each method was used as an indication of bias. Precision was defined as the root mean squared error (i.e., the square root of the mean squared prediction error).[15]

A two-tailed Student's *t* test with an adjustment for multiple comparisons was used to assess whether the mean prediction error was different from zero and thus indicated significant bias. The a priori level of significance was set at <0.05.

The bias and precision of the methods were compared by analysis of variance (ANOVA). If a significant difference was found, then Tukey's multiple-range test was used to isolate the source of the difference.

Results. *Naive Dosage Estimation Methods.* The mean ± S.D. age of the patients at the times of contact (n = 37 contacts with 13 patients) was 9.5 ± 3.7 years (median age, 10 years). Thirty of the contacts were with male patients.

Only estimates 3 and 9 were not significantly biased (Table 2). All the other estimates were significantly biased in either a positive direction (estimates 1, 2, 5, and 6) or a negative direction (4, 7, 8, and 10). ANOVA revealed a difference in both bias and precision among the estimates. However, estimates 3 and 9 did not differ significantly from one another in either regard. They rated third and second, respectively, in precision.

Feedback Methods Compared with the Best Naive Estimation Methods. The mean ± S.D. age of the patients at the

Table 2.
Bias and Precision of Naive Estimates of Phenytoin Sodium Dosage (mg/day)

Estimate	Mean Prediction Error[a]	Mean Squared Error	Root Mean Squared Error
1	96.9 ± 95.7 (+64 to +128), 0.000	18305.1	135.3
2	38.2 ± 73.6 (+13 to +63), 0.003	6734.4	82.1
3	6.3 ± 63.8 (−15 to +2), 0.550	4000.9	63.3
4	−21.4 ± 58.9 (−14 to −2), 0.034	837.7	62.0
5	31.0 ± 70.4 (+8 to +55), 0.011	5783.0	76.1
6	132.1 ± 108.8 (+95 to +168), 0.000	28972.9	170.2
7	−84.7 ± 61.7 (−105 to −64), 0.000	10912.2	104.5
8	−26.5 ± 61.9 (−47 to −6), 0.014	4431.8	66.6
9	−12.8 ± 62.1 (−34 to +8), 0.216	3910.5	62.5
10	−61.6 ± 58 (−81 to −42), 0.000	7052.0	84.0

[a] Reported as mean ± S.D. (95% confidence interval), *p*.

Table 3.
Bias and Precision of Phenytoin Sodium Dosage Estimates (mg/day) Made with Naive Estimation Methods 3 and 9 and Feedback Methods

Estimation Method	Mean Prediction Error[a]	Mean Squared Error	Root Mean Squared Error
Naive Estimation Methods			
Estimate 3	4.3 ± 50.0 (−19 to +28), 0.71	2363.6	48.6
Estimate 9	−13.3 ± 62.2 (−42 to +16), 0.40	3846.9	62.0
Feedback Methods			
Bayesian nomogram	10.2 ± 38.4 (−8 to +28), 0.25	1501.4	38.8
Population clearance nomogram	9.2 ± 34 (−8 to +25), 0.24	1179.9	34.4

[a] Reported as mean ± S.D. (95% confidence interval), *p*.

times of contact (n = 20 contacts with nine patients) was 11.1 ± 4.0 years (median age, 11.8 years). Eighteen of the contacts were with male patients.

Results of the comparison between the feedback methods and naive estimation methods 3 and 9 made in the 20 cases in which two pairs of concentration and dosage data were available are shown in Table 3. Neither the feedback methods nor the naive estimation methods were significantly biased. In addition, there was no significant difference in bias between them. However, there was a significant difference in precision (p = 0.009). The population clearance approach was the most precise, followed by the Bayesian approach. The precision of these two feedback methods was significantly different from that of naive estimation method 9 but not naive estimation method 3.

Discussion. The initial aim of this study was to select from published values the most appropriate V_{max} and K_m values to use in starting phenytoin therapy in a pediatric population. A review of the literature showed the available data for children, particularly black African and Indian children, to be limited. In addition, most pediatric V_{max} and K_m values have been derived in studies in which some of the patients received other anticonvulsants in addition to phenytoin.[6,8,16]

Of the nine sets of pediatric V_{max} and K_m estimates tested, five overestimated and four underestimated phenytoin dosage. However, only estimate 3, which overestimated dosage, and estimate 9, which underestimated dosage, were significantly unbiased at the 5% level. These two estimates did not differ from one another in terms of bias or precision.

Estimate 3 was based on K_m and V_{max} values of 3.6 μg/mL and 9.5 mg/kg/day, respectively, derived by Chiba et al.[6] for 24 Japanese children seven to nine years of age. Perhaps the reason why Chiba et al.'s values for this age group gave better estimates in our patients than did their other values may have been that of the 37 dosages estimated, 17 were for members of this particular age group.

Estimate 9 was based on V_{max} and K_m values computed from data for 104 Japanese children 0.5–16 years of age[6] by Grasela et al.[9] using NONMEM. The low K_m value of 2.2 may be especially appropriate to the population in question (73% black), as black adults have lower K_m values than other adults.[5] In addition, computation of V_{max} as a function of weight rather than age could be expected to be more appropriate when there is an imbalance in the representation of age groups, as in this study.

The only values for adults that were tested (in estimate 10) were included because they had been derived for patients of a similar population.[10] It is not surprising that this estimate was significantly negatively biased, as children can be expected to have a higher V_{max} than their adult counterparts.

Clearly, on initiating phenytoin treatment in these pediatric patients, the accuracy of dosage estimates based on published population values is sensitive to the source of the values used. Until sufficient data are available for computing V_{max} and K_m values for this patient population, a reasonable estimate of initial dosage can be expected to be achieved in most of the patients by using naive estimation method 3 or 9. The fact that the two best naive estimations (3 and 9) were not significantly more biased than the estimates made by using the feedback methods confirms that a reasonable estimate of phenytoin dosage can be made in these children by using either of these published sets of V_{max} and K_m values. In fact, the precision of naive estimate 3 was also not significantly different from that of the estimates made by using the two feedback methods.

Although the difference was not significant, both feedback methods were more precise than naive estimate 3, with the population clearance approach being slightly ahead of the Bayesian method. The Bayesian approach may have produced better estimates had V_{max} and K_m values appropriate to children been used in the nomogram. However, this possibility was not investigated because not only was the population clearance approach the most precise, it was more convenient in the study environment. While Bayesian forecasting cannot easily be performed, use of the population clearance nomogram requires only a programmable hand-held calculator. The population clearance nomogram provided an ideal means of individualizing phenytoin dosage irrespective of the patient's age, weight, or sex or the use of concomitant therapy.

As pointed out by Yuen et al.,[17] close monitoring of children receiving phenytoin is recommended, regardless of the method used to determine the dosage.

Conclusion. The most appropriate published V_{max} and K_m values can be used to initiate phenytoin treatment in the population of black African and Indian children studied, and dosages can subsequently be effectively individualized by using one pair of steady-state serum phenytoin concentration and dosage values and the population clearance nomogram of Graves et al.[12]

References

1. Gerber N, Wagner G. Explanation of dose-dependent decline of diphenylhydantoin plasma levels by fitting to the integrated form of the Michaelis-Menten equation. *Res Commun Chem Pathol Pharmacol.* 1972; 3:455-66.
2. Glazko AJ. Antiepileptic drugs: biotransformation, metabolism and serum half life. *Epilepsia.* 1975; 16:367-91.
3. Witkin KM, Buis DL, Teague BL et al. Determination of 5-(*p*-hydroxyphenyl)-5-phenylhydantoin and studies relating to the disposition of phenytoin in man. *Ther Drug Monit.* 1979; 1:11-34.
4. Goodman and Gilman's the pharmacological basis of therapeutics. 7th ed. Gilman AG, Goodman LS, Rall TW et al. New York: Macmillan; 1985.
5. Miller R, Rheeders M, Klein C et al. Population pharmacokinetics of phenytoin in South African black patients. *S Afr Med J.* 1987; 72:188-90.
6. Chiba K, Ishizaki MD, Miura H et al. Michaelis-Menten pharmacokinetics of diphenylhydantoin and application in the paediatric age patient. *J Pediatr.* 1980; 96:479-84.
7. Bruni J. Phenytoin. In: Taylor WJ, Diers Caviness MH, eds. A textbook for the clinical application of therapeutic drug monitoring. Irving, TX: Abbott Laboratories; 1986:253-67.
8. Garretson LK, Jusko WJ. Diphenylhydantoin elimination kinetics in overdosed children. *Clin Pharmacol Ther.* 1975; 17:481-91.
9. Grasela TH, Sheiner LB, Rambeck B et al. Steady-state pharmacocokinetics of phenytoin from routinely collected patient data. *Clin Pharmacokinet.* 1983; 8:355-64.
10. Miller R, Rheeders M. Effect of source of population data on phenytoin dosage predictions in black patients. *Clin Pharm.* 1989; 8:56-9.
11. Vozeh S, Muir JT, Sheiner LB et al. Predicting phenytoin dosage. *J Pharmacokinet Biopharm.* 1981; 9:131-47.
12. Graves NM, Leppik IE, Termond E et al. Phenytoin clearances in a compliant population: description and application. *Ther Drug Monit.* 1986; 8:427-33.
13. Bottorff MB, Stewart CF. Analytical techniques in quality control. In: Taylor WJ, Diers Caviness MH et al., eds. A textbook for the clinical application of therapeutic drug monitoring. Irving, TX: Abbott Laboratories; 1986:51-7.
14. Blain PG, Mucklow JC, Bacon CJ et al. Pharmacokinetics of phenytoin in children. *Br J Clin Pharmacol.* 1981; 12:659-61.
15. Sheiner LB, Beal SL. Some suggestions for measuring predictive performance. *J Pharmacokinet Biopharm.* 1981; 9:503-12.
16. Dodson WE. Nonlinear kinetics of phenytoin in children. *Neurology.* 1982; 32:42-8.
17. Yuen GJ, Latimer PT, Littlefield LC et al. Phenytoin dosage predictions in paediatric patients. *Clin Pharmacokinet.* 1989; 16:254-60.

Use of gentamicin clearance in estimating renal function

RANDALL K. NAKAHIRO, MARK P. OKAMOTO, ALFRED CHIN, MARK A. GILL, JOANNE S. CHAE, AND DAVID A. SCLAR

Clin Pharm. 1991; 10:931-4

Estimation of renal function is clinically important for adjusting dosage regimens of medications excreted by the kidney.[1-5] Creatinine clearance is often used in clinical practice to approximate glomerular filtration rate (GFR). Creatinine is produced at a relatively con-

RANDALL K. NAKAHIRO, PHARM.D., is Pharmacist Specialist–Drug Information, Kaiser Permanente, Downey CA. MARK P. OKAMOTO, PHARM.D., is Fellow in Infectious Disease Pharmacotherapy and Lecturer, School of Pharmacy; ALFRED CHIN, PHARM.D., is Assistant Professor of Clinical Pharmacy, School of Pharmacy; and MARK A. GILL, PHARM.D., is Associate Professor of Clinical Pharmacy and Director, Laboratory for Clinical Pharmacy Research, School of Pharmacy, University of Southern California, Los Angeles. JOANNE S. CHAE, PHARM.D., is Clinical Pharmacist, Los Angeles County/University of Southern California Medical Center, Los Angeles. DAVID A. SCLAR, PH.D., is Assistant Professor of Health Care Administration, College of Pharmacy, Washington State University, Pullman.

Address reprint requests to Dr. Gill at the School of Pharmacy, University of Southern California, 1985 Zonal Avenue PSC 208-A, Los Angeles, CA 90033.

stant rate by the liver and muscles. Creatinine clearance tends to reflect glomerular filtration because it is freely filtered by the glomerulus and is not extensively reabsorbed by the renal tubules; however, creatinine is also actively secreted and creatinine clearance cannot be assumed to be identical to GFR.[6]

Mathematical estimation of creatinine clearance has been used to estimate drug clearance by the kidney in adjusting the dosage of renally eliminated medications, because a 24-hour urine collection is costly in labor, time, and expense. The method of Cockcroft and Gault[2] is the most commonly used equation for estimating creatinine clearance.[3] An alternative method has been proposed by Jelliffe and Jelliffe.[1] These equations take into account sex, age, weight or body surface area, and serum creatinine concentration to estimate creatinine clearance, but they still have some faults in their predictive ability because of interpatient variability with regard to muscle mass, amount of body fat, diet, behavioral and cultural differences, and so forth.[3,7-9]

Because aminoglycosides are predominantly excreted by glomerular filtration (approximately 45–97% of the first dose is excreted unchanged in the urine within 24 hours) and the renal clearance of gentamicin is similar to that of endogenous creatinine, the total clearance of aminoglycosides can be calculated by using serum concentration data; this provides an estimate of renal clearance without having to take interpatient variables into account. When serum creatinine concentrations may not accurately approximate an individual's GFR[10] and a 24-hour urine collection cannot be obtained, estimating creatinine clearance by using measured serum aminoglycoside concentrations may be a more convenient indicator of renal function for patients receiving aminoglycoside therapy.

Twenty-four-hour urine collection is the standard in clinical practice for determining a patient's creatinine clearance. Other methods have been shown to be more accurate in estimating a patient's GFR, such as inulin clearance; however, these methods are not commonly used in clinical practice. The objective of this study was to determine the predictive ability of four methods for estimating creatinine clearance—gentamicin clearance calculated using actual body weight and ideal body weight, the Cockcroft and Gault formula, and the Jelliffe formula—as compared with the 24-hour urine collection taken from patients with perforated or gangrenous appendicitis.

Methods. Patients who received gentamicin for presumed appendicitis and who were subsequently diagnosed intraoperatively as having perforated or gangrenous appendicitis were analyzed retrospectively to estimate creatinine clearance. Patients were excluded from the study if they were less than 18 years or older than 70 years of age, were diagnosed as having septicemia, had serum creatinine concentrations greater than 1.5 mg/dL, or had received any other antimicrobial therapy 48 hours before or during hospital admission. All patients were started on gentamicin (as the sulfate salt) 1.5 mg/kg i.v. every eight hours plus clindamycin (as the phosphate salt) 900 mg i.v. every eight hours.

The gentamicin serum samples were drawn at steady state (defined as four or more half-lives into therapy). Each data set consisted of a peak (blood sample taken 30 minutes after the end of a 30-minute infusion), a trough (sample taken within one hour of the next dose), and a midpoint concentration (sample taken an estimated 1.66 half-lives after the dose). The samples were drawn within 48 hours postoperatively and were kept in ice until they were delivered to the chemistry laboratory for analysis. Serum creatinine and 24-hour urine creatinine samples were collected the same day the gentamicin concentrations were obtained. Hospital nursing staff collected all 24-hour urine samples. Research pharmacists prepared and administered the intermittent i.v. doses of gentamicin and collected all serum samples for gentamicin determination. Gentamicin concentrations were analyzed in batch by fluorescence polarization immunoassay (Abbott TDx) the day they were obtained. The cross-reactivity for other antibiotics used in this study was <1%. Sensitivity for gentamicin was 0.3 μg/mL. The average coefficient of variation over a three-month period was 8.9% at a concentration of 3.8 μg/mL and 5.2% at a concentration of 1.6 μg/mL. Urine creatinine was assayed by a colorimetric pitric acid reaction assay (DuPont Medical).

Creatinine clearance from the 24-hour urine collection was calculated as follows:

$$CL_{cr} = [(U_{cr} \times V_u)/(S_{cr} \times t)] \times (1.73/BSA)$$

where CL_{cr} = creatinine clearance (mL/min/1.73 sq m), U_{cr} = urine creatinine (mg/dL), S_{cr} = serum creatinine (mg/dL), t = urine collection time (min), BSA = body surface area (sq m), and V_u = urine volume (mL). Body surface area was calculated as follows[11]: BSA = $(wt^{0.425})(ht^{0.725})(0.007184)$, where weight is expressed as kilograms and height as centimeters.

Gentamicin clearance was determined from the pharmacokinetic data calculated by the USC Pack PC Bayesian computer software program (version 8.0)[12] as follows:

$$CL_{gent} = (k)(V)(1 \text{ hr}/60 \text{ min})(1000 \text{ mL/L})(1.73/BSA)$$

where CL_{gent} = gentamicin clearance (mL/min/1.73 sq m), k = elimination rate constant (hr^{-1}), and V = volume of distribution (L). The volume of distribution and elimination rate constant were calculated using the USC Pack PC. The program is based on a one-compartment model. Values for V(0.21 ± 0.03 L/kg) and k (0.53 ± 0.10 hr^{-1}) determined from a separate study of appendicitis patients at Los Angeles County/ University of Southern California Medical Center[13] were entered as a priori estimates. Patient data entered into the program included the dosing history, measured gentamicin concentrations, weight (ideal and actual), height, age, sex, and serum creatinine concentration (on day of gentamicin sampling). In men, ideal body weight equaled 50 kg + 2.3 (height in inches – 60); in women, ideal body weight equaled 45.5 kg + 2.3 (height in inches – 60).

Creatinine clearance was estimated by the Jelliffe method as follows:

E_{ss} (males) = wt [29.3 – 0.203 (age)]

E_{ss} (females) = wt [25.1 – 0.175 (age)]

where E_{ss} = steady-state urinary excretion rate, wt = patient's weight (kg), and age = patient's age (yr).

$E_{ss,\,corr} = E_{ss}R$

where $E_{ss,\,corr}$ = steady-state urinary excretion rate corrected for nonrenal creatinine clearance.

$R = 1.035 - 0.0337\,(S_{cr})$

$E = E_{ss,\,corr} - 4(wt)(S_{cr,\,2} - S_{cr,\,1})/t$

where $S_{cr,\,2}$ = current serum creatinine concentration, $S_{cr,\,1}$ = previous serum creatinine concentration, and t = number of days between serum creatinine determinations.

$CL_{cr} = [E/14.4 \times (S_{cr})] \times 1.73/BSA$

The Cockcroft and Gault method, with creatinine clearance normalized to a body surface area of 1.73 sq m, is as follows:

$CL_{cr} = [(140 - age) \times (wt)/(72) \times (S_{cr})] \times 1.73/BSA$

where wt = patient's weight (kg). Calculated creatinine clearance values for women were multiplied by 0.85.

Each patient's measured creatinine clearance (determined from the 24-hour urine collection) was compared with the creatinine clearances calculated by the gentamicin clearance method (using ideal body weight and actual body weight), the Jelliffe method, and the Cockcroft and Gault method. Measured and estimated creatinine clearance values were normalized to mL/min/1.73 sq m for comparison.

Because frequency distribution analysis indicated that the data used for the comparative analyses were not normally distributed, nonparametric tests were used. The Wilcoxon matched-pairs test was used to assess differences between the 24-hour creatinine collection and each of the four predictive methods. The level of significance was set at 0.05. Standard error of the mean was used to calculate 95% confidence intervals. Bias was calculated as the predicted creatinine clearance minus the observed creatinine clearance (mean prediction error).[14,15] Precision was defined as the root mean squared prediction error. All statistical analyses were performed with the BMDP statistical software package.[16]

Results. Data from 32 patients (25 men, 7 women) with a postoperative diagnosis of perforated appendicitis (23 patients) or gangrenous appendicitis (9 patients) were collected. The age range was 18–51 years (mean ± S.D., 28.7 ± 9.6 years). Actual body weight ranged from 41 to 90.9 kg (mean ± S.D., 65.6 ± 12.1 kg). The mean difference between ideal body weight and actual body weight was 10.1% (ideal body weight ranged from 46.1 to 55.6 kg) (mean ± S.D., 52.0 ± 2.86 kg). Thus, patients were considered not obese where obesity was defined as an actual body weight 20% or more above ideal body weight. Adjusted body weight (an intermediate value of actual and ideal body weight) was not used in any of the calculations of creatinine clearance because the mean difference between ideal and actual body weight was not more than 20%. Height ranged from 59 to 70 inches (mean ± S.D., 64.2 ± 2.9 inches). Serum creatinine concentration ranged from 0.6 to 1.4 mg/dL (mean ± S.D., 0.9 ± 0.2 mg/dL).

Measured creatinine clearance ranged from 67.4 to 227.8 mL/min/1.73 sq m (mean ± S.D., 126.13 ± 37.99 mL/min/1.73 sq m). All patients had stable renal function, determined by at least two consecutive serum creatinine concentration determinations within 48 hours of each other that did not differ by more than 7%. Gentamicin elimination rate constant ranged from 0.367 to 0.892 hr^{-1} (mean ± S.D., 0.526 ± 0.103 hr^{-1}), and volume of distribution ranged from 0.175 L/kg to 0.276 L/kg (mean ± S.D., 0.214 ± 0.025 L/kg).

Of all four methods employed, only gentamicin clearance calculated using actual body weight showed no significant difference from the measured creatinine clearance (p = 0.8088), as illustrated in Table 1. Gentamicin clearance calculated using actual body weight appeared to be the least biased method. The precision

Table 1.
Measured Creatinine Clearance Compared with Estimates from Cockcroft and Gault, Jelliffe, and Gentamicin Clearance Methods

Method	Mean ± S.D.[a] CL_{cr} (95% CI)[b]	p[c]	Mean Prediction Error ± S.D.[a]	Root Mean Squared Prediction Error ± S.D.[a]
24-Hour urine collection	126.13 ± 37.99 (112.4–139.8)	. . .	. . .	. . .
Cockcroft and Gault	111.24 ± 21.28 (103.6–118.9)	0.0318	−14.89 ± 37.46	31.59 ± 24.54
Jelliffe	102.77 ± 17.74 (96.4–109.2)	0.0009	−23.36 ± 36.03	33.05 ± 27.09
Gentamicin clearance (IBW)[d]	100.43 ± 25.87 (91.1–109.8)	0.0006	−25.70 ± 38.16	34.80 ± 29.79
Gentamicin clearance (ABW)[e]	124.39 ± 30.13 (113.5–135.3)	0.8088	−1.74 ± 40.27	30.53 ± 25.74

[a] Expressed as mL/min/1.73 sq m.
[b] CI = confidence interval.
[c] $p < 0.05$ indicates a significant difference from measurement obtained by 24-hour urine collection.
[d] Denotes clearance calculated using ideal body weight (IBW).
[e] Denotes clearance calculated using actual body weight (ABW).

for all four methods compared with zero was significantly different ($p < 0.0001$).

Discussion. Gentamicin clearance calculated using actual body weight was the least biased method, tended to slightly underpredict creatinine clearance, and did not differ significantly from the measured creatinine clearance. Values determined by the Cockcroft and Gault, Jelliffe, and gentamicin clearance based on ideal body weight methods were significantly different from the measured creatinine clearance and tended to underpredict creatinine clearance.

The Cockcroft and Gault and the Jelliffe methods have been shown to be reliable in determining creatinine clearance,[5,15,17,18] especially in young, nonobese adults; however, only gentamicin clearance calculated using actual body weight was shown not to be significantly different from the measured creatinine clearance. This difference could be attributable to the selection of patient populations. Gentamicin clearances were based on data from patients with perforated or gangrenous appendicitis. The Jelliffe method was based on data from renal transplant patients, and the Cockcroft and Gault method was based on data from a wide variety of patients.

One would expect similarity between gentamicin clearance values and the measured creatinine clearance because of the similar mechanisms of renal excretion of gentamicin and creatinine. The use of measured serum gentamicin concentrations would also minimize interpatient and intrapatient variables, which can affect the predictive ability of the Cockcroft and Gault and the Jelliffe methods.[3,6-8] However, this study did not investigate how accurate the gentamicin clearance method would be in estimating renal function in patients with fluctuating serum creatinine concentrations, in the elderly, or in patients with conditions (e.g., high fevers, burns, or morbid obesity) that could potentially alter the drug's pharmacokinetics.

Based on the data from appendicitis patients in this study, gentamicin clearance that is calculated using actual body weight appears to be more representative of the patient's creatinine clearance than estimates using the methods of Cockcroft and Gault or Jelliffe or gentamicin clearance that is calculated using ideal body weight. Creatinine clearance can be conveniently assessed from the gentamicin pharmacokinetic data if the patient has stable renal function. Serum sampling is routinely performed when patients are placed on aminoglycoside therapy because of the narrow therapeutic margin of these drugs, and such data would be readily available.

If gentamicin clearance is more indicative of creatinine clearance than are other estimation methods in patients with normal renal function, as shown in this postappendectomy population, one could possibly use the information for adjusting dosages of other renally eliminated drugs in patients already receiving gentamicin therapy. However, more studies are needed to determine the reliability of using gentamicin clearance to estimate creatinine clearance in patients with impaired or unstable renal function.

Conclusion. This study showed that gentamicin clearance based on actual body weight and stable renal function was not significantly different from a 24-hour measured urine creatinine collection in estimating creatinine clearance. Although the results are promising, it is difficult to extrapolate these findings to the general population because variables not examined in this study (e.g., changing renal function, changes in volume of distribution) might have an influence on the clearance of gentamicin.

References

1. Jelliffe RW, Jelliffe SW. A computer program for estimation of creatinine clearance from unstable serum creatinine levels, age, sex, and weight. *Math Biosci.* 1972; 14:17-24.
2. Cockcroft DW, Gault MH. Prediction of creatinine clearance from serum creatinine. *Nephron.* 1976; 16:31-41.
3. Drusano GL, Muncie HL, Hoopes JM et al. Commonly used methods of estimating creatinine clearance are inadequate for elderly debilitated nursing home patients. *J Am Geriatr Soc.* 1988; 36:437-41.
4. Ratain JS, Petri M, Hochberg MC et al. Accuracy of creatinine clearance in measuring glomerular filtration rate in patients with systemic lupus erythematosus without clinical evidence of renal disease. *Arthritis Rheum.* 1990; 33:277-80.
5. Boyce EG, Dickerson RN, Cooney GF et al. Creatinine clearance estimation in protein-malnourished patients. *Clin Pharm.* 1989; 8:721-6.
6. Coe FL. Alterations in urinary function. In: Wilson JD, Braunwald E, Isselbacher KJ et al., eds. Harrison's principles of internal medicine. Vol. 1 and 2. 12th ed. New York: McGraw-Hill; 1991:271.
7. James GD, Sealey JE, Alderman M et al. A longitudinal study of urinary creatinine and creatinine clearance in normal subjects. *Am J Hypertens.* 1988; 1:124-31.
8. Salazar DE, Corcoran GB. Predicting creatinine clearance and renal drug clearance in obese patients from estimated fat-free body mass. *Am J Med.* 1988; 84:1053-60.
9. Vree TB, Hekster YA, Hafkenscheid JCM et al. The influence of urine flow on renal clearance of creatinine in patients with normal and impaired kidney function. *DICP.* 1981; 15:194-8.
10. Robert S, Zarowitz BJ. Is there a reliable index of glomerular filtration rate in critically ill patients. *DICP.* 1991; 25:169-78.
11. Du Bois D, Du Bois EF. Clinical calorimetry: a formula to estimate the approximate surface area if height and weight be known. *Arch Intern Med.* 1916; 17:863.
12. D'Argenio DZ, Schumitzky A. A program package for simulation and parameter estimation in pharmacokinetic systems. *Comput Programs Biomed.* 1979; 9:115-34.
13. Hurst AK, Iseri KT, Gill MA et al. Comparison of four methods for predicting serum gentamicin concentrations in surgical patients with perforated or gangrenous appendicitis. *Clin Pharm.* 1987; 6:234-8.
14. Rhodes PJ, Rhodes RS, McClelland GH et al. Evaluation of eight methods for estimating creatinine clearance in men. *Clin Pharm.* 1987; 6:399-406.
15. Sheiner LB, Beal SL. Some suggestions for measuring predictive performance. *J Pharmacokinet Biopharm.* 1981; 9:503-12.
16. Dixon WJ, Brown MB, Engelman L et al., eds. BMDP statistical software program. Berkeley: University of California Press; 1988.
17. Luke DR, Halstenson CE, Opsahl JA et al. Validity of creatinine clearance estimates in the assessment of renal function. *Clin Pharmacol Ther.* 1990; 48:503-8.
18. Durakovic Z. Creatinine clearance in the elderly: a comparison of direct measurement and calculation from serum creatinine. *Nephron.* 1986; 44:66-9.

Effect of flurbiprofen and aspirin on platelet aggregation

KELLY T. PINCUS, WILLIAM J. SPRUILL, AND ROY C. PARISH

Clin Pharm. 1991; 10:935-8

Aspirin's effect as an irreversible inhibitor of platelet aggregation is well established.[1-3] The drug is given to patients with recurrent transient ischemic attacks and is used to prevent myocardial infarction in patients with previous infarction or unstable angina.[4-7] Aspirin's effectiveness in the primary prevention of adverse cardiovascular events has also been documented.[8,9]

The effects of nonsteroidal anti-inflammatory agents (NSAIAs) on platelet aggregation have been studied, and although results have been difficult to compare, conclusions from these investigations have been similar.[10-14] (In this article, aspirin is not considered an NSAIA.) NSAIAs appear to inhibit the enzyme cyclo-oxygenase, but the ability of an NSAIA to inhibit platelet aggregation appears to diminish as the plasma drug concentration decreases[15,16]; hence, inhibition is considered reversible. This reversibility is in direct contrast to aspirin's ability to inhibit platelet aggregation for the life of the platelet.

Data about the inhibition of platelet aggregation by the concurrent use of aspirin and an NSAIA in humans are minimal. Two studies performed in the early 1980s suggested a need to consider the timing of aspirin and NSAIA administration when the drugs are used in the same patient.[17,18] These studies, which indicated that the irreversible action of aspirin on platelet aggregation is blocked when the NSAIA is given 30–90 minutes before aspirin, suggest that the NSAIA and aspirin may be acting on the same enzyme site. The clinical relevance of these findings has not been established.

We studied (1) the in vitro ability of aspirin and the NSAIA flurbiprofen to inhibit platelet aggregation when added to plasma separately or together and (2) the in vivo ability of the two drugs to inhibit platelet aggregation when given separately, when given together, or when flurbiprofen is given one hour before aspirin.

KELLY T. PINCUS, PHARM.D., is Assistant Professor, School of Pharmacy and Allied Health Professions, Creighton University, Omaha, NE; at the time of this study she was Pharmacy Practice Fellow, University of Georgia, Athens. WILLIAM J. SPRUILL, PHARM.D., is Associate Professor, Pharmacy Practice, and ROY C. PARISH, PHARM.D., is Assistant Professor, Pharmacy Practice, College of Pharmacy, University of Georgia.

Address reprint requests to Dr. Pincus at the School of Pharmacy and Allied Health Professions, Creighton University, California at 24th Street, Omaha, NE 68178.

Supported by a grant from The Upjohn Company Pharmacy Sciences Liaison.

Presented at the 25th Annual ASHP Midyear Clinical Meeting, Las Vegas, NV, December 6, 1990.

Table 1.
Characteristics of Study Subjects

Age (yr)	Sex	Weight (lb)	Platelets/cu mm[a]
In Vitro Study			
27	M	160	369,000
In Vivo Study			
22	M	195	281,000
25	F	125	321,000
26	F	120	400,000
24	F	175	359,000
23	F	180	372,000
39	M	165	231,000

[a] Measured in platelet-rich plasma (normal = 200,000–400,000 cells/cu mm).[19]

Methods. *Subjects.* One nonsmoking adult volunteer was recruited for the in vitro study, and six more were recruited for the in vivo study (Table 1). No volunteer was pregnant or nursing or had a history of bleeding or clotting disorders, stroke, myocardial infarction, peptic ulcer disease, or allergy or adverse reactions to aspirin, flurbiprofen, or another NSAIA. Subjects were instructed not to take an aspirin-containing product within 10 days of study commencement or an NSAIA-containing product within 3 days of study commencement. Subjects were also instructed to avoid sulfinpyrazone and dipyridamole and to abstain from alcohol consumption for at least 24 hours before taking a study drug. The study was approved by the university's institutional review board, and all subjects gave written informed consent.

Turbidometric Determination of Platelet Aggregation. Platelet aggregation was studied by the turbidometric method described by Born.[19] In this method, light transmission through platelet-rich plasma is measured spectrophotometrically. Platelet-rich plasma is turbid because of the presence of platelets, which absorb light. When an agent that causes platelet aggregation is added to platelet-rich plasma, the platelets aggregate, turbidity decreases, and light transmission increases.

In this procedure, the aggregometer is calibrated, for each subject and each measurement, with the subject's platelet-rich plasma (with which the 0% light-transmission reading is set) and platelet-poor plasma (with which the 100% light-transmission reading is set). The aggregometer uses a magnetic stirrer to mix at 1000 rpm the sample of platelet-rich plasma whose platelet aggregation is to be measured. The temperature of the optical chamber containing the sample is maintained at 37 °C.

An aggregating agent (e.g., collagen, epinephrine, adenosine diphosphate [ADP]) is then added to the platelet-rich plasma. The resultant increase in light transmission, recorded as percentage of platelet aggregation (i.e., the percentage of all platelets that are aggregating), is plotted continuously over 10 minutes, and the maximum value reached during this time is recorded on the plotter.

Preparation of Plasma. Platelet-rich and platelet-poor plasma were freshly prepared after blood collection and were used within three hours. Blood was drawn from the antecubital vein into siliconized glass tubes containing the anticoagulant sodium citrate such that the final ratio of blood to anticoagulant was 9:1. The sample was then centrifuged at 100 *g* for 13 minutes at room temperature, and the platelet-rich plasma was removed and set aside. The remainder of the sample was then centrifuged at 1800 *g* for 13 minutes at room temperature, after which the platelet-poor plasma was removed. Platelet-rich and platelet-poor plasma were placed in labeled plastic containers and covered. A platelet count was performed on the platelet-rich plasma of each subject to determine that it was within normal limits[20] (Table 1).

In Vitro Study. An initial in vitro study was performed to compare the ability of therapeutic concentrations of aspirin (9 μg/mL) and flurbiprofen (3 and 8 μg/mL) to inhibit platelet aggregation.[21,22] Aspirin (Sigma Chemical Co., St. Louis, MO, lot 28F0878) and flurbiprofen (Sigma, lot 18F0913) were added to platelet-rich plasma from the volunteer recruited for the in vitro study. The plasma–drug mixtures were incubated for 12 minutes before the aggregating agent, ADP, was added. The ADP (Helena Laboratories, Beaumont, TX, lot 200767) was initially diluted with distilled water to a concentration of 100 μmol/mL. A 0.05-mL portion of the ADP solution was then added to 0.45 mL of platelet-rich plasma–drug mixture in the sample well; the final ADP concentration was 10 μmol/mL. Maximum percentage of platelet aggregation was determined in duplicate with an aggregometer and recorder (Monitor IV, Helena Laboratories).

In Vivo Study. After fasting for 8 hours, each volunteer recruited for the in vivo study took flurbiprofen 100 mg (Ansaid, Upjohn, lot 811dc) orally with a small amount of water and was allowed to eat a nonfatty meal 30 minutes later. Blood samples were collected immediately before and 2, 8, and 24 hours after drug administration, and platelet aggregation was measured for each subject and study time as described above (without the 12-minute incubation). After a five-day washout period, the procedure was repeated with the volunteers taking aspirin 325 mg (Bayer, lot 9c742) by mouth. After a nine-day washout period, the subjects were randomized such that three took flurbiprofen 100 mg and aspirin 325 mg at the same time, while the other three took flurbiprofen 100 mg and then aspirin 325 mg one hour later. Blood samples were collected immediately before and 2, 8, and 24 hours after aspirin was taken, and platelet aggregation was again measured.

Statistical Analysis. Differences among the in vivo treatments were evaluated with two-way analysis of variance with repeated measures (Abstat software, release 6, Anderson-Bell Co., Parker, CO). The a priori level of significance was <0.05.

Table 2.
In Vitro Effect of Flurbiprofen and Aspirin on Platelet Aggregation

Drug	Plasma Drug Concentration (μg/mL)	% Maximum Platelet Aggregation[a] Trial 1	Trial 2
None	. . .	92.1	92.9
Flurbiprofen	3	61.3	54.3
Flurbiprofen	8	60.4	55.4
Aspirin	9	62.6	49.9
Flurbiprofen, aspirin	8, 9	64.0	58.0

[a] Highest values recorded during the 10 minutes after the aggregating agent (adenosine diphosphate [ADP]) was added to platelet-rich plasma. Drug-containing plasma was incubated for 12 minutes before ADP was added. Low values suggest drug-induced inhibition of platelet aggregation.

Results. *In Vitro Study.* There was comparable inhibition of platelet aggregation in plasma samples containing aspirin, flurbiprofen, and both (Table 2).

In Vivo Study. There was no difference in inhibition of platelet aggregation among the treatments (aspirin alone, flurbiprofen alone, and aspirin plus flurbiprofen [either together or one hour apart]) (Table 3). In three subjects, blood was collected 48 hours after flurbiprofen was given alone; although inhibition of platelet aggregation was evident (i.e., the maximum percentage of platelet aggregation was less than the baseline [time 0] value) at 24 hours for these subjects, inhibition had returned or was returning to baseline at 48 hours. No subjects reported drug-related adverse effects.

Discussion. The inhibitory effects of aspirin on platelet aggregation were discovered more than 20 years ago.[3] Aspirin inhibits the platelet aggregation ordinarily triggered by arachidonic acid, collagen, and ADP. By acetylating cyclo-oxygenase, aspirin inhibits prostaglandin synthesis; this, in turn, inhibits the synthesis of thromboxane A_2, a substance vital for platelet aggregation. Aspirin inhibits aggregation for the platelets' eight- or nine-day life span because aspirin-exposed platelets cannot synthesize new cyclo-oxygenase.[1,15,16]

NSAIAs, as a group, also inhibit cyclo-oxygenase, but this effect is reversible because NSAIA-exposed platelets can recover their ability to produce cyclo-oxygenase; this recovery ability appears to be inversely related to the plasma NSAIA concentration.[15,16] Exactly how NSAIAs inhibit cyclo-oxygenase is not clearly understood.[1,21]

We designed this study, in part, to evaluate flurbiprofen's reversible inhibitory effect on platelet aggregation when the drug was given alone or an hour before aspirin. Previous studies have suggested that inhibition should be apparent as long as an appropriate plasma NSAIA concentration is present.[10-14] Al-

Table 3.
Platelet Aggregation in Subjects Given Flurbiprofen and Aspirin[a]

	Mean ± S.D. % Decrease in Maximum % Platelet Aggregation (MPPA)				
Time (hr)	Flurbiprofen Alone (*n* = 6)	Aspirin Alone (*n* = 6)	All Flurbiprofen with Aspirin (*n* = 6)	Flurbiprofen and Aspirin Together (*n* = 3)	Flurbiprofen before Aspirin (*n* = 3)
2	14.2 ± 7.8	17.5 ± 7.9	17.1 ± 13.5	6.6 ± 6.4	27.6 ± 9.2
8	17.9 ± 4.6	20.9 ± 9.6	20.7 ± 6.3	17.0 ± 4.6	24.5 ± 5.8
24	12.5 ± 24.3	15.9 ± 17.1	11.7 ± 11.0	8.9 ± 11.3	14.5 ± 12.36

[a] Plasma samples were obtained 2, 8, and 24 hours after drug administration. For each sample, the aggregometer determined the MPPA that occurred during the 10 minutes after adenosine diphosphate (ADP) was added. Table values represent percentage decreases in MPPA compared with the MPPA in plasma collected immediately before drug administration. Mean ± S.D. MPPA for samples collected before drug administration were as follows: flurbiprofen alone, 90.3 ± 5.8%; aspirin alone, 92.8 ± 9.2%; all flurbiprofen with aspirin, 93.3 ± 11.2%; flurbiprofen and aspirin together, 94.4 ± 12.9%; flurbiprofen before aspirin, 92.2 ± 11.9%. Because there was no significant difference between the treatment that used flurbiprofen and aspirin together and the treatment that used flurbiprofen before aspirin, these two treatments (each with *n* = 3) were combined for statistical comparison with the other two treatments. There was no statistical difference among treatments (flurbiprofen alone, aspirin alone, and all flurbiprofen with aspirin). Doses were flurbiprofen 100 mg and aspirin 325 mg by mouth.

though we did not measure actual plasma drug concentrations, we did use "therapeutic" doses of drugs (aspirin 325 mg and flurbiprofen 100 mg). Flurbiprofen doses as low as 4–10 mg have been reported to have platelet inhibitory properties.[23] We showed that the inhibitory effects of aspirin and flurbiprofen on platelet aggregation are similar.

If aspirin's effect on platelet aggregation accounts for the drug's benefit in cardiovascular disease, then further studies should investigate the effects of regular flurbiprofen administration (e.g., every eight hours) on platelet aggregation. If flurbiprofen's effects are maintained with multiple dosing, then the drug may prove to be an appropriate alternative to aspirin in aspirin-intolerant patients.

Another issue raised in our study is whether a patient who is taking flurbiprofen needs to take aspirin for the latter drug's antiplatelet effect. We found no difference among treatments in inhibition of platelet aggregation over 24 hours. In contrast, Rao et al.[18] showed that platelet aggregation returned or was returning to baseline values 24 hours after administration of ibuprofen alone or ibuprofen plus aspirin (90 minutes apart), whereas inhibition of aggregation continued 24 hours after administration of aspirin alone. These findings suggested that NSAIAs, such as ibuprofen, decrease the inhibitory effect of aspirin. The differences between our results and those of Rao et al. may stem from our crossover design and our use of flurbiprofen rather than ibuprofen.

Finally, we attempted to determine if platelet effects differed between patients taking flurbiprofen and aspirin together and those taking flurbiprofen an hour before aspirin. We found no differences, but there was no crossover for this portion of the study, and the sample size (three in each group) was small. This research question needs to be re-evaluated in a separate, larger study.

The use of aspirin for the primary and secondary prevention of cardiovascular and cerebrovascular disease is increasing. In addition, aspirin and NSAIAs are widely available to the public. Thus, it is important that clinicians gain a more complete understanding of the use of aspirin and of drugs considered similar to aspirin. This understanding should include a knowledge of the effect of aspirin and NSAIAs, when taken separately or together, on platelet function.

Conclusion. Aspirin, flurbiprofen, and an aspirin–flurbiprofen combination inhibited platelet aggregation to a similar degree in an in vitro and an in vivo investigation.

References

1. Reilly IAG, FitzGerald GA. Aspirin in cardiovascular disease. *Drugs*. 1988; 35:154-76.
2. Miller KP, Frishman WH. Platelets and antiplatelet therapy in ischemic heart disease. *Med Clin North Am*. 1988; 72:117-84.
3. O'Brien JR. Effects of salicylates on human platelets. *Lancet*. 1968; 1:779-83.
4. Boston Collaborative Drug Surveillance Group. Regular aspirin intake and acute myocardial infarction. *Br Med J*. 1974; 1:440-3.
5. Lewis HD, Davis JW, Archibald DG et al. Protective effects of aspirin against acute myocardial infarction and death in men with unstable angina. *N Engl J Med*. 1983; 309:396-403.
6. UK-TIA Study Group. United Kingdom transient ischaemic attack (UK-TIA) aspirin trial: interim results. *Br Med J*. 1988; 296:316-20.
7. Antiplatelet Trialists' collaboration. Secondary prevention of vascular disease by prolonged antiplatelet treatment. *Br Med J*. 1988; 296:320-31.
8. Peto R, Gray R, Collins R et al. Randomised trial of prophylactic daily aspirin in British male doctors. *Br Med J*. 1988; 296:313-6.
9. The Steering Committee of the Physicians' Health Study Research Group. Preliminary report: findings from the aspirin component of the ongoing physicians' health study. *N Engl J Med*. 1988; 318:262-4.
10. Rane A, Oelz O, Frolich JC et al. Relation between plasma concentration of indomethacin and its effect on prostaglandin synthesis and platelet aggregation in man. *Clin Pharmacol Ther*. 1987; 23:658-68.
11. Cockbill SR, Heptinstall S, Taylor PM. A comparison of the abilities of acetylsalicylic acid, flurbiprofen and indomethacin to inhibit the release reaction and prostaglandin synthesis in human blood platelets. *Br J Pharmacol*. 1979; 67:73-8.
12. Green D, Davies RO, Holmes GI et al. Effects of diflunisal on platelet function and fecal blood loss. *Clin Pharmacol Ther*.

1981; 30:378-84.
13. McIntyre BA, Philip RB, Inwood MJ. Effect of ibuprofen platelet function in normal subjects and hemophiliac patients. *Clin Pharmacol Ther.* 1978; 24:616-21.
14. Thebault JJ, Lagrue G, Blatrix CE et al. Clinical pharmacology of flurbiprofen: a novel inhibitor of platelet aggregation. *Curr Med Res Opin.* 1977; 5:130-4.
15. Peplow PV. Properties and action of non-steroidal antiinflammatory drugs, including their effects on prostaglandin and macromolecular biosynthesis. *Prostaglandins Leukot Essent Fatty Acids.* 1988; 33:239-52.
16. Patrono C, Ciabattoni G, Patrignani P et al. Clinical pharmacology of platelet cyclooxygenase inhibition. *Circulation.* 1985; 72:1177-84.
17. Livio M, Del Maschio A, Cerletti C et al. Indomethacin prevents the long-lasting inhibitory effect of aspirin on human platelet cyclo-oxygenase activity. *Prostaglandins.* 1982; 23:787-96.
18. Rao GH, Johnson GG, Reddy KR et al. Ibuprofen protects platelet cyclooxygenase from irreversible inhibition by aspirin. *Arteriosclerosis.* 1983; 3:383-8.
19. Born GV. Aggregation of blood platelets by adenosine diphosphate and its reversal. *Nature.* 1962; 4832:927-9.
20. Williams CE, Entwistle MB, Short PE. Platelet function tests: a critical review of methods. *Med Lab Sci.* 1985; 42:262-74.
21. Metz SA. Anti-inflammatory agents as inhibitors of prostaglandin synthesis in man. *Med Clin North Am.* 1981; 65:713-57.
22. Kaiser DG, Brooks CD, Lomen PL. Pharmacokinetics of flurbiprofen. *Am J Med.* 1986; 80(Suppl 3A):10-5.
23. Marsh CC, Schuna AA, Sundstrom WR. A review of selected investigational nonsteroidal antiinflammatory drugs of the 1980s. *Pharmacotherapy.* 1986; 6:10-25.

Effect of use of generic thioridazine products on clinical outcome and quality of life

ELENA BABLENIS, STANLEY S. WEBER, AND ROBERT L. DUFRESNE

Clin Pharm. 1991; 10:938-41

The availability of generic drugs often forces the pharmacist to face a dilemma. Generic products can reduce the pharmacy inventory budget, but some generic products may be associated with a need for more dosage adjustments, more physician visits, and rehospitalization.[1-7] These unfavorable outcomes may affect the cost of health care but are not usually included when the cost of a drug product is considered.

Some generic thioridazine products carry FDA's "AB" designation, which is applied to products that may not be bioequivalent to the innovator product but are considered therapeutically equivalent to the innovator product.[8-10] Case reports suggest that there may not be therapeutic equivalence among thioridazine products. Browning[11] described a patient who became increasingly agitated and uncontrollable one to two days after her brand of thioridazine was changed. The patient returned to her previous state after treatment with the original brand was reinstituted. Weber and Wagner[12] described two patients who had their brand of thioridazine changed. One patient became uncontrollable, and the other had new complaints of drowsiness. Both patients improved after treatment with another brand of thioridazine was started.

Alterations in behavior, in adverse effects, and in general clinical state may follow a change in the brand of thioridazine dispensed[13]; these alterations may be due to differences in bioavailability. The complexity of psychiatric illnesses sometimes makes it difficult to assess signs of therapeutic failure. When drug failures occur, patients may be unable or unwilling to allow their clinicians to make the appropriate clinical determinations. On the other hand, the clinician may misinterpret a patient's true report of symptoms as a manifestation of disease when the patient is really reporting the relative lack of effect of a generic drug.

Besides alterations in clinical response, changing the brand of thioridazine dispensed may cause other problems. Because not all tablet strengths are available in all brands, some patients might be required to take two different brands of the drug at the same time; this circumstance could lead to confusion and noncompliance. In addition, a patient might be reluctant to take a medication that does not look like what he or she was taking previously.

A deterioration in clinical condition that is caused by changing brands of an antipsychotic drug may lead to increased contact with mental health professionals and, consequently, an increase in the cost of health care. The intent of this study was to determine the effect of changing from Mellaril (Sandoz), the innovator product, to generic thioridazine products on indicators of clinical outcomes and quality of life. If changing products was found to affect these indicators, then we planned to examine whether health-care costs changed as well.

Methods. *Experimental Design.* Indicators of clinical outcome and quality of life were retrospectively as-

ELENA BABLENIS, PHARM.D., was, at the time of this study, Fellow in Psychiatric Pharmacotherapy, Institute of Mental Health, Cranston, RI. STANLEY S. WEBER, PHARM.D., is Associate Professor of Pharmacy, College of Pharmacy, University of Rhode Island, Kingston, and Clinical Pharmacist, Pharmacy Services, Department of Mental Health, Retardation, and Hospitals, Cranston, RI. ROBERT L. DUFRESNE, PH.D., is Assistant Professor of Pharmacy, College of Pharmacy, University of Rhode Island, and Clinical Pharmacist, Mental Health Services of Cranston, Johnston, and Northwestern Rhode Island, Johnston, RI.

Address reprint requests to Dr. Weber at the College of Pharmacy, University of Rhode Island, Kingston, RI 02881.

The assistance of Richard L. Wagner, M.D., Director of the Rhode Island Psychiatric Research and Training Center, and of Louis G. Roy, M.S., Chief of Pharmacy Services at the Rhode Island Department of Mental Health, Retardation, and Hospitals, is acknowledged.

Funded by the ASHP Research and Education Foundation Fellowship of Dr. Bablenis.

Presented at the 23rd Annual ASHP Midyear Clinical Meeting, Dallas, TX, December 6, 1988.

sessed in two groups of patients—one group whose brand of thioridazine had been changed and another group whose antipsychotic regimen, which did not include thioridazine, did not undergo a brand change. The study was approved by the appropriate institutional review board.

Potential subjects were identified from a list of patients who had used a pharmacy that filled prescriptions for a local community mental health center. This list included all patients who had had their mental health center prescriptions filled during a two-month period when that pharmacy started to dispense generic thioridazine products (Barr or Bolar) instead of Mellaril. Data supplied by the pharmacy included patients' names, dates of prescription filling, dosage, dates of original prescriptions, amounts of medication dispensed, prescribers' names, and numbers of refills. This information and knowledge of when the pharmacy started to dispense generic thioridazine products allowed us to determine, for any patient, when the brand change occurred and how long the various brands were used.

The thioridazine group consisted of all listed patients who had received Mellaril for at least one year and then received a generic brand for another year. The comparison group consisted of patients who had received an antipsychotic drug other than thioridazine whose regimen did not involve a brand change within the past year.

One investigator reviewed the mental health center medical records of all study patients for indicators of clinical outcome and quality of life. The investigator knew none of the patients and did not receive information personally from members of the mental health center staff. For the thioridazine group, medical records for one year preceding and following the generic change were reviewed for indicators of both clinical outcome and quality of life. For the comparison group, the medical records for one year (six months before and six months after the pharmacy started dispensing generic thioridazine) were reviewed for indicators of clinical outcome. Records for that and the preceding year were reviewed for the quality-of-life evaluation. Sources of information from the medical record included nurses' notes, physicians' notes, case managers' notes, emergency-service forms, and notes from staff members working in the day or vocational program. The investigator evaluated the medical records of the thioridazine group before examining those of the comparison group.

Outcome Indicators. Indicators of clinical outcome were the number of scheduled and unscheduled contacts with the mental health center, scheduled and unscheduled home visits by mental health center personnel, hospitalizations, and unkept appointments (Table 1). Quality of life was rated on a scale that considers the frequency of social contacts, the percentage of time employed, and the amount of time spent in the hospital (Table 2).[14-18]

Statistical Analysis. Monthly changes in thioridazine dosages were evaluated by analysis of variance with repeated measures. Student's *t* test for matched pairs and Hotelling's T^2 were used to analyze differences in the indicators of clinical response (1) between the thioridazine and comparison groups and (2) before and after the generic product in the thioridazine group. Quality-of-life data were evaluated by using Bowker's extension of McNemar's test of asymmetry.[19] Comparisons for which McNemar's test showed a *p* value of <0.05 were followed by tests for category changes. The a priori level of significance was ≤0.05.

Table 1.
Effect of Thioridazine Brand Change on Indicators of Clinical Response[a]

Indicator	Mean ± S.D. No. Occurrences (n = 34) Year before Brand Change	Year after Brand Change
Scheduled MHC contacts		
With nurse	9.6 ± 12.8	8.2 ± 10.1
With physician	3.7 ± 4.5	3.1 ± 4.5
With case manager	2.3 ± 6.1	2.0 ± 4.2
Unscheduled MHC contacts		
With nurse	0.4 ± 0.9	0.9 ± 2.0
With physician	0.2 ± 0.5	0.2 ± 0.6
With case manager	0.3 ± 0.9	0.2 ± 1.0
With emergency services	1.2 ± 3.8	1.2 ± 4.3
Scheduled home visits by MHC staff	1.1 ± 3.9	1.1 ± 2.9
Unscheduled home visits by MHC staff	0.2 ± 0.6	0.2 ± 0.5
Hospitalizations	0.1 ± 0.3	0.3 ± 0.7
Unkept appointments	0.4 ± 1.5	0.4 ± 1.0

[a] MHC = mental health center.

Results. Of the 134 patients identified as taking thioridazine, 34 (16 men, 18 women) met the inclusion criteria for the thioridazine group. Of the remaining 100 patients, medical records were unavailable for 5, and 95 had not taken Mellaril for an entire year. The alterations in antipsychotic medication regimens in the thioridazine group that occurred after the generic change are shown in Table 3. The comparison group included 62 patients (41 men, 21 women); 38 other patients were excluded because a change to a generic product had occurred in their drug regimen in the past year. The antipsychotic medications taken by the comparison group are shown in Table 4.

The thioridazine group had no significant change in clinical indicators after the transition to generic thioridazine (Table 1). In addition, there was no significant difference in clinical indicators between the comparison and thioridazine groups (either before or after the brand change in the latter group). There was no month-to-month difference in thioridazine dosage when Mellaril was compared with generic thioridazine. The mean ± S.D. daily dosage of thioridazine hydrochloride was 193 ± 143 mg for Mellaril and 185 ± 150 mg for the Barr and Bolar products.

The quality-of-life assessment showed no difference

Table 2.
Effect of Thioridazine Brand Change on Quality-of-Life Ratings[a]

Indicator	% Patients with Indicated Score[b]									
	First Year					Second Year				
	0	1	2	3	4	0	1	2	3	4
Thioridazine Group (*n* = 33–34)										
Duration of hospitalization	0	0	0	15	85	3	3	3	9	81
Frequency of social contacts[c]	0	0	18	29	53	0	6	33	42	18
Employment[d]	70		18		12	94		3		3
Comparison Group (*n* = 62)										
Duration of hospitalization	2	0	0	3	95	0	2	0	10	89
Frequency of social contacts	0	2	15	20	64	0	2	11	23	64
Employment	82		13		5	81		16		3

[a] Patients in the thioridazine group took Mellaril during the first year and a generic thioridazine product during the second year. Patients in the comparison group took antipsychotic drugs other than thioridazine. For these patients, the first year was the period 6 to 18 months before generic thioridazine began being used in the thioridazine group. The second year for the comparison group was the period ranging from six months before to six months after generic thioridazine began being used in the thioridazine group.

[b] Scores for duration of hospitalization in the past year: 0 = more than three months, 1 = two to three months, 2 = one to two months, 3 = up to one month, 4 = not hospitalized. Scores for frequency of social contacts (do not include contacts with nurses, physicians, or case managers): 0 = did not meet with friends under any conditions, 1 = met with friends only at work or school, 2 = met with friends about once a month, 3 = met with friends about once every two weeks, 4 = met with friends on average of at least once a week. Scores for employment status in the past year: 0 = unemployed, 2 = employed part-time (5–34 hr/wk) continuously or full-time (≥35 hr/wk) about half of the year, 4 = employed full-time continuously. Scale based on references 14–18.

[c] Significant difference between years (Bowker's extension of McNemar's test of asymmetry, $\chi^2 = 18$, d.f. = 6, $p < 0.01$).

[d] Significant difference between years ($\chi^2 = 18$, d.f. =6, $p < 0.05$).

Table 3.
Changes in Psychotropic Drug Regimen in Year after Brand Change in Patients Taking Thioridazine (*n* = 34)

No. Patients	Drugs Added	Drugs Discontinued
21	None	None
2	None	Lithium
1	Nortriptyline	Trazodone, desipramine
1	Amantadine, molindone	None
1	None	Diazepam
1	Trazodone, tryptophan	Benztropine, fluphenazine
1	Flurazepam, lorazepam, clorazepate	None
1	Diphenhydramine	None
1	Diazepam	None
1	Lorazepam	Amitriptyline
1	Chlorpromazine	None
1	Buspirone, diazepam	None
1	None	Fluphenazine

Table 4.
Antipsychotic Medications Taken by Comparison Group (*n* = 62)

No. Patients	Drug
32	Fluphenazine
6	Perphenazine
5	Haloperidol
5	Thiothixene
5	Fluphenazine and haloperidol
4	Trifluoperazine
2	Molindone
2	Fluphenazine and trifluoperazine
1	Fluphenazine and thiothixene

in the thioridazine group in the duration of hospitalization before and after the generic change (Table 2). (Second-year quality-of-life data were incomplete for one patient.) However, unemployment increased and the frequency of social contacts decreased significantly. Most of the change in employment was accounted for by six patients who had previously been partly employed and became fully unemployed. The change in social contacts was mostly accounted for by (1) nine patients who had met with friends at least once a week and decreased that frequency to once every two weeks and (2) four patients who had met with friends once a month and later limited contacts only to those with school or work acquaintances. No patient in the thioridazine group improved in employment or social contacts after the generic change.

There were no significant quality-of-life changes in the comparison group.

Discussion. The cost of medication is not simply the amount spent by a patient for a prescription. Other factors must be considered, such as the number and length of hospitalizations and the number of clinic visits. Any change in medication that changes the patient's clinical condition could affect these factors. Patients who experience clinical deterioration tend to require more health care services than those who are doing well. We intended to determine what impact brand change of thioridazine had on measures of clinical outcome. Because we did not detect changes in most measures, we did not proceed with a cost analysis.

Although there were no changes in the use of mental health resources after the brand shift, unemployment increased and social contacts decreased. These changes may not be directly reflected in the cost of health care, but there is a cost to society for an unemployed person. The changes may have resulted from a general worsening of clinical state after the product change. Patients in the comparison group did not experience an overall change in quality-of-life measures. Thus, the changes among the thioridazine group may have been caused by the change in thioridazine brand and not by the nature of the patients' illness.

Our study was not designed to detect early and transient clinical deterioration. It is possible that patients whose brand of thioridazine is changed may experience an initial worsening of symptoms that could be a consequence of a change in health care or a lack of bioequivalence in the newly used product. Such patients may return to their baseline state once they adjust to the change in products. Counseling by pharmacists who change the brand of medication may prevent some initial untoward reactions.

Although there may be a subset of patients whose quality of life is worsened by a brand change, we found that most patients had no such adverse effect. We were unable to detect changes in psychopathology that were too small to cause hospitalization or intervention by a health-care professional. Prospective, controlled studies with large samples are necessary to more closely examine whether brand change causes differences in clinical outcome and quality of life.

Conclusion. Change from the innovator product Mellaril to a generic thioridazine product did not affect indicators of clinical outcome but was associated with more unemployment and less social contact.

References

1. Barone JA, Colaizzi JL. Critical evaluation of thioridazine bioequivalence. *Drug Intell Clin Pharm.* 1985; 19:847-58.
2. Meyer HM Jr. Comment: thioridazine bioequivalence. *Drug Intell Clin Pharm.* 1986; 20:311. Letter.
3. Barone JA, Colaizzi JL. Author's reply: thioridazine bioequivalence. *Drug Intell Clin Pharm.* 1986; 20:312. Letter.
4. Barone JA, Byerly WG. Determination of bioequivalence of psychotropic drugs and concerns involving product interchange. *J Clin Psychiatry.* 1986; 47(Suppl):28-32.
5. Gottschalk LA. Clinical relevance of the bioavailability/bioequivalence controversy. *J Clin Psychiatry.* 1986; 47(Suppl):3-5.
6. Greenblatt DJ, Shader RI. Bioequivalence of generic drugs in clinical psychopharmacology. *J Clin Psychopharmacol.* 1987; 7:A21-3.
7. Seligman M. Generic substitution. *Biol Ther Psychiatry.* 1987; 10:17, 21-2.
8. USP Dispensing Information Volume III. Approved Drug Products and Legal Requirements. 9th ed. Rockville, Maryland: The United States Pharmacopeial Convention, Inc.; 1989.
9. Hammell MR, Martinez MN, Dighe S et al. Bioequivalence of generic thioridazine drug products. The FDA viewpoint. *Drug Intell Clin Pharm.* 1987; 21:362-9.
10. Barone JA, Colaizzi JL. Thioridazine bioequivalence—author's response. *Drug Intell Clin Pharm.* 1987; 21:369-72.
11. Browning G. Generic thioridazine failure. *Drug Intell Clin Pharm.* 1984; 18:738-9. Letter.
12. Weber SS, Wagner RL. Behavioral changes following generic thioridazine. *J Clin Psychiatry.* 1986; 47:277-8. Letter.
13. Chien CP. Bioequivalence of generic psychotropic drugs. *Integr Psychiatry.* 1985; 3:S58-62.
14. Wykes T, Sturt E. The measurement of social behavior in psychiatric patients: an assessment of the reliability and validity of the SBS schedule. *Br J Psychiatry.* 1986; 148:1-11.
15. Malm U, May PRA, Dencke SJ. Evaluation of the quality of life scale of the schizophrenic outpatient. *Schizoph Bull.* 1981; 7:477-87.
16. Strauss JS, Carpenter WT. The prediction outcome in schizophrenia. *Arch Gen Psychiatry.* 1974; 31:37-42.
17. Hawk AB, Carpenter WT, Strauss JS. Diagnostic criteria and five-year outcome in schizophrenia. *Arch Gen Psychiatry.* 1975; 32:343-7.
18. Strauss JS, Carpenter WT. The prediction outcome in schizophrenia. *Arch Gen Psychiatry.* 1972; 27:739-46.
19. Marascuilo LA, McSweeney M. Nonparametric and distribution-free methods for the social sciences. Monterey, CA: Brooks Cole Publishing Co. Inc.; 1977.

The Measles Epidemic

The nation has experienced a marked increase in measles cases during 1989 and 1990. Almost one half of all cases have occurred in unvaccinated preschool children, mostly minorities. The principal cause for the epidemic is failure to provide vaccine to vulnerable children on schedule. Major reasons for the low vaccine coverage exist within the health care system itself, which creates barriers to obtaining immunization and fails to take advantage of many opportunities to provide vaccines to children. . . . Essential changes can and should be made now. Specific recommendations include improved availability of immunization; improved management of immunization services; improved capacity to measure childhood immunization status; implementation of the two-dose measles vaccine strategy; and laboratory, epidemiologic, and operational studies to further define determinants of decreased vaccine coverage and to develop new combinations of vaccines that can be administered earlier in life. The measles epidemic may be a warning flag of problems with our system of primary health care.

—The National Vaccine Advisory Committee. The measles epidemic: the problems, barriers, and recommendations. *JAMA.* 1991; 266:1547-52.

Editorial

Succimer: Controversial issues involving the release of a new product

This issue of *Clinical Pharmacy* introduces a new therapeutic agent, succimer, for clinical use in the United States.[1] Although this agent is new as a legitimate prescription drug, the chemical, dimercaptosuccinic acid (DMSA), has been with us for many years as an experimental and occasional therapeutic agent for a variety of heavy metal exposures. It has also been available in Europe and has achieved a reputation for safety and efficacy among toxicologists overseas. This drug represents an important step forward in the rational management of heavy metal exposures. However, the process of FDA approval of succimer was in some respects atypical and warrants comment.

Succimer has potential clinical uses in both adults and children. With the exception of agents having uses unique to children, manufacturers have historically undertaken clinical studies and sought FDA approval in the often more accessible adult population. As a result of this and other factors, 91% of therapeutic drugs listed in the *Physicians' Desk Reference* have no labeling for pediatric use.[2] In view of succimer's potential health benefits in children, it is highly laudable that this drug was approved first for pediatric use. McNeil Consumer Products Company and the FDA deserve commendation for not taking the easy route and creating another pediatric orphan.

The second issue in the approval of this drug is likely to create confusion for health-care professionals. The FDA has chosen to limit the labeled indication for this agent on the basis of a blood lead concentration greater than 45 μg/dL. There is clearly nothing that discriminates patients with blood lead concentrations of 35–45 μg/dL from those with lead concentrations of greater than 45 μg/dL. Given the vagaries of sampling and measuring lead in blood and the inherent variability in the susceptibility of the human host to lead, the decision to treat an individual child must be based on a combination of patient and exposure circumstances. While it is appropriate to discourage the indiscriminate use of chelating agents, this regulation has traditionally been undertaken by physicians and pharmacists in collaboration. The FDA is setting a disappointing and counterproductive precedent by imposing regulations that mandate "cookbook" medicine and that cannot hope to keep pace with the changes in medical knowledge regarding this subject. This restriction does a disservice to succimer and also sets an unpleasant precedent for other drugs under development. In the very close future, reimbursement for medications may be limited to labeled uses and to off-label uses for which safety and efficacy are supported by selected drug monographs. It will be increasingly important for these monographs to consider departures from labeling based on chemical measures such as blood lead concentration. This may place a more difficult burden of proof on these publications to justify departures from labeling.

1. Mann KV, Travers JD. Succimer, an oral lead chelator. *Clin Pharm*. 1991; 10:914-22.
2. Final report of the Advisory Committee on the Food and Drug Administration, U.S. Department of Health and Human Services, May 1991.

William Banner, Jr., M.D., Ph.D.
Associate Professor of Pediatrics
Department of Pediatrics
The University of Utah
Salt Lake City, UT 84113

Commentary

Which lipid-lowering agent should be used first?

DAVID R. RUTLEDGE

Clin Pharm. 1991; 10:943-5

In the mid 1980s the National Heart, Lung, and Blood Institute launched the National Cholesterol Education Program, primarily because of the encouraging results of the Coronary Primary Prevention Trial.[1] Since that time, cholesterol screening and awareness of cholesterol concentrations have increased substantially in the United States. Most pharmacists know their own total cholesterol concentration. In January 1988 the program's expert panel published its recommendations on the detection, evaluation, and treatment of high blood cholesterol concentrations in adults.[2] These guidelines are supported by the results of clinical trials showing that modest reductions in total cholesterol and low-density lipoprotein (LDL) cholesterol concentrations significantly reduce cardiovascular morbidity and mortality.[1,3-5] The outcomes of six controlled angiographic trials of total cholesterol or LDL cholesterol lowering with or without increases in high-density lipoprotein (HDL) cholesterol provide evidence that treatment alters the natural history of atherosclerotic lesions.[6-11] Progression of lesions can be slowed, and existing lesions can regress.

These recommendations on lowering cholesterol have affected millions of Americans, and millions of dollars have been spent to carry out the recommendations that, in retrospect, have saved thousands of lives. But which cholesterol-lowering agent should we really be using as first-line therapy? The expert panel recommends bile acid sequestrants and nicotinic acid as first-line drugs.[2] Are these reasonable choices?

The estimated number of prescriptions for cholesterol-lowering drugs in the United States has increased fivefold, from 2.6 million in 1983 to nearly 13 million in 1988.[12] Most of this increase was due to the use of gemfibrozil and the hydroxymethylglutaryl-coenzyme A (HMG-CoA) reductase inhibitor lovastatin, which became the most prescribed cholesterol-lowering drug after only one year of marketing. Although the expert panel classifies lovastatin as a second-line drug,[2] it is being used as a first-line agent. It is reasonable to expect the second-generation HMG-CoA reductase inhibitor pravastatin to be used frequently as well.

There are many factors to consider when choosing a lipid-lowering agent, including efficacy, adverse effects, long-term safety, and cost. For example, niacin and lovastatin have both been shown to have the lowest ratios of cost per percent reduction in LDL cholesterol concentration.[13] However, niacin and gemfibrozil have the lowest ratios of cost per percent increase in HDL cholesterol concentration.[13] Nicotinic acid in relatively high dosages causes a deterioration of glycemic control in patients with diabetes. Since such patients represent a large group being treated with cholesterol- and triglyceride-lowering agents, lovastatin and gemfibrozil are considered by many clinicians to be lipid-lowering drugs of choice. However, gemfibrozil may also be associated with unfavorable effects in patients with diabetes because of the drug's deleterious effect in elevating LDL cholesterol concentrations in hypertriglyceridemic patients. Bile acid-sequestering agents are not cost-effective compared with niacin, lovastatin, and gemfibrozil for lowering high blood cholesterol concentrations. The constraints on the health-care dollar necessitate that the cost of cholesterol-lowering drugs be assessed in relation to their effectiveness before they are recommended.

Bile acid-binding resins historically have been used very frequently. They primarily affect LDL cholesterol and therefore have been recommended for most patients with heterozygous familial hypercholesterolemia. The bile acid-sequestering agents should not be used in patients with excessive plasma concentrations of chylomicrons, very-low-density lipoproteins, or intermediate-density lipoproteins because they have been reported to increase serum triglycerides. Cholestyramine, the first of the lipid-lowering agents shown to be effective in the primary prevention of coronary events,[1] is poorly tolerated.

DAVID R. RUTLEDGE, PHARM.D., is Associate Professor, Department of Pharmacy Practice, University of Florida College of Pharmacy, Box J-486, JHMHC, Gainesville, FL 32610-0486.

Most of the decrease in cholesterol concentrations seen with probucol is due to reductions in HDL cholesterol, the so-called "good cholesterol."

Gemfibrozil, a fibric acid derivative structurally related to clofibrate, is a relatively new drug whose long-term safety remains to be established. Gemfibrozil and bezafibrate have a greater effect on lowering triglyceride concentrations than on cholesterol, but they increase HDL cholesterol. In the Helsinki Heart Study, gemfibrozil was effective in the primary prevention of coronary events.[14]

The HMG-CoA reductase inhibitors are highly effective in lowering plasma LDL concentrations and will probably emerge as drugs of first choice pending the gathering of more long-term information. The first of these drugs to be discovered was mevastatin; lovastatin followed.

The ideal combination would appear to be a fibrate compound (e.g., gemfibrozil) and an HMG-CoA reductase inhibitor (e.g., lovastatin). The combination of gemfibrozil and lovastatin would appear to do all the right things, namely, lower LDL cholesterol, raise HDL cholesterol, and lower triglycerides. However, the frequency of myopathy and rhabdomyolysis increases when these two drugs are used together,[15] so I would not recommend this combination. A number of factors increase the frequency of these adverse effects, and as our knowledge increases, they may be preventable.

Once dietary therapy has proved ineffective, drug therapy must begin in conjunction with dietary restriction. It is likely that the drug regimen will be continued for a lifetime. Therefore the pharmacist must carefully examine the clinical and lipoprotein profiles of the patient. Factors such as cost, long-term safety, efficacy, and adverse effects should all be considered. Risk factors such as smoking, hypertension, obesity, and sedentary behavior should be eliminated or controlled. If the patient has diabetes, glycemic control must be maintained.

Epidemiologic studies in this country have consistently shown that lower concentrations of HDL cholesterol are associated with higher rates of coronary-artery disease. Which agent should the pharmacist recommend if the goal is to raise these low concentrations through pharmacotherapy? Nicotinic acid and gemfibrozil are the two agents that are most effective in this case. However, there are considerable differences of opinion on whether to use these agents in patients with normal LDL cholesterol and triglyceride concentrations. If these patients have coronary-artery disease, then some experts would recommend using these agents to raise the low HDL cholesterol concentration. In my conservative opinion, until we have positive results from prospective clinical trials that provide more information on the impact of drugs that mainly increase HDL cholesterol concentrations, nicotinic acid or gemfibrozil should be used only when there is an associated elevation in LDL cholesterol or triglyceride concentrations. Studies in relatively nonindustrialized countries, such as Mexico, suggest that a low HDL cholesterol concentration may not necessarily be an important risk factor in people whose diet is very low in fat.[16]

The HMG-CoA reductase inhibitors completely inhibit an enzyme that catalyzes cholesterol formation. They represent attractive drug regimens, and many pharmaceutical companies have invested heavily in these compounds. However, to date these drugs lack proven efficacy for reducing the risk of coronary-artery disease. For example, we have little information on the ability of the HMG-CoA reductase inhibitors to slow the progression of coronary lesions or cause regression of existing lesions and thereby lower coronary-artery-disease risk. This probably is why niacin and the bile acid-sequestering agents win out and receive the expert panel's formal recommendation as first-line agents, although they are primarily being used as second-line agents. Clinical trials are under way to address whether the HMA-CoA reductase inhibitors do in fact decrease the risk of coronary-artery disease. It will be very surprising to me if the results are negative.

Should the elderly be aggressively treated? Most of the information available from clinical trials demonstrates the efficacy of lowering cholesterol concentrations in middle-aged men. Given the potential cost of this therapy and the impact it would have on the pocketbooks of the elderly, clinical trials evaluating the efficacy of lowering cholesterol in elderly patients are urgently needed.

In summary, there is a dilemma as to which lipid-lowering agent to recommend first. As with most dilemmas, it depends on how confident you are in the data, both old and new. The National Cholesterol Education Program's expert panel makes it very clear which agent to use first: bile acid sequestrants (e.g., cholestyramine and colestipol) and nicotinic acid. These agents have been shown to lower the risk of coronary-artery disease in many large-scale clinical trials, and their long-term safety has been clearly established. There is a wealth of published data supporting this recommendation. It is safe, therefore, to follow the panel's guidelines. However, many clinicians disagree and are using HMG-CoA reductase inhibitors and fibric acid derivatives, even though their effects on coronary-artery disease and long-term safety have not been established. An assessment of their short-term safety and efficacy does make these agents an attractive first choice for many patients. But to date the expert panel disagrees with using them as first-line agents. I do too.

References

1. Lipid Research Clinics Program. The Lipid Research Clinics Coronary Primary Prevention Trials results. I. Reduction in the incidence of coronary heart disease. *JAMA*. 1984; 251:351-74.
2. The Expert Panel. Report of the National Cholesterol Education Program Expert Panel on Detection, Evaluation, and Treatment of High Blood Cholesterol in Adults. *Arch Intern*

Med. 1988; 148:36-69.

3. Frick MH, Elo O, Haapa K et al. Helsinki heart study: primary-prevention trial with gemfibrozil in middle aged men with dyslipidemia. *N Engl J Med*. 1975; 233:360-81.
4. Coronary Drug Research Project Group. Clofibrate and niacin in coronary heart disease. *JAMA*. 1984; 251:365-74.
5. Canner PL, Berge KG, Wenger NK et al. Fifteen year mortality in coronary artery drug project patients: long term benefit with niacin. *J Am Coll Cardiol*. 1986; 8:1245-55.
6. Brensike JF, Levy RI, Kelsey SF et al. Effects of therapy with cholestyramine on progression of coronary arteriosclerosis: results of the NHLBI Type II Coronary Intervention Study. *Circulation*. 1984; 69:313-24.
7. Blankenhorn DH, Nessim SA, Johnson RL et al. Beneficial effects of combined colestipol–niacin therapy on coronary atherosclerosis and coronary venous bypass grafts. *JAMA*. 1987; 257:3233-40.
8. Brown G, Albers JJ, Fisher LD et al. Progression of coronary artery disease as a result of intensive lipid-lowering therapy in men with high levels of apolipoprotein B. *N Engl J Med*. 1990; 323:1289-98.
9. Buchwald H, Varco RL, Matts JP et al. Effect of partial ileal bypass surgery on mortality and morbidity from coronary heart disease on patients with hypercholesterolemia: report of the Program on the Surgical Control of the Hyperlipidemias (POSCH). *N Engl J Med*. 1990; 323:945-55.
10. Kane JP, Malloy MJ, Ports TA et al. Regression of coronary atherosclerosis during treatment of familial hypercholesterolemia with combined drug regimens. *JAMA*. 1990; 264:3007-12.
11. Cashin-Hemphill L, Mack WJ, Pogoda J et al. Beneficial effects of colestipol–niacin on coronary atherosclerosis: a 4 year follow-up. *JAMA*. 1990; 264:3013-7.
12. Wysowski DK, Kennedy KL, Gross TP. Prescribed use of cholesterol-lowering drugs in the United States, 1978 through 1988. *JAMA*. 1990; 263:2185-8.
13. Schulman KA, Kinosian B, Jacobson TA et al. Reducing high blood cholesterol level with drugs. Cost-effectiveness of pharmacologic management. *JAMA*. 1990; 264:3025-33.
14. Frick MH, Elo O, Haapa K et al. Helsinki Heart Study. Primary prevention trial with gemfibrozil in middle-aged men with dyslipidemia. *N Engl J Med*. 1987; 317:1237-45.
15. Pierce LR, Wysowski DK, Gross TP. Myopathy and rhabdomyolysis associated with lovastatin–gemfibrozil combination therapy. *JAMA*. 1990; 264:71-5.
16. Connor WE, Cerqueira MT, Connor RW. The plasma lipids, lipoproteins, and diet of Tarahumara Indians of Mexico. *Am J Clin Nutr*. 1978; 31:1131-42.

ASHP Report

Acknowledgment to reviewers—October 1, 1990, to September 30, 1991

This year, approximately 128 manuscripts were submitted for publication consideration to *Clinical Pharmacy*, including papers solicited by the editors. Approximately 45% of the papers received were ultimately accepted. During this same period, we received critiques from 153 reviewers who evaluated the merit of *Clinical Pharmacy* submissions. Readers are indebted to these reviewers, who contributed their time in this advisory capacity. Their efforts have helped maintain the high standards of *CP*. Several referees reviewed more than one paper during the year, and their extra contributions are especially appreciated.

Bruce H. Ackerman
Jan Dalke Anderson
Philip O. Anderson
William H. Asbury
Arasb Ateshkadi
Brian A. Baker
William Banner
Joseph A. Barone
Eula D. Beasley
Diane E. Beck
Richard C. Berchou
Mary C. Birmingham
Kathryn V. Blake
Robert A. Blum
Michael B. Bottorff
Eric G. Boyce
Candace S. Brown
Bobby G. Bryant
Marcia L. Buck
Kelly Joan Burch
Henry I. Bussey
John F. Calvert
Donna J. Carroll
Peggy L. Carver
Daniel T. Casto
Robert B. Catalano
Betty J. Chaffee
John F. Cormier
M. Lynn Crismon
Michelle Crisp
Clarence E. Curry
Stephen L. Dahl
Larry H. Danziger
Lisa Davis
Marshall Dewell
Joseph T. DiPiro
Roland N. Dickerson
William D. Figg
Douglas Fish
Richard J. Fleck
Courtney V. Fletcher
Cynthia Foslien-Nash
Thomas S. Foster
Peter Gal
Douglas R. Geraets
Jamie Toback Gilman
Paul J. Godley
Barry R. Goldspiel
Ann Marie Greco
Elaine R. Green
S. Diane Goodwin
B. Joseph Guglielmo
Thomas C. Hardin
Erkan Hassan
Allen R. Hauser
Thomas K. Hazlet
Michael W. Horton
Paul R. Hutson
Domenic G. Iezzoni
Robert J. Ignoffo
Timothy J. Ives
Mary Ann Jenck
Martin L. Job
Cary E. Johnson
Curtis A. Johnson
Julie A. Johnson
Paul W. Jungnickel
Thomas P. Kanyok
John M. Kessler
Ujjaini Khanderia
Julienne K. Kirk
Rachel L. Kleiman-Wexler
Wayne A. Kradjan
Donna M. Kraus
Edward P. Krenzelok
Daniel W. Krichbaum
Calvin M. Kunin
Dustan G. Labreche
Clifton R. Lacy
Victor Lampasona
Ghassem E. Larijani
Eunmee Lee
Marc Levine
Edward Liao
Celeste M. Lindley
Thomas M. Ludden
Pierre A. Maloley
Henry J. Mann
Emory S. Martin III
Marc J. Massanari
Laurie S. Mauro
Vincent F. Mauro
Mary A. McCormick
Timothy R. McGuire
Patrick J. McNamara
Donald T. Miller
Michael A. Montwill
Bruce A. Mueller
Milap C. Nahata
Jean M. Nappi
Cheryl Nunn Thompson
Mary Beth O'Connell
Julie C. Oki
Frank P. Paloucek
Robert B. Parker
Michael D. Parr
John M. Patrias
Larry Patterson
Alice K. Pau
John G. Pearson
Frederic Penn
Stephanie J. Phelps
Roy A. Pleasants
Douglas A. Powers
Randy Pryka
Mark C. Pugh
Ralph H. Raasch
Marsha A. Raebel
Robert P. Rapp
Michael D. Reed
James M. Roberts
John H. Rodman
John C. Rotschafer
Ronald J. Ruggiero
Wayne L. Russell
David R. Rutledge
Michael J. Rybak
Jan V. Sahai
William T. Sawyer
Gary Schmidt
Arthur A. Schuna
Terry L. Schwinghammer
Amy L. Shafer
Steven L. Sheaffer
William Simonson
Pamela J. Sims
Ralph E. Small
Michael S. Soares
Ruth M. Steele
Robert L. Talbert
Kathleen M. Teasley-Strausberg
James E. Tisdale
Greg S. Umstead
Earl S. Ward
Sue H. Watson
Lynda S. Welage
Andrea Wendrow
Allison Winecoff
Michael E. Winter
Roberta Wong
Sun Dong Yoo
Barbara J. Zarowitz
Karin E. Zenk

DUE Criteria

The DUE Criteria *section of* Clinical Pharmacy *features model drug-use evaluation criteria that may be employed as a component of a comprehensive quality assurance program. The criteria sets are presented in the format used in the ASHP book* Criteria for Drug Use Evaluation. *Some of the criteria sets will have been originally published in that book; others will be presented here for the first time and published in future volumes of the ASHP book. The practitioners who developed a criteria set are acknowledged.*

In selecting drug products for coverage in DUE Criteria, *priority is given to products that have been recently marketed, those that are frequently prescribed, those that have high potential risk associated with their use, and those that are expensive. When feasible, a criteria set will be linked with a Drug Review that appears in the same issue.*

These criteria sets are a starting point for the development of DUE criteria for a specific practice setting. Readers are encouraged to modify the model criteria to fit their own circumstances.

Criteria for use of sargramostim (granulocyte–macrophage colony-stimulating factor) [a]

Element	Standard 100%	Standard 0%	Exception[b] or Critical Preventive/ Responsive Measure[c]	Sources of Information
Justification for Use				
1. Acceleration of myeloid recovery in patient with non-Hodgkin's lymphoma, acute lymphoblastic leukemia, or Hodgkin's disease undergoing autologous bone marrow transplant[1–6]	X		1A. None	1. History and physical (H&P), progress notes, physician orders
2. Sargramostim not administered to patient with acute myeloblastic leukemia, myelodysplastic syndrome, or excessive leukemic myeloid blasts (≥10%) in bone marrow or peripheral blood[1,6–8]	X		2A. None	2. H&P, physician orders, progress notes, laboratory reports
Critical (Process) Indicators				
3. No history of allergy to sargramostim or yeast-derived drugs or proteins[1,3,5–12]	X		3A. None	3. H&P, allergies
4. Complete blood count with differential (including examination for presence of blast cells) and platelet count done twice weekly during sargramostim treatment[1,4,6,7,9,10]	X		4A. None	4. Laboratory reports, progress notes, physician orders
5. Sargramostim not administered within 24 hr before or after cancer chemotherapy or within 12 hr before or after radiation therapy[1,6]	X		5A. None	5. Nursing notes, progress notes, physician orders, medication administration record (MAR)
6. Sargramostim discontinued if excessive leukemic myeloid blasts (≥10%) present in bone marrow or peripheral blood[1,6,8]	X		6A. None	6. Laboratory reports, progress notes, physician orders, MAR
7. Platelet count ≤500,000 cells/cu mm during sargramostim treatment[1,6]	X		7A. Sargramostim treatment interrupted 7B. Sargramostim dosage reduced by 50%[1] 7C. Sargramostim discontinued	7. Laboratory reports, progress notes 7A–C. MAR, nursing notes, progress notes, physician orders
8. Absolute neutrophil count (ANC) ≤20,000 cells/cu mm during sargramostim treatment[1,3,6]	X		8A. Sargramostim treatment interrupted 8B. Sargramostim dosage reduced by 50%[1]	8. Laboratory reports, progress notes 8A–C. MAR, nursing notes, progress notes, physi-

Prepared by J. Michael Burr, Director of Pharmaceutical Services, Selma Medical Center, Selma, AL, and Bruce B. McCall, Pharm.D., Clinical Coordinator, Department of Pharmacy, Tallahassee Memorial Regional Medical Center, Tallahassee, FL.

Element	Standard 100%	Standard 0%	Exception[b] or Critical Preventive/ Responsive Measure[c]	Sources of Information
			8C. Sargramostim discontinued	cian orders
9. In patient with pre-existing hepatic dysfunction, liver function (serum aspartate aminotransferase and alanine aminotransferase concentration, urine bilirubin concentration in presence of hyperbilirubinemia) monitored twice weekly during sargramostim treatment[1,5,6,8,9]	X		9A. None	9. H&P, laboratory reports, progress notes, physician orders
10. In patient with pre-existing renal dysfunction, renal function (serum creatinine and blood urea nitrogen concentration) monitored twice weekly during sargramostim treatment[1,5,6,8,9]	X		10A. None	10. H&P, laboratory reports, progress notes, physician orders
11. Appropriate dosage, 250 μg/sq m/day for 21 days[1,3,6]	X		11A. None	11. MAR, physician orders, progress notes
12. Daily dosage given as (a) continuous i.v. infusion[7,10] or (b) single subcutaneous injection[13] or (c) 2-hr i.v. infusion beginning 2 to 4 hr after autologous bone marrow transplant but not less than 24 hr after last cancer chemotherapy dose and not less than 12 hr after last dose of radiation[1,4,7,9]	X		12A. None	12. MAR, physician orders, progress notes, nursing notes
Complications				
13. Diarrhea, asthenia, malaise, nausea, fever, headache, chills, bone pain, myalgia, muscle cramps, deep vein thrombosis, facial flushing, vomiting[1,3–8,12]		X	13A. Identify other drug and nondrug causes 13B. Provide symptomatic and supportive therapy 13C. Discontinue sargramostim therapy	13. Nursing notes, progress notes, nursing flow sheets 13A–C. MAR, nursing notes, progress notes, physician orders
14. Peripheral edema, pleural or pericardial effusion[1,3,6,9]		X	14A. Identify other drug and nondrug causes 14B. Provide symptomatic and supportive therapy 14C. Reduce sargramostim dosage by 50%[1] 14D. Discontinue or interrupt sargramostim therapy	14. Nursing notes, progress notes, radiology reports 14A–D. MAR, nursing notes, physician orders, progress notes
15. Dyspnea[1,6,12]		X	15A. Identify other drug and nondrug causes 15B. Provide symptomatic and supportive therapy 15C. Reduce sargramostim dosage by 50%[1] 15D. Discontinue or interrupt sargramostim therapy	15. Nursing notes, progress notes 15A–D. MAR, nursing notes, physician orders, progress notes
16. Supraventricular arrhythmia[1,6]		X	16A. Identify other drug and nondrug causes 16B. Discontinue sargramostim therapy	16. Electrocardiographic reports, nursing notes, progress notes 16A, B. MAR, nursing notes, progress notes, physician orders
17. Rash or local reaction at the injection site[1,6,8,9]		X	17A. Identify other drug and nondrug causes 17B. Provide symptomatic and supportive therapy 17C. Discontinue or interrupt sargramostim therapy	17. Nursing notes, progress notes 17A–C. MAR, nursing notes, progress notes, physician orders
18. Anaphylactic reaction[1,6]		X	18A. Identify other drug and nondrug causes 18B. Provide symptomatic and supportive therapy 18C. Discontinue sargramostim therapy	18. Nursing notes, progress notes 18A–C. MAR, nursing notes, progress notes, physician orders

Element	Standard 100%	Standard 0%	Exception[b] or Critical Preventive/ Responsive Measure[c]	Sources of Information
19. Progression of the underlying neoplastic disease[1,6,8]		X	19A. Discontinue sargramostim therapy	19. Nursing notes, progress notes 19A. MAR, nursing notes, progress notes, physician orders
Outcome Measures				
20. Accelerated myeloid engraftment[1,3–6]	X		20A. Patient died 20B. Patient unable to tolerate sargramostim	20. Laboratory reports, progress notes, literature[d] 20A, B. Nursing notes, progress notes
or				
21. Reduction in duration or severity of ANC nadir[3–8,10,12]	X		21A. Patient died 21B. Patient unable to tolerate sargramostim	21. H&P, laboratory reports, progress notes, literature[d] 21A, B. Nursing notes, progress notes
22. Reduced incidence and severity of infection and decreased use of anti-infective agents[1,3–6,12]	X		22A. Patient died 22B. Patient and family request no additional medical treatment 22C. Patient unable to tolerate sargramostim	22. Physician orders, progress notes, MAR, laboratory reports, literature[d] 22A–C. Nursing notes, progress notes
or				
23. Reduced admission or length of hospitalization	X		23A. Patient died 22B. Patient and family request no additional medical treatment 23C. Patient unable to tolerate sargramostim	23. Progress notes, nursing notes, literature[d] 23A–C. Nursing notes, progress notes

[a] Criteria address justification for use (indications), critical (process) indicators, complications of therapy, and patient outcome. Each criterion consists of an element, a standard, exceptions to the standard, and sources of information. The element is the minimum level of evidence needed to show that patient care was optimal. The standard defines the deviation from an element that is acceptable. If no deviation is acceptable, the standard is 100%. Exceptions are circumstances in which deviation is allowable. Sources of information listed are the most reliable sources. Sources pertaining to an element or exception are identified by the number assigned to the element or exception (e.g., 7, 7A).

[b] For justification for use and critical (process) indicators.

[c] For complications and outcome measures.

[d] Outcome is relative to that of other patients of similar ages with the same disease state and treatment. Use the clinical literature or the institutional patient database as a basis for comparison.

References

1. Immunex Inc. Leukine package insert. Seattle, WA; 1991.
2. Brandt SJ, Peters WP, Atwater SK et al. Effect of recombinant human granulocyte–macrophage colony-stimulating factor on hematopoietic reconstruction after high-dose chemotherapy and autologous bone marrow transplantation. *N Engl J Med*. 1988; 318:869–76.
3. Nemunaitis J, Singer JW, Buckner CD et al. Use of recombinant human granulocyte–macrophage colony-stimulating factor in graft failure after bone marrow transplantation. *Blood*. 1990; 76:245–53.
4. Nemunaitis J, Singer JW, Buckner CD et al. Use of recombinant granulocyte–macrophage colony-stimulating factor in autologous marrow transplantation for lymphoid malignancies. *Blood*. 1988; 72:834–6.
5. Blazar BR, Kersey JH, McGlave PB et al. In vivo administration of recombinant human granulocyte/macrophage colony-stimulating factor in acute lymphoblastic leukemia patients receiving purged autografts. *Blood*. 1989; 73:849–57.
6. Hoechst-Roussel Pharmaceuticals Inc. Prokine package insert. Somerville, NJ; 1991 Mar.
7. Ganser A, Volkers B, Greher J et al. Recombinant human granulocyte–macrophage colony-stimulating factor in patients with myelodysplastic syndromes—a Phase I/II trial. *Blood*. 1989; 73:31–7.
8. Antin JH, Smith BR, Holmes W et al. Phase I/II study of recombinant human granulocyte–macrophage colony-stimulating factor in aplastic anemia and myelodysplastic syndrome. *Blood*. 1988; 72:705–13.
9. Welte K, Zeidler C, Reiter A et al. Differential effects of granulocyte–macrophage colony-stimulating factor and granulocyte colony-stimulating factor in children with severe congenital neutropenia. *Blood*. 1990; 75:1056–63.
10. Wing EJ, Magee DM, Whiteside TL et al. Recombinant human granulocyte/macrophage colony-stimulating factor enhances monocyte cytotoxicity and secretion of tumor necrosis factor alpha and interferon in cancer patients. *Blood*. 1989; 73:643–6.
11. Kaplan SS, Basford RE, Wing EJ et al. The effect of human granulocyte macrophage colony-stimulating factor on neutrophil activation in patients with refractory carcinoma. *Blood*. 1989; 73:636–8.
12. Herrman F, Schultz G, Lindemann A et al. Hematopoietic responses in patients with advanced malignancy treated with recombinant human granulocyte–macrophage colony-stimulating factor. *J Clin Oncol*. 1989; 7:159–67.
13. Vadhan-Raj S, Buescher S, Le Maistre A et al. Stimulation of hematopoiesis in patients with bone marrow failure and in patients with malignancy by recombinant human granulocyte macrophage colony-stimulating factor. *Blood*. 1988; 72:134–41.

Criteria for use of filgrastim (granulocyte colony-stimulating factor) [a]

Element	Standard 100%	Standard 0%	Exception[b] or Critical Preventive/ Responsive Measure[c]	Sources of Information
Justification for Use[d]				
1. Patient with nonmyeloid malignancy receiving myelosuppressive antineoplastic therapy[1,7–15]	X		1A. None	1. History and physical (H&P), medication administration record (MAR), physician orders, progress notes
Critical (Process) Indicators				
2. No history of allergy to *Escherichia coli*-derived drugs or proteins[1]	X		2A. None	2. H&P, allergies
3. Complete blood count (CBC) with differential and platelet count performed before initiation of cancer chemotherapy and twice weekly during filgrastim therapy[1]	X		3A. None	3. Laboratory reports, progress notes, physician orders
4. Initial filgrastim dose administered at least 24 hr after last dose of antineoplastic agent or last dose in cancer chemotherapy treatment cycle[1,8,12,14]	X		4A. None	4. MAR, nursing notes, progress notes, physician orders
5. Filgrastim discontinued at least 24 hr before next dose of antineoplastic agent or initiation of next cycle of cancer chemotherapy[1,8]	X		5A. None	5. MAR, nursing notes, progress notes, physician orders
6. Appropriate initial filgrastim dosage, 5 μg/kg/day[1]	X		6A. None	6. MAR, physician orders, progress notes
7. If absolute neutrophil count (ANC) below desired response after 5 to 7 days, dosage increased in increments of 5 μg/kg/day according to duration and severity of ANC nadir[1]	X		7A. None	7. Laboratory reports, MAR, nursing notes, progress notes, physician orders
8. Filgrastim continued through expected cancer chemotherapy-induced ANC nadir[e] until patient achieves ANC of ≥10,000 cells/cu mm[1]	X		8A. Dose-intensified cancer chemotherapeutic regimen (see element 9)	8. Laboratory reports, MAR, physician orders, progress notes 8A. MAR, progress notes, physician orders
9. In patient receiving dose-intensified cancer chemotherapeutic regimen, filgrastim continued through expected cancer chemotherapy-induced ANC nadir until ANC is ≥10,000 cells/cu mm on two consecutive occasions[14]	X		9A. None	9. Laboratory reports, MAR, progress notes, physician orders
10. Filgrastim discontinued when ANC is ≥10,000 cells/cu mm after cancer chemotherapy-induced ANC nadir[1]	X		10A. Dose-intensified cancer chemotherapeutic regimen (see element 9)	10. Laboratory reports, MAR, progress notes, physician orders 10A. MAR, progress notes, physician orders
11. Filgrastim given as single daily dose[1,3,4,6,7,10,12,16]	X		11A. None	11. MAR, physician orders, progress notes
12. Filgrastim administered as bolus subcutaneous injection or short (30-min) or continuous (24-hr) intravenous or subcutaneous infusion[16]	X		12A. None	12. I.V. flow sheet, MAR, nursing notes, physician orders, progress notes
13. Filgrastim administered within or infusion begun ≤6 hr after filgrastim removed from refrigerated storage[1]	X		13A. None	13. Institutional policies and procedures, nursing notes
Complications				
14. Bone pain (especially in sternum, pelvis, or lower back)[1,2,4,7,8,11,12,14,15]		X	14A. Identify other drug and nondrug causes 14B. Provide symptomatic and supportive care	14. Nursing notes, progress notes 14A–C. MAR, nursing notes, physician orders, prog-

Prepared by J. Michael Burr, Director of Pharmaceutical Services, Selma Medical Center, Selma, AL, and Bruce B. McCall, Pharm.D., Clinical Coordinator, Department of Pharmacy, Tallahassee Memorial Regional Medical Center, Tallahassee, FL.

 0278-2677/91/1201-0950$00.75.

Element	Standard 100%	Standard 0%	Exception[b] or Critical Preventive/ Responsive Measure[c]	Sources of Information
			14C. Discontinue filgrastim	ress notes
15. Exacerbation of pre-existing conditions, including alopecia, skin disorders, hematuria, proteinuria, thrombocytopenia (platelet count, <50,000/cu mm), osteoporosis, nausea, and anorexia[1,3,5,7]		X	15A. Identify other drug and nondrug causes 15B. Provide symptomatic and supportive care 15C. Discontinue filgrastim	15. H&P, laboratory reports, nursing notes, progress notes 15A–C. MAR, nursing notes, physician orders, progress notes
16. Splenomegaly (more frequent in pediatric patients and with long-term filgrastim use)[1,2,4]		X	16A. Identify other drug and nondrug causes 16B. Discontinue filgrastim	16. Radiology reports, nursing notes, progress notes 16A, B. MAR, nursing notes, progress notes, physician orders
Outcome Measures				
17. Decreased incidence and severity of infection, as manifested by febrile neutropenia, and decreased use of anti-infective agents[1,2,7–9,13,14] or	X		17A. Patient died 17B. Patient and family request no additional medical treatment 17C. Patient unable to tolerate filgrastim	17. Literature,[f] progress notes, physician orders, MAR, laboratory reports 17A–C. Nursing notes, progress notes
18. Planned doses of antineoplastics given as scheduled[7,9,10] or	X		18A. Patient died 18B. Patient refused treatment 18C. Patient unable to tolerate filgrastim	18. H&P, MAR, nursing notes, progress notes, physician orders 18A–C. Nursing notes, progress notes
19. Reduced admissions or length of hospitalization[1,7,13] or	X		19A. Patient died 19B. Patient unable to tolerate filgrastim 19C. Patient and family request no additional medical treatment	19. Literature,[f] progress notes, nursing notes 19A–C. Nursing notes, progress notes
20. Decreased incidence and severity of mucositis associated with cancer chemotherapy[7,13] or	X		20A. Patient died 20B. Patient unable to tolerate filgrastim	20. Literature,[f] nursing notes, progress notes 20A, B. Nursing notes, progress notes
21. Reduction in duration or severity of ANC nadir[1,7–11,13–15]	X		21A. Patient died 21B. Patient unable to tolerate filgrastim	21. Literature,[f] laboratory reports, progress notes, H&P 21A, B. Nursing notes, progress notes

[a] Criteria address justification for use (indications), critical (process) indicators, complications of therapy, and patient outcome. Each criterion consists of an element, a standard, exceptions to the standard, and sources of information. The element is the minimum level of evidence needed to show that patient care was optimal. The standard defines the deviation from an element that is acceptable. If no deviation is acceptable, the standard is 100%. Exceptions are circumstances in which deviation is allowable. Sources of information listed are the most reliable sources. Sources pertaining to an element or exception are identified by the number assigned to the element or exception (e.g., 8, 8A).

[b] For justification for use and critical (process) indicators.

[c] For complications and outcome measures.

[d] Although research involving the use of filgrastim in patients with congenital agranulocytosis, cyclic neutropenia, neutropenia associated with hairy cell leukemia, myelodysplastic syndromes (refractory anemias), and severe congenital neutropenia (Kostmann's syndrome) has been reported, the manufacturer does not recommend the use of filgrastim in patients with chronic neutropenic conditions, myelodysplastic syndromes, or AIDS.[1–6]

[e] The cancer chemotherapy-induced ANC nadir usually occurs two to three days earlier than expected during treatment with filgrastim.[1]

[f] Outcome is relative to that of other patients of similar ages with the same disease state and treatment. Use the clinical literature or the institutional patient database as a basis for comparison.

References

1. Amgen Inc. Neupogen package insert. Thousand Oaks, CA; 1991 Feb.
2. Bonilla MA, Gillio AP, Ruggeiro M et al. Effects of recombinant human granulocyte colony-stimulating factor on neutropenia in patients with congenital agranulocytosis. *N Engl J Med.* 1989; 320:1574–80.
3. Glaspy JA, Baldwin GC, Robertson PA et al. Therapy for neutropenia in hairy cell leukemia with recombinant human granulocyte colony-stimulating factor. *Ann Intern Med.* 1988; 109:789–95.
4. Hammond WP, Price TH, Souza LM et al. Treatment of cyclic neutropenia with granulocyte colony-stimulating factor. *N Engl J Med.* 1989; 320:1306–11.
5. Negrin RS, Haeuber DH, Nagler A et al. Treatment of myelodysplastic syndromes with recombinant human granulocyte colony-stimulating factor: a Phase I–II trial. *Ann Intern Med.* 1989; 110:976–84.
6. Welte K, Zeidler C, Reiter A et al. Differential effects of granulocyte–macrophage colony-stimulating factor and granulocyte colony-stimulating factor in children with severe congenital neutropenia. *Blood.* 1990; 75:1056–63.
7. Gabrilove JL, Jakubowski A, Scher H et al. Effect of granulocyte colony-stimulating factor on neutropenia and associated morbidity due to chemotherapy for transitional-cell carcinoma of the urothelium. *N Engl J Med.* 1988; 318:1414–22.
8. Morstyn G, Campbell L, Souza LM et al. Effect of granulo-

cyte colony-stimulating factor on neutropenia induced by cytotoxic chemotherapy, *Lancet*. 1988; 1:667–71.

9. Bronchud MH, Scarffe JH, Thatcher N et al. Phase I/II study of recombinant human granulocyte colony-stimulating factor in patients receiving intensive chemotherapy for small cell lung cancer. *Br J Cancer*. 1987; 56:809–13.
10. Bronchud MH, Howell A, Crowther D et al. The use of granulocyte colony-stimulating factor to increase the intensity of treatment with doxorubicin in patients with advanced breast and ovarian cancer. *Br J Cancer*. 1989; 60:121–5.
11. Taylor KM, Jagganath S, Spitzer G et al. Recombinant human granulocyte colony-stimulating factor hastens granulocyte recovery after high-dose chemotherapy and autologous bone marrow transplantation in Hodgkin's disease. *J Clin Oncol*. 1989; 7:1791–9.
12. Morstyn G, Campbell L, Lieschke G et al. Treatment of chemotherapy-induced neutropenia by subcutaneously administered granulocyte colony-stimulating factor with optimization of dose and duration of therapy. *J Clin Oncol*. 1989; 7:1554–62.
13. Sheridan WP, Morstyn G, Wolf M et al. Granulocyte colony-stimulating factor and neutrophil recovery after high-dose chemotherapy and autologous bone marrow transplantation. *Lancet*. 1989; 8:891–4.
14. Neidhart J, Mangalik A, Kohler W et al. Granulocyte colony-stimulating factor stimulates recovery of granulocytes in patients receiving dose-intensive chemotherapy without bone marrow transplantation. *J Clin Oncol*. 1989; 7:1685–92.
15. Groopman JE, Molina JM, Scadden DT. Hematopoietic growth factors: biology and clinical applications. *N Engl J Med*. 1989; 321:1449–59.
16. Duhrsen U, Villeval JL, Boyd J et al. Effects of recombinant human granulocyte colony-stimulating factor on hematopoietic progenitor cells in cancer patients. *Blood*. 1988; 72:2074–81.

hemodialysis. During hemodialysis, patients treated with EPOGEN® may require increased anticoagulation with heparin to prevent clotting of the artificial kidney.

Patients who are marginally dialyzed may require adjustments in their dialysis prescription. As with all patients on dialysis, the serum chemistry values [including blood urea nitrogen (BUN), creatinine, phosphorus, and potassium] in EPOGEN®-treated patients should be monitored regularly to assure the adequacy of the dialysis prescription.

Renal Function: In patients with CRF not on dialysis, renal function and fluid and electrolyte balance should be closely monitored, as an improved sense of well-being may obscure the need to initiate dialysis in some patients. In patients with CRF not on dialysis, placebo-controlled studies of progression of renal dysfunction over periods of greater than one year have not been completed. In shorter-term trials in patients with CRF not on dialysis, changes in creatinine and creatinine clearance were not significantly different in EPOGEN®-treated patients, compared with placebo-treated patients. Analysis of the slope of 1/serum creatinine vs. time plots in these patients indicates no significant change in the slope after the initiation of EPOGEN® therapy.

AZT-treated HIV-infected Patients

Hypertension: Exacerbation of hypertension has not been observed in AZT-treated HIV-infected patients treated with EPOGEN®. However, EPOGEN® should be withheld in these patients if pre-existing hypertension is uncontrolled, and should not be started until blood pressure is controlled. In double-blind studies, a single seizure has been experienced by an EPOGEN®-treated patient.

ADVERSE REACTIONS

Chronic Renal Failure Patients

Studies analyzed to date indicate that EPOGEN® is generally well-tolerated. The adverse events reported are frequent sequelae of CRF and are not necessarily attributable to EPOGEN® therapy. In double-blind, placebo-controlled studies involving over 300 patients with CRF, the events reported in greater than 5% of EPOGEN®-treated patients during the blinded phase were:

	Percent of Patients Reporting Event	
Event	EPOGEN®-Treated Patients (n=200)	Placebo-Treated Patients (n=135)
Hypertension	24%	19%
Headache	16%	12%
Arthralgias	11%	6%
Nausea	11%	9%
Edema	9%	10%
Fatigue	9%	14%
Diarrhea	9%	6%
Vomiting	8%	5%
Chest Pain	7%	9%
Skin Reaction (Administration Site)	7%	12%
Asthenia	7%	12%
Dizziness	7%	13%
Clotted Access	7%	2%

Significant adverse events of concern in patients with CRF treated in double-blinded, placebo-controlled trials occurred in the following percent of patients during the blinded phase of the studies:

Seizure	1.1%	1.1%
CVA/TIA	0.4%	0.6%
MI	0.4%	1.1%
Death	0	1.7%

In the U.S. EPOGEN® studies in patients on dialysis (over 567 patients) the incidence (number of events per patient-year) of the most frequently reported adverse events were: hypertension (0.75), headache (0.40), tachycardia (0.31), nausea/vomiting (0.26), clotted vascular access (0.25), shortness of breath (0.14), hyperkalemia (0.11), and diarrhea (0.11). Other reported events occurred at a rate of less than 0.10 events per patient per year.

Events reported to have occurred within several hours of administration of EPOGEN® were rare, mild and transient, and included flu-like symptoms such as arthralgias and myalgias.

In all studies analyzed to date, EPOGEN® administration was generally well-tolerated, irrespective of the route of administration.

Allergic Reactions: There have been no reports of serious allergic reactions or anaphylaxis associated with EPOGEN® administration. Skin rashes and urticaria have been observed rarely and when reported have been mild and transient in nature. There has been no evidence for development of antibodies to erythropoietin in patients tested to date, including those receiving intravenous EPOGEN® for over two years. Nevertheless, if an anaphylactoid reaction occurs, EPOGEN® should be immediately discontinued and appropriate therapy initiated.

Seizures: There have been 47 seizures in 1010 patients on dialysis treated with EPOGEN® with an exposure of 986 patient-years for a rate of approximately 0.048 events per patient-year. However, there appeared to be a higher rate of seizures during the first 90 days of therapy (occurring in approximately 2.5% of patients), when compared to subsequent 90-day time periods. The baseline incidence of seizures in the untreated dialysis population is difficult to determine; it appears to be in the range of 5-10% per patient-year.

Hypertension: Increases in blood pressure have been reported in clinical trials, often during the first 90 days of therapy. When data from all patients in the U.S. Phase III multicenter trial were analyzed, there was an apparent trend of more reports of hypertensive adverse events in patients on dialysis with a faster rate of rise of hematocrit (greater than 4 hematocrit points in any two week period). However, in a double-blind, placebo-controlled trial, hypertensive adverse events were not reported at an increased rate in the EPOGEN®-treated group (150 U/kg T.I.W.) relative to the placebo group. There do not appear to be any direct pressor effects of EPOGEN®.

Thrombotic Events: Clotting of the vascular access has occurred at an annualized rate of about 0.25 events per patient-year on EPOGEN® therapy.

Overall, for patients with CRF (whether on dialysis or not), other thrombotic events (e.g. myocardial infarction, cerebrovascular accident, transient ischemic attack) have occurred at an annualized rate of less than 0.04 events per patient-year of EPOGEN® therapy.

AZT-treated HIV-infected Patients

Adverse events reported in clinical trials with EPOGEN® in AZT-treated HIV-infected patients were consistent with the progression of HIV infection. In double-blind, placebo-controlled studies of 3-months duration involving approximately 300 AZT-treated HIV-infected patients, adverse events with an incidence of ≥ 10% in either EPOGEN®-treated patients or placebo-treated patients were:

	Percent of Patients Reporting Event	
Event	EPOGEN®-Treated Patients (n=144)	Placebo-Treated Patients (n=153)
Pyrexia	38%	29%
Fatigue	25%	31%
Headache	19%	14%
Cough	18%	14%
Diarrhea	16%	18%
Rash	16%	8%
Congestion, Respiratory	15%	10%
Nausea	15%	12%
Shortness of Breath	14%	13%
Asthenia	11%	14%
Skin Reaction, Medication Site	10%	7%
Dizziness	9%	10%

There were no statistically significant differences between treatment groups in the incidence of the above events.

In the 297 patients studied, EPOGEN® was not associated with significant increases in opportunistic infections or mortality. In 71 patients from this group treated with EPOGEN® at 150 U/kg T.I.W., serum p24 antigen levels did not appear to increase. Preliminary data showed no enhancement of HIV replication in infected cell lines in vitro.

Peripheral white blood cell and platelet counts are unchanged following EPOGEN® therapy.

Allergic Reactions: Two AZT-treated HIV-infected patients had urticarial reactions within 48 hours of their first exposure to study medication. One patient was treated with EPOGEN® and one was treated with placebo (EPOGEN® vehicle alone). Both patients had positive immediate skin tests against their study medication with a negative saline control. The basis for this apparent pre-existing hypersensitivity to components of the EPOGEN® formulation is unknown, but may be related to HIV-induced immunosuppression or prior exposure to blood products.

Seizures: In double-blind and open label trails of EPOGEN® in AZT-treated HIV-infected patients, ten patients have experienced seizures. In general, these seizures appear to be related to underlying pathology such as meningitis or cerebral neoplasms, not EPOGEN® therapy.

OVERDOSAGE

The maximum amount of EPOGEN® that can be administered in single or multiple doses has not been determined. Doses up to 1500 U/kg T.I.W. for three to four weeks have been administered without any direct toxic effects of EPOGEN® itself.

Therapy with EPOGEN® can result in polycythemia if the hematocrit is not carefully monitored and the dose appropriately adjusted. If the target range (hematocrit of 30-33%) is exceeded, EPOGEN® may be temporarily withheld until the hematocrit returns to the target range; EPOGEN® therapy may then be resumed using a lower dose (see "Dosage and Administration"). If polycythemia is of concern, phlebotomy may be indicated to decrease the hematocrit.

DOSAGE AND ADMINISTRATION

Chronic Renal Failure Patients

Starting doses of EPOGEN® over the range of 50-100 U/kg three times weekly (T.I.W.) have been shown to be safe and effective in increasing hematocrit and eliminating transfusion dependency in patients with CRF (see "Clinical Experience"). The dose of EPOGEN® should be reduced when the hematocrit reaches the target range of 30-33% or increases by more than 4 points in any two-week period. The dosage of EPOGEN® must be individualized to maintain the hematocrit within the target range. Dose changes should generally be in the range of 25 U/kg, T.I.W. The table below provides general therapeutic guidelines.

Starting Dose:	Reduce Dose When:	Increase Dose If:	Maintenance Dose	Target Hct. Range
50-100 U/kg T.I.W.; IV: Dialysis Patients IV or SC: Non-dialysis CRF patients	1) Target range is reached, or 2) Hct. increases > 4 points in any 2-week period	Hct. does not increase by 5-6 points after 8 weeks of therapy, and hct. is below target range	Individually titrate	30-33% (max: 36%)

In patients on dialysis, EPOGEN® usually has been administered as an IV bolus T.I.W. While the administration of EPOGEN® is independent of the dialysis procedure, EPOGEN® may be administered into the venous line at the end of the dialysis procedure to obviate the need for additional venous access. In patients with CRF not on dialysis, EPOGEN® may be given either as an intravenous or subcutaneous injection.

AZT-treated HIV-infected patients

Prior to beginning EPOGEN®, it is recommended that the endogenous serum erythropoietin level be determined (prior to transfusion). Avaliable evidence suggests that patients receiving AZT with endogenous serum erythropoietin levels > 500 mU/mL are unlikely to respond to therapy with EPOGEN®.

Starting Dose: For patients with serum erythropoietin levels ≤ 500 mU/mL who are receiving a dose of AZT≤ 4200 mg/week, the recommended starting dose of EPOGEN® is 100 U/kg as an intravenous or subcutaneous injection three times weekly (T.I.W.) for 8 weeks.

Increase Dose: During the dose adjustment phase of therapy, the hematocrit should be monitored weekly. If the response is not satisfactory in terms of reducing transfusion requirements or increasing hematocrit after 8 weeks of therapy, the dose of EPOGEN® can be increased by 50-100 U/kg T.I.W. Response should be evaluated every 4-8 weeks thereafter and the dose adjusted accordingly by 50-100 U/kg increments T.I.W. If patients have not responded satisfactorily to an EPOGEN® dose of 300 U/kg T.I.W., it is unlikely that they will respond to higher doses of EPOGEN®.

Maintenance Dose: After attainment of the desired response (i.e. reduced transfusion requirments or increased hematocrit), the dose of EPOGEN® should be titrated to maintain the response based on factors such as variations in AZT dose and the presence of intercurrent infectious or inflammatory episodes. If the hematocrit exceeds 40%, the dose should be discontinued until the hematocrit drops to 36%. The dose should be reduced by 25% when treatment is resumed and then titrated to maintain the desired hematocrit.

Manufactured by:

AMGEN®

Amgen Inc., Amgen Center, Thousand Oaks, California 91320-1789 Issue Date:8/7/91

Current Literature

Drug Reaction Alerts 966

Book Reviews

Patient Compliance in Medical Practice and Clinical Trials 970
Edited by Joyce A. Cramer and Bert Spilker
Reviewed by David A. Graves

Regional Antineoplastic Drug Delivery in the Management of Malignant Disease 976
By Maurie Markman
Reviewed by J. Kelly Martin, Jr.

Books Received 976

Drug Reaction Alerts

Drug Reaction Alerts focuses primarily on serious, unlabeled reactions to new chemical entities. The citations are compiled monthly from International Pharmaceutical Abstracts, *which covers over 800 pharmacy and health-related journals worldwide. An address for reprints (when available) follows the name of the corresponding author of each citation.*

Pharmacists may use the FDA Adverse Reaction Report form that appears in most issues of Clinical Pharmacy for submitting reports of adverse drug reactions directly to FDA.

Antivirals

Walter EB (Department of Pediatrics, Box 31273, Duke University Medical Center, Durham, NC 27710), Drucker RP, McKinney RE et al. Myopathy in human immunodeficiency virus-infected children receiving long-term **zidovudine** therapy. *J Pediatr*. 1991; 119:152-5. Case. (three-year-old girl with AIDS; received zidovudine 180 mg/sq m every six hours for two years; developed myopathy, generalized erythematous macular rash, and elevated serum creatine kinase concentration; withdrawal of zidovudine and therapy with vancomycin, gentamicin, and prednisone led to initial resolution of rash and fever within 48 hours; serum creatine kinase concentration as high as 25,945 IU/L on day 5)

Drug Abuse

Chen C, Duara S (University of Miami School of Medicine, Department of Pediatrics [R-131], P.O. Box 016960, Miami, FL 33101), Neto GS et al. Respiratory instability in neonates with in utero exposure to **cocaine**. *J Pediatr*. 1991; 119:111-3. Study. (case control; 11 in utero cocaine-exposed infants and 10 control infants; cocaine exposure identified by maternal drug history and results of urine screen; received facial air stream stimulation to induce respiratory pauses; 54.8% of stimulations to cocaine-exposed infants produced respiratory pauses while only 16.6% of stimulations to controls produced respiratory pauses [Fisher exact test, $p < 0.02$]; mean ± S.D. duration of respiratory pause was 4.9 ± 1.9 seconds in cocaine-exposed infants and 3.1 ± 0.7 seconds in controls)

Sempere AP, Posada I, Ramo C et al. (Cabello A, Neurology Department and Section of Neuropathology, Hospital University 12 de Octubre, 28041 Madrid, Spain). Spongiform leucoencephalopathy after inhaling heroin. *Lancet*. 1991; 338:320. Cases. (two patients, aged 40 and 43 years, who were addicted to **diacetylmorphine**; inhaled diacetylmorphine by smoking; developed spongiform leukoencephalopathy; one patient, whose cerebellar biopsy specimen showed vacuolation of white matter with hyperplastic astrocytes, showed improved cerebellar function three months later; other patient regressed

Continued on page 968

Continued from page 966

neurologically, became comatose, and died three weeks after hospital admission; examination at autopsy showed cerebral swelling with flattening of gyri and narrowing of sulci and small bilateral, symmetrical uncal herniations)

Erythromycins

Absher JR, Bale JF (Department of Pediatrics, University of Iowa Hospitals and Clinics, Iowa City, IA 52242). Aggravation of myasthenia gravis by **erythromycin.** *J Pediatr.* 1991; 119:155-6. Case. (15-year-old girl with suspected bacterial respiratory infection; received erythromycin 500 mg as i.v. infusion; developed acute respiratory failure during infusion; discontinuation of erythromycin infusion and therapy with racemic epinephrine, aminophylline by i.v. infusion, and albuterol by nebulization did not lead to improvement of dyspnea, bilateral facial weakness, and limb weakness; diagnosis of myasthenia gravis confirmed by elevated serum acetylcholine receptor antibody titer [>30 nM]; therapy with pyridostigmine bromide 45 mg six times daily led to gradual improvement; serum acetylcholine receptor antibody titer was within normal range two months later but elevated six months later; underwent thymectomy)

Hassel B (Norwegian Defense Research Establishment, N-2007 Kjeller, Norway). Hypothermia from **erythromycin.** *Ann Intern Med.* 1991; 115:69-70. Cases. (two first cousins, aged three and four years, with infections and rectal temperatures ≥39.0 °C; three-year-old boy received erythromycin 100 mg four times daily as oral solution for three doses; four-year-old girl received same dosage for two doses; rectal temperatures decreased to <35 °C; withdrawal of erythromycin led to resolution of hypothermia; four-year-old twin brother received same dosage of erythromycin but did not develop hypothermia)

Immunosuppressive Agents

Passfall J, Distler A, Riecken EO et al. (Zeitz M, Division of Nephrology and Gastroenterology, Department of Medicine, Klinikum Steglitz, Free University of Berlin, D-1000 Berlin 45, Germany). Onset of ulcerative colitis in a cyclosporin-treated patient. *Lancet.* 1991; 338:389. Case. (60-year-old kidney transplant recipient; received **cyclosporine** for six years at doses adjusted according to median blood concentrations of 140 µg/L; developed ulcerative colitis; therapy with oral methylprednisolone led to improvement)

Immunotherapy

de Vries EGE (Department of Medical Oncology, Haematology, and Rheumatology, University Hospital, 9713EZ Groningen, the Netherlands), Willemse PHB, Biesma B et al. Flare-up of rheumatoid arthritis during GM-CSF treatment after chemotherapy. *Lancet.* 1991; 338:517-8. Case. (57-year-old woman with stage III undifferentiated carcinoma of fallopian tube and rheumatoid arthritis; received carboplatin 300 mg/sq m and cyclophosphamide 750 mg/sq m on day 1 and **granulocyte–macrophage colony-stimulating factor** [GM-CSF] 6 µg/kg/day as s.c. injection on days 6-12; developed increased stiffness and joint pain by day 7; increased serum interleukin-6, tumor necrosis factor-α, C-reactive protein, and amyloid A concentrations; concomitant diclofenac; withdrawal of GM-CSF led to gradual resolution of clinical arthritic symptoms)

Psychotherapeutic Agents

Gerson SL (Department of Medicine and Psychiatry and Ireland Cancer Center of the University Hospital of Cleveland, Case Western Reserve University School of Medicine, Cleveland, OH 44106), Lieberman JA, Friedenberg WR et al. Polypharmacy in fatal **clozapine**-associated agranulocytosis. *Lancet.* 1991; 338:262-3. Case. (45-year-old man with refractory schizophrenia; received clozapine 200 mg twice daily for 10 weeks; hematocrit decreased from 42% to 37%; platelet count decreased from 175,000/µL to 104,000/µL; concomitant carbamazepine, lithium, benztropine, and clonazepam; became lethargic and developed fever; experienced respiratory arrest on second day in hospital and died)

Quinolones

Tham TC, Allen G, Hayes D et al. (Riddell JG, Department of Therapeutics and Pharmacology, Dermatology, and Pathology, Belfast City Hospital, Belfast BT9 7BL, Ireland). Possible association between toxic epidermal necrolysis and **ciprofloxacin.** *Lancet.* 1991; 338:522. Case. (72-year-old woman with urinary tract infection; received ciprofloxacin 500 mg twice daily for nine days; developed itchy, generalized erythematous confluent rash on right leg, chest, and back, and pyrexia, sweating, nausea, and vomiting seven days after completing course of ciprofloxacin; therapy with ciprofloxacin 200 mg twice daily by i.v. infusion and later addition of erythromycin did not lead to improvement; concomitant gliclazide, naproxen, ferrous fumarate, and temazepam; developed bullous lesions that sloughed easily on contact; diagnosed as toxic epidermal necrolysis; withdrawal of ciprofloxacin, erythromycin, naproxen, and gliclazide and therapy with cefotaxime, netilmicin, and methylprednisolone by i.v. infusion did not lead to improvement; deteriorated and died eight days after onset of illness; examination at autopsy showed epidermal necrosis consistent with drug-induced toxic necrolysis)

Continued on page 970

Statement of Ownership, Management and Circulation (Required by 39 U.S.C. 3685) 1. Title of publication, Clinical Pharmacy. 1A. Publication No. 02782677. 2. Date of filing, October 1, 1991. 3. Frequency of issue, Monthly. 3A. No. issues published annually, 12. 3B. Annual subscription price, $75.00. 4. Location of known office of publication, 4630 Montgomery Avenue, Bethesda, Montgomery County, MD 20814. 5. Location of the headquarters or general business offices of the publishers, 4630 Montgomery Avenue, Bethesda, MD 20814. 6. Publisher, American Society of Hospital Pharmacists, Inc., 4630 Montgomery Avenue, Bethesda, MD 20814. Editor, William A. Zellmer, 4630 Montgomery Avenue, Bethesda, MD 20814. Managing Editor, C. Richard Talley. 7. Owner, American Society of Hospital Pharmacists, Inc., 4630 Montgomery Avenue, Bethesda, MD 20814. 8. Known bondholders, mortgagees, and other security holders owning 1% or more of total amount of bonds, mortgages, and other securities, None. 9. For completion by nonprofit organizations authorized to mail at special rates (Section 132.122, PSM). The purpose, function, and nonprofit status of this organization and the exempt status for federal income tax purposes have not changed during preceding 12 months. 10. Extent and nature of circulation, A. Total no. copies printed, 9,751/9,690*; B. Paid circulation, 1. Sales through dealers and carriers, street vendors and counter sales, 300/300. 2. Mail subscriptions, 7,812/7,719; C. Total paid circulation, 8,112/8,019; D. Free distribution by mail, carrier or other means, samples, complimentary and other free copies, 507/522; E. Total distribution, 8,619/8,541; F. Copies not distributed, 1. Office use, left over, unaccounted, spoiled after printing, 1,132/1,149. Returns from news agents, 0, 0; G. Total, 9,751/9,690. I certify that the statements made by me are correct and complete, signed William A. Zellmer.
*First figure, average no. of copies each issue during preceding 12 months; second figure, actual no. of copies single issue published nearest to filing date.

Continued from page 968

Roentgenographic Agents

Bain PG, Colchester AC (Department of Neurology, Guy's Hospital, London SE1 9RT, England), Nadaraja D. Paraplegia after **iopamidol** myelography. *Lancet*. 1991; 338:252-3. Case. (57-year-old woman with sciatic pain; received 14 mL of iopamidol as intrathecal injection during lumbar myelography; immediately developed involuntary jerking of right leg, dry mouth, incoherent speech, and feeling of bilateral leg paralysis; flaccid paraparesis four months later; unable to walk or stand 14 months later)

Mallat Z, Vassal T, Naouri JF et al. (Offenstadt G, Intensive Care Unit and Department of Radiology and Rheumatology, Hôpital St. Antoine, 75012 Paris, France). Aseptic meningoencephalitis after **iopamidol** myelography. *Lancet*. 1991; 338:252. Case. (53-year-old man; received 14 mL of iopamidol 300 mg/mL during lumbar myelography; became agitated and confused and developed neck stiffness, mild facial palsy, and right hemiparesis 12 hours later; received empiric therapy with pefloxacin, rifampin, and methylprednisolone; therapy with pefloxacin and rifampin discontinued after blood and cerebrospinal fluid samples failed to grow bacteria; therapy with methylprednisolone by i.v. infusion for three days led to gradual improvement; neurological examination was normal five days after first symptoms appeared)

Skin and Mucous Membrane Preparations

Penneys NS (University of Miami School of Medicine, Miami, FL 33101), Hernandez D. Sticky problem with **etretinate**. *N Engl J Med*. 1991; 325:521. Case. (patient with severe psoriasis; received etretinate 75 mg/day; developed stickiness of palms and soles to the extent that material adhered to these skin surfaces; concentration of carcinoembryonic antigen [CEA] in stratum corneum scrapings from palmar surfaces, 143 ng/mL; dosage of etretinate decreased to 50 mg/day for one month, then decreased to 25 mg/day; palmar CEA concentration decreased to 16.8 ng/mL, and stickiness decreased)

Toxicity, Environmental

Dietemann-Molard A, Braun JJ, Sohier B et al. (Pauli G, Department of Respiratory Medicine, Hôpital Central, CHRU, 67091 Strasbourg, France). Extrinsic allergic alveolitis secondary to carmine. *Lancet*. 1991; 338:460. Case. (33-year-old male sales manager; worked in office near room where food additives were prepared and mixed in containers; developed recurrent episodes of spasmodic coughs followed by flu-like febrile syndrome when food additives containing **carminic acid** were prepared; positive clinical response to challenge with carminic acid; presence of precipitating serum antibodies)

Salom IL. Purpura due to inhaled **quinidine**. *JAMA*. 1991; 266:1220. Case. (35-year-old female employee at pharmaceutical distributor; repackaged quinidine tablets from bulk containers into smaller containers for three months; developed purpuric patches on arms, legs, and trunk; wore work gloves but did not wear mask or respirator; withdrawal from exposure to quinidine led to resolution of purpura; positive rechallenge)

Tranquilizers

Friedman LJ, Tabb SE, Worthington JJ et al. (Sved M, Dorothea Dix Hospital, Raleigh, NC 27603). **Clozapine**—a novel antipsychotic agent. *N Engl J Med*. 1991; 325:518. Case. (47-year-old woman with acute exacerbation of chronic paranoid schizophrenia; received single dose of clozapine 25 mg; became dizzy, weak, and apneic and had a weak pulse; cardiopulmonary resuscitation led to recovery; concomitant clonazepam, which had been changed from lorazepam during previous week)

Book Reviews

Patient Compliance in Medical Practice and Clinical Trials

Edited by Joyce A. Cramer and Bert Spilker.

Published by Raven Press, 1185 Avenue of the Americas, New York, NY 10036, 1991. xvii + 414 p. Price $65.

This book is organized into two basic parts: how to monitor patient compliance, and what to do with information about compliance once it has been collected. I think this book will serve as a much-needed educational tool and reference, because anyone who is a health-care professional has wanted answers to both questions. The book does not offer definitive answers; rather, numerous persons share their methods for dealing with these issues. Instead of creating a theoretical basis without follow-through, the text emphasizes observation and interpretation and follows with formulation of strategies based on real-life examples.

Widespread sophistication in the measurement and interpretation of compliance with treatment regimens is relatively new. The most obvious example of this sophistication is the use of miniature electronic monitoring devices, as well as ingenious physiologic markers of treatment, to enhance our true understanding of compliance. The authors describe an ample number of these approaches. Some are applicable to research only; however, a representative sampling of available approaches is described.

Most interesting to me was the way in which the data collected were applied to findings in clinical research; that is, what does one do with (presumably accurate) compliance data once they are collected? Some extremely valuable examples of interpretation are provided. There was some agreement that patients who are generally compliant are probably different in disease severity, and thus in pharmacologic responses, from poorly compliant patients. This suggests that studies that present data only on compliant patients may reduce the potential for generalizing results to all patients with a particular disease. The Food and Drug Administration has insisted on this interpretation of clinical trial results for quite some time, asking that an intent-to-treat analysis be a central part of a drug's approval in this country. Ironically, after all this work to measure compliance, one could suggest that the measurement of compliance is not worth the effort. After evaluating the contributions to this text, however, it is clear to me that an understanding of compliance (in the context of a specific disease and therapy) is alone informative. Further, differences between therapeutic studies might simply be differences in patient populations, as evidenced by the level of compliance.

The practitioner will find less of the book's information useful than will the researcher. Practitioners who routinely read the literature will gain somewhat from the discussions of how to apply compliance data to clinical results. On the whole, though, the text will be most helpful to persons responsible for conducting or analyzing clinical research; the text is one of the best available single references containing real-life examples.

Reviewed by David A. Graves, Pharm.D., Medical Affairs, Genentech, Inc., 460 Point San Bruno Boulevard, South San Francisco, CA 94080.

Continued on page 976

EXOSURF® Neonatal™
(COLFOSCERIL PALMITATE, CETYL ALCOHOL, TYLOXAPOL)
For Intratracheal Suspension / 10 mL vials

PLEASE CONSULT FULL PRODUCT INFORMATION BEFORE PRESCRIBING.

INDICATIONS AND USAGE: Exosurf Neonatal is indicated for:

1. **Prophylactic** treatment of infants with birth weights of less than 1350 grams who are at risk of developing RDS (see PRECAUTIONS),
2. **Prophylactic** treatment of infants with birth weights greater than 1350 grams who have evidence of pulmonary immaturity, and
3. **Rescue** treatment of infants who have developed RDS.

CONTRAINDICATIONS: There are no known contraindications to treatment with Exosurf Neonatal.

WARNINGS: Intratracheal Administration Only: Exosurf Neonatal should be administered only by instillation into the trachea. **General:** The use of Exosurf Neonatal requires expert clinical care by experienced neonatologists and other clinicians who are accomplished at neonatal intubation and ventilatory management. Adequate personnel, facilities, equipment, and medications are required to optimize perinatal outcome in premature infants. Instillation of Exosurf Neonatal should be performed **only** by trained medical personnel experienced in airway and clinical management of unstable premature infants. Vigilant clinical attention should be given to all infants prior to, during, and after administration of Exosurf Neonatal. **Acute Effects:** Exosurf Neonatal can rapidly affect oxygenation and lung compliance. **Lung Compliance:** If chest expansion improves substantially after dosing, peak ventilator inspiratory pressures should be reduced immediately, without waiting for confirmation of respiratory improvement by blood gas assessment. Failure to reduce inspiratory ventilator pressures rapidly in such instances can result in lung overdistention and fatal pulmonary air leak. **Hyperoxia:** If the infant becomes pink and transcutaneous oxygen saturation is in excess of 95%, FiO_2 should be reduced in small but repeated steps (until saturation is 90 to 95%) without waiting for confirmation of elevated arterial pO_2 by blood gas assessment. Failure to reduce FiO_2 in such instances can result in hyperoxia. **Hypocarbia:** If arterial or transcutaneous CO_2 measurements are <30 torr, the ventilator rate should be reduced at once. Failure to reduce ventilator rates in such instances can result in marked hypocarbia, which is known to reduce brain blood flow. **Pulmonary Hemorrhage:** In the single study conducted in infants weighing <700 grams at birth, the incidence of pulmonary hemorrhage (10% vs 2% in the placebo group) was significantly increased in the Exosurf Neonatal group. None of the five studies involving infants with birth weights >700 grams showed a significant increase in pulmonary hemorrhage in the Exosurf Neonatal group. In a cross-study analysis of these five studies, pulmonary hemorrhage was reported for 1% (14/1420) of infants in the placebo group and 2% (27/1411) of infants in the Exosurf Neonatal group. Fatal pulmonary hemorrhage occurred in three infants; two in the Exosurf Neonatal group and one in the placebo group. Mortality from all causes among infants who developed pulmonary hemorrhage was 43% in the placebo group and 37% in the Exosurf Neonatal group. Pulmonary hemorrhage in both Exosurf Neonatal and placebo infants was more frequent in infants who were younger, smaller, male, or who had a patent ductus arteriosus. Pulmonary hemorrhage typically occurred in the first 2 days of life in both treatment groups. In more than 7700 infants in the open, uncontrolled study, pulmonary hemorrhage was reported in 4%, but fatal pulmonary hemorrhage was reported rarely (0.4%). In the controlled clinical studies, Exosurf Neonatal treated infants who received steroids more than 24 hours prior to delivery or indomethacin postnatally had a lower rate of pulmonary hemorrhage than other Exosurf Neonatal treated infants. Attention should be paid to early and aggressive diagnosis and treatment (unless contraindicated) of patent ductus arteriosus during the first 2 days of life (while the ductus arteriosus is often clinically silent). Other potentially protective measures include attempting to decrease FiO_2 preferentially over ventilator pressures during the first 24 to 48 hours after dosing, and attempting to decrease PEEP minimally for at least 48 hours after dosing. **Mucous Plugs:** Infants whose ventilation becomes markedly impaired during or shortly after dosing may have mucous plugging of the endotracheal tube, particularly if pulmonary secretions were prominent prior to drug administration. Suctioning of all infants prior to dosing may lessen the chance of mucous plugs obstructing the endotracheal tube. If endotracheal tube obstruction from such plugs is suspected, and suctioning is unsuccessful in removing the obstruction, the blocked endotracheal tube should be replaced immediately.

PRECAUTIONS:

General: In the controlled clinical studies, infants known prenatally or postnatally to have major congenital anomalies, or who were suspected of having congenital infection, were excluded from entry. However, these disorders cannot be recognized early in life in all cases, and a few infants with these conditions were entered. The benefits of Exosurf Neonatal in the affected infants who received drug appeared to be similar to the benefits observed in infants without anomalies or occult infection. **Prophylactic Treatment-Infants <700 Grams:** In infants weighing 500 to 700 grams, a single prophylactic dose of Exosurf Neonatal significantly: improved FiO_2 and ventilator settings, reduced pneumothorax, and reduced death from RDS, but increased pulmonary hemorrhage (see WARNINGS). Overall mortality did not differ significantly between the placebo and Exosurf Neonatal groups (see Table 1 in full product information). Data on multiple doses in infants in this weight class are not yet available. Accordingly, clinicians should carefully evaluate the potential risks and benefits of Exosurf Neonatal administration in these infants. **Rescue Treatment-Number of Doses:** A small number of infants with RDS have received more than two doses of Exosurf Neonatal as rescue treatment. Definitive data on the safety and efficacy of these additional doses are not available. **Carcinogenesis, Mutagenesis, Impairment of Fertility:** Exosurf Neonatal at concentrations up to 10,000 μg/plate was not mutagenic in the Ames Salmonella assay. Long-term studies have not been performed in animals to evaluate the carcinogenic potential of Exosurf Neonatal. The effects of Exosurf Neonatal on fertility have not been studied.

ADVERSE REACTIONS:

General: Premature birth is associated with a high incidence of morbidity and mortality. Despite significant reductions in overall mortality associated with Exosurf Neonatal, some infants who received Exosurf Neonatal developed severe complications and either survived with permanent handicaps or died.

In controlled clinical studies evaluating the safety and efficacy of Exosurf Neonatal, numerous safety assessments were made. In infants receiving Exosurf Neonatal, pulmonary hemorrhage, apnea and use of methylxanthines were increased. A number of other adverse events were significantly reduced in the Exosurf Neonatal group, particularly various forms of pulmonary air leak and use of pancuronium. Tables 3 and 4 summarize the results of the major safety evaluations from the controlled clinical studies.

Table 3: Safety Assessments[a]—Prophylactic Treatment

Number of Doses: / Birth Weight Range:	Single Dose 500 to 700 grams		Single Dose 700 to 1350 grams		Single Dose 700 to 1100 grams		1 vs 3 Doses 700 to 1100 grams	
Treatment Group:	Placebo (Air)	EXOSURF	Placebo (Air)	EXOSURF	Placebo (Air)	EXOSURF	EXOSURF 1 Dose	EXOSURF 3 Doses
Number of Infants:	N=108	N=107	N=193	N=192	N=222	N=224	N=356	N=360
	% of Infants		% of Infants		% of Infants		% of Infants	
Intraventricular Hemorrhage (IVH)								
Overall	51	57	31	27	36	36	38	35
Severe IVH	26	25	10	8	13	14	9	9
Pulmonary Air Leak (PAL)								
Overall	52	48	16	11	32	25	29	27
Pneumothorax	23	10*	5	6	19	11*	14	12
Pneumopericardium	1	4	2	0	<1	1	1	1
Pneumomediastinum	2	1	2	3	7	1**	3	2
Pulmonary Interstitial Emphysema	43	44	13	7*	26	20	23	22
Death from PAL	4	6	<1	<1	2	1	2	1
Patent Ductus Arteriosus	49	53	66	70	50	55	59	57
Necrotizing Enterocolitis	2	4	11	13	3	4	6	2*
Pulmonary Hemorrhage	2	10**	2	4	1	4	4	6
Congenital Pneumonia	4	4	2	4	2	2	1	1
Nosocomial Pneumonia	10	10	2	4	4	7	14	15
Non-Pulmonary Infections	33	35	34	39	28	29	35	34
Sepsis	30	34	30	34	23	24	30	27
Death From Sepsis	4	4	3	3	1	2	3	2
Meningitis	4	6	3	1	2	3	1	2
Other Infections	7	4	5	3	6	10	10	11
Major Anomalies	3	1	2	4	7	4	4	4

Table 3: Safety Assessments[a]—Prophylactic Treatment (Cont.)

Number of Doses: / Birth Weight Range:	Single Dose 500 to 700 grams		Single Dose 700 to 1350 grams		Single Dose 700 to 1100 grams		1 vs 3 Doses 700 to 1100 grams	
Treatment Group:	Placebo (Air)	EXOSURF	Placebo (Air)	EXOSURF	Placebo (Air)	EXOSURF	EXOSURF 1 Dose	EXOSURF 3 Doses
Number of Infants:	N=108	N=107	N=193	N=192	N=222	N=224	N=356	N=360
	% of Infants		% of Infants		% of Infants		% of Infants	
Hypotension	70	77	52	47	59	62	54	50
Hyperbilirubinemia	22	21	63	61	27	31	20	21
Exchange Transfusion	4	3	1	2	2	2	3	1
Thrombocytopenia[b]	21	25	not available		9	8	12	10
Persistent Fetal Circulation	0	1	1	1	0	2*	1	<1
Seizures	11	8	2	2	11	9	6	5
Apnea	34	33	76	73	55	65*	62	68
Drug Therapy								
Antibiotics	96	99	98	96	98	99	>99	99
Diuretics	55	60	39	37	59	63	64	65
Anticonvulsants	14	18	23	24	20	16	9	8
Inotropes	46	40	20	20	26	20	28	27
Sedatives	62	71	65	64	63	57	52	52
Pancuronium	19	11	22	14*	19	13*	15	11
Methylxanthines	38	43	77	77	61	72*	75	82*

[a] All parameters were examined with "as-treated" analyses. * $p<0.05$
[b] Thrombocytopenia requiring platelet transfusion. ** $p<0.01$

Table 4: Safety Assessments[a]—Rescue Treatment

Number of Doses: / Birth Weight Range:	Two Doses 700 to 1350 grams		Two Doses 1250 grams and above	
Treatment Group:	Placebo (Air)	EXOSURF	Placebo (Air)	EXOSURF
Number of Infants:	N=213	N=206	N=622	N=615
	% of Infants		% of Infants	
Intraventricular Hemorrhage (IVH)				
Overall	48	52	23	18*
Severe IVH	13	9	5	4
Pulmonary Air Leak (PAL)				
Overall	54	34***	30	18***
Pneumothorax	29	20*	20	10***
Pneumopericardium	4	1	1	2
Pneumomediastinum	8	4	5	2**
Pulmonary Interstitial Emphysema	48	25***	24	13***
Death from PAL	7	3	<1	1
Patent Ductus Arteriosus	66	57	54	45*
Necrotizing Enterocolitis	3	3	1	2
Pulmonary Hemorrhage	3	1	<1	1
Congenital Pneumonia	2	3	2	2
Nosocomial Pneumonia	5	7	2	2
Non-Pulmonary Infections	19	22	13	13
Sepsis	15	17	8	8
Death From Sepsis	<1	<1	1	<1
Meningitis	1	<1	1	<1*
Other Infections	5	8	5	6
Major Anomalies	3	3	4	4
Hypotension	62	57	50	39**
Hyperbilirubinemia	17	19	12	10
Exchange Transfusion	3	4	1	2
Thrombocytopenia[b]	10	11	4	<1**
Persistent Fetal Circulation	1	1	6	2**
Seizures	10	10	6	3*
Apnea	48	65**	37	44*
Drug Therapy				
Antibiotics	100	99	98	98
Diuretics	60	65	45	34***
Anticonvulsants	17	17	10	5**
Inotropes	36	31	27	16***
Sedatives	72	68	76	64***
Pancuronium	34	17**	33	15***
Methylxanthines	62	74**	49	53

[a] All parameters were examined with "as-treated" analyses. * $p<0.05$ *** $p<0.001$
[b] Thrombocytopenia requiring platelet transfusion. ** $p<0.01$

Pulmonary Hemorrhage: See WARNINGS. **Abnormal Laboratory Values:** Abnormal laboratory values are common in critically ill, mechanically ventilated, premature infants. A higher incidence of abnormal laboratory values in the Exosurf Neonatal group was not reported. **Events During Dosing:** Data on events during dosing are available from more than 8800 infants in the open, uncontrolled clinical study (Table 5).

Table 5: Events During Dosing in the Open, Uncontrolled Study[a]

Treatment Type: / Number of Infants:	Prophylactic Treatment N=1127	Rescue Treatment N=7711
	% of Infants	% of Infants
Reflux of Exosurf	20	31
Drop in O_2 saturation ($\geq 20\%$)	6	22
Rise in O_2 saturation ($\geq 10\%$)	5	6
Drop in transcutaneous pO_2 (≥ 20 mm Hg)	1	8
Rise in transcutaneous pO_2 (≥ 20 mm Hg)	2	5
Drop in transcutaneous pCO_2 (≥ 20 mm Hg)	<1	1
Rise in transcutaneous pCO_2 (≥ 20 mm Hg)	1	3
Bradycardia (<60 beats/min)	1	3
Tachycardia (>200 beats/min)	<1	<1
Gagging	1	5
Mucous Plugs	<1	<1

[a] Infants may have experienced more than one event.
Investigators were prohibited from adjusting FiO_2 and/or ventilator settings during dosing unless significant clinical deterioration occurred.

Reflux: Reflux of Exosurf Neonatal into the endotracheal tube during dosing has been observed and may be associated with rapid drug administration. If reflux occurs, drug administration should be halted and, if necessary, peak inspiratory pressure on the ventilator should be increased by 4 to 5 cm H_2O until the endotracheal tube clears. ***>20% Drop in Transcutaneous Oxygen Saturation:*** If transcutaneous oxygen saturation declines during dosing, drug administration should be halted and, if necessary, peak inspiratory pressure on the ventilator should be increased by 4 to 5 cm H_2O for 1 to 2 minutes. In addition, increases of FiO_2 may be required for 1 to 2 minutes. ***Mucous Plugs:*** See WARNINGS.

DOSAGE AND ADMINISTRATION: See full product information.

Wellcome **BURROUGHS WELLCOME CO.**, Research Triangle Park, NC 27709

Printed in U.S.A. EX-Y01228

Continued from page 970

Regional Antineoplastic Drug Delivery in the Management of Malignant Disease

By Maurie Markman.
Published by The Johns Hopkins University Press, 701 West 40th Street, Suite 275, Baltimore, MD 21211, 1991. xii + 143 p. Price $50.

This thorough review of the current status of regional therapy of malignant disease is well written and extensively referenced. The author's research experience and expertise in this highly specialized field substantially add to the book. A complete evaluation of recent clinical studies helps the reader make valid conclusions about the state of the art in regional antineoplastic therapy.

The first chapter explains the general principles of regional antineoplastic drug delivery. Therapeutic goals, rationale, and pharmacokinetics are presented. This information sets the stage for the other chapters.

The next five chapters cover the major areas of clinical activity in regional antineoplastic drug delivery. These chapters include discussions on regional antineoplastic therapy of tumors confined to the liver; regional therapy of tumors outside the liver; intraperitoneal therapy of ovarian cancer, gastrointestinal malignancies, and peritoneal mesothelioma; intravesical therapy for superficial bladder cancer; and intrathecal therapy for leukemia, lymphoma, and meningeal carcinomatosis. Each chapter defines the clinical problem and provides a therapeutic rationale for the specific malignancy. Study design serves as the basis for discussing results of clinical studies. Each chapter also contains a summary of the data presented.

The last chapter of the book contains an interesting discussion of the cost-effectiveness of regional versus systemic cytotoxic drug therapy. The strengths and weaknesses of various therapeutic endpoints are presented, and a model for evaluating costs versus effectiveness in colon cancer metastatic to the liver is developed.

I have only one criticism of the book: It lacks technical information on the regional administration of antineoplastics. However, the exhaustive list of references provides the reader with the tools for obtaining further methodological details.

This book is well written and researched. It would be a worthwhile addition to the library of any pharmacist who specializes in oncology or works in a hospital that has an average-to-advanced oncology service or an emphasis on regional antineoplastic drug therapy.

Reviewed by J. Kelly Martin, Jr., Oncology Specialist, St. Joseph Hospital and Health Care Center, 1718 South I Street, P.O. Box 2197, Tacoma, WA 98401.

Books Received

Books are listed as soon as received; selected books may be reviewed in Book Reviews in subsequent issues.

Compendium of Drug Therapy, Eleventh Edition, edited by Excerpta Medica, Inc. Published by CORE Publishing Division, Excerpta Medica, Inc., 3131 Princeton Pike, Building 2A, Lawrenceville, NJ 08648, 1991. 1451 p. Price $49.95.

Neurotransmitters and Drugs, Third Edition, by Zygmunt L. Kruk and Christopher J. Pycock. Published by Chapman & Hall, 29 West 35th Street, New York, NY 10001, 1991. vii + 204 p. Price $25 (U.S.), $31.50 (Canada).

***N*-Oxidation of Drugs: Biochemistry, Pharmacology, Toxicology,** edited by P. Hlavica and L. A. Damani. Published by Chapman & Hall, 29 West 35th Street, New York, NY 10001, 1991. xx + 487 p. Price $165 (U.S.), $206.50 (Canada).

Advertising Index

American Lung Association
Institutional, 898
American Society of Hospital Pharmacists
AHFS Drug Information 92, 978
ASHP Membership, 979
ASHP Software, 967
CiteSearch, 913
Concepts in Clinical Pharmacokinetics, 969
Criteria for Drug Use Evaluation, Volumes 1 and 2, 952
Guidelines for Administration of Intravenous Medications to Pediatric Patients, 990
Safe Handling of Cytotoxic and Hazardous Drugs, 945
Amgen Inc.
Epogen, 961-965
Neupogen, 899-908
ASHP Research and Education Foundation
Institutional, 977
Burroughs Wellcome Company
Exosurf Neonatal, 971-975
Eisenhower Medical Center
Position Available, 954
National Foundation for Infectious Diseases
National Forum, 910
Roche Laboratories, Division of Hoffmann-La Roche, Inc.
Rocephin, inside back cover, outside back cover
Toledo Hospital
Position Available, 913
The Upjohn Company
Zefazone, 956-958
Wyeth-Ayerst Laboratories, Inc.
Ativan Injection, 894-896
Tubex, inside front cover

Index to Volume 10

The index to Volume 10 is composed of three parts: a subject index, an author index, and an advertising index.

The subject index is made up mainly of terms constructed by *International Pharmaceutical Abstracts*. The *IPA* index is an alphabetical, open-ended, controlled-vocabulary index that makes use of standardized headings. (The primary index terms for each article are listed routinely in *Clinical Pharmacy* as "index terms" after abstracts.) *IPA* covers all authored papers and editorials in *Clinical Pharmacy*, as well as selected letters and news reports. The subject index also notes all regular columns and, under the respective column headings, the titles of items in the "News," "Therapy Consultation," "Letters," "Editorials," and "Book Reviews" sections. The subject index also contains, under the heading "Correction Notices," the title and issue of publication of items for which corrections were printed, as well as the page numbers on which the corrections appear.

Issue	*Pages*	*Issue*	*Pages*
January	1–80	July	483–566
February	81–160	August	567–650
March	161–246	September	651–730
April	247–318	October	731–806
May	319–404	November	807–890
June	405–482	December	891–990

Subject Index

A

Absorption
glyburide; effects, age, 532
triazolam; interactions, ranitidine, 539
Acetaminophen
osteoarthritis; therapy, geriatrics, ulcer history, 740
pain; therapy, codeine allergies, 658
poisoning; overdose, acetylcysteine therapy, 765
Acetazolamide; epilepsy; therapy, review, 335
Acetimidoquinone; metabolites; acetaminophen, toxicity, 765
Acetylcholinesterase inhibitors; Alzheimer's disease; therapy, mechanism of action, review, 447
Acetylcysteine; therapy; acetaminophen overdose, 765
***N*-Acetylimidoquinone,** see **Acetimidoquinone**
***N*-Acetyl-D,L-penicillamine;** antidotes; mercury poisoning, pediatrics, 213
Achlorhydria; glutamic acid hydrochloride; effects, gastric pH, 866
***Acinetobacter* species;** resistance; ceftazidime, pneumonia, 49
Acquired immunodeficiency syndrome
aminoglycosides; pharmacokinetics, 784
pentamidine; toxicity, pancreatitis, hemophilia, 56
therapy; *Mycobacterium avium* complex, review, 280; research, AIDS conference, 809
Acyclovir; herpes zoster; and chickenpox, therapy, HIV infections, 301
Acyclovir sodium; herpes zoster; and chickenpox, therapy, HIV infections, 301
Adrenergic agents, see **Sympathomimetic agents**
Adsorbents; charcoal activated; therapy, impaired phenytoin metabolism, liver diseases, 711
Adverse drug reactions report form, 71, 151, 233, 311, 395, 479, 555, 641, 727, 801, 881, 959
Adverse reactions, see **Drugs, adverse reactions**
Advertising Index, 80, 160, 246, 318, 404, 482, 558, 650, 730, 806, 890, 976
Age; geriatrics; glyburide pharmacokinetics, 532
AIDS, see **Acquired immunodeficiency syndrome**
Albumin human; nutrition; parenteral, supplements, dosage predictions, pediatrics, 704
Alcohols, cetyl; combination, colfosceril palmitate, tyloxapol; vs. beractant, therapeutic equivalency, 909
Alfentanil; pharmacology; clinical uses, review, 581
Alfentanil hydrochloride; use; review, criteria, quality assurance programs, 635
Alglucerase; marketing; FDA approvals, 496
Allergies
codeine; alternative analgesics, 658
latex; adverse reactions, FDA recommendations, 417
Alteplase; comparison, anistreplase, streptokinase; myocardial infarction therapy, 486
Alzheimer's disease; therapy; mechanism of action, review, 447
Ambulatory care; hypertension; monitoring, devices, assessment, 175
Amikacin
Mycobacterium avium complex; therapy, AIDS, review, 280
resistance; gram-negative bacteria, in vitro, 544
Amino acids; Alzheimer's disease; therapy, mechanism of action, review, 447
Aminoglycosides
amikacin; *Mycobacterium avium* complex, AIDS, 280; resistance, gram-negative bacteria, in vitro, 544
gentamicin; dosage predictions, pharmacokinetics, methodology, 706; renal function estimation, 931; pharmacokinetics; AIDS, 784
Anabolic agents; steroids; reclassification, controlled substances, 417
Anabolic Steroids Act of 1990; laws; reclassification, controlled substances, 417
Analgesics and antipyretics
acetaminophen; osteoarthritis therapy, geriatrics, ulcer history, 740; overdose, acetylcysteine therapy, 765
alfentanil hydrochloride; DUE criteria, quality assurance programs, 635; review, 581
codeine; allergies, alternative therapies, 658
fentanyl; FDA approvals, transdermal patches, pain therapy, 9; review, 581
fentanyl citrate; DUE criteria, quality assurance programs, 635
ketorolac tromethamine; DUE criteria, 715
pain; postoperative, therapy, continuous epidural infusions, 745; therapy, pediatrics, 667
sufentanil; review, 581
sufentanil citrate; DUE criteria, quality assurance programs, 635
therapy; alternatives, codeine allergies, 658
Androgens; danazol; endometriosis therapy, 518
Anemia; epoetin; therapy, kidney failure, DUE criteria, 143, 303
Anesthetics, local
pain; postoperative, therapy, continuous epidural infusions, 745; therapy, pediatrics, 667
Angina pectoris; cardiac drugs; unstable, therapy, 825
Angiotensin-converting enzyme inhibitors
heart failure; congestive, therapy, diastolic dysfunction, 850
kidney diseases; therapy, 25
Anistreplase; comparison, alteplase, streptokinase; myocardial infarction therapy, 486
Antacids; use; evaluation, stress ulcer prophylaxis, criteria, 787
Antianemia drugs; epoetin; DUE criteria, quality assurance programs, 143, 303
Antiarrhythmic drugs, see **Cardiac drugs**
Antibiotics
Mycobacterium avium complex; therapy, AIDS, review, 280
imipenem; susceptibility, amikacin-resistant isolates, in vitro, 544
vancomycin; dosage guidelines, neonates, 129
vancomycin hydrochloride; blood levels, half-life, hepatic and renal dysfunction, 297
Antibodies; monoclonal; radionuclides, immunotherapy, neoplasms, 359
Anticoagulants
heparin; i.v. infusion sites, toxicity, 630; thromboembolism therapy, guidelines, 503
warfarin; interactions, ciprofloxacin, PT effects, lack, 136; nomograms, dosage, predictions, vs. computers, 923; thromboembolism therapy, guidelines, 503
Anticonvulsants
epilepsy; therapy, review, 335
phenytoin; blood levels, effects, ultrafiltration and freezing, 132; dosage calculations, black African and Indian children, 928
phenytoin sodium; impaired metabolism, liver diseases, activated charcoal therapy, 711
valproate sodium; syrups, availability, vs. valproic acid emulsions, 382
valproic acid; emulsions, availability, vs. valproate sodium syrup, 382
Antidepressants; tricyclic; panic disorders therapy, 893
Antidiabetic agents; glyburide; pharmacokinetics, effects, age, 532
Antidotes
acetylcysteine; acetaminophen overdose, 765
digoxin immune Fab; toxicity, digoxin, 823
heavy-metal antagonists; poisoning, pediatrics, 213
Antiemetics
ondansetron hydrochloride; DUE criteria, quality assurance programs, 471; pharmacology, review, 430; prophylaxis, chemotherapy toxicity, FDA approvals, 249
Antifungals
fluconazole; DUE criteria, quality assurance programs, 222; pharmacology, review, 179
ketoconazole; Cushing's syndrome therapy, 12
Anti-infective agents
Mycobacterium avium complex; combined therapy, AIDS, review, 280
pentamidine; toxicity, pancreatitis, AIDS, 56
pentamidine isethionate; infusions, adverse reactions, facial numbness, 257
Anti-inflammatory agents
aspirin; osteoarthritis therapy, geriatrics, ulcer history, 740
etodolac; osteoarthritis therapy, FDA approvals, 416

ibuprofen; interactions, misoprostol, ranitidine, lack, 870; osteoarthritis therapy, geriatrics, ulcer history, 740
nonsteroidal; pain therapy, codeine allergies, 658
salsalate; osteoarthritis therapy, geriatrics, ulcer history, 740
scleroderma; systemic, therapy, 14
Antilipemic agents
cholestyramine resin; palatability, oral formulations, vehicles, 138
colestipol hydrochloride; palatability, oral formulations, vehicles, 138
hyperlipidemia; therapy, protocols, 943
Antimanic agents
lithium; neutropenia therapy, HIV infections, review, 268
lithium carbonate; pharmacokinetics, methodology, models, 376
Antineoplastic agents
fludarabine phosphate; FDA approvals, 496
fluorouracil and levamisole; colonic neoplasms, combined therapy, 95
interleukin 2; renal cell carcinoma, single agent therapy, FDA denial, 141; therapy, review, 110
levamisole; colorectal neoplasms therapy, review, 95
toxicity; nausea and vomiting, ondansetron prophylaxis, 430; nausea and vomiting, ondansetron therapy, DUE criteria, 471; neutropenia, filgrastim prophylaxis, DUE criteria, 950; neutropenia, filgrastim prophylaxis, FDA approvals, 321; ondansetron prophylaxis, FDA approvals, 249
Antithyroid drugs; propylthiouracil; hyperthyroidism therapy, mercury poisoning, 742
Antivirals
acyclovir; chickenpox, herpes zoster therapy, HIV infections, 301
zidovudine; toxicity, neutropenia, HIV infections, review, 268
Anxiolytics, sedatives and hypnotics
chloral hydrate; interactions, furosemide, pediatrics, 385
lorazepam; dosage, pediatrics, 625
midazolam hydrochloride; DUE criteria, quality assurance programs, 388
triazolam; interactions, ranitidine, pharmacokinetics, 539
Arecoline; Alzheimer's disease; therapy, mechanism of action, review, 447
Arrhythmia
antiarrhythmic agents; therapy, blood levels, monitoring, 211
cardiac drugs; ventricular, therapy, review, 195
encainide hydrochloride; toxicity, product withdrawal, 897
moricizine; therapy, DUE criteria, 873
therapy; ventricular, pharmacists, monitoring, 210
Asians; psychotherapeutic agents; pharmacokinetics, vs. Caucasians, 467
Aspirin
alone and with flurbiprofen; effects, platelet aggregation, 935
and propoxyphene; pain therapy, codeine allergies, 658
and thrombolytic agents; myocardial infarction therapy, 486
myocardial infarction; prophylaxis, angina pectoris, 825
osteoarthritis; therapy, geriatrics, ulcer history, 740
Asthma; therapy; pediatrics, 685
Availability, drugs, see **Drugs, availability**

B

Barbiturates; delirium; therapy, intensive-care units, 456
Benazepril hydrochloride; marketing; FDA approvals, 739
Benzodiazepines
alone and with haloperidol; delirium therapy, intensive-care units, 456
epilepsy; therapy, review, 335
panic disorders; therapy, 893
pharmacokinetics; Asians vs. Caucasians, 467
Beractant; comparison, alcohols, cetyl, combination, colfosceril palmitate, tyloxapol; therapeutic equivalency, 909
Beverages; vehicles; cholestyramine, colestipol administration, palatability, 138
Bioavailability, see **Drugs, availability**
Blood derivatives; albumin human; dosage predictions, parenteral supplements, pediatrics, 704
Blood levels
acetaminophen; overdose, monitoring, 765
albumin human; dosage predictions, pediatrics, 704
antiarrhythmic agents; therapy, monitoring, 211
benzodiazepines; Asians vs. Caucasians, 467
cardiac drugs; ventricular arrhythmia therapy, 195
digoxin; toxicity, digoxin immune Fab retreatment, immunogenicity, 823
gentamicin; dosage, predictions, pharmacokinetics, 706
glyburide; pharmacokinetics, effects, age, 532
lead; succimer therapy, FDA restrictions, 942
lithium; pharmacokinetics, methodology, models, 376
mercury; poisoning, pediatrics, 213
phenytoin; dosage calculations, black African and Indian children, 928; effects, ultrafiltration and freezing, 132; high, impaired metabolism, 711
recainam hydrochloride; pharmacokinetics, computer programs, MS-DOS vs. Macintosh, 206
triazolam; interactions, ranitidine, 539
valproic acid; availability, stability, emulsions, 382
vancomycin; dosage guidelines, neonates, 129; half-life, hepatic and renal dysfunction, 297
Bloodletting; hemochromatosis; therapy, 775
Book Reviews, 80, 159, 239, 316, 649, 729, 805, 885, 970
Biopharmaceutics and Clinical Pharmacokinetics, Fourth Edition, 649
Cancer Chemotherapy by Infusion, Second Edition, 239
Clinical Pharmacology of Psychotherapeutic Drugs, Third Edition, 159
Diseases of the Nose, Throat, Ear, Head, and Neck, Fourteenth Edition, 729
Drug Interactions & Updates, 1991, 805
Drug Safety in Pregnancy, 650
Drugs in Pregnancy and Lactation, Third Edition, 316
Field Drug Reference for Emergency Care Providers, 80
Goodman and Gilman's The Pharmacological Basis of Therapeutics, 8th edition, 317
Handbook of Drug Therapy in Liver and Kidney Disease, 885
Handbook of Psychiatric Emergencies, 730
Infections in Intravenous Drug Abusers, 805
Manual of Clinical Microbiology, Fifth Edition, 885
Patient Compliance in Medical Practice and Clinical Trials, 970
Pharmacological Treatment of Endocrinopathies: Bone Disease, Kidney Stones and Related Disorders, 890
Poisoning and Drug Overdose, 243
Regional Antineoplastic Drug Delivery in the Management of Malignant Disease, 976
Books Received, 246, 318, 482, 650, 806, 890, 976
Botulinum toxin type A; dystonia; therapy, 88
Bristol Laboratories; encainide hydrochloride; product withdrawal, toxicity, 897
Bromocriptine; restless legs; therapy, nocturnal, 427
Bronchodilators; cromolyn sodium; asthma therapy, pediatrics, 685

C

Calcium antagonists
concomitant therapy, 630
heart failure; congestive, therapy, diastolic dysfunction, 850
proteinuria; therapy, diabetic nephropathies, 862
Calcium regulators; gallium nitrate; hypercalcemia therapy, FDA approvals, 573
Calculations; phenytoin; dosage, black African and Indian children, 928
Cancer, see **Antineoplastic agents**
Cancer drugs, see **Antineoplastic agents**
Candidiasis; fluconazole; therapy, DUE criteria, 222
Captopril
concomitant therapy, 500
kidney diseases; therapy, 25
Carbamazepine
epilepsy; therapy, review, 335
restless legs; therapy, nocturnal, 427
Carcinoma; interleukin 2; renal cell, single agent therapy, FDA denial, 141; renal cell, therapy, 110
Cardiac drugs
angina pectoris; unstable, therapy, 825
antiarrhythmic agents; therapy, blood levels, monitoring, 211; therapy, monitoring, pharmacists, 210
arrhythmia; ventricular, therapy, review, 195
digoxin; toxicity, digoxin immune Fab retreatment, immunogenicity, 823
encainide hydrochloride; product withdrawal, toxicity, 897
moricizine; arrhythmia therapy, DUE criteria, 873
recainam hydrochloride; pharmacokinetics, computer programs, MS-DOS vs. Macintosh, 206
Carisoprodol; muscle cramp; therapy, nocturnal leg cramps, 427
Caucasians; psychotherapeutic agents; pharmacokinetics, vs. Asians, 467
Ceftazidime
comparison, ciprofloxacin lactate; therapy, nosocomial pneumonia and urinary tract infections, 49
effects; amikacin-resistant isolates, in vitro, 544
Cephalosporins; ceftazidime; susceptibility, amikacin-resistant isolates, in vitro, 544; vs. ciprofloxacin, pneumonia and urinary tract infections therapy, 49
Charcoal activated; therapy; impaired phenytoin excretion, liver diseases, 711
Chickenpox; acyclovir; therapy, prophylaxis, HIV infections, 301
Chloral hydrate; interactions; furosemide, pediatrics, 385
Cholestyramine, see **Cholestyramine resin**
Cholestyramine resin
hyperlipidemia; therapy, protocols, 943
palatability; oral formulations, vehicles, preferences, 138
Choline; Alzheimer's disease; therapy, mechanism of action, review, 447
Ciprofloxacin; effects; amikacin-resistant isolates, in vitro, 544
Ciprofloxacin hydrochloride; interactions; warfarin, PT effects, lack, 136
Ciprofloxacin lactate; comparison, ceftazidime; therapy, nosocomial pneumonia and urinary tract infections, 49
Classification; steroids; anabolic, controlled substances, 417
Clearance, see **Excretion**
Clindamycin phosphate; concomitant therapy, 931
Clinical Pharmacy
acknowledgment to reviewers—October 1, 1990, to September 30, 1991, 946
instructions for submitting computer disks with revised manuscripts, 62
procedure for submission of manuscripts to journals published by the American Society of Hospital Pharmacists, 60
Clinical studies
meta-analysis; health data, applications and problems, 4
ondansetron hydrochloride; prophylaxis, antineoplastics toxicity, 430
Codeine; allergies; alternative analgesics, 658
Colestipol; hyperlipidemia; therapy, protocols, 943
Colestipol hydrochloride; palatability; oral formulations, vehicles, preferences, 138
Colfosceril palmitate; combination, alcohols, cetyl, tyloxapol; vs. beractant, therapeutic equivalency, 909
Colonic neoplasms
fluorouracil and levamisole; combined therapy, review, 95
levamisole and fluorouracil; combined therapy, review, 95
Colony-stimulating factors
filgrastim; DUE criteria, 950
neutropenia; therapy, HIV infections, review, 268
sargramostim; DUE criteria, 947
Colorectal neoplasms
interleukin 2; therapy, 110
levamisole; therapy, review, 95
Combined therapy
aspirin and thrombolytic agents; myocardial infarction, effects, mortality, 486
fluorouracil and levamisole; colonic neoplasms, review, 95
levamisole and fluorouracil; colonic neoplasms, review, 95
thrombolytic agents and aspirin; myocardial infarction, effects, mortality, 486
Commentary, 943
Compliance; patients; deferoxamine therapy, hemochromatosis, 775
Computers; programs; MS-DOS vs. Macintosh, recainam pharmacokinetics, 206; NONMEM, lithium pharmacokinetics, 376; warfarin dosage, predictions, vs. nomogram, 923
Contraceptives, oral; endometriosis; therapy, 518
Contraindications
botulinum toxin type A, 88
drugs; lactation, 594
Controlled substances; steroids; anabolic, reclassification, 417
Copper Cu 67; radionuclides; monoclonal antibodies, neoplasms, 359
Correction Notices, 261, 429, 501, 824, 913
Attention-deficit hyperactivity disorder (Aug 1990, Therapy Review), 261
Criteria for use of ketorolac tromethamine in adult

inpatients and outpatients (Sep 1991, DUE Criteria), 913
Current issues in the treatment of epilepsy (May 1991, Therapy Review), 501
Hypoprothrombinemic effect of warfarin not influenced by ciprofloxacin (Feb 1991, Research Notes), 429
Intravenous quinidine recommended for severe *Plasmodium falciparum* malaria; injectable quinine discontinued by CDC Drug Service (Sep 1991, News), 913
Management of postoperative pain by continuous epidural infusion of analgesics (Oct 1991, Therapy Review), 824
Olsalazine approved for use in ulcerative colitis (Dec 1990, News), 261
Costs
deferoxamine mesylate; hemochromatosis therapy, 775
filgrastim; prophylaxis, neutropenia, FDA approvals, 321
interleukin 2; renal cell carcinoma, single agent therapy, FDA denial, 141
pulmonary surfactants; respiratory distress syndrome therapy, 909
sargramostim, 411
thrombolytic agents; myocardial infarction therapy, 486
***CP* Continuing Education**, 68, 147, 228, 309, 392, 474, 552, 638, 718, 792, 876, 953
Creatinine; clearance; gentamicin excretion, renal function estimation, 931; predictions, lithium pharmacokinetics, models, 376
Cromolyn sodium; asthma; therapy, pediatrics, 685
Current Literature, 74, 154, 235, 313, 397, 478, 558, 644, 726, 803, 880, 966
Cushing's syndrome; ketoconazole; therapy, mechanism of action, 12
Cytokines; *Mycobacterium avium* complex; therapy, AIDS, review, 280
Cytotoxic agents, see **Antineoplastic agents**

D

Danazol; endometriosis; therapy, 518
Deferoxamine mesylate; hemochromatosis; therapy, 775
Delirium; therapy; review, intensive-care units, 456
Desmopressin acetate; dosage; high, mechanism of action, antidiuretic effects, 912
Devices
blood pressure; ambulatory care, monitoring, assessment, 175
infusion pumps; terbutaline, preterm labor, home therapy, 292
medical; latex, adverse reactions, FDA recommendations, 417
Diabetes mellitus; calcium antagonists; diabetic nephropathies, proteinuria therapy, 862
Diabetic nephropathies; calcium antagonists; proteinuria therapy, diabetes mellitus, 862
Digoxin; toxicity; therapy, digoxin immune Fab retreatment, immunogenicity, 823
Digoxin immune Fab; therapy; immunogenicity, retreatment, 823
Diltiazem
angina pectoris; unstable, therapy, 825
proteinuria; therapy, diabetic nephropathies, 862
Dimercaprol; antidotes; mercury poisoning, pediatrics, 213
Diuretics
and doxazosin mesylate; hypertension therapy, 9
furosemide; interactions, chloral hydrate, pediatrics, 385
heart failure; congestive, therapy, diastolic dysfunction, 850
Dosage
acyclovir; chickenpox, herpes zoster therapy, HIV infections, 301
albumin human; predictions, equations, parenteral supplements, pediatrics, 704
alfentanil hydrochloride; DUE criteria, 635
analgesics; pain therapy, pediatrics, 667
benazepril hydrochloride, 739
charcoal activated; multiple dose therapy, phenytoin toxicity, liver diseases, 711
desmopressin acetate; high, mechanism of action, antidiuretic effects, 912
digoxin immune Fab, 823
doxazosin mesylate; hypertension, therapy, 9
enalapril maleate; DUE criteria, 63
epoetin; DUE criteria, 143, 303
etodolac, 416
fentanyl; transdermal patches, pain therapy, 9
fentanyl citrate; DUE criteria, 635
filgrastim, 321; neutropenia prophylaxis, chemotherapy, DUE criteria, 950
fluconazole; DUE criteria, 222
fludarabine phosphate, 496
gallium nitrate, 573
gastrointestinal drugs; stress ulcer prophylaxis, DUE criteria, 787
gentamicin; predictions, pharmacokinetics, methodology, 706
heparin; thromboembolism therapy, guidelines, 503
hetastarch; DUE criteria, 549
interleukin 2; neoplasms therapy, 110
isradipine, 573
ketorolac tromethamine; DUE criteria, 715
levamisole; colorectal neoplasms therapy, 95
lorazepam; sedation, amnesia, pediatrics, 625
midazolam hydrochloride; DUE criteria, 388
misoprostol; DUE criteria, 307
moricizine; arrhythmia therapy, DUE criteria, 873
ondansetron hydrochloride, 249; DUE criteria, 471; review, 430
overdose; acetaminophen, acetylcysteine therapy, 765
phenytoin; calculations, black African and Indian children, 928
psychotherapeutic agents; Asians vs. Caucasians, 467
pulmonary surfactants; respiratory distress syndrome therapy, 909
radiopharmaceuticals; monoclonal antibodies, neoplasms, 359
ramipril, 573
sargramostim, 411; DUE criteria, 947
skeletal muscle relaxants; mechanically ventilated patients, 32
succimer; lead poisoning, therapy, 914
sufentanil citrate; DUE criteria, 635
terbutaline sulfate; preterm labor, home infusion therapy, 292
vancomycin; guidelines, neonates, 129
vancomycin hydrochloride; hepatic and renal dysfunction, 297
warfarin; predictions, nomograms vs. computers, 923; thromboembolism therapy, guidelines, 503
Dosage forms
etodolac, 416
filgrastim, 321
ondansetron hydrochloride, 249
sargramostim, 411
Dosage schedules
acetylcysteine; therapy, acetaminophen overdose, 765
analgesics; continuous epidural infusions, postoperative pain, 745
anticonvulsants; epilepsy therapy, long term, 335
aspirin and flurbiprofen; platelet aggregation effects, 935
flurbiprofen and aspirin; platelet aggregation effects, 935
interleukin 2; renal cell carcinoma, single agent therapy, FDA denial, 141
Doxazosin mesylate; hypertension; therapy, FDA approvals, 9
Drug administration
cholestyramine resin; beverages, palatability, 138
colestipol hydrochloride; beverages, palatability, 138
self-medication; terbutaline infusion, preterm labor therapy, 292
succimer; lead poisoning, therapy, 914
thrombolytic agents; comparisons, myocardial infarction therapy, 486
Drug administration rate; injections; continuous vs. intermittent infusion, toxicity, 630
Drug administration routes
asthma; acute vs. prophylactic therapy, pediatrics, 685
deferoxamine mesylate; s.c., i.v., hemochromatosis therapy, 775
epidural; analgesics, continuous epidural infusions, postoperative pain, 745
pentamidine isethionate; infusions, adverse reactions, facial numbness, 257
terbutaline sulfate; subcutaneous infusion, preterm labor therapy, 292
triazolam; oral vs. i.v., interactions, ranitidine, pharmacokinetics, 539
Drug administration sites; intravenous; toxicity, extravasation, phlebitis, 630
Drug interactions
chloral hydrate and furosemide; pediatrics, 385
ciprofloxacin hydrochloride and warfarin; PT effects, lack, 136
fluconazole; review, 179
flurbiprofen and aspirin; effects, platelet aggregation, lack, 935
furosemide and chloral hydrate; pediatrics, 385
ibuprofen and misoprostol or ranitidine hydrochloride; lack, 870
misoprostol and ibuprofen; lack, 870
ranitidine hydrochloride and ibuprofen; lack, 870
ranitidine hydrochloride and triazolam; pharmacokinetics, 539
triazolam and ranitidine hydrochloride; pharmacokinetics, 539
warfarin and ciprofloxacin hydrochloride; PT effects, lack, 136
Drug interactions therapy; aspirin and flurbiprofen; effects, platelet aggregation, lack, 935
Drug Reaction Alerts, 74, 154, 235, 313, 397, 478, 558, 644, 726, 803, 880, 966
Drugs, adverse reactions
codeine; allergies, alternative analgesics, 658
latex; allergies, FDA recommendations, 417
pentamidine isethionate; facial numbness, infusions, 257
vaccines; Vaccine Adverse Event Reporting System, 9
Drugs, availability
triazolam; interactions, ranitidine, 539
valproate sodium; syrups, vs. valproic acid emulsions, 382
valproic acid; emulsions, vs. valproate sodium syrup, 382
Drugs, body distribution
aminoglycosides; AIDS, 784
glyburide; effects, age, 532
lithium; pharmacokinetics, methodology, models, 376
Drugs, clinical effectiveness
antiarrhythmic agents; therapy, blood levels, monitoring, 211
drugs, nonprescription; lack, product withdrawal, FDA list, 88
meta-analysis; methodology, applications and problems, 4
thrombolytic agents; myocardial infarction therapy, 486
Drugs, nonprescription; product withdrawal; ingredients, FDA list, 88
Drug use
evaluation; filgrastim, neutropenia prophylaxis, criteria, 950; gastrointestinal drugs, stress ulcer prophylaxis, criteria, 787; ketorolac, criteria, 715; moricizine, arrhythmia therapy, criteria, 873; sargramostim, criteria, 947
review; alfentanil, fentanyl, sufentanil, criteria, quality assurance programs, 635; enalapril, criteria, quality assurance programs, 63; epoetin, criteria, quality assurance programs, 143, 303; fluconazole, criteria, quality assurance programs, 222; hetastarch, criteria, quality assurance programs, 549; midazolam, criteria, quality assurance programs, 388; misoprostol, criteria, quality assurance programs, 307; ondansetron, criteria, quality assurance programs, 471
DUE Criteria, 63, 143, 222, 303, 388, 471, 549, 635, 715, 787, 873, 947
enalapril maleate, 63
epoetin, 143, 303
fentanyl citrate, sufentanil citrate, and alfentanil hydrochloride, 635
filgrastim, 950
fluconazole, 222
hetastarch, 549
ketorolac tromethamine, 715
midazolam hydrochloride, 388
misoprostol, 307
moricizine, 873
ondansetron hydrochloride, 471
sargramostim, 947
stress ulcer prophylaxis in intensive-care patients, 787
Dystonia; botulinum toxin type A; therapy, 88

E

Edetate calcium disodium; therapy; mercury poisoning, 742
Editorials, 141, 210, 942
Antiarrhythmic monitoring: misplaced emphasis, 211
Recombinant interleukin-2 and the quest for FDA approval, 141
Succimer: controversial issues involving the release of a new product, 942
Trials and tribulations of evaluating ventricular arrhythmias, 210
Education
acquired immunodeficiency syndrome; therapy, re-

search, AIDS conference, 809
panic disorders; awareness, therapy, 893
Elimination, see **Metabolism**
Emulsions; valproic acid; stability, availability, vs. valproate sodium syrup, 382
Enalapril maleate
kidney diseases; therapy, 25
use; review, criteria, quality assurance programs, 63
Encainide hydrochloride; product withdrawal; toxicity, 897
Endometriosis; therapy, 518
Enterobacter cloacae; resistance; ceftazidime, pneumonia, 49
Enzymes; alglucerase; replacement therapy, Gaucher's disease, FDA approvals, 496
Epilepsy; therapy; review, 335
Epoetin; use; review, criteria, quality assurance programs, 143, 303
Equations
albumin human; dosage, predictions, pediatrics, 704
phenytoin; dosage, pediatrics, pharmacogenetics, 928
Equivalency
valproate sodium; syrups, availability, vs. valproic acid emulsions, 382
valproic acid; emulsions, availability, vs. valproate sodium syrup, 382
Equivalency, generic; thioridazine hydrochloride; brands, comparison, efficacy, quality of life, 938
Equivalency, therapeutic; pulmonary surfactants; comparison, respiratory distress syndrome therapy, 909
Ethnic groups; Hispanic Americans; psychotherapeutic agents, pharmacogenetics, 467
Ethosuximide; epilepsy; therapy, review, 335
Etodolac; marketing; FDA approvals, osteoarthritis therapy, 416
Excretion
aminoglycosides; AIDS, 784
benzodiazepines; clearance, Asians vs. Caucasians, 467
drugs; lactation, review, 594
gentamicin; renal function estimation, 931
glyburide; effects, age, 532
lithium; clearance, methodology, models, 376
phenytoin sodium; impaired, liver diseases, activated charcoal therapy, 711
vancomycin; hepatic and renal dysfunction, 297
Extravasation; injections; i.v. infusion sites, toxicity, 630

F

Fentanyl
patches transdermal; pain therapy, FDA approvals, 9
pharmacology; clinical uses, review, 581
Fentanyl citrate; use; review, criteria, quality assurance programs, 635
Filgrastim
approvals; FDA, prophylaxis, neutropenia, chemotherapy, 321
use; evaluation, neutropenia prophylaxis, criteria, 950
Filters; ultra; products, effects, phenytoin blood levels, 132
Filtration; ultra; methods, phenytoin blood levels, 132
Fluconazole
pharmacology; review, 179
use; review, criteria, quality assurance programs, 222
Fludarabine phosphate; marketing; FDA approvals, 496
Fluorouracil; and levamisole; colonic neoplasms, combined therapy, 95
Flurbiprofen; alone and with aspirin; effects, platelet aggregation, 935
Food and Drug Administration (U.S.)
approvals; alglucerase marketing, 496; benazepril marketing, 739; doxazosin, hypertension therapy, 9; etodolac marketing, 416; fentanyl, transdermal patches, marketing, pain therapy, 9; filgrastim marketing, 321; fludarabine marketing, 496; gallium marketing, 573; isradipine, ramipril, marketing, 573; ondansetron, 249; sargramostim marketing, 411; succimer marketing, controversies, 942
drugs, nonprescription; ingredients, product withdrawal, list, 88
interleukin 2; renal cell carcinoma, single agent therapy, FDA denial, 141
latex; medical devices, allergies, recommendations, 417
Formulations
cholestyramine resin; oral, palatability, vehicles, 138
colestipol hydrochloride; oral, palatability, vehicles, 138
Freezing; effects; phenytoin blood levels, ultrafiltration methods, 132
5-FU, see **Fluorouracil**
Furosemide; interactions; chloral hydrate, pediatrics, 385

G

Gallium nitrate; marketing; FDA approvals, 573
Gastrointestinal drugs
glutamic acid hydrochloride; effects, gastric pH, 866
histamine H_2 antagonists; use, evaluation, stress ulcer prophylaxis, criteria, 787
misoprostol; DUE criteria, quality assurance programs, 307; interactions, ibuprofen, lack, 870
ranitidine; peptic ulcers, prophylaxis, osteoarthritis, geriatrics, 740
ranitidine hydrochloride; interactions, ibuprofen, lack, 870; interactions, triazolam, pharmacokinetics, 539
scleroderma; systemic, therapy, 14
sucralfate; stress ulcer prophylaxis, DUE criteria, 787
Gaucher's disease; alglucerase; therapy, FDA approvals, 496
Gentamicin
dosage; predictions, pharmacokinetics, methodology, 706
excretion; renal function estimation, 931
Geriatrics; osteoarthritis; therapy, ulcer history, 740
Globulin immune; neutropenia; therapy, HIV infections, review, 268
Glutamic acid hydrochloride; effects; gastric pH, 866
Glyburide; pharmacokinetics; effects, age, 532
Goserelin agonists; nafarelin; endometriosis therapy, 518
Guidelines, treatment, see **Protocols**

H

Half-life
aminoglycosides; AIDS, 784
vancomycin; blood levels, hepatic and renal dysfunction, 297
Haloperidol; alone and with benzodiazepines; delirium therapy, intensive-care units, 456
Health-benefit programs; reimbursement; meta-analysis, 4
Health care; home; terbutaline infusion, preterm labor therapy, 292
Health professions; latex; medical devices, allergies, FDA recommendations, 417
Heavy metal antagonists
N-acetyl-D,L-penicillamine; mercury poisoning, pediatrics, 213
deferoxamine mesylate; hemochromatosis therapy, 775
dimercaprol; mercury poisoning, pediatrics, 213
edetate calcium disodium; therapy, mercury poisoning, 742
penicillamine; hepatolenticular degeneration therapy, 839
succimer; FDA approvals, controversies, 942; lead poisoning, therapy, 914
trientine; hepatolenticular degeneration therapy, 839
zinc; hepatolenticular degeneration, maintenance therapy, 839
Hemochromatosis; therapy, 775
Hemophilia; pentamidine; toxicity, pancreatitis, AIDS, 56
Heparin
injections; i.v. infusion sites, toxicity, 630
myocardial infarction; prophylaxis, angina pectoris, 825
thromboembolism; therapy, guidelines, 503
Hepatolenticular degeneration; heavy metal antagonists; therapy, 839
Herpes zoster; acyclovir; therapy, prophylaxis, HIV infections, 301
Hetastarch; use; review, criteria, quality assurance programs, 549
History; skeletal muscle relaxants; review, developments, 32
HIV infections
acyclovir; chickenpox, herpes zoster therapy, HIV infections, 301
therapy; neutropenia, review, 268; research, AIDS conference, 809
Hodgkin's disease; sargramostim; therapy, FDA approvals, 411
Hospitals; intensive-care units; delirium therapy, review, 456; patients, stress ulcer prophylaxis, DUE criteria, 787
Hyperalimentation, see **Nutrition; parenteral**
Hypercalcemia; gallium nitrate; therapy, cancer-related, FDA approvals, 573
Hyperlipidemia; therapy; protocols, National Cholesterol Education Program, 943
Hypertension
benazepril hydrochloride; therapy, FDA approvals, 739
calcium antagonists; therapy, diabetic nephropathies, 862
doxazosin mesylate; therapy, FDA approvals, 9
enalapril maleate; DUE criteria, 63
isradipine; therapy, FDA approvals, 573
labetalol hydrochloride; therapy, pediatrics, 500
ramipril; therapy, FDA approvals, 573
therapy; ambulatory care, monitoring, assessment, 175
Hyperthyroidism; mercury; toxicity, poisoning, 742
Hypotensive agents
benazepril hydrochloride; FDA approvals, 739
doxazosin mesylate; therapy, FDA approvals, 9
enalapril maleate; DUE criteria, quality assurance programs, 63
isradipine; FDA approvals, 573
labetalol hydrochloride; therapy, pediatrics, 500
ramipril; FDA approvals, 573

I

Iatrogenic diseases, see **Drugs, adverse reactions**
Ibuprofen
interactions; misoprostol, ranitidine, lack, 870
osteoarthritis; therapy, geriatrics, ulcer history, 740
Imipenem; effects; amikacin-resistant isolates, in vitro, 544
Immunogenicity; digoxin immune Fab; retreatment, digoxin toxicity, 823
Immunosuppressive agents; scleroderma; systemic, therapy, 14
Immunotherapy
colony-stimulating factors; neutropenia, HIV infections, review, 268
filgrastim; neutropenia prophylaxis, chemotherapy, DUE criteria, 950; prophylaxis, neutropenia, FDA approvals, 321
globulin immune; neutropenia, HIV infections, review, 268
interleukin 2; neoplasms therapy, 110
radionuclides; monoclonal antibodies, neoplasms, 359
sargramostim; DUE criteria, 947; FDA approvals, 411
Incompatibilities; ondansetron hydrochloride; review, 430
Infections; therapy; opportunistic, research, AIDS conference, 809
Infusion devices, see **Devices; infusion pumps**
Injections
analgesics; continuous epidural infusions, postoperative pain, 745
botulinum toxin type A; dystonia therapy, 88
furosemide; interactions, chloral hydrate, pediatrics, 385
gallium nitrate; hypercalcemia therapy, FDA approvals, 573
intravenous; toxicity, extravasation, phlebitis, 630
pentamidine isethionate; infusions, adverse reactions, facial numbness, 257
terbutaline sulfate; subcutaneous infusion, preterm labor therapy, 292
Interleukin 2
approvals; renal cell carcinoma, single agent therapy, FDA denial, 141
neoplasms; therapy, review, 110
Iodine I 125; radionuclides; monoclonal antibodies, neoplasms, 359
Iodine I 131; radionuclides; monoclonal antibodies, neoplasms, 359
Isradipine; marketing; FDA approvals, 573

K

Ketoconazole; Cushing's syndrome; therapy, mechanism of action, 12
Ketorolac tromethamine; use; evaluation, criteria, 715
Kidney diseases; angiotensin-converting-enzyme inhibitors; therapy, 25
Kidney failure; vancomycin hydrochloride; chronic, blood levels, half-life, 297
Klebsiella pneumoniae; resistance; ciprofloxacin, pneumonia, 49

L

Labetalol hydrochloride; hypertension; therapy, pediatrics, 500
Labor; terbutaline sulfate; preterm, home infusion therapy, 292
Lactation; drugs; patient information, excretion, review, 594
Latex; adverse reactions; allergies, FDA recommendations, 417
Laws; Anabolic Steroids Act of 1990; reclassification, controlled substances, 417
Lead; poisoning; succimer therapy, 914; succimer therapy, FDA approvals, controversies, 942
Lecithin; Alzheimer's disease; therapy, mechanism of action, review, 447
Letters, 177, 257, 333, 429, 500, 664, 742, 823, 912
Antimicrobial dosages in guidelines for prevention of bacterial endocarditis, 501
Correction to *AHFS Drug Information 91*, 913
Cryoprecipitate for uremic bleeding, 429
Dosage of antimycobacterial agents, 664
Ethnicity and clozapine-induced agranulocytosis, 743
Hyperthyroidism associated with mercury poisoning, 742
Interferon for genital warts, 177
Inverse relationship between desmopressin dosage and antidiuresis, 912
Labetalol for treatment of hypertension in a child, 500
Laboratory monitoring of heparin therapy, 824
Pentamidine-induced facial numbness, 257
Retreatment with digoxin immune Fab, 823
Valproic acid hepatoxicity in adults and older children, 665
Verapamil and left ventricular hypertrophy, 333
Leukemia
fludarabine phosphate; B-cell, chronic, therapy, FDA approvals, 496
sargramostim; lymphocytic, acute, therapy, FDA approvals, 411
Levamisole; colorectal neoplasms; therapy, review, 95
Lisinopril; kidney diseases; therapy, 25
Lithium; neutropenia; therapy, HIV infections, review, 268
Lithium carbonate; pharmacokinetics; methodology, models, 376
Liver cirrhosis; vancomycin hydrochloride; blood levels, half-life, 297
Liver diseases; phenytoin sodium; impaired metabolism, activated charcoal therapy, 711
Lorazepam; dosage; sedation, amnesia, pediatrics, 625
Lymphoma
radionuclides; monoclonal antibodies, 359
sargramostim; non-Hodgkin's, therapy, FDA approvals, 411

M

Magnesium sulfate; concomitant therapy, 292
Manufacturing; valproic acid; emulsions, availability, fresh vs. stored, 382
Marketing
alglucerase; FDA approvals, 496
benazepril hydrochloride; FDA approvals, 739
doxazosin mesylate; hypertension therapy, FDA approvals, 9
encainide hydrochloride; product withdrawal, toxicity, 897
etodolac; osteoarthritis therapy, FDA approvals, 416
fentanyl; transdermal patches, FDA approvals, pain therapy, 9
filgrastim; prophylaxis, neutropenia, FDA approvals, 321
fludarabine phosphate; FDA approvals, 496
gallium nitrate; FDA approvals, 573
isradipine; FDA approvals, 573
ondansetron hydrochloride; prophylaxis, chemotherapy toxicity, FDA approvals, 249
product withdrawal; nonprescription drugs, FDA list, 88
ramipril; FDA approvals, 573
sargramostim; FDA approvals, 411
succimer; FDA approvals, controversies, 942
Mechanism of action
acetylcholinesterase inhibitors; Alzheimer's disease therapy, review, 447
amino acids; Alzheimer's disease therapy, review, 447
analgesics; continuous epidural infusions, postoperative pain, 745; pain therapy, pediatrics, 667
calcium antagonists; proteinuria therapy, diabetic nephropathies, 862
desmopressin acetate; high dose, antidiuretic effects, 912
ketoconazole; Cushing's syndrome therapy, 12
parasympathomimetic agents; Alzheimer's disease therapy, review, 447
Melanoma; interleukin 2; therapy, 110
Memory disorders; therapy; Alzheimer's disease, review, 447
Meningitis; fluconazole; cryptococcal, therapy, DUE criteria, 222
Mercury
poisoning; dimercaprol, *N*-acetyl-D,L-penicillamine, antidotes, pediatrics, 213; toxicity, hyperthyroidism, 742
Metabolism
acetaminophen; acetimidoquinone metabolites, toxicity, 765
phenytoin sodium; impaired, liver diseases, activated charcoal therapy, 711
Metals; mercury; poisoning, hyperthyroidism toxicity, 742; poisoning, pediatrics, 213
Methodology
albumin human; dosage predictions, parenteral supplements, pediatrics, 704
antiarrhythmic agents; therapy, blood levels, monitoring, 211
cardiac drugs; monitoring, ventricular arrhythmia therapy, 195
creatinine; clearance, gentamicin excretion, renal function estimation, 931
gentamicin; dosage predictions, pharmacokinetics, 706
lithium carbonate; pharmacokinetics, models, 376
meta-analysis; health data, applications and problems, 4
pharmacokinetics; computer programs, MS-DOS vs. Macintosh, 206
phenytoin; dosage, pediatrics, pharmacogenetics, 928
warfarin; dosage predictions, nomograms vs. computers, 923
Midazolam hydrochloride; use; review, criteria, quality assurance programs, 388
Misoprostol
interactions; ibuprofen, lack, 870
use; review, criteria, quality assurance programs, 307
Models; pharmacokinetics; recainam, computer programs, MS-DOS vs. Macintosh, 206
Monoamine oxidase inhibitors; panic disorders; therapy, 893
Moricizine; use; evaluation, arrhythmia therapy, criteria, 873
Mortality; myocardial infarction; effects, thrombolytic agents and aspirin, 486
Muscle cramp; therapy; nocturnal leg cramps, 427
***Mycobacterium avium* complex;** therapy; AIDS, review, 280
Myocardial infarction
aspirin and thrombolytic agents; comparisons, therapy, 486
thrombolytic agents; comparisons, therapy, 486

N

Nafarelin; endometriosis; therapy, 518
National Cholesterol Education Program; protocols; hyperlipidemia therapy, 943
Nausea; ondansetron hydrochloride; therapy, DUE criteria, 471
Negroes; psychotherapeutic agents; pharmacogenetics, 467
Neoplasms
radionuclides; monoclonal antibodies, 359
therapy; research, AIDS conference, 809
Neutropenia
filgrastim; prophylaxis, chemotherapy, FDA approvals, 321
therapy; HIV infections, review, 268
News, 4, 88, 167, 249, 321, 411, 486, 569, 653, 733, 809, 893
American Academy of Pediatrics issues recommendations on treatment of Lyme disease, 738
Anabolic steroids reclassified as Schedule III controlled substances, 417
Benazepril approved for treatment of hypertension, 739
Bristol discontinues sales of encainide, 897
CAST II halted because of mortality trends, 897
CDC offers recommendations for folic acid prevention of neural tube defects, 898
CDC publishes guidelines for anergy testing in HIV-infected persons, 653
CDC revises mefloquine dosage recommendations, 417
Changes in federal programs for reporting suspected adverse reactions to vaccines announced, 9
Conference attendees told ISIS-3 shows equal efficacy, safety differences among thrombolytics, 486
Consensus panel considers uses of botulinum toxin, 88
Consensus panel stresses need for greater awareness of panic disorder and its treatment, 893
Consensus report focuses on hypertension during pregnancy, 93
Doxazosin approved as antihypertensive agent, 9
E5 antiendotoxin antibody reduces mortality among subset of patients with gram-negative sepsis, study finds, 897
Enzyme replacement therapy approved for Gaucher's disease, 496
Etodolac approved for marketing in the United States, 416
FDA advisory committee reviews data suggesting ethnic differences in response to zidovudine, recommends no changes in drug use, 326
FDA bans 223 ingredients in nonprescription drug products, 88
Fludarabine approved for marketing, 496
Gallium marketed for treatment of cancer-related hypercalcemia, 573
Guidelines for *Pneumocystis carinii* pneumonia prophylaxis in children issued, 569
Haemophilus b immunization recommendations updated by American Academy of Pediatrics, 733
Highlights of the Seventh International Conference on AIDS, 809
Intravenous quinidine recommended for severe *Plasmodium falciparum* malaria; injectable quinine discontinued by CDC Drug Service, 653
Latex in medical devices may cause severe reactions; extra care advised, 417
Marketing of recombinant granulocyte–macrophage colony-stimulating factor approved by FDA, 411
New method of analyzing health data stirs debate, 4
New recommendations for prevention of bacterial endocarditis include amoxicillin use, 168
News Briefs, 10, 94, 176, 253, 326, 417, 498, 573, 657, 739, 822, 898
Ondansetron granted marketing approval, 249
Recombinant granulocyte colony-stimulating factor approved by FDA, 321
Report assesses use of blood pressure monitoring devices for ambulatory patients, 175
Report on pain management in childhood cancer published, 93
Rubella prevention guidelines updated by CDC, 249
Single large dose of intravenous immune globulin more effective than four-day regimen in patients with Kawasaki disease, investigators report, 657
Study raises safety questions about β-agonist inhaler overuse, 822
Study shows effect of postmenopausal estrogen therapy on cardiovascular risk, 897
Study shows efficacy of monoclonal antibody in patients with sepsis and gram-negative bacteremia, 321
Transdermal fentanyl approved for chronic pain management, 9
Two cardiovascular agents, ramipril and isradipine, approved for U.S. market, 573
Two reports on hypertension available from National Heart, Lung, and Blood Institute, 253
Upcoming Specialty Meetings, 11, 94, 175, 326, 498, 574, 657, 739, 822, 898
Year-end review shows 23 new drugs approved, 14 important biologic licensing actions taken by FDA, 167
Niacin; hyperlipidemia; therapy, protocols, 943
Nicardipine; proteinuria; therapy, diabetic nephropathies, 862
Nicotinic acid, see **Niacin**
Nifedipine; angina pectoris; unstable, therapy, 825
Nitroglycerin; angina pectoris; unstable, therapy, 825
Nomograms; warfarin; dosage, predictions, vs. computers, 923
Nutrition; parenteral; albumin human, dosage predictions, pediatrics, 704

O

Ofloxacin; effects; amikacin-resistant isolates, in vitro, 544
Ondansetron hydrochloride
approvals; prophylaxis, chemotherapy toxicity, 249
pharmacology; review, 430
use; review, criteria, quality assurance programs, 471
Opiates

delirium; therapy, intensive-care units, 456
pain; postoperative, therapy, continuous epidural infusions, 745; therapy, pediatrics, 667
Osteoarthritis
etodolac; therapy, FDA approvals, 416
therapy; geriatrics, ulcer history, 740

P

Pain
analgesics; postoperative, continuous epidural infusions, 745
fentanyl; transdermal patches, therapy, FDA approvals, 9
ketorolac tromethamine; therapy, DUE criteria, 715
therapy; acute, pediatrics, 667
Pancreatitis; pentamidine; toxicity, AIDS, hemophilia, 56
Panic disorders; therapy, 893
Paralysis; skeletal muscle relaxants; mechanically ventilated patients, 32
Parasympatholytic agents; asthma; therapy, pediatrics, 685
Parasympathomimetic agents; Alzheimer's disease; therapy, mechanism of action, review, 447
Parenterals, see **Injections**
Patches transdermal; fentanyl; pain therapy, FDA approvals, 9
Patient education; hypertension; ambulatory care, monitoring, devices, 175
Patients
inpatients; gastrointestinal drugs, DUE criteria, 787; moricizine, DUE criteria, 873
latex; medical devices, allergies, FDA recommendations, 417
outpatients; fluconazole, DUE criteria, 222; ketorolac, DUE criteria, 715; moricizine, DUE criteria, 873; ondansetron therapy, DUE criteria, 471
Pediatrics
albumin human; dosage predictions, parenteral supplements, 704
analgesics; pain therapy, 667
asthma; therapy, 685
chloral hydrate; interactions, furosemide, 385
fluconazole; DUE criteria, 222
furosemide; interactions, chloral hydrate, 385
ketorolac tromethamine; DUE criteria, 715
labetalol hydrochloride; hypertension therapy, 500
lactation; drugs, excretion, review, 594
lorazepam; dosage, sedation, amnesia, 625
mercury; poisoning, 213
neonates; pulmonary surfactants, therapeutic equivalency, 909
ondansetron hydrochloride; therapy, DUE criteria, 471
phenytoin; dosage calculations, black African and Indian children, 928
succimer; therapy, FDA approvals, 942
vancomycin; neonates, dosage guidelines, 129
Penicillamine; hepatolenticular degeneration; therapy, 839
Pentamidine; toxicity; pancreatitis, AIDS, hemophilia, 56
Pentamidine isethionate; adverse reactions; facial numbness, infusions, 257
Pharmacists
antiarrhythmic agents; therapy, blood levels, monitoring, 211
arrhythmia; ventricular, therapy, monitoring, 210
Pharmacodynamics; glyburide; effects, age, 532
Pharmacogenetics
phenytoin; dosage calculations, pediatrics, 928
psychotherapeutic agents; race, ethnic groups, 467
Pharmacokinetics
alfentanil; review, 581
aminoglycosides; AIDS, 784
analgesics; continuous epidural infusions, postoperative pain, 745; pain therapy, pediatrics, 667
benazepril hydrochloride, 739
doxazosin mesylate; hypertension therapy, 9
drugs; lactation, excretion, review, 594
etodolac, 416
fentanyl; and derivatives, review, 581; transdermal patches, pain therapy, 9
filgrastim, 321
fluconazole; review, 179
fludarabine phosphate, 496
gallium nitrate, 573
gentamicin; dosage predictions, methodology, 706
glyburide; effects, age, 532
ibuprofen; interactions, misoprostol, ranitidine, lack, 870
interleukin 2; review, 110
isradipine, 573
levamisole; review, 95
lithium carbonate; methodology, models, 376
ondansetron hydrochloride, 249; review, 430
phenytoin; dosage calculations, pediatrics, 928
phenytoin sodium; impaired metabolism, excretion, liver diseases, 711
psychotherapeutic agents; race, ethnic groups, 467
ramipril, 573
recainam hydrochloride; computer programs, MS-DOS vs. Macintosh, 206
sargramostim, 411
skeletal muscle relaxants; review, mechanically ventilated patients, 32
succimer; lead poisoning, therapy, 914
sufentanil; review, 581
triazolam; interactions, ranitidine, 539
valproate sodium; syrups, availability, vs. valproic acid emulsions, 382
valproic acid; emulsions, availability, vs. valproate sodium syrup, 382
vancomycin hydrochloride; relation, creatinine clearance, 297
Pharmacy, institutional, hospital
quality assurance; programs, alfentanil, fentanyl, sufentanil, DUE criteria, 635; programs, enalapril, DUE criteria, 63; programs, erythropoietin, DUE criteria, 143, 303; programs, filgrastim, neutropenia prophylaxis DUE criteria, 950; programs, fluconazole, DUE criteria, 222; programs, hetastarch, DUE criteria, 549; programs, ketorolac, DUE criteria, 715; programs, midazolam, DUE criteria, 388; programs, misoprostol, DUE criteria, 307; programs, moricizine, arrhythmia therapy, DUE criteria, 873; programs, ondansetron, DUE criteria, 471; programs, sargramostim, DUE criteria, 947; programs, stress ulcer prophylaxis, DUE criteria, 787
Phenobarbital; epilepsy; therapy, review, 335
Phenytoin
blood levels; effects, ultrafiltration and freezing, 132
dosage; calculations, black African and Indian children, 928
epilepsy; therapy, review, 335
Phenytoin sodium; excretion; impaired, liver diseases, activated charcoal therapy, 711
Phlebitis; injections; i.v. infusion sites, toxicity, 630
Physostigmine; Alzheimer's disease; therapy, mechanism of action, review, 447
Pituitary hormones; desmopressin acetate; high dose, mechanism of action, antidiuretic effects, 912
Platelet aggregation inhibitors
aspirin; alone and with flurbiprofen, effects, 935
flurbiprofen; alone and with aspirin, effects, 935
Pneumonia
ceftazidime, comparison, ciprofloxacin lactate; nosocomial, therapy, 49
ciprofloxacin lactate, comparison, ceftazidime; nosocomial, therapy, 49
Poisoning
acetaminophen; overdose, acetylcysteine therapy, 765
lead; succimer therapy, 914; succimer therapy, FDA approvals, controversies, 942
mercury; dimercaprol, *N*-acetyl-D,L-penicillamine, antidotes, pediatrics, 213; toxicity, hyperthyroidism, 742
Prescriptions; anabolic agents; steroids, reclassification, controlled substances, 417
Primidone; epilepsy; therapy, review, 335
Product withdrawal
drugs, nonprescription; ingredients, FDA list, 88
encainide hydrochloride; toxicity, 897
Propoxyphene; and aspirin; pain therapy, codeine allergies, 658
Propylthiouracil; hyperthyroidism; therapy, mercury poisoning, 742
Proteinuria; calcium antagonists; therapy, diabetic nephropathies, 862
Prothrombin time
ciprofloxacin hydrochloride; interactions, warfarin, lack, 136
warfarin; interactions, ciprofloxacin, lack, 136
Protocols
alfentanil hydrochloride; DUE criteria, 635
algorithms; ventricular arrhythmia therapy, 195
enalapril maleate; DUE criteria, 63
epoetin; DUE criteria, 143, 303
fentanyl citrate; DUE criteria, 635
filgrastim; neutropenia prophylaxis, chemotherapy, DUE criteria, 950
fluconazole; DUE criteria, 222
gastrointestinal drugs; stress ulcer prophylaxis, DUE criteria, 787
heparin; thromboembolism therapy, 503
hetastarch; DUE criteria, 549
hyperlipidemia; therapy, National Cholesterol Education Program, 943
ketorolac tromethamine; DUE criteria, 715
midazolam hydrochloride; DUE criteria, 388
misoprostol; DUE criteria, 307
moricizine; arrhythmia therapy, DUE criteria, 873
ondansetron hydrochloride; DUE criteria, 471
sargramostim; DUE criteria, 947
sufentanil citrate; DUE criteria, 635
vancomycin; dosage, neonates, 129
warfarin; thromboembolism therapy, 503
Psychotherapeutic agents
haloperidol; delirium therapy, intensive-care units, 456
pharmacokinetics; race, ethnic groups, 467
Pulmonary surfactants
alcohols, cetyl, combination, colfosceril palmitate, tyloxapol; vs. beractant, therapeutic equivalency, 909
beractant; vs. cetyl alcohol–colfosceril–tyloxapol, therapeutic equivalency, 909

Q

Quality assurance
hospital pharmacy; programs, alfentanil, fentanyl, sufentanil, DUE criteria, 635; programs, enalapril, DUE criteria, 63; programs, epoetin, DUE criteria, 143, 303; programs, filgrastim, neutropenia prophylaxis, DUE criteria, 950; programs, fluconazole, DUE criteria, 222; programs, hetastarch, DUE criteria, 549; programs, ketorolac, DUE criteria, 715; programs, midazolam, DUE criteria, 388; programs, misoprostol, DUE criteria, 307; programs, moricizine, arrhythmia therapy, DUE criteria, 873; programs, ondansetron, DUE criteria, 471; programs, sargramostim, DUE criteria, 947; programs, stress ulcer prophylaxis, DUE criteria, 787
Quality of life; thioridazine hydrochloride; generic equivalency, brands, comparison, 938
Quinidine; concomitant therapy, 823
Quinolones
ciprofloxacin; susceptibility, amikacin-resistant isolates, in vitro, 544
ciprofloxacin hydrochloride; interactions, warfarin, PT effects, lack, 136
ciprofloxacin lactate; vs. ceftazidime, pneumonia and urinary tract infections therapy, 49
Mycobacterium avium complex; therapy, AIDS, review, 280
ofloxacin; susceptibility, amikacin-resistant isolates, in vitro, 544

R

Race
patients; psychotherapeutic agents, pharmacogenetics, 467
pediatrics; phenytoin dosage calculations, 928
Radionuclides; neoplasms; monoclonal antibodies, 359
Radiopharmaceuticals; neoplasms; monoclonal antibodies, 359
Ramipril; marketing; FDA approvals, 573
Ranitidine; ulcers; peptic, prophylaxis, osteoarthritis therapy, geriatrics, 740
Ranitidine hydrochloride; interactions; ibuprofen, lack, 870; triazolam, pharmacokinetics, 539
Rational therapy
cardiac drugs; ventricular arrhythmia therapy, 195
pharmacists; ventricular arrhythmia, monitoring, 210
Recainam hydrochloride; pharmacokinetics; computer programs, MS-DOS vs. Macintosh, 206
Reference books; lactation; drugs, patient information, review, 594
Regulations
Food and Drug Administration; nonprescription ingredients, withdrawal, 88
succimer; therapy, FDA restrictions, 942
Replacement solutions; hetastarch; DUE criteria, quality assurance programs, 549
Reports
botulinum toxin type A; dystonia therapy, 88
drugs, adverse reactions; and toxicity, Vaccine Adverse Event Reporting System, 9
hypertension; monitoring, devices, assessment, 175
Research
acquired immunodeficiency syndrome; therapy, AIDS conference, 809
hypertension; monitoring, devices, assessment, 175
Resistance
amikacin; gram-negative bacteria, in vitro, 544

ceftazidime, comparison, ciprofloxacin lactate; pneumonia and urinary tract infections, 49
ciprofloxacin lactate, comparison, ceftazidime; pneumonia and urinary tract infections, 49
Respiratory distress syndrome; pulmonary surfactants; therapy, therapeutic equivalency, 909
Respiratory smooth-muscle relaxants; theophylline; asthma therapy, pediatrics, 685
Restless legs; therapy; nocturnal, 427
Rhenium Re 188; radionuclides; monoclonal antibodies, neoplasms, 359
RS-86; Alzheimer's disease; therapy, mechanism of action, review, 447

S

Salsalate; osteoarthritis; therapy, geriatrics, ulcer history, 740
Sargramostim
marketing; FDA approvals, 411
use; evaluation, criteria, 947
Scleroderma; therapy; systemic, 14
Sex; patients; males, toxicity, i.v. infusion sites, 630
Skeletal muscle relaxants
delirium; therapy, intensive-care units, 456
pharmacology; review, mechanically ventilated patients, 32
therapy; nocturnal leg cramps, restless legs, 427
Sorbitol; vehicles; activated charcoal therapy, phenytoin toxicity, liver diseases, 711
Stability
ondansetron hydrochloride; review, 430
phenytoin; blood levels, freezing, ultrafiltration, 132
valproic acid; emulsions, availability, vs. valproate sodium syrup, 382
***Staphylococcus aureus*;** resistance; ciprofloxacin, pneumonia, 49
Steroids; anabolic agents; reclassification, controlled substances, 417
Steroids, cortico-; asthma; therapy, pediatrics, 685
Storage; effects; phenytoin blood levels, ultrafiltration methods, 132
Streptococcus species; resistance; ciprofloxacin, pneumonia, 49
Streptokinase; comparison, alteplase, anistreplase; myocardial infarction therapy, 486
Succimer
marketing; FDA approvals, controversies, 942
therapy; lead poisoning, 914
Sucralfate; use; evaluation, stress ulcer prophylaxis, criteria, 787
Sufentanil; pharmacology; clinical uses, review, 581
Sufentanil citrate; use; review, criteria, quality assurance programs, 635
Surgical supplies; latex; adverse reactions, FDA recommendations, 417
Sympatholytic agents
β blockers; and doxazosin, hypertension therapy, 9
scleroderma; systemic, therapy, 14
Sympathomimetic agents
asthma; therapy, pediatrics, 685
heart failure; congestive, therapy, diastolic dysfunction, 850
Syrups; valproate sodium; stability, availability, vs. valproic acid emulsions, 382

T

Tacrine hydrochloride; Alzheimer's disease; therapy, mechanism of action, review, 447
Taste; palatability; cholestyramine, colestipol, oral formulations, 138
Terbutaline sulfate; labor; preterm, home infusion therapy, 292
Tests, laboratory
phenytoin; blood levels, effects, ultrafiltration and freezing, 132
prothrombin; warfarin, interactions, ciprofloxacin, lack, 136
Theophylline; asthma; therapy, pediatrics, 685
Therapy Consultation, 12, 427, 658, 740, 909
Analgesic selection when the patient is allergic to codeine, 658
Comparing surfactant products, 909
Treatment of nocturnal leg cramps and restless leg syndrome, 427
Treatment options for a patient with osteoarthritis and a history of ulcer disease, 740
Use of ketoconazole in the treatment of Cushing's syndrome, 12
Thioridazine hydrochloride; equivalency, generic; brands, comparison, efficacy, quality of life, 938
Thromboembolism
heparin; therapy, guidelines, 503
warfarin; therapy, guidelines, 503
Thrombolytic agents; myocardial infarction; therapy, 486
Tissue levels; mercury; poisoning, pediatrics, 213
Tissue plasminogen activator, see **Alteplase**
Tocolytics; terbutaline sulfate; preterm labor, home infusion therapy, 292
Toxicity, environmental
mercury; poisoning, occupational exposure, hyperthyroidism, 742; spills, inhalation, poisoning, pediatrics, 213
meta-analysis; methodology, applications and problems, 4
Toxicity
see also **Drugs, adverse reactions**
acetaminophen; overdose, acetylcysteine therapy, 765
alfentanil hydrochloride; DUE criteria, 635
analgesics; side effects, continuous epidural infusions, 745; side effects, pain therapy, pediatrics, 667
anti-inflammatory agents; osteoarthritis therapy, geriatrics, ulcer history, 740
antineoplastic agents; nausea and vomiting, ondansetron prophylaxis, 430; neutropenia, filgrastim prophylaxis, FDA approvals, 321; ondansetron prophylaxis, FDA approvals, 249
benazepril hydrochloride, 739
botulinum toxin type A; side effects, 88
cardiac drugs; ventricular arrhythmia therapy, 195
chloral hydrate; interactions, furosemide, pediatrics, 385
deferoxamine mesylate; side effects, hemochromatosis therapy, 775
digoxin; therapy, digoxin immune Fab retreatment, immunogenicity, 823
doxazosin mesylate; side effects, hypertension therapy, 9
drugs; lactation, 594
enalapril maleate; DUE criteria, 63
encainide hydrochloride; side effects, product withdrawal, 897
epoetin; DUE criteria, 143, 303
etodolac; side effects, 416
fentanyl; side effects, transdermal patches, pain therapy, 9
fentanyl citrate; DUE criteria, 635
filgrastim; neutropenia prophylaxis, DUE criteria, 950; side effects, 321
fluconazole; DUE criteria, 222; side effects, review, 179
fludarabine phosphate; side effects, 496
furosemide; interactions, chloral hydrate, pediatrics, 385
gallium nitrate; side effects, 573
gastrointestinal drugs; stress ulcer prophylaxis, DUE criteria, 787
hetastarch; DUE criteria, 549
injections; i.v. infusion, extravasation, phlebitis, 630
interleukin 2; side effects, neoplasms therapy, 110
isradipine; side effects, 573
ketorolac tromethamine; DUE criteria, 715
labetalol hydrochloride; side effects, lack, pediatrics, 500
lead; poisoning, succimer therapy, 914
levamisole; side effects, colorectal neoplasms therapy, 95
lorazepam; side effects, high dose, pediatrics, 625
mercury; hyperthyroidism, long-term exposure, 742; poisoning, pediatrics, 213
midazolam hydrochloride; DUE criteria, 388
misoprostol; DUE criteria, 307
moricizine; arrhythmia therapy, DUE criteria, 873
ondansetron hydrochloride; DUE criteria, 471; side effects, 249; side effects, review, 430
pentamidine; pancreatitis, AIDS, hemophilia, 56
phenytoin sodium; impaired metabolism, liver diseases, 711
ramipril; side effects, 573
sargramostim; DUE criteria, 947; side effects, 411
skeletal muscle relaxants; side effects, mechanically ventilated patients, 32
succimer; side effects, lead poisoning therapy, 914
sufentanil citrate; DUE criteria, 635
terbutaline sulfate; side effects, preterm labor therapy, 292
thrombolytic agents; side effects, myocardial infarction therapy, 486
vaccines; side effects, Vaccine Adverse Event Reporting System, 9
zidovudine; neutropenia, HIV infections, review, 268
Toxins; botulinum toxin type A; dystonia therapy, 88
t-PA, see **Alteplase**
Tranquilizers; thioridazine hydrochloride; generic equivalency, comparisons, efficacy, quality of life, 938
Transplantation; bone marrow; acute lymphoblastic leukemia patients, sargramostim therapy, FDA approvals, 411; sargramostim therapy, DUE criteria, 947
Triazolam; interactions; ranitidine, pharmacokinetics, 539
Trientine; hepatolenticular degeneration; therapy, 839
Tyloxapol; combination, alcohols, cetyl, colfosceril palmitate; vs. beractant, therapeutic equivalency, 909

U

Ulcers
gastrointestinal drugs; stress, prophylaxis, DUE criteria, 787
misoprostol; gastric, therapy, DUE criteria, 307
prophylaxis; peptic, osteoarthritis, geriatrics, 740
Urinary tract infections
ceftazidime, comparison, ciprofloxacin lactate; therapy, 49
ciprofloxacin lactate, comparison, ceftazidime; therapy, 49
Urine levels; mercury; poisoning, pediatrics, 213

V

Vaccine Adverse Event Reporting System; vaccines; adverse reactions and toxicity, reports, 9
Vaccines; toxicity; and adverse reactions, Vaccine Adverse Event Reporting System, 9
Valproate sodium; comparison, valproic acid; stability, availability, emulsions vs. syrups, 382
Valproic acid
comparison, valproate sodium; stability, availability, emulsions vs. syrups, 382
epilepsy; therapy, review, 335
Vancomycin; dosage; guidelines, neonates, 129
Vancomycin hydrochloride; blood levels; half-life, relation creatinine, hepatic and renal dysfunction, 297
Vasodilating agents; heart failure; congestive, therapy, diastolic dysfunction, 850
Vehicles
cholestyramine resin; palatability, oral formulations, preferences, 138
colestipol hydrochloride; palatability, oral formulations, preferences, 138
sorbitol; activated charcoal therapy, phenytoin toxicity, liver diseases, 711
Ventilators; skeletal muscle relaxants; mechanical, patients, effects, 32
Verapamil
angina pectoris; unstable, therapy, 825
muscle cramp; therapy, nocturnal leg cramps, 427
Vitamin E; muscle cramp; therapy, nocturnal leg cramps, 427
Volume of distribution, see **Drugs, body distribution**
Vomiting; ondansetron hydrochloride; therapy, DUE criteria, 471

W

Warfarin
interactions; ciprofloxacin, PT effects, lack, 136
nomograms; dosage, predictions, vs. computers, 923
thromboembolism; therapy, guidelines, 503
Weight; patients; predictions, lithium clearance, models, 376

X

***Xanthomonas maltophilia*;** resistance; antibiotics, in vitro, 544

Y

Yttrium Y 90; radionuclides; monoclonal antibodies, neoplasms, 359

Z

Zidovudine; toxicity; neutropenia, HIV infections, review, 268
Zinc; hepatolenticular degeneration; maintenance therapy, 839

Author Index

A

Allen, Nancy M. Retreatment with digoxin immune Fab (letter), 823
Altman, Lawrence K. New method of analyzing health data stirs debate (News), 4
Anderson, Bruce D. see Smith, Leanne B., 132
Anderson, Philip O. Drug use during breast-feeding, 594
Antal, Edward J. see Schwinghammer, Terry L., 532
Ariano, Robert E. Inverse relationship between desmopressin dosage and antidiuresis (letter), 912
Asher, John P. Use of angiotensin-converting-enzyme inhibitors in the management of renal disease, 25

B

Bablenis, Elena Effect of use of generic thioridazine products on clinical outcome and quality of life, 938
Banner, William Jr. Succimer: controversial issues involving the release of a new product (editorial), 942
Barnett, Michael D. see McGee, Barbara A., 14
Basile, Sharon A. Criteria for use of hetastarch, 549
Baumann, Terry J. Analgesic selection when the patient is allergic to codeine (Therapy Consultation), 658
Beail, Barbara see Matsuyama, Joy R., 544
Bennett, Teresa A. Criteria for use of epoetin, 143, 303
Bennett, Teresa A. Criteria for use of moricizine in adult inpatients and outpatients, 873
Berardi, Rosemary R. see Knapp, Margaret J., 866
Bernard, Evelyne see Dellamonica, Pierre, 301
Bhatt-Mehta, Varsha Management of acute pain in children, 667
Billeter, Marianne see Rapp, Robert P., 49
Bombardt, Paul A. see Vanderveen, R. Pete, 539
Bond, William S. Ethnicity and psychotropic drugs, 467
Botha, Julia H. Estimating phenytoin dosages in black African and Indian children, 928
Bourne, David W. A. see Hampton, Edward M., 206
Bourne, Kimberly M. Criteria for use of fluconazole in adult and pediatric inpatients and outpatients, 222
Buck, Marcia L. Use of nondepolarizing neuromuscular blocking agents in mechanically ventilated patients, 32
Burwinkle, Joseph W. see Henry, David W., 625

C

Calis, Karim Anton see Kintzel, P. E., 110
Carles, Michel see Dellamonica, Pierre, 301
Carter, Barry L. Therapy of acute thromboembolism with heparin and warfarin, 503
Carver, Peggy L. see Knapp, Margaret J., 866
Chae, Joanne S. see Nakahiro, Randall K., 931
Chaffee, Betty J. Ondansetron—the first of a new class of antiemetic agents, 430
Check, William A. Conference attendees told ISIS-3 shows equal efficacy, safety differences among thrombolytics (News), 486
Chin, Alfred see Nakahiro, Randall K., 931
Clotz, Michael A. Clinical uses of fentanyl, sufentanil, and alfentanil, 581
Cochran, Emily B. Prediction of serum albumin concentration after albumin supplementation in pediatric patients receiving parenteral nutrition, 704
Coleman, Robert W. see Fredriks, Dean A., 923
Coley, Allison L. Criteria for use of enalapril maleate in adults, 63
Collins, Shelly Rainforth see Gabriel, Mariane Hardenbrook, 129
Comstock, Thomas J. Book review, 890
Coonce, Shannon L. see Murphy, Christine M., 685
Cortese, Linda M. Criteria for use of midazolam hydrochloride in adult patients, 388
Couch, Patricia Cryoprecipitate for uremic bleeding (letter), 429
Cox, Steven R. see Vanderveen, R. Pete, 539
Crismon, M. Lynn see Jermain, Donna M., 376

D

Davenport, Robertson Cryoprecipitate for uremic bleeding (letter), 429
Davis, Lisa E. see Spinler, Sarah A., 825
Dean, Roger P. Interaction of chloral hydrate and intravenous furosemide in a child, 385
Dellamonica, Pierre Preventing recurrent varicella and herpes zoster with oral acyclovir in HIV-seropositive patients, 301
Dempsey, Robert J. see Rapp, Robert P., 49
Dixon, Dennis M. see Kowalsky, Steven F., 179
Donnelly, Andrew J. see Shafer, Amy L., 745
Dressman, Jennifer B. see Knapp, Margaret J., 866
Dufresne, Robert L. see Bablenis, Elena, 938

E

Eaton, Virginia E. see Rathbun, R. Chris, 280

F

Fischer, Janet R. Continuous subcutaneous infusion of terbutaline for suppression of preterm labor, 292
Fish, Douglas N. Treatment of delirium in the critically ill patient, 456
Fish, Susan S. Book review, 730
Florentine, Mauro J. Elemental mercury poisoning, 213
Floriddia, Donald G. Book review, 649
Forrest, Alan see Weidle, Paul J., 711
Fredriks, Dean A. Nomogram for dosing warfarin at steady state, 923

G

Gabriel, Mariane Hardenbrook Prospective evaluation of a vancomycin dosage guideline for neonates, 129
Garabedian-Ruffalo, Susan M. see Saltiel, Emmanuel, 518
Garewal, Harinder S. see Rindone, Joseph P., 136
Garnett, William R. see Pugh, Carol B., 335
Gennrich, Jane L. see Gabriel, Mariane Hardenbrook, 129
Gill, Mark A. see Nakahiro, Randall K., 931
Gilman, Jamie T. Valproic acid hepatotoxicity in adults and older children (letter), 665
Goodwin, S. Diane see Bourne, Kimberly M., 222
Gora, Mary Lea Book review, 805
Graves, David A. Book review, 970
Green, Elaine R. Book review, 729

H

Hackimer, Mary E. see Schwinghammer, Terry L., 532
Hak, Lawrence J. see O'Neil, Michael G., 56
Hampton, Edward M. Comparison of MS-DOS and Macintosh pharmacokinetic analysis programs using a two-compartment, two-infusion dosing scheme, 206
Hartwig, Steven C. Criteria for use of ondansetron hydrochloride in adult and pediatric inpatients and adult outpatients, 471
Hasegawa, Guy R. Antiarrhythmic monitoring: misplaced emphasis (editorial), 211
Hatton, Jimmi see Rapp, Robert P., 49
Hatton, Randy C. see Veerman, Mark W., 382
Hecker, John see Wright, Alex, 630
Henry, David W. Determination of sedative and amnestic doses of lorazepam in children, 625
Hogue, Susan L. see Cochran, Emily B., 704
Housel, Ben F. see Ishisaka, Denis Y., 500
Hrdlicka, Kyle see Hampton, Edward M., 206
Hutson, Paul R. see Mutch, Rebecca S., 95

I

Ishisaka, Denis Y. Labetalol for treatment of hypertension in a child (letter), 500
Israel, Deb S. Neutropenia in patients infected with human immunodeficiency virus, 268
Ito, Matthew K. Acceptability of cholestyramine and colestipol formulations in three common vehicles, 138

J

Jacobi, Judith Book review, 80
Jermain, Donna M. Population pharmacokinetics of lithium, 376
Jirak, Jana L. see Vanderveen, R. Pete, 539
Johanson, Franck see Dellmonica, Pierre, 301
Johnson, Juli A. Diastolic dysfunction in congestive heart failure, 850
Johnston, Jann M. see Schwinghammer, Terry L., 532
Jones, Paul R. see McMorrow, Julie, 501
Jones, William N. see Rindone, Joseph P., 136

K

Kaatz, Brian L. see Fischer, Janet R., 292
Kelleher, Michael D. see Dean, Roger P., 385
Keller, James H. Book review, 239
Kelley, Catherine L. see Rindone, Joseph P., 136
Khanderia, Ujjaini Use of ketoconazole in the treatment of Cushing's syndrome (Therapy Consultation), 12
Kildoo, Carl W. III see Gabriel, Mariane Hardenbrook, 129
Kintzel, P. E. Recombinant interleukin-2: a biological response modifier, 110
Kirking, Marilyn H. Treatment of chronic iron overload, 775
Klutman, Neil E. see Henry, David W., 625
Knapp, Margaret J. Modification of gastric pH with oral glutamic acid hydrochloride, 866
Knight, Matthew E. see Veerman, Mark W., 382
Kolb, Kenneth W. see Walton, Ted, 427
Kowalsky, Steven F. Fluconazole: a new antifungal agent, 179
Kresel, James J. Book review, 243
Kubacka, Reneé T. see Schwinghammer, Terry L., 532

L

Lackner, Thomas E. A nonexponential, nonlogarithmic, pharmacokinetic dosing method for gentamicin, 706
Lewis, Richard K. Assessment and treatment of acetaminophen overdose, 765
Lin, Anne Y. F. Pentamidine-induced facial numbness (letter), 257
Lokiec, François see Dellamonica, Pierre, 301
Longley, Joyce M. Altered aminoglycoside volume of distribution in patients with acquired immunodeficiency syndrome, 784
Lopez, Larry M. Verapamil and left ventricular hypertrophy (letter), 333

M

Mann, Katherine V. Succimer, an oral lead chelator, 914
Martin, Emory S. III see Jermain, Donna M., 376
Martin, Emory S. III see also Rathbun, R. Chris, 280
Martin, J. Kelly Jr. Book review, 976
Matsuyama, Joy R. Susceptibility of *Xanthomonas maltophilia* and amikacin-resistant gram-negative bacteria to newer antimicrobials, 544
Matthew, Earl B. see Rathbun, R. Chris, 280
May, J. Russell Book review, 885
McCann, Michael Hyperthyroidism associated with mercury poisoning (letter), 742
McCollam, Patrick L. Evaluation and treatment of ventricular arrhythmias: an update, 195
McGee, Barbara A. Current options for the treatment of systemic scleroderma, 14
McGee, Barbara A. see also Small, Ralph E., 870
McMorrow, Julie Antimicrobial dosages in guidelines for prevention of bacterial endocarditis, 501
Medina, Richard A. see Peters, Mark D. II, 787
Mendel, Stephen Book review, 805
Michael, Katherine A. see Peters, Mark D. II, 787
Miller, Alan B. see Bennett, Teresa A., 873
Miller, Donald R. Treatment options for a patient with osteoarthritis and a history of ulcer disease (Therapy Consultation), 740
Miller, Raymond see Botha, Julia H., 928
Modanlou, Houchange D. see Gabriel, Mariane Hardenbrook, 129
Mondain, Véronique see Dellamonica, Pierre, 301
Moodley, Manikum see Botha, Julia H., 928
Morreale, Anthony P. see Ito, Matthew K., 138
Murphy, Christine M. Treatment of asthma in children, 685

Murray, Kim M. Calcium-channel blockers for treatment of diabetic nephropathy, 862
Murray, Kim M. see also Asher, John P., 25
Mutch, Rebecca S. Levamisole in the adjuvant treatment of colon cancer, 95

N

Nahata, Milap C. see Clotz, Michael A., 581
Nahata, Milap C. see also McMorrow, Julie, 501
Nakahiro, Randall K. Use of gentamicin clearance in estimating renal function, 931
Nappi, Jean Trials and tribulations of evaluating ventricular arrhythmias (editorial), 210
Newby, F. David see Longley, Joyce M., 784

O

O'Neil, Michael G. Pancreatitis during pentamidine therapy in patients with AIDS, 56
Okamoto, Mark P. see Nakahiro, Randall K., 931
Orlando, Patricia L. Book review, 885

P

Pachorek, Robert E. Vancomycin half-life in a patient with hepatic and renal dysfunction, 297
Paloucek, Frank P. see Lewis, Richard K., 765
Parish, Roy C. see Pincus, Kelly T., 935
Parker, Robert B. see McCollam, Patrick L., 195
Peloquin, Charles A. Dosage of antimycobacterial agents (letter), 664
Peters, Gary R. see Vanderveen, R. Pete, 539
Peters, Mark D. II Criteria for stress ulcer prophylaxis in intensive-care patients, 787
Pincus, Kelly T. Effect of flurbiprofen and aspirin on platelet aggregation, 935
Pittman, Donald G. see Longley, Joyce M., 784
Plaisance, Karen I. see Israel, Deb S., 268
Porter, Don R. Book review, 316
Prevost, Rebecca Rogers Comparing surfactant products (Therapy Consultation), 909
Price, Karen Overstreet Ethnicity and clozapine-induced agranulocytosis (letter), 743
Pugh, Carol B. Current issues in the treatment of epilepsy, 335
Pugh, Carol B. see also Smith, Leanne B., 132

R

Rapp, Robert P. Intravenous ciprofloxacin versus ceftazidime for treatment of nosocomial pneumonia and urinary tract infection, 49
Rathbun, R. Chris Current and investigational therapies for AIDS-associated *Mycobacterium avium* complex disease, 280
Reed, Michael D. see Buck, Marcia L., 32
Reilly, Raymond M. Radioimmunotherapy of malignancies, 359
Rider, Joan M. see Knapp, Margaret J., 866
Rindone, Joseph P. Hypoprothrombinemic effect of warfarin not influenced by ciprofloxacin, 136
Rosen, David A. see Bhatt-Mehta, Varsha, 667
Rudinsky, Brian F. see Dean, Roger P., 385
Rutledge, David R. Which lipid-lowering agent should be used first? 943

S

Saltiel, Emmanuel Pharmacologic management of endometriosis, 518
Sandroni, Stephen see Bennett, Teresa A., 143, 303
Sanfilippo, Dominic J. II see Florentine, Mauro J., 213
Satterlee, Grant B. Criteria for use of fentanyl citrate, sufentanil citrate, and alfentanil hydrochloride, 635
Scheckner, Stuart see McCann, Michael, 742
Scholten, Stephanie L. Correction to *AHFS Drug Information 91* (letter), 913
Schwinghammer, Terry L. Pharmacokinetics and pharmacodynamics of glyburide in young and elderly nondiabetic adults, 532
Sclar, David A. see Nakahiro, Randall K., 931
Selub, Steven E. see O'Neil, Michael G., 56
Seymour, Beverly see Ariano, Robert E., 912
Shafer, Amy L. Management of postoperative pain by continuous epidural infusion of analgesics, 745
Shepherd, Michele F. Criteria for use of ketorolac tromethamine in adult inpatients and outpatients, 715
Simon, Pamela A. see Murphy, Christine M., 685
Sjolander, Julie A. see Peters, Mark D. II, 787
Skiest, Daniel J. see Weidle, Paul J., 711
Skora, Irene A. see Satterlee, Grant B., 635
Small, Ralph E. Effects of misoprostol or ranitidine on ibuprofen pharmacokinetics, 870
Small, Ralph E. see also McGee, Barbara A., 14
Smith, Candace see Lin, Anne Y. F., 257
Smith, Leanne B. Effect of ultrafiltration product and ultrafiltration–freezing sequence on free phenytoin determination, 132
Spinler, Sarah A. Advances in the treatment of unstable angina pectoris, 825
Spruill, William J. see Pincus, Kelly T., 935
Stahl-Bayliss, Celine M. Interferon for genital warts (letter), 177
Swanson, Keith A. see Peters, Mark D. II, 787

T

Tami, Joseph A. Recombinant interleukin-2 and the quest for FDA approval, 141
Tankanow, Roberta M. Pathophysiology and treatment of Wilson's disease, 839
Tankanow, Roberta M. see also Chaffee, Betty J., 430
Tartaglione, Teresa see Matsuyama, Joy R., 544
Thom, Claire M. Verapamil and left ventricular hypertrophy (letter), 333
Tibbs, Phillip A. see Rapp, Robert P., 49
Todd, Mark W. Criteria for use of misoprostol, 307
Todd, Mark W. see also Bennett, Teresa A., 143, 303
Travers, John D. see Mann, Katherine V., 914
Trotter, J. Mark see Bennett, Teresa A., 873

U

Uden, Don Book review, 650

V

Vanderveen, R. Pete Effect of ranitidine on the disposition of orally and intravenously administered triazolam, 539
Veerman, Mark W. Relative bioavailability and stability of extemporaneously prepared valproic acid emulsion, 382
Volger, Burgunda W. Alternatives in the treatment of memory loss in patients with Alzheimer's disease, 447
Volger, Burgunda W. Book review, 317

W

Wallis, Carolyn see Matsuyama, Joy R., 544
Walton, Ted Treatment of nocturnal leg cramps and restless leg syndrome (Therapy Consultation), 427
Weber, Stanley S. see Bablenis, Elena, 938
Weidle, Paul J. Multiple-dose activated charcoal as adjunct therapy after chronic phenytoin intoxication, 711
Weiss, Peter D. see Lackner, Thomas E., 706
Welty, Timothy E. Book review, 159
Willis, Hayes E. see Small, Ralph E., 870
Wilmot-Pater, Melody G. see Small, Ralph E., 870
Wittkowsky, Ann K. Laboratory monitoring of heparin therapy (letter), 824
Wong, Roberta J. Highlights of the Seventh International Conference on AIDS (News), 809
Wood, Frederick see Pachorek, Robert E., 297
Wright, Alex Infusion failure caused by phlebitis and extravasation, 630

Y

Yamreudeewong, Weeranuj see Lackner, Thomas E., 706
Yonan, Charles D. see Ishisaka, Denis Y., 500
Young, A. Bryon see Rapp, Robert P., 49

Z

Zeleznik, Dee see Matsuyama, Joy R., 544

Advertising Index

A

Adria Laboratories
Idamycin, 5-7, Feb 160, IBC, OBC, Apr 318, IBC, OBC, Jun 482, IBC, OBC
American Diabetes Association
Institutional, 13, 739
American Lung Association
Institutional, 326
American Society of Hospital Pharmacists
AHFS Drug Information 91, 239, 334, 554
AHFS Drug Information 92, 978
American Journal of Hospital Pharmacy, 629
Aseptic Preparation of Parenteral Products, 67, 238
ASHP Membership, 212, 783, 979
CiteSearch, 256, 416
Clinical Pharmacy, 159, 221, 291, 401, 428, 738
Concepts in Clinical Pharmacokinetics, 317, 741, 969
Concepts in Immunology and Immunotherapeutics, 13, 400, 420
Criteria for Drug Use Evaluation, Volumes 1 and 2, Jan IFC, 261, 391, 476, 499, 640, 666, 952
European Drug Index, 315, 403, 559, 580
Guidelines for Administration of Intravenous Medications to Pediatric Patients, 548, 990
Handbook on Injectable Drugs, 6th Edition, 232, 302
International Pharmaceutical Abstracts, 231, 358
IV-EASE, 150
Medication Errors: A Closer Look, 744
Medication Teaching Manual, Fourth Edition, 178, 266
MedTeach, 531, 806
Pocket Guide to Injectable Drugs, 1991 Edition, 70, 236, 470, 574
Position Available, 744
QARx, 404, 725
Rx Triage, 267, 387
Safe Handling of Cytotoxic and Hazardous Drugs, 94, 253, 945
Software, 967
Amgen Inc.
Epogen, Sep IFC, Oct IFC, 961-965
Neupogen, 899-908
ASHP Research and Education Foundation
Anticoagulation Clinic Traineeship Program, 557
Awards Program, 75
Institutional, 89, 977

B

Baxter Healthcare Corporation, Hyland Division
Gammagard, 412-414, 488-490
Burroughs Wellcome Company
Exosurf Neonatal, 491-495, 575-579, 659-663, 795-799, 815-819, 971-975
Zovirax I.V., 76-78, 90-92, 240-242, 258-260, 322-324, 408-410, 560-562, 646-648

C

Charleston Area Medical Center
Position Available, 150

D

Department of Veterans Affairs (Richmond)
Positions Available, 73, 83, 163, 265, 325, 415, 563

E

Eisenhower Medical Center
Positions Available, 237, 416, 954

G

Glaxo Inc.
Antiemetic, Feb IFC
Ceptaz, 244-246, 254-256, 398-400
Zofran, 169-174, 327-332, 421-426

H

Harrisburg Hospital
Position Available, 11

I

International Pharmaceutical Federation (F.I.P.)
Membership, 643

K

Kent General Hospital
Position Available, 94

L

Eli Lilly and Company
Hospital Division, 3, 153, Mar IFC, Jun IFC, 485, 813
Lyphomed, Inc.
Amphotericin B, 84-86, 164-166, 262-264

M

Methodist Medical Center of Illinois
Position Available, 497

N

National Easter Seal Society
Institutional, 879
National Foundation for Infectious Diseases
National Forum, 910

P

The Pharmacy Council on Cholesterol
10 Cholesterol Battle Strategies, 502

R

Roche Laboratories, Division of Hoffmann-La Roche, Inc.
Rocephin, Aug IBC, OBC, Oct IBC, OBC, Dec IBC, OBC
Roerig, A Division of Pfizer Pharmaceuticals
Diflucan, 156-158, 250-252, May IFC, 407, Jul IFC, Aug IFC, 719-722
Unasyn, 418-420
Ross Laboratories
Survanta, 737-738, 883-884

S

San Francisco VA Medical Center
Position Available, 13
Schering-Plough Corporation
Position Available, 497
SmithKline Beecham
Tagamet, Jan IBC, OBC, Mar IBC, OBC, May IBC, OBC, Jul IBC, OBC, Sep IBC, OBC, Nov IBC, OBC
St. Jude Children's Research Hospital
Institutional, 11, 310, 665

T

Toledo Hospital
Positions Available, 649, 913

U

The University Hospital (Boston)
Position Available, 334
The University of Illinois College of Medicine at Peoria
Positions available, 499
The University of Rhode Island
Position Available, 11
The Upjohn Company
Zefazone, 810-812, 956-958
The Upjohn Company and Chugai-Upjohn, Inc.
Marogen 79, 87, Apr IFC

W

Wyeth-Ayerst Laboratories, Inc.
Ativan Injection, 564-566, 570-572, 654-656, 734-736, 886-888, 894-896
Position Available, 176
Tubex, Nov IFC, Dec IFC